Respiratory Medicine

Respiratory Medicine offers clinical and research-oriented resources for pulmonologists and other practitioners and researchers interested in respiratory care. Spanning a broad range of clinical and research issues in respiratory medicine, the series covers such topics as COPD, asthma and allergy, pulmonary problems in pregnancy, molecular basis of lung disease, sleep disordered breathing, and others.

The series editors are Sharon Rounds, MD, Professor of Medicine and of Pathology and Laboratory Medicine at the Alpert Medical School at Brown University, Anne Dixon, MD, Professor of Medicine and Director of the Division of Pulmonary and Critical Care at Robert Larner, MD College of Medicine at the University of Vermont, and Lynn M. Schnapp, MD, George R. And Elaine Love Professor and Chair of Medicine at the University of Wisconsin-Madison School of Medicine and Public Health.

Michael J. Lanspa • Andrew T. Levinson
Editors

Echocardiography and Ultrasonography in the ICU

A Comprehensive Text

Humana Press

ATS American Thoracic Society

Editors
Michael J. Lanspa
Pulmonary and Critical Care
Intermountain Medical Center
Murray, UT, USA

Andrew T. Levinson
Division of Pulmonary, Critical Care, and Sleep Medicine
The Warren Alpert Medical School, Brown University
Providence, RI, USA

ISSN 2197-7372 ISSN 2197-7380 (electronic)
Respiratory Medicine
ISBN 978-3-031-80037-5 ISBN 978-3-031-80038-2 (eBook)
https://doi.org/10.1007/978-3-031-80038-2

This Humana imprint is published by the registered company Springer Nature Switzerland AG
The registered company address is: Gewerbestrasse 11, 6330 Cham, Switzerland

Preface

The specialty of critical care echocardiography is in its adolescence, having grown considerably over the past two decades. Critical care ultrasound, previously used for procedural guidance or to make qualitative assessments for simple diagnoses, is now used to quantify hemodynamics, identify subtle abnormalities, and guide therapies. Over the same period, the specialties of critical care and echocardiography have evolved to include these new ultrasound advances. The development of a board examination in the field of critical care echocardiography underscores this growth. It is our hope that this textbook might spark insight in the next generation of clinicians and scientists, who might propel our field forward.

This textbook is an attempt to provide a comprehensive overview of the field of critical care echocardiography and ultrasound in its current state. The first chapters examine the fundamental principles and techniques that are the foundation of current critical care ultrasound techniques. The following chapters detail the echocardiographic skills and techniques pertinent to critical care practice. Lung, airway abdominal, vascular, and neurologic ultrasonography are then discussed in detail. The last third of the book explores complex scenarios, ultrasound education, and practical aspects of critical care ultrasound.

Throughout the text, we describe not only the current standard, but also areas of evolving evidence. These areas of evolving evidence are identified as such. It should be acknowledged that future investigation might invalidate those areas of evolving evidence. Additionally, the reader should recognize that the applications described herein presume a high-income and high-resource clinical environment. Clinical applications described in this text might require modification or additional considerations when used in resource-limited environments.

This book could not have come into existence without the generous contributions of countless national and international expert educators in echocardiography and ultrasound. One strength of this textbook is the diversity of the authors, who hail from multiple countries, disciplines, and specialties. We thank them for their generosity, diligence, and patience.

Murray, UT, USA — Michael J. Lanspa
Providence, RI, USA — Andrew T. Levinson

Contents

Contributors

Enyo Ablordeppey Emergency Medicine, Washington University School of Medicine, St. Louis, MO, USA

Stanley Abraham Zucker School of Medicine at Hofstra/Northwell, Hempstead, NY, USA

Tahir Ahmad Division of Critical Care Medicine, Department of Medicine, Montefiore Medical Center, Albert Einstein College of Medicine, Bronx, NY, USA

Taha Ahmed University of Kentucky, Gill Heart and Vascular Institute, Lexington, KY, USA

Gil Allen Division of Pulmonary and Critical Care, Department of Medicine, University of Vermont Medical Center and Larner College of Medicine, Burlington, VT, USA

Chris Allison Umass Chan Medical School—Baystate, Springfield, MA, USA

MaryEllen Antkowiak Division of Pulmonary and Critical Care, Department of Medicine, University of Vermont Medical Center and Larner College of Medicine, Burlington, VT, USA

Amit Arbune University of Kentucky, Gill Heart and Vascular Institute, Lexington, KY, USA

Gloria A. Ayuba Department of Medicine/Division of Cardiology, UT Southwestern, Dallas, USA

Sarah Bain Virginia Mason Franciscan Health, Seattle, WA, USA

Cristiana Baloescu Department of Emergency Medicine, Yale University School of Medicine, New Haven, CT, USA

Christopher F. Barnett Division of Cardiology and Critical Care Cardiology Section, Department of Medicine, University of California-San Francisco School of Medicine, CA, USA

Marcus Behrens Department of Anesthesiology and Pain Medicine, University of Washington, Seattle, WA, USA

Courtney Bennett Mayo Clinic College of Medicine and Science, Rochester, MN, USA

Ariel Bensimhon Department of Anesthesiology, University of Vermont, University of Vermont Medical Center, Burlington, VT, USA

Keith Boniface Department of Emergency Medicine, George Washington University, Washington, DC, USA

Tara Brakke, MD Department of Anesthesiology, University of Nebraska Medical Center, Omaha, NE, USA

Stephen Brannan, MD Department of Anesthesiology, University of Nebraska Medical Center, Omaha, NE, USA

Valeria Santibanez, MD Division of Pulmonary, Critical Medicine and Allergy, Thomas Jefferson University, Philadelphia, PA, USA

Drew Brotherston Department of Medicine, University of Toronto, Toronto, ON, Canada
Department of Medicine, St. Michael's Hospital, Unity Health Toronto, Toronto, ON, Canada
Zucker School of Medicine at Hofstra/Northwell, Hempstead, NY, USA

Hallie Brown Stanford University School of Medicine, Palo Alto, CA, USA

Becky Burk Renown Health, Reno, NV, USA

Mark Caridi-Scheible Emory University Hospital, Atlanta, GA, USA

Rachel Carlson Department of Anesthesiology, Perioperative, and Pain Medicine, Brigham and Women's Hospital, Boston, MA, USA
University of Vermont Medical Center, UVM Larner College of Medicine, Burlington, VT, USA

Stephanie Cha Department of Anesthesiology and Critical Care Medicine, Johns Hopkins University School of Medicine, Baltimore, MD, USA

Jen-Ting Chen Division of Critical Care Medicine, Department of Medicine, Montefiore Medical Center, Albert Einstein College of Medicine, Bronx, NY, USA

Jose L. Diaz-Gomez Department of Anesthesiology and Critical Care Medicine, Baylor College of Medicine, Texas Heart Institute at Baylor St. Luke's Medical Center, Houston, TX, USA

Aaran Drake Department of Emergency Medicine, George Washington University, Washington, DC, USA

Youyou Duanmu Department of Emergency Medicine, Stanford University School of Medicine, Palo Alto, CA, USA

Siddharth Dugar Department of Critical Care, Cleveland Clinic Lerner College of Medicine, Respiratory Institute, Cleveland Clinic, Cleveland, OH, USA
Department of Critical Care Medicine, Integrated Healthcare Institute (IHI), Cleveland Clinic, Cleveland, OH, USA

Renee Dversdal Department of Medicine, Division of Hospital Medicine, Oregon Health & Science University, Portland, OR, USA

Kristin Dwyer Emergency Medicine, Warren Alpert Medical School of Brown University, Providence, RI, USA

Karim El-Kersh Division of Pulmonary, Critical Care, and Sleep Medicine, Department of Medicine, University of Arizona College of Medicine, Phoenix, AZ, USA

Babar Fiza Division of Critical Care Medicine, Department of Anesthesiology, Emory School of Medicine, Atlanta, GA, USA

Saul Flores, MD, FACC, FCCM Adult Congenital Heart Disease ICU, Division of Critical Care Medicine in the Department of Pediatrics, Baylor College of Medicine at Texas Children's Hospital, Houston, TX, USA

Andrew Foderaro Warren Alpert Medical School, Brown University, Providence, RI, USA

Eli V. Gelfand Cardiovascular Division, Beth Israel Deaconess Medical Center, Harvard Medical School, Boston, MA, USA

Daniel Gerber Stanford University School of Medicine, Stanford, CA, USA

Shivani Ghoshal Department of Neurology, Columbia University, New York, NY, USA

Alberto Goffi Department of Medicine, University of Toronto, Toronto, ON, Canada
Department of Medicine, St. Michael's Hospital, Unity Health Toronto, Toronto, ON, Canada
Interdepartmental Division of Critical Care Medicine, University of Toronto, Toronto, ON, Canada
Department of Critical Care Medicine, St. Michael's Hospital, Unity Health Toronto, Toronto, ON, Canada

Ewan Goligher Interdepartmental Division of Critical Care Medicine, University of Toronto, Toronto, ON, Canada
Division of Respirology, Department of Medicine, University Health Network, Toronto, ON, Canada
Toronto General Hospital Research Institute, Toronto, ON, Canada

Matthew J. Griffee Department of Anesthesiology and Perioperative Medicine, School of Medicine, University of Utah, Salt Lake City, UT, USA

Pranjal Gupta Critical Care Fellow, Stanford University School of Medicine, Stanford, CA, USA

Mark Hamlin Department of Anesthesiology, University of Vermont, University of Vermont Medical Center, Burlington, VT, USA

Korbin Haycock Emergency Medicine and Pediatrics, Loma Linda University School of Medicine, Loma Linda, CA, USA
Department of Emergency Medicine, Riverside University Health System Medical Center, Moreno Valley, CA, USA
Department of Emergency Medicine, Loma Linda University Medical Center, Loma Linda, CA, USA
Department of Emergency Medicine, Desert Regional Medical Center, Palm Springs, CA, USA

Kathryn Hendrickson Pulmonary and Critical Care, The Oregon Clinic, Portland, OR, USA

Megan H. Hicks Wake Forest University School of Medicine, Winston-Salem, NC, USA

Ellie Hirshberg Intermountain, Salt Lake City, UT, USA

Maxwell Hockstein MedStar Washington Hospital Center, Washington, DC, USA

Christopher W. Hoeger Cardiovascular Division, Beth Israel Deaconess Medical Center, Harvard Medical School, Boston, MA, USA

Robert Jackson Interdepartmental Division of Critical Care Medicine, University of Toronto, Toronto, ON, Canada

Bilal Athar Jalil Divisions of Cardiovascular Critical Care and Advanced Heart Failure, Heart and Vascular Institute, West Virginia University, Morgantown, WV, USA

Jan Kasal Washington University School of Medicine, St. Louis, MO, USA

Christopher Kelly University of Utah, Salt Lake City, UT, USA

Sameer Khanijo Donald and Barbara Zucker School of Medicine at Hofstra/Northwell, New York, NY, USA

Mina Khorashadi Department of Anesthesia and Perioperative Care, University of California San Francisco, San Francisco, CA, USA

James N. Kirkpatrick Division of Cardiology, University of Washington School of Medicine, Seattle, WA, USA

John C. Klick Department of Anesthesiology, University of Vermont Medical Center, UVM Larner College of Medicine, Burlington, VT, USA

Christopher Koo Beth Israel Deaconess Medical Center, Boston, MA, USA

James Kornfield OHSU Pulmonary, Allergy and Critical Care Medicine, Portland, OR, USA

Danie Leahy Department of Anesthesiology and Critical Care Medicine, Johns Hopkins University School of Medicine, Baltimore, MD, USA

James Leatherman Division of Pulmonary and Critical Care, Hennepin County Medical Center, University of Minnesota, Minneapolis, MN, USA

Akiva Leibowitz Department of Anesthesia, Critical Care and Pain Medicine, Harvard Medical School, Beth Israel Deaconess Medical Center, Boston, MA, USA

Nicholas A. Leverone Division of Pulmonary, Critical Care, Sleep Medicine and Physiology, Department of Medicine, University of California, San Diego, La Jolla, CA, USA

Nicholas Levin Stanford University, Stanford, CA, USA

Andrew T. Levinson Division of Pulmonary, Critical Care, and Sleep Medicine, The Warren Alpert Medical School, Brown University, Providence, RI, USA

Flora Li University of Washington, Seattle, WA, USA

Erin J. Liang Department of Emergency Medicine, Kaiser Permanente San Diego, San Diego, CA, USA

Daniel A. Lichtenstein Medical intensivist, Ambroise-Paré hospital, Paris-West university, France

Viveta Lobo Stanford University School of Medicine, Palo Alto, CA, USA

Donald R. Maberry Division of Critical Care Medicine, Department of Anesthesiology, Emory School of Medicine, Atlanta, GA, USA

Nina Massad Department of Neurology, Columbia University, New York, NY, USA

John L. Maurer Department of Critical Care, University of Minnesota Physicians, Minneapolis, MN, USA

Paul H. Mayo Zucker School of Medicine at Hofstra/Northwell, Hempstead, NY, USA

Kimberly McPhearson Department of Critical Care Medicine, Mayo Clinic, Jacksonville, FL, USA

Taro Minami Division of Pulmonary, Critical Care, and Sleep Medicine, Care New England, Providence, RI, USA
Division of Pulmonary, Critical Care, and Sleep Medicine, Department of Medicine, The Warren Alpert Medical School of Brown University, Providence, RI, USA

Paul K. Mohabir Stanford University School of Medicine, Stanford, CA, USA

Amira Mohamed Critical Care Medicine Fellowship Program, Albert Einstein College of Medicine, Bronx, NY, USA
Division of Critical Care Medicine, Montefiore Medical Center, Bronx, NY, USA

Feroz Mohammed Intensive Care and Anaesthesia, Northampton, UK

Xavier Monnet AP-HP, Service de médecine intensive-réanimation, Hôpital de Bicêtre, DMU 4 CORREVE, Inserm UMR S_999, FHU SEPSIS, CARMAS, Université Paris-Saclay, Le Kremlin-Bicêtre, France

Idunn Morris Interdepartmental Division of Critical Care Medicine, University of Toronto, Toronto, ON, Canada
Division of Respirology, Department of Medicine, University Health Network, Toronto, ON, Canada
Department of Intensive Care Medicine, Nepean Hospital, Sydney, Australia

Aaron Murphy-Crews Division of Critical Care Medicine, Department of Anesthesiology, Washington University School of Medicine, St. Louis, MO, USA

Paul Musgrave Legacy Inpatient Medical Service, Legacy Health, Portland, OR, USA

Mangala Narasimhan Donald and Barbara Zucker School of Medicine at Hofstra/Northwell, New York, NY, USA

Linda Nguyen PeaceHealth St. Joseph Medical Center, Bellingham, WA, USA
Bellingham Anesthesia Associates, Bellingham, WA, USA

Sara Nikravan University of Washington, Seattle, WA, USA

Belal Noureddine Internal Medicine Group, Orlando Health, Orlando, FL, USA

Connor O'Brien Division of Cardiology and Critical Care Cardiology Section, Department of Medicine, University of California-San Francisco School of Medicine, CA, USA

Michael O'Neil Main Line Emergency Medicine Associates, West Chester, PA, USA

Brooks Ohlson Virginia Mason Franciscan Health, Seattle, WA, USA

Achikam Oren-Grinberg Department of Anesthesia, Critical Care and Pain Medicine, Harvard Medical School, Beth Israel Deaconess Medical Center, Boston, MA, USA

Nova Panebianco Department of Emergency Medicine, University of Pennsylvania, Philadelphia, PA, USA

Paru Patrawalla, MD Division of Pulmonary and Critical Care Medicine, Icahn School of Medicine at Mount Sinai (Mount Sinai West/Morningside/ Beth Israel), New York, NY, USA

Deepak Pradhan New York University Grossman School of Medicine, New York, NY, USA

Matthew E. Prekker Department of Medicine, Division of Pulmonary, Allergy, and Critical Care Medicine, Hennepin County Medical Center, Minneapolis, MN, USA

Karuna Puttur Rajkumar Wake Forest Baptist Health, Winston-Salem, NC, USA

Faisal S. Qadir Summa Health Medical Group, Akron, OH, USA

Nida Qadir Division of Pulmonary and Critical Care Medicine, David Geffen School of Medicine at UCLA, Los Angeles, CA, USA

Imrana Qawi Division of Pulmonary, Critical Care and Sleep Division, Tufts Medical Center, Boston, MA, USA

Mark M. Ramzy Multidisciplinary Critical Care Training Program, University of Pittsburgh Medical Center, Pittsburgh, PA, USA

Lisa Rapoport Emergency and Critical Care Medicine, Kaiser Permanente Santa Clara, Santa Clara, CA, USA
Department of Emergency Medicine, Stanford University School of Medicine, Santa Clara, CA, USA

Vera Rigolin Northwestern University Feinberg School of Medicine, Chicago, IL, USA
Department of Medicine, Bluhm Cardiovascular Institute, Northwestern University Feinberg School of Medicine, Chicago, IL, USA

Maha Salama Cardiothoracic ICU Lenox Hill Hospital NYC, Emergency Medicine Jacobi Medical Center/North Central Bronx, Bronx, NY, USA

Aarti Sarwal Division of Neurocritical Care Chief, Virginia Commonwealth University, Richmon, VA, USA

Ryota Sato The Queen's Medical Center, Honolulu, HI, USA
John A. Burns School of Medicine, University of Hawai'i Manoa, Honolulu, HI, USA

Monica Saxena Department of Emergency Medicine, Stanford School of Medicine, Stanford University, Stanford, CA, USA

Gregory A. Schmidt Division of Pulmonary Diseases, Critical Care, and Occupational Medicine, University of Iowa, Iowa City, IA, USA

Christopher K. Schott Critical Care Medicine and Emergency Medicine, VA Pittsburgh Healthcare Sciences and University of Pittsburgh, Pittsburgh, PA, USA

Ziad S. Shaman Case Western Reserve University, MetroHealth Medical Center, Cleveland, OH, USA

Christopher Shaw OHSU Pulmonary, Allergy and Critical Care Medicine, Portland, OR, USA

Manender Kumar Singla Fortis Hospital, Ludhiana, India

Meghan Snuckel Division of Pulmonary, Critical Care, and Sleep Medicine, The Warren Alpert Medical School, Brown University, Providence, RI, USA

Jacqueline Sohn Department of Anesthesiology and Critical Care Medicine, Texas Heart Institute at Baylor St. Luke's Medical Center, Houston, TX, USA

Vincent L. Sorrell University of Kentucky, Gill Heart and Vascular Institute, Lexington, KY, USA

Erik Su, MD, FAAP, FASE Adult Congenital Heart Disease ICU, Division of Critical Care Medicine in the Department of Pediatrics, Baylor College of Medicine at Texas Children's Hospital, Houston, TX, USA

David N. Suwondo Department of Emergency Medicine, Yale University School of Medicine, New Haven, CT, USA

Daniel A. Sweeney Division of Pulmonary, Critical Care, Sleep Medicine and Physiology, Department of Medicine, University of California, San Diego, La Jolla, CA, USA

Jordan Talan New York University Grossman School of Medicine, New York, NY, USA

Tonia Timperley Tauh Department of Anesthesiology and Pain Medicine, University of British Columbia, Vancouver, BC, Canada

Megan Trieu Department of Medicine, Division of Pulmonary, Critical Care, and Sleep Medicine, University of California, San Diego, La Jolla, CA, USA

Joel Turner Department of Emergency Medicine, Jewish General Hospital, McGill University, Montreal, QC, Canada

Saraschandra Vallabhajosyula Cardiology Division, Warren Alpert Medical School of Brown University, Providence, RI, USA

Carla Venegas Department of Critical Care Medicine, Mayo Clinic, Jacksonville, FL, USA

Chakra Venkata Saint Louis University/Mercy Hospital St. Louis, St. Louis, MO, USA

Daniel Walsh Beth Israel Deaconess Medical Center, Boston, MA, USA

Kathleen M. Waybill Division of Pulmonary, Critical Care and Sleep Division, Tufts Medical Center, Boston, MA, USA

Brandon M. Wiley Keck School of Medicine, University of Southern California, Los Angeles, CA, USA

Jonathan N. Wilkinson Intensive Care and Anaesthesia, Northampton, UK

Vidhushei Yogeswaran Division of Cardiology, University of Washington School of Medicine, Seattle, WA, USA

Part I

Ultrasound Basics

Physics of Ultrasound

1

Ziad S. Shaman and Faisal S. Qadir

I chose to pursue a career in physics because there the truth isn't so easily bent.

Angela Merkel

Learning Objectives

1. Understand the basic physical principles of sound waves
2. Demonstrate how an ultrasound image is formed
3. Review the different types of ultrasound
4. Describe the various *types of tissue interaction with the ultrasound beam*

Sound Waves

Sound, and ultrasound, waves are forms of mechanical energy propagated from one point to another by the effect of moving or vibrating the medium that transmits the sound. Sound is an example of a longitudinal wave oscillating back and forth in the direction of wave travel, and hence comprises areas of compressions alternating with areas of decompressions (rarefactions). If the sound wave strikes an object and cannot penetrate it (e.g., a wall), it may go around it by diffraction. If the beam encounters an object larger than the width of the beam (e.g., a mountain), it will be unable to go around it. The beam will bounce off (or reflect), creating an echo [1].

Z. S. Shaman (✉)
Case Western Reserve University, MetroHealth Medical Center, Cleveland, OH, USA
e-mail: zss@case.edu

F. S. Qadir
Summa Health Medical Group, Akron, OH, USA

Although sound is a longitudinal wave with energy traveling in the same direction as the propagation, it is usually represented graphically as a transverse wave. In this layout, the energy is depicted as waves drawn perpendicular to the direction of propagation (Fig. 1.1).

With this scheme in mind, a wave goes through a peak (compression) and a trough (rarefaction) to complete one cycle. A wave has a length that represents the distance the wave occupies in space or on the horizontal axis, called the wavelength. The time it takes the wave to complete one cycle is called the period. Each cycle has a frequency, which is the number of times the wave completes a cycle in 1 second. The product of the wavelength and the frequency determines the propagation speed of sound in a medium as in Fig. 1.1.

$$\text{The speed of sound} = \text{wavelength} \times \text{frequency}$$

Since the speed of sound depends on the medium it travels through, for a constant propagation speed the frequency and the wavelength of the ultrasound beam are inversely related.

On the vertical axis of the graphical representation of an ultrasound beam (Fig. 1.1), the strength of the compression/decompression is represented by the height of the wave and is referred to as the amplitude. While the strength of the sound wave is measured in units of sound energy, decibels, the effects of sound energy on the medium it travels through are described in terms of mechanical and thermal energy and will be addressed later.

M. J. Lanspa, A. T. Levinson (eds.), *Echocardiography and Ultrasonography in the ICU*, Respiratory Medicine, https://doi.org/10.1007/978-3-031-80038-2_1

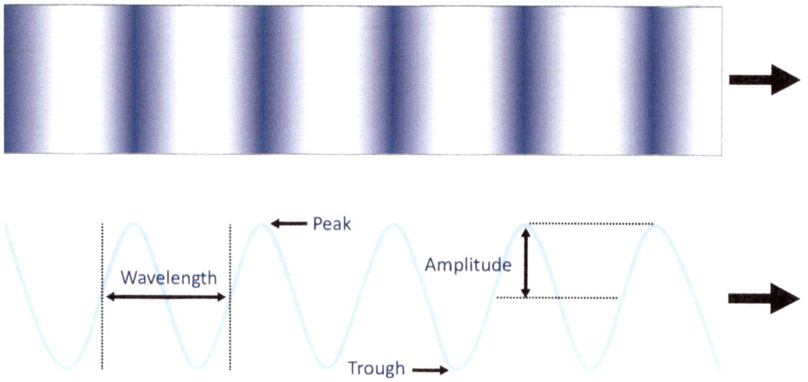

Fig. 1.1 Graphical depiction of a longitudinal wave such as sound traveling through a medium (upper panel), and a transverse wave representation of the longitudinal wave (lower panel) showing the locations of the peak (compression) and trough (rarefaction), in addition to the wavelength and the amplitude

Therefore, because the speed of sound in soft tissue is approximately 1540 m/s, in a typical cardiac transducer that generates an ultrasound beam of 3 MHz frequency, the period will be 0.33 μs and the wavelength of the beam will be approximately 0.513 mm.

However, a typical vascular transducer that generates an ultrasound beam of 10 MHz frequency will have a period of 0.1 μs. The beam wavelength will be 0.154 mm when traveling in soft tissue.

In both cases, the amplitude of the wave is determined by the transducer imaging modality and by other settings that allow tissue penetration to the desired depth of interrogation.

Ultrasound

Ultrasound waves are similar to audible sounds but have frequencies that are higher than audible sounds. The range of sound frequencies that humans can hear is 20 Hz–20 kHz. Therefore, frequencies >20 kHz are called ultrasound. Diagnostic ultrasound tends to be in the range of 2–12 MHz.

In diagnostic ultrasound transducers, ultrasound waveforms are generated by transforming electrical energy to pressure waves using crystals with piezoelectric properties. When these crystals are subjected to a high-voltage alternating current, they vibrate, and the vibration is translated into pressure waves [2] (Table 1.1).

The piezoelectric effect is known to naturally occur in quartz and in other materials such as lead-zirconate-titanate crystals which are currently in use in many commercial ultrasound transducers. New technologies use capacitive micromachined drums or use epoxy resin instead of piezoelectric crystals to perform similar conversions between electrical and mechanical energies. This allows lower production costs and may also reduce the electrical voltages required to operate transducers.

At appropriately high electrical frequencies, ultrasound waves are created through a series of compressions and rarefactions in the medium surrounding the vibrating elements. The same crystals that generate the ultrasound beam can act as receivers of reflected ultrasound energy, which results in the generation of electrical voltage that can be captured, processed, and presented on a screen as an image (Fig. 1.2).

Table 1.1 Characteristics, definitions, and examples of sound wave properties

Characteristic	Definition	Examples
Period (p)	Time required to complete one cycle Unit: any unit of time, usually in μs	Determined by the sound source Typically 0.5–0.083 μs
Frequency (f)	Number of cycles per second, which is also the inverse of the period f = cycles/s = $1/p$ Unit: per second, Hertz	Determined by the sound source Medical ultrasound frequency is typically 2–12 MHz
Propagation velocity (C)	Velocity of sound C = frequency (f) × wavelength (λ) Unit: m/s	Property of the medium varies according to the density and stiffness of the medium Velocity of sound in soft tissue is about 1540 m/s
Wavelength (λ)	Length of a single longitudinal wave Unit: any unit of length, usually mm	Determined by the sound source and medium Image resolution is inversely related to the wavelength
Amplitude	The strength or intensity of the sound beam Unit: dB	Determined by the sound source Decreases with propagation through the medium A wide range of amplitudes can be displayed on a gray-scale display for ultrasound imaging

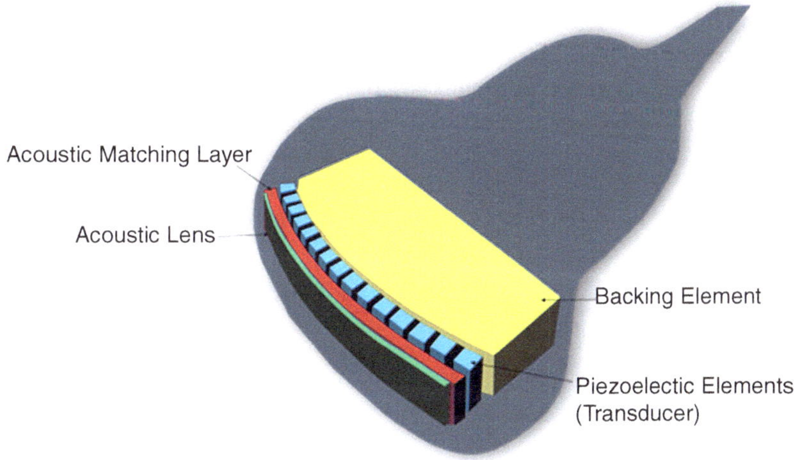

Fig. 1.2 A schematic depiction of the components of an ultrasound transducer. The piezoelectric elements are housed between a backing material on one side and an acoustic matching layer and lens on the other. The backing material dampens the vibrations. The acoustic matching layer allows ultrasound waves to travel to the face of the transducer. The acoustic lens focuses the beam coming out of the transducer

Velocity of Sound

The **velocity** of sound, in general terms, refers to the speed of sound through air in a particular direction. It is important to note that the speed of sound through a given medium is constant (at a certain temperature) and that the speed of sound varies across different media, depending on the density and stiffness of the medium (Table 1.2).

Table 1.2 The speed of sound in different tissue media

Medium	Sound velocity (m/s)
Lung	600
Adipose tissue	1450
Muscle	1580
Blood	1584
Liver	1590
Bone	2100–3500

Duck FA (1990) Acoustic properties of tissue at ultrasonic frequencies. Physical Properties of Tissues 73–135

In liquids, the velocity of sound is given by the Newton–Laplace equation:

$$\text{Sound velocity} = \sqrt{\frac{\text{stiffness}}{\text{density}}}$$

The velocity of sound through various media is shown in the table below.

For diagnostic medical sonography, the speed of sound is assumed to be constant at 1540 m/s, regardless of the tissue type being examined, ignoring the effect of sound on the tissue temperature.

Pulsed Ultrasound

For most applications of ultrasound, other than continuous wave ultrasound, the transducer sends signals as a collection of cycles separated by quiet, listening periods. Each set of cycles is called a pulse. The time the transducer is active, sending a pulse, is called the pulse duration, and the length of space that the pulse occupies is called the spatial pulse length (usually measured in mm) (Fig. 1.3). The time between the start of two pulses is called the pulse period (usually measured in ms), and the rate at which the pulse is repeated in 1 s is called the pulse repetition frequency (which is usually measured in kHz). Finally, the pulse duration relative to the pulse period, or the fraction of time that the transducer spends transmitting is called the duty factor (a unitless number), and it is usually <1%.

While the operator cannot change most of the pulse characteristics in two-dimensional imaging, as the operator attempts to examine deeper structures, the transducer will decrease the pulse repetition frequency, resulting in a lower duty factor, to allow for longer listening periods for returned echoes from deeper structures.

Not all modalities of ultrasound are pulsed (Table 1.3). A notable exception is **continuous wave Doppler** where some of the transducer vibrating elements generate a continuous beam (a duty factor of 100%) and other elements are used to continuously receive echoes (a duty factor of 0%). This imaging modality allows very accurate detection of signals at the expense of location (see Chap. 2).

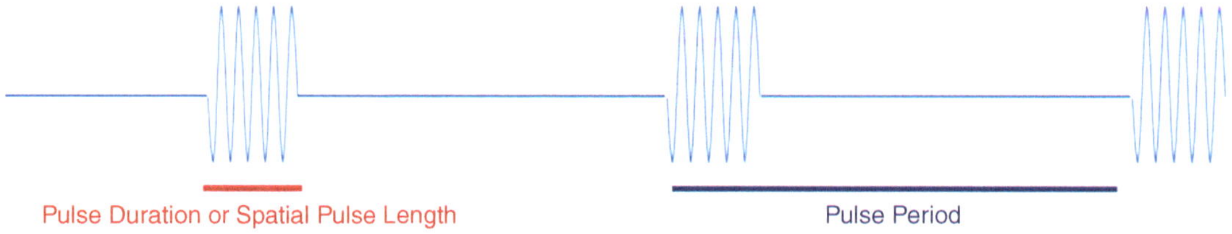

Fig. 1.3 Schematic showing the difference between pulse duration (which equals the spatial pulse length) and the pulse period

Table 1.3 Characteristics and definitions of the ultrasound beam and the pulsed nature of beam generation

Ultrasound beam characteristic		Pulsed beam characteristic	
Period (p)	Time required to complete one cycle, usually in μs	Pulse duration	Time from the start to the end of a pulse, usually in μs
		Pulse period or pulse repetition period (PRP)	Time from the start of one pulse to the start of the next pulse, usually in μs
		Duty factor	Pulse duration/pulse period, presented as a fraction
Frequency (f)	Number of cycles per second, usually in MHz	Pulse repetition frequency (PRF)	Number of pulses per second, usually in kHz (of note PRF = 1/PRP)
Wavelength (λ)	Length of a single wave, usually in mm	Spatial pulse length (SPL)	Distance from the start to the end of a pulse, usually in mm

The Range Equation

In diagnostic ultrasound, we can estimate the depth of a structure reflecting sound to generate two-dimensional images. Using the assumption that the velocity of sound is constant through various soft tissues, ultrasound systems measure the time it takes for an ultrasound pulse to travel from the transducer to the reflecting structure and back to the transducer. This **transit time** depends on both the velocity of the sound wave and on the depth of the reflecting structure. The "range equation" is used to calculate the depth:

$$\text{Distance to reflecting structure}(\text{mm}) = \text{Transit time}(\mu s) \times \text{speed}(\text{mm}/\mu s)/2$$

So, for a structure that is 30 mm in depth, it would take the ultrasound beam 39 μs to travel from the transducer to the structure and back. And here, the distance = (39 × 1.54)/2 = 30 mm.

However, if the ultrasound beam has a 130 μs transit time, the structure reflecting the beam must be (130 × 1.54)/2 = 100 mm away from the transducer.

A simplified "Rule of 13" states that for every 1 cm depth, the ultrasound beam takes 13 μs of round-trip travel time. Try the math on this. It works.

Interaction Between Ultrasound and Tissue

As ultrasound travels through the tissue, it is redirected through reflection, refraction, and scatter. Also, as ultrasound beams interact with the tissue, energy is lost as it converts into heat through a process called absorption. This loss of energy, called **attenuation**, results in dampening of the wave or reduction in its amplitude.

Reflection, refraction, and scatter occur because of differences in the acoustic properties of different tissues. This property is called **acoustic impedance**. Acoustic impedance depends on the density of the medium and the speed of sound. The bigger the difference in acoustic impedance of adjacent structures, the stronger the reflection, refraction, and scatter (Table 1.4).

Reflection and refraction occur when the ultrasound beam strikes a tissue boundary with a lateral dimension that is larger than the wavelength of the ultrasound beam. This happens, for example, when the ultrasound beam interacts with the diaphragm, with heart valves, or with vessel walls. These interfaces are referred to as "specular" reflectors. **Reflection** is the rebound of the beam from the interface. **Refraction** is the redirection of the transmitted beam at the interface. Both reflection and refraction increase as the angle of incidence deviates from 90° (Fig. 1.4).

Table 1.4 A summary of the terms, definitions, and examples of the effect of tissue interaction with the ultrasound beam

Term	Definition	Examples
Acoustic impedance (Z)	Tissue impedance = tissue density (ρ) × velocity of sound (*c*)	The boundaries between air and soft tissue and between soft tissue and bone make strong reflectors
Reflection	Return of ultrasound beam to the transducer from a boundary of media with different acoustic impedances of large width compared to the wavelength of the beam	Reflections are maximized when the incident ultrasound beam is perpendicular to the surface of the reflector
Scatter	Widespread redirection of the ultrasound beam due to interaction with a boundary of small width compared to the wavelength of the beam	Red blood cells fill the blood in cardiac chambers, but the chambers appear empty because the beam scatters when the beam hits the surface of the red blood cells
Absorption	Loss of energy of an ultrasound beam = tissue absorption coefficient (*a*) × distance × frequency (*f*)	Higher frequency ultrasound beam loses more energy than lower frequency beam for the same examination distance

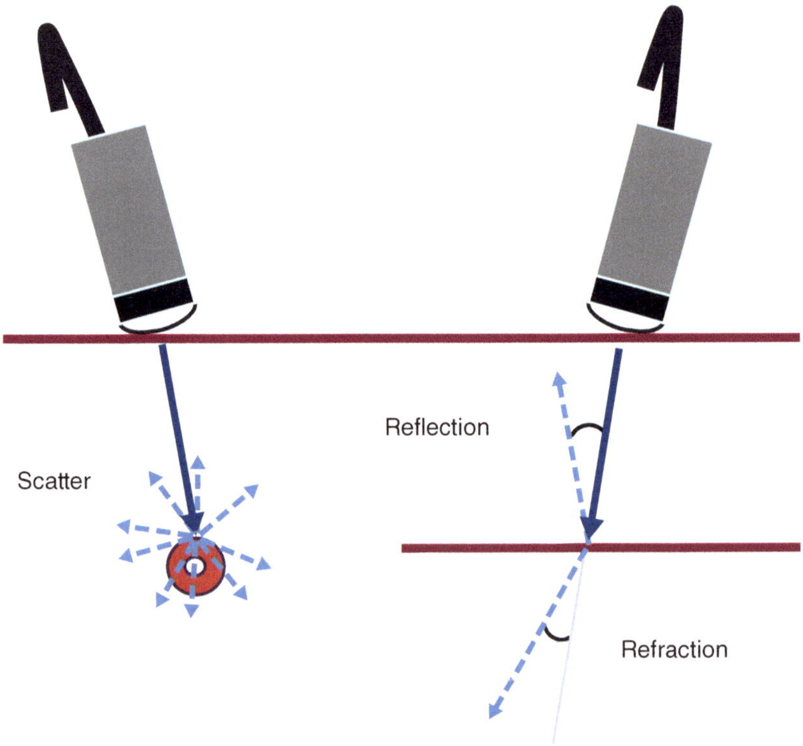

Fig. 1.4 Schematic showing reflection, refraction, and scatter as an ultrasound beam interacts with tissue boundaries

When the lateral dimension of the reflector is smaller than the wavelength of the ultrasound beam, the beam is scattered in all directions. This is called **Rayleigh scattering**. Scattering occurs, for example, at the surface of gas bubbles within the bowel lumen, at the edges of small granularities within tissues, or by red blood cell membranes within the blood. Scatter is used to detect flow when using the Doppler imaging modality, which is described later.

Signals returned to the transducer through reflection and scatter are used by ultrasound systems to generate two-dimensional images.

Unlike reflection that takes place only at the interfaces of two media with different properties, absorption occurs continuously throughout beam travel distance in any medium. Absorption depends on a tissue property, indicated by the **Attenuation Coefficient** (Table 1.5), and on the frequency of the ultrasound beam. The higher the coefficient, the more energy the tissue absorbs per unit of beam travel distance, and the higher the frequency, the greater the absorption of energy.

$$\text{Attenuation} = \text{Coefficient} \times \text{distance} \times \text{frequency}$$

As you can see from Table 1.5, water, or liquid media in general, is considered "ultrasound-friendly" where very little absorption occurs and the beam can travel generous distances with little attenuation, while air and bone are considered ultrasound-unfriendly because of significant degradation of signal in a very short travel distance.

For a clinical example, a 3 MHz cardiac ultrasound beam will lose 18 dB by absorption after traveling to a 6 cm deep reflector in soft tissue. Here, absorption = 0.5 dB/cm/MHz × 12 cm × 3 MHz = 18 dB. Of note, an 18 dB reduction in sound level corresponds to 63 times reduction in signal intensity because dBs are represented on a logarithmic scale.

However, setting the transducer to a frequency of 5 MHz will cause the beam to lose more energy examining the same structure. In this case, absorption = 0.5 dB/cm/MHz × 12 cm × 5 MHz = 30 dB. Here, a 30 dB reduction in sound level corresponds to 1000 times reduction in

Table 1.5 The attenuation coefficient of sound in different tissue media

Medium	Attenuation (absorption) coefficient (dB/cm/MHz)
Water	0.002
Blood	0.2
Spleen	0.45
Soft tissue	0.5 (on average)
Muscle	1.1
Fat	1.5
Bone	16
Lung	30

Duck FA (1990) Acoustic properties of tissue at ultrasonic frequencies. Physical Properties of Tissues 73–135

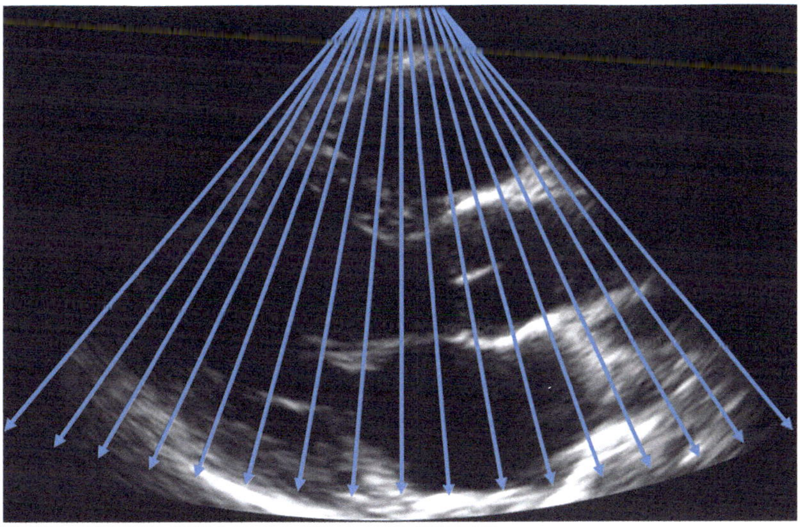

Fig. 1.5 An ultrasound image showing multiple scan paths. Each scan line detects reflections along its scan path

signal intensity due to the logarithmic nature of the sound intensity scale.

Ultrasound Image Formation

For diagnostic ultrasound, the differences in acoustic impedance within and between tissues cause echoes to return to the transducer allowing image formation [3]. The bigger the difference in acoustic impedance between two tissues, the larger the proportion of sound reflected, and the brighter the representation of the reflector on the ultrasound screen (Fig. 1.4). For each ultrasound beam (called "Scan Line"), multiple brightness signals can be represented on the screen vertically and this creates a single line on the screen. As multiple beams are transmitted through a swathe of tissue, and as multiple scan lines are presented on the screen, a two-dimensional image is formed (Fig. 1.5). After a two-dimensional image is created, the process is then repeated multiple times per second, each time creating a "frame." With multiple frames per second still images come to life, and a view of the underlying structures is created on the screen [4] (Fig. 1.6).

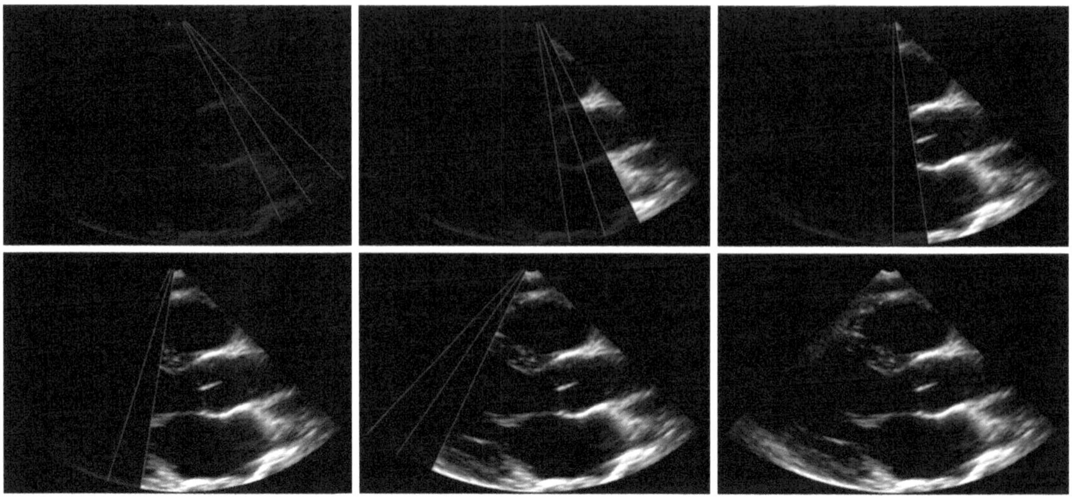

Fig. 1.6 A 2- dimensional ultrasound image is formed by running multiple scan lines through the width of the sector

Time Gain Compensation

Because attenuation weakens ultrasound beams as they travel through the tissue, the deterioration of echo signal strength returning from deeper structures needs to be taken into account to allow a homogeneous presentation of the reflectors on the screen. This post-processing is called "**Time Gain Compensation**" or Correction, or simply "**Gain**." Unfortunately, absorption will eventually make the signals returning from deeper structures too weak to be detected, and imaging depth is limited. This is particularly a problem with high-frequency beams because of the direct relationship between absorption and beam frequency.

Gaining an area can occur inappropriately, leading to acoustic enhancement artifacts (more in the artifact section). These artifacts occur when the beam traverses tissues with a higher or lower attenuation coefficient than expected by the machine algorithm. This anomaly causes the machine to inappropriately display reflections from deeper areas as dimmer or brighter than adjacent structures, leading to a misrepresentation of the tissue image on the screen.

Resolution

Resolution is defined as the smallest distance between two structures that can be distinguished using an ultrasound beam. The greater the resolution, the greater the detail of the image obtained.

The resolution of an ultrasound image can be described in terms of space and time as

- **Spatial Resolution**: Resolution relative to the ultrasound image plane, usually measured in mm, indicating the smallest distance between two structures that would still be recognizable as separate structures, therefore, a smaller number indicates better resolution (Fig. 1.7).
  - Axial: Resolution along/parallel to the ultrasound beam's main axis
  - Lateral: Resolution perpendicular to the ultrasound beam's main axis
  - Elevational: Resolution along the ultrasound image slice thickness
- **Temporal Resolution**: The ability to accurately locate moving structures over time, usually measured in milliseconds. A smaller number indicates more real-time imaging, where movement appears more smooth and less choppy.

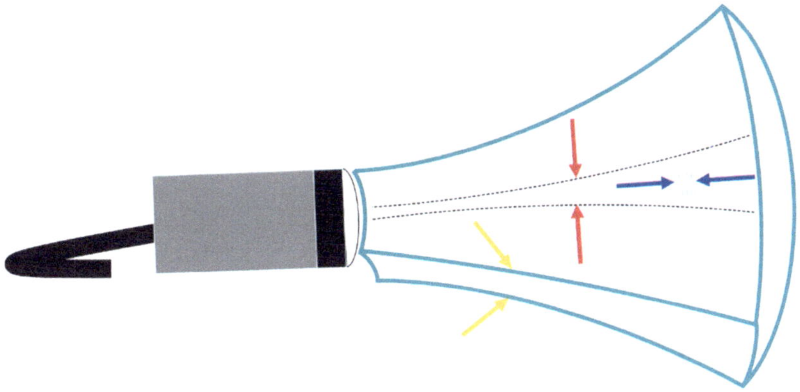

Fig. 1.7 Spatial resolution components are the axial resolution along the axis of the beam (blue arrows); lateral resolution perpendicular to the axis of the beam (red arrows); and elevational resolution (along the thickness of the imaging slice (yellow arrows))

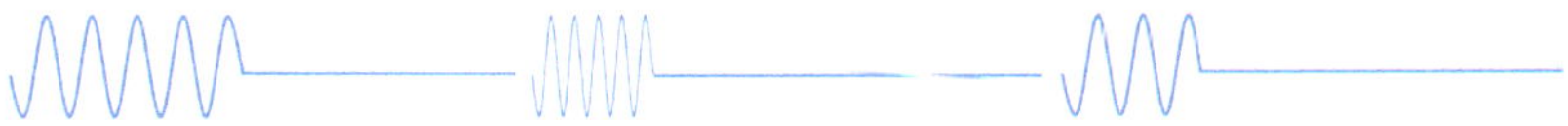

Fig. 1.8 Schematic showing multiple ultrasound beams. Beam A has an pulse of a particular length, the SPL, which determines the axial resolution of the beam. Beam B has a shorter SPL because the wave has a higher frequency although it has the same number of cycles per pulse. Beam C has a shorter SPL than beam A, as well, because it has fewer cycles in each pulse although it has the same frequency as beam A

There are multiple factors that affect each type of resolution. Some are modifiable by the operator, while others depend on the transducer type used and are not modifiable by the operator.

Axial Resolution

Of all resolution types, axial resolution is the most precise. This means that measurements are best obtained along the axis of the ultrasound beam (Fig. 1.8). Axial resolution is dependent on the length of the ultrasound pulse (the **spatial pulse length—SPL**).

$$\text{Axial resolution in mm} = \text{SPL in mm} / 2$$

The two factors that determine the SPL are the number of cycles per pulse and the wavelength (or frequency) of the beam. Therefore, axial resolution can be improved by using higher frequency beams (if modifiable by the operator). However, the number of cycles per pulse is intrinsic to each transducer and is not modifiable.

Of note, an ultrasound beam that is continuous and does not pulse, such as in continuous wave Doppler imaging, has no axial resolution at all.

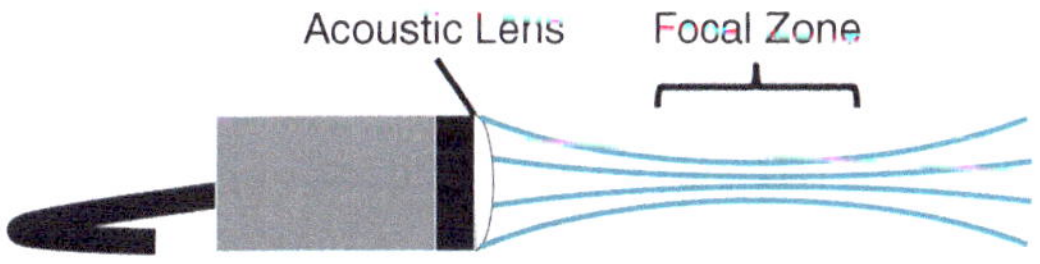

Fig. 1.9 The acoustic lens of the transducer lengthens the focused area of the beam, resulting in a focal zone that has higher lateral resolution than the zones proximal and distal to it

Lateral Resolution

Lateral resolution depends on the diameter of the ultrasound beam. Ultrasound beams tend to be more wide than long; therefore, lateral resolution is usually inferior to axial resolution. As the ultrasound beam exits the face of the transducer, the beam reaches a focal point and then widens (through divergence). The focal point is the narrowest area of the beam and has the best lateral resolution (Fig. 1.9). The focal point can be increased in length by focusing the beam, using an acoustic lens, and by electronic focusing of the beam, to create a focal zone. This improves the lateral resolution along more of the beam depth, rather than at just the focal point. The depth of the electronic focusing of the beam can be adjusted by the operator on some machines, however focusing that is achieved through the acoustic lens is not modifiable for each transducer. Of note, divergence is dependent on the beam frequency. The higher the frequency, the smaller the divergence angle and the better the lateral resolution in the area distal to the focal point or the focal zone.

Elevational Resolution

Elevational resolution is affected by the image slice thickness. A mechanical acoustic lens determines the slice thickness and is not modifiable by the user. So, similar to lateral resolution, elevational resolution is best at the acoustic focal point or focal zone for each transducer. While the acoustic lens is not modifiable by the user; divergence still depends on the beam frequency which is, in some machines, modifiable by the user. Here, the higher the frequency, the smaller the divergence angle, and the better the elevational resolution at the depth of the focal point.

Temporal Resolution

The ability of ultrasound images to track moving structures depends on the time it takes the system to generate a two-dimensional image. The time it takes an image to be formed depends on the image depth and the sector width. Both depth and width can be changed by the operator. Shallower imaging depth results in decreased transit time and less time is needed between ultrasound pulses. A narrow imaging sector requires a fewer number of scan lines per frame. In both cases, more frames can be generated per second resulting in a higher frame rate and better temporal resolution [5].

Certain imaging modalities, such as cardiac imaging, require high frame rates, while other modalities, such as abdominal imaging, do not. Therefore, frame rate ranges are usually set for each transducer for optimal performance for the area of predicted clinical use.

The Resolution—Penetration Interplay

Ultrasound beam frequency seems to play an important role in determining resolution (Table 1.6). A higher frequency improves both axial and lateral resolution. However, using high frequency ultrasound leads to higher attenuation of ultrasound energy and the inability to examine deeper structures. As ultrasound waves undergo attenuation in soft tissue with each wave cycle, attenuation becomes the limiting factor for the penetration of an ultrasound beam. Therefore, using lower frequency ultrasound transducers, and hence longer wavelengths, will undergo less attenuation. However, with the use of lower frequency, resolution suffers (for probe selection, see Chap. 2).

High frequency—shallow images with better overall resolution
Low frequency—deeper images with lower overall resolution

Table 1.6 Comparing different resolutions and the factors influencing each kind of resolution

Resolution	Factors	Adjustability	Resolution improves with
Axial	Frequency	Sometimes	Higher frequency
	Cycles per pulse	No	Fewer cycles per pulse
Lateral	Frequency	Sometimes	Higher frequency (less divergence)
	Focal zone	Sometimes	Scanning within the focal zone depth
Elevational	Frequency	Sometimes	Higher frequency (less divergence)
	Focal zone (fixed)	No	Scanning within the focal zone depth
Temporal	Image depth	Yes	Shallower scanning
	Sector width	Yes	Narrower sectors

Bioeffects of Ultrasound

Ultrasound is considered a relatively safe noninvasive diagnostic tool. However, that does not mean it comes without potential harm. There are bioeffects that result from the interaction of ultrasound energy with tissue. These can be classified as **Thermal** effects and **Mechanical** effects. Beginning in 1993, an output display standard that reports the bioeffects of ultrasound on tissue was required by the FDA. The standard display of the bioeffects of ultrasound was necessary to allow machines to operate at higher energy outputs, and to have greater diagnostic capabilities than previously possible. The display of the indices of thermal and mechanical effects of ultrasound is now standard, and they serve as a real-time alert to the operator so that they can implement the As Low As Reasonably Achievable (ALARA) principle and use this diagnostic tool safely.

Thermal Effects

As ultrasound propagates through tissue, it is converted from sound to other forms of energy through the process of attenuation. Most of this conversion is into heat energy, resulting in a thermal effect which can be harmful to sensitive tissues (e.g., fetal tissue). The heat-generating capacity of ultrasound is quantified and reported as the "Thermal Index."

The thermal index (TI) = power generated by the transducer/power required to raise tissue temperature by 1 °C.

Mechanical Effects

The mechanical effect of ultrasound refers to damage caused by the oscillation of tissue as a result of a sound wave passing through it. The most common mechanical effect on tissue is referred to as "cavitation." **Cavitation** is caused by the oscillation of small gas bubbles within the ultrasound field. In certain circumstances, these bubbles may grow in size or collapse, generating high energies that affect adjacent tissue, causing extreme temperature increases, free radical generation, and even tissue liquefaction. The mechanical effect of ultrasound on tissue is quantified and reported as the "Mechanical Index," which quantifies the likelihood of ultrasound exposure producing cavitation. The FDA requires the mechanical index to remain below 1.9 for safe diagnostic ultrasound use.

The mechanical index (MI) = Peak rarefactional pressure/sqrt of frequency

The mechanical effect of ultrasound has significant diagnostic benefits when using contrast media designed for ultrasound. There is also a potential therapeutic benefit of cavitation in intraocular drug delivery which is likely related to the transient, reversible cavitation effects of ultrasound on the cornea (evolving evidence).

Imaging Modes and Probes

Ultrasound imaging can be used in multiple ways to create different imaging modes. Each mode comes with unique characteristics that are well exploited in different clinical situations.

Two-Dimensional and Three-Dimensional Imaging

As mentioned in the prior section, diagnostic ultrasound imaging uses short pulses of sound to create representations of the anatomic structures. These pulses of sound interact with the tissue and are reflected back to the ultrasound system along individual scan lines. These scan lines "sweep" through a sector of tissue, and the reflections received by the system are analyzed and displayed using a gray scale. This scale is based on the intensity of the ultrasound beams returning to the system, ranging from black (no ultrasound signal) to white (maximum signal intensity). The location (or depth) of a reflecting structure on the image is determined by the transit time to and from the reflector.

Scan lines are then repeated and assembled into a frame, creating a two-dimensional (2-D) image. The process is then repeated to create more frames, making the image come to life. Two-dimensional imaging is the most used and easily recognizable mode of ultrasound imaging.

Other than being the most used imaging technique, 2-D imaging allows for a wide view of the underlying structures in addition to significant details of the examination area. This balance of breadth makes 2-D imaging useful for most clinical applications.

Three-dimensional (3-D) imaging is similar to 2-D imaging in concept, with the addition of multiple scan slices to create a three-dimensional image (Fig. 1.10). In 3-D imaging, multiple swaths of tissue are imaged along the perpendicular axis of the 2-D scan (the *z*-axis) and are reconstructed to be displayed on the screen using 3-D rendering. This can be achieved by using arrays of sound-generating elements or by mechanically moving regular linear arrays of elements. This imaging modality is most commonly used in cardiac and obstetric imaging.

M-Mode Imaging

In **motion mode** (M-Mode) imaging, the information from a single scan line is plotted against time to create an image. Structures along the scan line are displayed vertically according to their depth, while the horizontal axis on the screen represents time. Given that the signal is sent and received along a single scan line, multiple signals can be sent at a high rate, giving M-Mode imaging an excellent temporal, as well as axial resolution.

For optimal use of M-mode, it is important to start the examination in 2-D mode, and then to align the M-Mode scan indicator along the area of interest before activating M-Mode imaging.

While M-Mode imaging allows for higher resolution, it does sacrifice the breadth of the examination. When the details of movement along the axis of the beam are of significant interest, M-Mode imaging becomes very useful. Therefore, M-Mode is often used in evaluating the movement of heart valves and cardiac walls, in addition to applications related to vascular, diaphragmatic, and pleural changes relative to

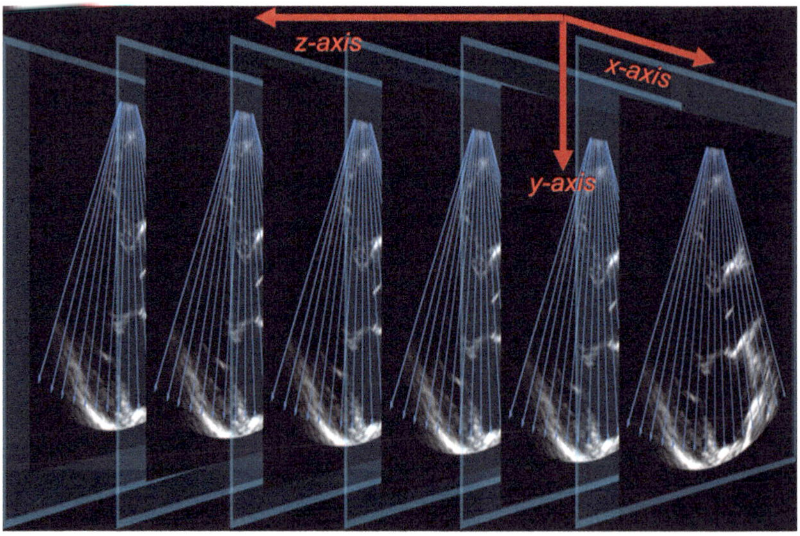

Fig. 1.10 Schematic of the way a three-dimensional image is created by adding multiple layers of the *x*-axis and *y*-axis two-dimensional scans along the *z*-axis

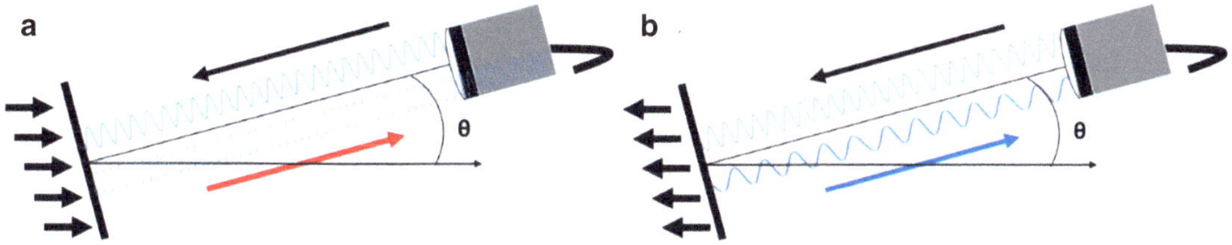

Fig. 1.11 Schematic showing the interaction of ultrasound with a moving reflector creating a positive and a negative Doppler shift. Panel A represents a positive shift (depicted as a red arrow) and panel B represents a negative shift (depicted as a blue arrow)

respirations. For example, M-Mode imaging is used to assess cardiac parameters such as tricuspid annular plane systolic excursion (TAPSE), assessing changes in large vessel caliber (respiratory variability of the IVC), and visceral pleural sliding against the parietal pleura during assessment for pneumothorax.

The Doppler Principle

So far, we have presented sound wave echoes bouncing off stationary reflectors. However, sometimes sound waves reflect after interacting with a moving reflector. Here, the reflector causes an additional effect on the wave, changing its frequency. This change in frequency is called the **Doppler shift** (Fig. 1.11). The term "Doppler effect" was coined by the Austrian mathematician and physicist Christian Doppler who described how light wave frequency depends on the relative speed of binary stars. Similarly, in ultrasound, the Doppler effect is defined as the change in frequency of a sound wave transmitted from a source that is in motion relative to the receiver.

By comparing the frequency of returned ultrasound waves relative to transmitted ones, the Doppler effect can be used to detect the motion of tissue and fluid being imaged and to measure their velocity. The velocity of the moving reflector can be calculated using this equation:

$$\text{Doppler shift} = \frac{2 \times \text{reflector speed} \times \text{source frequency} \times \text{cosine the angle of incidence}\,(\theta)}{\text{sound propagation speed}}$$

Therefore, the change in the frequency of the beam is proportional to the magnitude of the relative velocity of the source (reflector) and the receiver to each other. Also, if the direction of motion of the reflecting structure is at an angle (θ) to the ultrasound beam (angle of insonation), the Doppler shift will be a fraction (cosine θ) of the expected shift (Table 1.7). Hence, if the direction of motion is perpendicular to the incident beam (at 90 degrees), then the relative velocity of the reflector to the probe will be nil (cosine 90° = 0), leading to no Doppler shift, and no motion will be detected by the ultrasound system (Fig. 1.12).

Note that the Doppler shift is bidirectional. The shift is considered positive (resulting in a higher frequency) if the reflector and the receiver are moving toward each other, or negative (resulting in a lower frequency) if the reflector and the receiver are moving away from each other.

Doppler Imaging

Ultrasound systems use the Doppler principle to measure the velocity of reflectors in motion. This is done by continuous measurement (called **Continuous Wave Doppler**) or intermittent

Table 1.7 The values of the cosine of select angles

Insonation angle (θ)	Cosine θ
0°	1
15°	0.97
30°	0.87
45°	0.71
60°	0.5
75°	0.26
90°	0

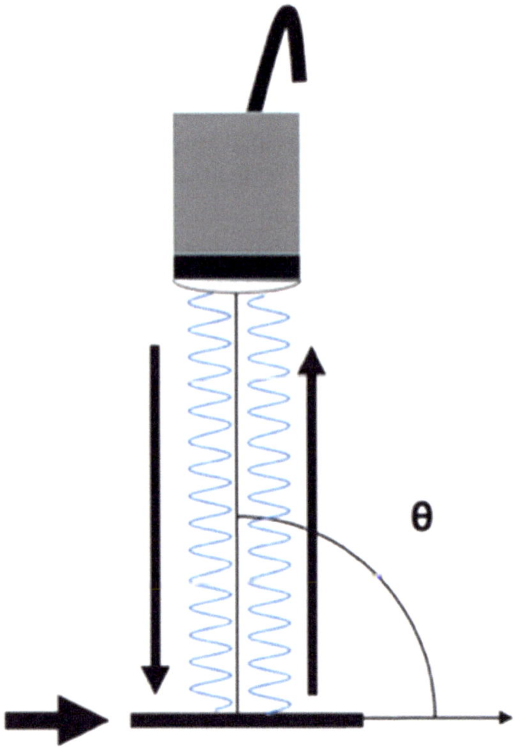

Fig. 1.12 Schematic showing the interaction of ultrasound with a moving reflector creating no Doppler shift. Panel C shows that when the sound beam interacts with a moving reflector at a right angle (90 degrees) there will be no frequency shift between the incident beam and the returned beam

measurement of the frequency of the reflected waves. When intermittent measurement is performed, the results are presented in a quantitative (called **Pulsed Wave Doppler**) or in a semiquantitative way (called **Color Flow Doppler**).

There are, of course, advantages and disadvantages to each of the three modes (Table 1.8).

Continuous Wave (CW) Doppler

In this mode, the ultrasound uses two crystals, one to continuously emit ultrasound signals, and one to continuously receive signals. This allows an accurate detection of Doppler shifts and therefore speed but lacks localization of the reflectors. CW Doppler imaging accurately measures high velocities such as regurgitant jets across heart valves; however, the location of movement along the length of the beam is unknowable. This depth uncertainty is called range ambiguity. Therefore, in CW Doppler, velocity is displayed most accurately while the location of the moving structures is now known.

Pulsed Wave (PW) Doppler

In this mode, one crystal alternates between emitting ultrasound pulses and receiving echoes. Ultrasound reflections from a specific area of interrogation, called "sample volume" or "gate," are analyzed. This localization of the area of interrogation is determined by the operator and is called "range gating" because the depth (or range) of frequencies that are analyzed is limited to a specific area (or gate). Range gating eliminates range ambiguity; however, high velocities may not be accurately detected, because of an artifact called aliasing, which is described below. Therefore, in PW Doppler there is information about both the velocity and the location of the movement, but both are somewhat limited in accuracy.

When using pulsed wave and continuous Doppler, the ultrasound system analyzes the frequency shift of the incoming sound waves, yielding a graphical representation of flow velocity over time, and is called spectral analysis. Spectral Doppler analysis allows measurements to be made of the flow velocity and the relationship of velocity to time. Spectral analysis of flow is often used in vascular and in cardiac ultrasound imaging.

Color Flow (CF) Doppler

This is a form of pulsed wave Doppler, in which the frequencies of the pulses of reflected sound, from multiple sample volumes, are analyzed. The flow at each sampling point is displayed as

Table 1.8 Comparing the accuracy of velocity measurement and the location of measurement of different Doppler modes of ultrasound

Doppler imaging mode	Velocity accuracy	Location of measurement
Continuous wave (CW)	Accurate, no aliasing at any speed	Along a single scan line but at all points of the line
	+++	+
Pulsed wave (PW)	Limited, may be affected by aliasing	Only at the sample volume of the single scan line
	++	++
Color flow (CF)	Semiquantitative, may be affected by aliasing	At multiple sample volumes along multiple scan lines
	+	+++

The benefits of each mode are presented as relative "+" signs

a color map of speed and direction. The color map is presented on the screen overlaying a conventional 2-D image. Color Doppler gives information about velocity in a semiquantitative way only. It is by convention that the color used to represent positive frequency shift is red and the color used to represent negative frequency shift is blue. Yellow hue color transitions from red and blue are used in a semiquantitative way to represent higher frequency shifts in both directions. The acronym "BART" is one way to remember that in CF Doppler "Blue" means the movement is "Away" from the transducer, and "Red" means the movement is "Toward" the transducer. Yellow color is used to represent higher positive, as well as, negative frequency shifts. While CF Doppler allows an accurate localization of flow, velocity determination is analyzed in a semiquantitative way only. Therefore, speed accuracy is sacrificed for information about location.

$$\text{BART} = \text{Blue} - \text{Away}, \text{Red} - \text{Toward}$$

Tissue Doppler Imaging (TDI)

Color flow, pulse wave, and continuous wave Doppler imaging are usually used to measure blood flow velocity [6]. Cardiac structures (the myocardium in particular) move at a much slower velocity when compared to blood flow, therefore, special Doppler settings are needed to detect relatively slower tissue motion. When the transducer is set to detect small shifts in frequency, myocardial motion speed can be detected. Tissue Doppler imaging is commonly used as PW and Color modalities.

Pulsed Wave TDI

This is similar to a traditional pulse wave doppler. The ultrasound system uses filters specifically designed to pick up low-velocity tissue structures and is therefore able to provide a precise measurement of tissue velocity within the designated sample volume. This modality is primarily used in the assessment of cardiac left ventricular diastolic dysfunction, where the sample volumes are set at the insertion points of the mitral valve annulus [7].

Color TDI

The ultrasound system superimposes color-coded tissue velocity images onto the 2-D image in real time. The system then displays the mean velocity of each pixel against time. This is useful in comparative assessment of regional velocity as well as direction but compromises on quantitative assessment. This is helpful, for example, in assessing regional wall motion abnormalities of the left ventricle.

Tissue Harmonics Imaging (THI)

When ultrasound energy interacts with the tissue, it returns to the transducer echoes of the original frequency as well as echoes of multiples of the original frequency (called harmonic frequencies). This occurs because of nonlinear propagation of ultrasound waves through tissue. These returning harmonic frequencies can be detected by the ultrasound system. Harmonic frequencies are then separated from the main beam frequency and are amplified to generate an image{Anvari, 2015 #12;Anvari, 2015 #12;Zderic, 2004 #23}. This mode of imaging offers several advantages [8]:

- Improved signal-to-noise ratio which results in better definition of subtle parenchymal details
- Improved lateral resolution because the effects of harmonic waves are most prominant at the center of the beam therefore resulting in a narrower imaging plane and improving lateral resolution
- Minimizing reverberation, side lobe, and grating lobe artifacts
- Minimize near-field noise because harmonic waves are not produced by superficial structures
- Improved imaging of deeper tissue because the effects of harmonic waves are most prominant at deeper structures

Because of the benefits above, harmonic imaging is standard in cardiac ultrasound examination

Probe Selection

There are many transducer types that are generally available in ultrasound systems. Each type is specifically designed for optimal imaging of a particular body region. The most commonly used transducers in the assessment of critically ill patients are three.

Curved Linear Array Transducers

Also known as convex transducers, these are designed for abdominal and pelvic ultrasonography. Sound emitting elements are arranged side by side along a curved surface, allowing for a cone-shaped, wide field of view, which gets wider at an increased depth. It also allows for good far-field resolution. The beam generated is generally of low frequency, which allows for greater penetration of tissue, and hence allows for an accurate assessment of deeper structures in the abdomen and pelvis.

Linear Array Transducers

Also known simply as linear transducers, these use crystals arranged along a straight line on the surface. These transducers generate high-frequency parallel beams, allowing for a greater and uniform near-field resolution, although at the expense of penetration. A rectangular 2-D image is formed by this probe. Linear probes are best utilized to assess vascular structures during ultrasound-guided vascular access [9].

Phased Array Transducers

Also known as sector array transducers, these are designed specifically for cardiac imaging. The crystals used are smaller and are arranged in a more compact arrangement, either horizontal or circular. The transducer utilizes variable timing of crystal activation, resulting in a fan-shaped image generation. The shape of the ultrasound beam, as well as the narrow footprint of the transducer, makes it ideal for imaging through narrow windows, such as the intercostal spaces, in cardiac imaging. These transducers allow imaging at increased depth, although that compromises significantly on near-field resolution [7].

Ultrasound Artifacts (See Chap. 3)

Ultrasound artifacts are images that do not accurately represent the structures underneath the transducer. Artifacts occur when the assumptions behind image generation deviate from the reality of space/time, attenuation, and/or frequency (Doppler) shifts.

Artifacts are frequently encountered in diagnostic ultrasound, and while some are unwanted, others may provide valuable information related to the structural features of the underlying tissue. Therefore, it is important to recognize and to understand common artifacts. This will help avoid image misinterpretation.

Once an artifact is detected, it is not too difficult to deduce how the artifact occurred. The

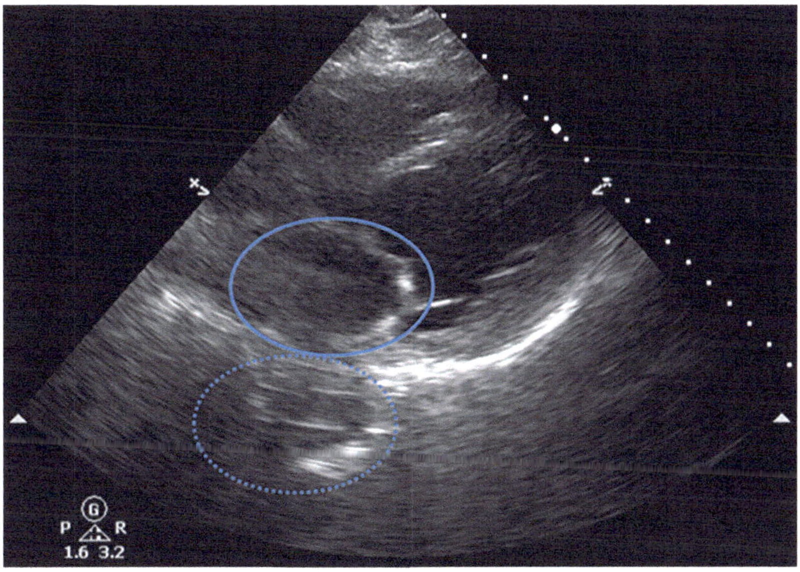

Fig. 1.13 A subcostal ultrasound view of the heart. The left atrium and the mitral valve (solid oval) are mirrored and appear deep to the pericardial line (dotted oval). This occurs because the ultrasound beam reflects between the pericardium and other structures in the heart

challenge, however, is to decide if an artifact exists to begin with. The general rule in two-dimensional imaging is to obtain multiple views of every area of interest, as most artifacts will not withstand the test of multiple views.

"One view is no view"; always obtain at least two (preferably perpendicular) views.

Space/Time Artifacts

Refraction

When the ultrasound beam encounters an interface at an angle, the difference in propagation velocities between the two media can cause refraction of the ultrasound beam. If the refracted beam reflects off a structure to the ultrasound system, this will result in that structure being assigned an incorrect location. This occurs because the ultrasound system assumes beams travel in straight lines. To resolve this artifact, the transducer can be adjusted to make the angle of the ultrasound beam perpendicular to the interface.

Mirror Image

Similar to refraction, when an ultrasound beam interacts with a structure on the way to a strong reflector, the primary beam may reflect back and forth between the structure and the strong reflector. This results in a second image of the structure being assigned a deeper location than the originalreflections (Fig. 1.13) because the ultrasound system assumes that the beam only reflected once and that the later echoes were generated from a deeper location. Examples of reflective surfaces that can produce a mirror image artifact are the pericardium and the diaphragm. The former is responsible for the appearance of cardiac mirror artifacts and the latter for the appearance of false pleural effusions in patients with ascites. Mirror imaging is type of reverberation artifact.

Reverberation

When the ultrasound beam encounters two strong reflectors that are usually (but not necessarily) parallel to one another, the beam may bounce continuously between the two reflectors. Here, the ultrasound system interprets the incoming signals as returning from deeper and deeper structures, due to the longer time it takes for the echoes to return to the transducer (Fig. 1.14). Examples of such strong reflectors include pacemaker leads in cardiac ultrasound, pleural surfaces, and procedural needles. This artifact is usually helpful in identifying strong reflectors.

Ring-down and Comet Tail

A type of resonance artifact that occurs when an ultrasound wave causes cholesterol crystals or

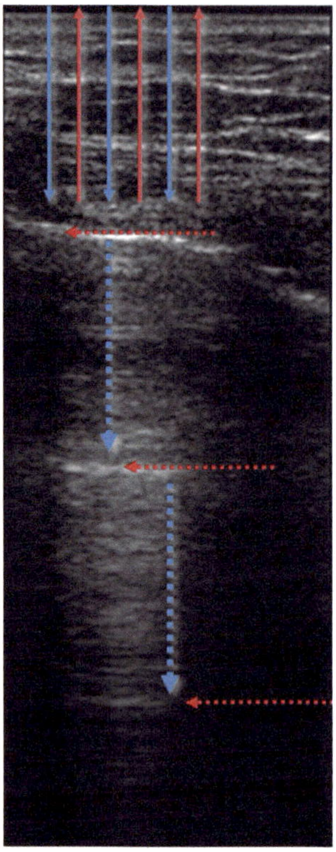

Fig. 1.14 Ultrasound view of the anterior chest showing the pleural line (top dotted red arrow) and reverberations of the pleural line (subsequent dotted red arrows). As the incident beam reflects back and forth between the pleural line and the transducer (solid blue and red arrows), the processor assumes the later signals to return from deeper and deeper structures

the fluid trapped between gas bubbles to resonate. The vibration of such crystals or bubbles will send a continuous signal back to the transducer. The ultrasound system will interpret this continuous signal of sound waves as a series of ladder-like bands in a straight line (Fig. 1.15). This artifact has important practical implications and is useful as a diagnostic tool in lung ultrasound where it is the mechanism by which vertical B-lines are created. Ringdown artifacts are similar in appearance to Comet Tail artifacts; however, the mechanism of Comet Tail artifacts is actually a reverberation between reflectors that are very close to each other. The returned echoes are presented on the screen as very short horizontal lines that stack up to create a bright vertical line [10].

Secondary Lobes and Beam Width

Whereas most of the ultrasound beam propagates along the central (main) beam, some low-intensity waves may be directed toward the sides of the central beam. Side lobes appear lateral to the central beam and the grating lobes usually appear lateral to the side lobes (Fig. 1.16). The energy from these lobes is usually inconsequential, but if there is a strong reflector present lateral to the central beam, reflections off these side beams would be displayed in the center of the image as if originating from the central beam. Side lobe artifacts create reflections of ghost images that can be reduced by obtaining images in planes perpendicular to each other. A similar spatial artifact may occur that relates to the width of the beam and is called the Beam Width artifact. In this case, as the beam widens in the far field, an echo returning from the edge of the wider beam is assumed to return from the center of the beam causing lateral structures to be superimposed on the central image.

Bayonet

This is a type of speed assumption error artifact. The ultrasound system calculates the depth of a structure by multiplying echo return time by the speed of ultrasound. Whereas sound velocity through soft tissue is assumed to be constant, there may be slight differences in adjacent tissues. The bayonet artifact is the appearance of bending of a straight structure like a needle being used for the vascular access procedure. When the needle traverses different tissues, the ultrasound beam may move at different speeds causing the needle to appear "bent" in shape (Fig. 1.17).

Edge

The edge of a structure may cause the ultrasound beam to refract and may not return to the transducer. This specific form of refraction causes areas immediately deep to the sides of vessels to appear dark and devoid of signal (Fig. 1.18). Not to be confused with shadowing (see below), an edge artifact occurs at boundaries that are nearly parallel to the beam direction while shadowing occurs at boundaries that are nearly perpendicular to the signal direction by attenuating the signal energy [11].

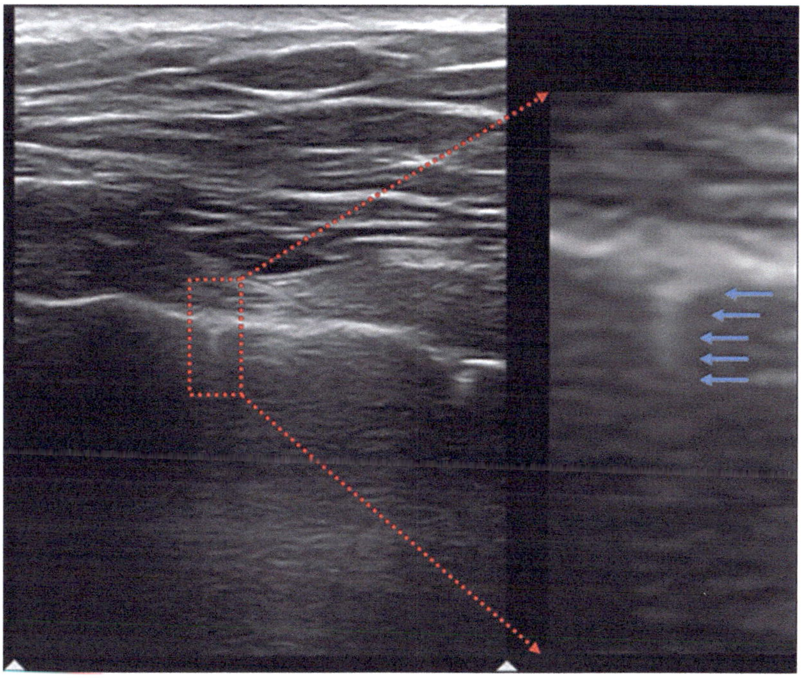

Fig. 1.15 Ultrasound view of the pleural surface showing ringdown generated by air/fluid boundaries in a secondary lobular septal insertion point. The inset (dotted red box) is expanded to show the effect of the continuous signal that is received by the transducer from the area of resonance

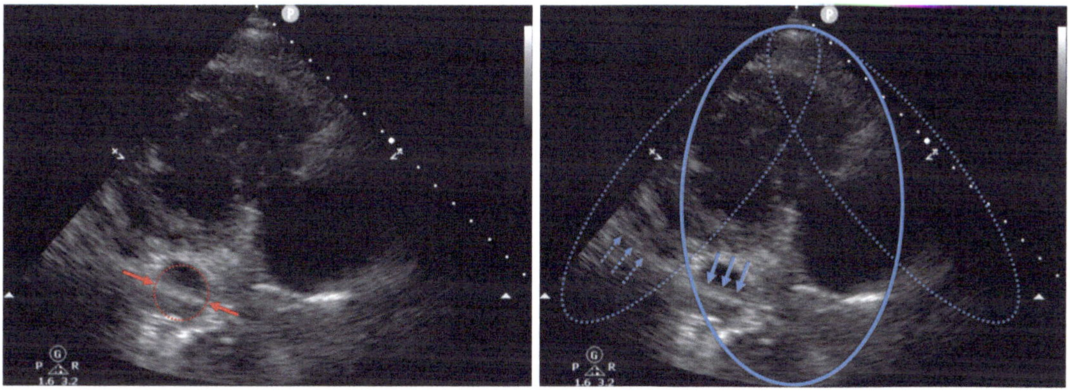

Fig. 1.16 A foreshortened parasternal long-axis ultrasound view of the heart. On the left side, a line (red arrows) is seen inside a short axis view of the descending aorta (dotted red circle). The explanation is shown on the right side image. Side lobe beams (dotted blue oval) are reflected by the pleura (dotted blue arrows) and return to the transducer. The echoes are misinterpreted as generated by the main beam (solid oval) and are therefore presented closer to the center of the image (solid arrows)

Attenuation Artifacts

Shadowing

This represents a signal void behind structures with high attenuation coefficients. This commonly occurs behind solid structures, such as bones and calcified masses (Fig. 1.19). Other examples include implants and prosthetic valves in the heart. Acoustic shadowing may be useful in identifying structures, such as gallstones, or to identify a needle in soft tissue during ultrasound-guided vascular access. Acoustic shadowing may also make it hard to identify structures directly behind the attenuating structure.

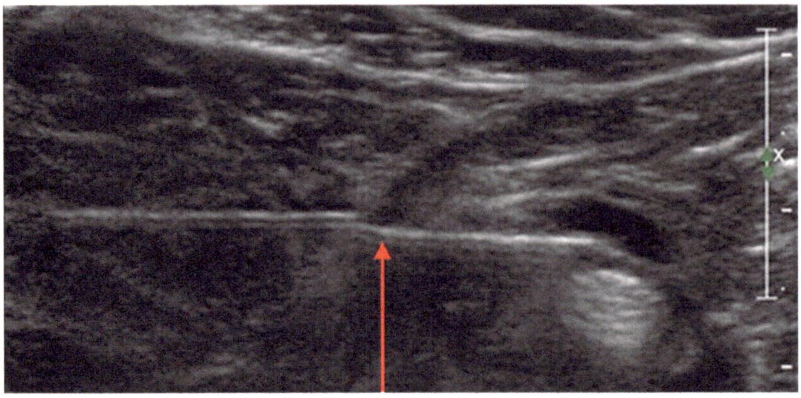

Fig. 1.17 Ultrasound image of a needle in soft tissue traversing two soft tissue media of different properties causing the speed of sound to be slightly different. This causes echoes from the needle to return slightly faster on one side and for the needle to appear broken or bent in shape (red arrow). Image adapted from Radiology key. In: Radiology Key. http://www.radiologykey.com/. Accessed 7 Mar 2022

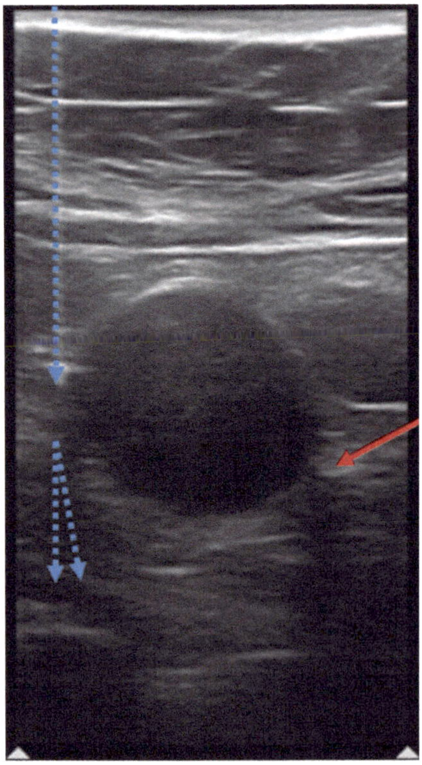

Fig. 1.18 An ultrasound view of a short axis of the carotid artery. The incident beam changes direction at the lateral borders of the vessel (dotted blue arrows) causing a signal void deep to the area. A similar pattern is indicated by the red arrow on the other side of the vessel

Enhancement

This represents unexpectedly strong signals returning from areas behind structures that are exceptional transmitters of sound waves, such as fluid. Enhancement can be seen with echoes deep to fluid-filled structures such as cysts, blood vessels, the urinary bladder, and the gallbladder (Fig. 1.20). Since ultrasound waves undergo little attenuation through fluid, higher amplitude ultrasound waves will be reflected from tissues deep into these structures. This will result in the appearance of higher echogenicity of deep tissues.

Doppler Artifacts

Aliasing

In Doppler modes that utilize intermittent pulses of signal (that is, in modes other than continuous wave Doppler), an artifact may arise that makes the speed and direction of the reflector ambiguous to the receiving transducer. This is called Aliasing (Fig. 1.21).

Aliasing occurs when the sampling rate from the specific gate is too slow as compared to the frequency shift. The magnitude of the frequency

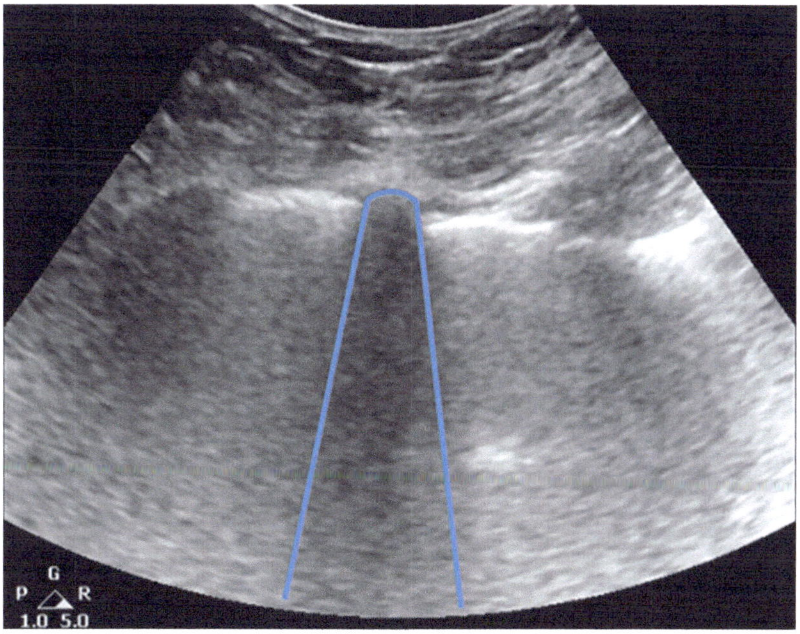

Fig. 1.19 Ultrasound image of the thorax, with multiple rib shadows creating areas of signal void. The central rib and shadow are outlined by a blue line

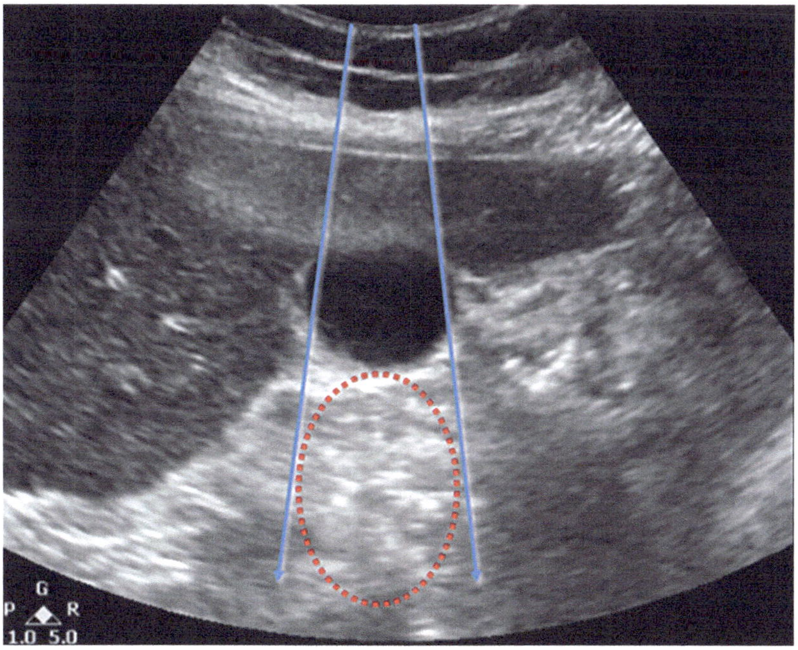

Fig. 1.20 Ultrasound view of the liver and gall bladder, showing the area deep to the gall bladder (dotted red oval) with a brighter signal than the areas to the side of it. The blue lines represent the path of the ultrasound beam

shift at which aliasing takes place is called the Nyquist Limit. The Nyquist limit is equal to half the pulse repetition frequency (PRF).

$$\text{Nyquist limit} = \text{Pulse Repetition Frequency} / 2$$

An example of aliasing is described here: If an observer of a fast-turning clock hand is unable to monitor the clock continuously but can take snapshots of the face of the clock at certain intervals (limited sampling rate), she may not be able to tell the direction of movement (clockwise or counter-clockwise) if the sampling rate is too slow. For the observer to be able to determine the direction of movement, she needs to take snap-

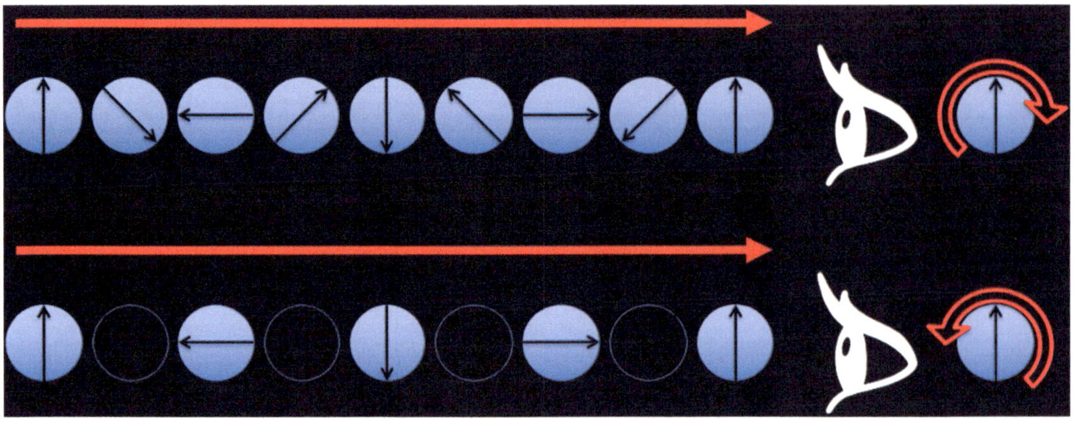

Fig. 1.21 A schematic of sampling rate and aliasing. In the upper panel, the sampling rate (clock face snapshots) occurs at more than twice the event rate (clock revolutions) which allows the observer to determine the rotation rate and direction accurately. In the lower panel, because the sampling rate is less than twice the event rate, the observer is unable to determine the direction of clock rotation accurately

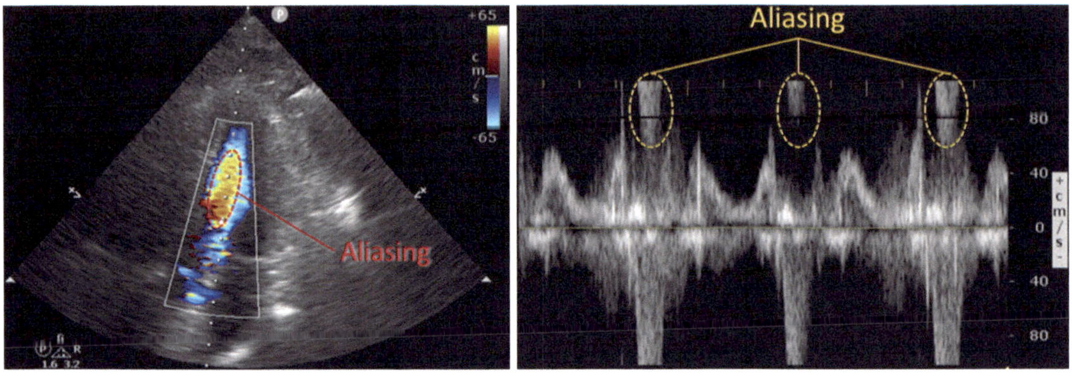

Fig. 1.22 Aliasing in CF Doppler (left panel) and in PW Doppler (right panel). In the left panel, the fast central flow of the left ventricular outflow in an apical view of the heart is designated a color that is the opposite in direction to the lower flow around it. In the right panel, the spectral flow of the same area is assigned a positive direction while it is generated by blood flow that is moving away from the transducer. In both cases, the fast flow velocity causes frequency phase shifts that exceed the Nyquist limit

shots at more than twice the frequency of a full revolution (see image below).

In ultrasound, aliasing shows as a reversal of (or the inability to determine) the direction of flow. In PW Doppler, the flow signal may appear below the baseline when blood flows toward the transducer at high speeds, such as in mitral valve stenosis. Aliasing may also cause CF Doppler to show a mix of colors in an arterial flow signal when the pulse repetition frequency is set to detect a slower venous flow (Fig. 1.22).

Because aliasing depends on the PRF, reducing aliasing is contingent on the ability of the operator to modify the PRF, and includes:

- Increasing the PRF, which is mostly possible, with certain limits
- Setting the sample volume at a shallower location, which increases the PRF
- Selecting a lower frequency transducer, which reduces the Doppler shift

- Shifting the spectral analysis view baseline, which applies a mathematical correction
- Using CW Doppler instead of PW or CF Doppler because CW Doppler suffers no aliasing

Questions

Please choose the best single answer

1. Traveling through soft tissue, which beam will lose most energy echoing back to the transducer from a 5 cm reflector?
   A. The beam that takes 65 μs for the round trip
   B. The beam with the shortest wavelength
   C. The beam with the highest amplitude
   D. The beam with the longest pulse duration
   E. The beam that has the longest period

   The correct answer is B: The beam with the shortest wavelength.

   Explanation: All beams are assumed to have the same speed of 1540 m/s in soft tissue. It is a good rule to remember that it takes an ultrasound beam 13 μs to make a round trip to and from a 1 cm deep reflector. Amplitude and pulse duration do not affect attenuation. Since attenuation = coefficient x distance x frequency, and since the medium and the distance are the same, the only factor affecting attenuation in this scenario is the frequency. Because frequency and wavelength are inversely related, the shortest wavelength beam will have the highest frequency and will suffer the most attenuation (option B is correct). The period is directly related to the wavelength, therefore long wave periods will result in lower frequency and lower attenuation.
2. Which of the following occurs as a result of decreasing the depth on the ultrasound image from 20 cm to 10 cm?
   A. The pulse period increases
   B. The pulse duration decreases
   C. The beam frequency increases
   D. The duty factor increases
   E. The spatial pulse length decreases

   The correct answer is D: The duty factor increases.

   Explanation: Decreasing the depth decreases the pulse period, which means that the pulse repetition frequency increases. Pulse duration (and spatial pulse length) are inherent characteristics of the transducer. Since the duty factor = pulse duration/pulse period, the duty factor increases as the depth of the scan is decreased (option D is correct). The beam frequency is not affected by the depth of the image.
3. Axial resolution in the far (deep) field can be improved by which of the following?
   A. Increasing the far-field time gain compensation
   B. Moving the electronic focal zone farther (deeper)
   C. Using higher wavelength options to scan
   D. Increasing the frame rate by narrowing the sector
   E. Switching to a higher frequency transducer

   The correct answer is E: Switching to a higher frequency transducer.

   Explanation: While higher gain will make distant structures appear brighter on the screen, post-processing manipulations do not affect resolution. The focal zone affects lateral resolution and the frame rate affects temporal resolution, but neither will affect axial resolution. Wave frequencies will affect the spatial pulse length, and axial resolution = SPL/2, so higher frequency transducers will have a better axial resolution (option E is correct). Longer waves mean lower frequency which is the opposite of what you need to improve axial resolution, although you will have better penetration into the tissue.
4. While examining the heart in an apical 5-chamber view using a phased array transducer, the structural details of the aortic valve (which is a deep structure) can be improved by which of the following maneuvers?
   A. Turning on M-Mode imaging
   B. Using tissue Doppler imaging
   C. Increasing the near-field time gain compensation
   D. Changing to a curvilinear transducer
   E. Turning on tissue harmonics imaging

The correct answer is E: Turning on tissue harmonics imaging.

Explanation: It is true that M-mode imaging offers great axial and temporal resolution; however, M-Mode imaging shows information from a single line of sight against time, and this information is not useful when examining the structure of a valve. Again, tissue Doppler imaging (in color tissue Doppler or in pulsed wave tissue Doppler) will show velocities but not structural details of the area of interest. Increasing the time gain compensation is post processing and will make the image brighter on the screen but does not add to the details. However, in this case, since the valve location is deep, changing the near field will not affect the area of interest. Because curvilinear transducers have more sound-emitting elements, they do offer better lateral resolution than phased array transducers, but in the case of an apical view of the heart, the large footprint of the curvilinear transducer will result in significant rib shadowing and image degradation. Tissue harmonics imaging is the standard in cardiac ultrasonography because it improves the signal-to-noise ratio particularly from deep structures, improves lateral resolution, and minimizes unwanted artifacts.

5. Using a 10 MHz linear transducer to examine the carotid artery, the measured speed of blood flow will be half the actual speed when the angle of insonation is:
   A. 15 degrees
   B. 30 degrees
   C. 45 degrees
   D. 60 degrees
   E. 75 degrees

   The correct answer D: 60 degrees.

   Explanation: Doppler shift = 2 × reflector speed × source frequency × cosine the angle of incidence (θ)/sound propagation speed. Therefore, when estimating the speed of blood flow using any particular ultrasound beam frequency, and since the speed of sound is assumed to be constant in soft tissue, the Doppler shift in the beam reflection will depend on the cosine of the angle of insonation. The table below show the cosine values of representative angles. Note that being "off" by 15 degrees results in an underestimation of velocity by 3% only (Table 1.7).

6. While examining the blood flow in the carotid artery using color flow Doppler, severe aliasing appears with mosaic color patterns that limit the ability to interpret the findings. How can aliasing be reduced?
   A. Increase transducer frequency
   B. Increase pulse repetition frequency
   C. Increase Doppler gain compensation
   D. Increase the depth of the interrogation field
   E. Increase the width of the interrogation field

   The correct answer is B: Increase pulse repetition frequency.

   Explanation: Color Doppler aliasing can be eliminated by elevating the Nyquist limit. This can be achieved by decreasing the transducer frequency therefore lowering the frequency shifts (option A is incorrect), or by increasing the pulse repetition frequency (option B is correct). Changing the Doppler gain will only change the color brightness on the screen but will not change the color itself (option C is incorrect). Increasing the size of the interrogation field will decrease the temporal resolution of the color flow Doppler but will not affect the Nyquist limit (options D and E are incorrect). Of note, decreasing the depth of the area of interest would allow for higher PRF and therefore decrease aliasing (the option not presented).

7. An operator notices a linear hyperechoic density in the lumen of the descending aorta in the short axis on a parasternal view of the heart. How can she minimize the possibility of an artifact causing the appearance of a dissection flap?
   A. Let the area of interest fall deeper than the focal zone
   B. Widen the imaging sector
   C. Turn off harmonics imaging
   D. Examine the area in a different plane
   E. Increase the Time Gain Compensation

The correct answer is D: Examine the area in a different plane.

Explanation: Side lobe and beam width artifacts are possible reasons for a lateral reflector to appear as if it is generated by the central beam. Decreasing scanning depth to the focal zone will decrease the beam width artifact (option A is incorrect). Narrowing the sector width will improve lateral resolution by increasing the number of scan lines in the area of interest but does not affect the beam width or side lobe artifacts (option B is incorrect). The nonlinear relationship between the harmonic generation and the original ultrasound wave can improve visualization and decrease the amount of side-lobe clutter (option C is incorrect). Viewing the structure of interest through multiple acoustic windows at different angles is unlikely to reproduce the same artifact in the same area (option D is correct). Increasing the gain is the opposite of what one should do because that will increase the brightness of the artifact (option E is incorrect).

8. When performing ultrasound-guided vascular access, when is the best time to image the target vessel, and make necessary adjustments to obtain an ideal image?
   A. During procedure planning, prior to taking sterile precautions
   B. After sterile precautions, prior to starting a procedure
   C. While performing the procedure, in real time
   D. Image adjustments are best done after the procedure
   E. None of the above. Machine default settings are optimal

The correct answer is A: During procedure planning, prior to taking sterile precautions.

When performing ultrasound-guided procedures, such as deep vascular access, procedural planning and setup are critical to the success of the procedure. Obtaining an ultrasound image of the target vessel is best done prior to taking sterile precautions and equipment set up (option A is correct). The proceduralist should use this time to identify the correct probe, obtain the image, and perform adjustments to the image parameters (e.g., depth and gain). These adjustments are usually needed to ensure a large, and clear field of view to visualize the blood vessel and the soft tissue around it (options D and E are incorrect). The proceduralist can also identify the sterile field and mark the site (if indicated). Importantly, the proceduralist can also use this time to assess the target vessel and surrounding tissue in detail and look for potential barriers (e.g., strictures and blood clots), prior to equipment set up. This task may be more difficult once sterile precautions have been taken, as the ultrasound machine may not always be within reach, and the machine controls will not be part of the sterile field (option B is incorrect). It is not recommended to perform image adjustments while performing the procedure, due to the risk of losing view of the needle and increasing risk of complications (option C is incorrect).

9. While attempting to obtain an ultrasound image of a patient's gall bladder, the sonographer encounters an air artifact. Which of the following maneuvers can help the sonographer obtain the desired image?
   A. Apply gentle pressure with the probe on the abdomen
   B. Slide the probe over the abdomen until an image is obtained
   C. Attempt to obtain the image from a different anatomical landmark
   D. Apply more ultrasound gel between the transducer and the skin
   E. All of the above

The correct answer is E: All of the above.

Explanation: During abdominal ultrasound, air artifacts are frequently encountered due to bowel gas. As discussed above, ultrasound waves are disrupted by air, and this is detrimental during abdominal imaging. All of the above-mentioned techniques can be helpful in attaining the desired image (Option E is correct). Applying gentle pressure on the abdomen can displace air-containing bowel loops between the probe and the target organ. Fine movements such as sliding the probe can change the angle of view and avoid the air containing bowel loops, as well as imaging from a different anatomic landmark (laterally, for example). Applying more ultrasound gel is always a good idea when unable to obtain a good image, as a lack of gel will prevent the ultrasound waves from transmitting from the probe into the soft tissue, resulting in poor image quality and artifacts.

References

1. Lau VI, Jaidka A, Wiskar K, et al. Better with ultrasound: transcranial Doppler. Chest. 2020;157:142–50.
2. NEMA. Standard for real-time display of thermal and mechanical acoustic output indices on diagnostic ultrasound equipment. Rockville, MD: The Institute; 1992.
3. Thomas JD, Rubin DN. Tissue harmonic imaging: why does it work? J Am Soc Echocardiogr. 1998;11:803–8.
4. Huang Q, Zeng Z. A review on real-time 3D ultrasound imaging technology. Biomed Res Int. 2017;2017:6027029.
5. Otto C. Textbook of clinical echocardiography. Philadelphia, PA: Elsevier, Inc.; 2018.
6. Ellens N, Hynynen K. Frequency considerations for deep ablation with high-intensity focused ultrasound: a simulation study. Med Phys. 2015;42:4896–10.
7. Klein AL. Clinical echocardiography review a self-assessment tool. Philadelphia, PA: Wolters Kluwer/Lippincott Williams & Wilkins Health; 2011.
8. Allison C, Cellum B, Karpinecz B, Nasrallah F, Zderic V. Ultrasound-enhanced transcorneal drug delivery for treatment of fungal keratitis. Cornea. 2022;41:894–900.
9. Anvari A, Forsberg F, Samir AE. A primer on the physical principles of tissue harmonic imaging. Radiographics. 2015;35:1955–64.
10. Radiopaedia. http://www.radiopaedia.org/. Accessed 7 Mar 2022. 2022.
11. Edelman S. Ultrasound physics and instrumentation. Woodlands, TX: Education for the Sonographic Professional; 1999.

Probes and Imaging Modes

2

Chris Allison

Learning Objectives
1. Describe the advantages and disadvantages of each type of probe by frequency
2. Describe the potential pitfalls of harmonic imaging
3. Identify strategies for obtaining optimal gain
4. Know the basic ultrasound imaging modes and the physical principles behind them
5. Understand how Doppler images are obtained

Probe Selection

There is a plethora of ultrasound probes available from various manufacturers. Probes generate ultrasound waves from an array of piezoelectric crystals at the surface, i.e., "footprint," of the probe.[1]

When selecting a probe, one should ask two simple questions: Is the structure you are visualizing superficial (for simplicity, less than about 5 cm) or deep? Is the sonographic window small, i.e., between ribs? If superficial, select a high-frequency, linear probe. High-frequency probes are capable of at least 10 MHz (note probes typically have their wavelength capabilities labeled on them).

At higher frequencies, and thus shorter wavelengths, the axial resolution is improved. However, the higher frequency ultrasound beams attenuate more per depth, preventing visualization of deep structures. Typical applications using a high-frequency linear probe include vascular access, lung pleura (e.g., pneumothorax), diaphragm thickness, DVT assessment, nerve blocks, ocular ultrasound, and some musculoskeletal/soft tissue studies. Within high-frequency linear probes, a higher frequency (e.g., 15 MHz) would be most useful for very small, superficial structures such as the radial artery; whereas a lower frequency (e.g., 8–10 MHz) would enable better visualization of the femoral and popliteal veins in a larger patient (Fig. 2.1).

For visualizing deep structures, users choose between a low-frequency curvilinear probe and a phased-array probe (commonly called a "cardiac"

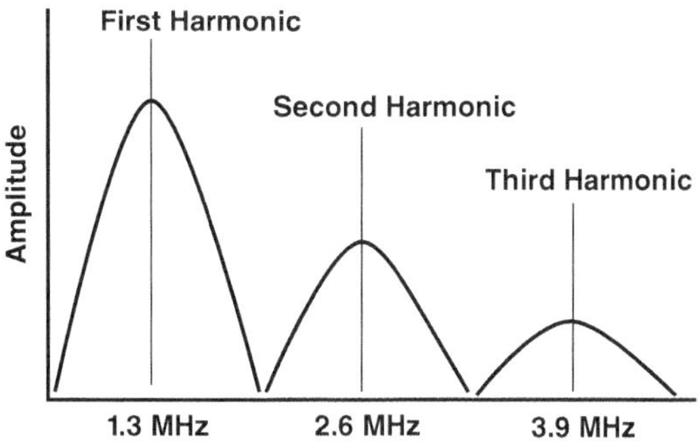

Fig. 2.1 A high-frequency linear probe (**a**) low-frequency curvilinear probe (**b**), and a phased-array probe (**c**)

[1]With the exception of some portable ultrasound devices that use an alternative to piezoelectric crystals.

C. Allison (✉)
Umass Chan Medical School—Baystate,
Springfield, MA, USA

M. J. Lanspa, A. T. Levinson (eds.), *Echocardiography and Ultrasonography in the ICU*,
Respiratory Medicine, https://doi.org/10.1007/978-3-031-80038-2_2

probe) . Phased-array probes differ from curvilinear and linear probes in that the piezoelectric crystals sequentially generate ultrasound waves with tiny delays along the probe, creating inference waves that steer the beam left and right; creating a larger field of view from a smaller footprint on the screen [1]. This allows for a transducer footprint that fits between ribs, making phased-array probes preferred for cardiac and other intrathoracic assessment. The curved arrangement of crystals on curvilinear probes allows for a broader field of view. Pragmatically, for the level of sophistication required for physician-performed point-of-care-ultrasound, a phased array probe can accomplish most studies that would often be performed with a curvilinear probe (FAST exam, gall bladder assessment).

An additional practical consideration is that modern ultrasound machines have presets available based on the transducer that optimizes the frequency and other settings for the selected study. Cardiac presets will typically only be available for phased-array probes.

Harmonic Imaging

Ultrasound transducers generate ultrasound waves at a set frequency termed the fundamental frequency. Unequal speeds of compression and rarefaction during ultrasound transmission through tissue result in the generation of additional higher frequency sound waves at multiples of the fundamental frequency, known as harmonics. Because of the distortion of the fundamental frequency, analyzing the harmonic frequencies returning to the probe can actually result in a higher resolution images with less noise [2, 3]. This is particularly useful when scanning through adipose tissue. The disadvantage is that the harmonics are not generated very close to the transducer, making this less useful for superficial imaging; also, the higher frequency harmonics attenuate more quickly with depth, limiting their use for imaging deep structures. Harmonic imaging mitigates reverberation artifacts, which generally improves image quality; however, assessment for extravascular lung water through sonographic B lines relies on artifact generation. Limited clinical data suggest B line visualization is improved with harmonic imaging [4].

Presets may use harmonic imaging. Some modern machines will include a "lung" preset with harmonics off to improve visualization of B lines. Users will note diminished image quality if such presets are used for other applications.

Imaging Modes

The default mode for ultrasound mode is known as "B" mode AKA "brightness" mode AKA 2D mode. (The naming has a historical basis in distinguishing this mode from "A" mode, which displays a graph of echo intensity at various depths) (Fig. 2.2). In the B mode, the ultrasound transducer footprint is displayed at the top of the screen, creating an "*x*-axis" of the position along the probe surface. The "*y*-axis" is time, but with the estimation of the speed with which ultrasound waves travel to and back from the tissue that reflects them, the *y*-axis is interpreted as depth. The intensity of the ultrasound waves that return at different time points (thus depths) is measured by the machine and then displayed in grayscale, with whiter being more intense and blacker less intense.

This leads us to the first two basic settings we modify to optimize images: depth and gain. Changing depth adjusts what amount of "ultrasound listening time" (thus depth) is displayed on the screen. It is a good practice to start with more depth than needed displayed on the screen to ensure important information/pathology is not missed in the far field, then reduce the depth such the entire structure of interest is visible without wasted space deep to it. Gain changes what grayscale values for displayed pixels correspond to absolute values of echo intensities received by the probe; practically making the image brighter or darker. Gain should be adjusted to optimize contrast between tissue densities; too little or too much gain reduces this (Fig. 2.3—too much and too little gain). A good rule of thumb is to have the gain lowered just until a structure known to be anechoic (thus black) such as the lumen of a

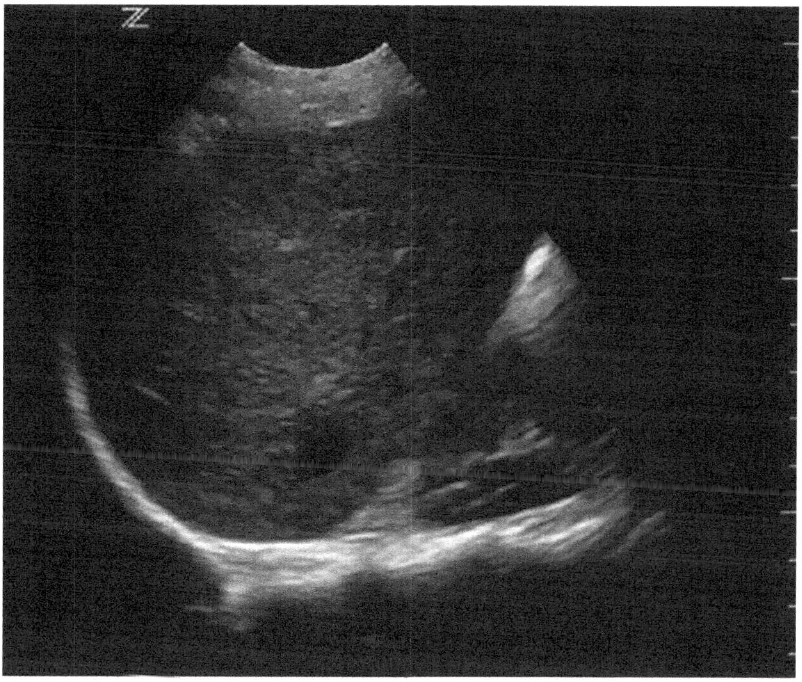

Fig. 2.2 In B mode, the transducer footprint is displayed. Intensities of echoes returning are displayed in grayscale

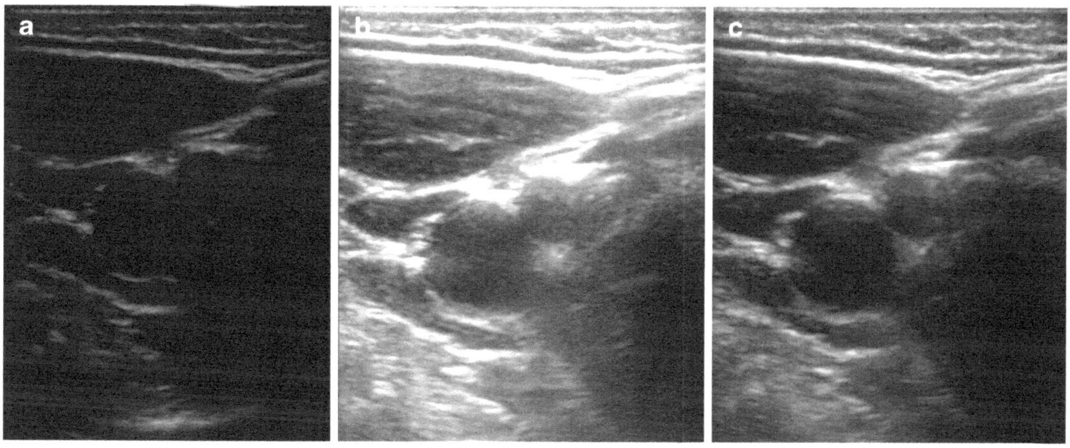

Fig. 2.3 Gain is optimized in B mode so images are not too dark (**a**) or too bright (**b**), maximizing contrast (**c**)

blood vessel becomes black without artifactual echoes within it. Time-gain compensation adjusts the gain at different depths, allowing a consistent image despite the attenuation of ultrasound intensity that has returned from the far field.

M mode can be used to visualize and measure moving structures. In this mode, pixels along a line originating from a single point on the probe surface are propagated over time (Fig. 2.4—M mode). The *x*-axis is time (in seconds, much longer than the time it takes ultrasound to travel to and from visualized tissue). The *y*-axis is depth. Care must be taken to not move the transducer during M mode to ensure that changes in the propagated line only represent movement of the visualized structure itself. M mode is used to measure the distances heart structures move during a cardiac cycle, fetal heart rates, and has been used for assessment of pleural sliding. M mode was particularly important historically when

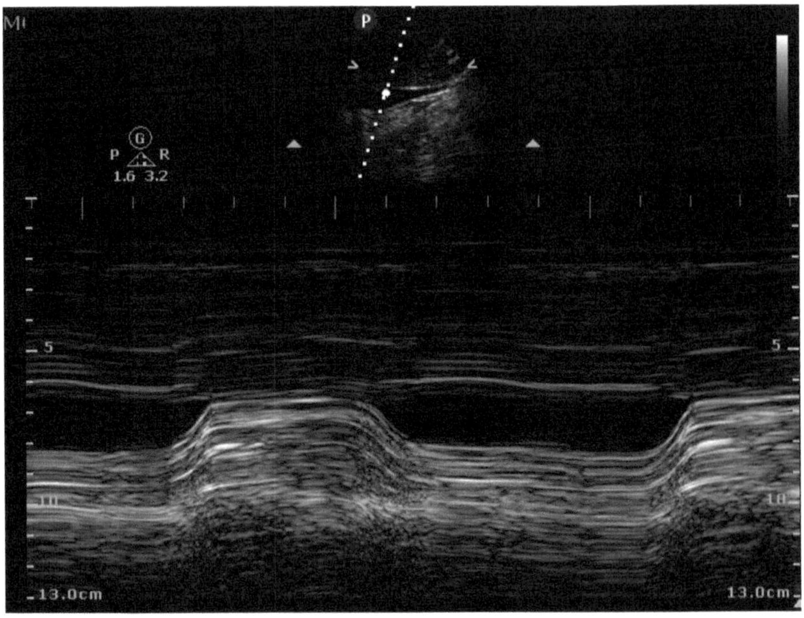

Fig. 2.4 M mode shows respiration variation in the inferior vena cava. The single line selected by the user is propagated over time, allowing visualization and measurement of moving structures. Here, a complete collapse of the IVC is seen

exporting videos (for example, to VHS) was cumbersome, as it allows movement to be displayed in a single still image. M mode remains useful for measuring the movement of cardiac structures, such as tricuspid annulus plane systolic excursion (TAPSE).

Doppler Imaging (See Chap. 7 for Echocardiographic Applications)

We are able to measure velocities of blood flow and moving tissue using ultrasound by taking advantage of the Doppler effect. If an object is stationary, echoes will return to the transducer with the same frequency. However echoes returning from a moving object after a change in frequency, known as the Doppler shift = $f_r - f_T$, where f_r is the frequency of reflected ultrasound waves and f_T is the frequency of transmitted sound waves. Echoes returning from an object moving toward the transducer have increased frequency, and those reflected from an object moving away from the transducer have decreased frequency (Fig. 2.5—showing Doppler shift, waves closer together).

The Doppler shift is predictable based on the speed of sound in tissue (c) and object velocities (v):

$$\text{Doppler shift} = 2 * f_T * \frac{v}{c}.$$

However, the Doppler shift also depends on the angle at which the ultrasound waves strike the moving object, known as the angle of insonation (θ). Doppler shift is directly proportional to the cosine of θ:

$$\text{angle-corrected Doppler shift} = 2 * f_T * \frac{v}{c} * \cos\theta.$$

Recall that cos 0° = 1, so the Doppler shift is unchanged if scanning a moving object "head-on" but this is usually impractical. cos 90° = 0, which corresponds to the intuitive fact that you cannot detect a Doppler shift if scanning perpendicularly to the moving object. However, if the angle of insonation exceeds 60°, these corrections become inaccurate to calculate velocities [5]. Users can manipulate angle correction on spectral Doppler studies [5] (Fig. 2.6—angle correction in spectral Doppler).

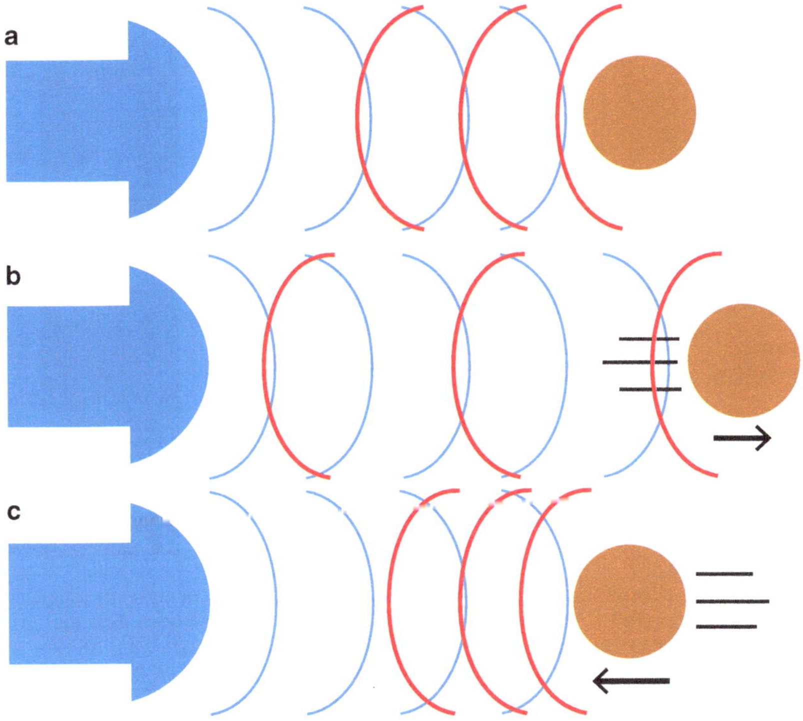

Fig. 2.5 (**a**) Echoes (red) from a stationary object return at the same frequency as the transmitted ultrasound (blue). (**b**) Echoes from an object moving away from the transducer have decreased frequency. (**c**) Echoes from an object moving toward the transducer have increased frequency

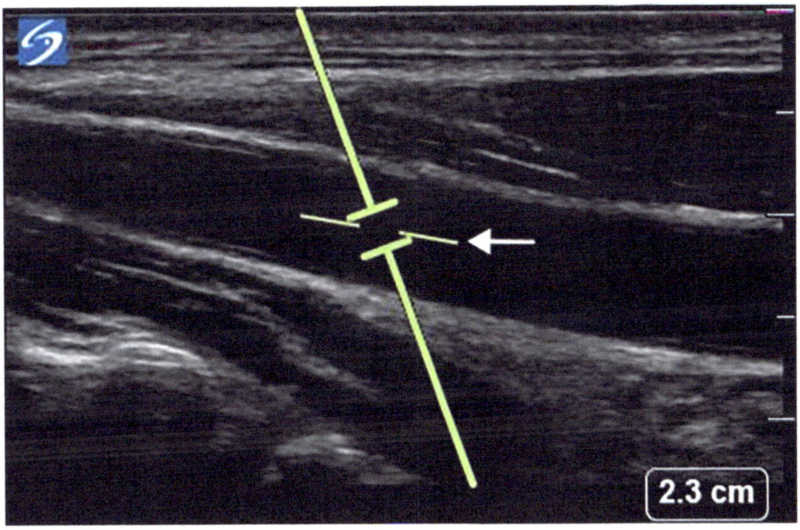

Fig. 2.6 Pulsed-wave Doppler of the carotid artery. The angle correction line (arrow) is adjusted to be parallel to blood flow to improve the accuracy of velocity calculation. Measurements are inaccurate at angles greater than 60°

In addition to constraints from the angle of insonation, there are limits to the maximum Doppler shift that can be measured. A waveform must be sampled at least twice its frequency to be accurately represented, according to the Nyquist-Shannon sampling theorem [6] (Fig. 2.7a—Nyquist limit). The sampling rate is the **pulse repetition frequency** (PRF), how many pulses of ultrasound are sent out per second. The maximum magnitude Doppler shift that can be accurately measured is PRF/2, known as the **Nyquist limit**. Velocities that produce a Doppler shift exceeding the Nyquist limit will be misinterpreted in a phenomenon known as **aliasing** and may appear as flow in the opposite direction (Fig. 2.7b—aliasing). This is analogous to the spinning wheels of a

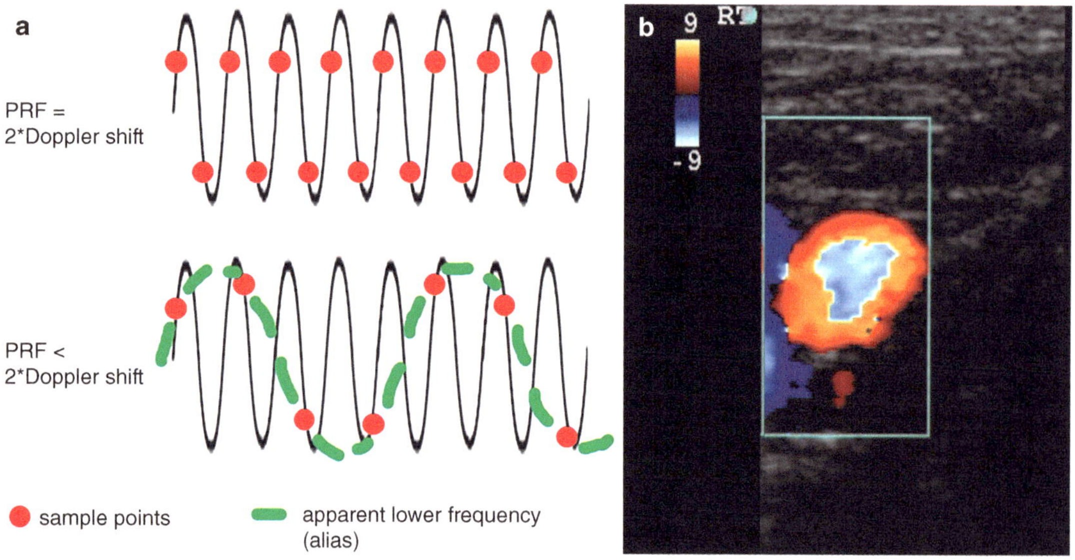

Fig. 2.7 (**a**) A waveform sampled at two different pulse rate frequencies (PRF). Above, the PRF is at the Nyquist limit, so the red dots at sampling points accurately recreate the original waveform. Shown below, at too low a PRF the red dots at too infrequent intervals create the appearance of a lower frequency waveform (an alias, green dashed line) than the original. (**b**) Color Doppler ultrasound showing aliasing resulting in the appearance of reversal of flow direction at the sites of higher velocity blood flow in the center of a blood vessel

car on a film appearing to rotate in reverse, which can happen when the sample rate of the camera is slower than twice the wheel rotation frequency (i.e., the camera's Nyquist limit).

Values derived from PRF include the **pulse repetition period** (PRP), which is the time between the beginning of the reach pulse: PRP = 1/PRF. Pulse duration is the length of time of each pulse. The **Duty factor** is the fraction of time that the transducer is generating sound, which is pulse duration/PRP.

In various Doppler modes, Doppler gain will adjust the sensitivity of the machine to flow. This should be adjusted until the artifact is not visible.

Machine presets are helpful for starting PRF, Doppler gain, etc. that are likely to work well for an application. For example, a cardiac preset will have a high PRF for the high flow velocities encountered in the heart.

Color Doppler

Color Doppler superimposes velocities calculated by Doppler shift in the form of color onto 2D images from B mode, also termed duplex scanning. Usually, velocities in a range consistent with blood flow are of interest, so filters are set so that low velocities that are likely artifactual or from probe movement are not displayed. Typical filters exclude frequencies below 50–100 MHz [5]. These may need to be adjusted if trying to detect low-velocity flow.

The color display provides information on velocity and direction. While the default convention is to represent the movement away from the probe as blue and toward the probe as red (leading to the mnemonic BART: blue-away, red-toward); this is sometimes reversed, and the user should refer to the legend displayed on the machine (Fig. 2.8—color Doppler).

The user can adjust the area of the 2D image being sampled for velocities, i.e., the color box. A larger color box requires more computing power, often resulting in a lower frame rate. Linear transducers often have available an angulated color box that steers the angle of insonation in addition to the angle of the probe contacting the skin, facilitating an angle of less than 60°.

Turbulent flow appears as a mix of colors representing different flow directions, but care should be taken that this has not been caused by

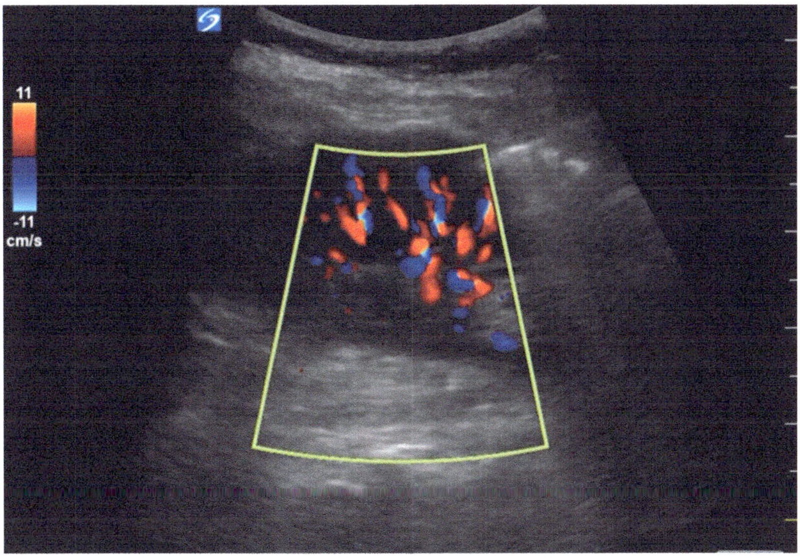

Fig. 2.8 Color Doppler ultrasound of a kidney, showing blood flow of intrarenal vasculature

aliasing from velocities causing Doppler shifts exceeding the Nyquist limit for the set PRF.

Spectral Doppler

Spectral Doppler imaging represents velocities as a spectrogram with time on the *x*-axis and velocities (calculated from Doppler shift) on the *y*-axis. This information is taken along a narrow line from the transducer surface. Note that multiple velocities are detected and displayed for one time point, representing the variation in flow in, for example, different locations within a single blood vessel. The brightness corresponds, qualitatively, to the number of blood cells moving at that velocity. The displayed brightness is adjusted with Doppler gain. The location of the baseline on the screen and the velocity scale for the *y*-axis are adjusted for optimal appearance (Fig. 2.9—spectrogram).

Two main forms of spectral Doppler imaging are pulsed-wave Doppler (PWD) and continuous-wave Doppler (CWD). In PWD, the transducer intermittently emits pulses of ultrasound, then "listens" between (Fig. 2.10—PW vs. CW Doppler).The user specifies the depth from which to sample velocities in the form of a range gate. This allows the measurement of velocities in a specific area, for example from only the left ventricular outflow tract, despite other blood flow occurring along the same line of measurement. Because ultrasounds are sent in pulses, aliasing will occur when velocities exceed the Nyquist limit for the set PRF. In contrast, CWD has separate transmitters continuously emitting and "listening" for ultrasound. This eliminates aliasing at velocities encountered clinically but does not allow the assessment of depth along the line of measurement [6]. CWD is used for measuring the highest velocities encountered clinically with accuracy, such as those of a stenotic heart valve.

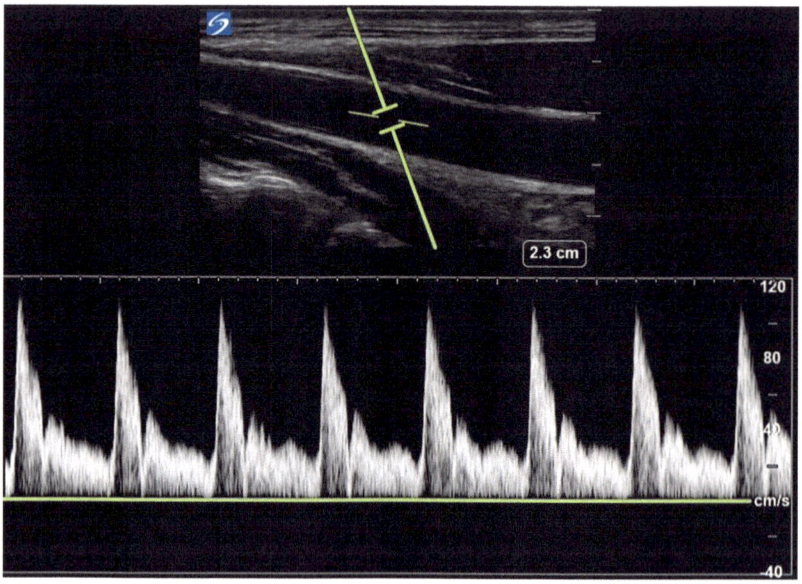

Fig. 2.9 Pulsed wave ultrasound of the carotid artery demonstrating velocities within the gated area over multiple cardiac cycles

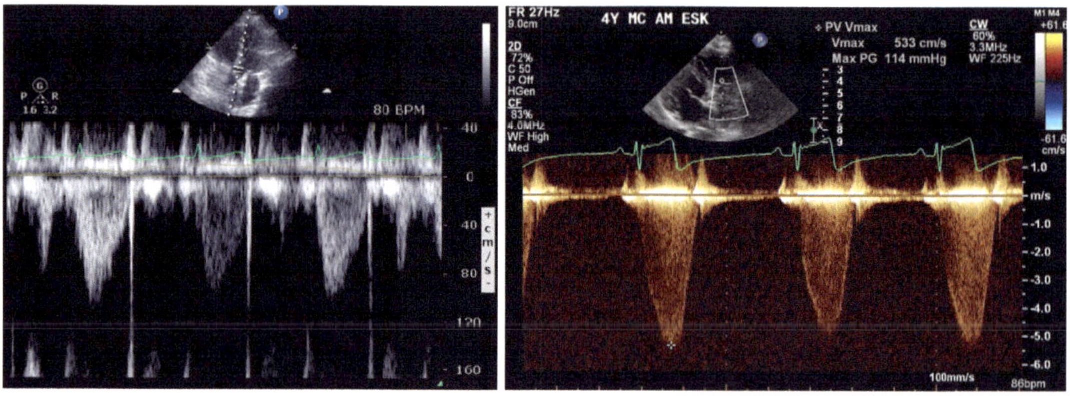

Fig. 2.10 Comparison of pulsed wave (left) and continuous wave Doppler (right). Note the aliasing present in pulsed wave Doppler. Continuous wave Doppler has no aliasing and can measure high velocities

Tissue Doppler

Tissue Doppler is a subtype of spectral Doppler imaging that is optimized for moving soft tissue, usually myocardium, instead of blood cells. Filters for slower velocity, but higher amplitude movement allow Doppler shifts from moving tissue to be isolated from those of blood [7].

Pro-tips

In spectral Doppler the brightness corresponds, qualitatively, to the number of blood cells moving at that velocity. The displayed brightness is adjusted with Doppler gain. Two main forms of spectral Doppler imaging are pulsed-wave Doppler (PWD) and continuous-wave Doppler (CWD).

Evolving Evidence

Cardiac presets often use harmonic imaging. Some modern machines will include a "lung" preset with harmonics off to improve visualization of B lines. Users will note diminished image quality if such presets are used for other applications.

Summary Points

- For superficial structures, select a high-frequency, linear probe
- For visualizing deep structures, choose a low-frequency curvilinear (abdominal)probe or a phased-array (cardiac) probe

Questions

1. Which of the following is most appropriate for ultrasound guidance of radial arterial line placement?
   A. 3.5 MHz, curvilinear probe
   B. 13 MHz, linear probe
   C. 5 MHz, phased array probe
   D. 8 MHz, linear probe

   Answer: (B). Visualization of a small, superficial structure like the radial artery is optimized with a higher resolution linear probe
2. Which of the following is true of harmonic imaging?
   A. Interpretation echoes at higher frequencies generated at multiples of the fundamental frequency can generally provide higher-resolution images.
   B. It provides better axial resolution for very deep structures.
   C. Limited evidence suggests it improves visualization of sonographic B lines.
   D. It facilitates wide-angle imaging from a smaller footprint, for example, through rib spaces.

   Answer: (A). The harmonic frequencies generally improve resolution and image quality, but visualization of deep structures is limited, and it can reduce the generation of useful artifacts used in lung ultrasound. Harmonic imaging can reduce the axial resolution. Harmonic imaging will have minimal to no effect on the angle of the image.
3. On Color Doppler of the abdominal aorta, blood flow velocities away from the probe are seen as blue color around the periphery of the vessel lumen, but velocities in the center of the lumen appear red corresponding to flow toward the probe. Which of the following explains this artifact?
   A. The Doppler gain is set too high
   B. Edge artifact causing acoustic shadowing at the edges of the vessel
   C. The pulse repetition frequency is less than the Nyquist limit required to measure the velocities of the blood in the center of the lumen
   D. Aortic calcifications causing reverberation artifact, leading to misinterpretation of velocity direction

   Answer: (C). This is an example of aliasing occurring at the higher velocities at the center of the artery lumen. Likely the pulse repetition frequency was inappropriately decreased to less than what was needed for this application.

References

1. Bushberg JT. The essential physics of medical imaging. 3rd ed. Wolters Kluwer Health/Lippincott Williams & Wilkins; 2012.
2. Desser TS, Jeffrey RB. Tissue harmonic imaging techniques: physical principles and clinical applications. Semin Ultrasound CT MR. 2001;22(1):1–10. https://doi.org/10.1016/s0887-2171(01)90014-9.
3. Hedrick WR, Metzger L. Tissue harmonic imaging: a review. J Diagn Med Sonogr. 2005;21(3):183–9. https://doi.org/10.1177/8756479305276477.
4. Matthias I, Panebianco NL, Maltenfort MG, Dean AJ, Baston C. Effect of machine settings on ultrasound assessment of B-lines. J Ultrasound Med. 2020;40(10):2039–46. https://doi.org/10.1002/jum.15581.
5. Rumack CM, Wilson SR, Charboneau JW, Levine D. Diagnostic ultrasound. 4th ed. Mosby; 2011.
6. Rubin JM. Spectral Doppler US. Radiographics. 1994;14(1):139–50. https://doi.org/10.1148/radiographics.14.1.8128046.
7. Ho CY, Solomon SD. A clinician's guide to tissue Doppler imaging. Circulation. 2006;113(10):e396–8. https://doi.org/10.1161/CIRCULATIONAHA.105.579268.

3 Ultrasound Artifacts

Taro Minami

Learning Objectives

1. Define a radiographic image artifact
2. Describe common image artifacts
3. Examine how ultrasound image artifacts arise

An ultrasound machine creates images based on assumptions from the physical properties of the ultrasound wave. For example, the sound travels in the human body, hits the target, and returns to the probe. If we know the time it takes to return to the probe, we can calculate the distance between the probe and the target as the sound travels at a fixed speed of 1540 m/s in the human body. Based on the intensity of the ultrasound wave returning to the probe and the time it takes to travel, a machine can draw a dot on the screen with a color ranging from white to black.

An ultrasound machine assumes many things to create images. It assumes that the ultrasound beam moves at a fixed speed in a human body at 1540 m/s. It also assumes that the beam goes straight, hits the target, and returns once. In the ideal world, ultrasound follows these assumptions.

However, realities often differ from our assumptions. Sound travels much faster in the bone and much slower in the air. The ultrasound beam may not propagate as expected, sometimes going back and forth between the probe and the target multiple times.

Artifacts arise from such deviations. For example, if the sound travels twice between the probe and the object, the ultrasound machine would assume it came back from twice as deep a position. It may also assume that the ultrasound came back from the shallower location if it travels much faster and thus takes less time. Understanding ultrasound artifacts stems from understanding ultrasound properties and assumptions the ultrasound machines make.

Why It Is Important to Understand Ultrasound Artifacts

Ultrasound artifacts happen often, and we encounter them daily: Artifacts may confuse us daily if we do not recognize them properly. They may give clinicians wrong impressions of the structure they are observing, thus leading them to the wrong diagnosis and, ultimately, the wrong treatment. On the other hand, recognizing specific image artifacts can help us make a particular

Supplementary Information The online version contains supplementary material available at https://doi.org/10.1007/978-3-031-80038-2_3.

T. Minami (✉)
Division of Pulmonary, Critical Care, and Sleep Medicine, Department of Medicine, The Warren Alpert Medical School of Brown University, Providence, RI, USA

M. J. Lanspa, A. T. Levinson (eds.), *Echocardiography and Ultrasonography in the ICU*, Respiratory Medicine, https://doi.org/10.1007/978-3-031-80038-2_3

diagnosis. For example, we make diagnoses based on artifact patterns in lung ultrasound. Since we cannot observe the lung structures directly, as we do for heart or vascular structures, we assume lung pathophysiology through artifact patterns, owing much to the presence of air that attenuates and dissipates ultrasound signals. We utilize reverberation artifacts (A-lines or A-profile) to assume the presence of air and ring-down artifacts (B-lines) to assume the presence of water. Understanding ultrasound artifacts is thus vital as we must (1) avoid confusion by the false structures or functions created by artifacts that do not exist and (2) deepen our understanding of the pathophysiologies artifacts imply.

Types of Artifacts

There are many image artifacts under different mechanisms which can confuse learners. To simplify image artifacts, we can classify them into three major categories: artifacts associated with sound reflections, artifacts associated with ultrasound attenuation, and artifacts associated with ultrasound beam characteristics [1]. For additional specific examples of cardiac artifacts, refer to Chap. 10.

1. Reflections: reverberation, ring-down, comet tail, mirror
2. Attenuation: shadow artifact, enhancement artifact
3. Beam characteristics: side-lobe artifacts

> **Pro-tip**
> Be on the lookout for artifacts when dealing with strong reflectors (pericarditis, mechanical valve, etc.).

Artifacts Associated with Reflections

An ultrasound machine creates an image based on the assumption that ultrasound travels once straight to the target before returning to the probe at a constant speed through the human body, i.e., 1540 m/s. The ultrasound machine translates the time the ultrasound takes to return and the strength of the sound coming back into an image [2]. The more time it takes, the location at which it reflects should be located deeper (thus, the dot is drawn at the lower part of the screen), and the stronger the signal coming back, the whiter it appears on the screen. Conversely, if the coming back signal is weak, it will appear darker on the screen. In other words, the traveling time determines the location and the attenuation determines the location. That is why water appears black, bones, air, lungs, and membranes appear white, and the liver and spleen, soft tissues, appear gray.

> **Pro-tip**
> Different authors may refer to the same or similar artifacts by different names: ring-down vs. reverberation artifact.

Reverberation Artifacts

The amount of ultrasound reflected off a tissue surface depends on the difference in acoustic impedance of the two tissues. If the difference is small, the reflection is small; if the difference is large, the reflection is large. A typical example of multiple reflections is the A-line caused by reflections from the pleural surface of the lungs

First, ultrasound waves emitted from the ultrasound probe are reflected by the pleura, then some of the ultrasound waves are reflected back to the skin/probe surface, then again to the pleura, and so on. Since the ultrasound machine cannot tell the difference between the sound traveling once, twice, or sometimes three times, it thinks that the sound traveling twice or three times is coming back from a deeper location.

A famous example would include A-lines seen in lung ultrasounds (Image 3.1, Lung ultrasound with regularly spaced horizontal A-lines indicating aerated lung or pneumothorax).

> **Pro-tip**
> Doppler, including color flow, is susceptible to artifacts as well.

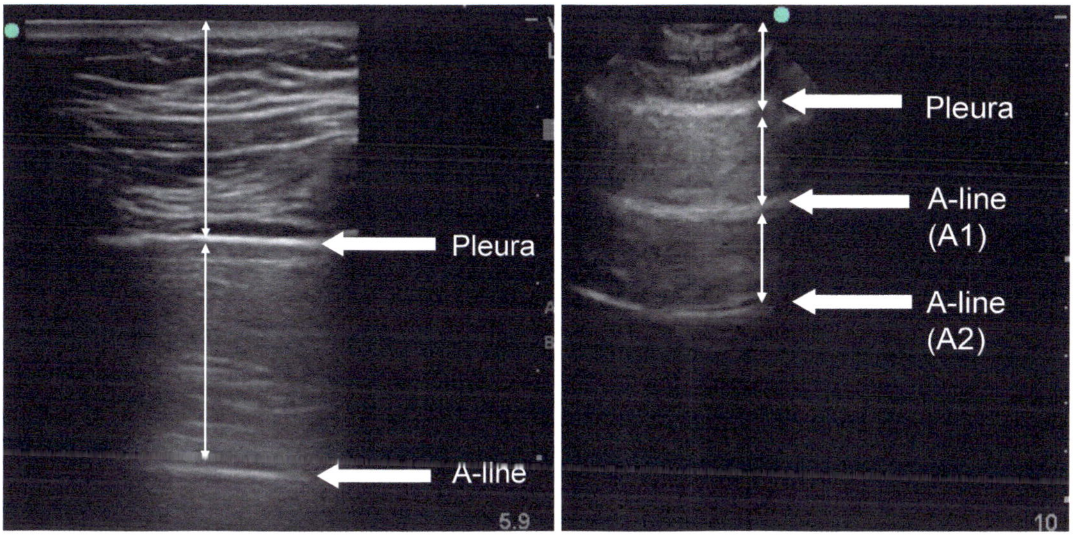

Image 3.1 Examples of reverberation artifact: A-lines. Please note that A-lines are artifacts created from the pleura and hence note that the distance of the surface-pleura and pleura-A-line is same. Also note although it may seem subtle, the pleura is the most echogenic (most white) line, followed by A1, then by A2 (less white)

Comet-Tail Artifact

There is a lot of confusion about this artifact. First, the comet-tail artifact—though it looks similar—is not the ring-down artifact as its mechanism is quite different. Comet-tail artifact is a variation of a reverberation artifact and, thus, not the same as a ring-down artifact.

Ring-Down Artifact

Ultrasonic energy transmitted from the probe causes resonant vibrations within the fluid surrounded by air. This vibration produces a continuous sound wave toward the probe, which the ultrasound device interprets as a backward-facing linear structure, which looks like a white line extending down from the air-enclosed structure. This is the B-line, a common finding on lung echo. This is a common B-line finding on a lung echo because water comes from an air-filled space.

A famous example of the ring-down artifact is seen in lung ultrasound as B-lines (Image 3.2, Lung ultrasound with vertical B-lines indicating extravascular lung water).

Mirror Image Artifacts

A typical example of a mirror image artifact is that of the liver, which is in front of the diaphragm on the image, and appears as if it is reflected in a mirror behind the diaphragm. This is caused by the strong reflection of ultrasound waves from the diaphragm, which causes the ultrasound waves emitted from the probe to travel in the following order: diaphragm, liver, diaphragm, and probe. In addition to the diaphragm, similar images across a strongly reflecting surface, such as the pericardium or bladder wall, may be mirror images. Color flow and Spectral Doppler can also be susceptible to mirror artifacts.

Artifacts Associated with Attenuation

The further ultrasound travels, the more its energy lessens. This is called attenuation. The higher the ultrasound frequency, the more the energy attenuates over the same distance. Some tissues (e.g., water (blood)) retain more energy than others (e.g., bones and lungs). The attenuation unit is Db/cm, and the higher the number, the more attenuation the ultrasound has over the same distance.

High attenuation (bone, lungs, and air) means more ultrasound is reflected at the site, while low attenuation (water, blood) means little ultrasound is reflected at the site. Ultrasound waves pass

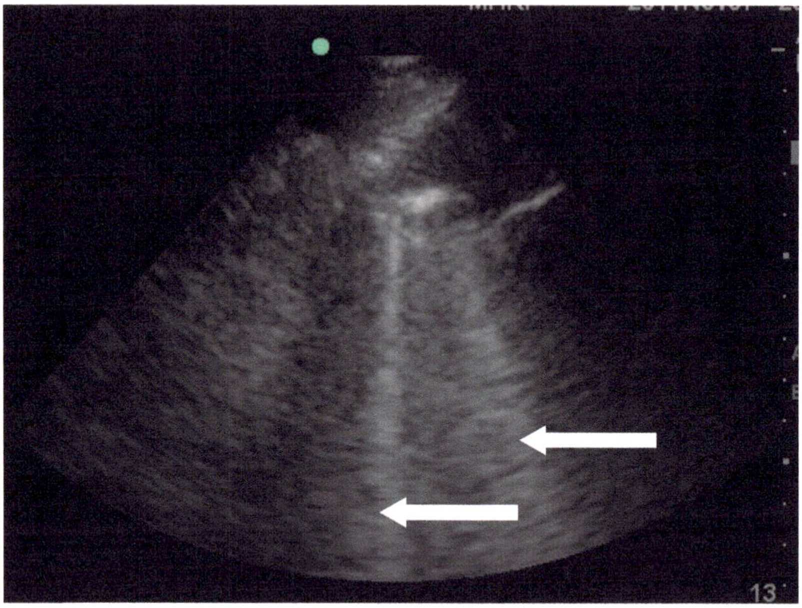

Image 3.2 Lung ultrasound with vertical B-lines. Examples of ring-down artifact. B-lines can be observed which arise from the pleura surface

through water without much attenuation (or, conversely, with almost no reflection). In contrast, in bone and air, ultrasound waves are so attenuated (mostly reflected) that they cannot pass beyond a certain distance. Soft tissues, such as the liver, transmit a portion of the ultrasound and reflect the rest [3].

If the ultrasound is not reflected and passes through the area unimpeded (e.g., fluid), the ultrasound signal that is reflected back is less and appears black. On the other hand, if ultrasound waves are only reflected off the surface of a material (e.g., bone surface and membranes) more ultrasound waves will be returned to the probe, and the brightness on the screen will be higher. In the case of parenchymal organs such as the liver and kidneys, some ultrasound waves pass through, and some are reflected, which is why they appear gray on the screen [4].

Shadowing Artifact

When ultrasound passes through a target with high attenuation (e.g., bone and air), the ultrasound is reflected from the surface, making it difficult for an ultrasound to reach the area behind the target, resulting in a black shadow beneath the target on the image. In this case, the black shadow does not mean that water is present, but rather it means that there is no signal coming back beyond the target (Image 3.3).

Enhancement Artifact

Conversely, when ultrasound travels through a target with low attenuation (e.g., water), it maintains relatively high energy compared to other locations. In such cases, the signal reflected back will be higher than in other areas because of the higher energy. This is called Enhancement Artifact (Image 3.4).

Artifacts Associated with Ultrasound Beam Properties

The type of assumption discussed here is that there is only one ultrasound beam: However, there are other beams, such as side lobes and grating lobes. These beams could, from time to time, generate ultrasound reflection strong enough to be detected by the probe and create artifacts.

Side-Lobe Artifacts

Side lobe beams are often generated in linear array transducers; they could generate a detectable reflection of ultrasound beam by an object

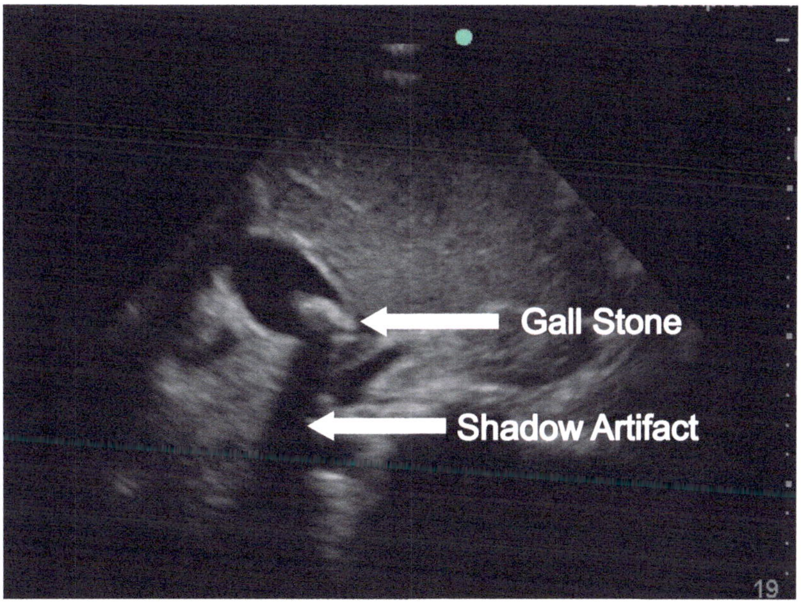

Image 3.3 Example of the shadow artifact. You can observe shadow artifact behind the gall stone, which has a highly echogenic surface

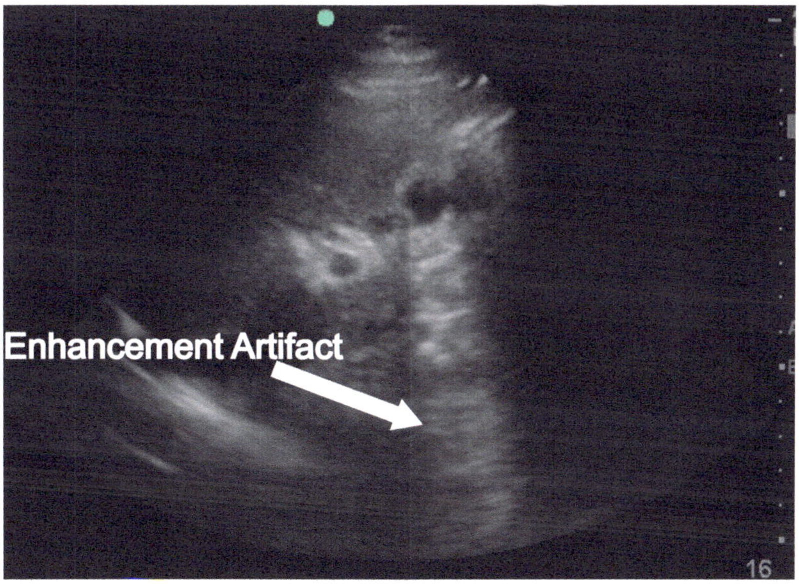

Image 3.4 Enhancement artifact. Note the high echogenic zone behind the gall bladder, which itself is anechoic

with strong reflector properties but does not exist in the path of the main beam. Since the ultrasound machine assumes there only exists one beam, thus it will display the reflector in the position it should not exist.

Pro-tip
Image from multiple windows and views to better recognize artifacts.

Refraction Artifacts

When a sound wave encounters another medium with a different propagation speed at an oblique angle, it can refract, or bend. We see this property in light as well, when an image is distorted when seen through water compared to air [5].

> **Pro-tip**
> Blood flow can be useful to identify artifacts. Artifacts should not affect blood flow.

Summary Points

- An ultrasound machine creates images based on the physical properties of the ultrasound wave, with assumptions of its expected behavior.
- Artifacts arise when the actual behaviors of the ultrasound deviate from these assumptions.
- Understanding US artifacts is essential as we can avoid making erroneous conclusions from the artifacts. It is also important as we recognize specific pathophysiology from specific image artifacts.
- There are three types of US artifacts.
  - Reflection: reverberation, ring-down, comet tail, mirror image
  - Attenuation: shadow artifact, enhancement artifact
  - Beam properties: side-lobe artifact

Question

1. A 51-year-old obese male is admitted with septic shock. A right internal jugular hemodialysis catheter is placed, and dialysis is underway. You perform a transesophageal echocardiogram. You see the following on mid-esophageal long-axis (Video 3.1). What is the appropriate next step in management?
   A. Remove the catheter, it is arterially placed
   B. Image the SVC and aorta in the short axis
   C. CT scan of the chest with contrast to confirm aortic dissection
   D. Plan for pericardiocentesis

   Answer: B. Image the SVC and aorta in the short axis (Video 3.2).

   The image seen prior is an artifact of the catheter in the SVC creating a side-lobe artifact into the ascending aorta. Side lobe artifacts can occur both in the imaging plane and outside the image plane. In the question, the SVC is not visualized and out of the imaging plane. When there is suspicion for artifacts, image for multiple planes. Color Flow imaging may also help determine if a finding is real, as both aortic dissection and an intra-aortic catheter will likely affect blood flow. The other advice is that it is usually good to be thorough and complete an exam rather than rush to treatment based one image. Because this is an artifact, there is no dissection or intra-aortic catheter. There is no evidence for tamponade physiology.

References

1. Feldman MK, Katyal S, Blackwood MS. US artifacts. Radiographics. 2009;29:1179–89.
2. Edelman S. Understanding ultrasound physics. 3rd ed. Texas: ESP; 2004.
3. Lichtenstein DA, Meziere GA. Relevance of lung ultrasound in the diagnosis of acute respiratory failure: the BLUE protocol. Chest. 2008;134:117–25.
4. Walz-Flannigan AI, Brossoit KJ, Magnuson DJ, Schueler BA. Pictorial review of digital radiography artifacts. Radiographics. 2018;38:833–46.
5. Kremkau F. Sonography instruments and principles. 10th ed. Philadelphia: Elsevier; 2021.

Positioning, Safety, Manipulation of Probe

4

Sameer Khanijo and Mangala Narasimhan

Learning Objectives

1. Suitable patient positioning is essential when performing all ultrasound scans
2. Optimal patient positioning for cardiac ultrasound involves the patient supine, and if possible, in the left lateral decubitus position
3. The probe should be grasped with the first three fingers of the dominant hand
4. The ultrasonographer should be seated on the same side of the patient as the ultrasound machine, so they can operate the machine while scanning
5. Five basic probe movements: sliding, rocking, tilting, rotating, and compression

Point-of-care ultrasound involves medical provider acquisition and interpretation of ultrasound images at the patient's bedside to diagnose and guide medical therapies [1]. The time-consuming step in this focused use of ultrasound is often the image acquisition as it involves appropriate positioning of the patient and sonographer and manipulation, and fine-tuning, of the transducer in multiple directions, to obtain the ideal image [2]. In this chapter we will review patient positioning and safety, ergonomics, practitioner positioning, and holding and manipulation of the ultrasound probe.

Patient and sonographer positioning and ergonomics are important in the quest for obtaining optimal imaging. Poor positioning affects scan time and can cause chronic injuries in ultrasound practitioners [3]. Optimal patient positioning for cardiac ultrasound involves the patient supine, or in the left lateral decubitus position, with arms raised above their head as this brings the heart closest to the chest wall [4]. In critical care echocardiography, patient positioning may be restricted due to the clinical condition (intubation, pacing, or central access sites), room space with lots of equipment present, and the inability to move patients. Mechanical ventilation may alter hemodynamics and therefore scan position in the critically ill [5].

Ultrasonographers should be positioned to the side of the patient and in a comfortable position, seated when feasible. The ultrasound machine should be on the same side as the scanner. Transthoracic evaluation can be performed with the sonographer sitting on either the patient's left or right side and this is often a matter of personal preference, custom, and comfort. However, when scanning with the right hand the sonographer is often seated on the right side of the patient and the machine is manipulated with the left hand. If scanning on the left side of the patient, the left hand is used to scan, and the machine is adjusted with the right hand (Image 4.1). Your arms should

S. Khanijo · M. Narasimhan (✉)
Donald and Barbara Zucker School of Medicine at Hofstra/Northwell, New York, NY, USA
e-mail: skhanijo2@northwell.edu; mnarasimhan@northwell.edu

M. J. Lanspa, A. T. Levinson (eds.), *Echocardiography and Ultrasonography in the ICU*, Respiratory Medicine, https://doi.org/10.1007/978-3-031-80038-2_4

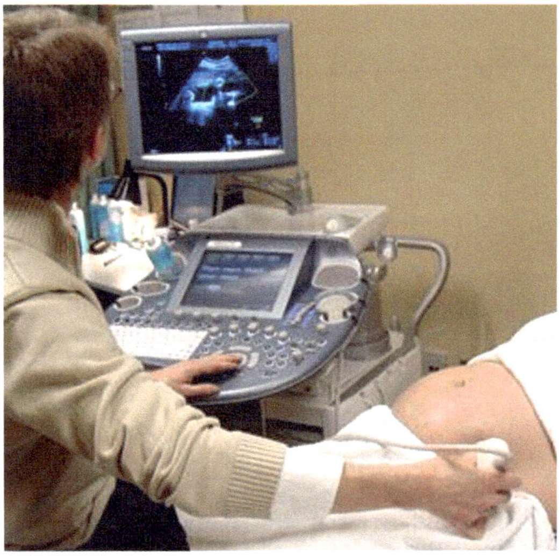

Image 4.1 The machine should be placed on the same side as the operator so they can adjust the machine

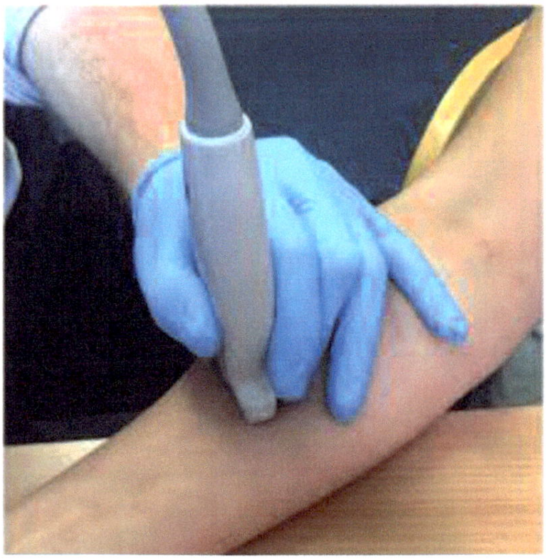

Image 4.2 Best hand position for the probe

be as close to your side as possible and not crossing over your body with the patient positioned close to you. Make sure you are positioned appropriately to reach onto, and when necessary, over the patient. Standing may help provide better posture. Sonographers should move down the bed rather than contorting their bodies to reach behind them. It is best to keep all joints in a neutral position when able. Developing the ability to scan from both sides minimizes the risk of repetitive use injuries and prepares the sonographer for circumstances where only one side of the patient is available for scanning. One important note is that patient positioning may influence the findings on lung ultrasonography, particularly in the heart failure population, and so a consistent approach to patient positioning during point-of-care ultrasonography may be important to monitor dynamic changes [6].

Once the patient and provider are appropriately positioned ultrasonography can begin. Generally, the probe should be held like a pen, although it can be held in the overhand position when imaging the heart in subcostal. Ultrasonographers should not be afraid of getting gel on their hands or making physical contact with the patient. The probe, also known as the transducer, should be grasped with the first three fingers of the dominant hand. This is enough to hold and maneuver the probe and leaves the pinkie, finger, and heel of the palm, to stabilize the probe on the patient (Image 4.2). Direct contact with the patient is particularly important for obtaining quality images. Direct contact allows one to properly stabilize the transducer on the patient without having to use excessive pressure, thus making the patient more comfortable and decreasing fatigue on the hand. Appropriate probe holding technique will allow one to obtain optimal images without sliding around too much and without applying too much pressure: this becomes even more important when the probe is being used for procedural guidance. Remember to clean the probe immediately after scanning and prior to use on a new patient and to use a sterile probe cover if performing a sterile procedure (Image 4.3).

Ultrasound probe manipulation is important in point-of-care ultrasound as patient anatomy and clinical conditions vary greatly. Often, the transducer placement illustrated in textbooks does not work in real time. While experienced clinicians will naturally adjust the probe, new sonographers will often move the transducer in multiple planes simultaneously resulting in repeated suboptimal image acquisition and frustration [2]. Slow fine movements should be made, and evaluation of the changes seen on the screen should be continuous.

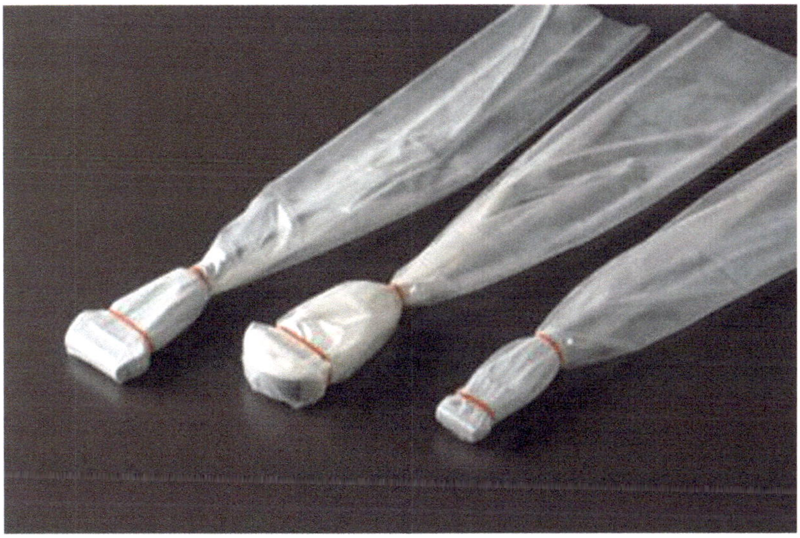

Image 4.3 Three probe types: (**a**) linear probe (**b**) abdominal probe (**c**) Smaller linear probe

Initially, there was no consistent terminology for the manipulation of the ultrasound probe to obtain high-quality images. In 1999, the American Institute of Ultrasound in Medicine published a technical bulletin, which described five basic movements: sliding, rocking, tilting, rotating, and compression [7]. While this nomenclature is standardized, there remain substantial inconsistencies in terminology describing transducer motion. Some frequently used, nonstandard terms, include move, angle, fan, rock, and heel-toe [2].

Understanding, and mastering, the transducer manipulation techniques will allow practitioners to obtain the desired images. These movements are [8] (Image 4.4):

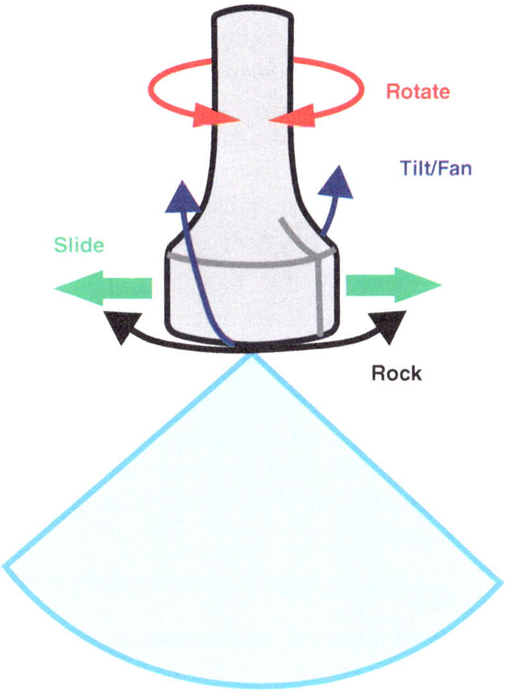

Image 4.4 Probe movements

- **Sliding** involves moving the transducer along the long axis of the probe across the body with a consistent angle against the body. Sliding will move the target structure from side to side on the screen. This moves the entire probe in a specific direction to find a better imaging window.
- **Rocking** involves motion in the long axis of the probe at a fixed point on the body while changing the angle against the body. This allows you to help center the area of interest and keeps the desired image in plane throughout the manipulation.
- **Tilting**, also called fanning, involves a side-to-side motion along the short axis of the probe. This allows multiple cross-sectional images of a structure of interest. The axis is unchanged while tilting.
- **Rotation** is most used to move between short-axis and long-axis views of a desired structure.
- **Compression** involves direct pressure on the transducer onto the body causing compression of the area of interest by the transducer.

With all of these tools, scanning can be done consistently, safely, and comfortably. Teaching can also be done consistently and using standard terminology.

Summary Points

- Patient and ultrasonographer positions can greatly affect the quality of the images obtained.
- In critical care scanning, optimal positioning may not be possible.
- Ideally, the ultrasonographer should be seated on the same side as the ultrasound machine in order to be able to operate the machine while scanning.
- The probe should be held like a pen with contact made with the patient's body with the hypothenar eminence.
- Slow movements should be made while altering an image or changing an angle.
- Use standardized nomenclature. There are five basic movements described: sliding, rocking, tilting, rotating, and compression.

Pro-tips

The probe should be grasped with the first three fingers of the dominant hand. This leaves the pinkie, finger, and heel of the palm free to stabilize the probe on the patient.

In 1999, the American Institute of Ultrasound in Medicine described five basic probe movements: sliding, rocking, tilting, rotating, and compression.

Questions

1. Optimal position for the scanner is:
   A. On the same side as the machine
   B. On the opposite side of the machine
   C. Either side is fine

   Answer: (A) On the same side as the machine

   For point-of-care ultrasonography, the scanner must be on the same side as the machine as the operator must work with machines as they are scanning. There is usually only one scanner and no technician or other person to operate the machine. Adjustments must be made to optimize the image to fix gain, depth, and to make measurements.
2. To go from the parasternal long axis view of the heart to the short axis view of the heart the motion employed is:
   A. Tilting
   B. Rocking
   C. Rotating
   D. Sliding

   Answer: (C) Rotating

   Rotating is moving the probe around the transducer axis, on a fixed point on the body, in a clockwise or counterclockwise direction. This motion is the most common one used when going from a long-axis view of a structure to a short-axis view of the same structure. When moving from the parasternal long-axis view to short-axis view the rotation is clockwise with the pointer starting at the right shoulder and ending at the left shoulder (approximately).

References

1. Moore CL, Copel JA. Point-of-care ultrasonography. N Engl J Med. 2011;364:749–57.
2. Bahner DP, Blickendorf JM, Bacbrader M, et al. Language of transducer manipulation: codifying terms for effective teaching. J Ultrasound Med. 2016;34:183–8.
3. Claes F, Berger J, Stassijns G. Arm and neck pain in ultrasonographers. Hum Factors. 2015;57:238–45.
4. Bauman DJ. Position of patient for echocardiography. Chest. 1977;72(1):132.
5. Kirkpatrick JN, Grimm R, Johri AM, Kimura BJ, Kort S, Labovitz AJ, Lanspa M, Phillip S, Raza S, Thorson K, Turner J. Recommendations for echocardiography laboratories participating in cardiac point of care cardiac ultrasound (POCUS) and critical care echocardiography training: report from the American Society of Echocardiography. J Am Soc Echocardiogr. 2020;33(4):409–22.e4.
6. Frasure SE, Matilsky DK, Siadecki SD, Platz E, Saul T, Lewis RE. Impact of patient positioning on lung ultrasound findings in acute heart failure. Eur Heart J Acute Cardiovasc Care. 2015;4:326–32.
7. American Institute of Ultrasound in Medicine. AIUM technical bulletin: transducer manipulation. J Ultrasound Med. 1999;18:169–75.
8. Ramsingh D, Gatling J. Teaching point-of-care ultrasound (POCUS) to the perioperative physician. In: Bowe E, Schell R, DiLorenzo A, editors. Education in anesthesia: how to deliver the best learning experience. Cambridge: Cambridge University Press; 2018. p. 131–50.

Part II

Echocardiography

5 Transthoracic Windows and Views

Nova Panebianco and Michael O'Neil

Learning Objective

1. Describe the surface anatomy, sonographic anatomy, imaging tips, and common pearls and pitfalls for each of the transthoracic echocardiography views.

Parasternal Window: PLAX, PSAX, RV Inflow, RV Outflow Views

The parasternal window is useful in the assessment of left ventricular ejection fraction, the presence of pericardial effusion and tamponade physiology, the right ventricle to left ventricle ratio, pulmonary inflow and outflow anatomy, as well as valvular anatomy and function.

Parasternal Long Axis (PLAX)

See Fig. 5.1.

Supplementary Information The online version contains supplementary material available at https://doi.org/10.1007/978-3-031-80038-2_5.

N. Panebianco (✉)
Department of Emergency Medicine, University of Pennsylvania, Philadelphia, PA, USA
e-mail: nova.panebianco@uphs.upenn.edu

M. O'Neil
Main Line Emergency Medicine Associates, West Chester, PA, USA
e-mail: Michael.O'neil@pennmedicine.upenn.edu

External Surface Anatomy

For the parasternal long-axis view, the patient should be placed in the supine or left lateral decubitus position. Place the probe on the patient's left chest just lateral to the sternum in the third to fifth intercostal space with the probe marker facing the right shoulder.

Sonographic Anatomy

In this image, the right ventricle, interventricular septum, left ventricle, aortic outflow tract, aortic root, and the left atrium should be visualized. Deep into the cardiac structures and pericardium, the descending thoracic aorta may be visualized in the transverse plane (Fig. 5.1, Video 5.1).

Imaging Tips

If no clear cardiac image is seen in this window, slide the probe cephalad or caudal until the heart is encountered. The probe may need to be rotated clockwise or counter-clockwise to match the axis of the patient's heart.

An image is in the plane when the mitral and aortic valves are seen clearly. To visualize more of the base of the heart, slide or rock the probe toward the sternum. To see more of the LV, slide or rock the probe toward the apex.

The gain should be set so that the fluid in the heart is black, but not so low that the endocardium is difficult to see. Place the focal zone in the center of the heart.

M. J. Lanspa, A. T. Levinson (eds.), *Echocardiography and Ultrasonography in the ICU*, Respiratory Medicine, https://doi.org/10.1007/978-3-031-80038-2_5

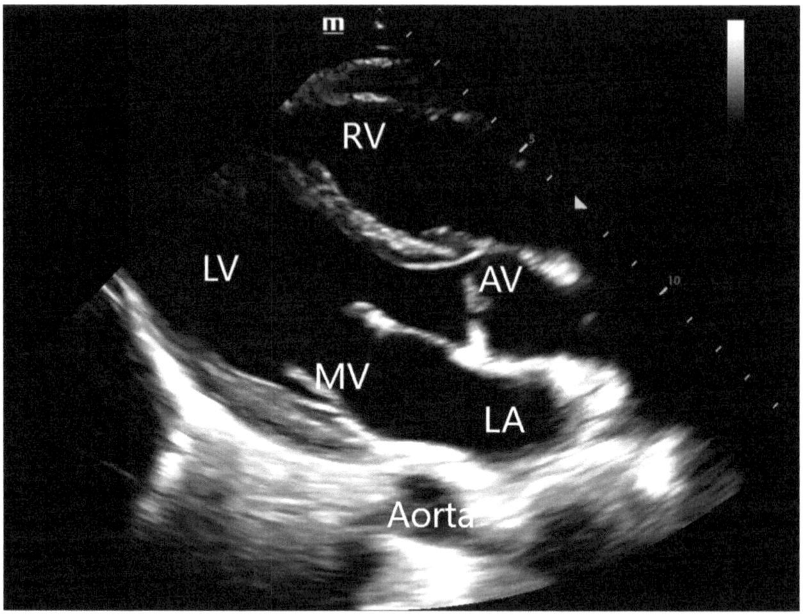

Fig. 5.1 Parasternal long axis (PLAX)

Pearls and Pitfalls

- Oblique views can overestimate the EF.
- Patients with COPD/asthma may have midline hearts with images obstructed by the sternum. To improve imaging, have the patient roll into the left-lateral position (if possible), which may drop the heart into view.
- Pregnant patients may need significantly more rotation to match their heart's axis.
- Pleural effusion can be mistaken for pericardial effusion. To distinguish the two conditions, it is important to identify the descending thoracic aorta. In a circumferential pericardial effusion, pericardial fluid will tract anterior to the descending thoracic aorta and may cross the midline. The fluid in a pleural effusion will track posterior to the descending thoracic aorta and not cross the midline.
- In a patient where the lung is obscuring relevant cardiac anatomy having the patient fully exhale may provide a brief opportunity to obtain diagnostic images.
- The strategies described above to locate the heart are starting points; however, what you see on the screen will dictate how to move your hand when optimizing images.

Right Ventricular (RV) Inflow

See Fig. 5.2.

External Surface Anatomy

From the parasternal long-axis view, the probe is tilted caudally and toward the right hip to assess the right ventricle and give an image of the inflow of the right ventricle (Fig. 5.2, Video 5.2).

Sonographic Anatomy

The right ventricle, anterior and posterior leaflets of the tricuspid valve, right atrium, SVC, and IVC are seen in this sonographic view. The left ventricle should not be visible if appropriately in the plane.

Imaging Tips

To optimize the image, roll the patient into the left-lateral decubitus position and have them fully exhale.

Pearls and Pitfalls

- Abdominal distention, bowel gas, and stomach contents can interfere with quality images.
- Patients with COPD and asthma may have limited right ventricular views in this window.

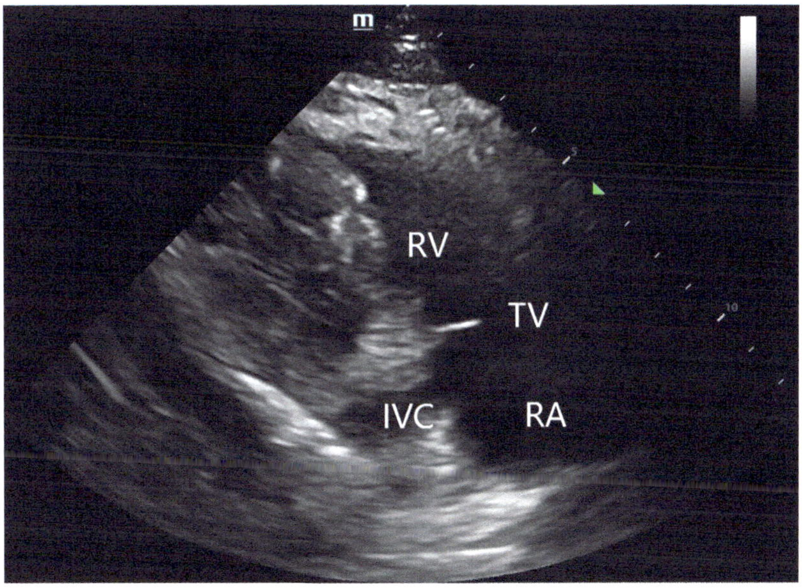

Fig. 5.2 Right ventricular (RV) inflow view

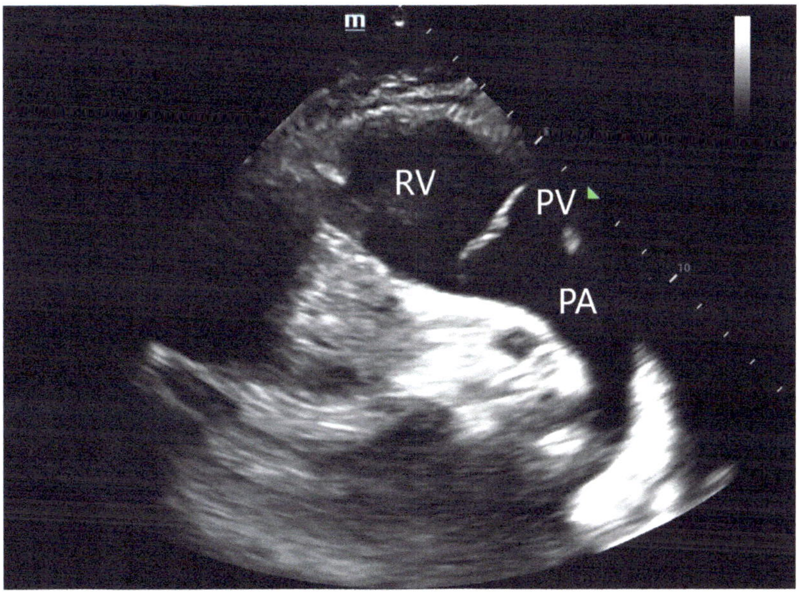

Fig. 5.3 Right ventricular (RV) outflow view

RV Outflow

See Fig. 5.3.

External Anatomy

In this view, the probe should then be tilted from the PSLA window toward the left shoulder to visualize the right atrium and pulmonary artery.

Sonographic Anatomy

In this view, the right atrium, pulmonary valve, and pulmonary artery should be visualized (Fig. 5.3, Video 5.3).

Imaging Tip

To ensure the image is in the plane, slight rotation or tilt of the probe may be necessary.

Pearls and Pitfalls

- In an awake and cooperative patient, having them take a deep breath and then completely exhale may remove artifacts caused by a lung curtain.
- Left lateral decubitus positioning is also helpful for this view.

Parasternal Short Axis (PSAX)

The PSAX view, depending on the plane being visualized, is useful in assessing LV ejection fraction, regional wall motion abnormalities, aortic valvular structure, mitral valvular structure, RV/LV ratio, and septal movement abnormalities caused by increased pulmonary pressures or volumes.

External Anatomy

For the PSAX view, the ultrasound probe is placed in the third to fifth intercostal space with the patient in the supine or left lateral decubitus position. The probe marker in this instance should be directed toward the patient's left shoulder. From the PSLA axis view, the PSSA view is obtained by rotating the probe 90° clockwise.

Sonographic Anatomy

At the mid-ventricular (or papillary muscle) level, the papillary muscles are clearly visualized in the O-shaped left ventricle. This axis is particularly useful for assessing LV ejection fraction, regional wall motion abnormalities, increased RV volume/pressure, and pericardial effusion (Fig. 5.4, Video 5.4).

From the mid-ventricular view, the mitral valve short-axis view is obtained by fanning or tilting the beam of the probe toward the right shoulder. In this view, the right ventricle and left ventricle are visualized. The thin anterior and posterior leaflets of the mitral valve are visualized within the short-axis view of the left ventricle. The axis is particularly useful for assessing the anatomy of the mitral valve.

To obtain the basilar short view, the probe is tilted further toward the right shoulder. In this plane, the base of the heart, right ventricular inflow and outflow, aortic valve, and left atrium are visualized. The three aortic valvular leaflets should be clearly visible giving the "Mercedes-Benz" sign. This plane is commonly used to assess for valvular anatomy/abnormalities and to assess the gradients across the tricuspid valve and pulmonary valves (Fig. 5.5, Video 5.5).

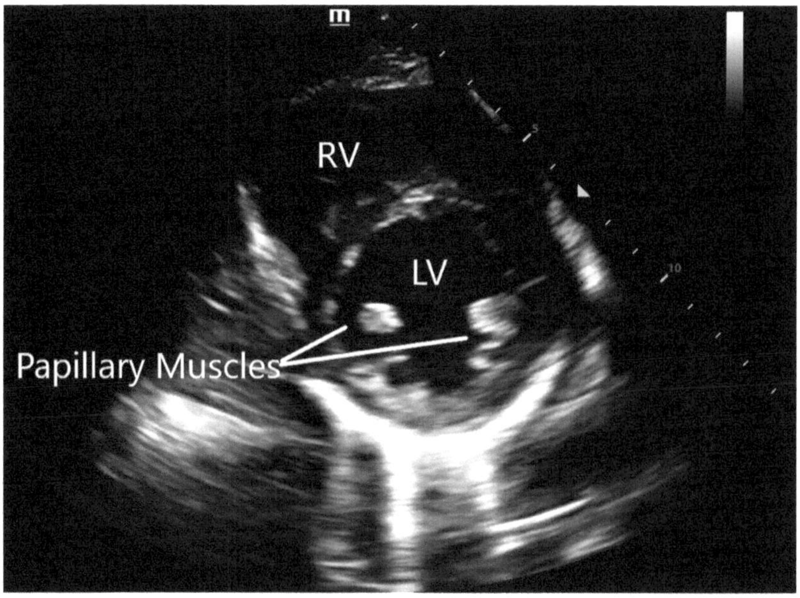

Fig. 5.4 Parasternal short-axis (PSAX) at the level of the papillary muscles

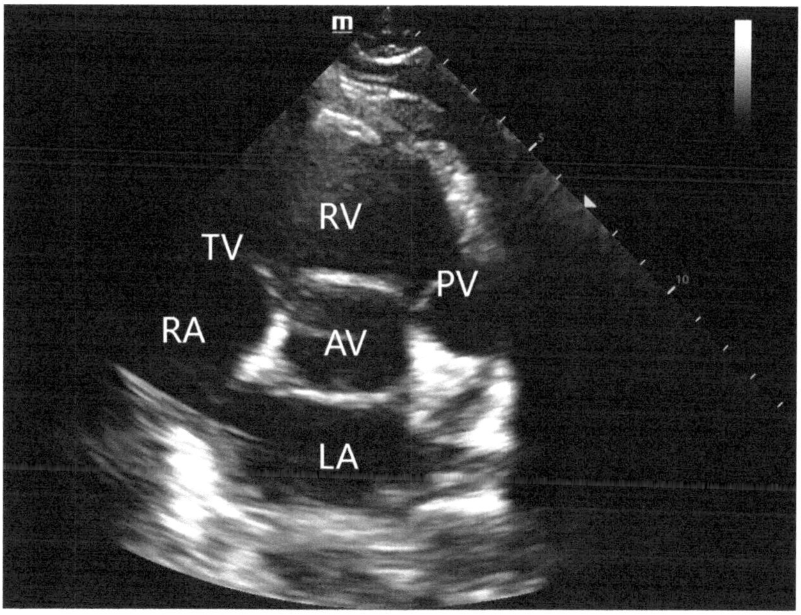

Fig. 5.5 Parasternal short-axis (PSAX) aortic valve level

The apical short-axis view at the level of the aorta is obtained by fanning or sliding the probe toward the base of the heart (toward the right shoulder). This view is helpful when assessing for aortic or pulmonary valve pathology.

Imaging Tips

As with the PLAX view, gently sliding or tilting the probe up or down rib spaces and slight rotation of the probe may be needed to optimize the correct anatomical view.

Pearls and Pitfalls

- If the beam traverses the heart obliquely, the LV can be transected obliquely, making the cavity appear oval or D-shaped which may give an inaccurate EF.

Apical: A4C, A5C, A2C, A3C

The apical viewing windows give attention to flow through the valves, as well as comparisons and evaluations for ventricular and atrial sizes. In these views, the entire atria and ventricle should be in view. These viewing windows are generally best seen in the left lateral position, although most patients in the supine position will have adequate viewing windows.

Apical Four-Chamber View (A4C)

External Anatomy

To obtain the A4C view, the ultrasound probe is traced laterally along the left fifth intercostal space to the anterior axillary line with the probe marker facing the patient's left side (3 o'clock) position. Slight rotation or fanning may need to be utilized to optimize the correct anatomical view. In some patients, the probe may have to slide more medially or laterally to fully view the examined structures. The point of maximum impulse (PMI), if palpable, is also a useful landmark to start with before placing the transducer on the chest.

Sonographic Anatomy

In this view, the ultrasound beam passes through the apex of the heart with the right and left ventricles, tricuspid valve, mitral valve, and right and left atria fully in view. The septum should be lined up vertically in the center of the screen (Fig. 5.6, Video 5.6).

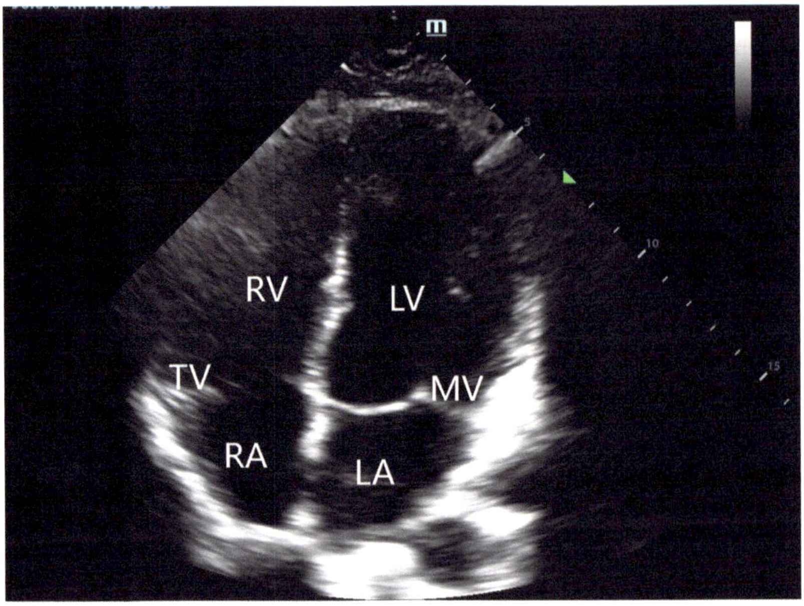

Fig. 5.6 Apical four-chamber view (A4C)

Scanning Tips

If the four chambers are visible but the septum is not vertical, fan the probe so that the beam is pointing toward the right shoulder (and the tail of the probe is pointing toward the left hip). If the ventricles are visualized but the atria are not, try decreasing the angle of the probe (flatten out the probe) relative to the chest wall. If the atria are well seen but the ventricles are not, try the opposite maneuver just described. If one side of the heart dominates the image (right or left) try rotating the probe to even out the cavities.

Pearls and Pitfalls

- As with the parasternal windows, if the lung is obstructing the echocardiography window, attempt to roll the patient onto their left side.
- If the probe marker is inadvertently flipped, one could falsely diagnose right heart strain because the right side of the heart will appear larger than the left side. There are several anatomic structures that should be noted to prevent this mistake.
  - First, the right heart will have the moderator band seen at the RV apex.
  - Second, the tricuspid valve annulus is slightly more anterior than the left.
  - Lastly, sliding slightly cephalad should reveal the aortic valve outflow tract, which will confirm the location of the left ventricle.
  - When breast tissue is encountered, place the probe under it rather than trying to scan through it. Supportive garments and EKG stickers should be removed, and monitor leads should be relocated outside the scanning window. Remember to drape your patient with towels to preserve modesty.

Apical Five-Chamber View (A5C)

External Anatomy

The AC5 view is often obtained at the same anatomic location as the AC4, in the left fifth intercostal space in the mid-axillary line or just inferior to the nipple by simply fanning the probe cephalad. If rib shadows are encountered, move the probe cephalad one rib space.

Sonographic Anatomy

The image obtained in this view is similar to the A4C; however, the left ventricular outflow tract and aortic valve will be seen connecting to the left ventricle. The left atrium view may be foreshortened when obtaining the image in this window (Fig. 5.7, Video 5.7).

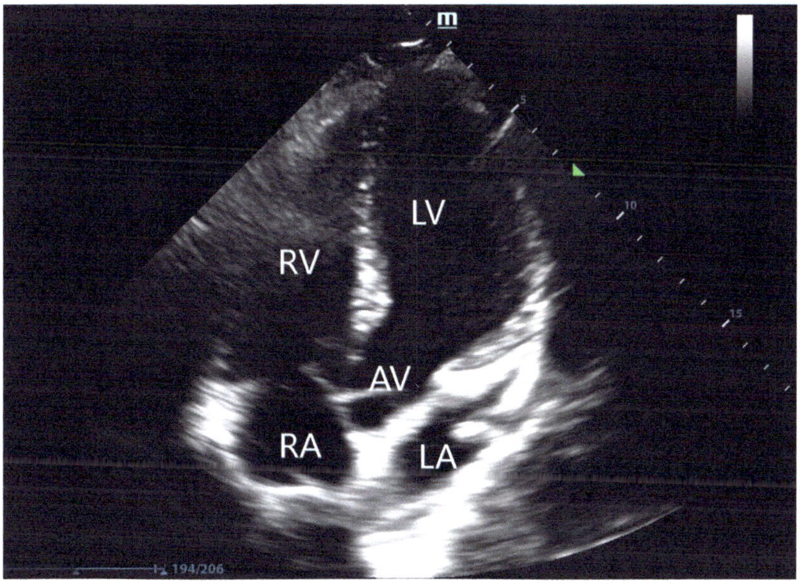

Fig. 5.7 Apical five-chamber view (A5C)

Scanning Tips

The tips for this view are similar to those for the A4C. If a rib shadow is encountered when fanning the cephalad to obtain the image, consider moving the probe up one rib space. This movement may cause the ventricles to be cut short and the atria to come out of view.

Pearls and Pitfalls

- This view is commonly used to calculate the cardiac stroke volume and output. Being off-plane can cause variability in serial Doppler measurements and erroneous calculations.
- In patients with a low body mass index, it may be challenging to obtain enough skin contact to generate an adequate image. In this scenario, use more gel or a step-off to get better skin contact.

Apical Two-Chamber View (A2C)

External Anatomy

Same as the AC4 view.

Sonographic Anatomy

From the A4C view, rotate the probe 90° counterclockwise so that the indicator is toward the head. In this view, the ultrasound beam passes through the apex of the heart, the left ventricle, the mitral valve, and the left atria. In the A4C view, the left ventricular septum and lateral wall are seen. In the A2C view, the left ventricular inferior wall is seen on screen left, and the anterior wall is seen on screen right. The right ventricle should not be visualized in this view (Fig. 5.8, Video 5.8).

Scanning Tips

The scanning tips for this window are similar to those for the A4C view.

Pearls and Pitfalls

- Over- or under-rotation can yield inadequate visualization of the pertinent structures.

Apical Three-Chamber View (A3C)

External Anatomy

The external anatomy is often the same as for the A4C and A2C views.

Sonographic Anatomy

To obtain this view, rotate the probe counterclockwise from the A2C view (about 60°) until the aortic outflow tract is seen connecting to the left ventricle. When in plane, this view should look very similar to the PSLA image, however

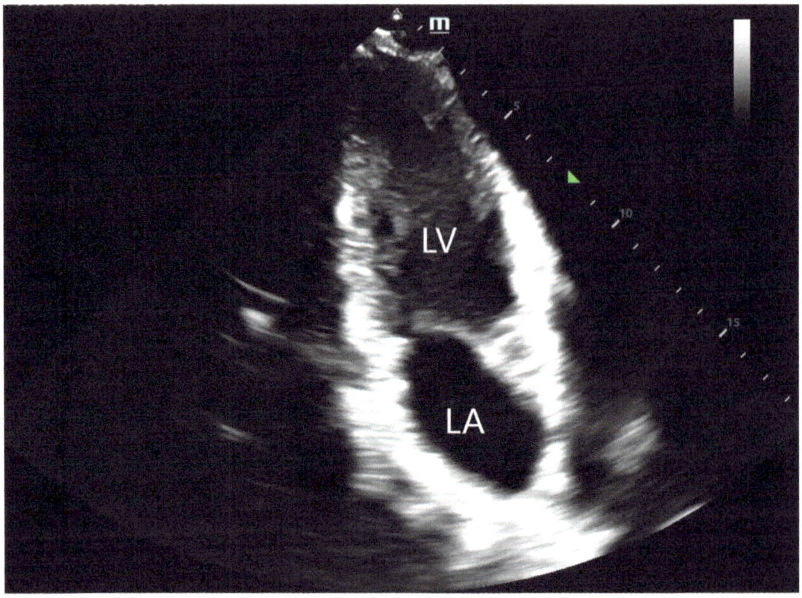

Fig. 5.8 Apical two-chamber view (A2C)

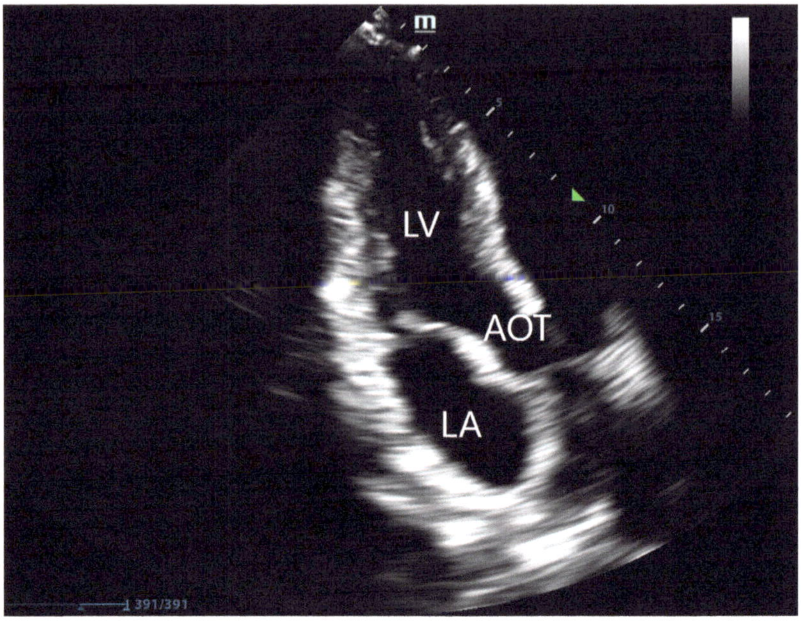

Fig. 5.9 Apical three-chamber view (A3C)

visualized from the apex of the heart. The sonographic anatomy will include the left ventricle, right ventricle, interventricular septum, left ventricular outflow tract, and left atrium (Fig. 5.9, Video 5.9).

Scanning Tips

The scanning tips for this view are similar to those of the A4C and A2C. Over-rotation can cause inadequate imaging. Similarly, if not on the plane, the size of the LV and RV can be misinterpreted.

Pearls and Pitfalls

- This view is particularly helpful when assessing the left ventricular outflow tract.
- If lung artifact obscures, the view has the patient exhale completely.

Subcostal: SC4, SC Long Access, IVC

Many of the cardiac views described in the parasternal and apical windows can also be obtained in the subcostal window. In patients with COPD or asthma, cardiac structures may be elongated and midline, leaving the subcostal window as the only window for adequate cardiac imaging. This window is unique from the other windows previously described because it includes anatomy below the diaphragm such as the inferior vena cava (IVC), liver, and peritoneum.

Subcostal Four-Chamber View (SC4)

External Anatomy

The subcostal four-chamber view is obtained by placing the probe with the probe marker to the patient's left (3 o'clock position), just below the bony xiphoid process, and often slightly to the patient's right using the liver as a sonographic window. The probe should be pressed almost flat against the abdomen to clear the bony structures, and the operator may need to overhand the probe to apply the appropriate amount of pressure and angle to obtain adequate images.

Sonographic Anatomy

In this view, the ultrasound beam first passes through the liver, then both the right atria and right ventricle, and subsequently the left atria and left ventricle. The echogenic pericardium should be flush against the myocardium and indistinguishable from adjacent structures. Physiologic pericardial effusion may be seen anteriorly by the right atrium. This view is useful for assessing pericardial effusion and tamponade. Additionally, it is often the best location to assess the right ventricular free wall thickness (Fig. 5.10, Video 5.10).

Scanning Tips

Unlike the other views, images in the subcostal window are often best obtained when the patient is completely supine and not rolled. If a patient cannot tolerate a supine position, consider placing the patient in reverse Trendelenburg to let gravity bring the heart closer to the probe. Chest and abdominal wounds and bandages may interfere with this window and should be removed when appropriate. In patients who are gravid, and have significant abdominal distention, ascites, or abdominal tenderness, this view may not be obtainable.

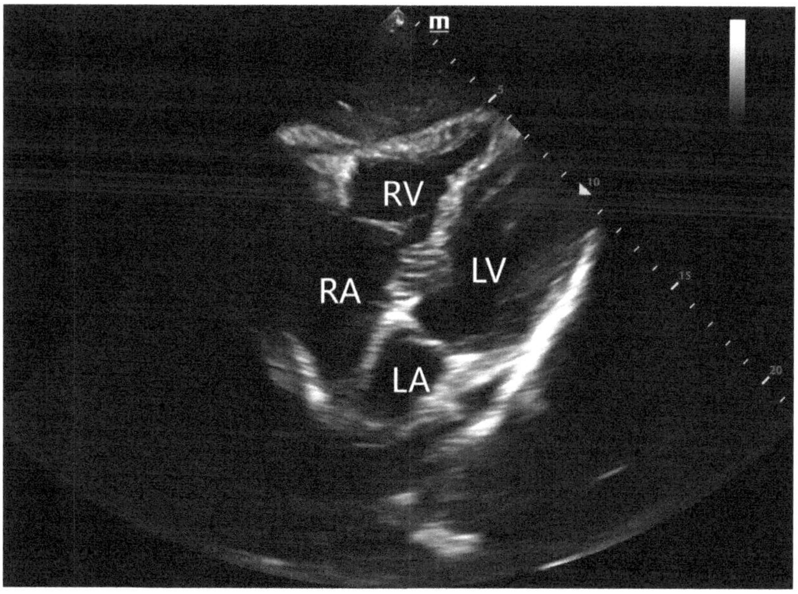

Fig. 5.10 Subcostal four-chamber view (SC4)

Pearls and Pitfalls

- In an awake patient, having them take a deep breath and hold it may improve imaging.
- Having the patient bend their knees may loosen the abdominal musculature and allow the examiner to press hard enough to get under the bony sternum.
- An image is in the plane when the four cardiac chambers, tricuspid, and mitral valves are in view. Off-axis images can over or underestimate the size of chambers.
- An epicardial fat pad can be mistaken as a pericardial effusion. Epicardial fat will not be circumferential, moves with the cardiac cycle, and often has internal echoes.
- Abdominal ascites can be mistaken for pericardial effusion.

Subcostal Long Axis IVC

External Anatomy

The external anatomy for the long-axis view of the IVC is the same as for the subcostal view of the heart. The probe is rotated so that the marker is facing the cephalad (12 o'clock position) and tilted upward toward the heart.

If bowel gas, wounds, or other factors limit this window, scanning through the liver may provide an adequate view of the IVC. To do this, line the probe up with the xiphoid process and then slide laterally to the right toward the midclavicular line, between the ribs, angled cephalad, with the liver as the sonographic window.

Sonographic Anatomy

In this view, the IVC is visualized passing through the diaphragm into the right atrium. The hepatic veins converge with the IVC just before the vessel enters the thoracic cavity. Once the appropriate imaging level has been identified, the hand should be held still to assess the morphology and collapsibility of the great vessel (Figs. 5.11 and 5.12, Videos 5.11 and 5.12).

Scanning Tips

As described above, if the subcostal window is inadequate, the right intercostal window may be useful. If bowel gas is preventing, adequate imaging gentle pressure may be applied with the transducer to move it out of the scanning field; however, attention must be paid to not press so hard to cause collapse of the IVC. Adjusting the frequency, depth, gain, and dynamic range machine settings may be necessary to visualize the abdominal IVC. To quantify the IVC variation through the respiratory cycle, M-Mode may be useful.

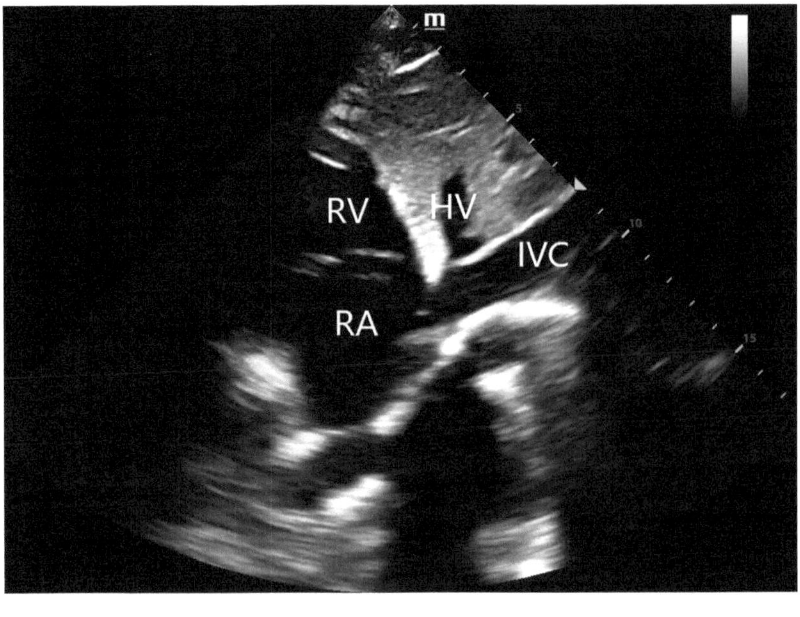

Fig. 5.11 Subcostal long axis IVC

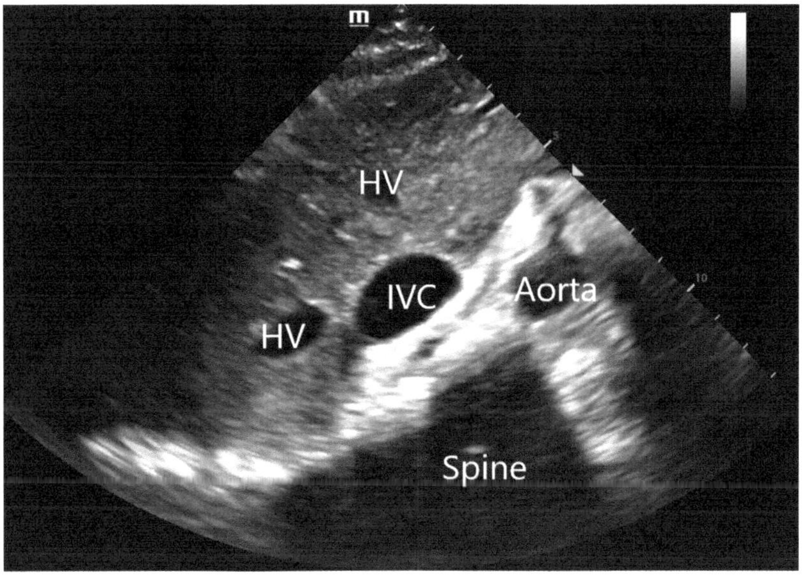

Fig. 5.12 Subcostal short axis IVC

Pearls and Pitfalls

- The abdominal aorta can be mistaken for the IVC, particularly in patients with hypovolemia. There are several strategies to distinguish the abdominal aorta from the IVC. The hepatic veins course through the liver and join the IVC just before the vessel passes through the diaphragm, while the celiac trunk and superior mesenteric arteries branch from the aorta. The IVC is on the patient's right relative to the abdominal aorta, which may be more easily recognized when scanning in the transverse plane. The walls of the aorta are generally thicker than that of the IVC; however, this relative size may be difficult to distinguish on ultrasound.
- The IVC pulsates and this finding cannot be used to distinguish the IVC from the aorta.
- In patients with intra-abdominal hypertension, the IVC may be compressed.
- Increased right heart pressures and tamponade physiology will dilate the IVC. For this reason, the IVC alone cannot be used to assess the volume status.

Suprasternal/Supraclavicular View

This sonographic window is valuable for the assessment of the great vessels that are typically obscured by the bones of the anterior chest. It is often one of the more challenging windows to obtain images from because of patient anatomy, patient discomfort, and transducer size. When setting up for the exam, placing a pillow or prop behind the shoulders and having the patient turn their head gently to the left may open the window and make more room for the transducer and its cord. Suprasternal imaging may not be possible in patients in cervical traction or with a tracheostomy or prior tracheostomy scar tissue. If the patient is orally intubated, be mindful to position equipment away from the scanning window so as not to dislodge any items.

External Anatomy

Apply copious gel to the suprasternal notch to reduce the amount of pressure needed on the neck. Place the probe in the suprasternal notch with the probe indicator toward the 1 o'clock position. If imaging is inadequate, the right supraclavicular is an alternative location for scanning.

Sonographic Anatomy

A long-axis view of the ascending aorta, aortic arch, descending thoracic aorta, and the origins of the right brachiocephalic, left common carotid, and left subclavian artery may be seen. The corresponding venous structures are positioned superior to the aortic arch. The superior vena

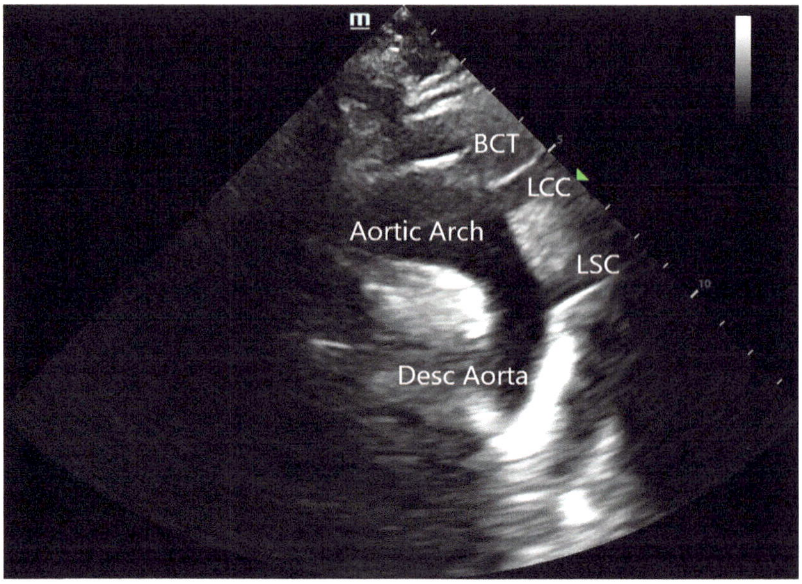

Fig. 5.13 Suprasternal aortic arch

cava may be visualized on the left of the ascending aorta, while the right pulmonary artery is identified as inferior to the aortic arch.

The short-axis view is obtained by rotating the probe 90° from the position where the optimized long-axis image was obtained (Fig. 5.13, Video 5.13).

Imaging Tips

As described above, attention to patient positioning and copious gel can greatly improve imaging in this location. Once the aorta is visualized, the probe may need to be rotated clockwise or counterclockwise to bring the anatomy into the plane. In an awake patient, if the lung is obscuring the image, have the patient completely exhale and hold their breath.

Pearls and Pitfalls

- Mirror and side-lobe artifacts can confound the interpretation of thoracic aorta imaging and create the appearance of pathology (particularly a dissection flap) when there isn't one. Optimize depth, gain, and the focal zone to reduce artifacts. Pathologic findings should persist when assessed in orthogonal planes.
- Small dissections and other aortic pathology may be difficult to see on transthoracic echocardiography. Consider using alternative imaging modalities, such as computed tomography and transesophageal echocardiography, given the limitations of this exam.

Key Points

- This chapter describes the fundamental two-dimensional views of echocardiography with a systematic description of the patient's external surface anatomy, sonographic anatomy, scanning tips, and pearls and pitfalls.
- The information in this chapter provides insight into commonly encountered difficulties in obtaining views and strategies for troubleshooting them when they arise.

6 Transthoracic M-Mode Echocardiography

Becky Burk

Learning Objectives

1. Know the advantages m-mode has over 2D imaging in specific instances and applications.
2. Be familiar with common m-mode images in echocardiography.

Introduction to M-Mode

M-mode, or "motion" mode, records ultrasound data from a single scan line and plots it sequentially over time. The displayed image shows time on the x-axis versus depth on the y-axis. Thus, the change in the depth of cardiac structures along the scan line is observed over time. The use of ultrasound to characterize the heart began in the 1950s. M-mode was the original echocardiogram modality, and it was dominant until the 1970s when 2D imaging was developed [1]. Some echocardiographers consider m-mode an historical relic, but it has two key advantages which make it a relevant part of the modern echocardiogram.

The first and major advantage of m-mode is its high temporal resolution. This characteristic makes it the mode of choice to analyze rapidly moving structures, such as cardiac valves. Temporal resolution is defined by the **frame rate**, which is the number of images displayed per second. A higher frame rate results in more granular and smoother imaging over time. A single image, or "frame," is generated once ultrasound waves have been emitted and "listened to" for each scan line. Therefore, the frame rate is inversely proportional to the number of scan lines. Unlike 2D imaging, which requires many scan lines, m-mode only has a single scan line, so the frame rate is very high (Fig. 6.1, artist figure showing frame rate). M-mode frame rates are typically around 1000–2000 frames/s, as compared to 2D imaging in which a typical frame rate is 40–80 frames/s [1]. For rapidly moving structures, such as valves, a few milliseconds may result in a meaningful change in position which can be reliably depicted by the high frame rate of m-mode.

The second advantage of m-mode is that the movements of cardiac structures over time are displayed in a single image. This contrasts with 2D imaging, in which the echocardiographer scrolls through a cine loop comprising multiple images to observe movement over time. Thus, m-mode is well suited for examining cardiac changes throughout the respiratory cycle, such as the collapse of the inferior vena cava.

To obtain an m-mode image on modern equipment, the echocardiographer starts with a 2D "scout" image. The echocardiographer then moves the cursor over the structures of interest and m-mode is initiated. Precise cursor place-

B. Burk (✉)
Renown Health, Reno, NV, USA

M. J. Lanspa, A. T. Levinson (eds.), *Echocardiography and Ultrasonography in the ICU*, Respiratory Medicine, https://doi.org/10.1007/978-3-031-80038-2_6

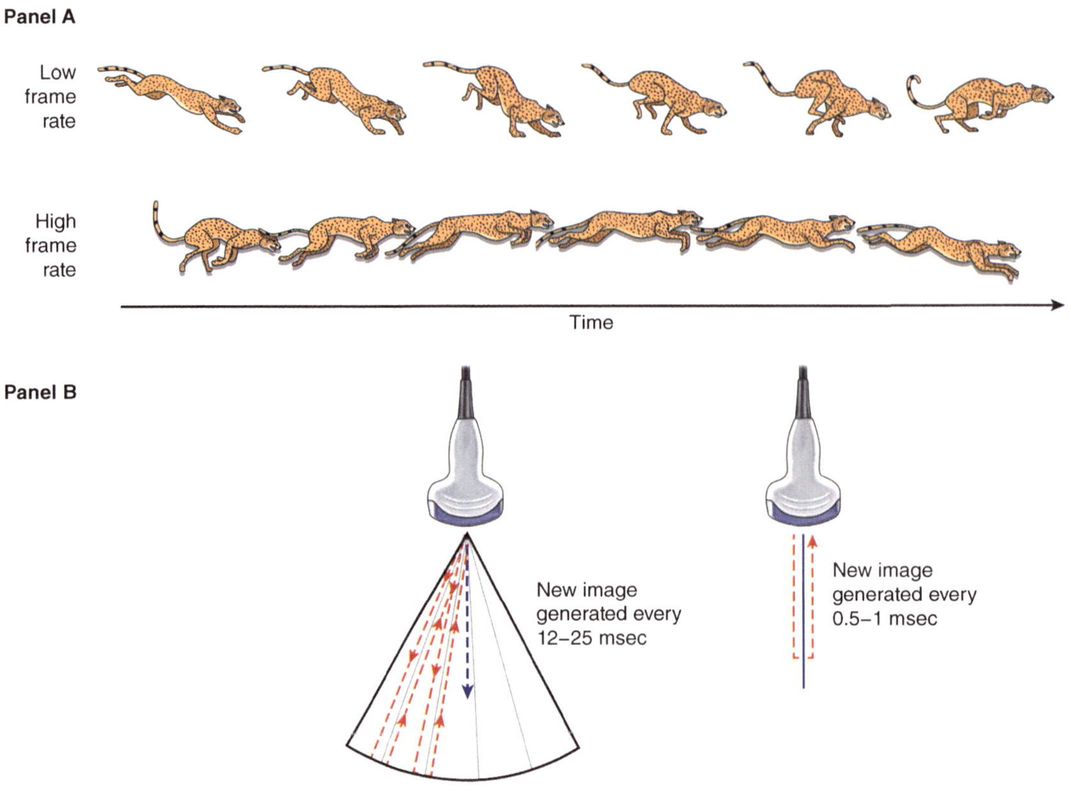

Fig. 6.1 Temporal resolution. Frame rate is the number of images displayed per second. A low frame rate (panel **a**, top row) results in a choppy video with poor temporal resolution. A high frame rate (panel **a**, bottom row) results in a smooth video that clearly shows cardiac movement over time. A single frame is generated once ultrasound waves have been emitted and received for each scan line, so the number of scan lines and frame rate are inversely proportional. 2D imaging has many scan lines, so the frame rate is lower while m-mode has a single scan line, so the frame rate is higher (panel **b**)

ment is critical. If the cursor is placed incorrectly, measurements made using m-mode tracings are inaccurate. Once m-mode is initiated, the display of depth vs. time is generated. The display is frozen and analyzed once the movements of interest have been captured.

One limitation of m-mode is that the m-mode scan line is parallel to the angle of insonation, which does not necessarily align with the cardiac structures of interest. "Anatomic m-mode" is a digital postprocessing technique that eliminates this problem by allowing an m-mode cursor to be oriented in any direction [2]. However, because anatomic m-mode relies on 2D images, it also eliminates the main benefit of m-mode, which is high temporal resolution (Box 6.1).

Box 6.1 Benefits of M-Mode

1. High temporal resolution. M-mode is ideal for assessing rapidly moving structures.
2. Shows depth vs. time on a single image. Observations can be made about cardiac changes throughout the respiratory cycle without cycling through a cine loop.

Color Doppler can be overlayed onto m-mode to create "color m-mode." Color m-mode has various applications, but it can be particularly helpful in identifying the precise time that a valve opens or closes. Therefore, color m-mode can be used to calculate time intervals such as isovolumic relaxation or contraction time.

The benefits of m-mode, described above, make it an advantageous mode for specific applications, which will be described below. See Box 6.2 for a list of m-mode parameters used in a comprehensive TTE and in specific clinical situations.

Box 6.2 M-Mode Uses

1. For a comprehensive TTE: Aortic and mitral valve in PLAX, TAPSE, IVC with respiratory variation.
2. Specific situations:
   (a) LV-FS, EPSS, and MAPSE: Use as an adjunct for the LV systolic function with difficult windows.
   (b) RVOT-FS: Use as an adjunct for the RV systolic function with difficult windows.
   (c) Velocity of propagation (V_p): Use when a (relatively) load-independent metric of the diastolic function is needed.
   (d) MV in PLAX looking for SAM: Assess if there is clinical concern for outflow obstruction.
   (e) RV cavity diastolic collapse: Use when there is pericardial fluid and clinical concern for tamponade.

M-Mode Echocardiography

Left Ventricular (LV) Function

The assessment of LV systolic function is one of the most common reasons to perform echocardiography. Suboptimal imaging is extremely common in the critically ill due to factors such as difficult patient positioning, patient inability to cooperate, and medical devices that interrupt access to the chest. Frequently, a complete echocardiogram and assessment of LV function are impossible. If only limited views are available, m-mode may be used to supplement the evaluation of the LV function. M-mode-derived parameters, including LV fractional shortening, E-point septal separation, and the mitral annular plane systolic excursion (MAPSE), all correlate with the LV ejection fraction.

Diastolic LV function, or the filling of the left ventricle, is a complex phenomenon. Active and passive LV relaxation as well as left atrial pressure dictate how the LV fills. One limitation of current echocardiographic diastolic function guidelines [3] is that many patients are deemed to have "indeterminate diastolic function." Additional echocardiogram parameters can be used to supplement the understanding of diastolic function in those indeterminate cases. One of these parameters is the propagation velocity (V_p), which is acquired using color m-mode through the mitral valve. V_p describes how rapidly blood flow propagates from the mitral valve to the LV apex and is thought to be relatively load independent. This means that it primarily describes the relaxation of the ventricle independent of preload and afterload [4]. Multiple methods have been described for acquiring V_p and studies have correlated it with various diastology metrics. One proposed "normal" cutoff is 45 m/s, with values below that velocity representing an abnormal diastolic function [5] (Fig. 6.2 showing V_p measurement).

Right Ventricular (RV) Systolic Function

Unlike the bullet-shaped LV, the RV is not a typical geometric structure. This makes quantification of RV systolic function more difficult. Tricuspid annular plane systolic excursion (TAPSE) is a commonly used and quantifiable metric of RV function [6]. TAPSE uses m-mode to assess the vertical motion of the lateral tricuspid annulus and provides information about the function of longitudinal RV myocardiocytes. Right ventricular outflow tract fractional shortening (RVOT FS), which is measured using m-mode in either the parasternal long- or short-axis, is an emerging metric to evaluate RV systolic function. RVOT FS correlates well with the RV function when compared to cardiac MR images [7] (Fig. 6.3 showing TAPSE and RVOT FS).

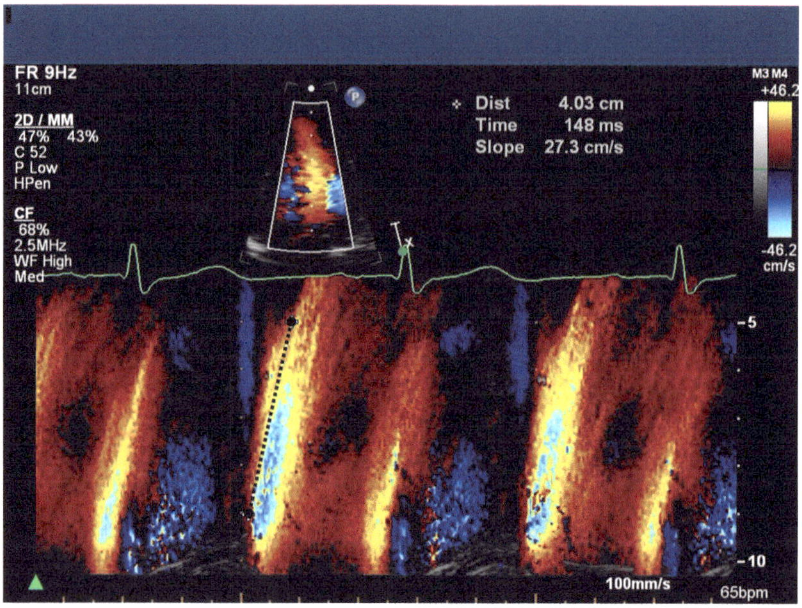

Fig. 6.2 Velocity of propagation (V_p). Color m-mode is obtained through the mitral valve from an apical four-chamber view. The Nyquist limit is set at 75% of the E velocity, the sweep speed is typically set at 100 mm/s, and the V_p slope is measured at the aliasing velocity (black dotted line)

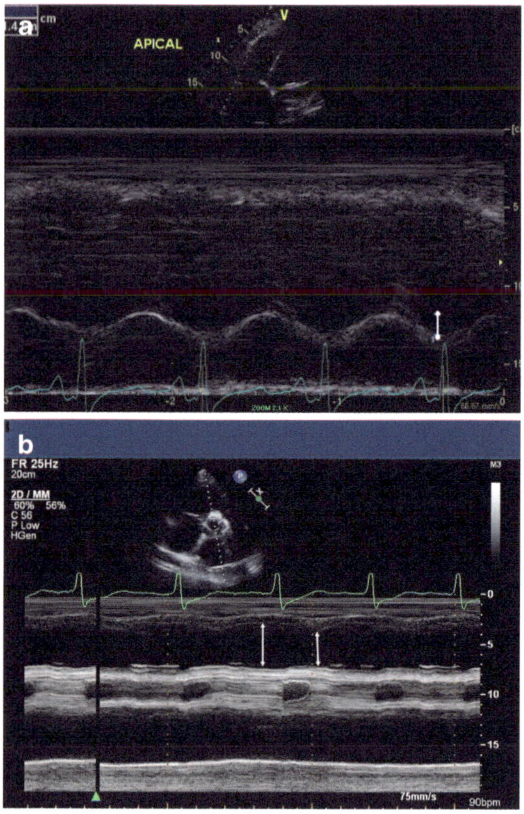

Fig. 6.3 M-mode indicators of the right heart function. TAPSE uses m-mode to show the vertical displacement of the lateral tricuspid annulus. A value of 17 mm or greater is normal. Panel (**a**) shows a reduced TAPSE suggesting reduced RV function. Panel (**b**) shows the measurements for RVOT fractional shortening in a patient with severe pulmonary hypertension. This m-mode tracing was obtained from the PLAX and the RV internal diameters are measured at the end systole and end diastole (white arrows)

Cardiac Valves

Until the advent of 2D and Doppler echocardiography, m-mode was relied on for the assessment of valvular function [8]. In the modern era, 2D and Doppler echocardiography have largely replaced m-mode for the evaluation of cardiac valves. However, the recognition of normal m-mode patterns allows the echocardiographer to notice when an abnormal pattern is present. This can alert them to the need for a more detailed valve assessment.

M-mode is commonly performed on the aortic and mitral valves in the parasternal long-axis. When it is visualized well, m-mode may also be performed on the pulmonic valve in the parasternal short or long axis. Tricuspid valve m-mode is uncommon.

To perform m-mode of the mitral valve, the echocardiographer places the m-mode cursor through the mitral valve in a parasternal long-axis view. Alternatively, one may utilize the parasternal short-axis at the mitral valve level, or the "fish mouth" view. Ideally, the m-mode cursor traverses both the anterior and posterior leaflets of the mitral valve. When normal sinus rhythm is present, the E and A waves are identified by the anterior motion of the anterior mitral valve leaflet. These represent the opening of the valve leaflet during early diastolic filling (E) and the atrial kick (A). There may be a flat space between the E and A waves, which represents diastasis, the mid-portion of diastole during which mitral flow is diminished or absent. During systole, the mitral valve remains passive or moves slightly anteriorly due to ventricular movement (Fig. 6.4 showing normal m-mode and m-mode with mitral stenosis).

Aortic valve m-mode is also obtained from the parasternal long-axis view. The right coronary cusp is seen anteriorly and either the left or the noncoronary cusp are seen posteriorly. The sonographer places the m-mode cursor through both visualized leaflets and m-mode is activated. Coaptation of the valve leaflets is seen during diastole and during systole the aortic valve leaflets open creating the appearance of rectangles on a string (Fig. 6.5 shows a normal AoV m-mode). Abnormal coaptation and opening are indicators of valvular dysfunction and should prompt additional evaluation of the valve.

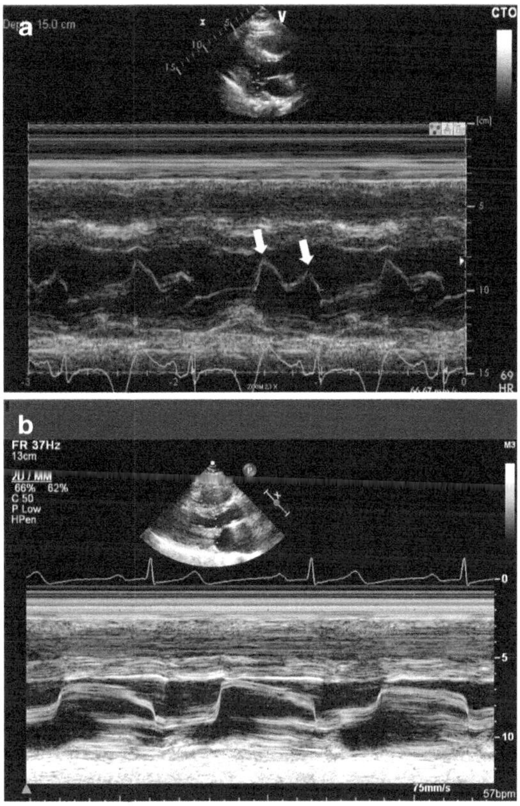

Fig. 6.4 Mitral valve m-mode. Panel (**a**) shows a normal E and A wave (white arrows). Panel (**b**) shows the m-mode appearance of severe mitral stenosis. If abnormalities are noted, such as thickened valves or perturbations in the normal E and A pattern, the valve should be evaluated more fully

The pulmonic valve is more difficult to see on transthoracic echo. If windows allow for it, the pulmonic valve may be seen either in the parasternal long or short axis. From a standard parasternal long axis, tilt the probe so that the ultrasound beam aims more cranially and to the patient's left, which allows visualization of the pulmonic valve and main pulmonary artery. From the parasternal short axis at the level of the aortic valve, the pulmonic valve may be seen in the 2 o'clock position. Small probe adjustments are often required from this view to optimize the visualization of the pulmonic valve. In a normal heart, the right atrial contraction causes a rise in

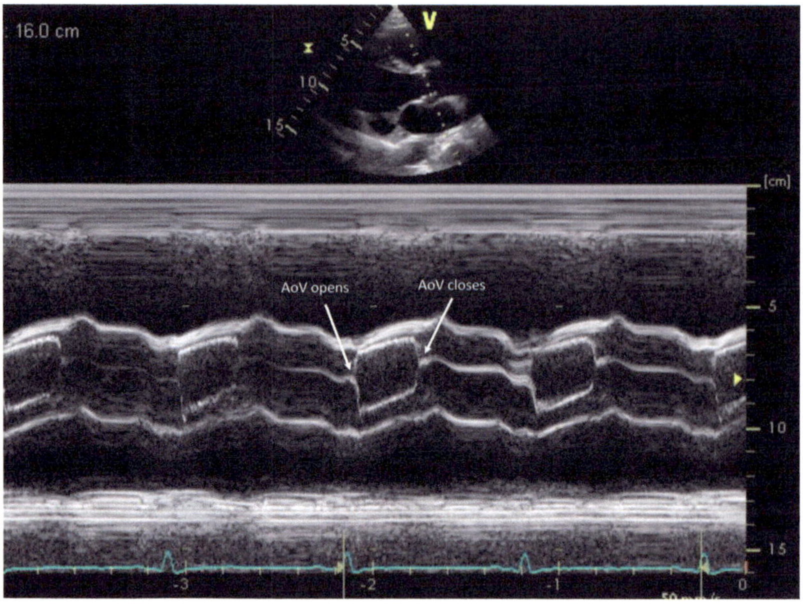

Fig. 6.5 Normal m-mode through the aortic valve with the appearance of rectangles (valve open) on a string (valve closed). Note the thin leaflets that open and close quickly. Thickened leaflets or abnormalities in opening or closing suggest the need for further investigation of the valve

right ventricular pressure resulting in a small posterior displacement of the pulmonic valve (A), followed by a larger posterior movement that represents valve opening. This typical pattern may be disrupted in abnormal physiologic states, such as pulmonary hypertension or pulmonic stenosis.

Outflow Obstruction

Outflow obstruction is a relatively frequent occurrence in the critically ill. Improper management can lead to profound shock and death. Thus, identification with echocardiography is essential. In the latter stages of outflow obstruction, high-velocity flow in the left ventricular outflow tract causes a Bernoulli effect that pulls open the anterior mitral leaflet during systole. This mitral opening further obstructs blood flow in the outflow tract and results in significant mitral regurgitation. This phenomenon is termed "systolic anterior motion of the mitral valve," or SAM. Mitral valve motion is very rapid and these patients are typically tachycardic, so SAM is difficult to identify with the unaided human eye watching a 2D cine loop. M-mode can be essential in identifying SAM because of its high temporal resolution. As compared to the usual mitral valve m-mode tracing, when SAM is present, anterior movement of the mitral valve is seen during systole in addition to the E and A waves (Fig. 6.6).

Pericardial Tamponade

Pericardial tamponade occurs when pressure in the pericardium exceeds pressure in the right heart, causing the right heart chambers to collapse during filling. This impaired filling results in poor cardiac output. RV collapse is seen on the echocardiogram during the latter stages of tamponade. The RV appropriately moves inward during systole due to contraction, therefore it can be difficult to differentiate this appropriate contraction from an inappropriate diastolic collapse when viewing a 2D cine loop. M-mode shows the timing of ventricular inward movement during the cardiac cycle (Fig. 6.7 showing RV collapse in diastole). M-mode images through the pericardial effusion and RV may be obtained from either the parasternal long axis, parasternal short axis, or the subcostal four-chamber view with the m-mode cursor perpendicular to the long axis of the RV.

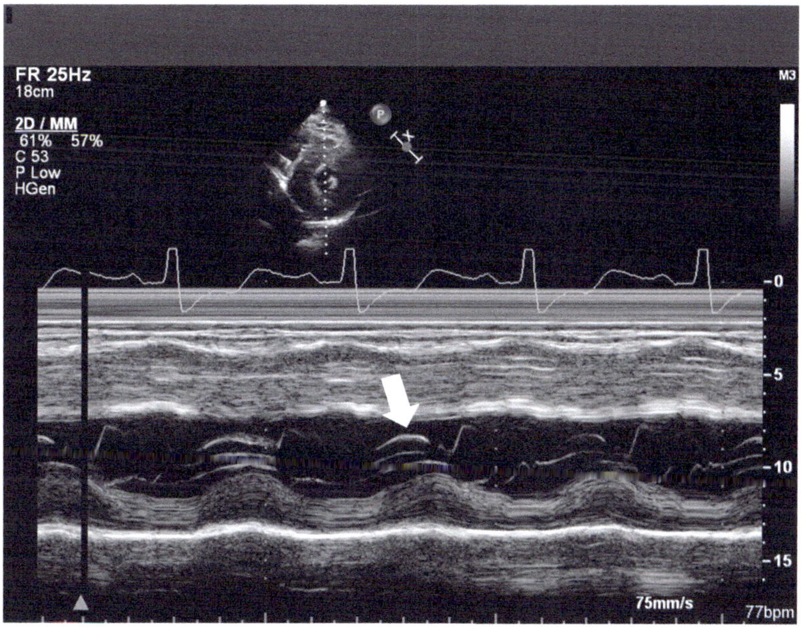

Fig. 6.6 Systolic anterior motion of the mitral valve (SAM, white arrow) due to hypertrophic cardiomyopathy. Compare this to the normal mitral valve movement in Fig. 6.4, panel (**a**)

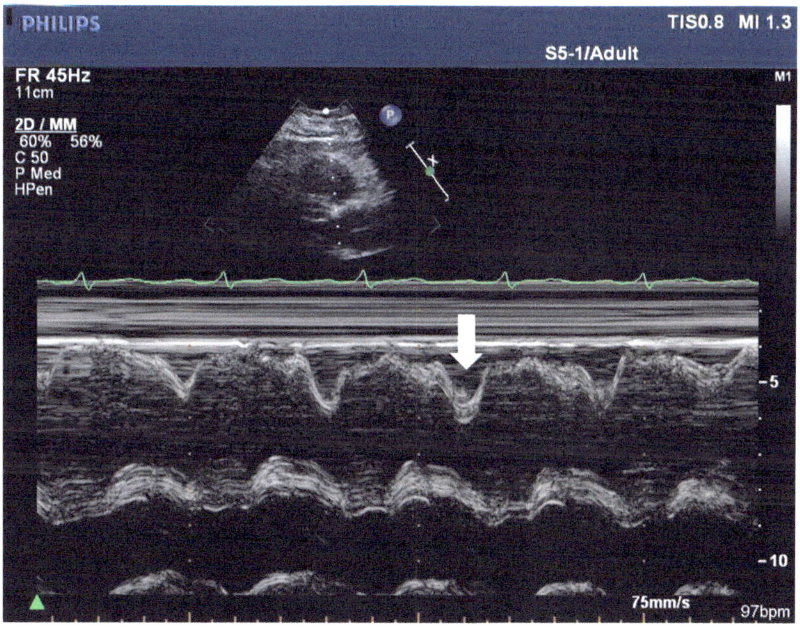

Fig. 6.7 RV-free wall collapse (white arrow) during diastole due to tamponade. This image was obtained in the parasternal long axis, but a parasternal short axis or a subcostal view may also be used

Inferior Vena Cava (IVC) Collapsibility

Analysis of the IVC is a common application of point-of-care echocardiography in the critically ill. In the appropriate clinical context, fluid responsiveness may be predicted by vena cava collapse. RA pressure can be estimated using a combination of the IVC size and collapsibility [9]. Respirophasic variation in IVC diameter can be assessed using m-mode either in the IVC long axis or short axis. One drawback of the long-axis view is that during inhalation, the movement of the diaphragm may cause the IVC to move out of the plane of the ultrasound beam, thus invalidating measurements

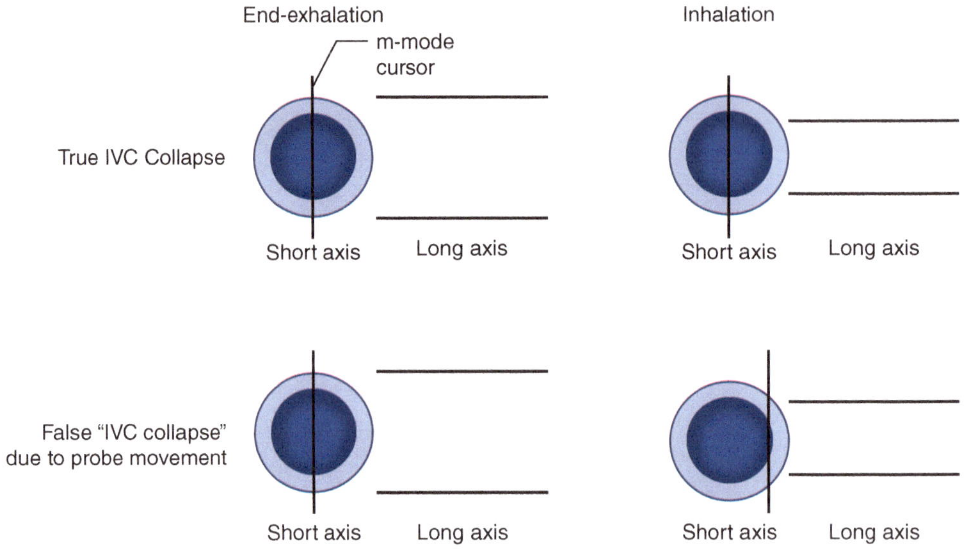

Fig. 6.8 True IVC collapse versus the false appearance of IVC collapse in the long axis due to lateral probe movement during inhalation. This problem can be solved using the short axis as the scout view so the sonographer can ensure the m-mode cursor stays in the middle of the vessel

(Fig. 6.8). This problem may be overcome by switching to a short-axis view of the vena cava. The m-mode cursor is seen traversing the center of the IVC in the scout image, so the sonographer can ensure that respiratory movement does not affect the position of the ultrasound beam in the IVC.

In the long-axis view, the echocardiographer places the m-mode cursor just upstream of the hepatic vein junction with the IVC. Care must be taken to ensure that the m-mode cursor is as perpendicular to the long axis of the IVC as possible. In the short-axis view, a similar location should be selected, although it can be more challenging to identify the hepatic inflow in the short axis. Ideally, a respirometer tracing is used to identify inspiration, but this is often not possible in the point-of-care setting. The m-mode tracing should be frozen and captured once a full respiratory cycle has occurred. The expiratory diameter is measured at end-exhalation. There is no consensus on when to measure during inhalation, but the smallest diameter during the inhale is frequently used.

Summary Points

- M-mode has two major advantages over 2D imaging: (1) high temporal resolution and (2) the ability to show cardiac movement over the respiratory cycle.
- These benefits put m-mode at an advantage in specific clinical situations to show fast-moving and respirophasic phenomena.
- While 2D imaging is the workhorse of echocardiography, m-mode is still a key tool that the echocardiographer must be familiar with.

References

1. Armstrong WF, Ryan T. Feigenbaum's echocardiography. 8th ed. Philadelphia: Wolters Kluwer; 2019.
2. Carerj S, Micari A, Trono A, Giordano G, Cerrito M, Zito C, et al. Anatomical M-mode: an old-new technique. Echocardiography. 2003;20(4):357–61.
3. Nagueh SF, Smiseth OA, Appleton CP, Byrd BF 3rd, Dokainish H, Edvardsen T, et al. Recommendations for the evaluation of left ventricular diastolic function by echocardiography: an update from the American Society of Echocardiography and the European Association of Cardiovascular Imaging. J Am Soc Echocardiogr. 2016;29(4):277–314.
4. Garcia MJ, Smedira NG, Greenberg NL, Main M, Firstenberg MS, Odabashian J, et al. Color M-mode Doppler flow propagation velocity is a preload insensitive index of left ventricular relaxation: animal and human validation. J Am Coll Cardiol. 2000;35(1):201–8.

5. De Boeck BW, Oh JK, Vandervoort PM, Vierendeels JA, van der Aa RP, Cramer MJ. Colour M-mode velocity propagation: a glance at intra-ventricular pressure gradients and early diastolic ventricular performance. Eur J Heart Fail. 2005;7(1):19–28.
6. Kaul S, Tei C, Hopkins JM, Shah PM. Assessment of right ventricular function using two-dimensional echocardiography. Am Heart J. 1984;107(3):526–31.
7. Srinivasan A, Kim J, Khalique O, Geevarghese A, Rusli M, Shah T, et al. Echocardiographic linear fractional shortening for quantification of right ventricular systolic function—a cardiac magnetic resonance validation study. Echocardiography. 2017;34(3):348–58.
8. Chang S. M-mode echocardiographic techniques and pattern recognition. London: Lea & Febiger; 1976.
9. Rudski LG, Lai WW, Afilalo J, Hua L, Handschumacher MD, Chandrasekaran K, et al. Guidelines for the echocardiographic assessment of the right heart in adults: a report from the American Society of Echocardiography endorsed by the European Association of Echocardiography, a registered branch of the European Society of Cardiology, and the Canadian Society of Echocardiography. J Am Soc Echocardiogr. 2010;23(7):685–713; quiz 86–8.

7 Transthoracic Doppler Echocardiography

Enyo Ablordeppey and Aaron Murphy-Crews

Learning Objectives

1. Understand the basic principles of Doppler ultrasound.
2. Be able to optimize the acquisition of Doppler images and measurements.
3. Become familiar with specific Doppler applications, indications, and clinical relevance.
4. Optimizing spectral and color Doppler by minimizing aliasing and adjusting the pulse repetition frequency.
5. Understand Doppler measurements from the LV inflow (mitral valve) and LV outflow (aortic valve).
6. Understand Doppler measurements from the RV inflow (tricuspid valve) and RV outflow (pulmonic valve).
7. Understand venous flow patterns from the pulmonary and hepatic veins.
8. Be able to describe color Doppler for valvular regurgitation and stenosis.

Doppler is an essential tool for the echocardiographer looking to expand their skill set beyond basic views and interpretation. Color, pulse wave, and continuous wave Doppler allows for the visualization and measurement of blood flow through the heart, thereby unlocking the ability to assess valvular abnormalities, noninvasive measurement of pulmonary arterial pressure, diastolic functioning, stroke volume, and much more. In this chapter, we will discuss techniques for optimizing the use of Doppler tools and provide an overview of individual clinical applications of Doppler during a focused echocardiography. Artifacts and pathology associated with Doppler will be discussed in separate chapters.

General Approach

The convention for a comprehensive TTE is to apply Doppler modality over each valve in the same order, starting with color, then pulse wave, continuous wave, and lastly tissue Doppler. This approach is efficient for the sonographer as it obtains all the relevant data at each view for an economy of scanning. However, bedside clinicians are typically more focused on simultaneously obtaining and interpreting views to answer focused and immediate clinical questions. Thus, we have organized the material in this chapter around specific clinical questions rather than a comprehensive anatomical approach. An overview of clinical questions and related Doppler applications can be found in Table 7.1. At the end of this chapter, the reader will have a framework

E. Ablordeppey (✉)
Emergency Medicine, Washington University School of Medicine, St. Louis, MO, USA
e-mail: ablordeppeye@wustl.edu

A. Murphy-Crews
Division of Critical Care Medicine, Department of Anesthesiology, Washington University School of Medicine, St. Louis, MO, USA

M. J. Lanspa, A. T. Levinson (eds.), *Echocardiography and Ultrasonography in the ICU*, Respiratory Medicine, https://doi.org/10.1007/978-3-031-80038-2_7

Table 7.1 Clinical questions and related doppler applications

Clinical assessment	Doppler applications
Cardiac output	LVOT VTI (PW Doppler)
Fluid responsiveness	Variability in SV via LVOT VTI in response to respiratory cycle or fluid bolus/passive leg raise
Focused RV assessment	TR max for PASP (CW Doppler)
	PAAT (PW Doppler)
	RV S′ for RV function (TDI)
LV diastolic function	MV e/a (PW Doppler)
	Septal and lateral e′ (TDI)
	Pulmonary vein (PW Doppler)

for moving toward a more comprehensive skill set with Doppler applications that can be easily tailored to focused exams when indicated.

Principles of Doppler Echocardiography

The use of Doppler echocardiography relies on the Doppler effect, which is the principle that waves will change in frequency when an observer is moving relative to the wave source. You have experienced the Doppler effect, perhaps without realizing it. Imagine standing on a street as an ambulance passes you. As the ambulance approaches, the siren has a higher pitch (frequency), which changes to a lower pitch as it heads away. Similarly, ultrasound waves emitted by the probe change speed when they encounter blood cells or tissue and are reflected at higher or lower speeds as a result, which can be measured by the ultrasound machine. The relationship between frequency and velocity is quantified in the **Doppler shift equation** (Fig. 7.1)

There are multiple types of Doppler ultrasound that vary in their function and application (Fig. 7.2).

Color Doppler displays the mean velocities of blood flow by visual color. Traditionally, blood moving toward the probe is in the red spectrum, and blood moving away from the probe is in the blue spectrum. Faster velocities of flow are brighter shades of red or blue.

Spectral Doppler plots velocity on the Y-axis relative to time on the X-axis. Spectral Doppler includes three subtypes.

a $$\Delta f = 2\frac{v}{c} f_0 \cos\theta$$

b $$v = \frac{\Delta f * c}{2f \ \cos\theta}$$

Fig. 7.1 Doppler shift equation (**a**), which can be rearranged to calculate blood velocity (**b**). The Doppler shift is a change in frequency (Δf) calculated from the speed of blood (v), the speed of ultrasound waves through the tissue (c), the original US frequency (f_0), and the cosign of the angle ($\cos\theta$) between the direction of blood flow and the ultrasound probe

Pulse wave Doppler (PWD): The ultrasound alternates between sending and receiving pulses, which allows the machine to measure the velocity of blood at a precise location that is controlled by moving the gate. This precision of location, known as *range specificity*, comes at the cost of limiting the frequencies that can be measured.

Continuous wave Doppler (CWD): The ultrasound is continuously sending and receiving signals, which removes the limit to measurable frequency but lacks range specificity.

Tissue Doppler imaging (TDI): Similar to PWD, but with a filter to remove high-frequency signals (typically blood moving fast) to focus on the slower movement of cardiac tissues.

Power Doppler averages the amplitude of flow for more sensitive detection of flow. It does not measure the direction of flow.

Information obtained with Doppler about the speed of blood in the heart can reveal a tremendous amount of relevant clinical data in both

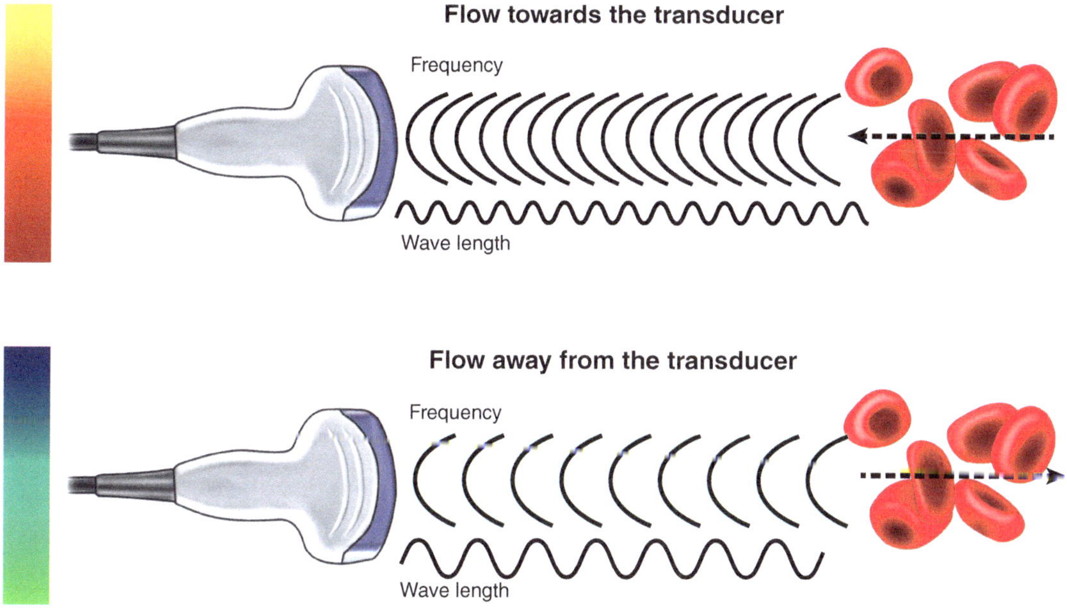

Fig. 7.2 Frequency and wavelength, inverse relationship relative to the observer

static and dynamic assessments. This information is highly dependent, however, on the quality of our images and measurements. There are functionally two major contributors to image quality: those relating to the physics of image acquisition and those relating to machine processing power. In the next section, we will address strategies to optimize our Doppler images.

Optimization of Spectral Doppler

Window Selection and Probe Positioning

Note that the Doppler shift (see Fig. 7.1) is dependent on the angle between the moving object and the receiver. The accuracy of speed measurements via the Doppler effect will be best when the movement is directly parallel to the beam. As the angle becomes more oblique, the accuracy drops off steeply. For example, at an angle of 20°, there is only a 6% difference between the measured and actual speed. At 60°, the measurement is off by 50%. Thus, window selection and optimal Doppler interrogation are essential in Doppler echocardiography to obtain accurate results. For this reason, many measurements are best obtained through specific windows in order to align the probe as parallel to the direction of blood flow as possible.

Spectral Broadening

When measuring laminar blood flow with PWD, the blood cells move with relatively uniform velocities, thus the spectral envelope should appear narrow with a clear window underneath. The loss of this clear window is referred to as spectral broadening (Fig. 7.3). Spectral broadening can be secondary to user technique as well, such as with unnecessarily high gain, wide PWD, or misplacement of the gate along the edge of a structure where nonlaminar flow is expected. This is commonly seen when attempting measurements with challenging windows, and the presence of spectral broadening can be useful feedback to the sonographer that the acquisition should be optimized if possible, or if not, that the measurements may be of limited quality. Of note, even with optimal technique, spectral broadening may be seen as an indicator of nonlaminar flow in cases of valvular stenosis.

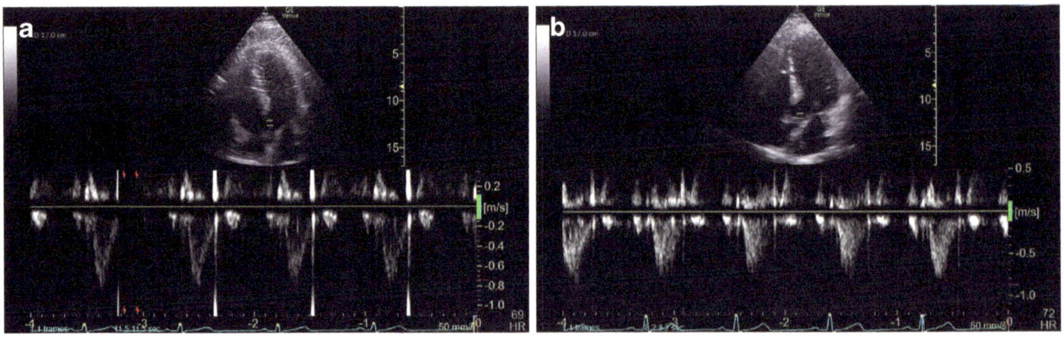

Fig. 7.3 Pulse wave Doppler velocities with and without spectral broadening. (**a**) Shows the ideal without spectral broadening. Image in (**b**) has spectral broadening, which can affect velocity accuracy

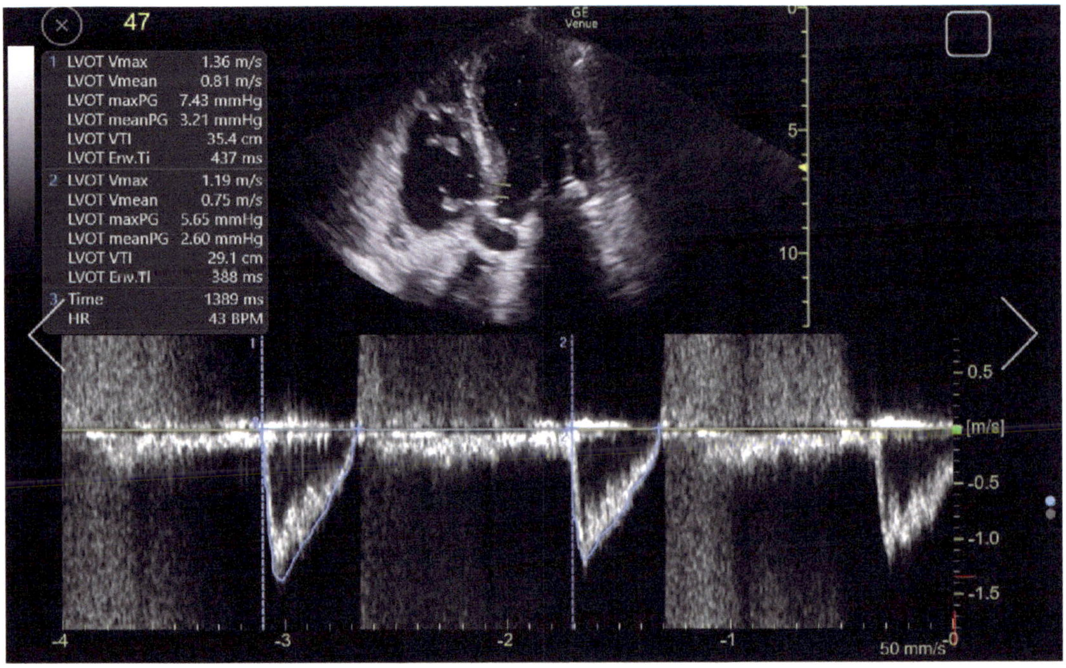

Fig. 7.4 Aliasing occurs when Doppler shift exceeds the Nyquist limit. In this example, high-velocity aortic regurgitation (which should only be seen above the baseline) appears coming from the bottom of the plot. When using PWD and Doppler shift exceeds the Nyquist limit, aliasing will occur. Aortic insufficiency velocity seen above the baseline is "wrapping around" and coming from the opposite direction toward the baseline

Aliasing (PRF and Nyquist Limit)

Range specificity is a significant advantage of PW Doppler modalities, allowing for the measurement of blood flow at a precise intracardiac location. The disadvantage of this is a limitation in the frequencies that can be measured. In PW mode, transducers alternate between transmitting and receiving pulses, which puts a limit on the maximum Doppler shift that can be measured. This limit is known as the **Nyquist limit** and is a function of the pulse repetition frequency (PRF) and is depicted in the following equation, Nyquist limit = PRF/2. When the Doppler shift exceeds the Nyquist limit, aliasing will occur (see Fig. 7.4). In PWD, aliasing presents as a spectral signal "wrapping around" and coming from the opposite direction toward the baseline. There are a few strategies to remove aliasing when present.

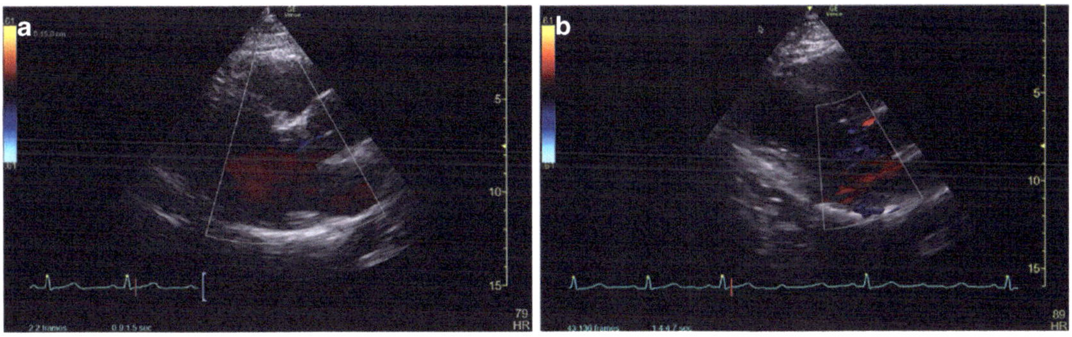

Fig. 7.5 Parasternal long-axis view with color Doppler to look for mitral and aortic valvopathies. Note that the color box in (**a**) is unnecessarily large, which will require more machine processing and lower resolution than (**b**)

The sonographer can lower the baseline (though this is for appearances only and does not change the characteristics of the signal), increase the scale (if not already maximal), or find a view with a shallower sample volume. Lastly, changing the Doppler mode to CWD will eliminate aliasing and allow for the measurement of unlimited Doppler shift; however, the range specificity of PWD will be lost.

Pulse Repetition Frequency

The PRF is the number of pulses that are sent and received in 1 s. The temporal resolution is improved as a function of the pulse repetition frequency. Given that the speed of the sound in the medium cannot be controlled, the PRF is dependent on how far the pulses have to travel, i.e., the depth of the gate. Using the appropriate window and setting the gate as shallow as possible will maximize the PRF.

Optimization of Color Doppler (Frame Rate and Zoom)

Color Doppler is based on the principles of PWD and is therefore subject to similar constraints relating to aliasing and dependence of angle of incidence. Recall from Chap. 1 that color wave Doppler is created by a series of scan lines, each with multiple pulse gates, the data being overlayed with color to show the direction and speed of moving blood. With color Doppler, aliasing will appear as a shift in color from red to blue (or vice versa) when the velocities exceed the Nyquist limit. The quality and utility of visual images created with color Doppler is dependent on the frame rate, which is a function of how many frames or images can be produced by the ultrasound machine, measured in frames per second (FPS). The frame rate for color Doppler is dependent on the pulse repetition frequency, the number of scan lines, and the number of pulses per scan line. The PRF is a function of the depth of the color sector, once again highlighting the importance of selecting an appropriate depth for the area of interest. The scan lines and pulses per scan line are a function of the size of the color sector. The larger the sector (color box), the lower the frame rate and detail. In general, it is best to limit the size of the color sector as small as possible while covering the necessary area of interest (see Fig. 7.5).

Pro-tip
In general, color sectors should be as small as possible to optimize temporal resolution.

Now that we have discussed tactics to optimize image acquisition, let us turn our discussion to specific applications of Doppler echocardiography.

Clinical Applications for Doppler Echocardiography

LV Outflow/Inflow

LV Outflow Tract Velocity Time Integral (LVOT VTI)

TTE can be used to quantitatively assess stroke volume and cardiac output by measuring the integral of the velocity through the LVOT over time (Fig. 7.6).

To measure the velocity of blood in the left ventricular outflow tract (LVOT), we start in the apical five- or three-chamber view with PWD. Optimize the depth and sector width to provide the best resolution for the LVOT. Align the PWD gate in the LVOT on the ventricle side of the aortic valve. It is important to keep the Doppler beam as parallel to the LVOT as possible for accurate measurements. Of note, some machines have an option for angle correction on Doppler; however, this should be avoided, and better imaging alignment should be attempted instead. With settings optimized, activate the PWD to record the velocity over time. Note that we are interested in the speed of blood flow through the LVOT (away from the probe), so the area of interest will be below the baseline. Move the baseline up to provide maximum room to see the data of interest. The flow velocity is measured over time and called the velocity-time integral (VTI; Fig. 7.4 demonstrates a VTI with tracing). In a laminar flow state, the column of blood moving through the LVOT should be moving at the same speed, thus the tracing should have a well-defined and tightly grouped line with no spectral broadening. Deviations from this may suggest interference from poor image quality or gate positions, or nonlaminar flow, such as in the case of dynamic outflow obstruction.

$$Stroke\ Volume = \pi * \left(\frac{LVOT\ diameter}{2}\right)^2 * LVOT\ VTI$$

Fig. 7.6 Stroke volume calculated by measuring an LVOT VTI and the LVOT diameter. For a shortcut, the average LVOT is 2 cm, so SV ≈ π * LVOT VTI. Cardiac output is the product of SV*HR

> **Pro-tip**
> The VTI is affected by the angle of the probe. When doing serial measurements, it is important to keep the probe angle consistent.

Compared to estimates of ejection fraction, CO is often a more directly relevant clinical variable to the intensivist and is less susceptible to interpretation bias from tachycardia or mitral regurgitation. The VTI can also be used to assess volume responsiveness. Recall that volume responsiveness means that additional preload will lead to an increase in SV. By taking serial VTI measurements before and after a passive leg raise or fluid bolus, changes in SV can be directly measured. In addition, respirophasic variability in LVOT VTI morphology can also be used as a surrogate for fluid responsiveness. A temporary increase in stroke volume with increased venous return from spontaneous inspiration (or during exhalation in the mechanically ventilated patient) may signal that a patient will be responsive to volume. It is important to note that VTI measurement of CO does require sinus rhythm, as beat-beat variability will make the generalization of any given measurement unreliable.

> **Pro-tip**
> Sometimes respirophasic variability in VTI may be a reflection of cardiac translation or change in angle with breathing. If the heart is moving substantially with respiration, interpret VTI variation with caution.

LV Inflow for Diastolic Function

Diastolic function is the ability of the heart to recoil and relax to receive blood in preparation for ventricular systole. One modality for assessing diastolic dysfunction is based on patterns in the velocity of blood flowing from the left atrium to the left ventricle during early and late diastole. To obtain LV inflow velocities, start with the apical four-chamber view and place PWD with the gates in the ventricle at the tips of the mitral valve (MV) coaptation point. Color Doppler can be overlaid to visualize the path of blood flow and help optimize the angle for a more accurate measurement. Blood flowing into the ventricle will appear as peaks above the baseline as blood is flowing toward the direction of the probe. The first peak, known as the E-wave, is formed by early diastolic blood flow and is reflective of LV relaxation. This is followed by the A-wave, which is caused by additional blood flow into the ventricle from atrial contraction (if present). The relative speed of blood during early diastole versus during atrial contraction can be used to characterize a spectrum of impaired LV relaxation (see Chap. 15 on diastolic function). LV inflow is used in conjunction with LV tissue relaxation in many standard approaches to diastolic assessment.

MV E′, A′ and S′

The term prime (denoted " ′ ") is added to describe tissue movement velocity. In an A4C view, place PWD with activated tissue Doppler index (TDI) on the septal and lateral insertion of the mitral valve and record tissue velocities during early diastole and atrial contraction. The early and late diastolic waves are called e' and a' and are seen below the baseline (as the tissue is moving away from the probe during diastole) and correspond to LV relaxation and atrial contraction (see Fig. 7.7). Tissue movement of the LV during systole is represented in the S′ wave, which is seen above the baseline from the A4C view. MV S′ is a less commonly used tool to estimate LV systolic function. Due to the relatively good performance of TDI even with limited views, TDI can contribute to the assessment of both diastolic and systolic functioning in patients with relatively poor echo windows.

> **Pro-tip**
> Doppler imaging, including tissue Doppler, can often provide information when 2D image quality is limited.

RV Inflow/Outflow

TR Max for PASP

The modified Bernoulli equation (Fig. 7.8) allows us to calculate the pressure gradient across a valve by measuring the maximum velocity of regurgitant flow.

Fig. 7.7 Measuring velocities at the mitral annulus with tissue Doppler

Mitral annular dynamics and corresponding tissue Doppler echocardiogram spectral display

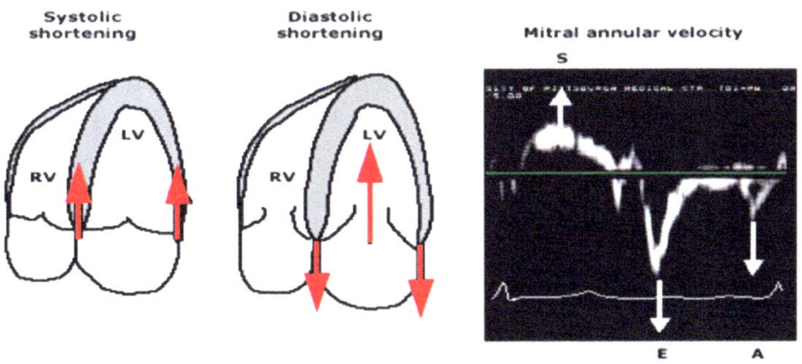

Panels A and B show the movement of the mitral annulus during systole and diastole; panel C shows the corresponding pulsed-tissue Doppler echocardiogram spectral display.

S: peak systolic velocity; E: peak early diastolic velocity; A: peak atrial velocity.

a

$$\Delta P = 4 * V_{max}^2$$

b

$$PASP = RVSP = 4 * TR_{max}^2 + RAP$$

Fig. 7.8 The modified Bernoulli equation (**a**) yields the pressure gradient (ΔP) across a valve as a function of maximal regurgitant velocity (V_{max}). This can be modified (**b**) to determine RVSP (which is assumed to equal PASP in the absence of PS) by measuring the maximal TR velocity and adding right atrial pressure (RAP)

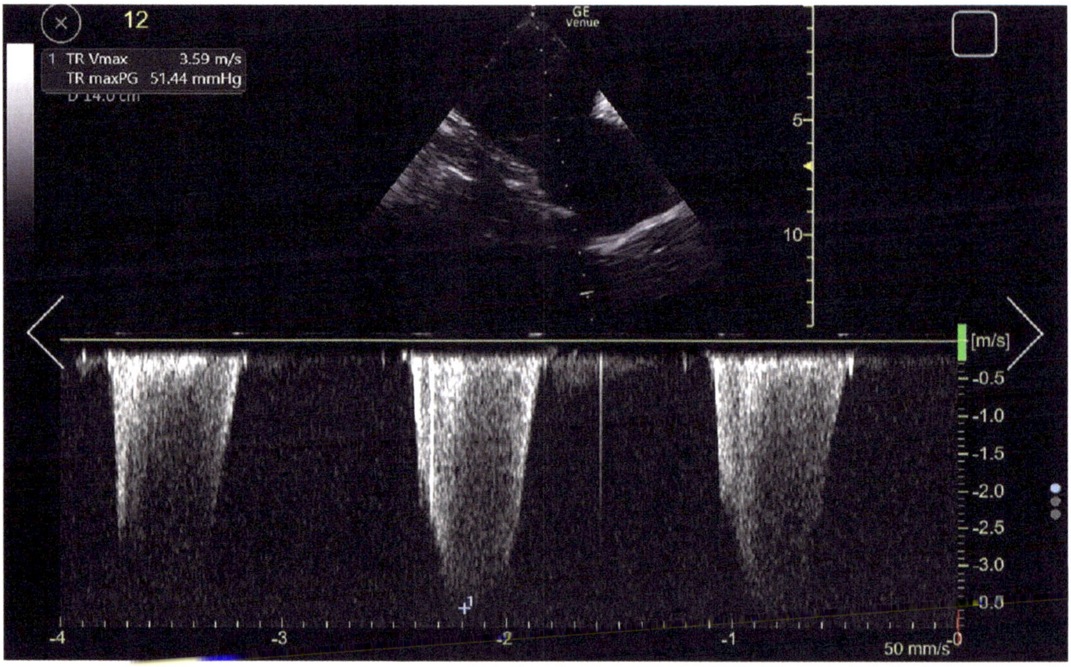

Fig. 7.9 CWD across the TV in RV inflow view with measurement of TRmax. The calculated pressure gradient, when added to the CVP (measured or estimated from IVC characteristics), will give an estimated PASP

The most useful application of this is estimating the pulmonary artery systolic pressure (PASP) using tricuspid regurgitation (TR). To determine if TR is present, place the color Doppler over the tricuspid valve in any view. A4C view often allows for the best Doppler alignment of the TR jet, though parasternal RV inflow or PSX basal views may also be used. Use continuous wave Doppler (CWD) over the most visible areas of high velocity through the tricuspid valve to capture flow away from the probe during ventricular systole. The maximum velocity (TR max) will give us the pressure gradient between the RV and RA. By adding the right atrial pressure (either from CVP tracing or an estimate based on IVC), we can estimate the right ventricular systolic pressure, which is a good surrogate for PASP in the absence of significant pulmonic stenosis (Fig. 7.9).

Pulmonary Artery Acceleration Time (PAAT)

Pulmonary artery acceleration time (PAAT) is the time it takes from the beginning of flow through the pulmonic valve to peak velocity. This time reflects the gradient pressure between the right ventricular outflow and the pulmonary artery. Short PAAT is seen when there is elevated pulmonary artery pressure. From the RVOT view or PSAX basal view, place the PWD gate proximal to the pulmonary valve in the RVOT (see

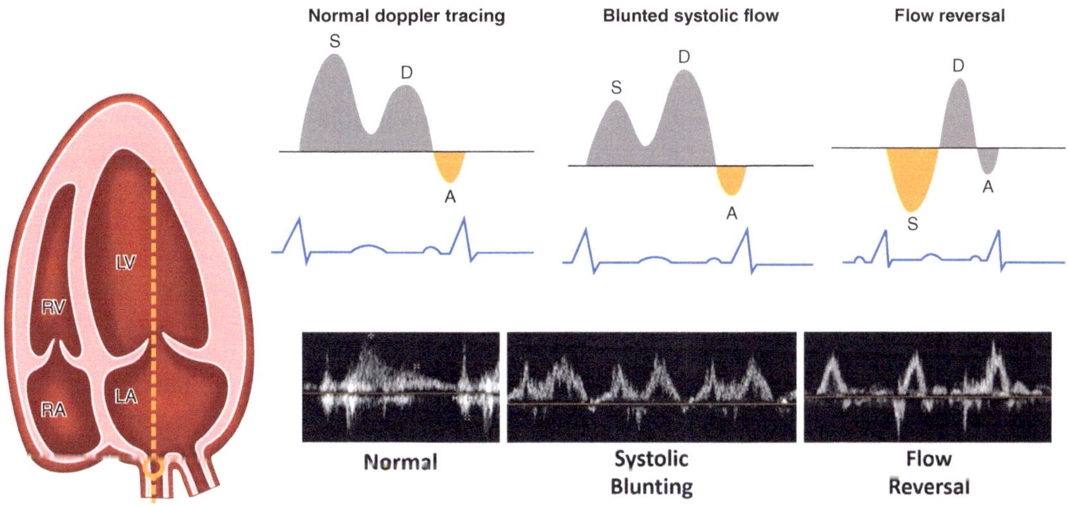

Fig. 7.10 PWD of pulmonary vein flow from normal evidence of high left atrial pressures

Fig. 7.10). The time from PV opening to peak velocity is correlated with PA pressure (see Chap. 55 on pulmonary embolism and acute cor pulmonale for more on this).

RV S′ for RV Systolic Function

Tissue Doppler can be used to measure the speed of the right ventricle during systole, which has been shown to correlate with RVEF and has very similar test characteristics to TAPSE (see Chap. 13 on RV assessment). To measure RV S′, obtain an A4C view and place the TD on the RV lateral wall at the junction of the lateral tricuspid annulus. The peak systolic velocity (above the baseline, as the ventricle moves toward the probe in an A4C during systole) is measured, with velocities >10 cm/s correlating with RVEF >50%.

Pulmonary Venous Flow (Diastolic Function)

Doppler measurements through the pulmonary veins allow an understanding of the speed of blood flow during diastole from the pulmonary veins into the left atrium. Normal flow has characteristic features, and abnormalities in flow patterns are present when there is impedance from the left atrium. PWD is used to characterize flow during early and late ventricular systole, when the left atrium is being filled. PWD placed in any of the pulmonary veins (at least 1 cm) with the best Doppler alignment will generate a waveform with three peaks. During ventricular systole, there are two systolic inflections referred to as S1 and S2. Frequently, these two peaks are fused and indistinguishable, then they are referred to as the S-wave. The first (S1) component denotes atrial relaxation (diastole) with suction of blood into the left atrium and is affected by LA pressure, contraction, and relaxation. The second (S2) component occurs when the mitral annulus is apically displaced with ventricular systole, decreasing left atrial pressure and creating a gradient for forward flow. The second group of deflections that occur during ventricular diastole is known as the D-wave. The downstroke of the D-wave will dip beyond the baseline, indicating flow away from the transducer, and is referred to as the AR wave (atrial reversal). This wave corresponds to atrial contraction and “reversal” of flow.

A progressive increase in left atrial pressure (from severe mitral regurgitation or diastolic dysfunction for example) will blunt the systolic flow velocities in the pulmonary veins, with the majority of forward flow increasingly occurring during diastole. The elevation in left ventricular end-diastolic pressure will exaggerate the flow reversal that occurs with atrial contraction, prolonging the AR wave. Normal filling patterns are predominantly systolic, with an S/D ratio > 1. A pathologic increase in mean left atrial pressure will reverse this pattern, resulting in an S/D ratio < 1 and a diastolic filling predominance. Atrial reversal velocity and duration abnormalities can also suggest elevated filling pressures, for example, AR peak velocity > 35 cm/s implies elevated left atrial pressures. Similarly, pulmonary venous AR should be similar in duration to the trans-mitral A-wave. Large discrepancies between the two suggest elevated filling pressures. It is, however, important to recall that in young or very healthy patients, pulmonary vein flow may have an appearance similar to elevated filling pressures because of the vigorous LV function that generated elevated peak D-wave velocities. There are some abnormal pulmonary vein flow patterns from benign etiology such as elevated S/D ratio and peak AR velocity with age and tachycardia. Whereas atrial fibrillation causes decreased peak S1 and AR velocity because of the lack of organized atrial contraction. See Fig. 7.11 for possible cardiac pathology seen in various abnormal pulmonary vein flows.

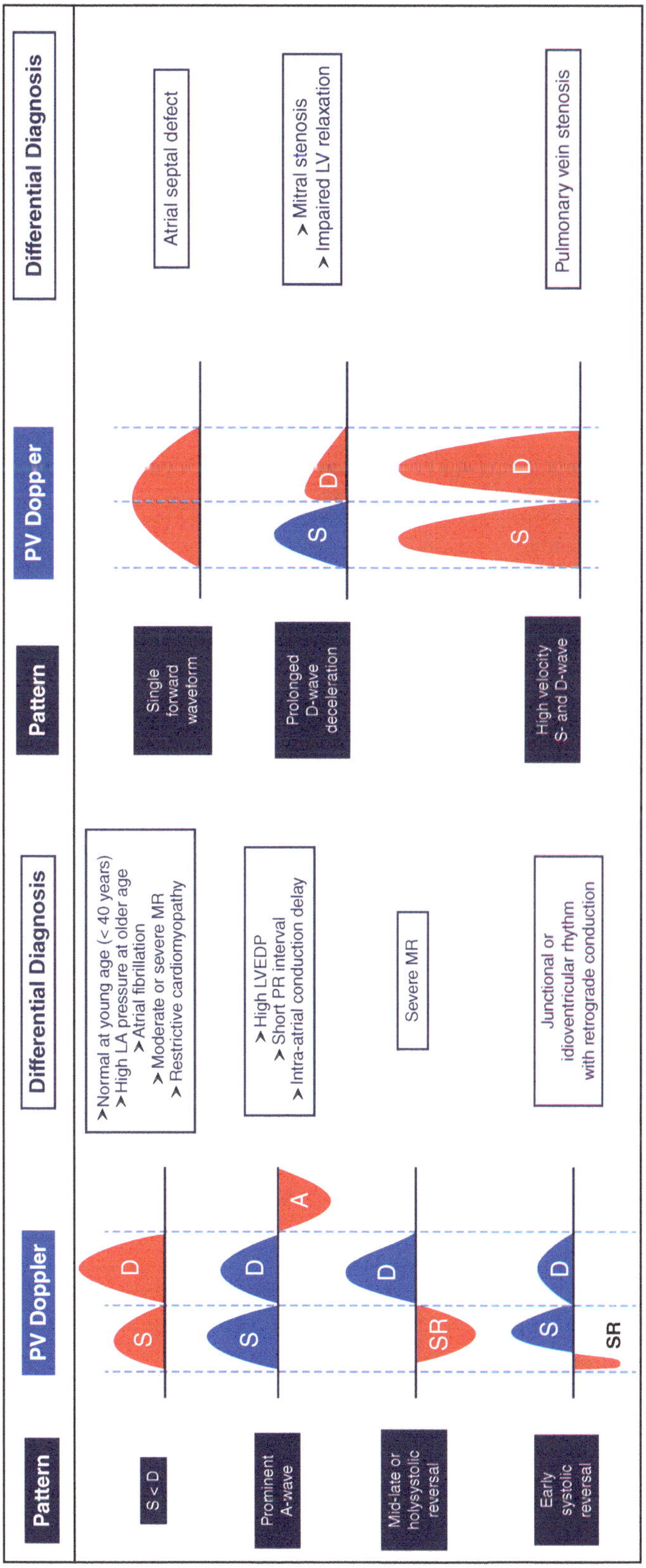

Fig. 7.11 Cardiac pathology differential for abnormal pulmonary vein flow

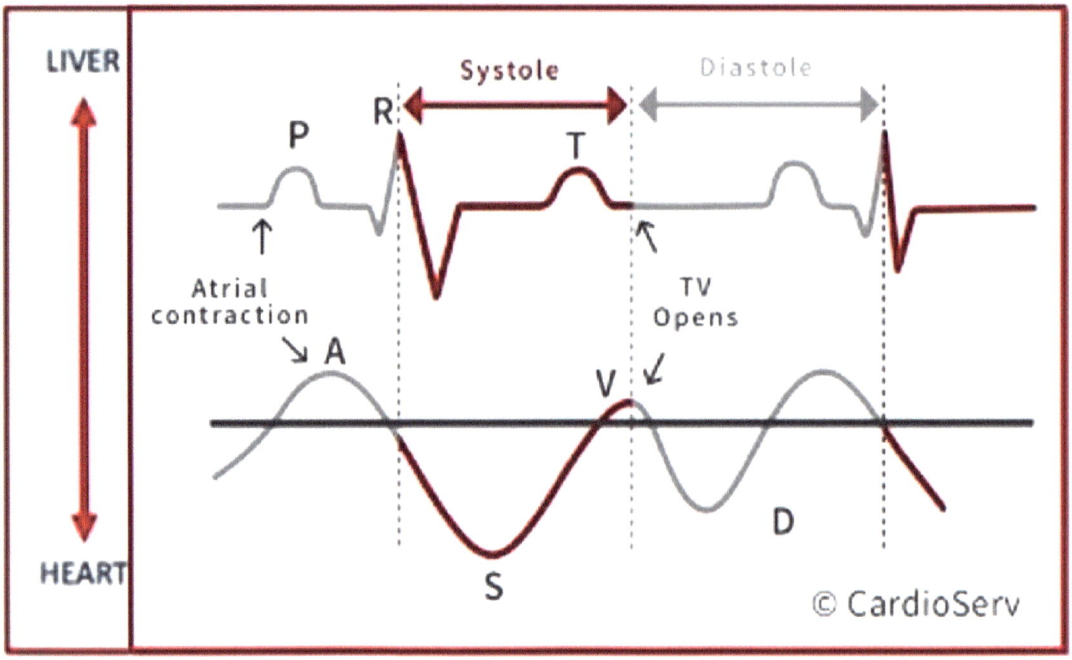

Fig. 7.12 Hepatic vein flow waveforms during the normal cardiac cycle

Hepatic Vein Flow

Right heart-sided disease severity, including tricuspid valve, pericardial disease, and cardiomyopathy can be evaluated by hepatic vein flow. When discussing the flow pattern for the *hepatic veins*, we must consider the blood flow pathway in regard to the circulatory system and transducer. Antegrade is flow *toward* the heart. Retrograde is flow *away* from the heart, toward the liver. The hepatic veins are considered phasic waveforms and are predominately antegrade. They are composed of four parts (Fig. 7.12).

A-wave occurs during *Atrial Systole and is* generated by the increase in RAP from an open tricuspid valve.

S-wave occurs during *Ventricular Systole where the* largest amount of blood flows from hepatic veins into RA. The RV walls contract, pushing blood out into the right ventricular outflow tract (RVOT).

V-wave is a *Transitional Phase that occurs from atrial overfilling when the tricuspid annulus returns to resting position.*

D-wave occurs in *Ventricular Diastole when the tricuspid valve is open and there is the passive filling of the RA from hepatic veins. This velocity is less than the S-wave because of decreased RAP from the rapid diastolic filling of RV.*

Hepatic vein flow abnormalities, most commonly from tricuspid regurgitation (TR) and/or RV failure, begin with triphasic waveforms and progress to a biphasic waveform and an increased V-wave. When severe pathology is present, one fused retrograde flow is seen during diastole. The more severe the regurgitation, the more pulsatile the waveform becomes.

Color Doppler for Valvular Regurgitation and Stenosis

As described in Chap. 1, there are several modes of Doppler yet each has the same goal. Doppler shift is an angle-dependent measurement of blood or tissue velocity. When color is used, velocities within the frame are averaged but the direction is noted. By convention, on TTE, the color box is typically red or blue. Red demonstrates blood flow toward your ultrasound probe and blue is blood flow away from the ultrasound probe. When determining if there is valvular regurgitation or stenosis, color flow Doppler can be useful in visually identifying the high-velocity signals or jets that are going toward or away from the probe. Whether the valve is regurgitant or stenotic is based on the characteristics of the valve and the native direction of blood flow. Slightly atypical views may help to align the jets in a more parallel fashion which is always the goal. The color box can be moved back and forth between valves, depending on assessment priority. Moving a sector box back and forth is much better than using a large color box that covers both valves and where the color resolution is poor.

Pulse-Wave/CW Doppler (Aorta Flows)

Because of the properties of PWD and CWD, interrogation can be made through the aortic valve to understand and diagnose multiple valvular conditions. PWD in front of the aortic valve will measure velocities in the left ventricular outflow tract (LVOT). These velocities can be used to estimate left ventricular stroke volume. CWD through the aortic valve will measure velocities through the aortic valve. The ratio between in front of the aortic valve and through the aortic valve can used to evaluate aortic valve stenosis. In addition, the shape and speed of the velocities through the aortic valve can help determine if there is left ventricular outflow obstruction.

Summary Points

- The velocity of blood and tissue in the heart can be determined by changes in the emitted ultrasound waves according to the Doppler shift principle.
- Doppler echo is essential for measuring cardiac output, noninvasive measurement of intracardiac pressures, diastolic function, and more.
- Doppler measurements can be optimized with proper technique. Align the probe with the direction of blood flow (less than 20° angles) and minimize depth, sector width, and color boxes to focus on the areas of clinical interest.
- Abnormalities in velocities of flow through the pulmonary veins and hepatic veins can demonstrate pathologic conditions that affect ventricular filling pressure.

Questions

1. Which of the following is true regarding spectral Doppler imaging?
   A. TDI filters out low-velocity signals to measure tissue rather than blood
   B. All modes of spectral Doppler are subject to aliasing artifacts
   C. PWD is ideal for measuring high-velocity flows
   D. PWD offers range specificity

   Answer: D. PWD offers range specificity.

   TDI filters high-velocity, low-intensity signals to measure blood. Continuous wave Doppler is not subject to aliasing. PWD is typically unsuitable for high-velocity flows, although there are additional settings that can improve assessments of high-velocity flows.
2. Which of the following can be determined about intracardiac blood flow with spectral Doppler?
   A. Velocity only
   B. Direction only
   C. Direction and velocity
   D. Neither direction nor velocity

   Answer: C. Direction and velocity.

   The spectral Doppler waveform assesses the vector of blood velocity parallel to the probe. It can only assess the direction in one dimension (either moving toward or away from the probe). It will underestimate velocity as the direction becomes less parallel.
3. Which of the following variables are required to estimate RVSP via the modified Bernoulli method?
   A. Pulmonary artery acceleration time
   B. Maximal velocity of the tricuspid regurgitation jet
   C. Right atrial pressure
   D. B & C
   E. A & C

   Answer: D. B&C.

While pulmonary artery acceleration time can be used to estimate mean pulmonary artery pressure, the calculation does not use the modified Bernoulli equation. The modified Bernoulli equation calculates a pressure gradient from a velocity. One needs to know the pressure in one of the chambers in order to calculate the pressure in the other.

4. Which of the following is true regarding spectral Doppler imaging?
   A. Pulmonary veins can be useful in diagnosing additional pathologies such as TR and right heart failure
   B. An abnormal hepatic waveform pattern is demonstrated showing S/D < 1 indication of elevated RAP
   C. The more severe the tricuspid regurgitation, the less pulsatile the hepatic waveform becomes
   D. Flow reversal through hepatic veins means that the pattern cannot be used to assess right atrial pressure

   Answer: B. An abnormal hepatic waveform pattern is demonstrated showing S/D < 1 indication of elevated RAP.

   Pulmonary vein hemodynamics are typically more informative of left-sided diastolic function. Normal hepatic waveforms (and pulmonary vein waveforms) are systolic dominant in adults. Severe TR can increase hepatic vein pulsatility. Flow reversal associated with diastolic dysfunction can offer some information about right atrial pressures, while flow reversal associated with tricuspid regurgitation may be less clear.

References

1. Mottram PM, Marwick TH. Assessment of diastolic function: what the general cardiologist needs to know. Heart. 2005;91(5):681–95. https://doi.org/10.1136/hrt.2003.029413.
2. Kamp O. Advanced systolic and diastolic function: beyond the E-and A-wave. Semin Cardiothorac Vasc Anesth. 2016;10(1):63–5. https://doi.org/10.1177/108925320601000111.
3. Echocardiographic assessment of diastolic function. Digestive Dis Sci. 2019;63(12):119.
4. Garcia MJ. Comprehensive echocardiographic assessment of diastolic function. Heart Failure Clin. 2006;2(2):163–78. https://doi.org/10.1016/j.hfc.2006.01.005.
5. Scheinfield MH, Bilali A, Koenigsberg M. Understanding the spectral Doppler waveform of the hepatic veins in health and disease. Radiographics. 2009;29:2081–98. https://doi.org/10.1148/rg.297095715.
6. Rudski LG, MD. Guidelines for echocardiographic assessment of the right heart in adults: a report from the American Society of Echocardiography. J Am Soc Echocardiogr. 2010;23:685–713.
7. Miller D, Farah MG, Liner A, Fox K, Schluchter M, Hoit BD. The relation between quantitative right ventricular ejection fraction and indices of tricuspid annular motion and myocardial performance. J Am Soc Echocardiogr. 2004;17(5):443–7. https://doi.org/10.1016/j.echo.2004.01.010.
8. Fadel BM, Pibarot P, Kazzi BE, Al-Admawi M, Galzerano D, Alhumaid M, Alamro B, Mahjoub H, Echahidi N, Mohty D. Spectral Doppler interrogation of the pulmonary veins for the diagnosis of cardiac disorders: a comprehensive review. J Am Soc Echocardiogr. 2021;34(3):223–36.
9. www.cardioserv.net.

Transesophageal Echocardiography: Insertion, Manipulation, Risks, Complications

8

Christopher Koo and Daniel Walsh

Learning Objectives

1. Understand the indications and risks of TEE.
2. Know the complications of TEE.
3. Understand how to insert and manipulate the TEE probe.

Indications

Point of care ultrasound (POCUS) is becoming rapidly embraced as a noninvasive and portable way of evaluating and directing management of patients in the hospital setting. With the advent of readily accessible ultrasound equipment, echocardiography has become an invaluable tool for assessing the presence of a wide range of pathology. More specifically, in the ICU, echocardiography can be used to assess hemodynamic instability and to evaluate ventricular function, valvular anatomy, post-surgical complications, pericardial effusions, undiagnosed congenital heart disease, cardiopulmonary thrombosis, and the integrity of the aorta [1, 2].

TEE may be preferred over TTE when patients are not suitable candidates for adequate transthoracic imaging. TTE may be inadequate in almost 40% of patients in the ICU [2]. Limitations can include dressings or other superficial objects, unconducive body habitus, edema, and severe lung disease. A change in body weight of >10% from admission, usage of PEEP > 15 cm H_2O, and the presence of chest tubes are all risk factors for an inadequate TTE examination [2–5].

Despite this potential difficulty in obtaining satisfactory exams, several studies report that up to 32–79% of patients who received echocardiography in the ICU had some form of their management changed including changes in fluid administration, treatment limitations, surgical intervention, or adjustments to inotropes and vasopressors [6–8].

Post Cardiac Surgery

TEE has proven to be immensely useful in the post-cardiac surgery patient when the potential for accurate transthoracic echocardiograms may be significantly limited. Usage of TEE in the post-cardiac surgery patient has been shown to alter the clinical management 49–59% (medical and surgical) of the time when compared to conventional clinical bedside assessments. Changes in surgical management were affected by a TEE examination approximately 10–38% of the time with the most common indication being to re-explore for potential bleeding [9].

A potential advantage of TEE in this patient population is the identification of pericardial tamponade. Different studies have shown that

C. Koo · D. Walsh (✉)
Beth Israel Deaconess Medical Center, Boston, MA, USA
e-mail: dpwalsh@bidmc.harvard.edu

M. J. Lanspa, A. T. Levinson (eds.), *Echocardiography and Ultrasonography in the ICU*, Respiratory Medicine, https://doi.org/10.1007/978-3-031-80038-2_8

TTE alone may miss the diagnosis of tamponade in 25–59% of patients, diagnosed later by TEE and confirmed with surgery [10–12].

Acute Cardiopulmonary Disease

Left ventricular failure is the most common cause of cardiogenic shock. Evaluation of the left atrium, ventricular anatomy, contractility, and left-sided valvular defects can help quickly diagnose cases of cardiogenic shock and guide appropriate therapy [13, 14]. While "eyeballing" is a common way of estimating potential issues with valvular regurgitation or poor contractility, more objective assessment can be useful in quantifying severity of valvular pathology or the severity of reduced ventricular function. Furthermore, quick identification of wall motion abnormalities on TEE exam can further help clarify the need for revascularization therapy in a patient suffering from cardiogenic shock.

Compared to pulmonary artery catheters and thermodilution, TEE showed no significant difference in estimations of cardiac output. Furthermore, TEE can help clarify cardiac function in patients with significant tricuspid regurgitation or intracardiac shunts, a significant limitation to the thermodilution method [15]. Using aortic velocity time index (VTI) helps improve the accuracy of TEE readings of cardiac output in patients that may not have regular symmetrical blood flow. In the case of patients with atrial fibrillation, averaging approximately 13 heart beats could provide mean values of CO similar in accuracy to those in sinus rhythm.

In addition, acute cor pulmonale (ACP) as seen in patients with acute respiratory distress syndrome (ARDS) or pulmonary embolus can also be evaluated with TEE. In the case of ARDS, the presence of ACP has been associated with worse outcomes. Early recognition of RV dysfunction can help guide the course of treatment. It should be kept in mind however that a complementary TTE examination may be needed in order to fully measure pulmonary artery systolic pressure due to difficulty in anatomic alignment and positioning with TEE [16, 17].

Hypovolemia, Fluid Responsiveness

Unexplained hypotension is often the most commonly cited reason for performing a TEE examination in the critically ill. Colreavy et al. found that an underlying cause was found 2/3 of the time for patients who received a TEE for unexplained hypotension, 22% leading to surgery without further diagnostic workup [4].

Accurate prediction of whether or not a patient will be responsive to additional volume resuscitation continues to be a topic of debate especially for those in the ICU. Intravascular depletion can be assessed using TEE depending on whether or not the patient is spontaneously breathing or reliant on ventilatory support. Usage of the inferior vena cava (IVC) and superior vena cava (SVC) change in diameter are common metrics for determining a patient's fluid responsiveness. In the fully ventilator-dependent patient, a ratio of the change in IVC diameter called the distensibility index has a reported sensitivity and specificity of 90%. Changes in the SVC during mechanical ventilation of >36% during inspiration has a sensitivity of 90% and specificity of 100% [13, 14].

A therapeutic response to volume resuscitation can then be subsequently assessed via a change in SV or CO of >15% using TEE. Measurements using VTI and CSA can quantify stroke volume and cardiac output then approximated using the classic CO = SV × HR equation [14].

A study using esophageal Doppler and passive leg raise reported that a >10% aortic blood flow predicted fluid responsiveness with a sensitivity of 97% and specificity of 94% [18].

It is important, however, to consider the effect of RV function as well as the rate and volume of mechanical ventilation before relying on these measures to guide fluid resuscitation.

Endocarditis

One of the major criteria for the diagnosis of endocarditis is identification of a characteristic finding on echocardiogram with TEE being the preferred modality in patients with prosthetic valves or potential paravalvular abscesses [19, 20]. While TTE is noninvasive and can be logistically preferred in patients with potential infective endocarditis, as discussed previously in this chapter, adequate imaging via a transthoracic evaluation may not always be accurate or even feasible in the ICU.

Bai et al. compared TTE detection of vegetations on prosthetic valves against TEE and found a sensitivity of 46% and specificity of 79%. When used to detect intracardiac abscesses, the results showed a wide range of reported sensitivity for TTE of anywhere between 29% and 100% [21]. Another report showed that while TTE was able to identify correctly 80% of the patient without vegetations, 44% of patients who were found to have false positives when re-examined with TEE. Furthermore, 37% of patients with prosthetic valves and inconclusive results on TTE were found to have vegetations on TEE examination [22].

While TTE may be satisfactory screening tests in patients with native valves and low likelihood of infective endocarditis, indeterminate TTE imaging, or the presence of valvular prostheses highlights the advantage of TEE to definitively assess the critically ill patient for potential infective endocarditis.

Aortic Pathology

Use of TEE in assessing disease of the aorta in the ICU setting can be considered in those with suspected dissection, intramural hematomas, or penetrating atherosclerotic ulcers (PAUs) and contraindications to contrast CT imaging. With regard to aortic dissections, TEE has been found to have both high sensitivity and specificity for aortic dissections reaching 99% and 89%, respectively. Localization of intimal tears can be found using TEE up to 78–100% of the time. Sensitivity is 100% for detecting aortic regurgitation as a complication of dissection. Impressively, by adding the use of small amounts of peripherally injected contrast, TEE has reportedly shown almost perfect sensitivity and specificity for detecting aortic dissection, intramural hematoma, and penetrating aortic ulcers [23, 24]. TEE can however be limited in its ability to assess the distal ascending aorta as well as proximal aortic arch where interference by the trachea and bronchus can limit image quality [23].

In the post aortic surgery patient, TEE can also assess the integrity of aortic arch repairs or grafting, trauma, or the presence of endoleaks after endovascular intervention of aneurysms. In fact, color flow Doppler TEE has been shown to be superior to angiography in detecting graft leaks [25].

Assessment of Embolism Risk

A common indication for TEE is to assess for presence of a potential cardiac source of embolism, particularly in the setting of atrial fibrillation or flutter. TTE is not sufficient to rule out the presence of thrombus in the left atrium in the setting of atrial fibrillation and can facilitate decision making in regards to anticoagulation and cardioversion [26].

Risks and Complications

Risks of TEE can be separated into risks related to the procedure itself and risks related to any necessary sedation required to perform the procedure. Understandably, these risks may be reduced in the ICU where many patients are already intubated and sedated compared to the ambulatory setting. This discussion will focus on the risks related to the procedure itself.

Studies of TEE safety in general report 0.5% complication rates and a mortality rate of <0.01% [5, 27]. Similarly, TEE in the ICU is generally low risk in relation to major complication or mortality. From 2508 reported cases of TEE, specifically in ICU patients, no incidents of oropharyngeal, esophageal, or gastric perforations occurred. No mortalities were reported. The most common complications included nasogastric tube removal, abrasion of oropharyngeal surfaces, transient hypotension from increased sedation, and sometimes transient hypoxemia.

Table 8.1 TEE complications and incidences

Complication	Incidence (%)
Hemodynamic instability	0.8
Arrhythmias	0.2–0.9
Significant bleeding	0.03–0.8
Oropharyngeal bleeding	0.01–0.7
Hypoxia	0.2
Esophageal perforation	0.01–0.3
Endotracheal tube displacement	0.03
Mortality	<0.01

These less serious complications typically occurred approximately <1–2% of the time, with transient hypotension and trauma to the oropharyngeal surfaces occurring most commonly [5].

Even in special populations such as those with thrombocytopenia or esophageal varices (grade 1 or 2) have reportedly underwent TEE without significant rates of adverse events [28, 29].

Table 8.1: Complications from TEE are listed with the most frequent events listed in descending order. Because of a lack of data specific to the ICU population, the numbers are primarily from studies looking at both ICU and perioperative settings [5, 27].

Contraindications to TEE

Absolute contraindications to TEE include the presence of a perforated viscus, esophageal abnormalities such as strictures, tumors, lacerations, or diverticula, as well as active upper gastrointestinal bleeding. Physical defects and deformities can lead to difficulty placing the device safely and potentially worsen already existing lesions further jeopardizing the patient.

Relative contraindications should be carefully considered against a risk versus benefit analysis of the patient's current clinical status and potential diagnostic value. Examples of relative contraindications to consider before performing TEE on a critically ill patient include prior radiation to the neck and mediastinum, prior gastrointestinal surgery, recent upper gastrointestinal bleeding, Barrett's esophagus, active esophagitis or peptic ulcer disease, a reported history of dysphagia, reduced cervical range of motion (atlantoaxial instability, severe arthritis), symptomatic hiatal hernias, esophageal varices, coagulopathy, and severe thrombocytopenia [5, 26, 30].

Insertion

Prior to insertion of the transesophageal echocardiography probe, it is important to ensure adequate preparation, positioning, and resources to perform the exam safely. Performing clinicians should review the patient's unique circumstances and assess any potential contraindication to examination. Consideration of any pertinent history, exam findings, lab results, and prior imaging findings should be done. The presence of an endotracheal tube and mechanical ventilatory support, oral or nasogastric tube, use of vasopressors or inotropes, and sedating medications should also be taken into account prior to examination. Depending on the indication, paralysis prior to insertion of the probe may be helpful. The ability of the patient to tolerate repositioning should be also clarified. Last, ensure that all equipment has been cleaned and safe for use in a new patient and that additional assistance can be quickly called for should it be required [26, 30, 31].

For Insertion of the TEE Probe

1. The operator should be at the head of the bed with the patient ideally in the left lateral decubitus position. The height of the bed should be adjusted based on the operator's comfort.
2. If there is an endotracheal tube in place, it should be carefully secured to the left corner

of the patient's mouth to allow for easier passage of the TEE probe.
3. If the patient is sedated, consider additional sedation during initial passage of the TEE probe from the mouth into the esophagus as this may be particularly stimulating. Careful monitoring of vital signs is recommended.
4. A bite block can be placed, being careful not to push the patient's tongue posteriorly and occlude the hypopharynx.
5. Topical lubricant should be applied to the probe.
6. After ensuring the probe is not in the locked position, the probe can be inserted into the patient's mouth, midline, to avoid placement into the piriform fossae. An assistant can help thrust the mandible forward or to flex the patient's neck while the operator lightly anteflexes the probe to help follow the natural curvature of the hypopharynx into the esophagus.
7. If resistance is met while inserting the probe, efforts to insert the probe should stop to prevent injury to the pharynx, esophagus, or stomach.
8. Direct or videolaryngoscopy can be used to help visualize and guide the TEE probe down the esophagus if there is continued difficulty.[1]
9. When advancing the probe, it is important to generally avoid ante- or retroflexion of the probe head as this may cause injury.

Manipulation

Standardized terminology provided by the American Society of Echocardiography is commonly used to describe handling and operation of a TEE probe. The patient is assumed to be in the standard anatomic position and supine. The imaging plane from the probe is thus anterior pointing from the esophagus towards the heart and sternum while posterior directs the user towards the spine. In this position, superior is meant to refer towards the head and inferior towards the feet. Right and left are in relation to the patient's right and left. It is important to keep in mind that the image displayed from the TEE probe is typically inverted from anatomic position with structures located on the patient's right viewed on the left side of the TEE image.

Advancement is used to describe further insertion of the TEE probe into the esophagus and withdrawal to mean retraction of the probe out of the esophagus. Rotation along the parallel axis of the esophagus is turning to the right and left. Movement of the probe tip out of the axis parallel to the esophagus or "curving" the probe can be performed by most standard TEE probes by a large control wheel with anterior and posterior movement of the probe tip described as anteflexing and retroflexing, respectively. Lateral flexion to the right and left is performed via a smaller control knob that typically sits atop of the larger counterpart.

Altering the angle of the imaging plane from 0° to 180°, or the horizontal/transverse plane, is called rotating forward. Rotating from 180° back to 0 is rotating backward. When the imaging plane is at 90°, it is referred to a vertical or longitudinal plane. These movements can be performed typically by buttons on the probe that increase or decrease the angle. Keep in mind that due to the horizontal inversion from the patient's anatomic position and the image displayed, movement from 0° to 90° of the imaging plane will cause the left side of the image to now display inferior structures instead of anatomy on the patient's right side [26, 30, 33] (Fig. 8.1).

An example using the midesophageal four chamber view for assessment of MV and TV function, global LV and RV systolic function, and regional LV inferoseptal and anterolateral wall motion is provided:

1. Advance the probe to 30–35 cm until immediately posterior to the left atrium.
2. Turn the probe to the left or right to center the patient's mitral valve and left ventricle in the imaging display.

[1] *Currently, while some studies have shown a decreased number of insertion attempts and mechanical trauma with the use of direct or videolaryngscopy for TEE insertion, the evidence is not robust* [32].

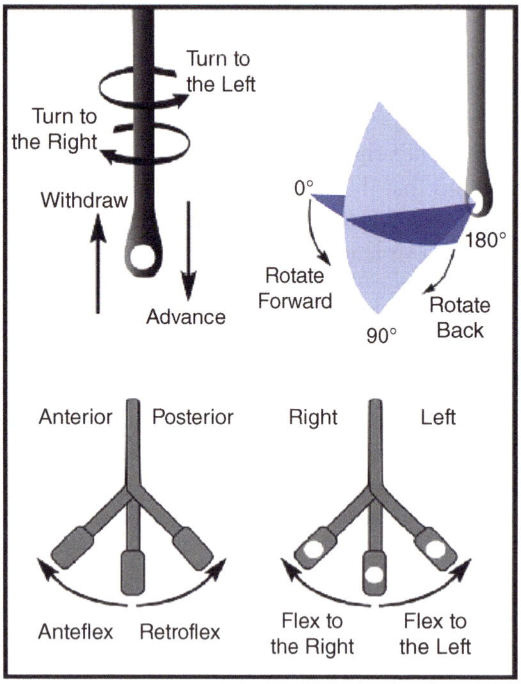

Fig. 8.1 Manipulation terminology. (Illustration from Hahn et al. [26])

3. If necessary, adjust the multiplane angle up to about 10–20°.
4. Slight retroflexion of the probe can be used to further align the MV and LV apex.

Summary Points

- TEE can be useful when TTE is nondiagnostic or not sufficiently diagnostic.
- TEE is a low-risk procedure with complication rates generally 0.5% incidence or lower.
- Complications can include bleeding, esophageal damage, airway or hypoxia issues, or hemodynamic instability.
- There are very few absolute contraindications to TEE but they include severe esophageal pathology such as perforations, strictures, diverticula, or bleeding.
- Considerations for insertion include patient positioning, patient sedation, placement of bite block, and probe position.
- Use of standardized terminology allows for discussion of probe manipulation to systematically obtain views and make assessments.

Questions

1. You would like to perform a TEE in order to evaluate a patient with a history of prosthetic valve replacement who continues to have unexplained hemodynamic instability. Before performing the exam, you review the patient's chart to identify any possible contraindications. Which of the following is neither a relative nor absolute contraindication to performing TEE?
   A. Symptomatic hiatal hernia
   B. Scleroderma
   C. Therapeutic anticoagulation
   D. Esophagitis

   Answer: C. Therapeutic anticoagulation. While active GI bleeding is an absolute contraindication and coagulopathy and recent GI bleeding are both relative contraindications, the use of therapeutic anticoagulation is not. The risk of oropharyngeal or esophageal trauma should always be considered when considering the use of TEE, but serious injury or complication is rare even in critically unstable patients.
2. On a mid-esophageal four chamber view, you note that you have a foreshortened ventricle and would like to manipulate the probe to optimize your image. You would like to retroflex the probe by:
   A. Adjusting the large wheel on the probe
   B. Pressing the down button on the probe
   C. Pushing on the midshaft of the probe while leaning forward
   D. Adjusting the small wheel on the probe

   Answer: A. Adjusting the large wheel on the probe. The large wheel on the probe allows the probe to flex anteriorly or posteriorly, described as anteflexing and retroflexing, respectively. The smaller wheel on the probe allows the probe to move in a lateral motion. The buttons on the probe rotate the imaging plane and do not move the probe itself.

References

1. Reeves ST, Finley AC, Skubas NJ, Swaminathan M, Whitley WS, Glas KE, Hahn RT, Shanewise JS, Adams MS, Shernan SK. Basic perioperative transesophageal echocardiography examination: a consensus statement of the American Society of Echocardiography and the Society of Cardiovascular Anesthesiologists. J Am Soc Echocardiogr. 2013;26(5):443–56. https://doi.org/10.1016/j.echo.2013.02.015.
2. Vieillard-Baron A, Millington SJ, Sanfilippo F, Chew M, Diaz-Gomez J, McLean A, Pinsky MR, Pulido J, Mayo P, Fletcher N. A decade of progress in critical care echocardiography: a narrative review. Intensive Care Med. 2019;45(6):770–88. https://doi.org/10.1007/s00134-019-05604-2.
3. Beaulieu Y. Bedside echocardiography in the assessment of the critically Ill. Crit Care Med. 2007;35(5 Suppl):S235–49. https://doi.org/10.1097/01.ccm.0000260673.66681.af.
4. Colreavy FB, Donovan K, Lee KY, Weekes J. Transesophageal echocardiography in critically ill patients*. Crit Care Med. 2002;30(5):989–96. https://doi.org/10.1097/00003246-200205000-00007.
5. Hutteman E. Critical care transesophageal echocardiography. Minerva Anestesiol. 2006;72:891–913.
6. Arntfield R, Lau V, Landry Y, Priestap F, Ball I. Impact of critical care transesophageal echocardiography in medical–surgical ICU patients: characteristics and results from 274 consecutive examinations. J Intensive Care Med. 2018;35(9):896–902. https://doi.org/10.1177/0885066618797271.
7. Orme RM, Oram MP, McKinstry CE. Impact of echocardiography on patient management in the intensive care unit: an audit of district general hospital practice. Br J Anaesth. 2009;102(3):340–4. https://doi.org/10.1093/bja/aen378.
8. Poelaert JI, Everaert J, Colardyn FA, Trouerbach J, De Buyzere M. Evaluation of transesophageal echocardiography as a diagnostic and therapeutic aid in a critical care setting. Chest. 1995;107(3):774–9. https://doi.org/10.1378/chest.107.3.774.
9. Heiberg J, El-Ansary D, Royse CF, Royse AG, Alsaddique AA, Canty DJ. Transthoracic and transoesophageal echocardiography: a systematic review of feasibility and impact on diagnosis, management and outcome after cardiac surgery. Anaesthesia. 2016;71(10):1210–21. https://doi.org/10.1111/anae.13545.
10. Ellenbroek DF, van Kessel L, Compagner W, Brouwer T, Bouwman RA, van Straten BA, Otterspoor LC, De Bie AJ. Diagnostic performance of echocardiography to predict cardiac tamponade after cardiac surgery. Eur J Cardiothorac Surg. 2022;62(1):ezab468. https://doi.org/10.1093/ejcts/ezab468.
11. Grumann A, Baretto L, Dugard A, Morera P, Cornu E, Amiel J-B, Vignon PP. Localized cardiac tamponade after open-heart surgery. Ann Thorac Cardiovasc Surg. 2012;18(6):524–9. https://doi.org/10.5761/atcs.oa.11.01855.
12. Imren Y, Tasoglu I, Oktar GL, Benson A, Naseem T, Cheema F, Unal Y. The importance of transesophageal echocardiography in diagnosis of pericardial tamponade after cardiac surgery. J Card Surg. 2008;23(5):450–3. https://doi.org/10.1111/j.1540-8191.2008.00581.x.
13. Boissier F, François B, Dessap AM. Hemodynamic monitoring using trans esophageal echocardiography in patients with shock. Ann Transl Med. 2020;8(12):791. https://doi.org/10.21037/atm-2020-hdm-23.
14. McLean AS. Echocardiography in shock management. Crit Care. 2016;20(1):275. https://doi.org/10.1186/s13054-016-1401-7.
15. Wetterslev M, Møller-Sørensen H, Johansen RR, Perner A. Systematic review of cardiac output measurements by echocardiography vs. thermodilution: the techniques are not interchangeable. Intensive Care Med. 2016;42(8):1223–33. https://doi.org/10.1007/s00134-016-4258-y.
16. Poth JM, Beck DR, Bartels K. Ultrasonography for haemodynamic monitoring. Best Pract Res Clin Anaesthesiol. 2014;28(4):337–51. https://doi.org/10.1016/j.bpa.2014.08.005.
17. Vignon P, Begot E, Mari A, Silva S, Chimot L, Delour P, Vargas F, Filloux B, Vandroux D, Jabot J, François B, Pichon N, Clavel M, Levy B, Slama M, Riu-Poulenc B. Hemodynamic assessment of patients with septic shock using transpulmonary thermodilution and critical care echocardiography. Chest. 2018;153(1):55–64. https://doi.org/10.1016/j.chest.2017.08.022.
18. Monnet X, Rienzo M, Osman D, Anguel N, Richard C, Pinsky MR, Teboul J-L. Passive leg raising predicts fluid responsiveness in the critically ill. Crit Care Med. 2006;34(5):1402–7. https://doi.org/10.1097/01.ccm.0000215453.11735.06.
19. Baddour LM, Wilson WR, Bayer AS, Fowler VG, Tleyjeh IM, Rybak MJ, Barsic B, Lockhart PB, Gewitz MH, Levison ME, Bolger AF, Steckelberg JM, Baltimore RS, Fink AM, O'Gara P, Taubert KA. Infective endocarditis in adults: diagnosis, antimicrobial therapy, and management of comp. Circulation. 2015;132:1435–86. https://doi.org/10.1161/CIR.0000000000000296.
20. Mourvillier B, Trouillet J-L, Timsit J-F, Baudot J, Chastre J, Régnier B, Gibert C, Wolff M. Infective endocarditis in the intensive care unit: clinical spectrum and prognostic factors in 228 consecutive patients. Intensive Care Med. 2004;30(11):2046–52. https://doi.org/10.1007/s00134-004-2436-9.
21. Bai AD, Steinberg M, Showler A, Burry L, Bhatia RS, Tomlinson GA, Bell CM, Morris AM. Diagnostic accuracy of transthoracic echocardiography for infective endocarditis findings using transesophageal echocardiography as the reference standard: a meta-analysis. J Am Soc Echocardiogr. 2017;30(7):639–646.e8. https://doi.org/10.1016/j.echo.2017.03.007.

22. Kini V, Logani S, Ky B, Chirinos JA, Ferrari VA, St. John Sutton MG, Wiegers SE, Kirkpatrick JN. Transthoracic and transesophageal echocardiography for the indication of suspected infective endocarditis: vegetations, blood cultures and imaging. J Am Soc Echocardiogr. 2010;23(4):396–402. https://doi.org/10.1016/j.echo.2009.12.017.
23. Baliga RR, Nienaber CA, Bossone E, Oh JK, Isselbacher EM, Sechtem U, Fattori R, Raman SV, Eagle KA. The role of imaging in aortic dissection and related syndromes. JACC Cardiovasc Imaging. 2014;7(4):406–24. https://doi.org/10.1016/j.jcmg.2013.10.015.
24. Patil TA, Nierich A. Transesophageal echocardiography evaluation of the thoracic aorta. Ann Card Anaesth. 2016;19(5):44. https://doi.org/10.4103/0971-9784.192623.
25. Nowak-Machen M. The role of transesophageal echocardiography in aortic surgery. Best Pract Res Clin Anaesthesiol. 2016;30(3):317–29. https://doi.org/10.1016/j.bpa.2016.05.003.
26. Hahn RT, Abraham T, Adams MS, Bruce CJ, Glas KE, Lang RM, Reeves ST, Shanewise JS, Siu SC, Stewart W, Picard MH. Guidelines for performing a comprehensive transesophageal echocardiographic examination: recommendations from the American Society of Echocardiography and the Society of Cardiovascular Anesthesiologists. J Am Soc Echocardiogr. 2013;26(9):921–64. https://doi.org/10.1016/j.echo.2013.07.009.
27. Hilberath JN, Eltzschig HK, D'Ambra MN, Bulwer BE, Shernan SK, Oakes DA. Safety of transesophageal echocardiography. Am Soc Echocardiogr. 2010;23:1115–11127. https://doi.org/10.1016/j.echo.2010.08.013.
28. Kitkungvan D, Kalluru D, Lunagariya A, Sanchez L, Yusuf SW, Hassan S, Palaskas N, Mouhayar E, Banchs J. Safety of transesophageal echocardiography in patients with thrombocytopenia. J Am Soc Echocardiogr. 2019;32(8):1010–5. https://doi.org/10.1016/j.echo.2019.04.421.
29. Liu E, Guha A, Dunleavy M, Obarski T. Safety of transesophageal echocardiography in patients with esophageal varices. J Am Soc Echocardiogr. 2019;32(5):676–7. https://doi.org/10.1016/j.echo.2019.01.013.
30. Mayo PH, Narasimhan M, Koenig S. Critical care transesophageal echocardiography. Chest. 2015;148(5):1323–32. https://doi.org/10.1378/chest.15-0260.
31. Leitman M, Fuchs S, Ilgiyaev E. How to facilitate the placement of a transesophageal probe in a ventilated patient? J Crit Care. 2019;50:66–8. https://doi.org/10.1016/j.jcrc.2018.11.020.
32. Namekawa M, Tsujimoto Y, Banno M, Kataoka Y, Tsujimoto H, Inaba Y, Fujiwara T. Videolaryngoscopy for transesophageal echocardiography probe insertion: a systematic review and meta-analysis of randomized controlled trials. J Anesth. 2020;34(3):453–63. https://doi.org/10.1007/s00540-020-02759-x.
33. Prabhu M, Pauli H, Raju D. Transesophageal echocardiography: instrumentation and system controls. Ann Card Anaesth. 2012;15(2):144. https://doi.org/10.4103/0971-9784.95080.

9 Transesophageal Windows and Views

Mark Hamlin and Ariel Bensimhon

Abbreviations

2D	Two-dimensional
3D	Three-dimensional
AA	Ascending aorta
Ao	Aorta
AV	Aortic valve
CS	Coronary sinus
DTG	Deep transgastric
IAS	Interatrial septum
IVS	Interventricular septum
LA	Left atrium
LIPV	Left inferior pulmonary vein
LSPV	Left superior pulmonary vein
LV	Left ventricle
LVOT	Left ventricular outflow tract
ME	Mid esophageal
MV	Mitral valve
PA	Pulmonary artery
PV	Pulmonic valve
RA	Right atrium
RAA	Right atrial appendage
RIPV	Right inferior pulmonary vein
RSPV	Right superior pulmonary vein
RV	Right ventricle
RVOT	Right ventricular outflow tract
TEE	Transesophageal echocardiography
TG	Transgastric
TV	Tricuspid valve
UE	Upper esophageal

2D Transesophageal Imaging

The transesophageal echocardiographic (TEE) exam for adults with structurally normal hearts, i.e., those without profound congenital heart malformations, will consist of images obtained in the upper esophageal (UE), mid esophageal (ME), transgastric (TG), and deep transgastric (DTG) esophageal probe positions. Image optimization will utilize probe manipulations seen in Fig. 9.1. Image acquisition sequences are based on anatomy, echo view, or cardiac segment and are influenced by clinical situation and institutional protocols. Figure 9.2 offers a pictorial representation of probe movements used to complete an exam. Within each image, structure morphology and function should be noted, with interrogation including color flow and spectral Doppler where applicable [1–3].

Supplementary Information The online version contains supplementary material available at https://doi.org/10.1007/978-3-031-80038-2_9.

M. Hamlin (✉) · A. Bensimhon
Department of Anesthesiology, University of Vermont, University of Vermont Medical Center, Burlington, VT, USA
e-mail: Mark.Hamlin@uvmhealth.org

M. J. Lanspa, A. T. Levinson (eds.), *Echocardiography and Ultrasonography in the ICU*, Respiratory Medicine, https://doi.org/10.1007/978-3-031-80038-2_9

Pro-tip
Small probe movements may yield larger than expected image alterations. Furthermore, while patients are similar, they are not the same. As such, the described omniplane angles are relative and may need adjustment for each patient.

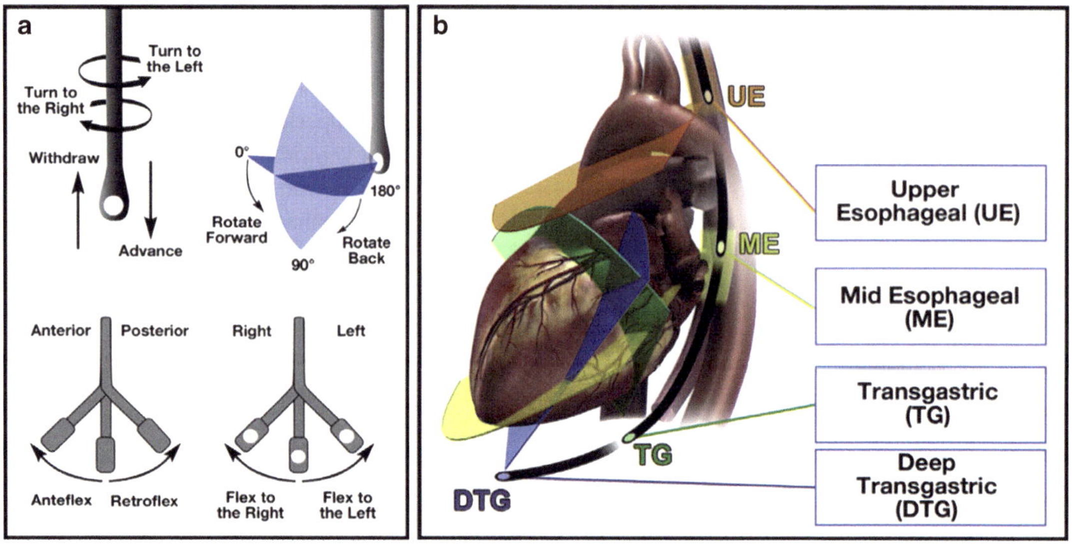

Fig. 9.1 Schematic displaying probe manipulations and positions utilized in image acquisition [1]

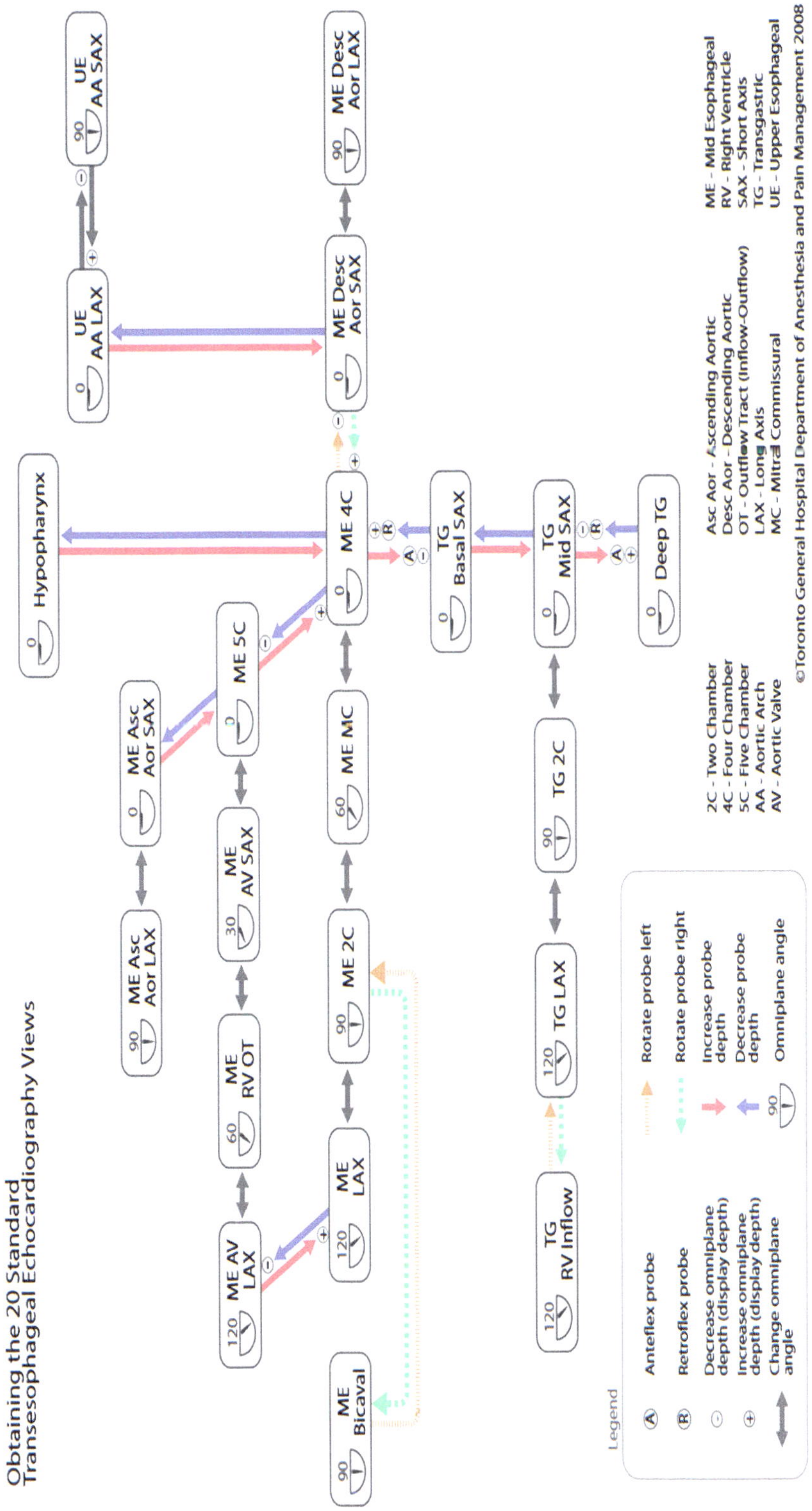

Fig. 9.2 Pictorial representation of probe movements used to shift between TEE views [4]

Mid-esophageal four chamber (ME 4C) 0–20°

The probe is positioned in the mid esophagus with an omniplane angle of 0–20°, behind the left atrium (LA) and utilizing the LA as the acoustic window. In a left ventricular (LV) centered view, the LA and LV are aligned in the center of the imaging plane. Optimization will include retroflexion and omniplane angle adjustment to visualize the LV from base to apex, attempting to eliminate foreshortening. Rightward probe rotation will better align the right atrium (RA) and right ventricle (RV) with imaging plane center for a right heart centric view. Visible structures include the LA, LV (anterolateral and inferoseptal walls), MV (mitral valve—A3, A2, P2, P1 scallops), RA, RV, TV (tricuspid valve), interatrial septum (IAS), and interventricular septum (IVS) (Image/Video 9.1) [1, 3]

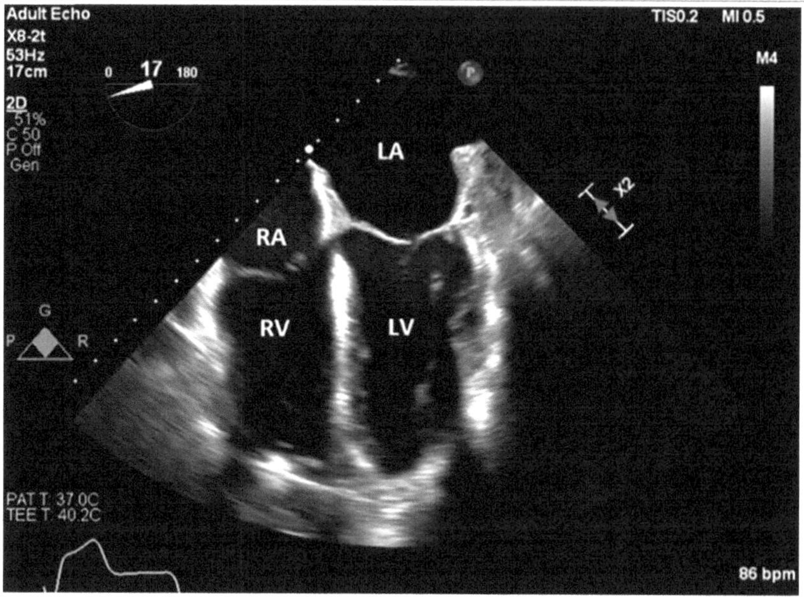

Image/video 1. ME 4C view.

Image/Video 9.1 ME 4C view

Mid esophageal five chamber (ME 5C) 0–20°

From the ME 4C, slight probe withdrawal will bring the aortic valve (AV) and left ventricular outflow tract (LVOT) into view. Visible structures include the LA, LV (anterolateral and inferoseptal walls), AV, MV (mitral valve—A2, A1, P1 scallops), RA, RV, TV, IAS, IVS (Image/Video 9.2) [1, 3]

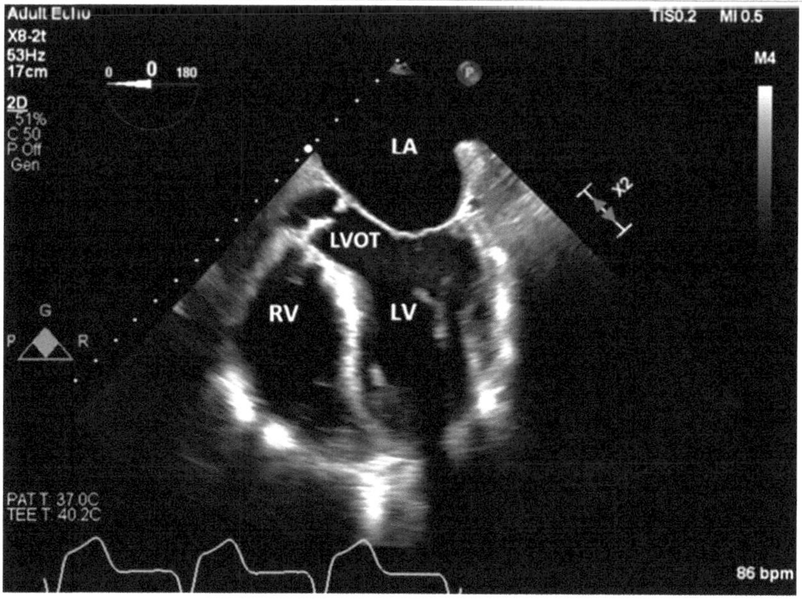

Image/video 2. ME 5C view.

Image/Video 9.2 ME 5C view

(continued)

Mid-esophageal mitral commissural (ME MC) 50–70° From an appropriate LV-centered ME 4C view, increase the omniplane to 60°, visualizing the LA, LV, and MV (P1, A2, P3 scallops from right to left). Additionally, the anterolateral and posteromedial papillary muscles and associated chordae, as well as the coronary sinus, may be seen. Color flow Doppler can assist with localization of MV regurgitation (Image/Video 9.3) [1, 3]	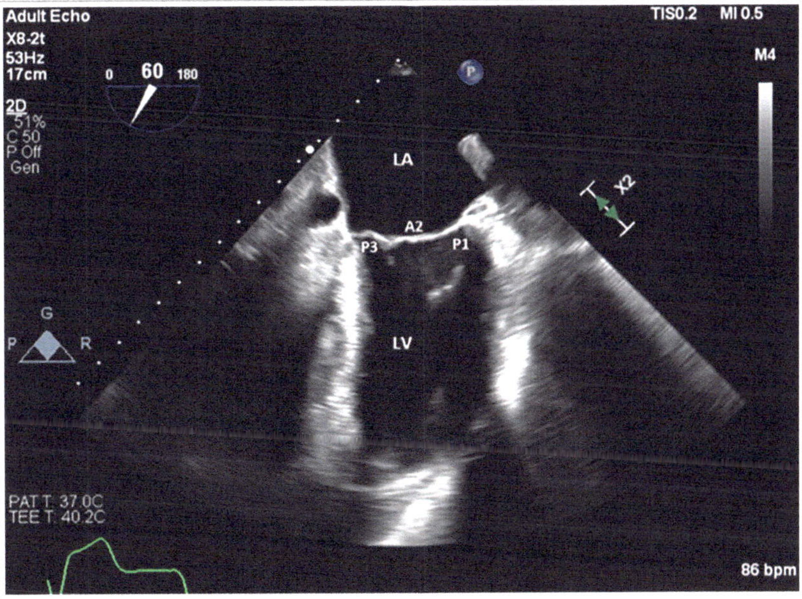 Image/video 3. ME MC view. Image/Video 9.3 ME MC view
Mid-esophageal two chamber (ME 2C) 80–100° Increasing the omniplane to 90° from either the ME 4C or ME MC views will yield the ME 2C view. This is an orthogonal view to ME 4C and seen when placing biplane imaging through a LV-centered ME 4C image. In the ME 2C plane, visible structures include the LA, LA appendage (LAA), LV (anterior and inferior walls), MV, and coronary sinus. With regard to the MV, the amount of withdrawal/insertion and probe rotation will determine which scallops are visualized. A more anterior position may capture A2, A3, and P3 while a more posterior position may visualize P1, P2, and P3, both from screen right to left (Image/Video 9.4) [1, 3]	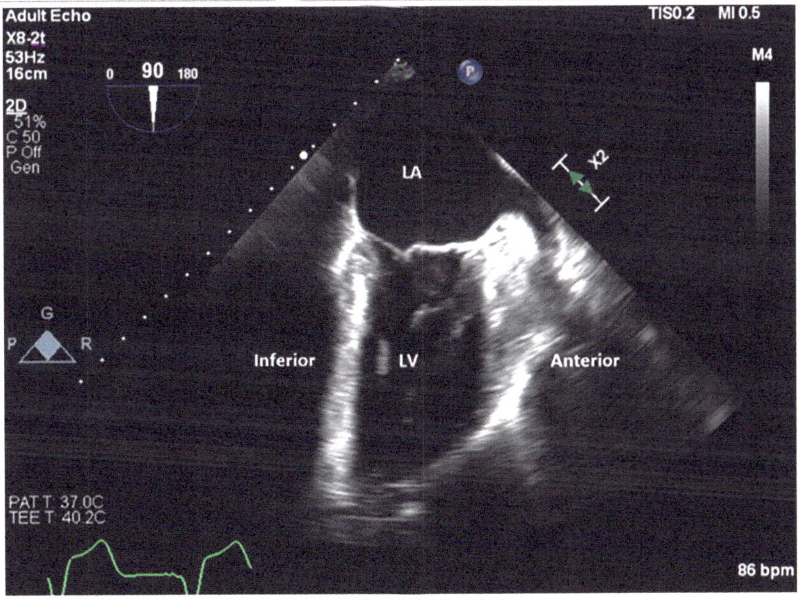 Image/video 4. ME 2C view. Image/Video 9.4 ME 2C view

(continued)

Mid-esophageal long Axis (ME LAX) 120–150°

From the ME 4C, ME MC, or ME 2C views, increase the omniplane to 120–150°, until the LVOT and AV are seen in a long axis orientation at screen right, ensuring capture of the full LV. The ME LAX displays the LA, LV (anteroseptal and inferolateral walls), MV (A2 and P2 scallops), LVOT, AV, aortic root and proximal ascending aorta, IVS, and RV. See Fig. 9.3 for further delineation of mitral valve segments (Image/Video 9.5) [1, 3]

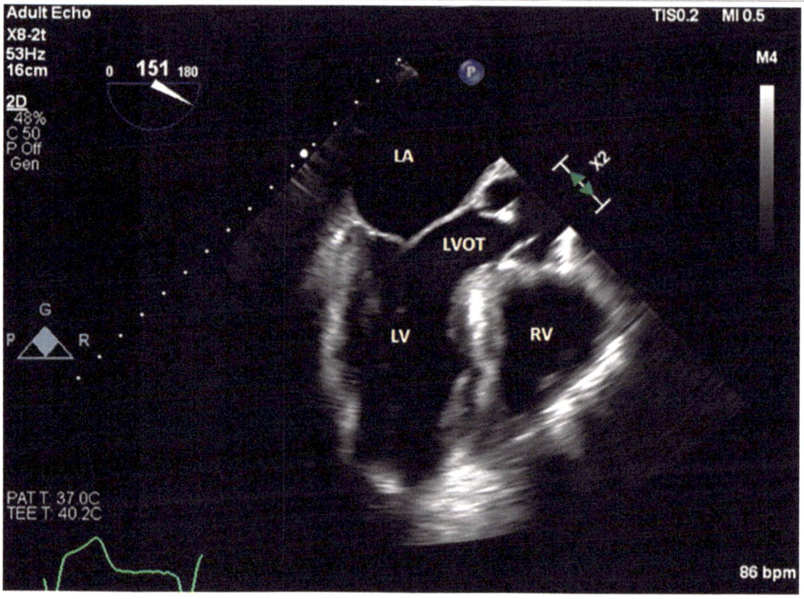

Image/video 5. ME LAX view.

Image/Video 9.5 ME LAX view

Mid-esophageal left atrial appendage (ME LAA) 80–110°

Returning to the ME 2C view at 90° and adding slight probe withdrawal, anteflexion, and/or rightward rotation, will bring the LAA into view, adjacent to the MV. The left superior pulmonary vein (LSPV) may be seen to the right of the LAA. Alternatively, from the ME RV inflow–outflow view, decrease the omniplane to 50–70° and rotate leftward with slight withdrawal to image the LAA to the right of the AV. multiplane imaging, color flow Doppler, and pulse wave Doppler are used to interrogate the LAA. Alterations in the omniplane angle may be necessary to fully visualize all LAA lobes (Image/Video 9.6) [1, 3]

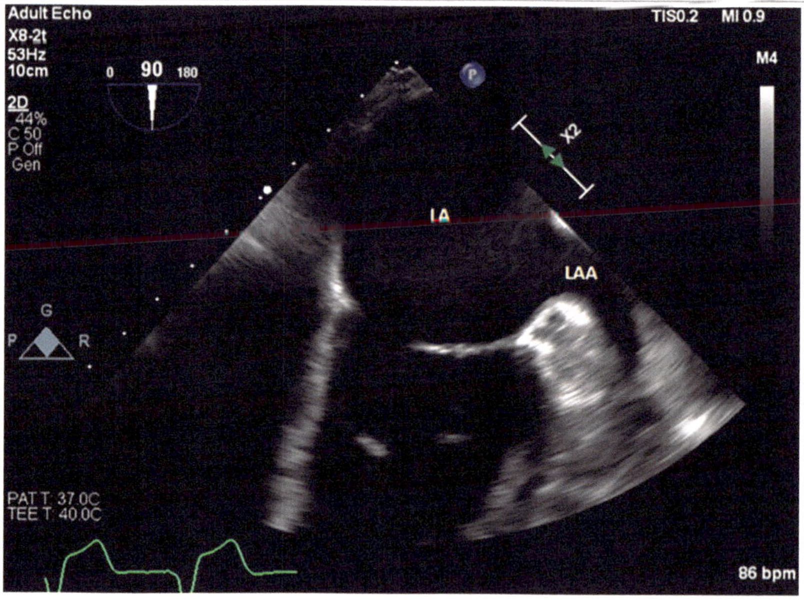

Image/video 6. ME LAA view.

Image/Video 9.6 ME LAA view

(continued)

Mid-esophageal Bicaval 80–100° Centering on the IAS at 0° and increasing the omniplane to 80–100°, then rotating the probe to the right, will visualize the LA, RA, right atrial appendage (RAA), IAS, superior vena cava (SVC), and inferior vena cava (IVC). Depending on probe alignment, the coronary sinus (CS) may be seen between the IVC and IAS. Alternatively, the ME bicaval view is obtained when rotating the probe rightward from the ME 2C view. The IAS can be evaluated for aneurysm and perforation. A Eustachian valve, crista terminalis, and/or device wires/cannulas may be seen. A further increase in rightward probe rotation or omniplane will allow for imaging of the right pulmonary veins adjacent to the SVC (Image/Video 9.7) [1, 3]	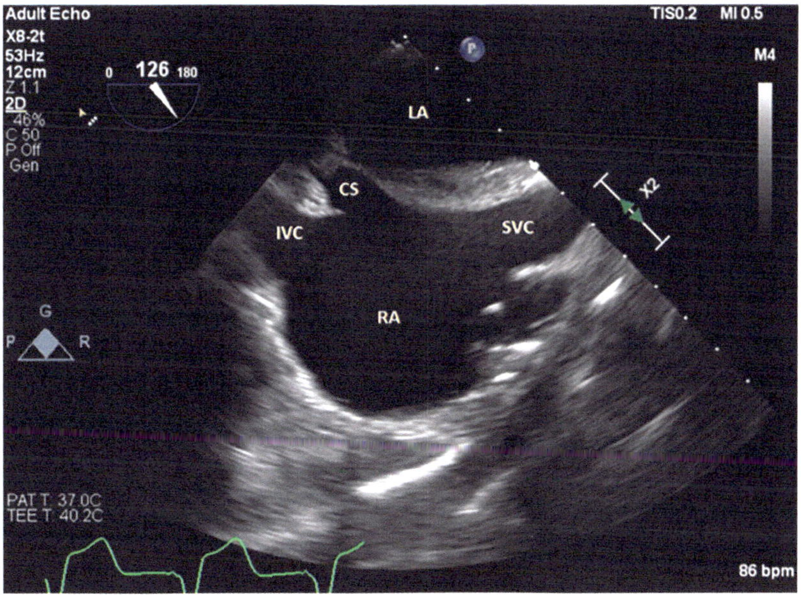 Image/video 7. ME bicaval view. Image/Video 9.7 ME bicaval view
Mid-esophageal modified Bicaval Continuing to increase the omniplane from the ME Bicaval view to 110–140° will align the TV inflow with the Doppler beam (Image/Video 9.8) [3]	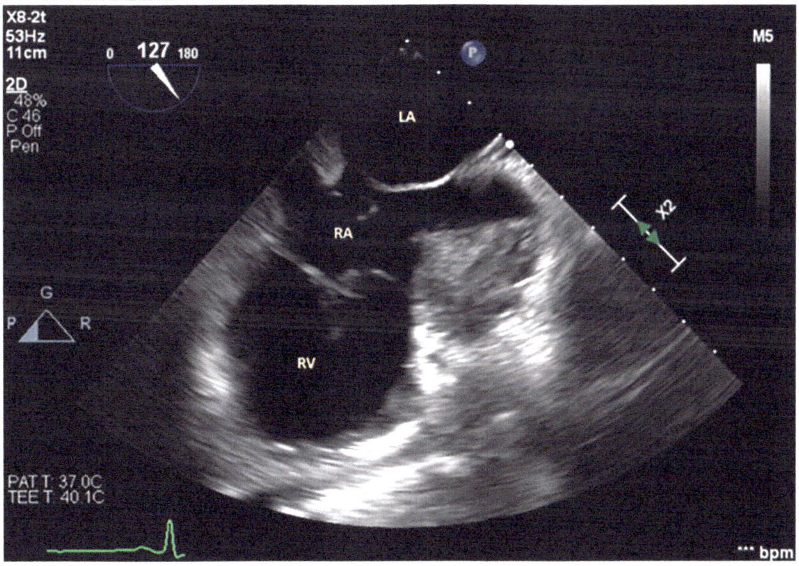 Image/video 8. ME Modified bicaval view. Image/Video 9.8 ME modified bicaval view

(continued)

Mid-esophageal left pulmonary veins 80–100° From the ME LAA view, slight probe withdrawal and/or leftward rotation will position the left pulmonary vein (either the LSPV or the left superior and inferior pulmonary vein confluence) to the right of the LAA. Alternatively, rotating leftward from the ME bicaval view will bring the LAA and left pulmonary veins into view (Image/Video 9.9) [1, 3]	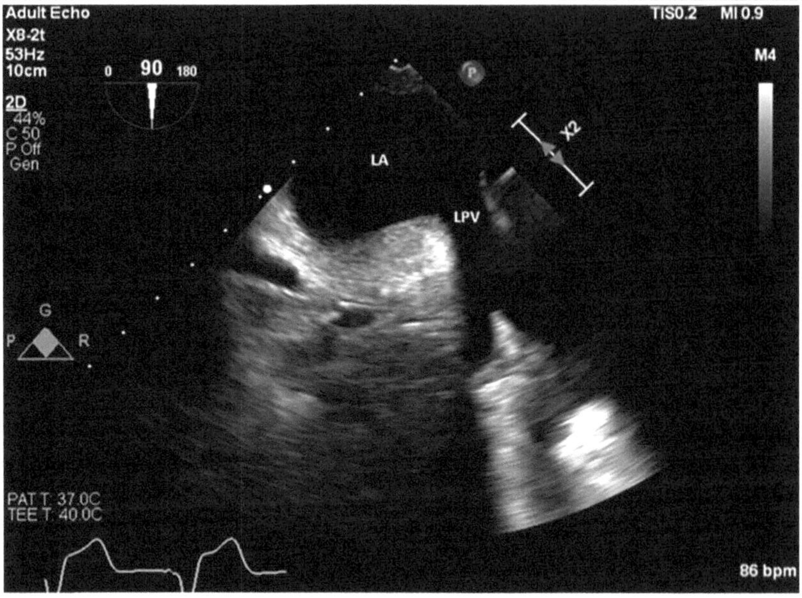 Image/video 9. ME Left pulmonary vein view. Image/Video 9.9 ME left pulmonary vein view
Mid-esophageal right pulmonary veins 0° or 80–100° From the ME 4C view, slight probe withdrawal and rightward rotation will position the right pulmonary veins in the left upper portion of the screen. Alternatively, from the ME bicaval view, rightward rotation and/or an increase in omniplane angle will place the right superior pulmonary vein on screen right, flowing into the LA (Image/Video 9.10) [1, 3]	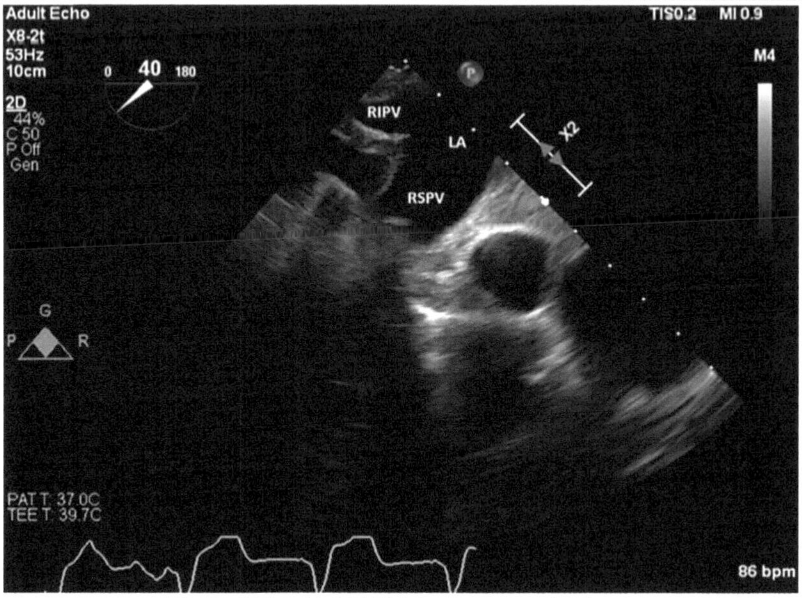 Image/video 10. ME Right pumonary vein view. Image/Video 9.10 ME right pulmonary vein view

(continued)

Mid-esophageal aortic valve short-Axis (ME AV SAX) 30–50° Beginning at the ME 4C view, withdraw the probe slightly to bring the AV into view. Then increase the omniplane to about 40°, utilizing slight probe rightward rotation and/or anteflexion may improve the short axis alignment. The right coronary cusp of a trileaflet valve will be seen in the far field. The non-coronary cusp will be adjacent to the IAS and the left coronary cusp will be on screen right. Visualization of the left main and right coronary arteries is possible with slight probe withdrawal (Image/Video 9.11) [1, 3]	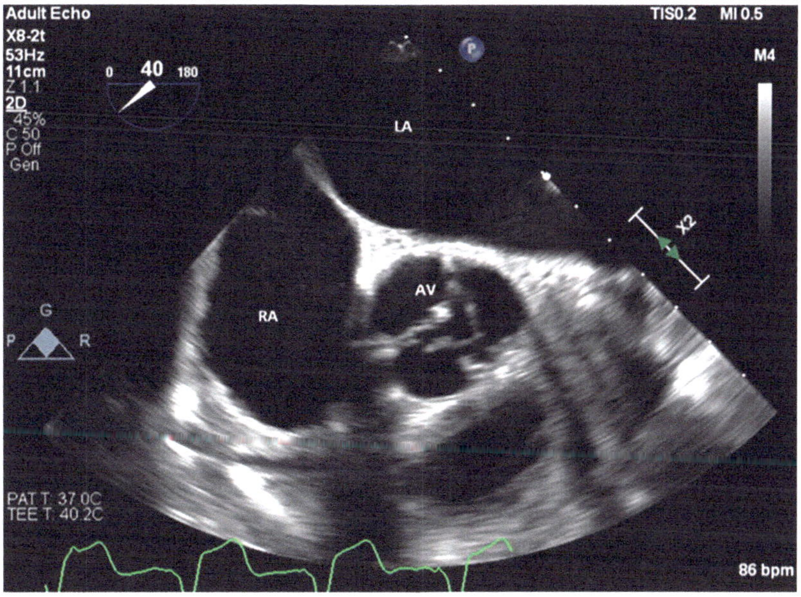 Image/video 11. ME AV SAX view. Image/Video 9.11 ME AV SAX view
Mid-esophageal aortic valve long-Axis (ME AV LAX) 120–150° This is the orthogonal view to the ME AV SAX and is obtained by increasing the omniplane to 120–150° from the ME AV SAX view. Alternatively, from the ME LAX, decreasing the imaging depth and slightly withdrawing the probe and/or adding rightward rotation centers the aortic valve. Structures imaged include: LVOT, aortic valve annulus, right (anterior) and either left and/or non-coronary aortic valve leaflets, sinuses of Valsalva, sinotubular junction, and ascending aorta. (Image/Video 9.12) [1, 3]	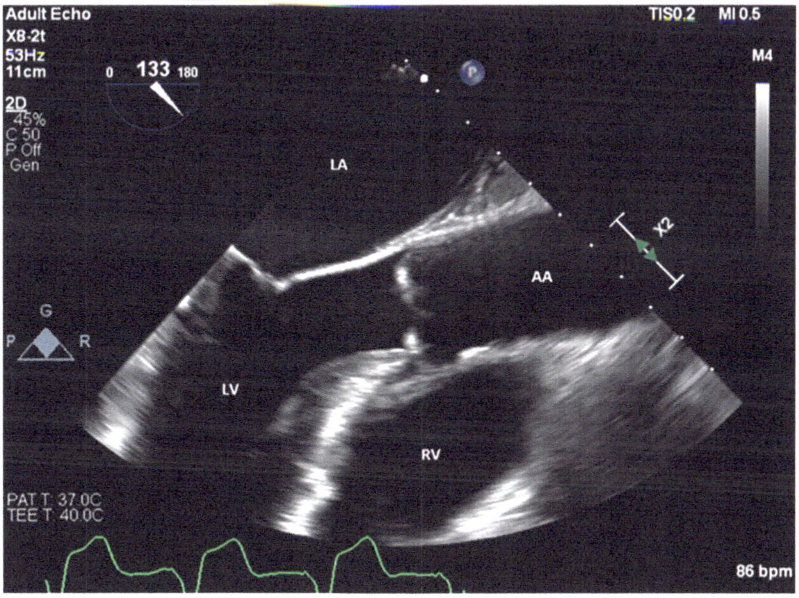 Image/video 12. ME AV LAX view. Image/Video 9.12 ME AV LAX view

(continued)

Mid-esophageal right ventricular inflow outflow 50–70° Begin with a ME 4C view and rotate rightward to obtain an RV centric image. Then, increase the omniplane angle to 60° thereby visualizing the LA, RA, IAS, TV, RVOT, and PV. On the left side of the TV will be the posterior leaflet, while on the right side of the TV will be either the anterior or septal leaflet (Image/Video 9.13) [1, 3]	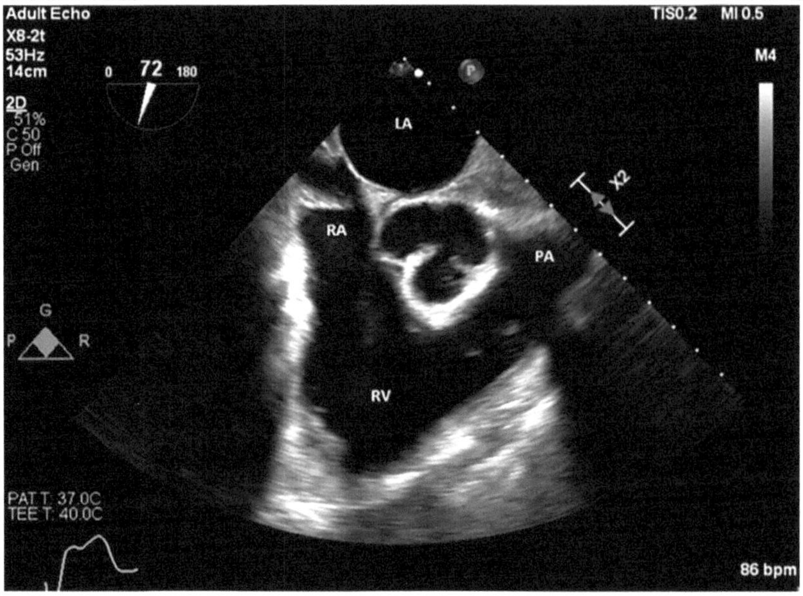 Image/video 13. ME RV inflow outflow view. Image/Video 9.13 ME RV inflow outflow view
Deep Transgastric five chamber/long Axis (DTG 5C) 0° Advance the probe from the ME 4C view, following the LV, into the stomach and to the DTG position. Always yield to resistance in order to avoid patient injury. Once in the DTG position, anteflex, left flex, rotate rightward, and withdraw the probe to center the aortic valve in the screen while keeping the LV apex at the top of the imaging sector. Alternatively, advance the probe into the stomach, rotate leftward, then anteflex and withdraw the probe. Parallel alignment between the LVOT/AV and spectral Doppler allows for less inaccurate calculations than less parallel measurements (Image/Video 9.14) [1, 3]	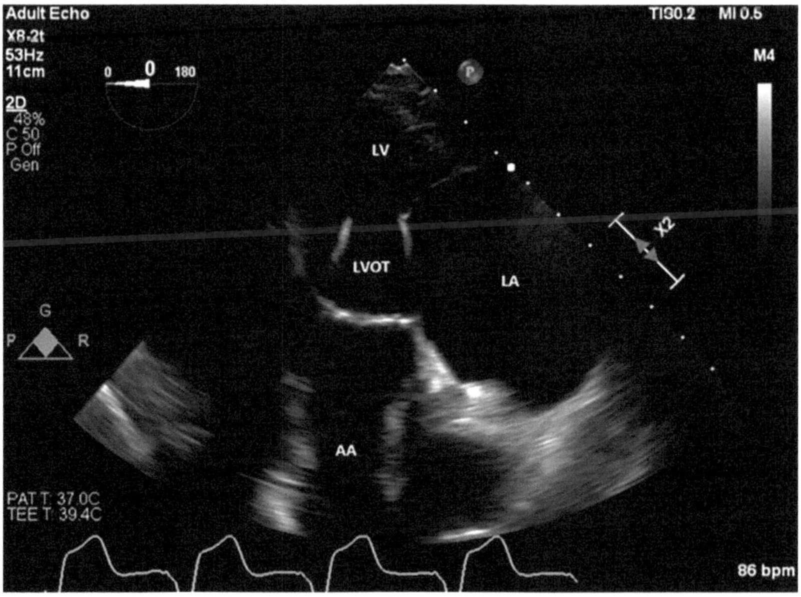 Image/video 14. DTG 5C view. Image/Video 9.14 DTG 5C view

(continued)

Transgastric mid-papillary short Axis (TG mid SAX) 0° Insert the probe from the ME 4C view or withdraw the probe from the DTG 5C, both at 0–20° until the imaging sector is at the mid-papillary level. Slight anteflexion may enhance contact with the LV and improve image quality. Biplane imaging assists in recognizing a foreshortened image. This view enables simultaneous visualization of LV wall segments perfused by the left anterior descending, circumflex, and right coronary arteries (Image/Video 9.15) [1, 3]	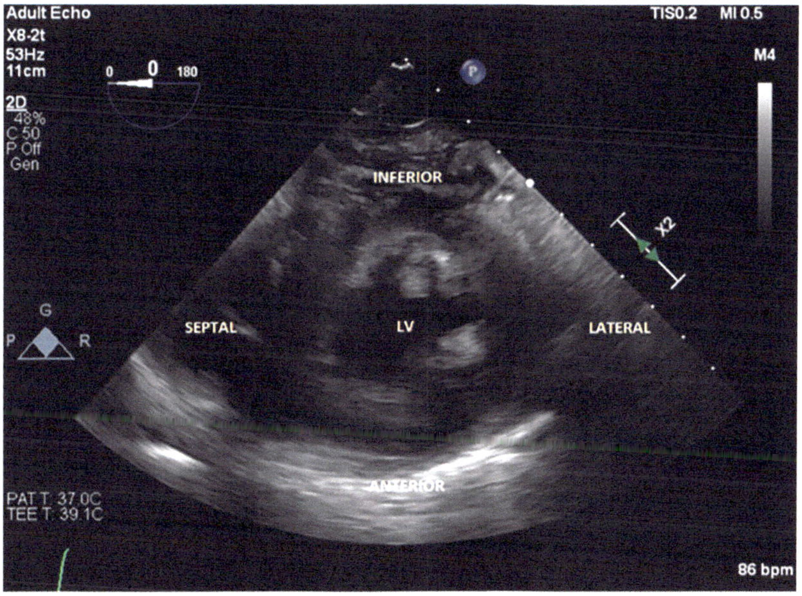 Image/video 15. TG mid papillary SAX view. Image/Video 9.15 TG mid-papillary SAX view
Transgastric basilar short Axis (TG basal SAX) 0° Slight probe withdrawal, and/or anteflexion, from the TG mid SAX allows for evaluation of the basilar LV segments. Also visualized is a short axis view of the MV with the anterior leaflet on the left and posterior leaflet on the right (Image/Video 9.16) [1, 3]	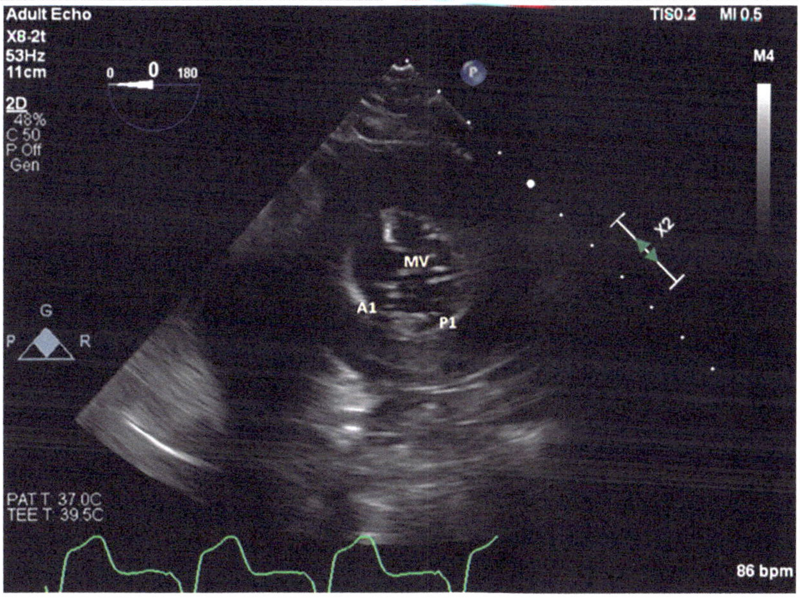 Image/video 16. TG basilar SAX view. Image/Video 9.16 TG basilar SAX view

(continued)

Transgastric apical short Axis (TG apical SAX) 0°

Slight probe insertion, or retroflexion, from the TG mid SAX allows for assessment of the LV apical segments (Image/Video 9.17) [1, 3]

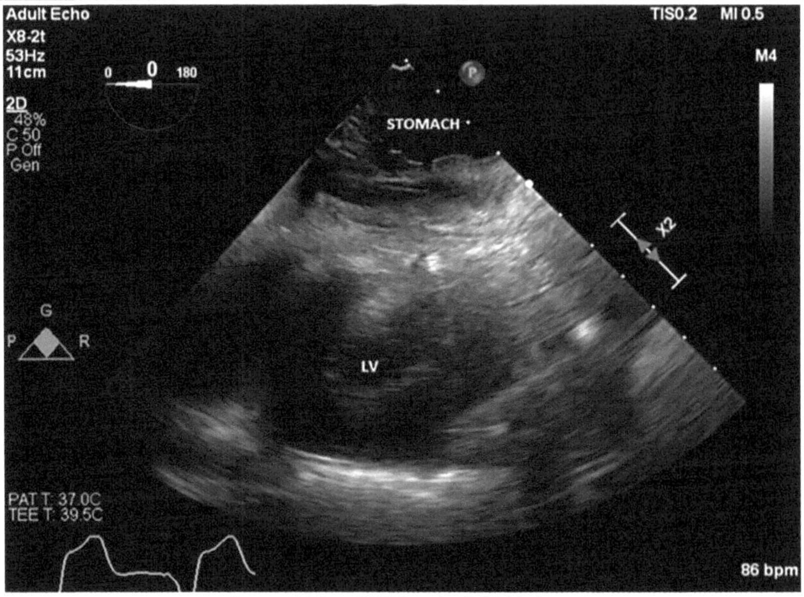

Image/video 17. TG apical SAX view.

Image/Video 9.17 TG apical SAX view

Transgastric two chamber (TG 2C) 80–100°

From the TG mid SAX, increase the omniplane to 90°. This places the anterior LV wall at image bottom (far field) and the LV inferior wall at image top (near field). The MV apparatus is also visualized (Image/Video 9.18) [1, 3]

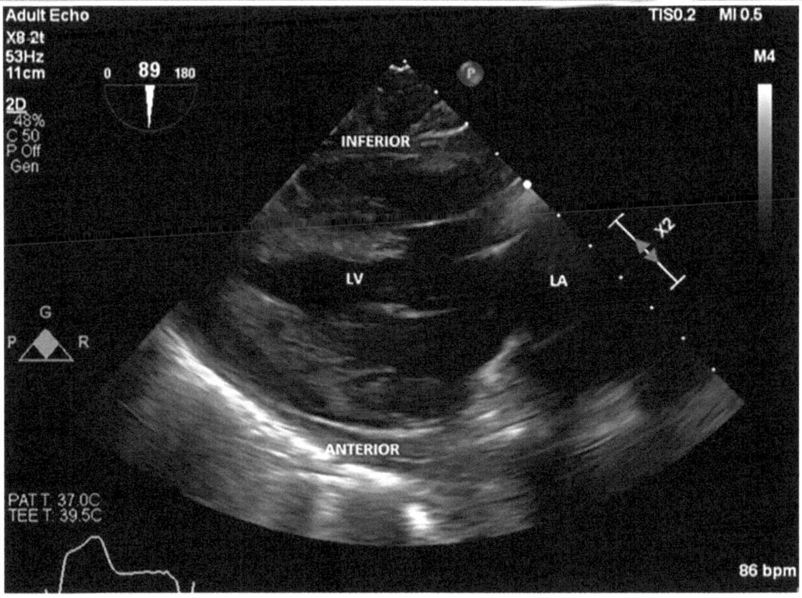

Image/video 18. TG 2C view.

Image/Video 9.18 TG 2C view

(continued)

Transgastric long Axis (TG LAX) 120–140°

From the TG 2C, increasing the omniplane angle to 120–140°, with or without slight rightward rotation, will obtain the TG LAX view. For patients with a difficult to obtain DTG 5C, the TG LAX may align the AV and LVOT appropriately for Doppler interrogation (Image/Video 9.19) [1, 3]

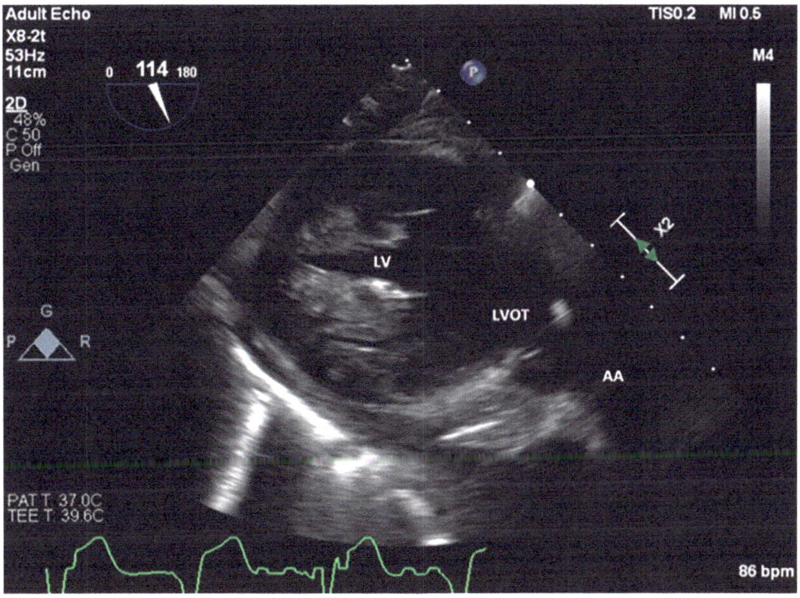

Image/video 19. TG LAX view.

Image/Video 9.19 TG LAX view

Descending aortic short Axis 0°

With the probe in the TG position at 0°, rotate leftward until the descending aorta appears in short axis at the imaging vector apex. Decrease the image depth and utilize biplane imaging to best interrogate the descending aorta. The descending aorta can be followed retrograde in a cephalad movement, from TG to ME and UE probe positions, to the distal portion of the aortic arch (Image/Video 9.20) [1, 3]

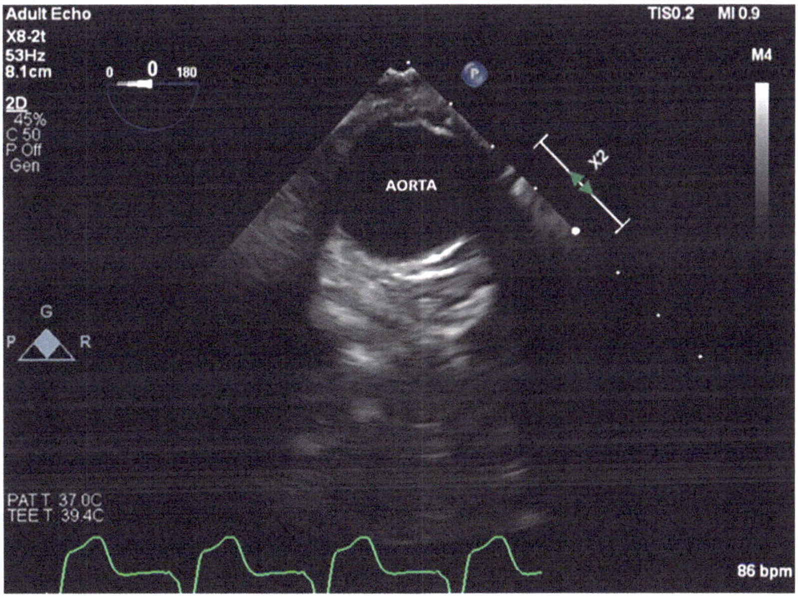

Image/video 20. Descending aorta SAX view.

Image/Video 9.20 Descending aorta SAX view

(continued)

Descending aortic long Axis 90° After localizing the descending aorta in short axis, rotate the omniplane to 90° to view the aorta in long axis. Proximal aorta will be on screen right and distal aorta will be on screen left. Alternatively, utilize biplane imaging to simultaneously view the descending aorta in both short and long axes (Image/Video 9.21) [1, 3]	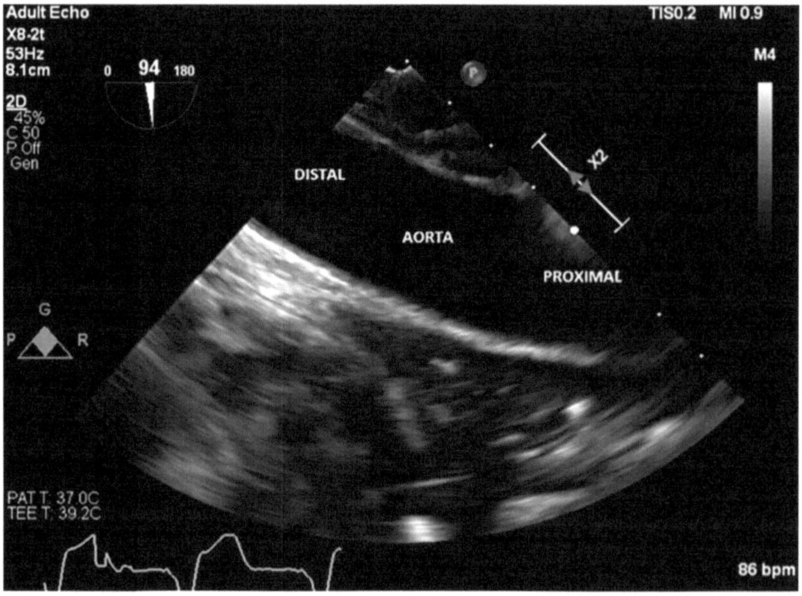 Image/video 21. Descending Aorta LAX view. Image/Video 9.21 Descending aorta LAX view
Upper esophageal aortic arch long Axis 0° As the descending aorta is viewed in short axis from the TG to UE probe positions, the aorta will change from a circular descending aorta to an elliptical aortic arch. The left subclavian, left common carotid, and innominate arteries may be visualized with rightward probe rotation and increased omniplane toward 90°. Part of the aortic arch will likely be obscured by the left main bronchus as it passes between the esophagus and aorta (Image/Video 9.22) [1, 3]	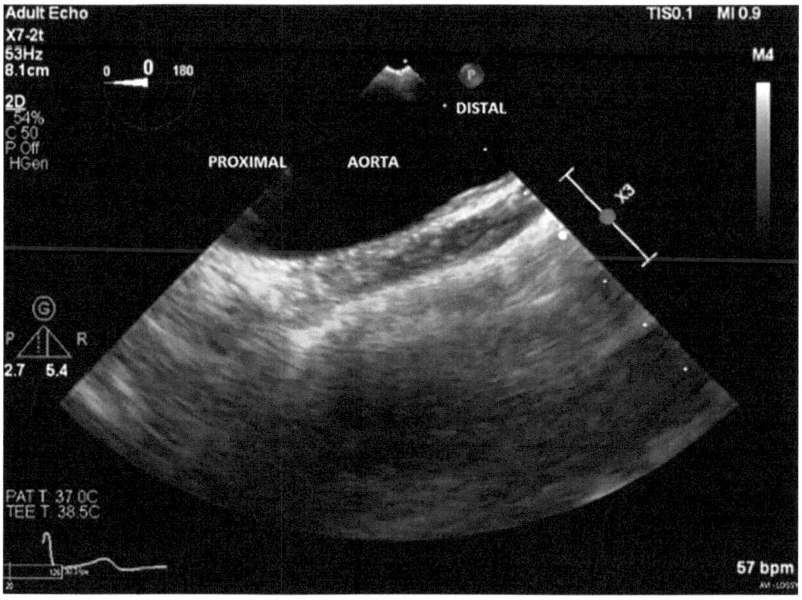 Image/video 22. UE aortic arch LAX view. Image/Video 9.22 UE aortic arch LAX view

(continued)

Upper esophageal aortic arch short Axis 90°

From the upper esophageal aortic arch short axis view, increase the omniplane angle to 90° to view the aortic arch in short axis. Alterations of probe depth and omniplane angle will bring the main pulmonary artery and pulmonic valve into view (Image/Video 9.23) [1, 3]

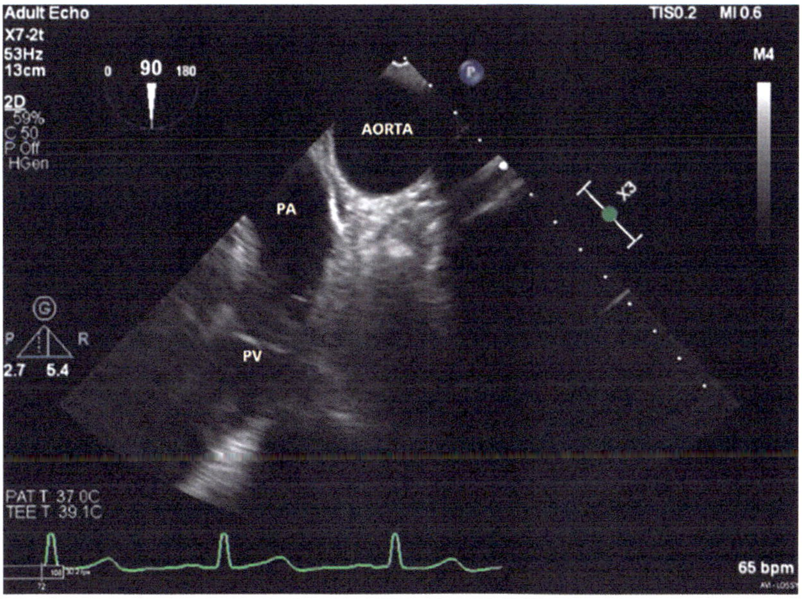

Image/video 23. UE aortic arch SAX view.

Image/Video 9.23 UE aortic arch SAX view

Mid-esophageal ascending aorta short Axis 0–20°

Beginning with the ME 5C or ME AV SAX view, adjust the omniplane angle to 0–20° and withdraw the probe slightly, visualizing the ascending aorta and SVC in short axis and main pulmonary artery (PA) in long axis. The right PA is seen interposed between the probe and aorta. The left PA is obscured by the left main bronchus. This view can be used to identify the position of a PA catheter tip during catheter placement or identify a proximal "saddle" pulmonary embolism (Image/Video 9.24) [1, 3]

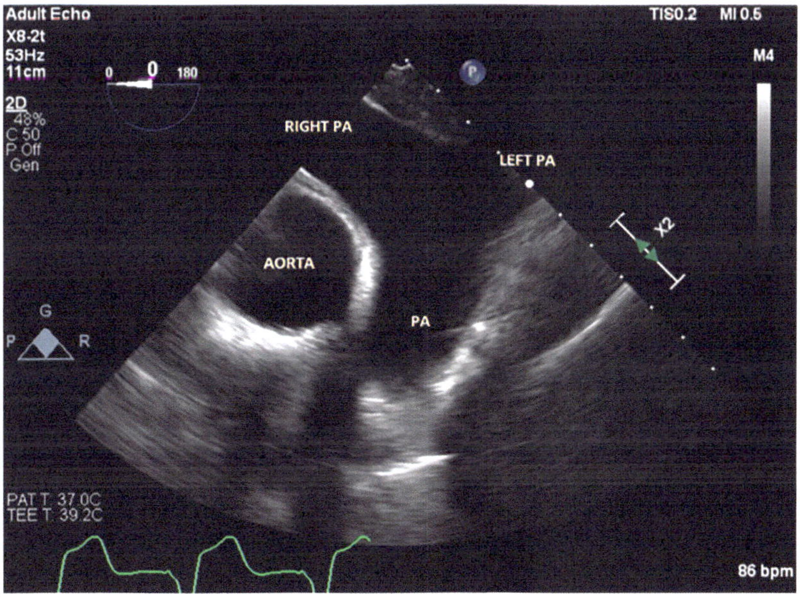

Image/video 24. ME ascending aorta SAX view.

Image/Video 9.24 ME ascending aorta SAX view

(continued)

Mid-esophageal ascending aorta long axis 90–110°

This view is orthogonal to the mid-esophageal ascending aorta short axis view and can be obtained by increasing the omniplane from that position. Alternatively, from the ME AV LAX view, slight omniplane decrease and probe withdrawal will display the PA in short axis again interposed between the probe and the ascending aorta in long axis (Image/Video 9.25) [1, 3]

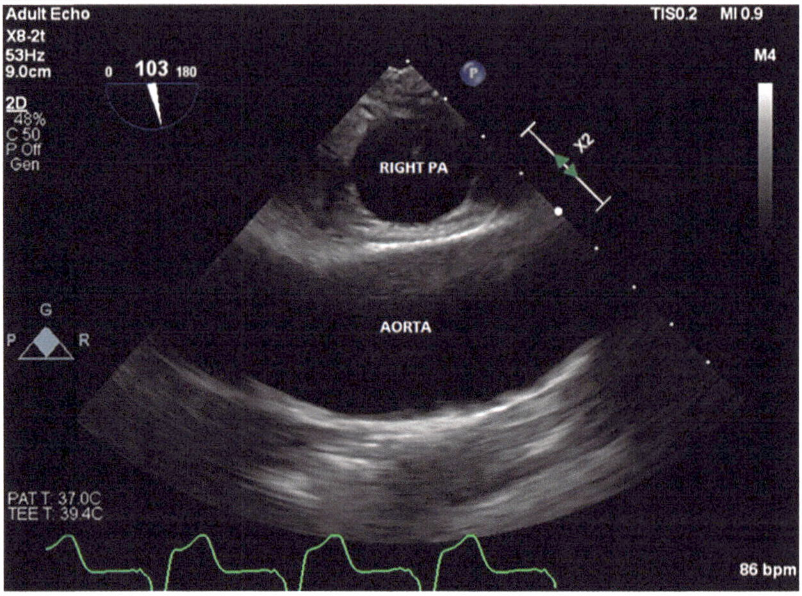

Image/video 25. ME ascending aorta LAX view.

Image/Video 9.25 ME ascending aorta LAX view

3D transesophageal imaging

While 2D imaging acquires individual sector scans to produce a planar image, three-dimensional (3D) imaging utilizes pyramidal volume data sets to display an image capable of being manipulated in the X, Y, and Z axes. Usable 3D images begin with a quality 2D image as any limitation within the 2D sector will be present in the 3D image.

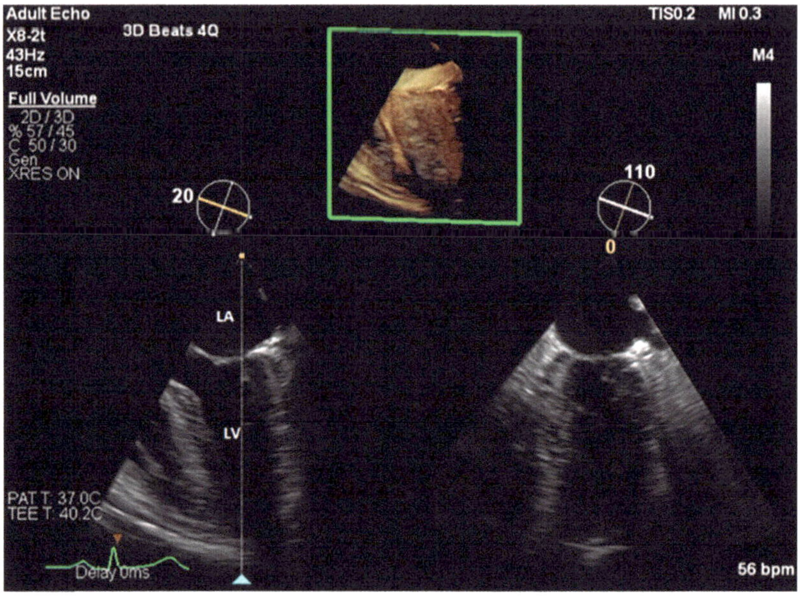

Image/video 26. 3D full volume.

Image/Video 9.26 3D full volume

(continued)

3D image displays range from multiplane to full volume modes, with the acquired volume size altered based on the structure(s) to be imaged. Image acquisition can be in real time or over multiple beats, the latter of which will allow for a higher temporal resolution, but also the introduction of stitching artifact.

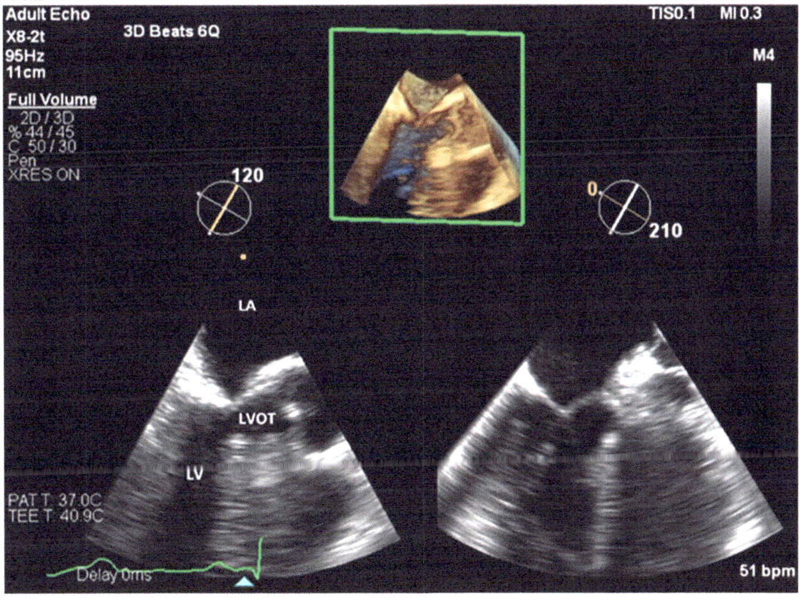

Image/video 27. 3D AV LAX.

Image/Video 9.27 3D AV LAX

Quality 3D images can be used for examining chamber morphology and calculating ventricular volumes and ejection fractions, assessing valve structure and abnormal flow patterns, and visualizing structural heart interventions including transcatheter valve therapies and left atrial appendage occlusion devices (Images/Videos 9.26, 9.27, and 9.28) [5, 6]

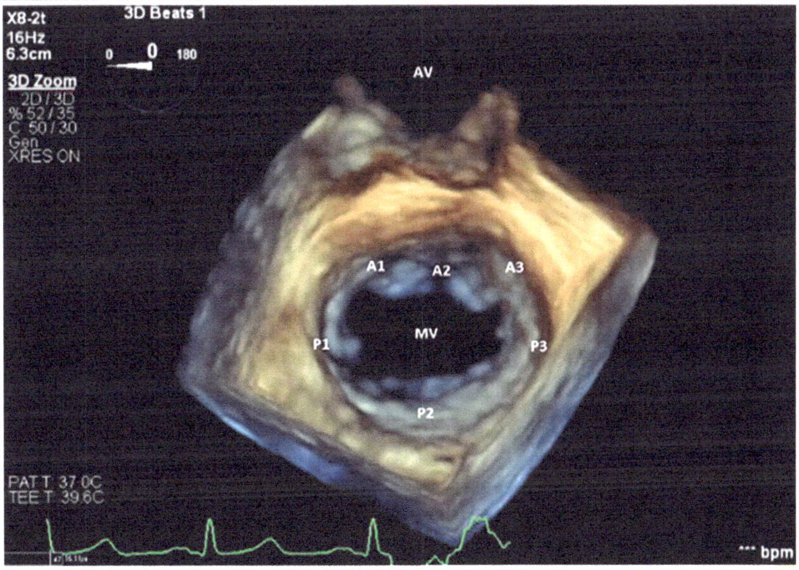

Image/video 28. 3D MV surgeon's view.

Image/Video 9.28 3D MV surgeon's view

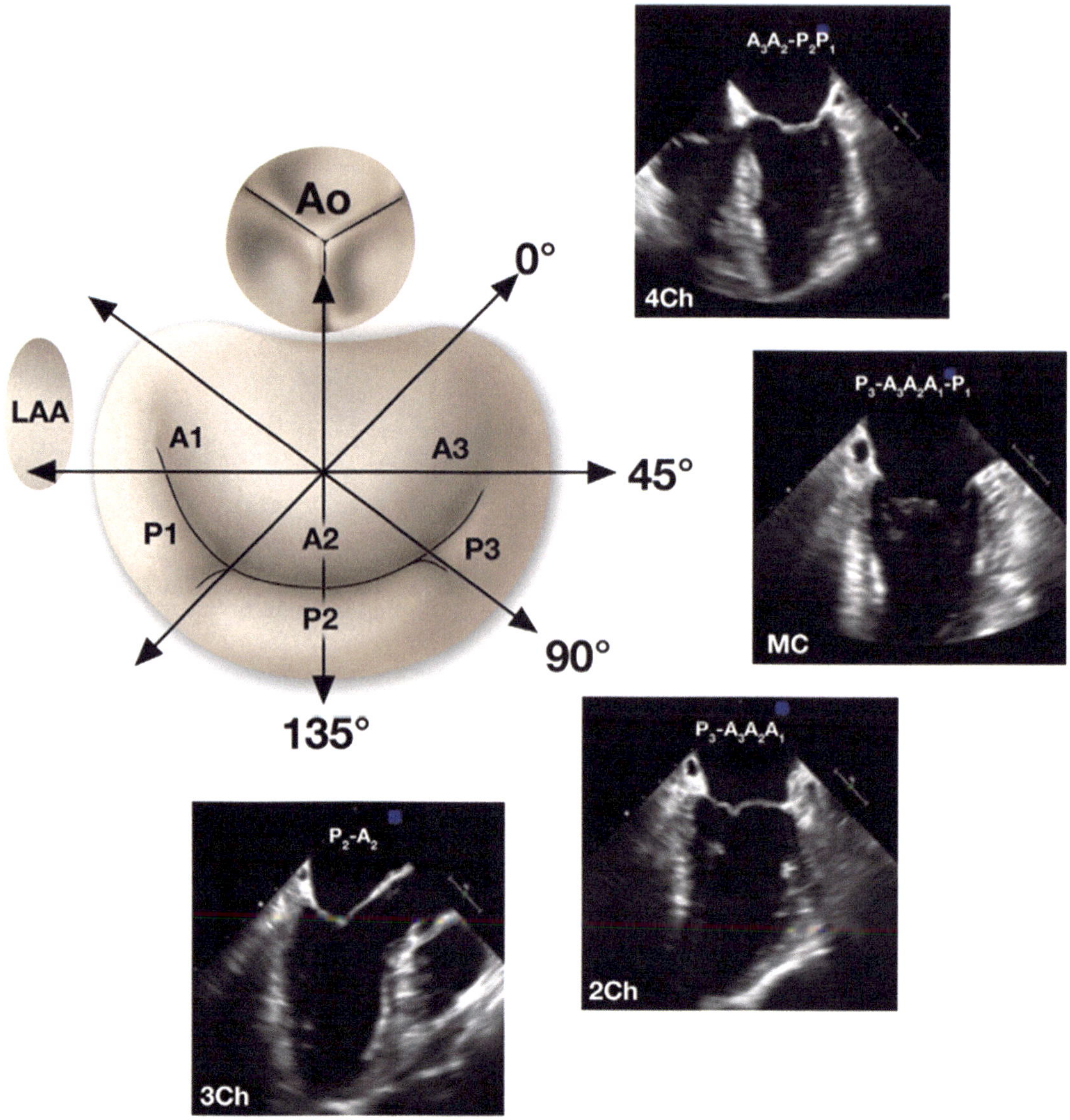

Fig. 9.3 Diagram of MV segments potentially visualized within standard ME views. The actual segments viewed, however, will vary with probe position and movements [1]

Summary Points

- The TEE exam consists of images obtained in the UE, ME, TG, and DTG esophageal positions
- Imaging sequence will be determined by clinical situation and institutional protocols
- Cardiac structure and function can be evaluated with 2D and 3D images, in combination with color flow and spectral Doppler, enabling diagnosis of pathology and guidance of cardiac interventions

Questions

1. Transesophageal echocardiography utilizes which structure as the acoustic window for mid-esophageal views?
   A. Right atrium
   B. Right ventricle
   C. Left atrium
   D. Left ventricle

Answer: Transesophageal echocardiography utilizes the left atrium as the acoustic window in mid-esophageal views.

2. Which image contains myocardium perfused by the left anterior descending, circumflex, and right coronary arteries?
   A. Mid-esophageal four chamber
   B. Deep transgastric
   C. Transgastric long axis
   D. Transgastric mid-papillary short axis

Answer: The transgastric mid-papillary short axis view allows simultaneous imaging of left ventricular myocardium perfused by the left anterior descending, circumflex, and right coronary arteries.

3. At 120° which mitral valve scallops are most likely visualized?
   A. P1, P2, P3
   B. A2, P2
   C. P1, A2, P3
   D. A2, A1, P1

Answer: The mitral valve scallops most likely visualized around 120° are A2, P2, selection b. P1, P2, and P3 scallops may be visualized in a posteriorly directed mid-esophageal two chamber view. P1, A2, and P3 are seen in the mid-esophageal mitral commissural view. A2/A1, P1 are imaged in a mid-esophageal five/four chamber view.

References

1. Hahn RT, Abraham T, Adams MS, et al. Guidelines for performing a comprehensive transesophageal echocardiographic examination: recommendations from the American Society of Echocardiography and the Society of Cardiovascular Anesthesiologists. J Am Soc Echocardiogr. 2013;26:921–64.
2. Puchalski MD, Lui GK, Miller-Hance WC, et al. Guidelines for performing a comprehensive transesophageal echocardiographic: examination in children and all patients with congenital heart disease: recommendations from the American Society of Echocardiography. J Am Soc Echocardiogr. 2019;32:173–215.
3. Vegas A. Perioperative two-dimensional transesophageal echocardiography: a practical handbook. Springer; 2018. https://doi.org/10.1007/978-3-319-60902-7.
4. Virtual TEE: Standard views, transesophageal echocardiography, cardiac, education, interactive guide. http://pie.med.utoronto.ca/tee/TEE_content/TEE_guideSheet.html. Accessed 23 Dec 2021.
5. Vegas A, Meineri M, Jerath A. Real-time three-dimensional transesophageal echocardiography. Springer; 2012. https://doi.org/10.1007/978-1-4614-0665-5.
6. Lang RM, Badano LP, Tsang W, et al. EAE/ASE recommendations for image acquisition and display using three-dimensional echocardiography. Eur Heart J Cardiovasc Imaging. 2012;13:1–46.

10 Artifacts and Pitfalls in Transesophageal Echocardiography

Marcus Behrens and Tonia Timperley Tauh

Ultrasound Assumptions

Ultrasound images are created by the return of emitted ultrasound pulses that have interacted with targeted structures. These returning signals are then received by the probe and processed thereby producing an image. Unfortunately, the machine is limited by certain assumptions, listed below [1].

1. Ultrasound travels in straight lines
2. Ultrasound pulses are infinitely thin and pulses are extremely small
3. The depth of an object is directly related to the travel time for an ultrasound pulse to return to the transducer; speed = 1540 m/s
4. Echos originate only from objects located on the main transducer axis
5. Echos return to the transducer after a single reflection
6. Pulses and echos are attenuated uniformly by all tissues

Artifacts, defined as "an ultrasound image that does not correlate directly with the actual structure being visualized" [2], are produced when these assumptions are violated. Spatial resolution is the ability of the ultrasound system to detect and display structures that are close together in space. Spatial resolution is a combination of both lateral and axial resolution. Conceptually, artifacts exist due to violation of the ultrasound imaging assumptions occurring in either of these planes [3]. Echocardiographic imaging artifacts can be grouped into either the violation of ultrasound imaging assumptions, equipment malfunction, and finally interactions within an external device (Table 10.1).

M. Behrens (✉)
Department of Anesthesiology and Pain Medicine, University of Washington, Seattle, WA, USA
e-mail: mab221@uw.edu

T. T. Tauh
Department of Anesthesiology and Pain Medicine, University of British Columbia, Vancouver, BC, Canada

M. J. Lanspa, A. T. Levinson (eds.), *Echocardiography and Ultrasonography in the ICU*, Respiratory Medicine, https://doi.org/10.1007/978-3-031-80038-2_10

Table 10.1 A list of the ultrasound assumptions, the corresponding artifacts linked to violations of the assumptions, a description of why the artifact is created, and a clinical example of each artifact

Assumption	Artifact	Violations	Example
Artifacts in the lateral direction			
1. Ultrasound travels in a straight line	Refraction Reflection	Ultrasound travels in broken lines and is redirected in different angles	Double aortic valve
2. Ultrasound pulses are extremely small and pulses are extremely thin	Beam width	Echos originate from objects located off the transducer axis	Thickened or blurred valves
3. The depth of an object is directly related to the travel time for an ultrasound pulse to return to the transducer; speed = 1540 m/s	Refraction	Different mediums conduct sound at various speeds, echos return from alternative angles which will result in refracted images	Pseudoaneurysm of aorta
4. Echos originate only from the main transducer axis	Side lobe, grating lobe	Echos originate from objects located off the transducer axis	Dissection flap ascending aorta
Artifacts in the axial direction			
5. Echos return to the transducer after a single reflection	Reverberation, mirror image	Echos are reflected multiple times and will take longer before it returns to echo probe	Double barrel aorta
6. Pulses and echos are attenuated uniformly by all tissues	Shadowing, enhancement	Brightness of an object is related to not only the reflective properties, but also to the acoustic shadow and enhancement of nearby structures	Areas of heavy calcification and presence of external device such as guidewire, valve implant, and catheters

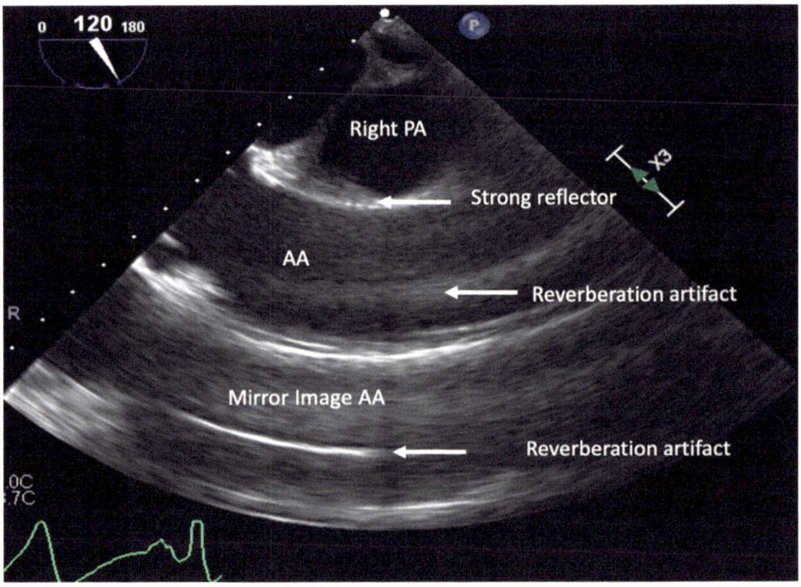

Fig. 10.1 Mid-esophageal ascending aortic long axis with an example of both mirror image and reverberation artifact. *PA* pulmonary artery

Reverberation Artifact

The reverberation artifact violates the assumption that the ultrasound beam returns to the transducer after a single reflection. This occurs when an ultrasound beam encounters two strong parallel reflectors, for example, such as the pulmonary artery and aorta interface, mimicking an intimal flap (Fig. 10.1).

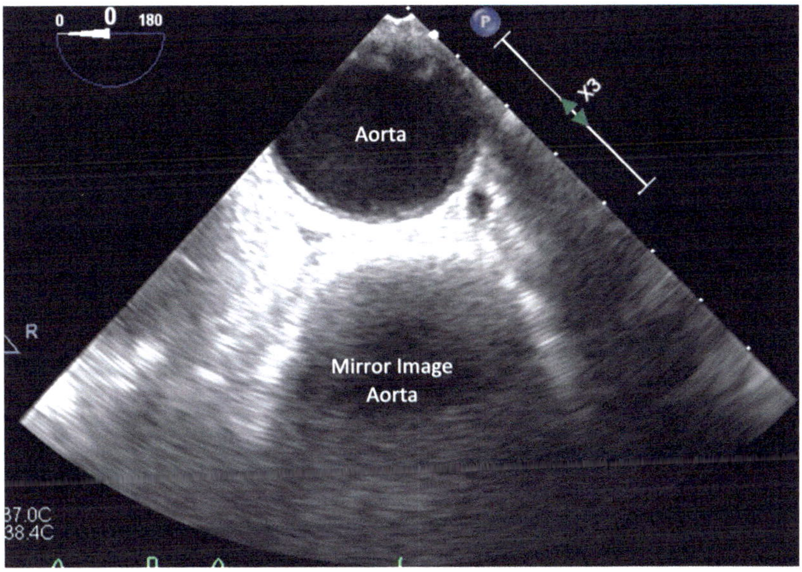

Fig. 10.2 Descending aortic short axis with an example of a mirror image artifact of the descending aorta

To generate an image, a sound beam is emitted and travels through tissues. Normally, the sound is then reflected by the structure and travels back to the probe unaltered and uninterrupted. Some of the ultrasound beam, however, can be reflected by a second reflector (i.e., vessel wall, pericardium). The beam returns for the second time towards the original reflector before reflecting back again towards the probe. The processing software locates this second signal as an object located twice the distance from the probe because it listened for twice the transit time before receiving the ultrasound beam [4, 5].

Common reflectors in clinical echo include the anterior wall of the aorta, the left atrial–aortic wall interface, and the pulmonary artery–aortic interface. The two figures in this section show two examples of the aortic wall (the first reflector) and the resulting artifact. Mirror artifact can manifest a whole mirror image below the anatomical aorta resulting in a double barrel aortic artifact (Fig. 10.1) or an artifact aorta below the real one in cross section (Fig. 10.2). Reverberation artifacts always occur as a reoccurring structures equidistant from each other below the real object.

Side-Lobe Artifact

A side-lobe artifact violates the assumption that all echoes originate from objects located on the transducer axis. Typically, ultrasound generation occurs from excitation of piezoelectric crystals within the probe, which contract and expand as an acoustic wave in the direction of the probe. The piezoelectric elements also contract and expand radially and produce secondary beams. These are unwanted but will be present. These radial beams are called side-lobe beams and are low-intensity beams surrounding the central beam. Side-lobe artifacts occur when enough side lobe hit a highly reflective surface and get interpreted as returning with the main beam. Figure 10.3 visually demonstrates side-lobe artifact. The intensity of the side-lobe beams are usually less than the main beam, so the artifact is often less echogenic on screen and can be linear or curvilinear [4, 6].

[There are three things to look for in an ultrasound image when a side-lobe artifact is suspected; (1) A strong reflector with an (2) acoustic shadow below it and (3) lateral displacement of the side-lobe artifact from the strong reflector.]

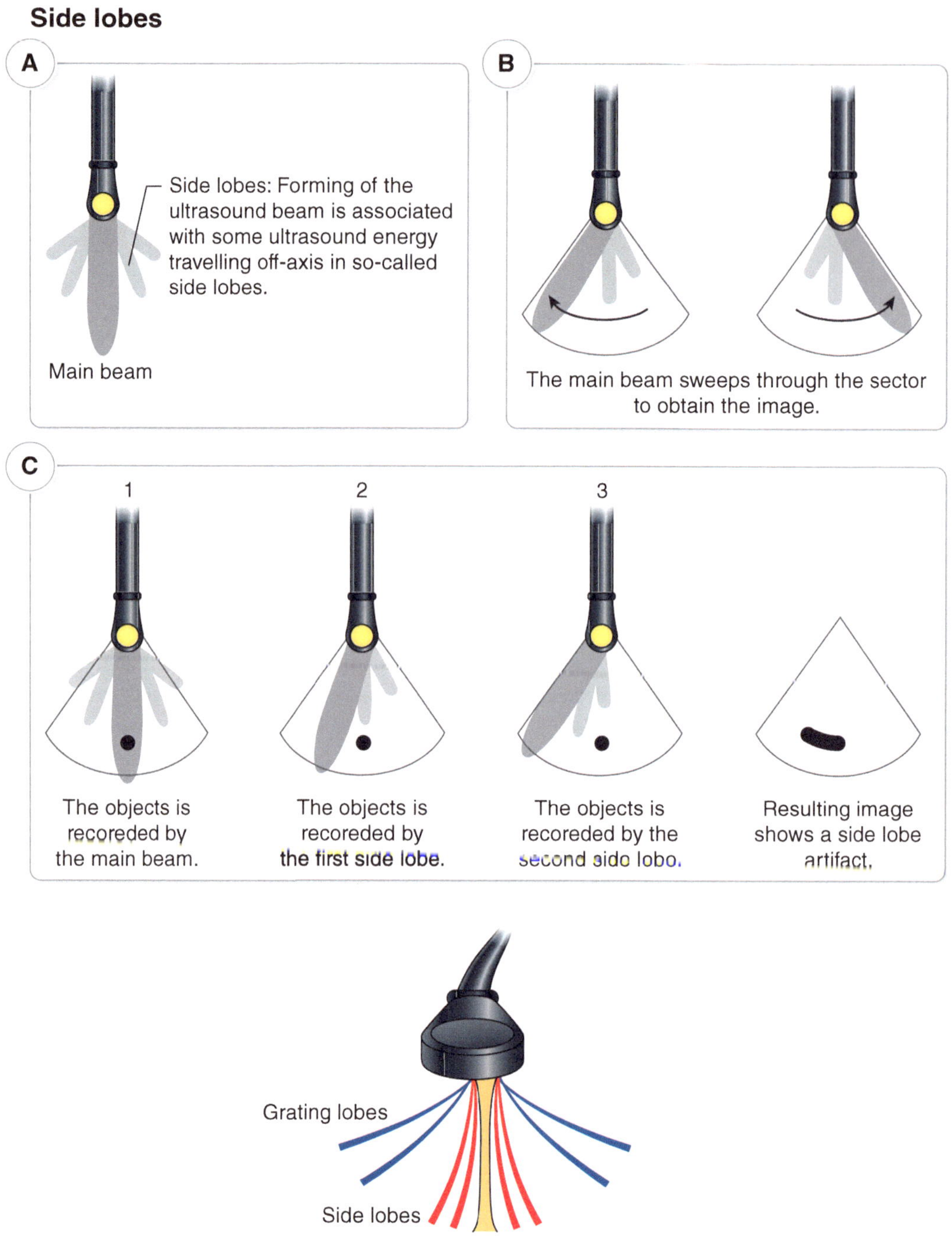

Fig. 10.3 Part (**a**) demonstrates how the ultrasound beam actually forms a focal point, creating a main lobe with side lobes fanning radially. Part (**b**) demonstrates how the main beam continuously sweeps through the sector during image acquisition. Part (**c**) demonstrates how side lobe artifact is created

Grating artifacts tend to occur at more oblique angles (90°), more echogenic and are transducer dependent. Side lobe is another artifact that can clinically mimic an aortic dissection intimal flap as seen in Fig. 10.4.

Reverberation and side-lobe artifacts at the ascending aorta are predictable and expected. Particularly at the pulmonary arterial–aortic interface or the left atrial–aorta interface. Tips to identify artifacts and solutions to avoiding them are summarized in Table 10.2.

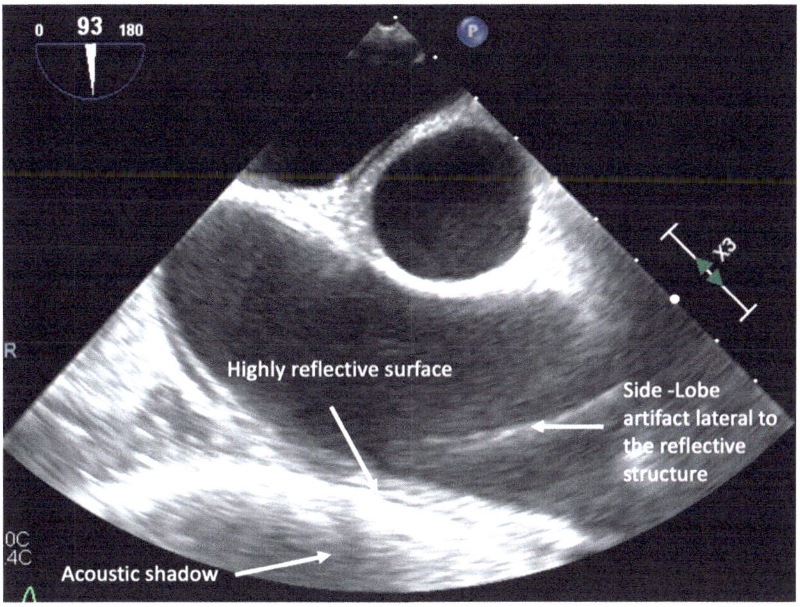

Fig. 10.4 Starting at the midesophageal aortic valve long axis view, the echocardiographer has withdrawn the probe and is demonstrating the ascending aorta in a nonstandard view. A side-lobe artifact mimicking a dissection flap is visualized

Table 10.2 Tips for identifying and overcoming artifacts in the ascending aorta [7]

1	Optimize spatial resolution by decreasing gain and field of view
	Optimize temporal resolution by setting the depth to just below the structure of interest
2	Look for strong reflectors above the reverberation artifact, this is usually the left atrial-aortic interface or pulmonary artery–aorta interface
3	Both reverberation and side-lobe artifacts do not obey anatomical boundaries and can be seen extending beyond the aorta
4	Both reverberation and side-lobe artifacts usually have ill-defined borders
5	Use color flow doppler to establish if flow are the same in both lumens. The presence of similar blood flow velocities on both sides of the flap suggests linear artifact rather than dissection
6	Aortic dissection intimal flaps often oscillate with the cardiac cycle and blood flow whereas a linear artifact will be relatively fixed with respect to the aortic wall
7	Harmonic imaging mode can limit the side lobes threshold and decrease both side-lobe and grating artifacts
8	Change the echocardiographic view to remove the strong reflector interface. E.g., move to a trans-gastric view from mid esophageal
9	Use multiplane imaging with a systematic approach
10	Clinical correlation and pretest probability should be considered if a pathology is suspected

Intravascular Devices

The echocardiographer will encounter a plethora of intravascular devices in the ICU patient. While not exhaustive this list may include central venous catheters, pulmonary artery catheters, transvenous pacing wires, prosthetic valves, percutaneous microaxial circulatory support, extracorporeal membrane oxygenator (ECMO) cannulas, and intraortic balloon pumps (IABP).

Identifying the type of devices will be based on clinical scenario, anatomic location, size, and structure. It is not uncommon for critical care patients to have multiple devices in situ. Any of the listed devices can be linear structures and can create both acoustic shadowing and artifacts.

Prosthetic valves, since they have a combination of graft and metallic components, produce acoustic shadowing. This will limit visualization distal to the prosthesis. One of the artifacts unique to intravascular devices is the ring down effect. This artifact is very common from mechanical prosthetic valves. The mechanism of ringdown artifact is the same as reverberation artifact. This time instead of having only a second reflected sound beam, there are multiple re-reflected sound waves each producing an artifact below the device. An example of reverberation artifact from a percutaneous microaxial pump can be seen in Fig. 10.5 [8, 9].

3D Ultrasound

The modern transesophageal echocardiography (TEE) probe is composed of electrically independent matrix array transducer allowing for imaging of cardiac structures in either two-dimensional (2D) multiplane imaging, "live" or "real time" imaging in three-dimensional (3D), or electrocardiogram-gated multi-beat 3D imaging. While a 2D image is acquired via axial images, 3D images include the addition of "depth" or the "Z" plane that allows for real-time volumetric imaging and acquisition of pyramidal data sets. ECG-gated 3D acquisitions are multiple sub-volumes added together to complete an entire 3D image (Fig. 10.6). Technological advances have improved making it a viable modality in the clinical setting [10, 11].

3D imaging requires high-quality 2D imaging and is still governed by the same physics and constraints of ultrasound. Artifacts exist in 3D as well. The mechanism of artifact creations are similar between both modalities. Additional artifacts are unique to how 3D images are acquired and postprocessed.

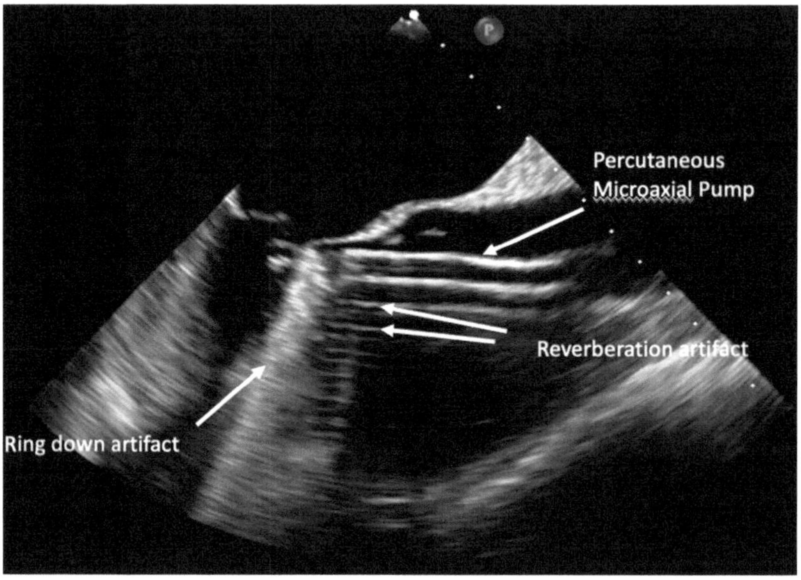

Fig. 10.5 Midesophageal long axis view of a percutaneous microaxial pump with both ring down and reverberation artifact

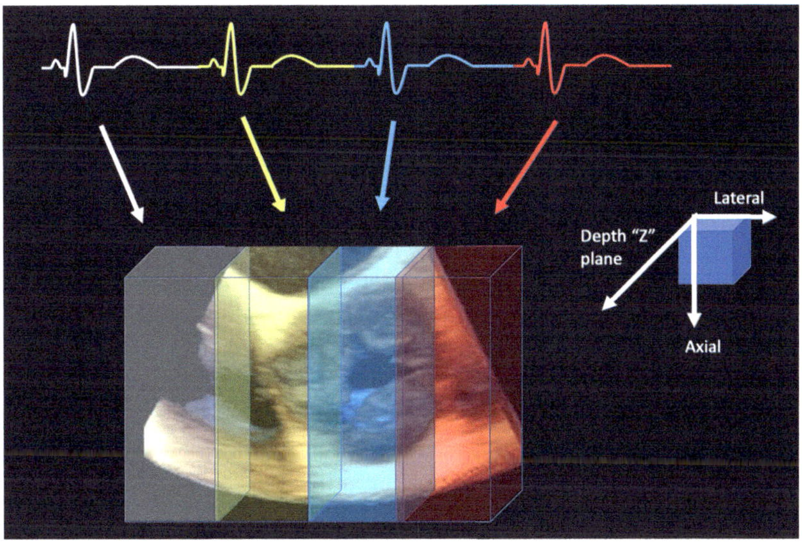

Fig. 10.6 Multi-beat 3D acquisition of an aortic valve. Appreciate how each beat, a sub-volume of the structure, is acquired and "stitched" together to form the entire 3D volume and final image

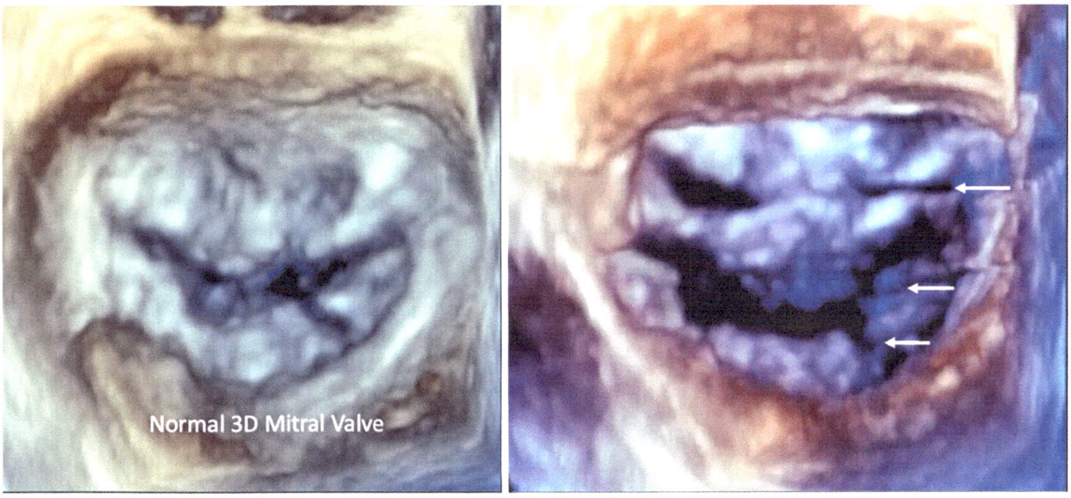

Fig. 10.7 Three-dimensional image of the mitral valve from the surgeons view acquired with multi-beat acquisition showing a complete 3D volume on the left compared with a 3D volume with these linear artifacts called stich artifacts

Stitch Artifact

Stitch artifacts, otherwise known as reconstruction artifact, are misalignment of two or more contiguous sub-volumes created during ECG-gated acquisitions in post processing. In acquiring multi-beat 3D images, sequential volumes of data are acquired with each beat and then "stitched" together (Fig. 10.7). The misalignments are most commonly secondary to arrythmia, electrocautery, patient movement including the patient's respiratory cycle, or transducer movement. Stich artifact appears as shifting or oscillating sliced segments with demarcated lines due to the improper merging of the pyramidal sub-volumes. In an irregular rhythm, multi-beat ECG-gated 3D acquisition is seldom practical. Reverting back to single-beat 3D acquisition or 2D multiplane mode are ways to circumvent this limitation while still taking advantage of technology afforded on modern echo probes.

Blurring and Blooming Artifacts

Blurring artifacts occur as a result of side-lobe ultrasound beams emitting radially, reflecting and being misinterpreted as part of the main ultrasound beam (Fig. 10.5). The side-lobe echoes are then "added" onto the central beam resulting in objects appearing thicker than they really are and with indistinct and blurring edges. In 2D imaging, we are able to adjust axial and lateral resolution, as well as the focus to minimize side-lobe and beam-width artifacts. In 3D echocardiography, the elevation (Z plane) is fixed and commonly causes this blurring artifact. Blooming artifacts are when a blurring artifact occurs secondary to metallic structures interacting with the ultrasound beam (Fig. 10.8). Decreasing gain will mitigate blurring or blooming artifact at the expense of resolution and increase risk of dropout artifact.

Dropout and Railroad Artifacts

Dropout artifacts occur most commonly to thin structures, such as valve leaflets or the inter-atrial septum when imaged in a non-perpendicular orientation (Fig. 10.9). This oblique interrogation with the ultrasound beam coupled with a poor reflector results in scattering of the ultrasound beam and suboptimal signals. Dropout artifact appears as transparent tissues, holes, or perforations on the 3D image due to a paucity of returning signals. While increasing gain can reduce the artifact, it can compromise global image sharpness and worsening blurring or blooming artifact. Conversely, over gain artifact in 3D echocardiography appear as brown speckles with blood signal typically obscuring any structure of interest below.

Railroad artifact is created by vascular catheters or cannulas with large lumens, for example, ECMO cannulas or pulmonary artery catheters. Similar to dropout artifact, the sections of the device that interact with the ultrasound beam at an oblique angle return weak or without signal (Table 10.3).

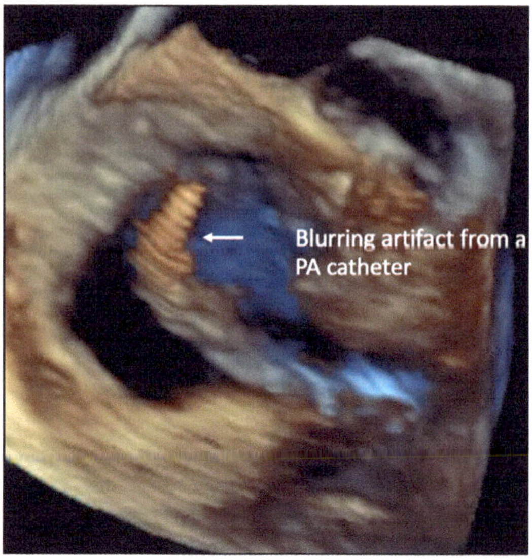

Fig. 10.8 Three-dimensional full volume showing an example of a blurring artifact from a pulmonary artery (PA) catheter

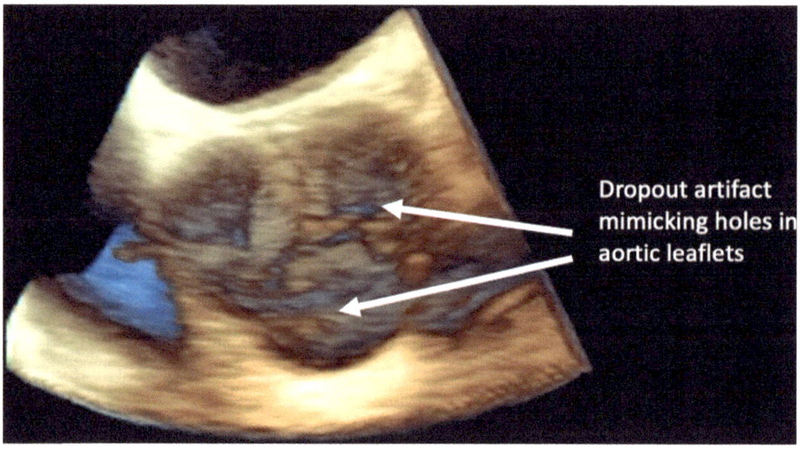

Fig. 10.9 Three-dimensional short axis of the aortic valve with an example of drop out artifact at the level of the aortic leaflets

Table 10.3 Artifacts in three-dimensional (3D) echocardiography

Artifact	Description	Tips
Stitch	Reconstruction artifact due to improper merging of multiple beat sub-volumes	• Arrythmia, electrocautery, patient movement worsen artifact
		• Respiratory artifact, hold ventilator
		• Decrease the number of multi-beats acquired
		• If unable to acquire 3D, then trial 2D multiplane
Blurring and blooming	Side-lobe beams adding to the main beam inappropriately	• Adjust the focus point to the structure of interest to minimize wide beam artifact
	The focus is not at the area of interest	• Optimize spatial resolution by decreasing gain and field of view
		• Optimize temporal resolution by setting the depth to just below the structure of interest
		• Harmonic imaging mode can limit the side lobe's threshold and decrease side-lobe and grating artifacts
Drop-out and railroad	Thin structures with oblique angles to the ultrasound beam	• Optimize gain to bring in drop-out areas while minimizing blurring
		• Change the viewing window to optimize reflecting angle as close to 90° as possible

Common Anatomical Variants and Pitfalls

Anatomic variants typically are either normal anatomy or remnants of embryologic gestation that are misinterpreted for pathology. Classification of anatomic variants is easiest via anatomic location. A complete list of common anatomical variants is organized in Table 10.4. While a complete list of all the possible variants is beyond the scope of this chapter, the highest yield structures both clinically and for examination are discussed below in more detail.

Right Atrium: Crista Terminalis, Eustachian Valve, Chiari Network

The crista terminalis is located at the junction of the superior vena cava (SVC) and the right atrium near the right atrial appendage. Anatomically, it separates the smooth and trabeculated layers of the atrial wall. The crista terminalis is typically seen by the SVC in the mid-esophageal bicaval view and can be misinterpreted as a tumor or thrombus (Fig. 10.10).

The eustachian valve is seen in approximately a quarter of adults as a 1–2 cm crescent-shaped thin band of tissue originating at the posterior junction of the inferior vena cava (IVC) and the right atrium, and extends both anteriorly and superiorly (Fig. 10.11). As a remnant, its purpose was to preferentially direct blood flow towards the patent foramen ovale. The eustachian valve is most commonly seen near the IVC in the mid-esophageal bicaval view or the right ventricular inflow outflow view. The eustachian valve typically does not directly cause flow acceleration on color flow doppler. Rarely, it has been mistaken for thrombus. However, the eustachian valve can complicate IVC cannulation or be a site for endocarditis or thrombosis [7].

Another anatomical variant, the Chiari network, can arise anterior to the orifice of the IVC. This network is a thin filamentous, fenestrated, mobile structure and is an embryological remanent of the sinus venosus (Fig. 10.12). It commonly originates at the IVC and RA junction; however, it can originate from other structures including the right atrium, inter-atrial septum, or the coronary sinus. Similar to the Eustachian valve, the Chiari network most commonly arises from the orifice of IVC, but the Chiari network is

Table 10.4 Common anatomic variants grouped by anatomical location

Right atrium	Right ventricle	Left atrium	Left ventricle
Chiari network	Moderator band	Coumadin ridge	Calcified chordae tendineae
Crista terminalis		Left atrial appendage	False tendons and LV bands
Dilate coronary sinus and persistent SVC		Trabeculations and pectinate muscles	Lambl's excrescence
Eustachian valve		Transverse sinus	
Fossa ovalis			
Interatrial septum aneurysm			
Lipomatous interatrial septum			
Right atrial appendage			
Thebesian valve			
Trabeculations and pectinate muscles			

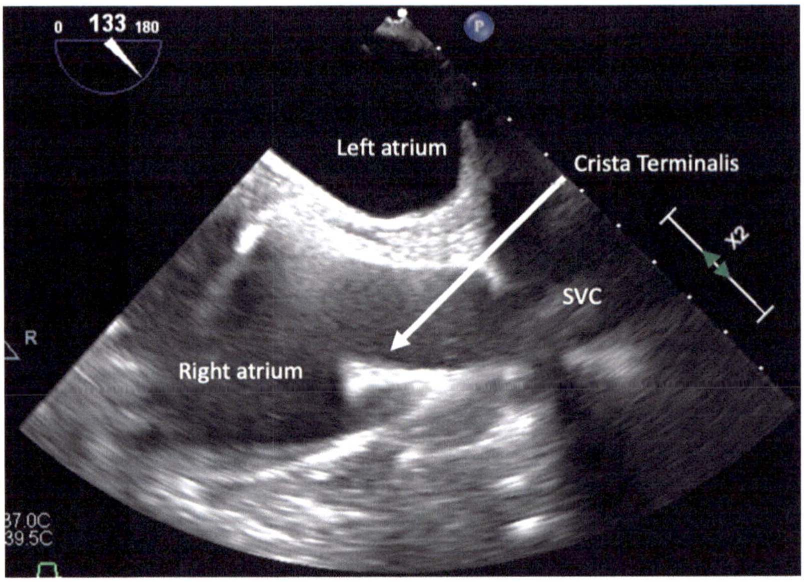

Fig. 10.10 Crista terminalis is labeled in a modified bicaval view

thinner and more mobile. In echocardiography, the Chiari network may be mistaken for tricuspid vegetation, flail tricuspid valve, free RA thrombus, and tumors. Thorough investigation can trace its attachment most commonly to the IVC and rarely the interatrial septum and coronary sinus.

Right Ventricle-Moderator Band

The moderator band is a prominent myocardial trabeculation seen in the mid to apical right ventricle and can be found in much of the population. Functionally, it is involved in the cardiac conduction system. The moderator band is commonly seen in the mid-esophageal four chamber view. To distinguish it from tumor, thrombus, or catheter, the band is a hyperechoic linear structure on ultrasound that originates on either wall of the right ventricle (Fig. 10.13).

Left Ventricle: Fibroelastoma Versus Lambl's Excrescence

Lambl's excrescence are thin structures typically arising from the aortic valve leaflet tips. Historically, there has been a thought that they

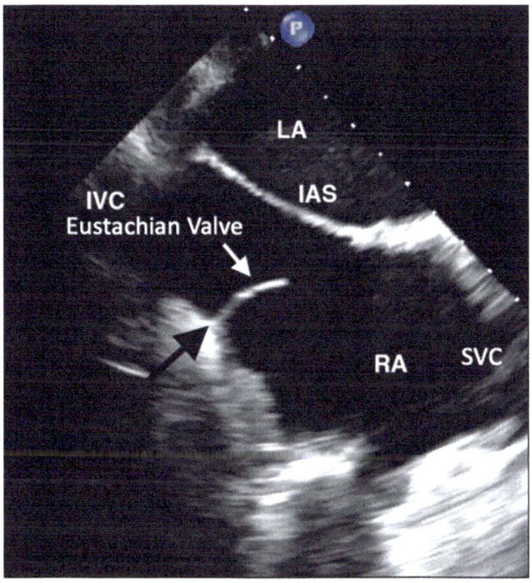

Fig. 10.11 Midesophageal bicaval view with an example of an eustachian valve (labeled with white arrow) at the inferior vena cava (IVC) and right atrial (RA) junction (black arrow). Appreciate how the eustachian valve would direct blood through the foramen ovale of the intra-atrial septum (IAS). *LA* left atrium

develop from repeated shear forces on the heart valves at the lines of closure. It has also been suggested that Lambl's excrescence could be a variant of papillary fibroelastoma. A papillary fibroelastoma is pedunculated, speckled pattern, independent in its motion and is associated with either side of the valve surface. Lambl's excrescence is more filiform, moves with undulating motion and has the highest density at valve leaflet tips (Fig. 10.14). Lambl's excrescence have very rarely been associated with ischemic stroke, making surgical removal of incidentally found Lambl's excrescence quite controversial. Lambl's excrescence are best seen in the midesophageal aortic valve long-axis view [7].

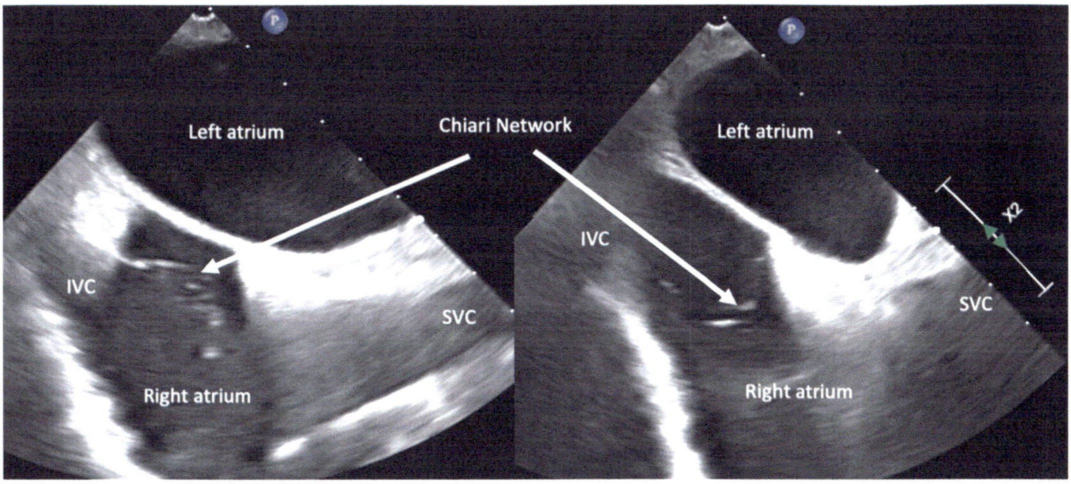

Fig. 10.12 Chiari network shown in two different views at the inferior vena cava (IVC) and right atrial (RA) junction

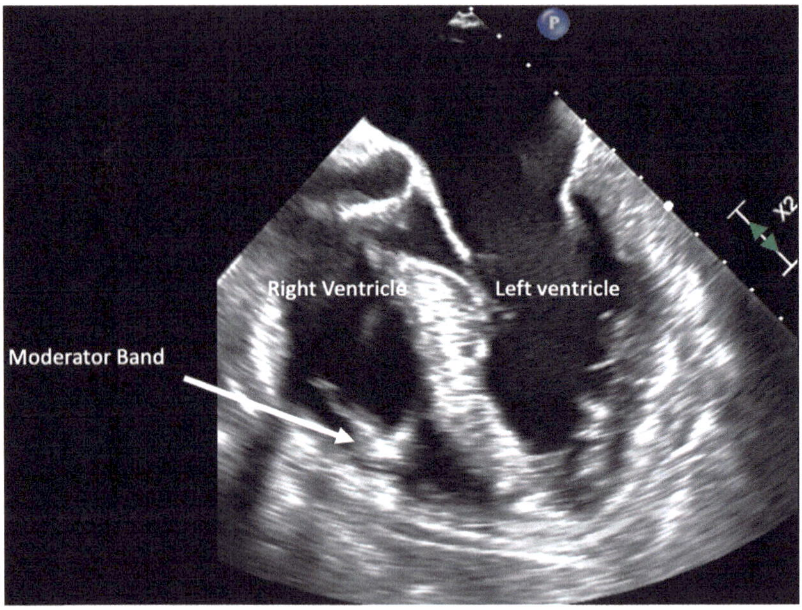

Fig. 10.13 Mid-esophageal four chamber demonstrating an example of the moderator band

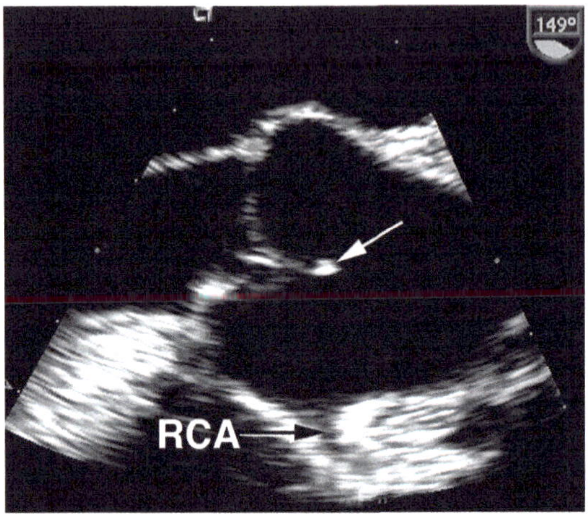

Fig. 10.14 A zoomed in midesophageal aortic valve long-axis view with a Lambl's excrescence, labeled with a white arrow. *RCA* right coronary artery

Summary Points

- Ultrasound images are generated by receiving reflecting echoes and by the machine utilizing certain assumptions, see Table 10.1. After post processing creates an image.
- Artifacts occur for three reasons: the violation of ultrasound imaging assumptions, equipment malfunction, and interactions within an external device.
- Artifacts do not obey anatomical boundaries.
- Artifacts usually need a strong reflector. In TEE, this reflector is usually the left atrial–aortic interface, the pulmonary artery–aortic interface, or an intravascular device.
- Interrogating the structure of interest from an alternative view or multiplane imaging will clinically help avoid erroneous classification as pathology versus artifact.
- The pretest probability and clinical correlation of an aortic dissection should be made and care should be taken to rule out an artifact on TEE mimicking an aortic intimal flap.
- 3D echo also has artifacts including stich, blurring, blooming, and those seen in 2D echo cardiography.
- There are many anatomical variants that should not be mistaken for artifacts or pathology.

Questions

1. What artifact is identified by the arrow in the following image?

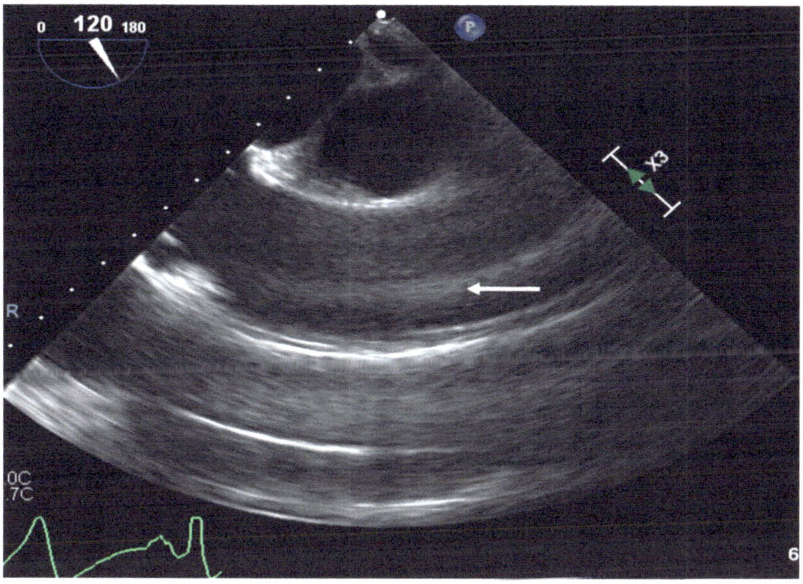

A. Side-Lobe Artifact
B. Stich Artifact
C. Mirror Artifact
D. Reverberation Artifact
E. Ring down Artifact

Answer: D. This is an example of reverberation artifact. The left atrial–aortic wall interface is a strong reflector allowing for echoes to be re-reflected before reaching the ultrasound probe. The reverberation artifact can mimic an intimal flap. With a reverberation artifact, there should be decreasing intensity with increasing distance from the probe. The artifact also should lack independent movement.

2. What structure is identified by the arrow in the following image?

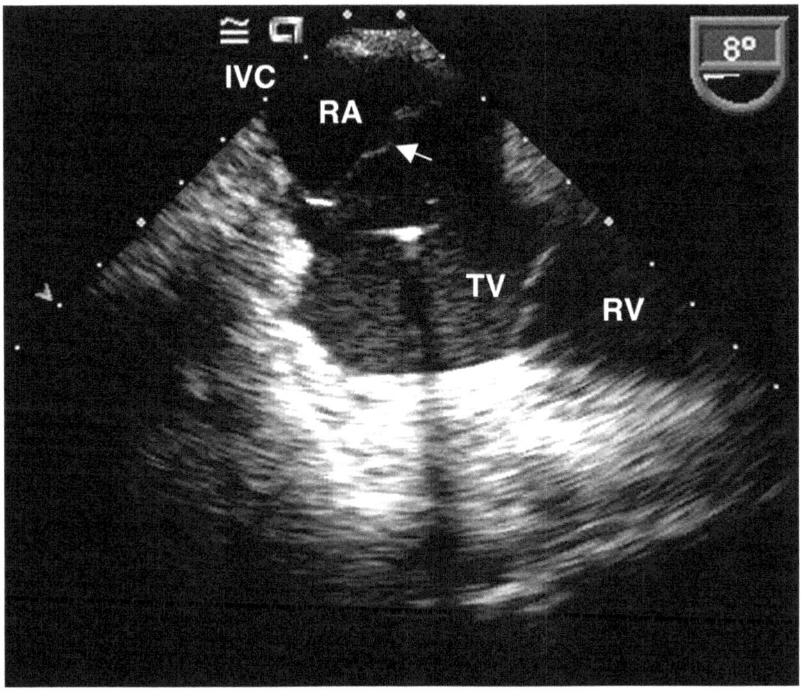

A. Eustachian Valve
B. Chiari Network
C. Cor Triatriatum Dexter
D. Pulmonary Artery Catheter
E. Crista Terminalis
F. Moderator Band

Answer: B. This is a TEE image with an example of a Chiari network labeled with the white arrow. The operator has pushed the probe in from the mid-esophageal four chamber and is showing the inferior vena cava (IVC) and right atrial (RA) junction. This anatomic location helps narrow the differential of the structure being a Chiari network versus an eustachian valve. The very thin, filamentous, and mobile nature of the structure make it a Chiari network.

3. What structure is identified by the arrow in the following image?

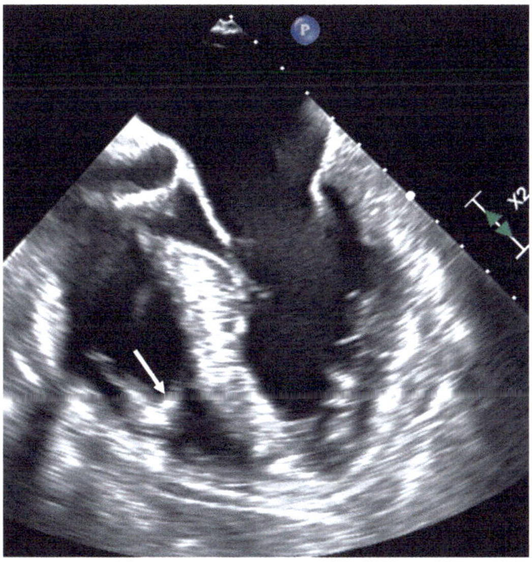

A. Eustachian Valve
B. Chiari Network
C. Cor Triatriatum Dexter
D. Pulmonary Artery Catheter
E. Crista Terminalis
F. Moderator Band

Answer: F. This an example of a moderator band. As a review, this is a prominent myocardial trabeculation seen in the mid to apical right ventricle and can be found in much of the population. Most of the time this test question will present an image in the midesophageal four chamber view similar to the above and Image 14. It possible that a deep transgastric five-chamber view in TEE or apical four-chamber view from TTE could be used to show this structure. Remember the moderator band is a normal anatomical variant.

References

1. Le HT, Hangiandreou N, Timmerman R, Rice MJ, Smith WB, Deitte L, Janelle GM. Imaging artifacts in echocardiography. Anesth Analg. 2016;122(3):633–46.
2. Hykes DL, Hedrick WR, Starchman DE. Ultrasound physics and instrumentation. Mosby; 1992.
3. Quien M, Saric M. Ultrasound imaging artifacts: how to recognize them and how to avoid them. Echocardiography. 2018;35(9):1388–401.
4. Bertrand PB, Levine RA, Isselbacher EM, Vandervoort PM. Fact or artifact in two-dimensional echocardiography: avoiding misdiagnosis and missed diagnosis. J Am Soc Echocardiogr. 2016;29(5):381–91.
5. Allen MN, editor. Echocardiography. Lippincott Williams & Wilkins; 1999.
6. Scanlan KA. Sonographic artifacts and their origins. AJR Am J Roentgenol. 1991;156(6):1267–72.
7. Oxorn D, Otto CM. Intraoperative and interventional echocardiography: atlas of transesophageal imaging E-book. Elsevier Health Sciences; 2016.
8. Klopman MA, Chen EP, Sniecinski RM. Positioning an intraaortic balloon pump using intraoperative transesophageal echocardiogram guidance. Anesth Analg. 2011;113(1):40–3.
9. Otto CM. Textbook of clinical echocardiography. Elsevier Health Sciences; 2018.
10. Lang RM, Badano LP, Tsang W, Adams DH, Agricola E, Buck T, Faletra FF, Franke A, Hung J, de Isla LP, Kamp O. EAE/ASE recommendations for image acquisition and display using three-dimensional echocardiography. Eur Heart J Cardiovasc Imaging. 2012;13(1):1–46.
11. Pamnani A, Skubas NJ. Imaging artifacts during transesophageal echocardiography. Anesth Analg. 2014;118(3):516–20.

LV Systolic Function

11

Jonathan N. Wilkinson and Feroz Mohammed

Learning Objectives

1. Understand multiple methods of quantifying left ventricular systolic function.
2. Recognize the limitations of these methods.
3. Correlate regional wall motion abnormalities with the coronary distribution.

Assessment of left ventricular systolic function is a core application of critical care echocardiography. In critically ill patients, most assessments of left ventricular function can be done qualitatively to facilitate a decision at the bedside. One can recognize profound dysfunction without quantification. However, familiarity with quantification may develop one's qualitative heuristics for the "eyeballing" function. This chapter will review some common methods of quantifying LV systolic function used in critical care. Throughout this chapter, we will employ reference standards in accordance with the American Society of Echocardiography and the European Association of Cardiovascular Imaging [1].

Supplementary Information The online version contains supplementary material available at https://doi.org/10.1007/978-3-031-80038-2_11.

J. N. Wilkinson (✉) · F. Mohammed
Intensive Care and Anaesthesia, Northampton, UK

Structural Anatomy

The left ventricle has three parts: The inlet, containing the mitral valve; the apex, containing a trabeculated network, and the outlet, containing the aortic valve. The orientation of the cardiac muscles provides the basis for the heart to function as a pump. The ellipsoid shape of the left ventricle is a result of the laminar layering of spiraling bundles of cardiac muscles. The muscle bundles are longitudinal in the subepicardial myocardium, circumferential in the middle segment and become longitudinal again in the subendocardial myocardium.

This muscular configuration results in a more complex contraction profile than is first apparent on 2D ultrasound (pure up-down movement). At the apex and base, there is vertical contraction, whereas in the middle, there is circumferential contraction. Movement therefore occurs in a fashion more akin to the ringing of a wet cloth with the LV ejecting blood in a corkscrew-type motion. It begins at the base and ends at the apex.

The architecturally complex structure of the LV allows maximal shortening of myocytes, which results in increased wall thickness and the generation of force during systole. Moreover, the release of the twisted LV may provide a suction mechanism facilitating the filling of the LV during diastole.

M. J. Lanspa, A. T. Levinson (eds.), *Echocardiography and Ultrasonography in the ICU*, Respiratory Medicine, https://doi.org/10.1007/978-3-031-80038-2_11

Chamber Dimensions and Size

Left ventricular size is commonly assessed using the internal linear dimension from the parasternal long-axis view. The internal diameter is measured at the level of the mitral valve leaflet tips. Measurement should be performed using two-dimensional (2D) images rather than M-mode images, as the internal diameter may be nonorthogonal to the ultrasound, although M-mode can provide high temporal resolution. The measurement should be perpendicular to the long axis of the ventricle. Care should be taken to avoid confusing the chordae or papillary muscle with the inferolateral wall. The endpoints of the linear segment should be positioned at the endocardial border. Measurement should occur at end-diastole (LVIDd, Fig. 11.1) and end-systole (LVIDs, Fig. 11.2). Table 11.1 demonstrates the normal values of LV internal dimensions. These linear measurements are assumed to be representative of the entire ventricle. In the case where the mid-ventricle or apex is enlarged, the LVIDd may not be accurate.

LV end-diastolic area (LVEDA), obtained from the parasternal short-axis view at the mid-ventricle, is less commonly quantified in standard echocardiography, as volumetric assessments are preferred (Fig. 11.3). However, various studies in critical care have used LVEDA from the trans-esophageal short-axis view at the mid-chamber, tracing the endocardial border and taking care to exclude the papillary muscles [2, 3]. One study exploring intraoperative hypovolemia found that LVEDA was 9.5–22 cm^2 in normal patients, with an indexed LVEDA <5.5 cm^2/m^2 suggestive of hypovolemia [2].

LV volumetric measurements can be obtained from 2D echo and 3D echo. Volume should not be calculated from linear dimensions given their inaccuracies with approximating the shape of the LV cavity. Rather, volume is calculated using Simpson's biplane method of disks, which traces the compacted endocardial border from the apical four-chamber and apical two-chamber views. 3D echo may offer improved accuracy as it does not rely on any geometric assumptions of the LV cavity. Imaging the apical views with 2D echo should attempt to maximize the LV area and avoid foreshortening of the LV. The imaging depth should be shortened to maximize the LV area on the screen. Outpatient echocardiography is typically performed with the patient in the left lateral decubitus position, which improves both image quality and reduces foreshortening. Critical care echocardiography is often performed with a suboptimal position, which may foreshorten the left ventricle. Additionally,

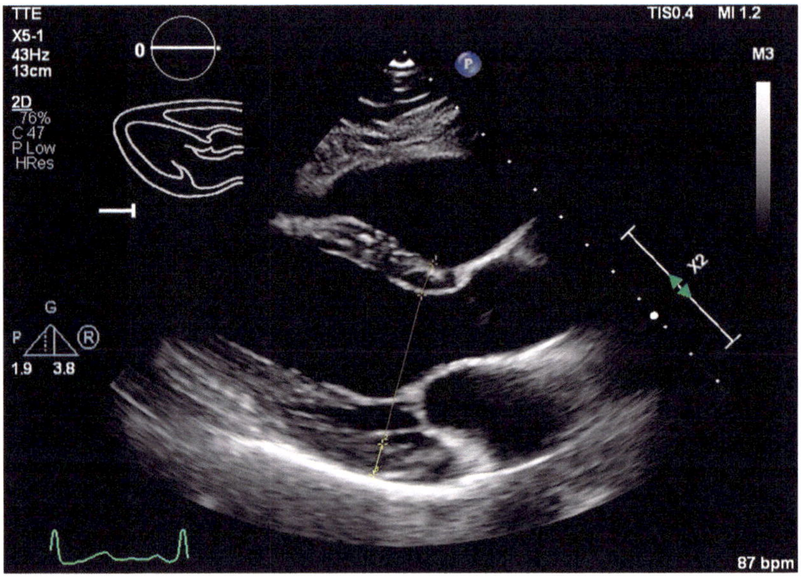

Fig. 11.1 Parasternal Long Axis view, showing a mid LV cavity view at the end-diastolic phase of contraction (Mitral valve closed and aortic valve about to open)

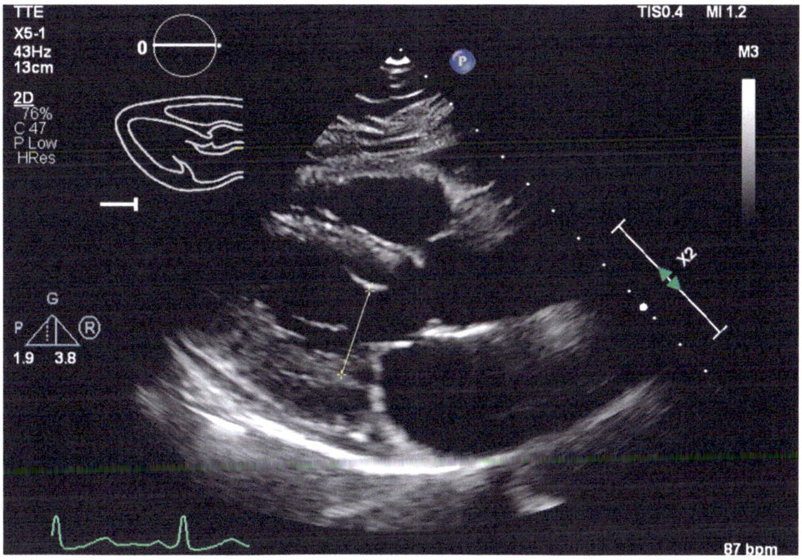

Fig. 11.2 Parasternal Long Axis view, showing a mid LV cavity view at the end-systolic phase of contraction (Aortic valve open)

Table 11.1 Reference ranges for common echocardiographic parameters of LV size and function

	Male	Female
LV internal diameter, diastolic (cm)	4.2–5.8	3.8–5.2
LV internal diameter, systolic (cm)	2.5–4.0	2.2–3.5
LV wall thickness (cm)	0.6–0.9	0.6–1.0
LV end-diastolic volume (mL)	62–150	46–106
LV end-systolic volume (mL)	21–61	14–42
LV ejection fraction (%)	52–72	54–74

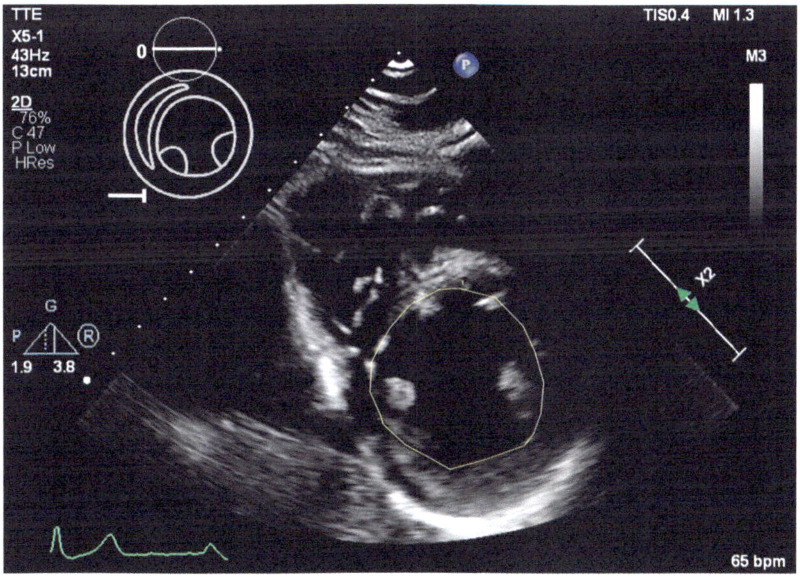

Fig. 11.3 Measurement of end-diastolic area on a short axis view of the heart. The Mid Papillary view is seen here

increased intrathoracic pressure from mechanical ventilation or obstructive lung disease may medially displace the heart apex, which may result in foreshortened imaging. Contrast echocardiography (see Chap. 12) may improve assessment when image quality is poor.

After optimizing an image for acquisition, the measurement is performed by starting at the mitral annulus and tracing the compacted endocardial border to the other side of the mitral annulus. The papillary muscle should be excluded. Viewing the cine loop or the frames immediately before or after may help with discriminating the endocardial border. The tracing should occur at end-diastole (LVEDV) (Figs. 11.4 and 11.5) and end-systole (LVESV) (Figs. 11.6 and 11.7). Although the electrocardiogram can aid in this process, the timing is based on ventricular size

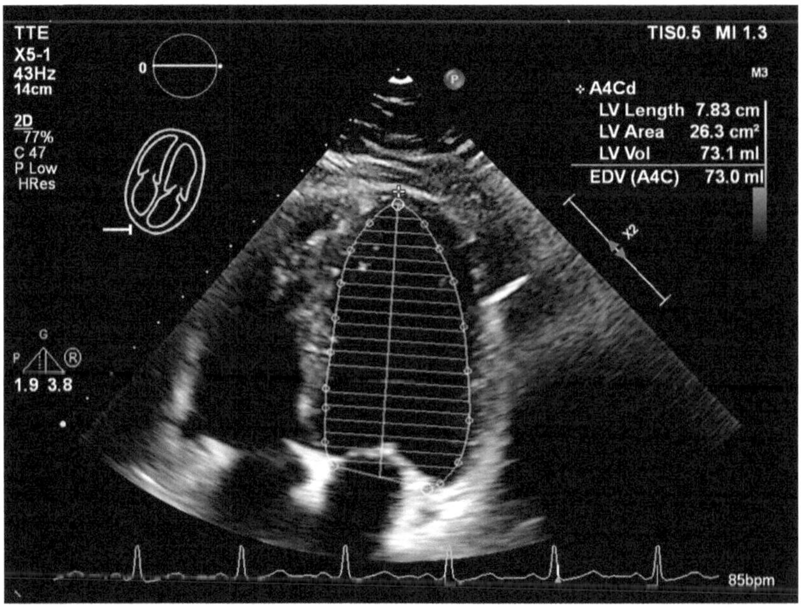

Fig. 11.4 Apical 4 chamber image at end diastole. Demonstrates Simpson's biplane measurement of LV cavity volume

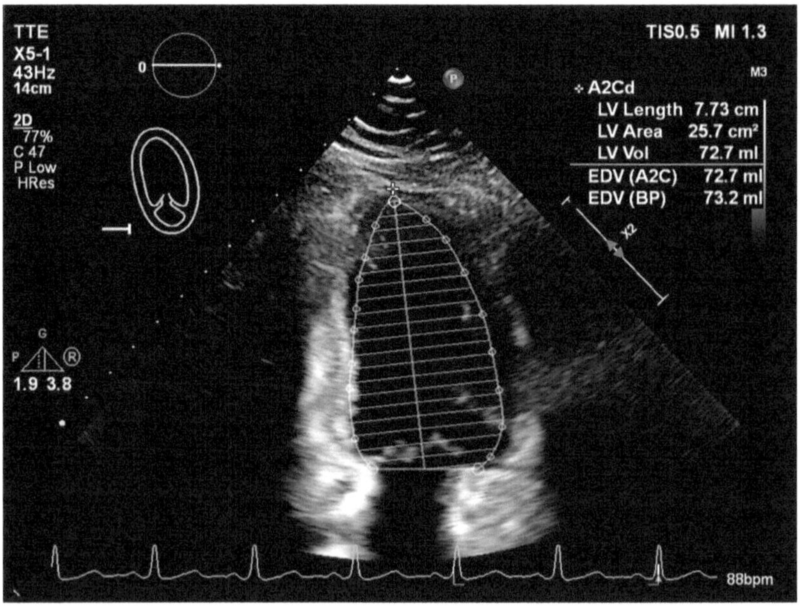

Fig. 11.5 Apical 4 chamber image at end diastole. Demonstrates Simpson's biplane measurement of LV cavity volume

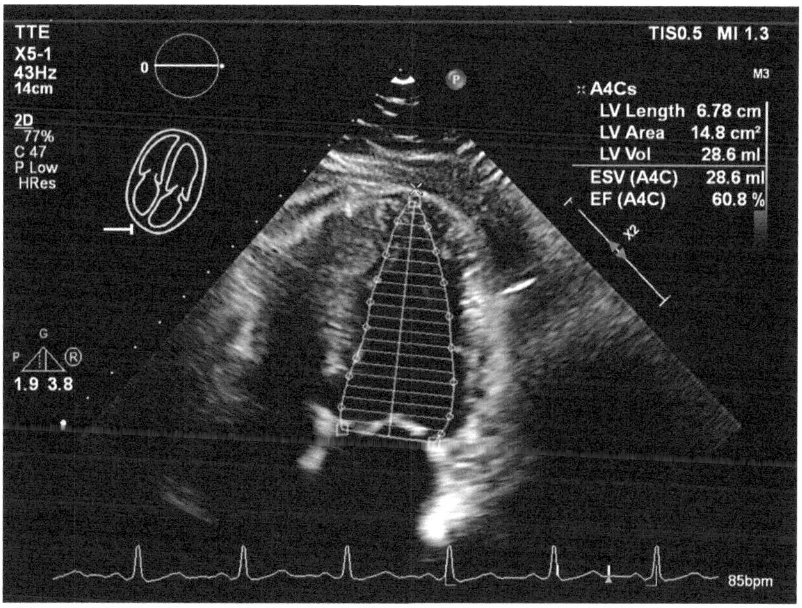

Fig. 11.6 Apical 4 chamber image at end systole. Demonstrates Simpson's biplane measurement of LV cavity volume

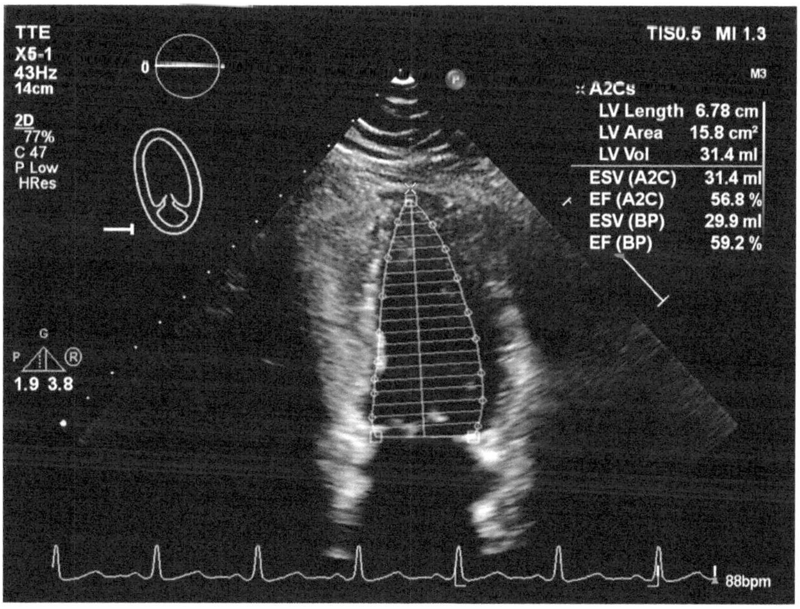

Fig. 11.7 Apical 4 chamber image at end systole. Demonstrates Simpson's biplane measurement of LV cavity volume

rather than electrocardiographic signal. In most software applications, the tracing can be adjusted to conform with the endocardial walls after initial placement.

This technique should be repeated for the Apical two-chamber view. Simpson's method calculates ellipses from both the apical four-chamber and apical two-chamber. One cannot simply average the two volume calculations. Additionally, if one image is substantially foreshortened, the software may identify an error, as the disks will not align. The biplane method of disks should not be used for calculating stroke volume. Minor errors in foreshortening and measurement can result in inaccurate stroke volume calculation.

Left Ventricular Hypertrophy

Left ventricular hypertrophy (LVH) is a condition in which there is an increase in left ventricular mass. This is either due to an increase in wall thickness, or secondary to left ventricular cavity enlargement, or both. Most commonly, left ventricular wall thickening occurs in response to pressure overload, whereas chamber dilatation often occurs in response to volume overload.

The etiology can often be ascertained on an echocardiogram, this being the test of choice in establishing the diagnosis of LVH. The patient's height and weight are considered along with left ventricular end-diastolic diameter, posterior wall thickness, and interventricular septum thickness, to determine the LV mass index.

LVH is defined as an increased left ventricular mass index (LVMI) of: >95 g/m in women and >115 g/m in men, which is calculated from wall thickness and size. There are multiple methods to calculate mass, including the use of three-dimensional echocardiography [1, 4]. In practice, however, LVH is more commonly assessed using LV wall thickness due to its simplicity.

The left ventricle wall thickness is typically measured in the parasternal long-axis view, along the same plane as the inner diameter: at the level of the mitral valve leaflet tips. Measurement of the anteroseptal wall should be located at the myocardial border. Measurement of the inferolateral wall should be located at the myocardial border and should exclude the pericardium. As with LV chamber size, 2D echocardiography is preferred over M-mode, as the walls may be nonorthogonal or oblique. Measurement should occur at end-diastole (Fig. 11.1). Normal values are in Table 11.1. In some elderly individuals, the upper interventricular septum might be prominent, a finding called discrete upper septal thickening (DUST, Video 11.1). This finding is associated with hypertension and is not independently associated with cardiovascular disease, mortality risk, or adverse prognosis [5]. Athletes may also demonstrate mild LV hypertrophy. The athlete's heart typically exemplifies eccentric hypertrophy, with a maintained or large chamber diameter, while pathologic hypertrophy is often concentric, demonstrating reduced chamber diameter. Another simple way to differentiate these phenotypes is to assess diastolic function: the athlete's heart will typically have normal diastolic function with a low E/e'. Hypertrophic heart disease, which occurs with hypertension, valvulopathy, and cardiovascular disease is often erroneously conflated with hypertrophic cardiomyopathy (see Chap. 16). Hypertrophy from hypertension or aortic stenosis will typically be uniform in distribution, while hypertrophic cardiomyopathy typically has a nonuniform presentation of severe hypertrophy in some regions and sparing in others.

LV Function: Linear Measurements

One of the earlier methods of assessing LV function in the critical care literature was the E-point Septal Separation (EPSS). This method was adopted as it was simple and reproducible with minimal training [6]. The concept of underpinning this measurement is that the amplitude of mitral valve opening is dependent on the pressure gradient between the left atrium and left ventricle: with decreased ejection fraction, the pressure gradient between the left atrium and ventricle is diminished during diastole, resulting in the smaller opening of the valve. The measurement of EPSS can be done from M-mode or 2D echocardiography from the parasternal long-axis view (Figs. 11.8 and 11.9). M-mode can provide greater temporal resolution. An EPSS >7 mm is associated with LV ejection fraction <30% [6]. This method of assessment can be inaccurate in mitral stenosis. Although EPSS is reproducible among novices, it is not commonly reported.

EPSS Method

- Obtain a parasternal long-axis view.
- Place the M-mode tracer over the distal tip of the anterior leaflet of the mitral valve.
- Measure during the early diastolic phase of the cardiac cycle.
- Place a caliper between the E point of the anterior mitral valve leaflet and the septum.

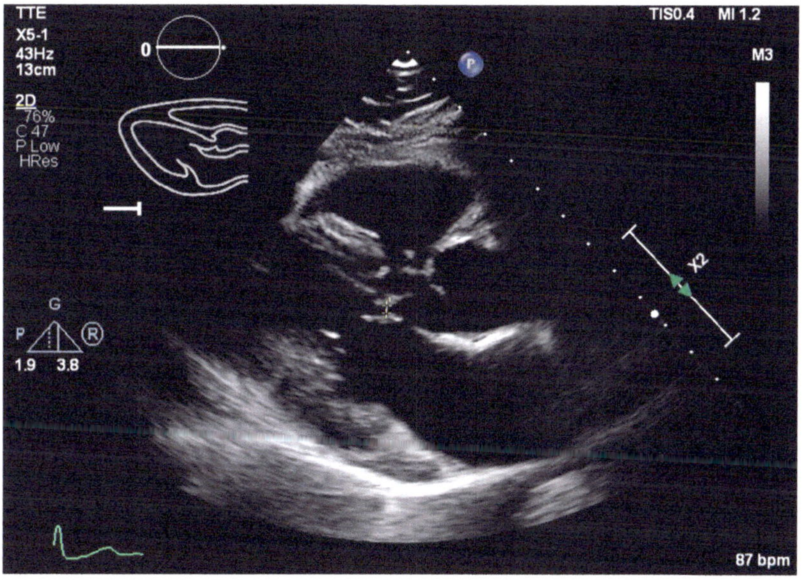

Fig. 11.8 Measurement of E-point Septal Separation (EPSS), in the parasternal longf axis view. Calipers are placed across the mitral valve leaflets, tip-to-tip

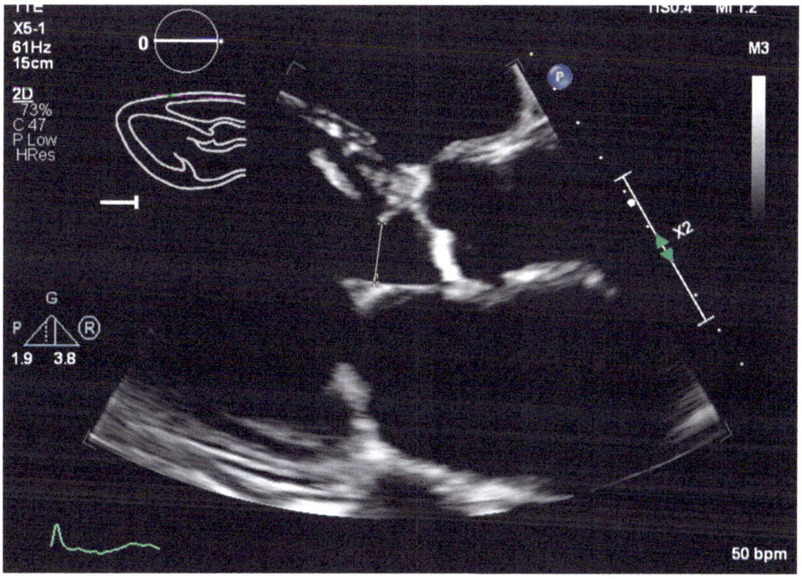

Fig. 11.9 Measurement of E-point Septal Separation (EPSS), in the parasternal longf axis view. Calipers are placed across the mitral valve leaflets, tip-to-tip

- EPSS <6 mm = normal LVEF
- EPSS >7 mm = reduced LVEF
- EPSS ≥13 mm = severely decreased function, with an estimated LVEF of ≤35% 0.3

Caution

- Mitral stenosis results in decreased excursion of their mitral valve with normal LV function.
- Severe Aortic Regurgitation may impair forward anterior leaflet movement.
- Atrial fibrillation results in beat-to-beat variation. Averaging several EPSS readings is recommended to improve accuracy under this circumstance.

Another linear measurement of function is fractional shortening, which is the difference of LVIDd and LVIDs, divided by the LVIDd. The fractional shortening can correlate with LV systolic function but can be inaccurate when there are regional wall motion abnormalities or conduction abnormalities [7].

LV Function: Ejection Fraction

The most common method of assessing LV systolic function is the ejection fraction (EF) from the biplane method of disks. This method measures LV systolic and diastolic volumes in two different planes. Utilizing the apical four-chamber view and apical two-chamber views, the endocardial borders are traced, then the cavity is divided into approximately 20 discs. The EF is calculated by taking the difference of LVEDV and LVESV, divided by the LVEDV.

$$\text{EF} = (\text{LVEDV} - \text{LVESV}) / \text{LVEDV}$$

Normal EF values are presented in Table 11.1, although as with all values in Table 11.1, it is important to remember that these ranges constitute a continuum rather than a discrete threshold between normal and abnormal. Reference values also vary with age [1]. It is important to remember the clinical context when interpreting EF. Ejection fraction is affected by preload and afterload, as well as by vasoactive medications. A patient who has an EF of 52% while on high doses of vasopressors may have abnormal contractility. Similarly, a patient who has an EF of 75% in the setting of low preload may decrease their EF substantially upon receipt of intravenous fluid. A patient's ejection fraction may change over the course of hours or days in response to critical illness or treatment [8]. These frequent changes imply three conclusions especially relevant for the critically ill: (1) EF is not always the best marker of intrinsic cardiac function, (2) assessing ventricular function may require alternative methods, and (3) repeated measurements may be needed to track changes in EF.

Patients with high ejection fractions (>70–75%) are classified as hyperdynamic. These patients are often tachycardic, and often hypovolemic. When interpreting these images, it is important not to conflate tachycardia with hyperdynamic contractility—it is easy to do so when assessing qualitatively. Ejection fraction does not always correspond to stroke volume or cardiac output. In the setting of hyperdynamic hypovolemia, a patient may have very high EF with a low stroke volume. In the setting of dilated cardiomyopathy or dilated ischemic heart disease, a patient may have a relatively preserved stroke volume despite having a profoundly low EF. The use of EF also requires adequate image quality to measure LVEDA and LVESA.

EF (Simpson's Biplane) Method

- Perform the following in BOTH the apical two-chamber and four-chamber views.
- Trace the endocardial borders of the LV, excluding any sub-valvular apparatus/papillary muscles.
- Ensure the axis line is placed as perpendicular to the LV cavity as possible, running from the LV apex to the base.
- Record one series in LV diastole.
- Record another in LV systole.

Cautions

- When performing any Simpson's biplane measurements for EF, axis measurements should be as identical as possible between the A4c and A2c views (<10% difference). Large differences may highlight off-axis views, or measurements performed that were not truly perpendicular to the LV cavity.
- If the views are foreshortened, then EF measurements may be over-estimated.

LV Function: Cardiac Output

Ironically, stroke volume is typically not measured using volumetric assessments, as minor errors in image acquisition and tracing can lead to inaccurate measurement. The preferred method of calculating stroke volume is the product of the left ventricular outflow tract (LVOT) cross-sectional area and the velocity time integral (VTI) of blood flow exiting the LVOT during systole. This method is also used in the continuity equation calculation for valve areas among other applications (see Chap. 17) [9]. The LVOT diameter is measured from an apical five-chamber view. The diameter is measured from the inner edge of the septal myocardium to the inner edge of the anterior mitral leaflet in mid-systole. The diameter is measured approximately 0.3–1.0 cm from the aortic valve orifice (Fig. 11.10). The diameter should be parallel to the aortic valve, and perpendicular to the outflow tract walls. The cross-sectional area is calculated from the LVOT diameter as:

$$A = \pi r^2$$

where the radius, r, is one-half the diameter.

The second component of the calculation of stroke volume is the velocity time integral from the apical five-chamber or apical long-axis (three-chamber) view. This waveform is obtained by placing the sample gate of a pulsed wave Doppler proximal to the aortic valve, ideally the same distance as where the LVOT diameter was measured. The angle of the jet should be aligned to be parallel to the ultrasound. The operator should adjust the baseline, scale, and sweep speed to optimize the waveform for measurement. The waveform should demonstrate laminar flow with a bright narrow band and a black interior, with a well-defined peak. The waveform is traced using the modal velocity (the middle of the dense signal, Fig. 11.11), not the black-white edge (Fig. 11.12). The imaging software should calculate the area above the curve or the integral. The integral of velocity and time is distance, therefore the VTI is reported in cm. The VTI can be thought of as the average distance blood travels through the LVOT during systole. Multiplying the VTI with the LVOT cross-sectional area yields the stroke volume in cubic centimeters or milliliters. Multiplying the stroke volume by the heart rate will yield cardiac output in milliliters. Dividing the cardiac output by body surface area will yield a cardiac index.

$$\text{Cardiac Index} = \frac{\pi\left(\dfrac{\text{LVOT Diameter}}{2}\right)^2 \times \text{LVOT VTI} \times \left(\dfrac{1\,\text{L}}{1000\,\text{mL}}\right) \times \text{Heart Rate}}{\text{Body Surface Area}}$$

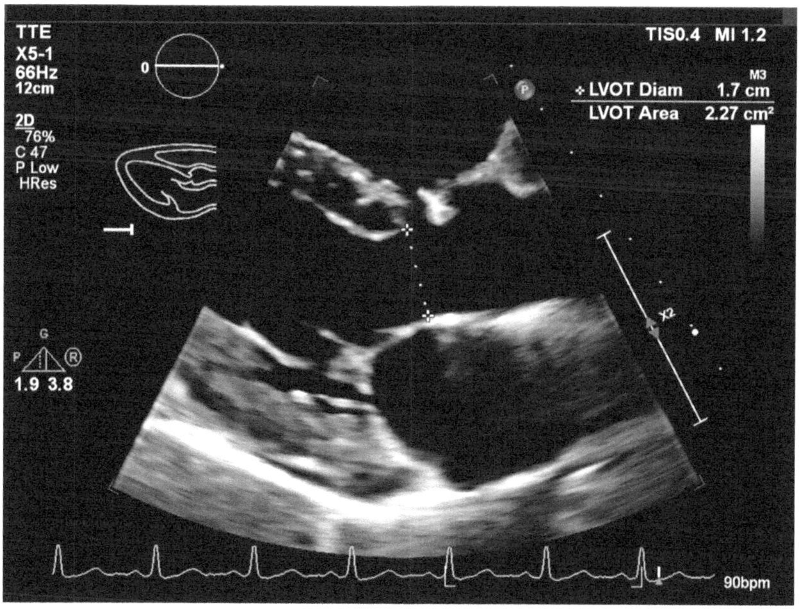

Fig. 11.10 Measurement of the diameter of the left ventricular outflow tract in mid systole, 0.3–1.0 cm from the aortic valve orifice. Calipers can be seen. A normal measurement is around 2 cm

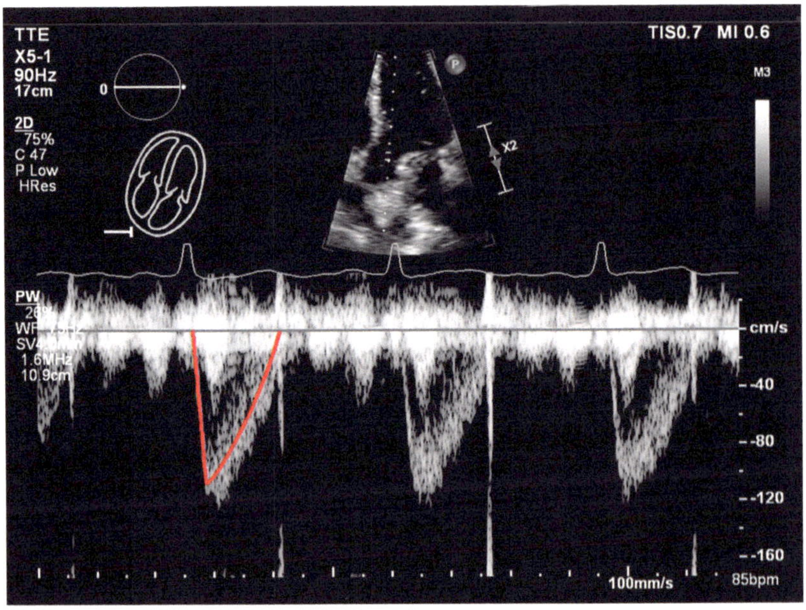

Fig. 11.11 An apical 5-chamber view. Pulsed wave doppler is placed into the LVOT, proximal to the aortic valve, at the point the LVOT was measured. The correct mid part of the dense black waveform is traced, using the modal velocity

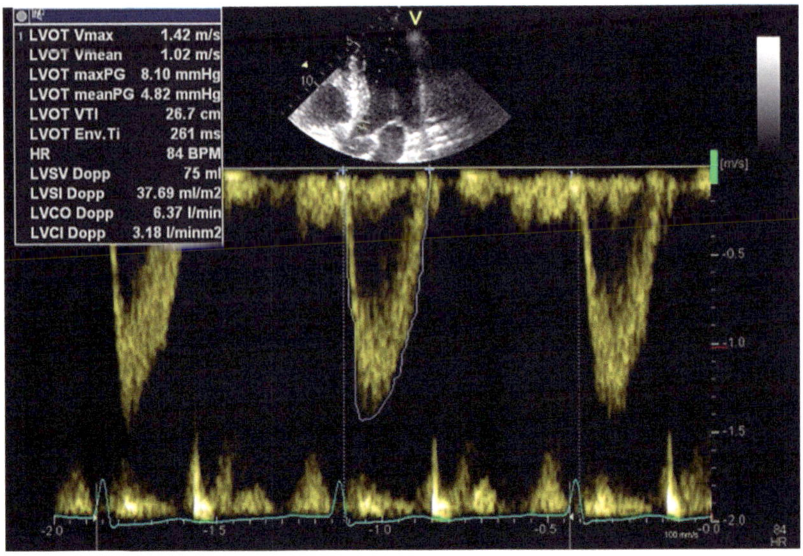

Fig. 11.12 An apical 5-chamber view. Pulsed wave doppler is placed into the LVOT, proximal to the aortic valve, at the point the LVOT was measured. The incorrect black/white edge of the trace has been measured here

There are multiple potential errors that may arise when measuring the stroke volume. The LVOT diameter is an imperfect measurement for the LVOT cross-sectional area, as the LVOT is not truly circular. Additionally, any minor imprecision in the measurement of the LVOT will be squared and multiplied. When performing serial measurements of cardiac output, it is unnecessary to measure the LVOT diameter multiple times, as each time will introduce unnecessary variation. As many decisions in critical care rely on relative changes in stroke volume or cardiac output rather than absolute measurements, many intensivists may forgo the measurement of the LVOT diameter altogether, instead of assessing changes in LVOT VTI and/or heart rate. Additional errors can occur when the pulsed wave Doppler is not aligned with the outflow jet. The greater the angle, θ, between the true jet and the ultrasound beam, the greater the inaccuracy in measuring velocity. Measured velocity is the true velocity multiplied by cosineθ. One could correct this error by dividing the velocity by cosineθ, but this introduces another potential error in measuring θ. In practice, it is preferred to not attempt correction but to attempt to align the jet so θ is <15°, which would mean the measured jet is >97% of the true jet. For repeated measurements of stroke volume, consistency is essential. Changing the angle of the probe will affect the measurement of stroke volume. Arrhythmia is another potential source of inaccuracy. If the VTI is not representative of the average VTI or the heart rate, the cardiac output will be inaccurate. One should not select the VTI occurring in relationship to a premature ventricular complex. In the setting of atrial fibrillation, one may take an average of several consecutive cardiac cycles to estimate stroke volume or cardiac output. Respiratory variation will also affect cardiac output, as it may affect preload. Measuring cardiac output from a VTI at end-inspiration may be substantially different from one measured at end-expiration. Severe aortic insufficiency will also result in inaccuracy. The VTI will measure blood exiting the ventricle, but will not account for blood reentering the ventricle, thus overestimating cardiac output. In such a case, it may be preferable to either calculate the regurgitant fraction, if possible (see Chap. 18) or to calculate stroke volume from another area of the heart, such as mitral inflow or right-sided cardiac output.

Regional Wall Motion Abnormalities

The left ventricle is divided into segments. Although 16- and 18-segment models exist, the 17-segment model is the most commonly used (Fig. 11.13, regional abnormalities in contractile function). This model correlates with the segments used in other imaging modalities. The base and mid-chamber are each divided into six segments: anteroseptal, anterior, anterolateral, inferolateral, inferior, and inferoseptal, while the apex is divided into five segments: anterior, lateral, inferior, septal, and apical. The standard assessment of these segments is visual estimation, although newer technologies such as strain (see below) may quantify function with greater reproducibility and accuracy. Regional wall motion abnormality is an indicator of ischemic heart disease, but it may also be present in other conditions, including myocarditis, stress cardiomyopathy, and septic cardiomyopathy.

When assessing each segment, it is important to evaluate wall thickening rather than wall movement. Translation of diseased myocardium may still occur when that region is tethered to an adjacent segment or when the entire heart is displaced during the cardiac cycle. Each segment should be assessed in multiple views. The short-axis view, when scanned from base to apex, will image all segments

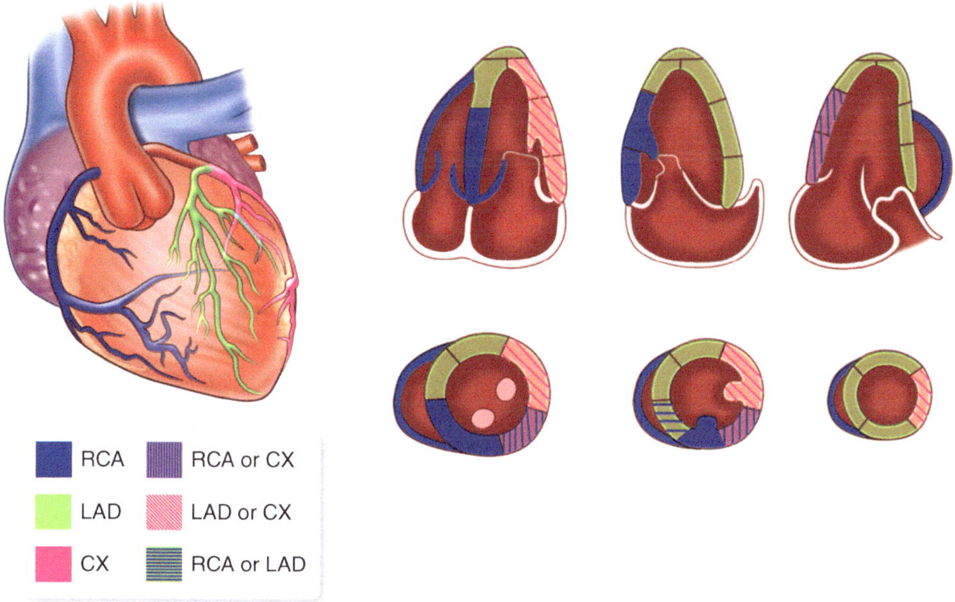

Fig. 11.13 Coronary artery territories associated with anatomical areas of the heart

of the heart. The parasternal or apical long axis will image the anteroseptal and inferolateral walls. The apical four-chamber will image the anterolateral and inferoseptal walls, and the apical two-chamber will image the anterior and inferior walls.

Each segment is assigned a wall motion score based on the visualized thickening of the myocardium. Normokinesis should thicken ≥5 mm or >40%; Hypokinesis should thicken 2–4 mm or 10–40%; Akinesis should thicken 0–1 mm or <10%; and dyskinesis is akinesis with expansion of the segment during systole. These scores are graded 1–4 from normokinesis to akinesis for each segment. The wall motion score is the sum of all these scores. The wall motion score index is the sum of these scores divided by the number of visualized segments. Although global assessments are useful, regional wall motion assessments are more useful when they are correlated with coronary artery territories (Fig. 11.14). As mentioned above, regional wall motion abnormalities may occur in the absence of coronary

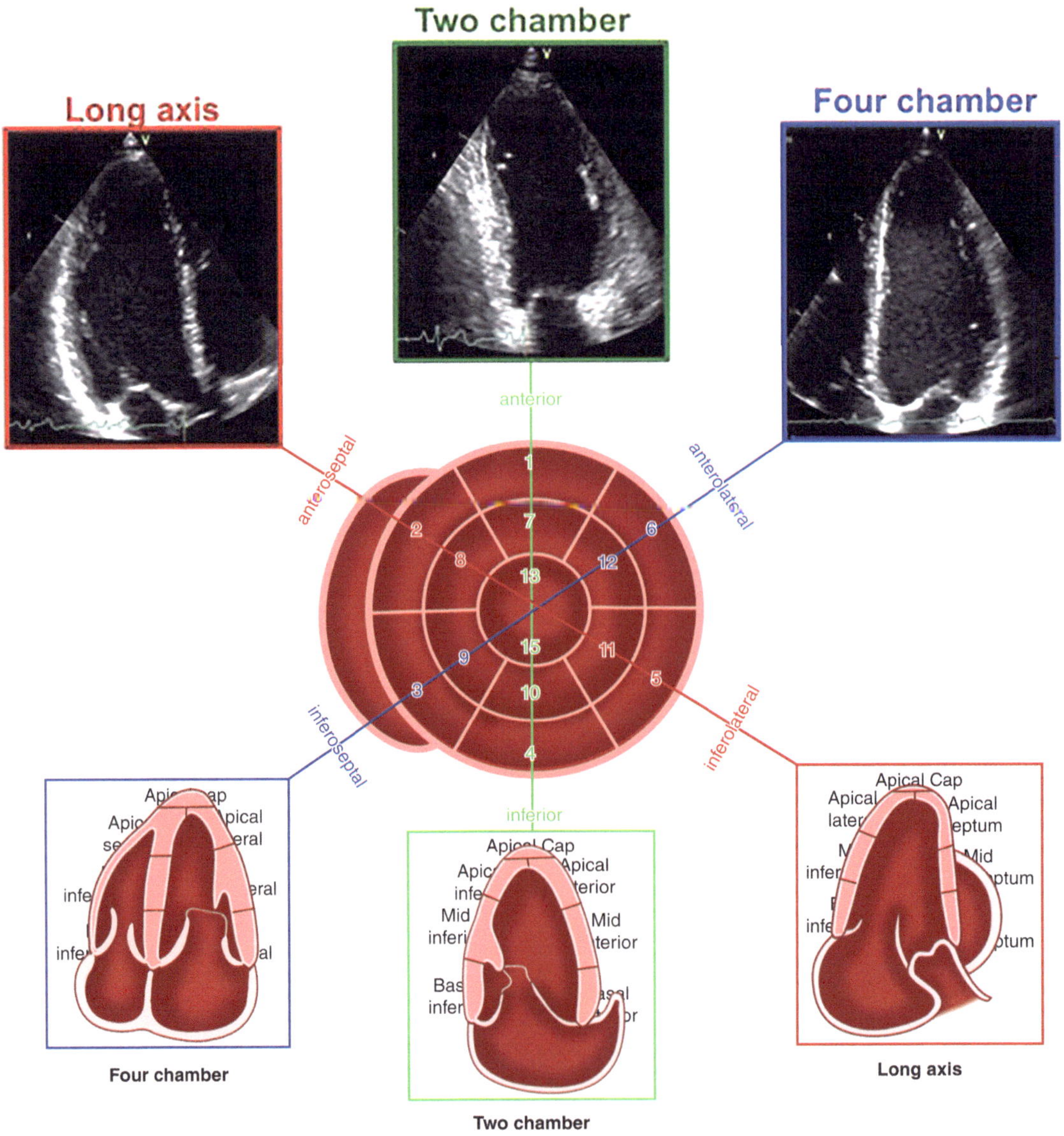

Fig. 11.14 Detailed anatomical area descriptions of the transthoracic echo views

artery disease. Bundle branch block, other conduction delays, and right or left ventricular pacing may result in abnormal regional wall motion. Right ventricular pressure or volume overload may also result in abnormal septal motion.

Methods

- Obtain the following views
  - Parasternal Short-axis view
  - Apical four-chamber view
  - Apical two-chamber view
  - Parasternal long-axis view
- Assess wall thickening during systole
  - **Normal**: >40%, ≥5 mm
  - **Hypokinetic**: 10–40%
  - **Akinetic**: <10%
  - **Dyskinetic**: Akinesis and expansion during systole

Strain

Strain is a newer assessment of ventricular function that measures the amount of deformation in a region of the myocardium. Strain is the percent change in length relative to its baseline.

$$\text{Strain}(\varepsilon) = \left[(\text{instantaneous length} - \text{baseline length}) / \text{baseline length}\right]$$

Strain rate is the rate at which deformity occurs.

$$\Delta\varepsilon / \Delta\,\text{time} = \Delta\,\text{myocardial velocity gradient} / \text{baseline length}$$

Strain may represent different axes of contraction. Radial strain represents the thickening of the myocardium in the short axis. Circumferential strain represents the shortening of the short axis during systole, and longitudinal strain represents the myocardial shortening from base to apex. During systole, the ventricular wall contracts, resulting in a negative longitudinal strain value. Discussion of strain can be confusing, as a change from −15% to −20% is described as an improvement in strain, and the literature is inconsistent with describing this change as an increase or a decrease in strain. Strain is typically assessed using specialized software that employs frame-by-frame tracking of unique speckle "fingerprints" within the myocardium. The method of assessment is semi-automated. The operator typically selects an appropriate image and traces the myocardium. The software will track the tracing throughout the cardiac cycle (Fig. 11.15, Video 11.2, Strain). Strain imaging requires high-quality images and high frame rates (40–90 Hz). For global longitudinal strain, the apical four-chamber, apical two-chamber, and apical long-axis (three-chamber) are all measured, and the software will create a composite 17-segment ventricle, with strain values for each region as well as a global value. The role of strain imaging is well established in conventional echocardiography, as it may detect subtle dysfunction that is otherwise missed in conventional assessment. Strain may herald changes in cardiac function well before it is reflected by changes in EF. Strain is influenced by preload (it increases as LV size increases) and afterload (decreases as blood pressure rises) [10]. Strain rate may be less dependent on load than strain. One potential application of strain is that it may be less preload or afterload dependent than ejection fraction, and global longitudinal strain might identify patients with septic cardiomyopathy that might otherwise be missed [11]. Despite this, the role of strain in critical care is still evolving, with insufficient evidence at present to justify its routine application in the critically ill. Normal reference values may depend on the software version and vendor. Healthy persons may have a global longitudinal strain of around −20%.

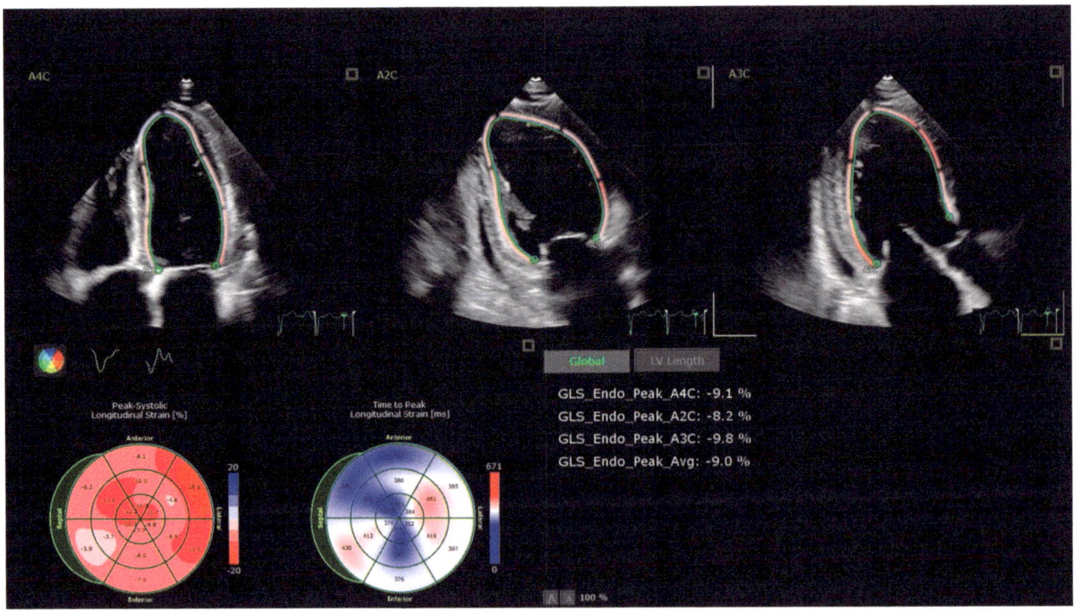

Fig. 11.15 Strain measurement of the LV cavity

Strain Methods

- Strain measurement method may be software-dependent
- Normal longitudinal systolic strain
  - -16% to -22% with values closer to 0 being abnormal
- Normal resting longitudinal strain rate
  - 1.0/s (s) to 1.4/s

Global Longitudinal Strain measurement can detect:

- Left ventricular Hypertrophy
- Degree of cardiotoxicity
- Ischemic heart disease
- Regional strain
- Chamber function
- Diastolic dysfunction
- Valve disease
- Atrial Fibrillation risk
- Pulmonary hypertension

Cautions

- When regional tracking is suboptimal in more than two myocardial segments in a single view, the calculation of GLS should be avoided.
- Intervendor and intersoftware variability exist, therefore the serial assessment of GLS in individual patients should be performed using the same vendor's equipment and the same software.

(a) Measuring LVOT diameter parallel to the aortic valve during each assessment of cardiac output.
(b) Ensuring that the pulsed wave Doppler is aligned <15° from the outflow jet during each assessment of cardiac output.
(c) Measuring velocity time integral tracings at end-expiration for each assessment of cardiac output.
(d) Selecting velocity time integral tracings during periods without arrhythmia for each assessment of cardiac output.

Questions

1. A 67-year-old male presents to the intensive care unit in septic shock for community-acquired pneumonia. Prior to admission, he had complained of 3 days of dyspnea and 1 day of pleurisy. He is receiving mechanical ventilation, norepinephrine, and epinephrine. A troponin-I level is measured at 3.2 ng/mL (normal range < 0.04 ng/mL). An echocardiogram is performed (Video 11.3). Which of the following is most correct?
   A. The patient has global hypokinesis from septic cardiomyopathy.
   B. The patient has takotsubo cardiomyopathy with apical ballooning and compensatory basal hyperkinesis.
   C. Vasopressors may worsen contractility in this setting.
   D. The patient is experiencing a myocardial infarction in the circumflex distribution.

   Answer: C. Vasopressors may sometimes worsen contractility in this setting. This patient has septic cardiomyopathy with regional wall motion abnormality: a hypokinetic inferoseptal wall. The pathophysiology of septic cardiomyopathy is complicated. One proposed mechanism for dysfunction is circulating endogenous or exogenous catecholamines. In some cases, additional vasopressors can worsen function [8]. A is incorrect. Although septic cardiomyopathy can present with global hypokinesis, this patient is demonstrating a normokinetic anterolateral wall. B is incorrect. Although septic cardiomyopathy and stress cardiomyopathy may have similar pathophysiology, the reason this answer is incorrect is because the takotsubo pattern describes a specific type of stress cardiomyopathy with apical ballooning and basal hyperkinesis (Video 11.4) not seen here. D is incorrect. Myocardial infarction is a possible complication of septic shock, but this distribution of regional wall motion abnormality demonstrates inferoseptal hypokinesis, consistent with right coronary or left anterior descending coronary distribution. The circumflex is more likely to perfuse the anterolateral wall. Troponin elevation and regional wall motion abnormalities in the absence of coronary artery disease are common findings in septic shock.

2. A 17-year-old male presents to the emergency department in hemorrhagic shock after a motor vehicle collision. Massive transfusion protocol is initiated. The heart rate is 124 beats/min. Blood pressure is 68/44 mmHg. An echocardiogram is performed to measure cardiac output. The velocity time integral from this image is measured at 60 cm (Fig. 11.16). The LVOT diameter is measured at 1.95 cm. Which of the following is true:
   A. The cardiac output is 22.2 L/min.
   B. The VTI is an underestimate because the ultrasound angle of insonation is not aligned with the LVOT jet.
   C. The cardiac output is high because of severe aortic insufficiency.
   D. The VTI is high because its corresponding cross-sectional area is severely reduced.

   Answer: D. The VTI is high because its corresponding cross-sectional area is severely reduced. This patient has dynamic outflow obstruction. The Doppler waveform is very high because the ventricular cross-sectional area is extremely small during mid—to late systole. The image reveals that the sample gate is positioned mid-chamber rather than at the LVOT. The late-peaking waveform is suggestive of dynamic outflow obstruction. A is incorrect. Although the calculation of cardiac output from the numbers provided yields an answer of 22.2 L/min, the VTI is not the VTI of the LVOT, but of the LV mid-ventricle, which has a different cross-sectional area, and is likely much smaller than 1 cm^2 during systole. B is incorrect. Although the ultrasound angle is not aligned with the outflow jet, the sample gate is also not positioned in the LVOT. C is incorrect. There is no evidence of severe aortic insufficiency in the provided image, although this image is not useful to ascertain the presence or absence of aortic insufficiency. Cardiac output may be overestimated in the setting of aortic insufficiency, as the calculation for cardiac output from VTI does not typically account for the regurgitant

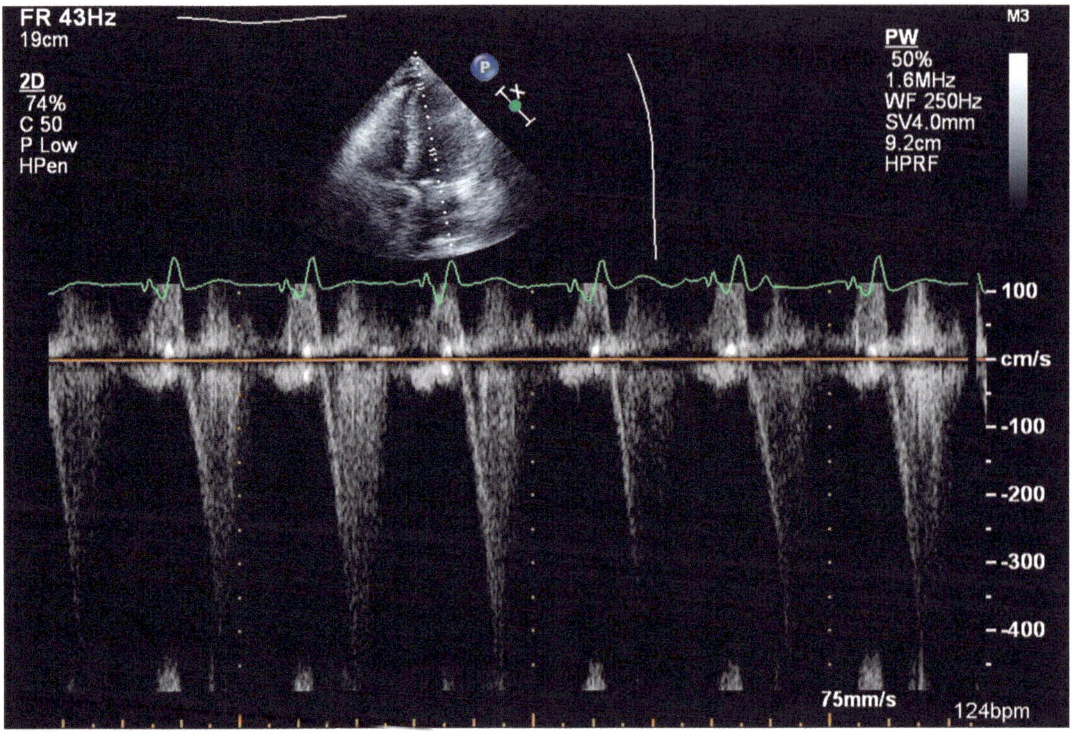

Fig. 11.16 Question 2 LVOT VTi measurement

volume. In such a case, the cardiac output would be lower than calculated. Regardless, aortic insufficiency would not explain the Doppler pattern seen in this patient.

3. A 58-year-old woman presents to the emergency department in cardiogenic shock after an out-of-hospital arrest with the return of spontaneous circulation. The patient continues to have frequent premature ventricular complexes. The ICU team monitors her status with serial echocardiography. Which of the following may worsen accuracy for repeated measures calculation of cardiac output:
   A. Measuring LVOT diameter parallel to the aortic valve during each assessment of cardiac output.
   B. Ensuring that the pulsed wave Doppler is aligned <15° from the outflow jet during each assessment of cardiac output.
   C. Measuring velocity time integral tracings at end-expiration for each assessment of cardiac output.
   D. Selecting velocity time integral tracings during periods without arrhythmia for each assessment of cardiac output.

Answer: A. Measuring LVOT diameter parallel to the aortic valve during each assessment of cardiac output. LVOT diameter is not expected to change during these assessments, but the potential imprecision in measuring the LVOT can result in significant errors. For example, a measurement of 20 mm versus 19 mm results in an 11% difference in cardiac output. When making serial measurements, consistency is important. It is reasonable to use a single high-quality measurement of LVOT diameter for repeated assessments of stroke volume. All the other answers will improve the accuracy of the cardiac output.

References

1. Lang RM, Badano LP, Mor-Avi V, et al. Recommendations for cardiac chamber quantification by echocardiography in adults: an update from the American Society of Echocardiography and the European Association of Cardiovascular Imaging. J Am Soc Echocardiogr. 2015;28(1):1–39.e14.
2. Leung JM, Levine EH. Left ventricular end-systolic cavity obliteration as an estimate of intraoperative hypovolemia. Anesthesiology. 1994;81(5):1102–9.
3. Feissel M, Michard F, Mangin I, Ruyer O, Faller JP, Teboul JL. Respiratory changes in aortic blood velocity as an indicator of fluid responsiveness in ventilated patients with septic shock. Chest. 2001;119(3):867–73.
4. Mizukoshi K, Takeuchi M, Nagata Y, et al. Normal values of left ventricular mass index assessed by transthoracic three-dimensional echocardiography. J Am Soc Echocardiogr. 2016;29(1):51–61.
5. Diaz T, Pencina MJ, Benjamin EJ, et al. Prevalence, clinical correlates, and prognosis of discrete upper septal thickening on echocardiography: the Framingham Heart Study. Echocardiography. 2009;26(3):247–53.
6. McKaigney CJ, Krantz MJ, La Rocque CL, Hurst ND, Buchanan MS, Kendall JL. E-point septal separation: a bedside tool for emergency physician assessment of left ventricular ejection fraction. Am J Emerg Med. 2014;32(6):493–7.
7. Weekes AJ, Reddy A, Lewis MR, Norton HJ. E-point septal separation compared to fractional shortening measurements of systolic function in emergency department patients: prospective randomized study. J Ultrasound Med. 2012;31(12):1891–7.
8. Beesley SJ, Weber G, Sarge T, et al. Septic cardiomyopathy. Crit Care Med. 2018;46(4):625–34.
9. Baumgartner H, Hung J, Bermejo J, et al. Recommendations on the echocardiographic assessment of aortic valve stenosis: a focused update from the European Association of Cardiovascular Imaging and the American Society of Echocardiography. J Am Soc Echocardiogr. 2017;30(4):372–92.
10. Dandel M, Lehmkuhl H, Knosalla C, Suramelashvili N, Hetzer R. Strain and strain rate imaging by echocardiography—basic concepts and clinical applicability. Curr Cardiol Rev. 2009;5(2):133–48.
11. Sanfilippo F, Corredor C, Fletcher N, et al. Left ventricular systolic function evaluated by strain echocardiography and relationship with mortality in patients with severe sepsis or septic shock: a systematic review and meta-analysis. Crit Care. 2018;22(1):183.

12 Assessment of Left Ventricular Systolic Function in Patients with Difficult or Poor Acoustic Windows

Brandon M. Wiley

Patient Positioning and Alternative Acoustic Windows

The optimization of patient positioning is the initial approach for improving visualization of the left ventricle. The parasternal and apical windows are usually optimized by placing the patient in the left lateral decubitus position with the left arm raised to expand the intercostal spaces. Intubated, postsurgical, or other intensive care patients with limited mobility can be slightly tilted into a left lateral decubitus position by using pillows placed under the right shoulder and thorax (Fig. 12.1). The subcostal imaging window is a simple and high-yield view that is optimized with the patient supine and the knees bent to relax the abdominal muscles (Video 12.1). In spontaneously breathing patients, apical imaging may be improved withheld expiration. Whereas subcostal imaging is optimized with forceful inspiration.

In addition to patient repositioning and respiratory control, the use of alternative acoustic windows may be valuable in patients with challenging imaging. For example, in patients with moderate to large left pleural effusions and nondiagnostic transthoracic echocardiograms using traditional acoustic windows, the left posterior thoracic window has been shown to provide improved visualization of the left ventricle [1, 2]. In patients with left ventricular assist devices (LVAD), the right transhepatic view has been shown to improve the delineation of right and left ventricular systolic function [3].

Supplementary Information The online version contains supplementary material available at https://doi.org/10.1007/978-3-031-80038-2_12.

B. M. Wiley (✉)
Keck School of Medicine, University of Southern California, Los Angeles, CA, USA
e-mail: brandon.wiley@med.usc.edu

M. J. Lanspa, A. T. Levinson (eds.), *Echocardiography and Ultrasonography in the ICU*, Respiratory Medicine, https://doi.org/10.1007/978-3-031-80038-2_12

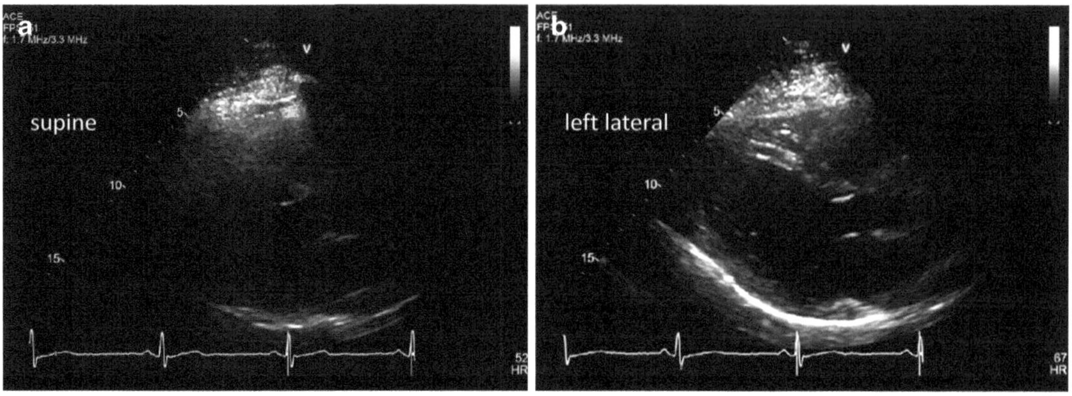

Fig. 12.1 Patient positioning improves acoustic window (Video 12.1). (**a**) This hospitalized ICU patient is imaged in the supine position and the resulting parasternal long-axis view is poor which precludes assessment of LV function. (**b**) The same patient is now turned onto the left-side by placing towels under the right shoulder and thorax. This repositioning significantly improves the acoustic window providing adequate endocardial border definition for LV function assessment

Ultrasonic Enhancement Agents (UEAs)

Ultrasonic enhancement agents (UEAs), previously termed ultrasound contrast agents, are composed of microbubbles that contain inert high-molecular weight gas. These microbubbles are smaller than red blood cells which allow them to pass through the pulmonary circulation. UEAs undergo volumetric oscillation when exposed to an ultrasound field and as a result, opacify the blood pool during echocardiography which provides a strong contrast to the myocardium and improves endocardial definition (Fig. 12.2). Three commercially available UEAs in the United States are approved for left ventricular opacification (LVO) (Table 12.1).

In practice, these agents are given intravenously either diluted in normal saline or as a tiny bolus with a saline flush (Table 12.1). Dilution and slow infusion of UEAs help avoid attenuation of the LV cavity. Additionally, B-mode imaging with UEAs should be performed using harmonic imaging at a low mechanical index (MI < 0.3) which prevents the destruction of the microbubbles.

UEAs are safe and large studies have not shown increased mortality in a variety of patient populations [4]. The most common side effects of UEA appear to be headaches. There is a low incidence of transient back pain associated with Definity that spontaneously resolves. The most serious potential complication is an anaphylactoid reaction which occurs at a rate of about 1 in 10,000 [4]. The contraindications for each UEA are listed in Table 12.1. Notably, in 2021, the Food and Drug Administration removed hypersensitivity to blood and blood products as a contraindication for the use of Optison. Additionally, studies have demonstrated safety in patients with LVADs and those supported by extracorporal membrane oxygenation (ECMO) [5, 6]. These agents can also be used in patients with right-to-left intracardiac shunts and in those patients with pulmonary hypertension. Finally, the American Society of Echocardiography states that UEA-assisted echocardiography "should not be withheld on the basis of any particular diagnosis or comorbidity" in ICU or emergency room patients with technically difficult imaging [4].

Clinical studies have shown that the use of ultrasound enhancement agents greatly reduces the number of suboptimal or nondiagnostic transthoracic echocardiograms (Video 12.2) [7]. In addition to improved endocardial border delineation, LVO has been demonstrated to yield more accurate and reproducible measurement of left ventricular size and systolic function [8]. The American Society of Echocardiography and the European Association of Echocardiography rec-

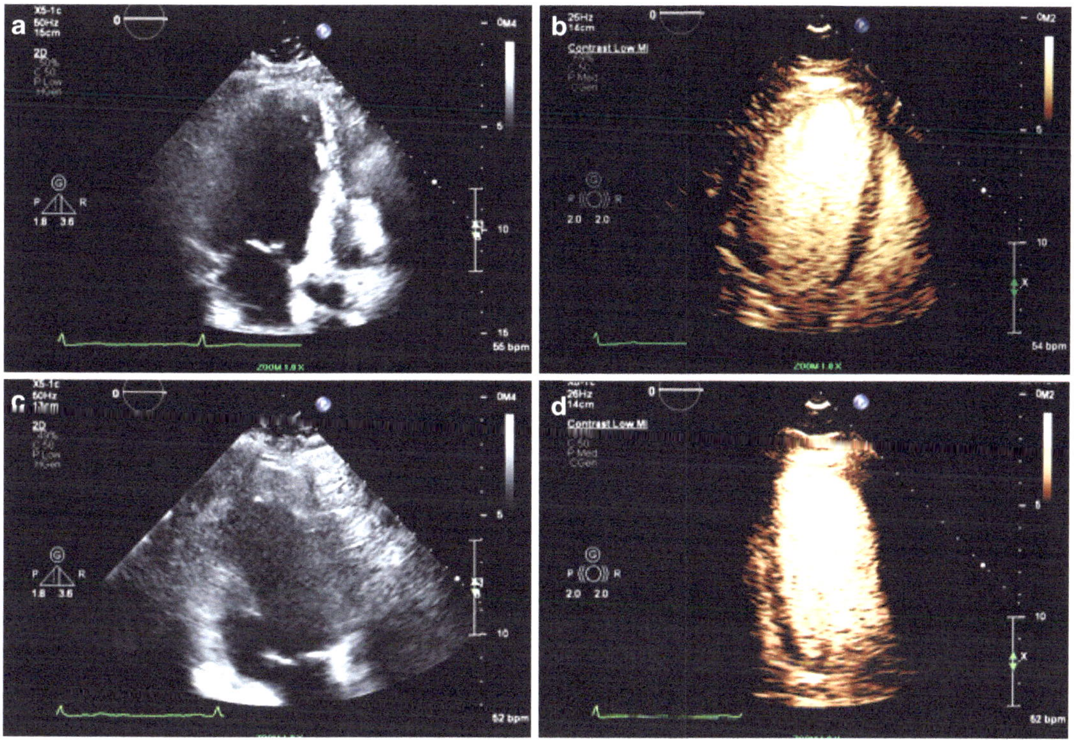

Fig. 12.2 Echocardiogram with ultrasound enhancement agent (UEA) (Video 12.2). Example of improvement in endocardial border delineation with UEA. (**a**) and (**c**) are apical 4-chamber and apical 2-chamber views without UEA. (**b**) and (**d**) are the same views after the addition of intravenous UEA. The UEA imaging is performed with low mechanical index (MI 0.16). (Note the left ventricle is on the left in image **a** and **b**)

Table 12.1 Ultrasound enhancement agents approved for clinical use in the United States

Ultrasound enhancement agents (UEAs)			
Brand name	Manufacturer	Important points	Contraindications
Lumason	Bracco Diagnostics	• Requires refrigeration prior to use • Requires mechanical agitation prior to use • Given as 0.5 mL bolus with slow saline flush	Allergy to sulfur hexafluoride
Definity	Lantheus Medical Imaging	• Stored as dry powder • Requires manual agitation prior to use • Given as infusion diluted with normal saline	Allergy to perflutren
Optison	GE Healthcare	• Requires refrigeration prior to use • Requires resuspension prior to use • Given as infusion diluted with normal saline	Allergy to perflutren

ommend that ultrasound enhancement agents should be used to improve left ventricular endocardial visualization when ≥2 contiguous wall segments are not seen, to increase accuracy of LV ejection fraction or to increase the physician confidence in the interpretation of LV size and function [8, 9].

The ability of ultrasound enhancement agents to improve LV visualization is of particular importance in the intensive care unit where a significant percentage of patients have suboptimal or difficult acoustic windows (Fig. 12.1, Video 12.2). A study of 632 consecutive patients (180 ICU patients) with technically difficult echocardiograms showed that the greatest benefit of UEAs was in ICU patients where nondiagnostic studies decreased from 16.7% to 0.5% and technically difficult studies decreased from 82.7% to 13.8%. The use of ultrasound enhancement agents averted the need for a transesophageal echocardiogram in 16.7% of the medical ICU patients and 31.4% of the surgical ICU patients. In addition, 9% of the medical ICU patients and 25.5% of the surgical ICU patients had a change in their medication regimen (hemodynamically active medications or anticoagulation) as a result of the ultrasound enhancement agent [10]. These findings were supported by a larger study that retrospectively analyzed 1,538,864 patients who underwent transthoracic echocardiography in an ICU setting [11]. Only 3.3% of these critically ill patients had an echocardiogram with an UEA. However, after multivariate adjustment, those patients who underwent TTE with UEAs were statistically more likely to have a change in inotropic therapy, vasopressor therapy, and anticoagulant therapy. Additionally, patients who underwent TTE with UEA had a 10% shorter ICU length of stay and were less likely to undergo additional TTE or TEE studies.

M-Mode

Motion mode (M-mode) ultrasound demonstrates a line of motion over time. Although this one-dimensional mode of imaging has limitations, it provides simple and reproducible parameters for assessing LV systolic function when endocardial definition by 2D echocardiography is suboptimal.

Mitral Annular Plane Systolic Excursion

Mitral annular plane systolic excursion (MAPSE), also referred to as atrioventricular plane displacement (AVPD), describes the descent of the mitral annulus toward the apex during LV systole. This displacement distance is a measure of longitudinal shortening of the LV cavity and correlates with LV systolic function [12]. MAPSE can be assessed at the septal, anterior, lateral, or inferolateral aspects of the mitral annulus. The measurement is highly angle-dependent and therefore must be performed using the apical acoustic window to ensure parallel alignment of the M-mode cursor with the LV walls. The average systolic excursion distance varies between 12 and 15 mm and is typically lowest at the anterior and septal points [13, 14]. In general, MAPSE >10 mm is associated with normal systolic function (LVEF $\geq$ 55%), and a value of <8 mm is associated with abnormal systolic function (LVEF < 50%) (Fig. 12.3) [13]. A large study using the average of septal and lateral MAPSE found that normal LVEF corresponded to $\geq$13 mm in men (sensitivity 92%, specificity 85%) and $\geq$11 mm (sensitivity 92%, specificity 72%) in women [14]. A reduced MAPSE of <6 mm (sensitivity 73–100%, specificity 99–100%), regardless of gender, was associated with severely reduced LV systolic function (ejection fraction $\leq$30%) [14].

It is important to note that MAPSE, like ejection fraction, is pre—and afterload dependent. MAPSE reflects global LV longitudinal systolic function but does not reflect regional wall motion abnormalities. The correlation of MAPSE with ejection fraction is best in patients with normal or dilated cardiomyopathies and may be limited in the presence of severe LV hypertrophy or the elderly. The reduced LV longitudinal function in elderly or severely hypertrophied ventricles may be compensated for by augmentation of radial and circumferential contraction [13, 15]. Additionally, significant mitral annular calcification may reduce LV longitudinal annular motion in the presence of normal LVEF.

E-Point to Septal Separation

The mitral valve E point-to-septal separation (EPSS) is the distance between the interventricular septum and the anterior leaflet of the mitral valve during early diastole. This parameter is

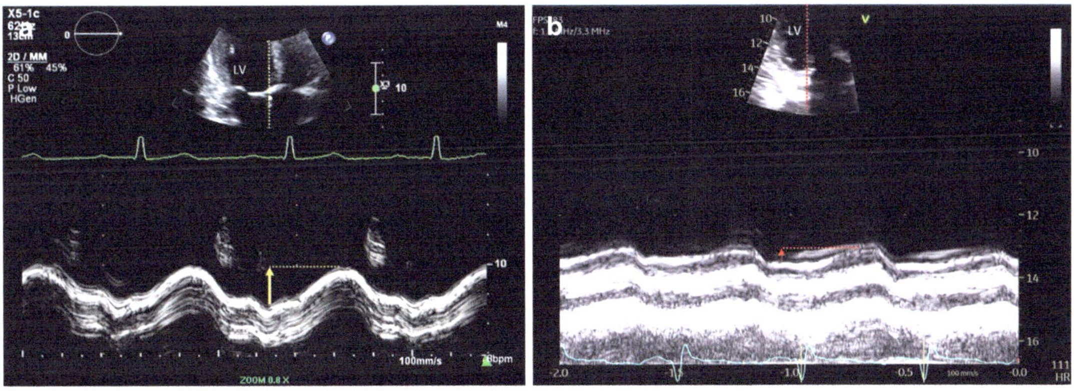

Fig. 12.3 M-Mode mitral annular plane systolic excursion (MAPSE). MAPSE is the measurement of mitral annular apical displacement during systole and reflects longitudinal shortening of the ventricle. This measurement is typically performed using the septal or lateral aspect of the mitral annulus. The M-mode cursor is placed on the mitral annulus and aligned in parallel to the left ventricular wall. The measurement is made from the diastolic nadir of the M-mode tracing to the peak at end systole. (**a**) Normal left ventricular systolic function, MAPSE 15 mm (measured on septal aspect of annulus). (**b**) Dilated cardiomyopathy with severely reduced systolic function, MAPSE 5 mm (measured on lateral aspect of annulus). (*LV* left ventricle)

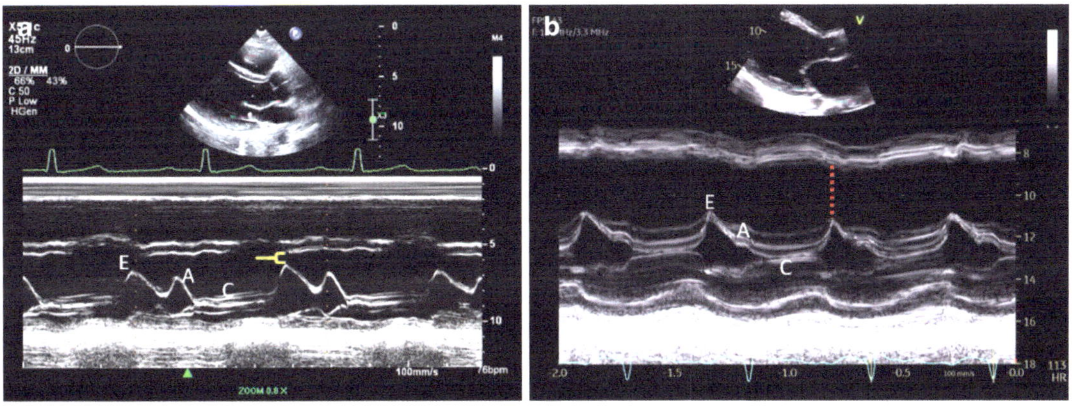

Fig. 12.4 M-Mode mitral valve E-point septal separation (EPSS). The normal M-mode profile of the mitral valve includes opening of the leaflets in early diastole (E-point) followed by atrial contraction (A-point) and then valve closure during systole (C-point). (**a**) The tracing of normal-sized left ventricle with normal systolic function. There is brisk excursion of the mitral valve anterior leaflet during early diastole and as a result the distance between the tip of the anterior leaflet and ventricular septum is small (EPSS <7 mm, yellow bars). (**b**) The tracing from a patient with a dilated cardiomyopathy and severely reduced left ventricular systolic function. The EPSS distance is markedly increased (25 mm, red line)

assessed using the parasternal long-axis view with the M-mode cursor perpendicular to the interventricular septum and directed through the tip of the anterior leaflet of the mitral valve. Normal LV size and systolic function are associated with a small EPSS distance (0–5 mm) due to the brisk early diastolic excursion of the mitral leaflets which causes the anterior leaflet to contact, or nearly contact, the interventricular septum (Fig. 12.4). The EPSS distance increases progressively with worsening LV systolic dysfunction and dilation. An EPSS >7–8 mm is a highly sensitive threshold for the presence of LV systolic dysfunction [16, 17].

It is important to note that EPSS is not valid in patients with prosthetic mitral valves. Overestimation of left ventricular systolic function can occur when a small EPSS distance is the result of asymmetric septal hypertrophy or in the presence of severe mitral regurgitation. Severe aortic regurgitation or restricted excursion of the mitral leaflets due to intrinsic valvular disease can cause a large EPSS that may lead to an underestimation of LVEF. The presence of atrial fibrillation may cause beat-to-beat variability in EPSS which can confound its association with LV systolic function.

Pulse Wave and Continuous Wave Doppler Echocardiography

Pulse wave Doppler echocardiography and continuous wave Doppler echocardiography measure the velocity of red blood cells and provide a beat-to-beat assessment of cardiac hemodynamics that correlate well with invasive measures.

Stroke Volume and Cardiac Output

Pulse wave (PW) Doppler echocardiography provides a noninvasive measurement of forward flow which can be used to calculate stroke volume and cardiac output. PW Doppler-derived stroke volume is calculated using the left ventricular outflow (LVOT) velocity-time integral (VTI) and the LVOT cross-sectional surface area (CSA) [18]. The LVOT VTI is measured through PW Doppler interrogation of systolic flow in the LVOT. The assessment is performed using the apical five-chamber or three-chamber acoustic window which enables the PW Doppler sample volume to be placed in LVOT, just proximal to the aortic valve annulus, with the angle of interrogation aligned parallel to the flow. The LVOT systolic PW Doppler spectral envelop should demonstrate laminar flow and therefore appear smooth with a discrete band of velocities. The LVOT systolic PW Doppler signal should also include the closure click of the aortic valve. Tracing area under the LVOT systolic PW Doppler signal yields the LVOT VTI or systolic stroke distance (the distance the red blood cells travel during systole). LVOT VTI is directly proportional to stroke volume with normal values of 17–24 cm [19]. The LVOT CSA = πr^2 since it is assumed to be circular and unchanging during systole [18]. The radius (r) is derived from the LVOT diameter (normal 2.1 ± 2.2 cm) which is measured in the parasternal long-axis view at the same level the PW Doppler sample volume was placed for the LVOT VTI [20]. The final calculation of LV stroke volume is a product of LVOT VTI (cm) and LVOT CSA (cm^2) which yields a volume (cm^3 = mL) [18]. The LV stroke volume is multiplied by the heart rate to provide the cardiac output (Fig. 12.5).

The PW Doppler-derived stroke volume and cardiac output correlate well with invasively derived measurements in critically ill patients [21, 22]. PW Doppler-derived stroke volume index correlates with shock severity and improves risk stratification for in-hospital mortality [23]. It is important to note that the LVOT diameter is a fixed parameter whereas the LVOT VTI is variable and therefore the change in LVOT VTI can be used to monitor dynamic hemodynamics and assess relative changes in stroke volume [24]. For example, the likelihood of fluid responsiveness can be evaluated by simply using the percentage change in LVOT VTI elicited by fluid challenge or passive leg raise [25]. Furthermore, LVOT VTI has been shown to be a powerful predictor of hospital mortality in patients with cardiogenic shock [26].

The LVOT diameter (d) requires special attention since the value is squared (CSA = $\pi(d/2)^2$) which magnifies any error in measurement. Therefore, the LVOT diameter should be measured using a focused, zoomed view to maximize accuracy. The PW Doppler sample volume interrogation angle must be parallel to LVOT flow (apical five-chamber or three-chamber view) to avoid underestimation of stroke volume. Overestimation of the LVOT VTI and calculated stroke volume can occur in the presence of abnormal flow acceleration or turbulence in the LVOT caused by the systolic anterior motion of the mitral valve or subaortic stenosis. It is important to average several [1, 2, 27] PW Doppler LVOT VTI signals in patients with irregular rhythms to account for beat-to-beat variation in stroke volume. It is important to note that low

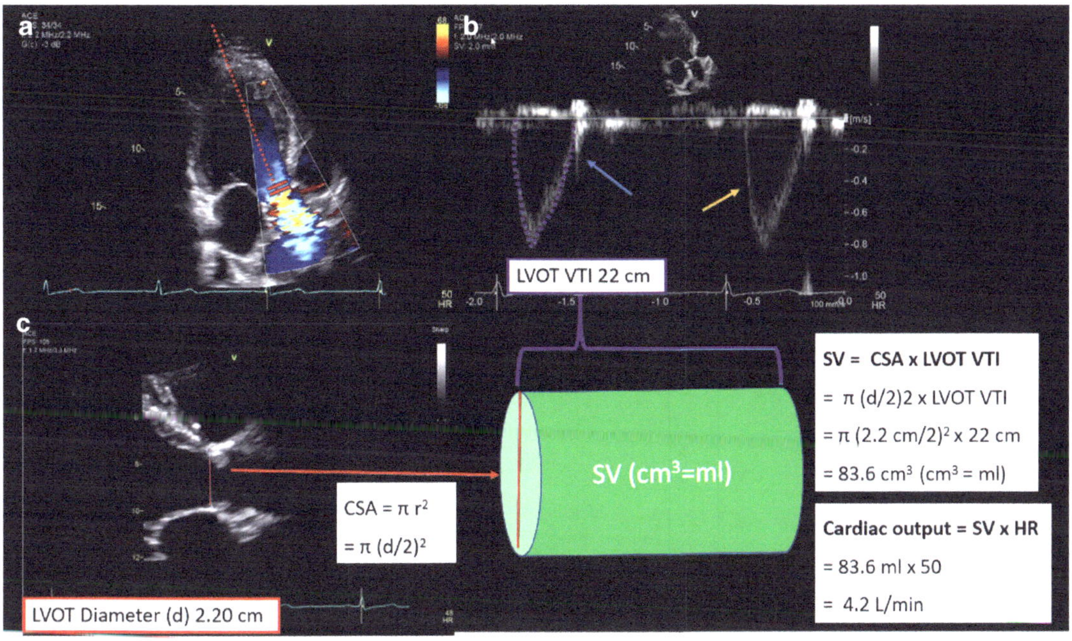

Fig. 12.5 Example of PW Doppler LV stroke volume and cardiac output calculation. (**a**) The systolic flow in the LVOT is interrogated by PW Doppler. The sample volume is placed in the LVOT just proximal to the aliasing of color Doppler caused by turbulence and flow acceleration through the aortic valve. (**b**) The PW Doppler signal of LVOT systolic flow should be smooth, reflecting laminar flow, with a discrete band of red blood cell velocities (orange arrow). The closure click of the aortic valve should be visible (blue arrow). Tracing the area under the curve of the signal yields the LVOT VTI (22 cm). (**c**) The LVOT diameter (2.20 cm) is measured just at the annulus of the aortic valve using a zoomed view. SV is approximated using the volume of a cylinder. The base of the cylinder is the CSA of the LVOT. The height of the cylinder is the LVOT VTI. (*PW* pulse wave, *LV* left ventricle, *LVOT* left ventricular outflow tract, *VTI* velocity time integral, *SV* stroke volume, *CSA* cross-sectional surface area, *HR* heart rate)

LV stroke volume may not reflect primary LV systolic dysfunction and instead be the result of reduced LV preload caused by right ventricular failure, obstructive shock, hemorrhagic shock, or reduced forward flow due to severe mitral regurgitation.

d*P*/d*t*

Continuous wave (CW) Doppler echocardiography can be utilized to evaluate the rate of pressure rise in the LV during isovolumic contraction. This rate of pressure rise (d*P*/d*t*) is a marker of LV contractility that is less affected by loading conditions [28]. Normal LV systolic function is characterized by a short isovolumic contraction period with the concomitant rapid increase in LV pressure. The isovolumic contraction period prolongs and the rise of LV pressure is attenuated with progressive worsening of LV contractility. The CW Doppler-derived d*P*/d*t* is calculated by measuring the time interval between the mitral regurgitant velocity at 1 and 3 m/s. This method has been shown to correlate well with catheter-derived invasive measurements of d*P*/d*t* [29, 30]. Normal LV contractility is associated with a d*P*/d*t* > 1200 mmHg/s (steep pressure/time slope) and severe LV systolic dysfunction is associated with d*P*/d*t* < 800 mmHg/s [28] (Fig. 12.6).

The accuracy of d*P*/d*t* evaluation by Doppler echocardiography is angle-dependent and accurate measurements require a parallel alignment of the CW Doppler cursor with early systolic mitral regurgitation signal. An increased CW Doppler cursor intercept angle will result in an underestimation of d*P*/d*t*. The feasibility of d*P*/d*t* measurements is limited with inadequate mitral regurgitation or in the

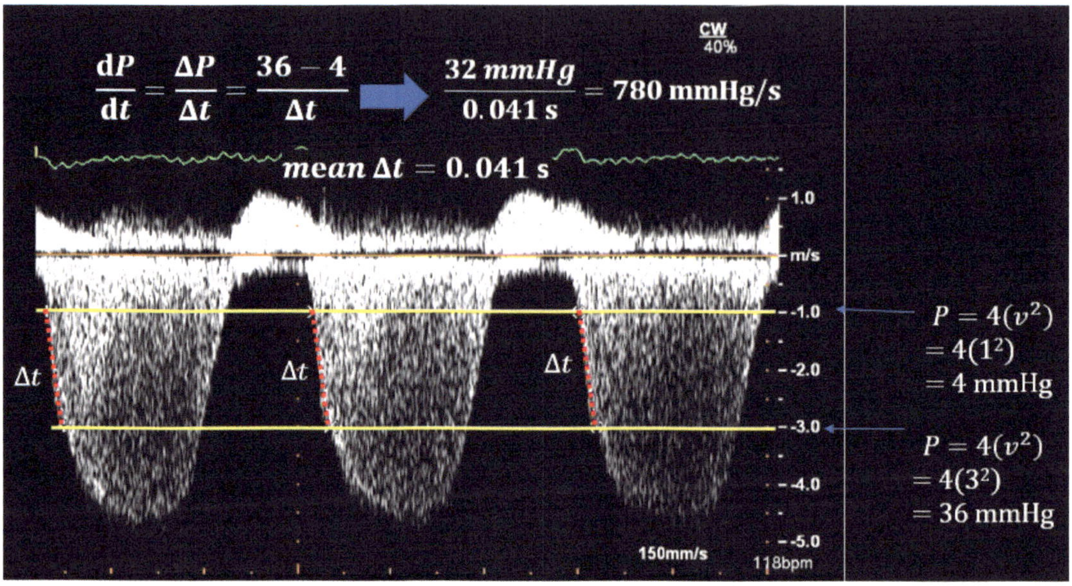

Fig. 12.6 d*P*/d*t* (rate of pressure rise). This illustrates the calculation of d*P*/d*t* using the CW Doppler tracing of mitral regurgitation in a patient with an ischemic cardiomyopathy and severely reduced LV systolic function. The red dashed line represents the time interval (Δt) required for an increase in mitral regurgitation velocity from 1 to 3 m/s. The mitral regurgitation velocity is a surrogate for the change in LV pressure since the left atrial pressure is relatively stable during early systole. As LV contractility worsens, the rate of rise of LV pressure is attenuated and the time interval (Δt) prolongs. Normal LV contractility is associated with a d*P*/d*t* > 1200 mmHg and severe LV systolic dysfunction is associated with a d*P*/d*t* < 800 mmHg

presence of an eccentric regurgitant jet that precludes parallel alignment of the CW Doppler cursor during the target time interval.

Tissue Doppler Imaging (TDI)

TDI measures the velocity of the myocardium in contrast to conventional PW and CW Doppler which measure the velocities of red blood cells. TDI can be performed using both pulsed wave (PW-TDI) and color modes. PW-TDI measures the peak velocity and the color-TDI mode measures the mean velocity. TDI provides a sensitive assessment of regional systolic and diastolic myocardial mechanics [31].

Systolic Mitral Annular Velocity (s′)

The TDI-derived systolic mitral annular velocity (s′ or s_m) is analogous to MAPSE, an indicator of LV systolic longitudinal function. The s′ velocity is measured using PW-TDI with the sample volume placed at the medial or lateral aspects of the mitral annulus in the apical four-chamber view. The s′ measurement is angle-dependent and the PW-TDI cursor must be parallel to the apical descent of the mitral annular plane. The peak s′ velocity has been correlated to LV ejection fraction and d*P*/d*t* [32]. The mean s′ velocity is 8.9 cm/s in healthy controls with the septal s′ velocity usually lower than that of the lateral [33]. Additionally, the mean s′ velocity decreases with age [33]. An s′ value <8 cm/s has a sensitivity of 86% and specificity of 93% for mild to moderately reduced LV systolic function (LVEF 30–50%). An s′ < 6 cm/s has a sensitivity of 92% and specificity of 84% for severely reduced LV systolic function (LVEF <30%) [34] (Fig. 12.7).

It is important to note that TDI interrogates myocardial velocity and as a result, it can be affected by tethering and translational forces which may mask regional hypokinesis. The presence of a mitral prosthesis or significant mitral

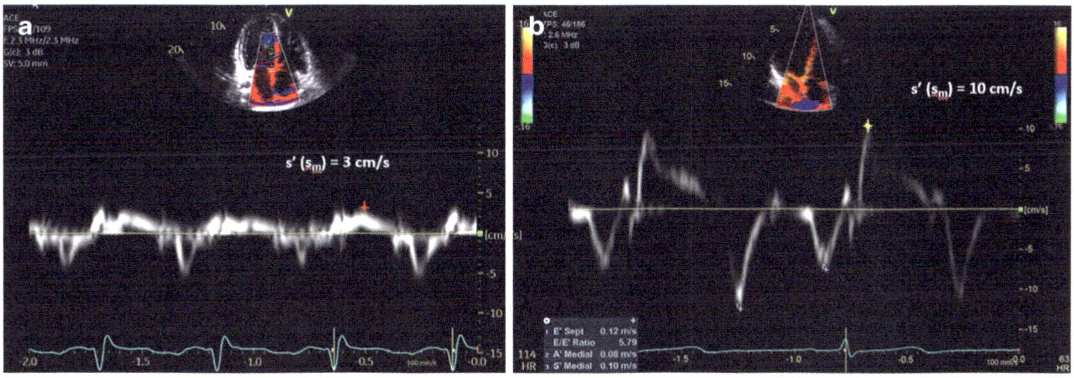

Fig. 12.7 TDI mitral annular systolic velocity (s′). TDI mitral annular systolic velocity provides a measure of myocardial velocity. The s′ velocity, similar to MAPSE, is a measure of LV systolic longitudinal function. The measurement is the peak positive velocity during systole and can be made using the medial (s_m) or lateral (s_l) aspect of the mitral annulus. (**a**) This patient with acute decompensated had left ventricular ejection fraction of 15% and a s′ velocity of 3 cm/s. (**b**) The s′ velocity of 10 cm/s correlated with normal left ventricular systolic function and ejection fraction of 65%. (*TDI* tissue Doppler imaging, *MAPSE* mitral annular plane systolic excursion)

annular calcification precludes the correlation of s′ velocity with LV systolic function.

Cardiac Cycle Time Intervals and Myocardial Performance Index

The myocardial performance index (Tei index) is a parameter that enables the assessment of global LV function [35]. Tei index is performed by using Doppler echocardiography (conventional PW or TDI-PW) to define cardiac cycle time intervals and is founded in the principle that LV dysfunction is characterized by prolongation of LV isovolumetric contraction and isovolumetric relaxation with concomitant shortening of the LV ejection time. TDI-PW is the simplest method for calculating the Tei index in patients with challenging acoustic windows since the entire cardiac cycle time can be captured using a single view of the medial or lateral aspect of the mitral annulus in the apical four-chamber window [36] (Fig. 12.8). Additionally, the TDI-PW method simultaneously provides the medial s′ velocity parameter for LV systolic function assessment. The measurement of the Tei index using conventional PW Doppler requires imaging of both the mitral inflow pattern and LVOT systolic flow signal [35]. The Tei index has been shown to be highly reproducible and independent of blood pressure, heart rate, and mitral regurgitation [35]. Normal mean LV Tei index is >0.40 and studies have correlated increased values with worse clinical outcomes in patients with congestive heart failure, acute myocardial infarction, and transcatheter aortic valve replacement [35–39]. It is important to note that the myocardial performance index can also be used to assess right ventricular function. The evaluation of right ventricular index of myocardial performance (RIMP) is analogous to the PW-TDI left ventricular method but uses the lateral aspect of the tricuspid annulus (normal RIMP PW-TDI is >0.54) [40].

The application of the Tei index is limited in patients with variable rhythms (atrial fibrillation or significant ectopy). The assessment is precluded in patients with significant intraventricular dyssynchrony, paced rhythms, and prosthetic mitral valves.

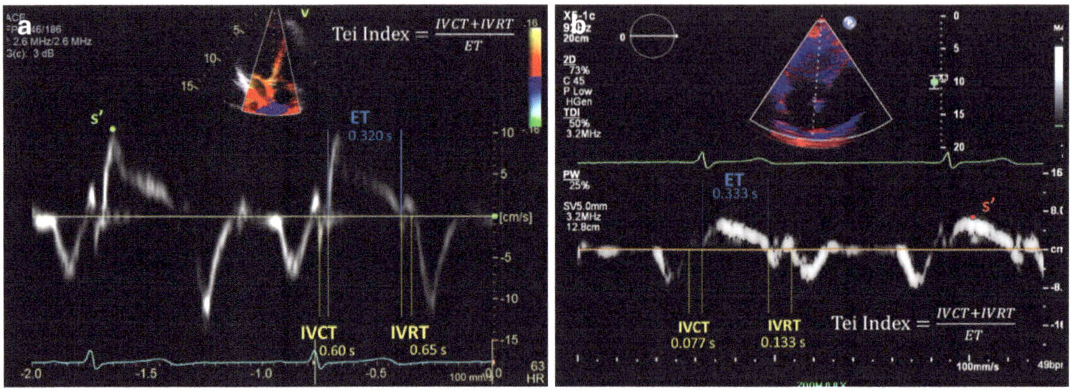

Fig. 12.8 Tissue Doppler imaging—Tei index (myocardial performance index). (**a**) The Tei index can be assessed using Tissue Doppler imaging (TDI) of the medial annulus of the mitral valve. This patient has normal LV diastolic and systolic function with short IVCT and IVRT intervals. The Tei index in this patient is 0.39 (normal <0.40). Note that the s′ velocity is also normal (10 cm/s). (**b**) This is a 25-year-old patient with a dilated cardiomyopathy and severe LV systolic dysfunction. The isovolumetric contraction and relaxation times are prolonged. The Tei index in this patient is 0.63. Note the s′ velocity is also reduced at 6.8 cm/s. (*IVCT* isovolumetric contraction time, *IVRT* isovolumetric relaxation time, *LV* left ventricle)

Summary Points

- Delineation of left ventricular systolic function using traditional 2D-echocardiography can prove challenging in critically ill patients due to poor acoustic windows.
- Ultrasound enhancement agents improve visualization of the endocardium and have been demonstrated to be effective at salvaging technically challenging or nondiagnostic echocardiograms in the intensive care unit.
- Pulse wave Doppler-derived stroke volume and cardiac output are key parameters that correlate well with invasive measurements in critically ill patients.
  - LVOT VTI can be monitored to assess dynamic changes in hemodynamics.
- Mitral annular plane systolic excursion (MAPSE) is an M-mode parameter that correlates with LV systolic function.
  - MAPSE >10 mm is associated with normal LV systolic function.
  - MAPSE <6 mm is associated with severely reduced LV systolic function (LVEF <30%).
- Pulse wave Doppler-derived dP/dt is a measure of LV contractility that correlates with invasive measurements.
  - dP/dt > 1200 mmHg/s correlates with normal LV systolic function.
  - dP/dt < 800 mmHg/s correlates with severely reduced LV systolic function.
- Tissue Doppler mitral annular systolic velocity (s′) correlates with LV systolic function.
  - s′ > 8 correlates with normal LV systolic function.
  - s′ < 6 has high sensitivity and specificity for severely reduced LV systolic function.
- Myocardial performance index (Tei index) is a parameter that assesses global LV function.
  - Tei index <0.40 is associated with normal LV systolic function.

Questions

1. A 45-year-old male with no prior medical history presents to the cardiac intensive care unit after undergoing emergent percutaneous intervention for acute ST-elevation myocardial infarction. He is tachycardiac (heart rate 114) with a blood pressure of 95/65 mmHg. What is his cardiac index if his body surface area is 2.2 m^2?

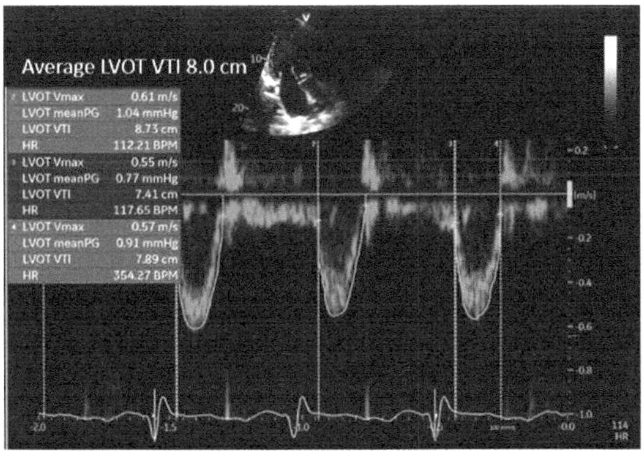

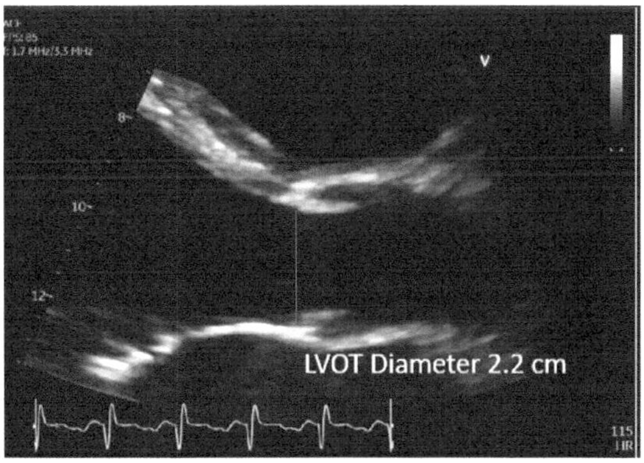

A. 1.5 L/min/m^2
B. 3.5 L/min/m^2
C. 7.0 L/min/m^2
D. 6.3 L/min/m^2

Answer: A

The stroke volume is calculated by multiplying the cross-sectional surface area of the LVOT by the stroke distance (LVOT VTI).

$\pi(d/2)^2 \times$ LVOT VTI [d = LVOT diameter (2.2 cm); LVOT VTI = 8.0 cm]

Therefore, the stroke volume is 30.4 mL and the cardiac output is 30.4 mL × 114 BPM = 3.465 L/min.

The cardiac index is 3.465 L/min divided by the body surface area (2.2 m^2) which equals 1.5 L/min/m^2.

(LVOT, left ventricular outflow tract; VTI, velocity time integral)

2. A 55-year-old female presents to emergency room with hypotension and fever. She receives 30 cc/kg of IV fluids but remains hypotensive. Bedside cardiac ultrasound is performed, but the acoustic windows are technically challenging. M-mode assessment of the mitral valve is performed (**A**). Based on the M-mode tracing, what is the next best step?

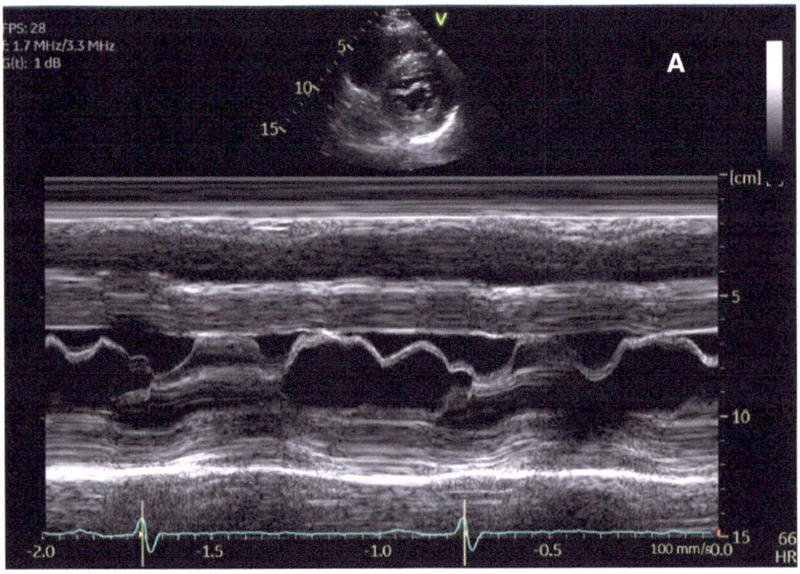

A. Start epinephrine
B. Start dobutamine
C. Start milrinone
D. Start phenylephrine

Answer: D

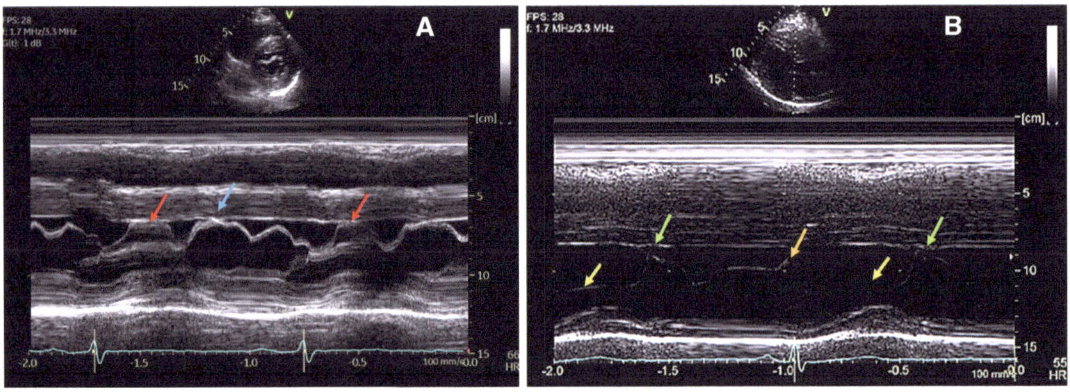

The M-mode mitral valve tracing demonstrates a negligible EPSS distance (blue arrow) in early diastole suggestive of normal LV systolic function. However, note that the anterior leaflet of the mitral valve also touches the ventricular septum during systole (red arrow). This is a classic M-mode tracing of systolic anterior motion of the mitral valve causing left ventricular outflow tract obstruction in a patient with hypertrophic obstructive cardiomyopathy. The administration of inotropic agents in this patient can worsen the outflow obstruction and cause worsening hypotension. The best agent for hypotension in this situation is a vasopressor such as phenylephrine (or vasopressin) that will increase the systemic vascular resistance without concomitant increase in heart rate. Figure B demonstrates a normal M-mode of the mitral valve with negligible EPSS distance (green arrows). However, note that the mitral leaflets stay on the closure line (yellow arrows) during systole. The orange arrow is the A-point that reflects mitral anterior leaflet motion due to atrial contraction (EPSS, E-point septal separation; LV, left ventricle)

3. The pulse wave Doppler tracings of the LVOT are from a patient with a dilated cardiomyopathy that was admitted to the cardiac intensive care unit with oliguria and elevated lactate. The blood pressure at the time of admission was 135/80 mmHg. What was the intervention that was performed to cause the change from image A to image B?

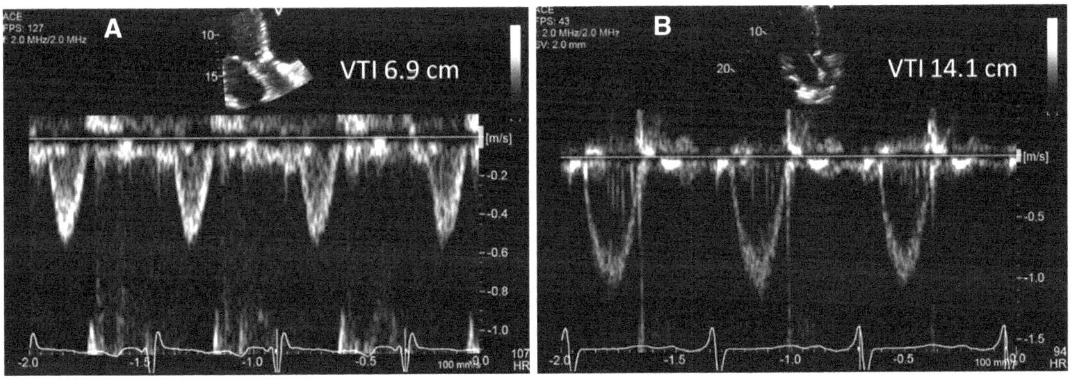

A. Started phenylephrine
B. Started vasopressin
C. Started nitroprusside
D. Started esmolol

Answer: C

This was patient admitted to the cardiac intensive care unit with normotensive cardiogenic shock (mean arterial pressure 98 mmHg). The initial LVOT VTI (6.9 cm) is consistent severely reduced stroke volume. The patient was started on a nitroprusside infusion to target a mean arterial pressure of 65–70 mmHg. Image B is the repeat LVOT VTI after reaching target mean arterial pressure. The LVOT VTI has increased to 14.1 cm which correlates with a doubling of stroke volume. (LVOT, left ventricular outflow tract; VTI, velocity time integral).

References

1. Naqvi TZ, Huynh HK. A new window of opportunity in echocardiography. J Am Soc Echocardiogr. 2006;19(5):569–77.
2. Waggoner AD, Baumann CM, Stark PA. "Views from the back" by subscapular retrocardiac imaging: technique and clinical application. J Am Soc Echocardiogr. 1995;8(3):257–62.
3. Strachinaru M, Hirsch A, Bowen D, Caliskan K. Echocardiography from a transhepatic approach in left ventricular assist device patients with difficult transthoracic imaging. Eur Heart J Case Rep. 2021;5(4):ytab108.
4. Porter TR, Mulvagh SL, Abdelmoneim SS, Becher H, Belcik JT, Bierig M, et al. Clinical applications of ultrasonic enhancing agents in echocardiography: 2018 American Society of Echocardiography guidelines update. J Am Soc Echocardiogr. 2018;31(3):241–74.
5. Bennett CE, Tweet MS, Michelena HI, Schears GJ, Mulvagh SL. Safety and feasibility of contrast echo-

cardiography for ECMO evaluation. JACC Cardiovasc Imaging. 2017;10(5):603–4.
6. Fine NM, Abdelmoneim SS, Dichak A, Kushwaha SS, Park SJ, Mulvagh SL. Safety and feasibility of contrast echocardiography for LVAD evaluation. JACC Cardiovasc Imaging. 2014;7(4):429–30.
7. Bhatia VK, Senior R. Contrast echocardiography: evidence for clinical use. J Am Soc Echocardiogr. 2008;21(5):409–16.
8. Mulvagh SL, Rakowski H, Vannan MA, Abdelmoneim SS, Becher H, Bierig SM, et al. American Society of Echocardiography consensus statement on the clinical applications of ultrasonic contrast agents in echocardiography. J Am Soc Echocardiogr. 2008;21(11):1179–201.
9. Senior R, Becher H, Monaghan M, Agati L, Zamorano J, Vanoverschelde JL, et al. Clinical practice of contrast echocardiography: recommendation by the European Association of Cardiovascular Imaging (EACVI) 2017. Eur Heart J Cardiovasc Imaging. 2017;18(11):1205–1205af.
10. Kurt M, Shaikh KA, Peterson L, Kurrelmeyer KM, Shah G, Nagueh SF, et al. Impact of contrast echocardiography on evaluation of ventricular function and clinical management in a large prospective cohort. J Am Coll Cardiol. 2009;53(9):802–10.
11. Main ML, Fu JW, Gundrum J, LaPointe NA, Gillam LD, Mulvagh SL. Impact of contrast echocardiography on outcomes in critically ill patients. Am J Cardiol. 2021;150:117–22.
12. Mondillo S, Galderisi M, Ballo P, Marino PN. Left ventricular systolic longitudinal function: comparison among simple M-mode, pulsed, and M-mode color tissue Doppler of mitral annulus in healthy individuals. J Am Soc Echocardiogr. 2006;19(9):1085–91.
13. Hu K, Liu D, Herrmann S, Niemann M, Gaudron PD, Voelker W, et al. Clinical implication of mitral annular plane systolic excursion for patients with cardiovascular disease. Eur Heart J Cardiovasc Imaging. 2013;14(3):205–12.
14. Matos J, Kronzon I, Panagopoulos G, Perk G. Mitral annular plane systolic excursion as a surrogate for left ventricular ejection fraction. J Am Soc Echocardiogr. 2012;25(9):969–74.
15. Otto CM. The practice of clinical echocardiography. 6th ed. Philadelphia: Elsevier; 2021.
16. McKaigney CJ, Krantz MJ, La Rocque CL, Hurst ND, Buchanan MS, Kendall JL. E-point septal separation: a bedside tool for emergency physician assessment of left ventricular ejection fraction. Am J Emerg Med. 2014;32(6):493–7.
17. Oh JK, Maleszewski JJ. Transthoracic M-mode and two-dimensional echocardiography. In: The echo manual. 4th ed. Lippincott Williams and Wilkins. p. 1–24.
18. Quiñones MA, Otto CM, Stoddard M, Waggoner A, Zoghbi WA. Recommendations for quantification of Doppler echocardiography: a report from the Doppler quantification task force of the nomenclature and standards committee of the American Society of Echocardiography. J Am Soc Echocardiogr. 2002;15(2):167–84.
19. Rusinaru D, Bohbot Y, Djelaili F, Delpierre Q, Altes A, Serbout S, et al. Normative reference values of cardiac output by pulsed-wave Doppler echocardiography in adults. Am J Cardiol. 2021;140:128–33.
20. Kou S, Caballero L, Dulgheru R, Voilliot D, De Sousa C, Kacharava G, et al. Echocardiographic reference ranges for normal cardiac chamber size: results from the NORRE study. Eur Heart J Cardiovasc Imaging. 2014;15(6):680–90.
21. Mercado P, Maizel J, Beyls C, Titeca-Beauport D, Joris M, Kontar L, et al. Transthoracic echocardiography: an accurate and precise method for estimating cardiac output in the critically ill patient. Crit Care. 2017;21(1):136.
22. McLean AS, Needham A, Stewart D, Parkin R. Estimation of cardiac output by noninvasive echocardiographic techniques in the critically ill subject. Anaesth Intensive Care. 1997;25(3):250–4.
23. Jentzer JC, Wiley BM, Anavekar NS, Pislaru SV, Mankad SV, Bennett CE, et al. Noninvasive hemodynamic assessment of shock severity and mortality risk prediction in the cardiac intensive care unit. JACC Cardiovasc Imaging. 2021;14(2):321–32.
24. Porter TR, Shillcutt SK, Adams MS, Desjardins G, Glas KE, Olson JJ, et al. Guidelines for the use of echocardiography as a monitor for therapeutic intervention in adults: a report from the American Society of Echocardiography. J Am Soc Echocardiogr. 2015;28(1):40–56.
25. Lamia B, Ochagavia A, Monnet X, Chemla D, Richard C, Teboul J-L. Echocardiographic prediction of volume responsiveness in critically ill patients with spontaneously breathing activity. Intensive Care Med. 2007;33(7):1125–32.
26. Jentzer JC, Tabi M, Wiley BM, Singam NSV, Anavekar NS. Echocardiographic correlates of mortality among cardiac intensive care unit patients with cardiogenic shock. Shock. 2021;57(3):336–43.
27. Reilly JP, Tunick PA, Timmermans RJ, Stein B, Rosenzweig BP, Kronzon I. Contrast echocardiography clarifies uninterpretable wall motion in intensive care unit patients. J Am Coll Cardiol. 2000;35(2):485–90.
28. Loutfi H, Nishimura RA. Quantitative evaluation of left ventricular systolic function by Doppler echocardiography techniques. Echocardiography. 1994;11(3):305–14.
29. Chung N, Nishimura RA, Holmes DR, Tajik AJ. Measurement of left ventricular dp/dt by simultaneous Doppler echocardiography and cardiac catheterization. J Am Soc Echocardiogr. 1992;5(2):147–52.
30. Bargiggia GS, Bertucci C, Recusani F, Raisaro A, de Servi S, Valdes-Cruz LM, et al. A new method for estimating left ventricular dP/dt by continuous wave Doppler-echocardiography. Validation studies at cardiac catheterization. Circulation. 1989;80(5):1287–92.

31. Abraham TP, Dimaano VL, Liang H-Y. Role of tissue Doppler and strain echocardiography in current clinical practice. Circulation. 2007;116(22):2597–609.
32. Ho CY, Solomon SD. A clinician's guide to tissue Doppler imaging. Circulation. 2006;113(10):e396–8.
33. Caballero L, Kou S, Dulgheru R, Gonjilashvili N, Athanassopoulos GD, Barone D, et al. Echocardiographic reference ranges for normal cardiac Doppler data: results from the NORRE study. Eur heart J Cardiovasc Imaging. 2015;16(9):1031–41.
34. Duzenli MA, Ozdemir K, Aygul N, Altunkeser BB, Zengin K, Sizer M. Relationship between systolic myocardial velocity obtained by tissue Doppler imaging and left ventricular ejection fraction: systolic myocardial velocity predicts the degree of left ventricular dysfunction in heart failure. Echocardiography. 2008;25(8):856–63.
35. Tei C, Ling LH, Hodge DO, Bailey KR, Oh JK, Rodeheffer RJ, et al. New index of combined systolic and diastolic myocardial performance: a simple and reproducible measure of cardiac function—a study in normals and dilated cardiomyopathy. J Cardiol. 1995;26(6):357–66.
36. Tekten T, Onbasili AO, Ceyhan C, Unal S, Discigil B. Value of measuring myocardial performance index by tissue Doppler echocardiography in normal and diseased heart. Jpn Heart J. 2003;44(3):403–16.
37. Asami M, Pilgrim T, Lanz J, Heg D, Franzone A, Piccolo R, et al. Prognostic relevance of left ventricular myocardial performance after transcatheter aortic valve replacement. Circ Cardiovasc Interv. 2019;12(1):e006612.
38. Lakoumentas JA, Panou FK, Kotseroglou VK, Aggeli KI, Harbis PK. The Tei index of myocardial performance: applications in cardiology. Hellenic J Cardiol. 2005;46(1):52–8.
39. Bennett S, Wong CW, Griffiths T, Stout M, Khan JN, Duckett S, et al. The prognostic value of Tei index in acute myocardial infarction: a systematic review. Echo Res Pract. 2020;7(4):49–58.
40. Lang RM, Badano LP, Mor-Avi V, Afilalo J, Armstrong A, Ernande L, et al. Recommendations for cardiac chamber quantification by echocardiography in adults: an update from the American Society of Echocardiography and the European Association of Cardiovascular Imaging. J Am Soc Echocardiogr. 2015;28(1):1–39.e14.

The Right Ventricle

13

Siddharth Dugar
and Saraschandra Vallabhajosyula

Learning Objectives
1. Describe techniques for the assessment of right ventricular function
2. Discuss the utility of TAPSE (Tricuspid annulus plane systolic excursion) to assess right ventricular function
3. Examine echocardiography-derived estimates of pulmonary pressure including RVSP, SPAP, DPAP, and mean PAP

The Right Ventricle

The right ventricle (RV) is the most anteriorly positioned thin-walled cardiac chamber supplying blood to the highly compliant pulmonary circulation. It is crescentic shaped, wrapping around the left ventricle in a U-shaped manner [1, 2]. The late adoption and incorporation of RV as part of the comprehensive cardiac assessment are partly due to its unique shape and retrosternal position limiting image acquisition and quantitative assessment. There is no single echocardiographic view that completely encompasses the entire RV [3, 4]. Hence, a comprehensive echocardiographic assessment of the RV requires multiple windows including the conventional apical four-chamber (A4C), parasternal long- (PLAX) and short-axis (PSAX), RV inflow and subcostal views, and RV-focused view. On transesophageal echocardiogram (TEE), mid-esophageal four-chamber, RV inflow-outflow views, and the trans-gastric short- and long-axis views are utilized for RV assessment. In addition, the pronounced trabeculations compromise accurate endocardial delineation. Despite the challenges of evaluating the RV using echocardiography, it remains the most widely utilized imaging modality for RV assessment.

Echocardiographic Evaluation of the Right Ventricle

The comprehensive examination of the RV includes the parasternal long-axis (PLAX), RV inflow view, RV outflow view, parasternal short-axis (PSAX) view, standard apical four-chamber

Supplementary Information The online version contains supplementary material available at https://doi.org/10.1007/978-3-031-80038-2_13.

S. Dugar
Department of Critical Care, Cleveland Clinic Lerner College of Medicine, Respiratory Institute, Cleveland Clinic, Cleveland, OH, USA
e-mail: dugars@ccf.org

S. Vallabhajosyula (✉)
Cardiology Division, Warren Alpert Medical School of Brown University, Providence, RI, USA
e-mail: svallabhajosyula@brownhealth.org

M. J. Lanspa, A. T. Levinson (eds.), *Echocardiography and Ultrasonography in the ICU*, Respiratory Medicine, https://doi.org/10.1007/978-3-031-80038-2_13

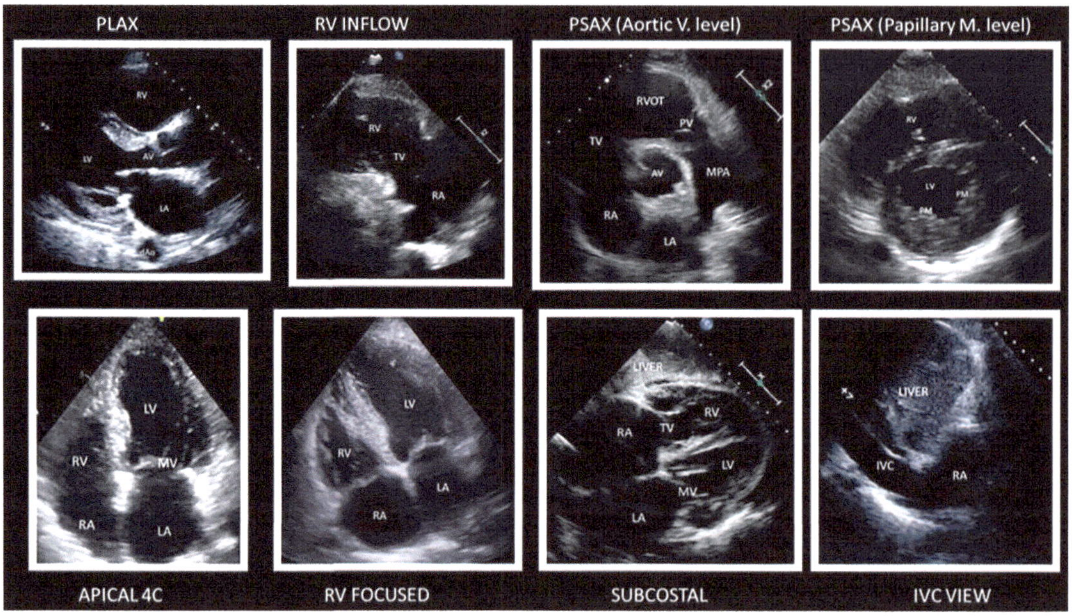

Fig. 13.1 The routinely used echocardiographic views to assess right ventricle size and function. *PLAX* parasternal long axis, *RV* right ventricle, *PSAX* parasternal short axis, *IVC* inferior vena cava

view, and subcostal views (Fig. 13.1) [3, 5]. The PLAX view produces views of the proximal RVOT, and the PSAX view allows assessment of the proximal and distal RVOT in the RV outflow view and RA and tricuspid valve in the RV inflow view. The linear dimension and area measurements of the RV along with regional and global functional assessment of the RV are mostly performed in apical views. Traditionally, the subcostal view is utilized for the assessment of inferior vena cava (IVC) size and collapsibility to estimate right atrial pressures. In a critically ill patient, the subcostal view is more frequently obtainable than the apical view, a more comprehensive assessment of the RV in the subcostal view has been suggested including a strain with promising results [6–9].

Right Ventricular-Focused View

The conventional apical four-chamber view (A4C) is obtained with the cardiac apex in the center of the screen to avoid left ventricle (LV) foreshortening (Video 13.1). This results in significant variability of the RV dimension and functional assessment. In addition, the RV-free wall may be obscured by lateral artifacts limiting precise RV assessment in a significant proportion of critically ill patients. The RV-focused view is obtained by lateral displacement of the transducer from the conventional A4C view position together with a probe rotation to obtain the largest RV dimension in its long axis (Video 13.2) [3, 4, 10]. The RV-focused view enhances RV cavity and free wall visualization without foreshortening. The visualization of the entire RV both during systole and diastole in this view has been shown to improve accuracy, hence is being recommended as the ideal view to assess the RV. In a recent study, the RV size was larger and the RV function quantified using RV Fractional area change (FAC), Tricuspid annulus plane systolic excursion (TAPSE), and Tricuspid annular systolic velocity (TASV) to be higher in the RV-focused view in comparison to conventional A4C view. Importantly, the authors established RV-focused view had higher intra-rater and inter-rater accuracy for RV dimensions [10]. This is especially important in critically ill patients, where these measurements may be used in a dynamic manner to determine response to interventions [11].

Semi-Quantitative Right Ventricular Assessment

RV dimensions may be challenging to obtain and inaccurate when the RV-free wall is not well visualized. In such cases, qualitative measurement of RV dilation by comparing it to LV size in an A4C view has been described.

- Normal (RV ≤ 2/3 LV size)
- Mildly dilated (RV ≥ 2/3 but <LV size)
- Moderately dilated (RV = LV area)
- Severely dilated (RV > LV area)

Orde et al. [12] showed a visual assessment of RV size and function can be used as an initial screening tool for the detection of RV pathology in critical care settings when performed by an intensivist with expertise in critical care echocardiography. One must be careful in cases of LV size abnormality, as it may lead to an incorrect assessment of RV dimension. However, if one is to use RV assessment for dynamic monitoring, quantitative assessment is recommended. In a study by Vallabhajosyula et al., quantitative parameters failed to show any benefit or semi-quantitative assessment in predicting outcomes [13]. One can also assess the apex to determine the presence of RV dilation. The LV usually forms the apex. As the RV enlarges, it displaces the LV and occupies the apex, which can act as an indirect marker of RV enlargement. RV can also be evaluated from the subcostal view, where if the RV appears larger than LV, RV dilatation is likely to be present. One has to be careful to confirm subcostal findings in other views. McConnell's sign is another visually characteristic echocardiographic pattern with dyskinesia of the mid-RV-free wall with relative sparring of the RV apex observed in acute RV dysfunction from increased afterload as in the case of pulmonary embolism and ARDS (Video 13.3).

Interventricular Septum

The interventricular septum functions as part of the LV in the normal heart. A qualitative examination of the septal motion in the PSAX view at the papillary muscles level may help to distinguish normal RV dysfunction from RV dysfunction due to volume and pressure overload. In the absence of RV dysfunction, the LV chamber appears circular during both systole and diastole. RV pressure overload (RV hypertrophy with a nondilated chamber) results in a leftward shift of septal motion throughout the cardiac cycle with the maximum reversed curvature at end-systole, while RV volume overload (RV dilatation) results in septal flattening (D-shaped pattern) at end-diastole [3, 14, 15].The abnormal pattern of septal motion can be easily appreciated in 2D imaging. In cases, where the pattern is not clear, M-mode imaging with higher temporal resolution can be utilized (Video 13.4) [16].

Right Ventricular Dimensions

One of the challenges in the uniform calculation of RV dimension stems from the absence of specific right-sided anatomic landmarks to be used as a reference point (Table 13.1). One must be careful in assessing RV dimension in standard apical view as small probe manipulations may result in significant variation in linear dimension and chamber size, hence RV-focused view is recommended for linear dimension and area measurement [10]. RV basal dimensions are measured at the base of RV at the point of insertion of a tricuspid leaflet to RV-free wall and interventricular septum (IVS) at end-diastole. It comprises the maximal short-axis dimension in the basal one-third of the RV. RV mid-cavity dimension is obtained on RV-free wall at the level of completely open anterior tricuspid leaflet tip and routinely corresponds to LV papillary muscle level. The longitudinal dimension is drawn from the plane of the tricuspid annulus to the RV apex. In the RV-focused view, RV enlargement is identified when RV basal diameter >41 mm, mid-cavity dimension >35 mm, or longitudinal dimension >86 mm. Proximal RV outflow diameter (RVOT prox) is measured in PLAX or PSAX at the aortic valve level from the RV-free wall to the interventricular septal-aortic junction (PLAX) or the aortic valve (PSAX) at end-diastole with normal

Table 13.1 Measurement of right ventricular function in critical care echocardiography

Linear dimension		
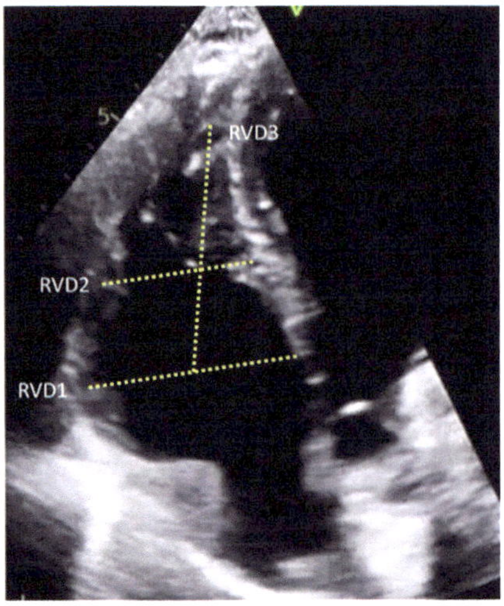	Normal 33 ± 4 mm (basal) 27 ± 4 mm (mid) 71 ± 6 mm (long) Abnormal >41 mm (basal) >35 mm (mid) >83 mm (long)	• Measured in A4C or preferably in RV-focused view • End-diastole • Inner edge to inner edge • Avoid foreshortening • Significant variability in obtained measurement with minimal probe rotation
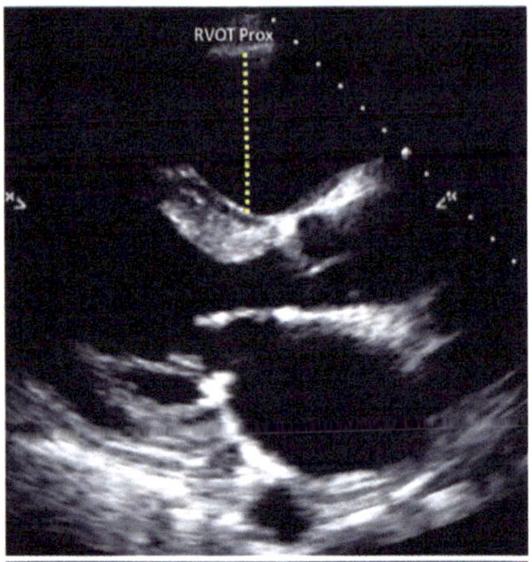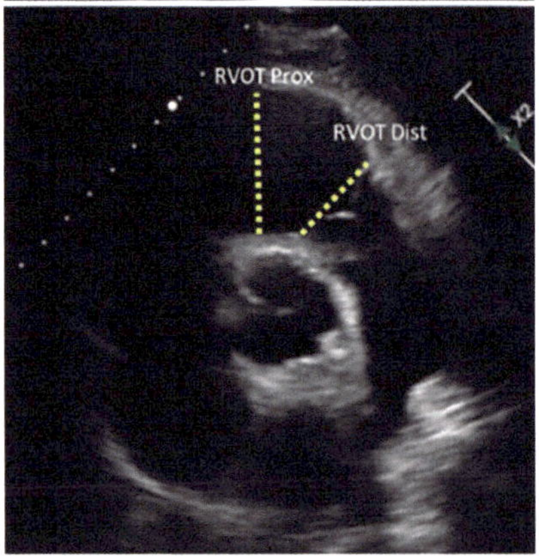	Normal 28 ± 3.5 mm (Prox) 22 ± 2.5 mm (Dist) Abnormal >35 mm (Prox) >27 mm (Dist)	• RVOT proximal is measured in PLAX and PSAX view • RVOT distal is measured in PSAX and RV outflow view • End-diastole • Inner edge to inner edge • Avoid obliquely oriented image • Inner edge to inner edge • Limited data on normal values

(continued)

Table 13.1 (continued)

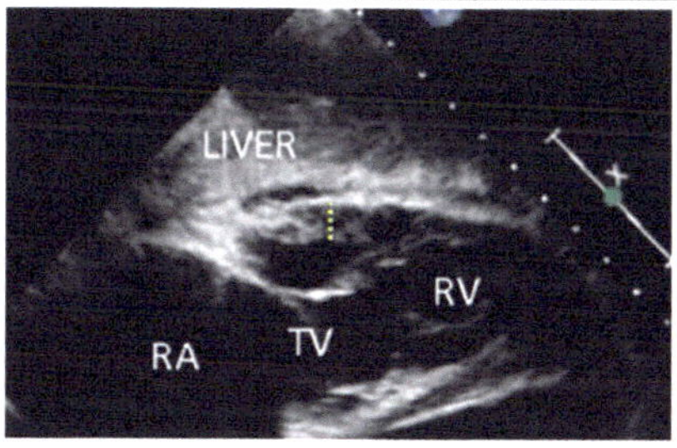	Normal 3 ± 1 mm Abnormal >5 mm	• Measured in zoomed-in subcostal view using M-mode or B-mode imaging • At the level of tip of open anterior tricuspid leaflet on RV free wall • End-diastole • Exclude trabeculae, papillary muscles, and epicardial fat • Single site measurement may limit accuracy
Area		
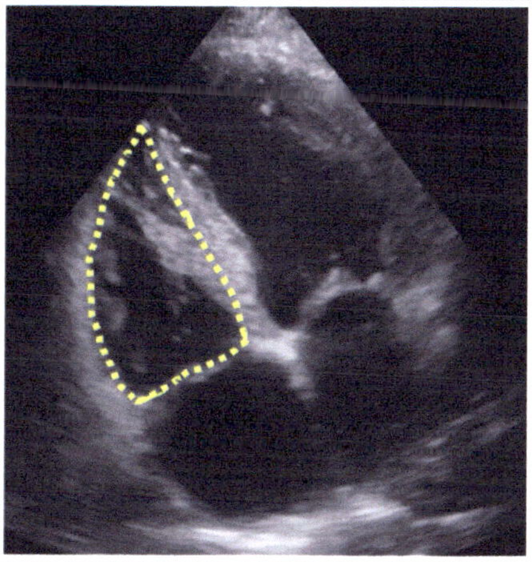	Normal 18 ± 7 cm^2 Abnormal >23 cm^2	RV end-diastolic area • Measured by tracing endocardium in RV-focused view • End-diastole • Trabeculations, papillary muscles, and moderator band are included in the cavity area • Needs optimal image with a clear definition of the endocardial border • Avoid foreshortening
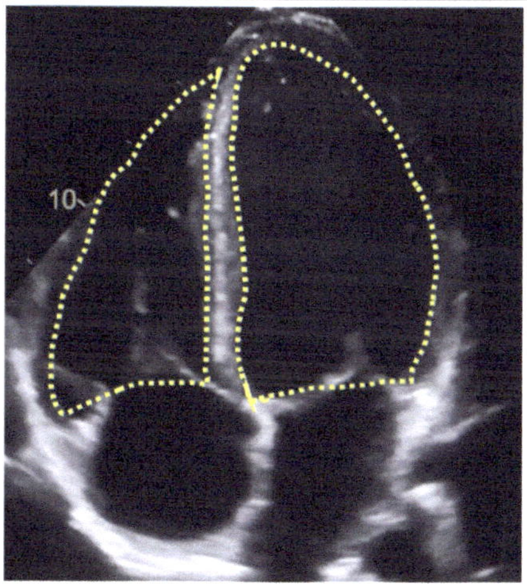	Normal RVEDA/LVEDA >0.6 Abnormal RVEDA/LVEDA ≥0.6	RV end-diastolic area/LV end-diastolic area • Measured by tracing endocardium in A4C view • End-diastole • Needs optimal image with a clear definition of the endocardial border • Avoid foreshortening • Established prognostic values in critically ill patients

(continued)

Table 13.1 (continued)

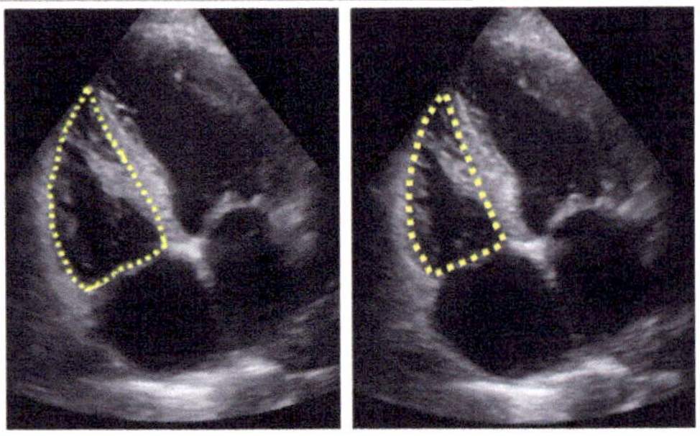	Normal 49 ± 7% Abnormal <35%	• Measured by tracing endocardium in RV-focused view • End-diastole and end-systole • Needs optimal image with clear definition of endocardial border • Incorporates both longitudinal and radial components of RV contraction • Established prognostic value in critically ill patients including sepsis, PH, pulmonary embolism, ARDS, and heart failure • Limited inter-rater reliability and reproducibility
Regional measurement		
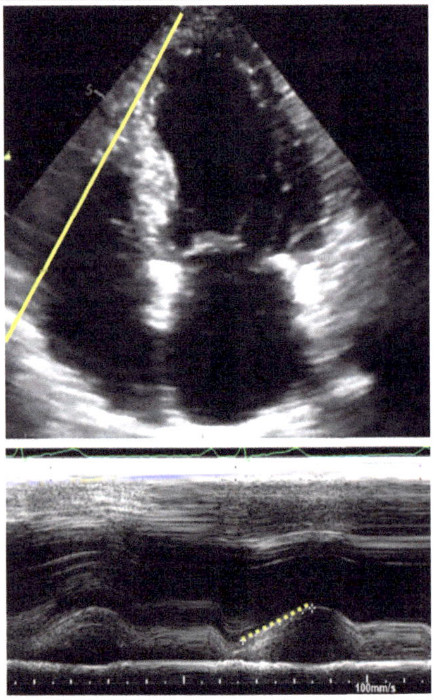	Normal 24 ± 3.5 mm Abnormal <17 mm	• Measures displacement of lateral tricuspid annulus toward cardiac apex in systole • Can be acquired in suboptimal images • Excellent inter-rater reliability and reproducibility • Established prognostic value in critically ill patients including sepsis, PH, pulmonary embolism, ARDS, and heart failure • Regional measurement • Angle dependent

(continued)

Table 13.1 (continued)

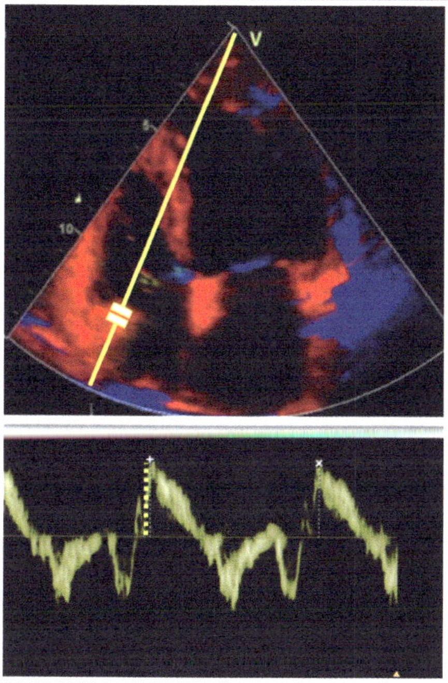	Normal 14.1 ± 2.3 cm/s Abnormal <9.5 cm/s	• Measures peak tissue velocity of lateral tricuspid annulus movement toward cardiac apex in systole • Can be acquired in suboptimal images • Excellent inter-rater reliability and reproducibility • Established prognostic value in critically ill patients including sepsis, PH, pulmonary embolism, ARDS, and heart failure • Regional measurement • Angle dependent
Global measurement		
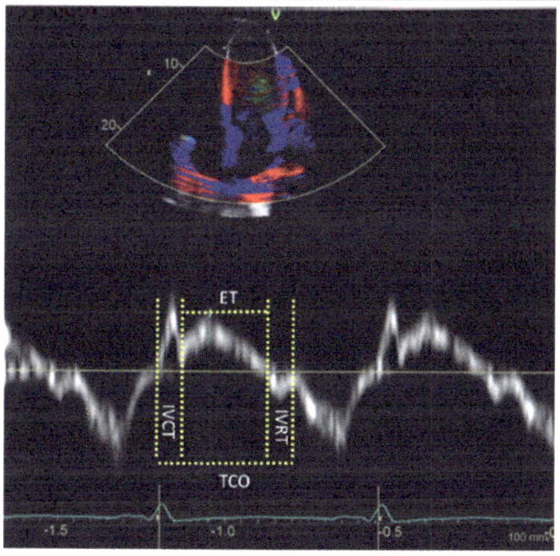	Normal 0.38 ± 0.08 Abnormal >0.54	• Measures time spent in nonejection time of total ejection time • Measured in A4C view using tissue Doppler or pulsed wave Doppler • Avoid geometric assumptions • Limited literature on critical illness • Angle dependent • Not accurate in severe TR and elevated RA pressure

(continued)

Table 13.1 (continued)

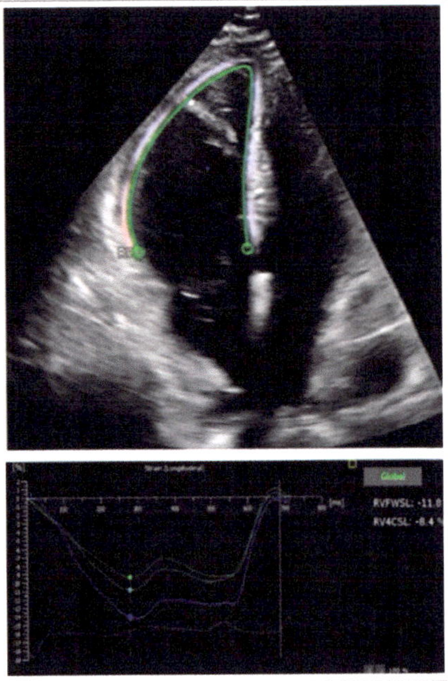	Normal −29 ± 4.5% Abnormal >−20%	• Measures movement of speckles toward each other in systole • Angle independent • Needs optimal image with a clear definition of the endocardial border • Needs strain analysis platform • Emerging prognostic value in critically ill patients including sepsis, PH, pulmonary embolism, ARDS, and heart failure • May have a role in the identification of subclinical dysfunction
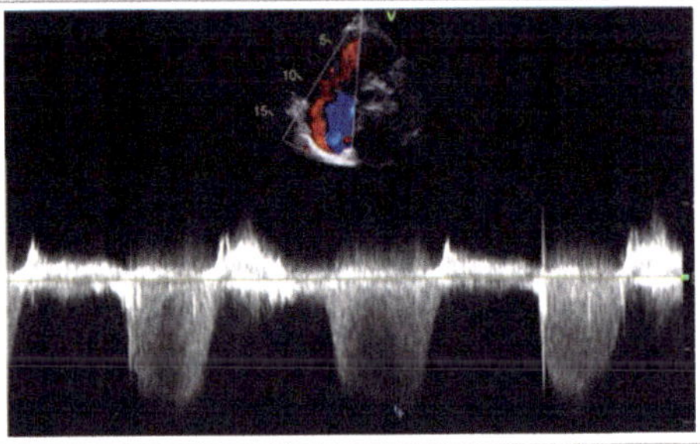	Normal ≤2.8 m/s Abnormal >2.8 m/s	• Measured from RV inflow, PSAX, A4C views • Measures the RV-RA gradient • Utilized to measure SPAP • Highest value is considered Angle dependent

A4C apical four-chamber view, *RV* right ventricle, *RVOT* right ventricle outflow tract, *PLAX* parasternal long axis, *PSAX* parasternal short axis, *LV* left ventricle, *PH* pulmonary hypertension, *ARDS* acute respiratory distress syndrome, *TR* tricuspid regurgitation, *RA* right atrium, *SPAP* systolic pulmonary arterial pressure

reference range of 21–35 mm. Distal RV outflow diameter (RVOT distal) is measured just proximal to the pulmonic valve at end-diastole with a normal reference range of 17–27 mm [3, 4].

Right Ventricular Wall Thickness

In the setting of chronically elevated right-sided pressure, adaptive RV hypertrophy ensues which can be identified by RV-free wall thickness of >0.5 cm. The measurement is performed in subcostal view using either M-mode or 2D image on the free wall at the tip of the fully open tricuspid leaflet at end-diastole [4, 17]. The accuracy of measurement can be improved with a zoomed image of RV mid-wall with the endocardium and epicardium perpendicular to the ultrasound beam and the exclusion of trabeculations, papillary muscle, and epicardial fat pad from the measurement.

Right Ventricular Area/Volume

LV volumes are routinely measured to determine the presence of LV dilation and to obtain LV ejection fraction. Volumetric assessments are limited due to the complex RV anatomy. The disk summation method has been applied for RV volume and RVEF similar to LVEF in A4C but remains technically challenging and has limited data to support its routine use. RV EF < 44% is considered abnormal [4].

Given the complexity of obtaining RV volume, Jardin and colleagues proposed comparing the area measurement of both ventricles and using the ratio to diagnose RV dilation [18]. The ventricular areas are traced at end-diastole in the A4C view. RV end-diastolic area to left ventricular end-diastolic area (RVEDA: LVEDA) >0.6 to be highly suggestive of moderate RV dilation, while area of (RVEDA: LVEDA) ≥1 suggests severe RV dilation. RVEDA/LVEDA ≥1 has been shown to be associated with high morbidity and mortality in pulmonary embolism and acute respiratory distress syndrome (ARDS) patients [19–21]. In the study, the authors noted RVEDA/LVEDA may be not feasible in 1/4th of ARDS patients with TTE, as area measurement requires complete visualization of ventricles and suggested routine use of TTE. RV end-diastolic dimension to left ventricular end-diastolic dimension (RVEDD: LVEDD), a more easily measured value above 1 has also been studied in pulmonary embolism and may be an alternative to more complex RVEDA/LVEDA ratio [20].

Regional Systolic Functional Assessment

TAPSE (Tricuspid Annulus Plane Systolic Excursion)

Traditionally, the longitudinal fiber shortening has been postulated to account for most of the RV contraction [22]. TAPSE or TAM (tricuspid annular motion) is a simple and easily obtainable quantitative measurement of RV systolic function [3–5]. The contraction of these longitudinally oriented RV muscle fibers results in systolic displacement of the tricuspid annulus toward the RV apex providing one of the most visible estimations of RV systolic function. TAPSE is obtained by measuring the distance of this excursion at peak systole. M-mode cursor is placed on the junction of the tricuspid valve plan along the RV-free wall in orientation toward the cardiac apex in A4C and RV-focused view [3, 4, 10]. The normal value is >17 mm based on 46 studies with over 2300 patients; a lower value is suggestive of RV systolic dysfunction [3]. Reduced TAPSE has been shown to be a poor prognostic maker in inferior wall myocardial infarction, pulmonary embolism, ARDS, sepsis, and in the general patient population [21, 23–27]. TAPSE has also been validated as an accurate measurement of RV systolic function to gold standard measures including radionuclide angiography, biplane Simpson RV ejection fraction, and RV fractional area shortening [28, 29]. In addition to ease of measurement with minimal training, high inter-rater and intra-rater reliability and repeatability are the main reasons for its widespread use [30].

SEATAK (Systolic Excursion Assessment of Tricuspid Annular Kick) or sTAPSE (Subcostal TAPSE)

Subcostal echocardiographic assessment of tricuspid annular kick (SEATAK) or subcostal TAPSE (sTAPSE) has recently been proposed as an alternative to conventional TAPSE in critically ill patients with morbid obesity, chronic lung disease, mechanical ventilation, or in patients where apical view may be inadequate [8, 9]. Studies have shown SEATAK and sTAPSE from a subcostal view to be more easily obtainable in these cohorts. M-mode or B-mode can then be used to measure the linear displacement of tricuspid annulus from end-diastole to end-systole. Both SEATAK and sTAPSE have been shown to have excellent correlation to conventional TAPSE [8, 9] and other echocardiographic markers of RV function. Subcostal TAPSE was shown to accurately detect abnormal longitudinal shortening with a sensitivity of 97.8% and specificity of 87.5% in critically ill.

Tricuspid Annular Systolic Velocity (Right Ventricular S′)

Tricuspid annular systolic velocity (TASV) or RV S′ measures the peak myocardial tissue velocity of systolic displacement of the tricuspid annulus toward the RV instead of distance as measured with TAPSE. It is measured at the tricuspid annulus on the RV-free wall (same as TAPSE) using tissue Doppler (TDI). In a conventional A4C or RV-focused view, TDI is activated highlighting the RV-free wall with pulsed wave Doppler sample volume placed at the lateral tricuspid annulus [4]. The highest resultant tissue velocity at the tip of the clear signal is measured. A value of <9.5 cm/s indicates RV systolic dysfunction [3]. Validation studies comparing pulsed TASV with radionuclide angiograph have shown good correlation and excellent discriminative ability of TASV to differentiate normal and abnormal RV systolic function [4, 31].

Unlike volumetric assessments, TAPSE and TASV do not require distinct endocardial border definitions. However, it assumes that the displacement of the tricuspid annulus is representative of the function of the entire RV, an assumption that is not valid in many disease states or with regional RV wall motion abnormalities. These measurements are also angle-dependent.

Global Systolic Functional Assessment

Right Ventricular Fractional Area Change

Fractional area change (FAC) is the percentage change in RV area at the end of systole from the end of diastole and is calculated as:

$$\text{RV FAC} = \frac{\text{RVEDA} - \text{RVESA}}{\text{RVEDA}} * 100$$

RVFAC is usually measured in conventional A4C or RV-focused view in transthoracic echocardiography and the mid-esophageal 4C view in transesophageal echocardiography. A key requirement for accurate RVFAC is a well-defined endocardial border definition, limiting its application and reproducibility in a critically ill patient. The heavy trabeculations in RV should also be excluded during tracing the true apex and RV-free wall. The major benefit of RVFAC over other measurements is it is not angle-dependent and accounts for both the longitudinal and radial components of RV contraction. RVFAC has also been validated against cardiac magnetic resonance (CMR) obtained RV ejection fraction and 3D EF [32, 33]. An FAC <35% is considered abnormal. A reduced RV FAC is associated with poor outcome in ARDS, pulmonary embolism, sepsis, and myocardial infarction [32, 34–36].

Right Ventricular Index of Myocardial Performance

Right ventricular index of myocardial performance (RIMP) also known as *Tei* index is a global estimate of RV systolic and diastolic function. It is the ratio of time spent during nonejection time (isovolumetric contraction and isovolumetric relaxation) to total ejection time. RIMP being the ratio of time intervals, is independent of the complex RV geometry. The measurement can be obtained using either tissue Doppler at the lateral annulus or pulsed wave Doppler at the tricuspid leaflet tips. The benefit of using the tissue Doppler technique is that the isovolumetric contraction time (IVCT), the isovolumetric relaxation time (IVRT), and ejection time (ET) can be obtained from the same heartbeat. The pulsed Doppler-derived RIMP is obtained over two separate cardiac cycles; hence one needs to make sure the RR interval of the cardiac cycle used is the same length for accurate results.

$$\text{RIMP} = \frac{\text{IVRT} + \text{IVCT}}{\text{ET}}$$

$$\text{RIMP} = \frac{\text{TCO} + \text{ET}}{\text{ET}}$$

As the RV decompensates, the time spent during nonejection of total ejection time increases [37]. The upper reference limits for RIMP obtained using the pulsed wave technique are 0.43 and 0.54 when calculated by tissue Doppler imaging. RIMP is affected by pressure and loading conditions, which limits its utilization in the presence of severe TR and elevated RA pressure (RAP), conditions frequently observed in critically ill patients.

Right-Sided Hemodynamics

RV systolic pressure (RVSP) is the most frequently documented right-sided pressure in the critically ill cohort and general population. RVSP is calculated from peak TR jet velocity, using the simplified Bernoulli equation and combining this value with an estimate of the RA pressure

$$\text{SPAP} = \text{RVSP} = 4(\text{Peak TR jet velocity})^2 + \text{RAP}$$

Peak TR jet velocity is usually obtained by continuous-wave Doppler from the RV inflow or the A4C view and is reflective of the pressure difference between RV and RA during systole. Hence, the addition of RA pressure to the equation to obtain RVSP. In spontaneously breathing patients, the RA pressure can be estimated from IVC diameter and collapsibility. However, no echocardiographic measurements have been validated for RA pressure measurement in patients on positive pressure ventilation. During the use of positive pressure, the RA pressure should be obtained from central venous access with a tip located in the right atrium. RVSP and Systolic pulmonary artery pressure (SPAP) are equal in the absence of pulmonary stenosis or RVOT obstruction. The velocity measurements are angle-dependent, hence it is recommended to gather TR signals from several windows and to use the signal with the highest velocity. In cases of weak or incomplete TR signal, enhancement of signal with agitated saline or blood-saline contrast has been shown to improve measurement accuracy. One has to be careful to avoid overestimation of the spectral envelope by ensuring that only the well-defined, dense spectral profile is measured. In patients with severe TR, the Doppler envelope may be cut off early due to the equalization of RV and RA pressures. The simplified Bernoulli equation assumes the proximal velocity to be small and is ignored, in the situation of severe TR with elevated RA pressure, the equation underestimates the RV-RA gradient. The normal cutoff value for mean PA pressure is 25 mmHg, which correlates to a peak TR gradient of 2.8–2.9 m/s. TR gradients higher than 2.9 m/s are highly suggestive of pulmonary hypertension. The development of pulmonary hypertension has been shown to independently predict mortality in sepsis [38], ARDS [39], and myocardial infarction [40].

Diastolic pulmonary artery pressure (DPAP) is estimated from the velocity of the end-diastolic pulmonary regurgitant jet using the modified Bernoulli equation. The systolic and diastolic pulmonary artery pressure can then be utilized to obtain mean pulmonary artery pressure (mPAP).

$$\text{DPAP} = 4\begin{pmatrix}\text{pulmonary} \\ \text{regurgitant end} - \text{diastolic} \\ \text{velocity}\end{pmatrix}^2 + \text{RAP}$$

$$\text{mPAP} = \frac{\text{PASP} + 2\,\text{PADP}}{3}$$

Right Ventricular Outflow Tract (RVOT) Pulse Wave (PW) Doppler Indices

RV outflow tract (RVOT) pulse wave (PW) Doppler has been studied as a surrogate for RV function and (RV-pulmonary artery) RV-PA interaction. It can be imaged from multiple transthoracic views including the PSAX, RV outflow view, modified PLAX view, or a modified subcostal approach interrogating the RVOT [41]. The PW gate is placed just below the pulmonic cusp in the middle of the RVOT. Normal RVOT VTI shows a slower acceleration, a longer time from the onset of flow to peak flow, and a more "rounded" velocity curve. As pulmonary vascular resistance increases, the shape of the RV ejection curve resembles more closely to the LVOT VTI curve, with a shorter time to peak velocity from downstream resistance or impedance. A value below 105 ms is very suggestive of significant pulmonary hypertension [4]. Mean pulmonary artery pressure can also be estimated from pulmonary artery acceleration [42].

$$\text{mPAP} = 79 - (0.45 * \text{AT})$$

$$\text{mPAP} = 90 - (0.62 * \text{AT}), \text{if AT} < 120\,\text{ms}$$

Right Ventricular-Pulmonary Artery Coupling

In physiological conditions, the right heart is "coupled" to the pulmonary circulation as a single cardiopulmonary unit, keeping a relative matching between contractility and afterload. As pulmonary hypertension (PH) develops, the vascular bed becomes a high-resistance, and low-compliance system adding additional load on the ventricular contraction and altered RV-PA coupling. Right heart catheterization is the gold standard for assessment of RV-PA coupling, yet echocardiography is increasingly being used due to its noninvasive nature. Composite echo-variables incorporating RV systolic function and loading condition have been suggested to overcome the load dependency of most echocardiographic variables in assessing RV-PA coupling. One of them is the TAPSE/SPAP ratio, which assesses RV systolic function as a ratio of RV longitudinal shortening in relation to loading condition and has been an important prognostic marker in critical illness [43, 44]. Hemodynamically significant acute PE can be diagnosed by using a combination of PASP <60 mmHg and PVAT <60 ms (the "60/60 sign") with high positive predictive value. TAPSE/PVR incorporates the relationship between afterload increase and RV function and is termed as RV ejection efficiency (RVEe) and has been used for early identification of RV-PA uncoupling in pulmonary hypertension [45, 46].

Right Ventricular Diastolic Function

An emerging concept in the field of cardiology and critical care is assessment of RV diastolic dysfunction. It stems from multiple studies showing RV diastolic dysfunction to precede RV systolic dysfunction and may serve as an early and easily available quantifiable variable of subclinical RV dysfunction [47, 48]. The assessment is similar to LV diastolic function; however, the numerical value may differ due to the greater area of the tricuspid valve and lower velocity of trans-tricuspid blood flow. One can obtain E (Early diastolic filling velocity) and A (Late diastolic filling velocity) by placing a pulse wave Doppler at the tip of the tricuspid leaflet in the A4C view at end-expiration. RV E′ velocity is then obtained by TDI at the level of the tricuspid lateral annular plane. One can calculate E/E′ and E/A ratios to identify and quantify RV diastolic dysfunction. An E/E′ ratio > 4 has been shown to have good sensitivity and specificity for predicting an RAP ≥10 mmHg in critically ill patients. The presence of moderate to severe TR, atrial fibrillation, and tachycardia may confound diastolic parameters [4].

Grading of RV diastolic dysfunction

- Impaired relaxation: E/A ratio < 0.8
- Pseudo-normal filling: E/A ratio of 0.8–2.1 and E/E′ > 6 or diastolic flow predominance in the hepatic veins
- Restrictive filling: E/A ratio > 2.1 with a DCT < 120 ms

Right Ventricular Strain

Myocardial deformation (strain) imaging is a relatively novel echocardiographic technique to assess RV myocardial function and, unlike other echo techniques can identify subtle RV dysfunction [6, 20, 49–51]. Speckle tracking (STE) tracks the movement of grayscale-based "speckles" (known as "kernels"); an ultrasound artifact evaluates the degree of deformation of the kernels relative to each other. The closer the speckles move toward each other, the higher the deformation. Since STE evaluates how close the speckles move toward each other from their original position, the more negative the value of strain, the higher the systolic function. The most commonly performed RV strain is a longitudinal strain (in the base to apex direction) measured from apical windows assessing the RV-free wall with the exclusion of the interventricular septum. For proper strain assessment, the entire myocardium should be clearly visualized throughout the cardiac cycle with a frame rate of the image ranging between 60 and 80 frames/s. Foreshortening of the echocardiographic image may further compromise the accuracy of the measurement. These image requirements for strain analysis are challenging to meet in critically ill patients, limiting its widespread use in clinical decision-making.

Conclusion

The integration of RV assessment using echocardiography is vital in the appropriate management of critically ill patients. Echocardiography allows rapid qualitative or in-depth quantitative assessment of RV including dimensions, septal morphology, regional and global RV systolic function, and an estimation of RV hemodynamics. This chapter details various echocardiographic assessments that are easy to obtain providing comprehensive insight into the underlying pathophysiology. The emergence and increased accessibility to novel tools including strain imaging, trans-esophageal echocardiogram, and 3-D echocardiography have the potential to provide more precise assessments of the RV with higher reliability in critically ill patients.

Summary Points

- RV dysfunction is routinely observed in patients with critical illness.
- RV dysfunction has been shown to be independently associated with poor outcomes in sepsis, acute respiratory failure, COVID-19, myocardial infarction, and heart failure.
- Echocardiography is the preferred modality to assess RV in the critically ill patient population.
- The complex geometry of RV requires assessment of RV in multiple views for an accurate assessment of both size and function.
- A RV size >2/3 size of the left ventricle in apical four-chamber is suggestive of RV dilation.
- TAPSE <16.5 mm, TASV <9.5 cm/s, and RVFAC <35% are suggestive of RV dysfunction.
- Echocardiography-derived pulmonary pressure including RVSP, SPAP, DPAP, and mean PAP have been validated against RHC and found to have high accuracy except in extreme cases.
- RV-PA coupling incorporates assessment of RV systolic function in relation to loading conditions.
- RV strain imaging may be able to recognize subclinical RV dysfunction.

References

1. Kamperidis V, Nihoyannopoulos P, Bax JJ, Delgado V. Assessing the right ventricle. In: Echocardiography. Springer; 2018. p. 373–95.
2. Ho SY, Nihoyannopoulos P. Anatomy, echocardiography, and normal right ventricular dimensions. Heart. 2006;92(Suppl 1):i2–13.
3. Lang RM, Badano LP, Mor-Avi V, Afilalo J, Armstrong A, Ernande L, et al. Recommendations for cardiac chamber quantification by echocardiography in adults: an update from the American Society of Echocardiography and the European Association of Cardiovascular Imaging. J Am Soc Echocardiogr. 2015;28(1):1–39.e14.
4. Rudski LG, Lai WW, Afilalo J, Hua L, Handschumacher MD, Chandrasekaran K, et al. Guidelines for the echocardiographic assessment of the right heart in adults: a report from the American Society of Echocardiography. J Am Soc Echocardiogr. 2010;23(7):685–713.
5. Zaidi A, Knight DS, Augustine DX, Harkness A, Oxborough D, Pearce K, et al. Echocardiographic assessment of the right heart in adults: a practical guideline from the British Society of Echocardiography. Echo Res Pract. 2020;7(1):G19–41.
6. Bleakley C, de Marvao A, Morosin M, Androulakis E, Russell C, Athayde A, et al. Utility of echocardiographic right ventricular subcostal strain in critical care. Eur Heart J Cardiovasc Imaging. 2021;23(6):820–8.
7. López-Candales A, Vallurupalli S. Right ventricular free wall contractility in subcostal views: a proof-of-concept study to assess right ventricular systolic function. Echocardiography. 2021;38(12):2052–9.
8. Main AB, Braham R, Campbell D, Inglis AJ, McLean A, Orde S. Subcostal TAPSE: a retrospective analysis of a novel right ventricle function assessment method from the subcostal position in patients with sepsis. Ultrasound J. 2019;11(1):19.

9. Diaz-Gomez JL, Alvarez AB, Danaraj JJ, Freeman ML, Lee AS, Mookadam F, et al. A novel semiquantitative assessment of right ventricular systolic function with a modified subcostal echocardiographic view. Echocardiography. 2017;34(1):44–52.
10. Genovese D, Mor-Avi V, Palermo C, Muraru D, Volpato V, Kruse E, et al. Comparison between four-chamber and right ventricular-focused views for the quantitative evaluation of right ventricular size and function. J Am Soc Echocardiogr. 2019;32(4):484–94.
11. Vieillard-Baron A, Millington SJ, Sanfilippo F, Chew M, Diaz-Gomez J, McLean A, et al. A decade of progress in critical care echocardiography: a narrative review. Intensive Care Med. 2019;45(6):770–88.
12. Orde S, Slama M, Yastrebov K, McLean A, Huang S. Subjective right ventricle assessment by echo qualified intensive care specialists: assessing agreement with objective measures. Crit Care. 2019;23(1):70.
13. Vallabhajosyula S, Kumar M, Pandompatam G, Sakhuja A, Kashyap R, Kashani K, et al. Prognostic impact of isolated right ventricular dysfunction in sepsis and septic shock: an 8-year historical cohort study. Ann Intensive Care. 2017;7(1):94.
14. Kossaify A. Echocardiographic assessment of the right ventricle, from the conventional approach to speckle tracking and three-dimensional imaging, and insights into the "right way" to explore the forgotten chamber. Clin Med Insights Cardiol. 2015;9:65–75.
15. Ryan T, Petrovic O, Dillon JC, Feigenbaum H, Conley MJ, Armstrong WF. An echocardiographic index for separation of right ventricular volume and pressure overload. J Am Coll Cardiol. 1985;5(4):918–27.
16. Prada G, Vieillard-Baron A, Martin AK, Hernandez A, Mookadam F, Ramakrishna H, et al. Echocardiographic applications of M-mode ultrasonography in anesthesiology and critical care. J Cardiothorac Vasc Anesth. 2019;33(6):1559–83.
17. Jurcut R, Giusca S, La Gerche A, Vasile S, Ginghina C, Voigt JU. The echocardiographic assessment of the right ventricle: what to do in 2010? Eur J Echocardiogr. 2010;11(2):81–96.
18. Jardin F, Dubourg O, Bourdarias JP. Echocardiographic pattern of acute cor pulmonale. Chest. 1997;111(1):209–17.
19. Mekontso Dessap A, Boissier F, Charron C, Begot E, Repesse X, Legras A, et al. Acute cor pulmonale during protective ventilation for acute respiratory distress syndrome: prevalence, predictors, and clinical impact. Intensive Care Med. 2016;42(5):862–70.
20. Khemasuwan D, Yingchoncharoen T, Tunsupon P, Kusunose K, Moghekar A, Klein A, et al. Right ventricular echocardiographic parameters are associated with mortality after acute pulmonary embolism. J Am Soc Echocardiogr. 2015;28(3):355–62.
21. Sato R, Dugar S, Cheungpasitporn W, Schleicher M, Collier P, Vallabhajosyula S, et al. The impact of right ventricular injury on the mortality in patients with acute respiratory distress syndrome: a systematic review and meta-analysis. Crit Care. 2021;25(1):172.
22. Brown SB, Raina A, Katz D, Szerlip M, Wiegers SE, Forfia PR. Longitudinal shortening accounts for the majority of right ventricular contraction and improves after pulmonary vasodilator therapy in normal subjects and patients with pulmonary arterial hypertension. Chest. 2011;140(1):27–33.
23. Vallabhajosyula S, et al. Impact of right ventricular dysfunction on short-term and long-term mortality in sepsis: a meta-analysis of 1,373 patients. Chest. 2021;159(6):2254–63.
24. Lobo JL, Holley A, Tapson V, Moores L, Oribe M, Barrón M, et al. Prognostic significance of tricuspid annular displacement in normotensive patients with acute symptomatic pulmonary embolism. J Thromb Haemost. 2014;12(7):1020–7.
25. Forfia PR, Fisher MR, Mathai SC, Housten-Harris T, Hemnes AR, Borlaug BA, et al. Tricuspid annular displacement predicts survival in pulmonary hypertension. Am J Respir Crit Care Med. 2006;174(9):1034–41.
26. Modin D, Møgelvang R, Andersen DM, Biering-Sørensen T. Right ventricular function evaluated by tricuspid annular plane systolic excursion predicts cardiovascular death in the general population. J Am Heart Assoc. 2019;8(10):e012197.
27. Vishram-Nielsen JK, Foroutan F, Ross HJ, Gustafsson F, Buchan TA, Alba A. Association between serial measurements of tricuspid annular plane systolic excursion and mortality post heart transplant. J Heart Lung Transplant. 2019;38(4):S209.
28. Barthélémy R, Roy X, Javanainen T, Mebazaa A, Chousterman BG. Comparison of echocardiographic indices of right ventricular systolic function and ejection fraction obtained with continuous thermodilution in critically ill patients. Crit Care. 2019;23(1):312.
29. Miller D, Farah MG, Liner A, Fox K, Schluchter M, Hoit BD. The relation between quantitative right ventricular ejection fraction and indices of tricuspid annular motion and myocardial performance. J Am Soc Echocardiogr. 2004;17(5):443–7.
30. Huang SJ, Nalos M, Smith L, Rajamani A, McLean AS. The use of echocardiographic indices in defining and assessing right ventricular systolic function in critical care research. Intensive Care Med. 2018;44(6):868–83.
31. Meluzín J. Pulsed Doppler tissue imaging of the velocity of tricuspid annular systolic motion. A new, rapid, and non-invasive method of evaluating right ventricular systolic function. Eur Heart J. 2001;22(4):340–8.
32. Anavekar NS, Skali H, Bourgoun M, Ghali JK, Kober L, Maggioni AP, et al. Usefulness of right ventricular fractional area change to predict death, heart failure, and stroke following myocardial infarction (from the VALIANT ECHO study). Am J Cardiol. 2008;101(5):607–12.
33. Anavekar NS, Gerson D, Skali H, Kwong RY, Kent Yucel E, Solomon SD. Two-dimensional assessment of right ventricular function: an echocardiographic? MRI correlative study. Echocardiography. 2007;24(5):452–6.

34. Lanspa MJ, Cirulis MM, Wiley BM, Olsen TD, Wilson EL, Beesley SJ, et al. Right ventricular dysfunction in early sepsis and septic shock. Chest. 2021;159(3):1055–63.
35. Chotalia M, Ali M, Alderman JE, Kalla M, Parekh D, Bangash MN, et al. Right ventricular dysfunction and its association with mortality in coronavirus disease 2019 acute respiratory distress syndrome. Crit Care Med. 2021;49(10):1757–68.
36. Dahhan T, Siddiqui I, Tapson VF, Velazquez EJ, Sun S, Davenport CA, et al. Clinical and echocardiographic predictors of mortality in acute pulmonary embolism. Cardiovasc Ultrasound. 2016;14(1):44.
37. Tei C, Dujardin KS, Hodge DO, Bailey KR, McGoon MD, Tajik AJ, et al. Doppler echocardiographic index for assessment of global right ventricular function. J Am Soc Echocardiogr. 1996;9(6):838–47.
38. Vallabhajosyula S, Geske JB, Kumar M, Kashyap R, Kashani K, Jentzer JC. Doppler-defined pulmonary hypertension in sepsis and septic shock. J Crit Care. 2019;50:201–6.
39. Villar J, Blazquez MA, Lubillo S, Quintana J, Manzano JL. Pulmonary hypertension in acute respiratory failure. Crit Care Med. 1989;17(6):523–6.
40. Haeck MLA, Hoogslag GE, Boden H, Velders MA, Katsanos S, Al Amri I, et al. Prognostic implications of elevated pulmonary artery pressure after ST-segment elevation myocardial infarction. Am J Cardiol. 2016;118(3):326–31.
41. Hockstein MA, Haycock K, Wiepking M, Lentz S, Dugar S, Siuba M. Transthoracic right heart echocardiography for the intensivist. J Intensive Care Med. 2021;36(9):1098–109.
42. Dabestani A, Mahan G, Gardin JM, Takenaka K, Burn C, Allfie A, et al. Evaluation of pulmonary artery pressure and resistance by pulsed Doppler echocardiography. Am J Cardiol. 1987;59(6):662–8.
43. Guarracino F, Bertini P, Pinsky MR. Right ventriculo-arterial coupling in the critically ill. Springer International Publishing; 2017.
44. Jentzer JC, Anavekar NS, Reddy YNV, Murphree DH, Wiley BM, Oh JK, et al. Right ventricular pulmonary artery coupling and mortality in cardiac intensive care unit patients. J Am Heart Assoc. 2021;10(7):e019015.
45. Dandel M, Hetzer R. Echocardiographic assessment of the right ventricle: impact of the distinctly load dependency of its size, geometry and performance. Int J Cardiol. 2016;221:1132–42.
46. Todaro MC, Carerj S, Zito C, Trifirò MP, Consolo G, Khandheria B. Echocardiographic evaluation of right ventricular-arterial coupling in pulmonary hypertension. Am J Cardiovasc Dis. 2020;10(4):272–83.
47. Tavazzi G, Bergsland N, Alcada J, Price S. Early signs of right ventricular systolic and diastolic dysfunction in acute severe respiratory failure: the importance of diastolic restrictive pattern. Eur Heart J Acute Cardiovasc Care. 2020;9(6):649–56.
48. Zochios V, Lau G, Conway H, Parhar KKS. Protecting the right ventricle network (PRORVNet): time to defend the "forgotten ventricle"? J Cardiothorac Vasc Anesth. 2021;35(6):1565–7.
49. Bleakley C, Singh S, Garfield B, Morosin M, Surkova E, Mandalia MS, et al. Right ventricular dysfunction in critically ill COVID-19 ARDS. Int J Cardiol. 2021;327:251–8.
50. Bonizzoli M, Cipani S, Lazzeri C, Chiostri M, Ballo P, Sarti A, et al. Speckle tracking echocardiography and right ventricle dysfunction in acute respiratory distress syndrome a pilot study. Echocardiography. 2018;35(12):1982–7.
51. Sachdev A, Villarraga HR, Frantz RP, McGoon MD, Hsiao JF, Maalouf JF, et al. Right ventricular strain for prediction of survival in patients with pulmonary arterial hypertension. Chest. 2011;139(6):1299–309.

Atrial Size and Function

14

Taha Ahmed, Amit Arbune, and Vincent L. Sorrell

Learning Objectives

1. Discuss how the left atrium is a critically important modulator of left ventricular filling, a volume sensor, and a barometer of diastolic function.
2. Review optimal TTE techniques for assessing LA structure and function.

Left Atrium

The left atrium (LA) is an oval-shaped structure visualized posterior to the aortic root and superior to the left ventricle (LV) forming a large part of the base of the heart. Anatomically, the anterosuperior wall is adjacent to the ascending aorta and pulmonary trunk and the posteroinferior wall is adjacent to the esophagus and typically has four pulmonary vein orifices. The posteroinferior wall corresponds to the diaphragmatic face; the mitral valve is positioned at the anteroinferior wall; the medial wall corresponds to the interatrial septum and contains the fossa ovalis; and the lateral wall contains the left atrial appendage (LAA) [1]. The walls are mostly composed of smooth muscle fibers but contain prominent trabeculae in and near the LAA [1]. The atrioventricular orifice is positioned lower anteriorly and is intimately related to the mitral valve.

Imaging assessment of atrial size and function can be performed using cardiac computed tomography (CCTA) and cardiovascular magnetic resonance (CMR); however, transthoracic echocardiography (TTE) is conventionally the initial diagnostic modality given its safety profile, portability, comprehensive capabilities with high temporal and spatial resolution. Complete assessment of the LA includes the use of real-time two-dimensional (2D) and three-dimensional (3D) TTE, Doppler techniques, and off-line analysis of quantitative volumes, function, and novel speckle-tracking determination of mechanical properties [2]. Although not exploited in clinical practice, TTE is well suited to provide a detailed assessment of LA structure and function.

The LA functions as a *reservoir* draining from the pulmonary veins during ventricular systole, a *conduit* during early diastole, and a *contractile pump* during late diastole to complete left ventricular filling just prior to the LV contraction and mitral valve closure [2]. An alteration in the LA dimension and function may impact any one of these three components of the LA function.

Supplementary Information The online version contains supplementary material available at https://doi.org/10.1007/978-3-031-80038-2_14.

T. Ahmed · A. Arbune · V. L. Sorrell (✉)
University of Kentucky, Gill Heart and Vascular Institute, Lexington, KY, USA
e-mail: Taha.Ahmed@uky.edu; amitarbune@uky.edu; v.sorrell@uky.edu

M. J. Lanspa, A. T. Levinson (eds.), *Echocardiography and Ultrasonography in the ICU*, Respiratory Medicine, https://doi.org/10.1007/978-3-031-80038-2_14

Left Atrial Size, Dimensions, and Volumes

Left atrial (LA) size quantification is complicated by the complex LA geometry, intricate fiber orientation, and the variable contributions of the left atrial appendage and pulmonary veins. LA volume determination is one of the rare circumstances in which TTE is preferred over transesophageal echocardiogram (TEE) due to the intimate esophageal/LA relationship that limits visualization in the immediate near-field [2].

Due to the challenges of securing an accurate scan plane and the variable patterns of LV dilation, linear dimensions using M-mode or 2D-TTE have been replaced by estimation of LA volumes from visualization in multiple views [3].

Utilizing apical two- and four-chamber views in orthogonal planes to the left atrial long axis, phasic measurements of the LA are performed (Figs. 14.1 and 14.2). Carefully tracing the maximally visualized border of the LA in two orthogonal views allows you to apply the ultrasound system's biplane Simpson's method of disc formula to determine the LA volume (LAV) (Fig. 14.3).

Once calculated, the LAV is indexed to the body surface area (LAVI) to correct for changes related to physical stature and categorized by sex (Table 14.1) [2]. Importantly, given the current ubiquitous prevalence of obesity in society, the normal relationship of LAV to BSA is altered and the optimal method to index the LAV is being scrutinized [4]. To better understand this relationship, the maximal ($LAVI_{max}$) and minimal ($LAVI_{min}$) are being carefully investigated and matched to clinical outcomes. The $LAVI_{max}$ is strongly associated with predicting cardiovascular outcomes. However, its prognostic value is lower in atrial fibrillation (AF) [2]. Recent findings suggest that LAV_{min} is more strongly associated with AF than LAV_{max} regardless of using isometric or allometric height-indexation [5].

Call Out

In a retrospective assessment of >300 patients in sinus rhythm, $LAVI_{max}$ measured in the biplane 2-D apical views was found superior to four-chamber LA area alone or LA dimension in predicting the development of first atrial fibrillation (AF), congestive heart failure (CHF), cerebrovascular accident, acute myocardial infarction, coronary revascularization, and cardiovascular death over a 3.5-year follow-up [6].

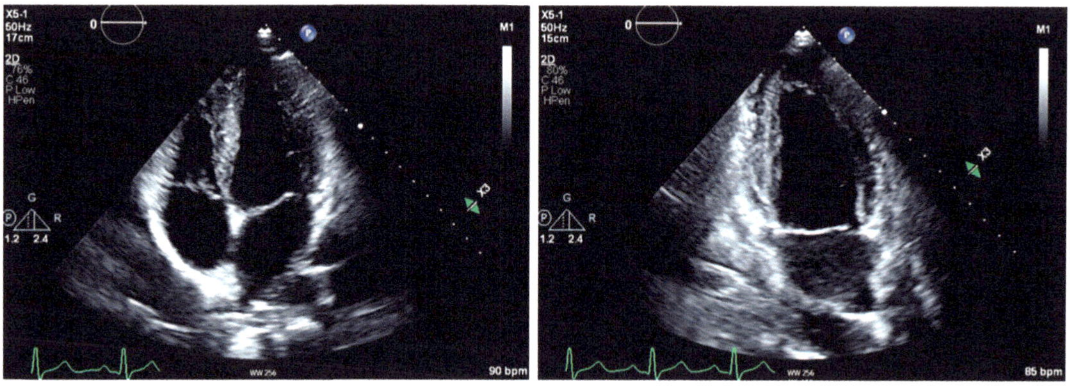

Fig. 14.1 LV four-chamber and two-chamber views with long axis along the LV where LA is not well visualized

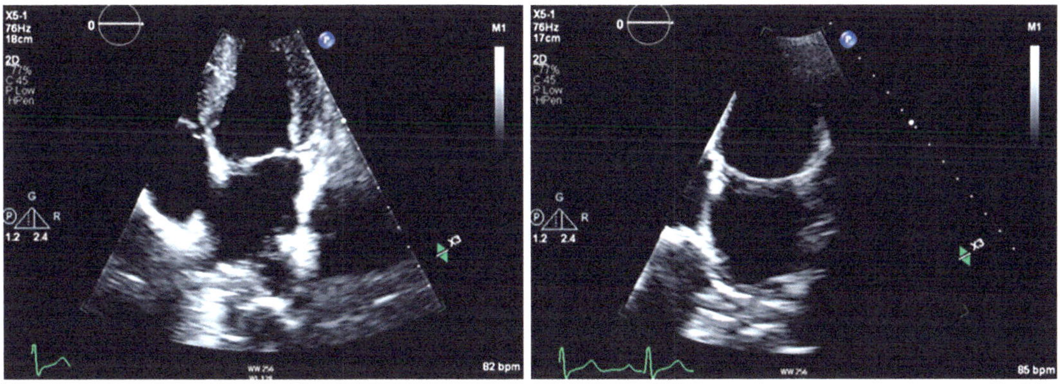

Fig. 14.2 Dedicated LA views in four-chamber and two-chamber orientation demonstrating better visualization of the LA and foreshortening of the LA

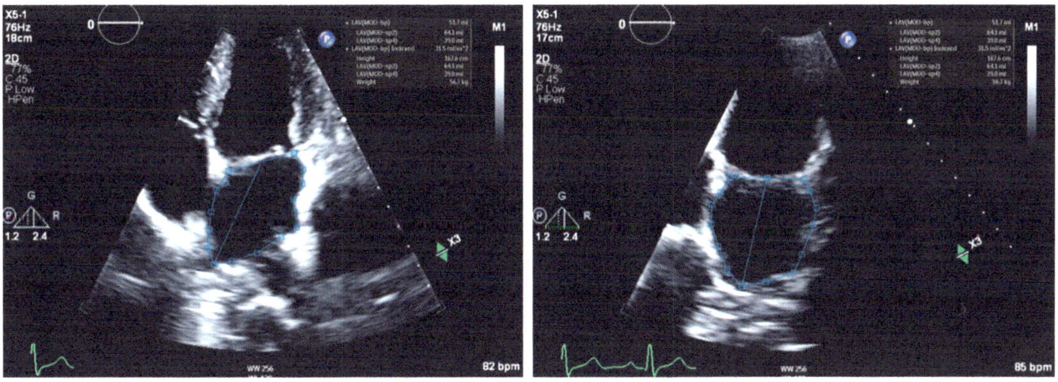

Fig. 14.3 Biplane measurement of the LA volumes in the four-chamber and two-chamber views on dedicated LA views

Table 14.1 LA size gradation as per the recommendations for cardiac chamber quantification by echocardiography in adults: an update from the American Society of Echocardiography and the European Association of Cardiovascular Imaging [2]

LAVI	Males and females
Normal (mL/m^2)	<34
Mild (mL/m^2)	34–41
Moderate (mL/m^2)	42–48
Severe (mL/m^2)	>48

Technical Considerations

While assessing the LA using TTE, the following technical considerations are vital [2, 3]:

- LA size should be measured when the chamber is at its greatest dimension (typically, end-systolic).
- Apical TTE images dedicated to the LA chamber should be obtained to avoid LA foreshortening that may occur with conventional LV-aligned apical TTE images.
- The lengths of the LA measured in the two orthogonal views should be similar (e.g., within 5.0 mm) and provide a quality measure to minimize foreshortening.
- While tracing LA borders, the confluences of the pulmonary veins and the LAA should be excluded.
- The atrioventricular interface should be represented by the mitral annulus plane, not by the tip of mitral leaflets.

Call Out

A systematic underestimation of 2DE-acquired $LAVI_{max}$ *compared to CCT and CMR is observed, likely due to foreshortening and difficult endocardial border visualization.*

Where CCT and CMR have their own limitations, real-time 3DE is gaining popularity as the modality of choice to accurately measure cardiac chamber volumes with lower interobserver variability and higher test-retest reproducibility compared with 2DE [7].

LAVI is a predictor of the development of heart failure and poor clinical outcomes, irrespective of LV systolic function. In patients with heart failure with preserved ejection fraction (HFpEF), the relevance of LAVI is perhaps even greater. Although normative data and prognostic utility of 3DE are warranted, evaluation of LA parameters will likely be included in future guidelines (Figs. 14.4 and 14.5, Video 14.1).

Evolving Evidence

There is recent evidence suggesting that $LAVI_{min}$ *may be a more important prognostic indicator using either 2DE or 3DE* [8]. *Current recommendations encourage the reporting of the maximum and minimum LAVI.*

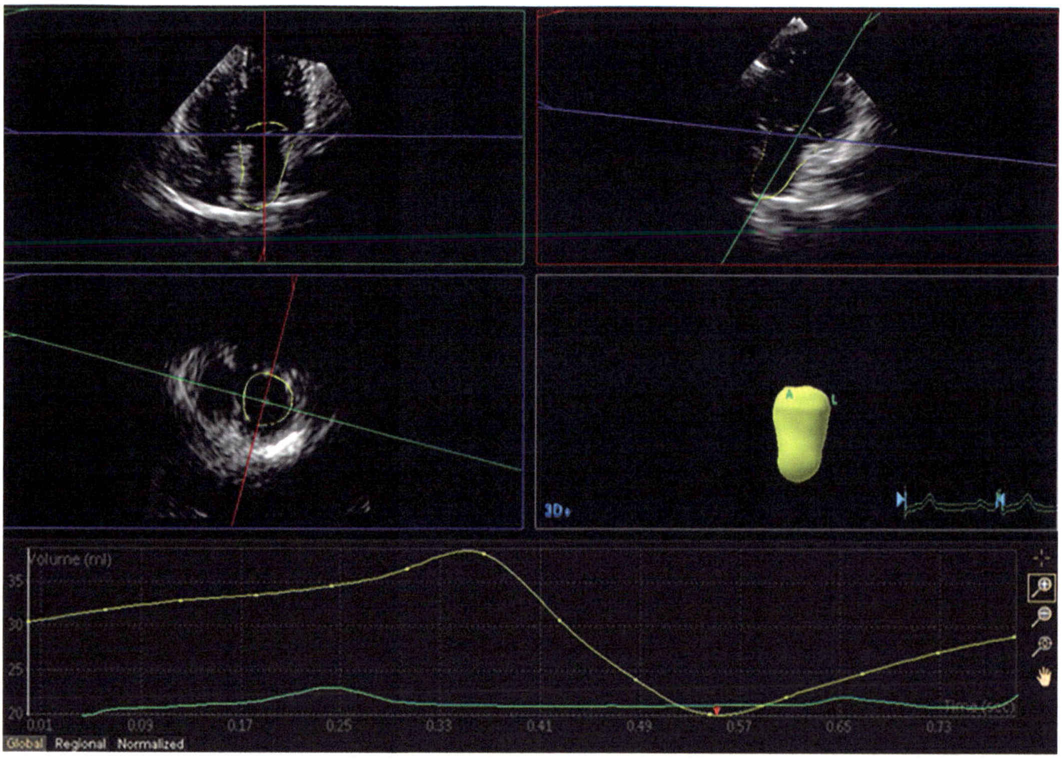

Fig. 14.4 3D-TTE, apical four-chamber, two-chamber, and short-axis views providing the volumetric assessment of the LA size and function. The bottom lines represent the time-volume curves for LA physiology

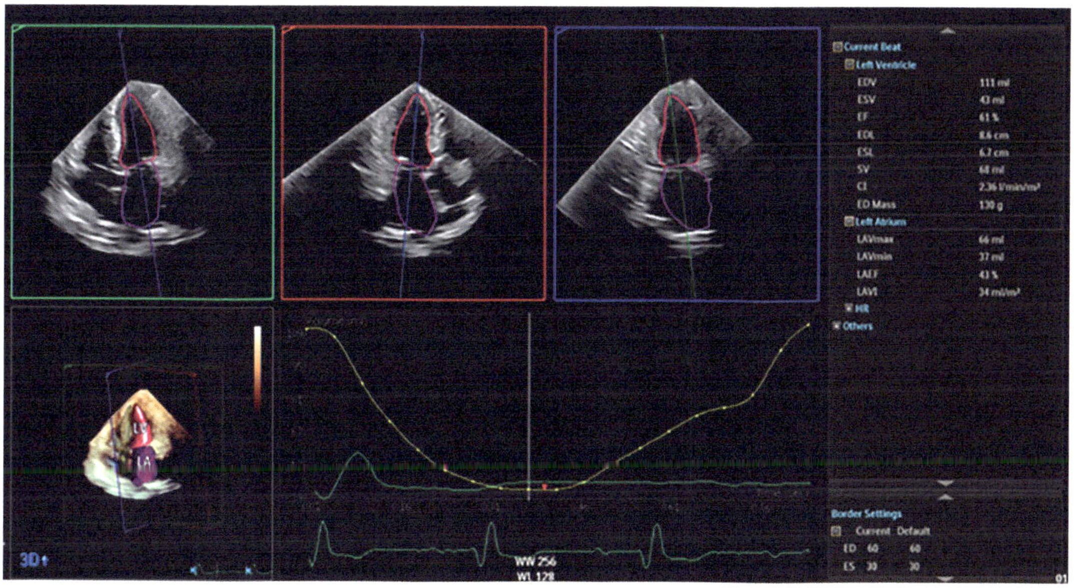

Fig. 14.5 3D-TTE captured as a full volume loop, showing the apical four-chamber, three-chamber, and two-chamber views for the LV and volumetric rendering of both LV and LA along the LA and LV volume curves at the bottom calculated on the Philips EPIQ machine utilizing the Heart Model A.I. 3D tool. The tool calculates the LA volumes, LAVI, and LAEF as well. This eliminates the need for dedicated LA views for accurately obtaining LAVI

Summary Points

- *LA chamber dimensions often dilate asymmetrically with the disease, should be measured using biplane LAVI, and 3DE is superior to 2DE and allows the determination of $LAVI_{max}$ and $LAVI_{min}$ which may offer additional prognostic value compared with LAVI alone.*
- *Accurate LAVI determination requires careful acquisition is confounded in AF and mitral valve disease and is underutilized in routine clinical practice.*

Left Atrial Function

Left atrial function holds significance and can be assessed using conventional 2D and Doppler techniques, as well as more contemporary 3D volumetric and speckle-tracking deformation analysis.

A **volumetric assessment** of LA function can aid in assessing total, passive, and active emptying (ejection) fractions, representative of the reservoir, conduit, and booster pump function, respectively.

Doppler waveforms of pulmonary venous flow (LA filling) and trans-mitral flow (LA emptying) can be used to estimate relative atrial functions. The ratios of peak trans-mitral early (E) and late (A) velocities (or their velocity time integrals [VTIs]) and the atrial filling fraction ($A_{VTI}/[E_{VTI} + A_{VTI}]$) estimate the relative contribution of atrial booster pump function. The ratio of systolic (S) to diastolic (D) pulmonary venous flow estimates relative reservoir to conduit function (Fig. 14.6). The magnitude and duration of pulmonary vein flow reversal during atrial contraction (PVa) are used to estimate atrial contractility and LV diastolic pressure [9]. Atrial ejection force is the force exerted by LA to accelerate blood into LV and is, yet another Doppler parameter studied for atrial systolic function [6].

Call Out

Interpretations of pulsed wave spectral Doppler indices are challenging in patients with sinus tachycardia, conduction system disease, and arrhythmia (especially AF), and obtaining high-quality pulmonary venous recordings may be difficult. A disadvantage of spectral Doppler is its lack of specificity [6].

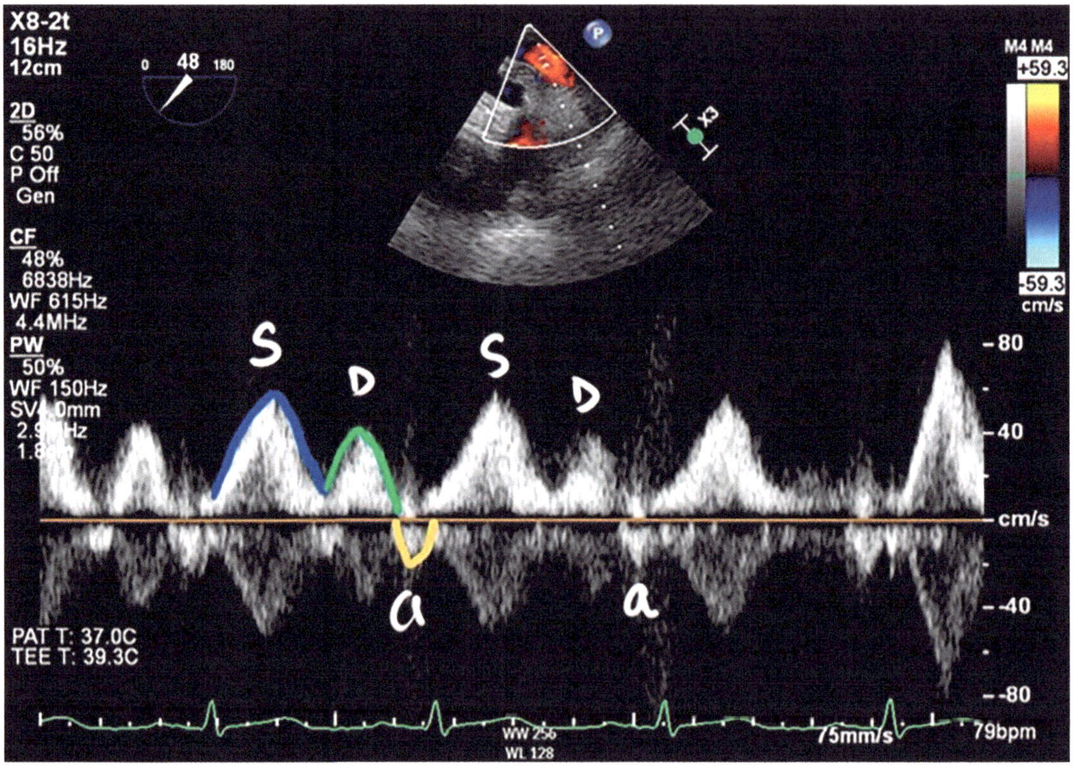

Fig. 14.6 2D TEE, mid-esophageal window, 48-degree display of the pulsed wave spectral Doppler analysis with the sample volume positioned in the left superior pulmonary vein demonstrating the LA phases—S corresponding with the reservoir (blue contour), D corresponding with conduit (green contour) and PVa (yellow contour) corresponding with LA pump function

Deformation analysis utilizing atrial strain and strain rates (SR) representing the magnitude and rate, respectively, of myocardial deformation have been applied in an effort to better understand left atrial mechanics. This was initially assessed using tissue Doppler velocities (TDI) but has more recently been evaluated with 2D speckle-tracking echocardiography (STE) techniques (Fig. 14.7). STE analyzes myocardial motion through frame-by-frame tracking of natural acoustic speckles, from interactions between ultrasound and myocardial tissue, within a user-defined region [6]. Frame rates of approximately 50–70 frames/s are needed to prevent speckle decorrelation, and good image quality is crucial for accurate tracking.

An LA-focused **apical four-chamber view** is recommended to generate longitudinal strain and strain rate curves throughout the cardiac cycle out of which regional and average values can be calculated [6]. The myocardial region of interest is defined by the inner and outer LA wall contours. The tracing should start at the endocardial border of the mitral annulus with extrapolation of the contour across the pulmonary veins and the LAA orifices. Global longitudinal strain is defined as strain in the direction **tangential to the endocardial atrial border in the apical view** [6].

The left atrial appendage is rarely optimal using TTE and therefore TEE is considered standard to assess emptying velocities and assess for the presence of thrombus (Fig. 14.8).

2D strain and strain rate imaging overcome much of the subjectivity and variability inherent in assessing endocardial motion. A recent small report suggests that LA reservoir strain can be reproducibly measured with a standardized methodology which incorporates self-directed education [10]. However, these methods fail to address the complexities of 3D cardiac geometry and

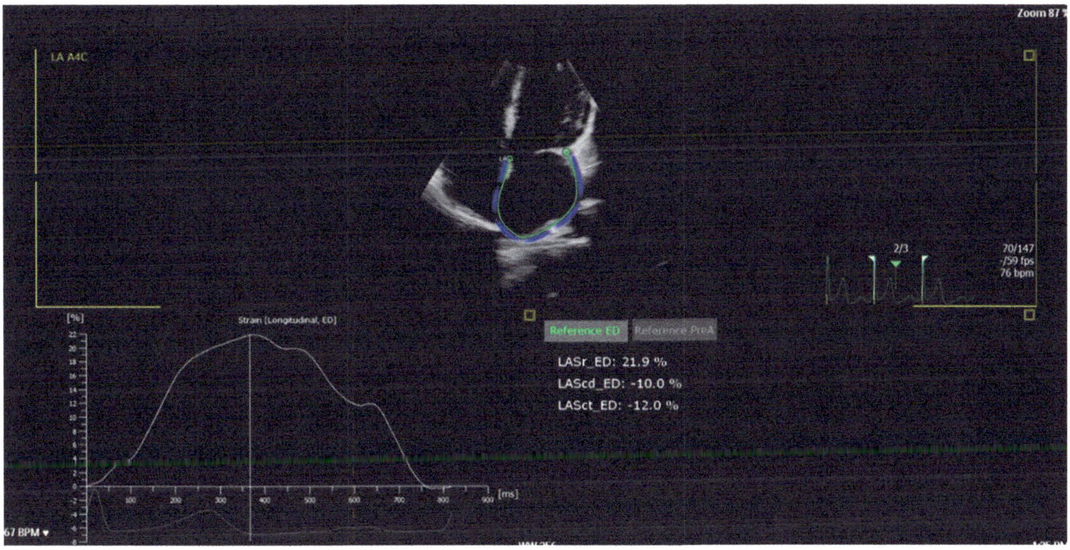

Fig. 14.7 2D apical four-chamber view demonstrating 2D LA strain measurement

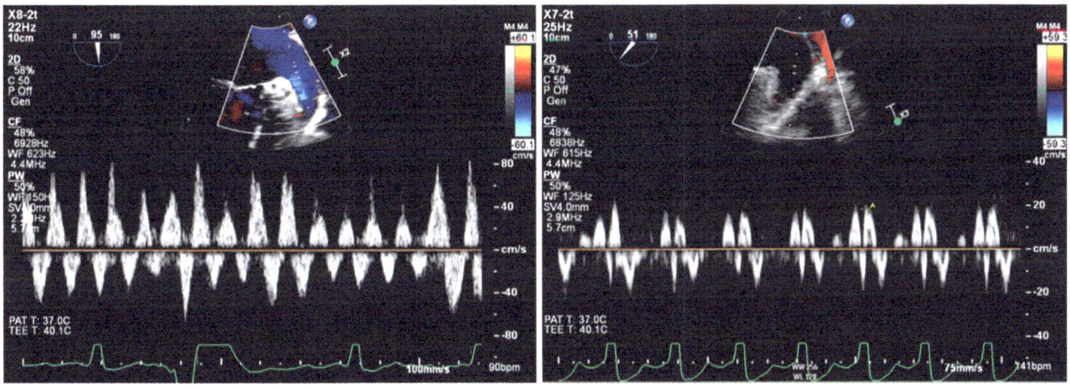

Fig. 14.8 2D TEE orthogonal 95- and 51-degree imaging planes from the mid-esophageal window demonstrating pulsed wave spectral Doppler velocities of the LAA. LAA exit velocities in a patient with organized atrial flutter (>40 cm/s) are seen on the left, and abnormal LAA exit velocities in a patient with sinus rhythm, but low flow (<20 cm/s) are seen on the right panel

motion. Data suggest that **3D speckle-tracking echocardiography (3D STE)** overcomes these limitations because it eliminates the effects of through-plane motion that may occur with 2D imaging [11]. By design, one can measure longitudinal and circumferential strains from a single 3D dataset. Moreover, the evaluation of LA endocardial area strain is possible. To date, this is not available in clinical practice.

Another very important consideration in the assessment of LA size and function is recognizing the differences associated with aging where it is known that the LA dilates despite normal aging and a compensatory rise in booster function, which serves to compensate for the age-associated changes in LV function, is expected [12].

Evolving Evidence
Normal values for 3D STE are available but are limited in the number of patients studied. Although time and expertise in analyzing 3D LA datasets have raised concerns, advancements in artificial intelligence with automated analysis can potentially resolve these issues.

Caveats in Sick Patients

Recognition of LA structural and functional abnormalities is essential in critically ill patients. In response to stressors such as diastolic dysfunction (DD), tachycardia, ischemia, and valvular disease, the LA adapts to a spectrum of complex structural changes, often referred to as "LA remodeling."

In a prospective cohort study, the LAVI was found to be the best predictor of MACE and prognosis [13]. In ischemic heart disease and MI, an exponential increase in mortality in patients' post-MI is observed with increasing $LAVI_{max}$ [14]. Another study showed a $LAVI_{max}$ > 32 mL/m [2] to be an independent predictor of 5-year mortality [15]. More recently, the ASE guidelines for LAVI upper limits of normal were increased from 28 to 34 mL/m [2] for added specificity and a better risk-based cutoff [2].

In patients with systolic heart failure, a $LAVI_{max}$ > 50 mL/m [2] showed a similar predictive value as LVEF <45%. Unarguably, an enlarged LA is a marker for both the severity and chronicity of LV DD and the magnitude of LA pressure elevation. A graded response of LAVI is observed as the severity of DD increases and evaluating LAVI is key in evaluating DD in current guidelines [16]. However, an important caveat is that it cannot be used in AF or significant MV disease.

In a multicenter study of >350 patients, an LA strain (LAS) value of >23% was considered normal, when this cutoff was applied to patients with DD, interestingly reduced LAS was observed in patients with normal volumetric measures, indicating strain to be more sensitive marker of DD [17].

In patients with diastolic heart failure, one study showed LA strain to correlate with wedge pressure and provided a discriminatory value between HFrEF, HFpEF, and DD [18]. In a Korean study of 300 patients with paroxysmal AF evaluated longitudinally, an LA global strain of <30.9% was associated with a fourfold risk of permanent AF [19]. Another study in AF patients showed global LAS provided incremental value when added to $CHA_2DS_2VAS_C$ score, presence of OAC, and LA volumetric function in separating patients at risk of developing and mortality from embolic stroke [20]. Moreover, in AF, LAS has been shown to predict the maintenance of sinus rhythm after cardioversion and pulmonary vein isolation [21, 22].

In patients with severe mitral regurgitation undergoing MV surgery, LAS is found to be a more powerful predictor of adverse outcomes even compared to left ventricular strain [23].

In critically ill COVID-19 patients, acutely reduced LA function has been observed with a significantly reduced LAS associated with AF development [24]. In orthotropic heart transplantation recipients, a significant correlation is found between LA and RA size (and donor and recipient remnants) and overall survival [25].

Summary Points
LA function can be accessed via *multiple parameters and has particular use in patients with HFpEF. It is more sensitive than LA volume change and holds prognostic value. LA function assessment requires training and expertise, there is vendor variability with no standardized normal values and for the past 15 years and to date, still we use an LV algorithm for LA strain assessment.*

Atrial Septum

Abnormalities of the interatrial septum include a patent foramen ovale (PFO), atrial septal defect (ASD), and atrial septum aneurysm (ASA). PFO is prevalent in 25–30% of the population and results in the probability of intermittent bidirectional flow between the atria [26]. An atrial septum that is hypermobile and protrudes >1.0 cm rightward or leftward or >1.5 cm bidirectionally, is considered an ASA [27]. An ASA is usually seen with 2D TTE, commonly associated with a PFO, and can be more precisely interrogated with TEE. A thorough assessment of the atrial septum can be performed with the aid of contrast echocardiography, color Doppler imaging, or both. The ability to visualize right-to-left (R-L) shunting is dependent on interatrial pressure gradients which can be provoked by physiologic parameters (e.g., Valsalva release) [26]. During an agitated saline echocardiographic bubble study, an R-L shunt is typically observed within three to four cardiac cycles from when bubbles are first seen in the RA. However, a better method to assess for a PFO would be to more temporally search for R-L shunting associated with transient atrial septal leftward deviation which would confirm an R > L interatrial pressure gradient [28].

Fatty infiltration of the atrial septum, mostly in the superior and inferior portions is called lipomatous hypertrophy, giving the septum a dumbbell-shaped appearance since the fossa ovalis (in the center of this dumbbell) is never involved.

Right Atrium

The Right Atrium (RA) receives deoxygenated blood from the superior and inferior vena cava (IVC) as well as the coronary sinus. It is a thin-walled ovoid structure. A dilated and diseased RA frequently accompanies right ventricular volume and pressure overload. RA size and function are less well studied compared to the LA. For RA size assessment on TTE, apical-four chamber or subcostal views are utilized at the end-systole, measuring the RA area and RA volume index similar to LA for enhanced accuracy [29]. Visually enlarged RA compared to LA in apical four-chamber view is qualitative evidence of chamber enlargement. The RA can be at risk of compression by mediastinal or herniating abdominal structures, e.g., the liver. Distinguishing extra cardiac compression from intracardiac masses may at times be difficult.

Certain anatomic variants within the RA require consideration. The Eustachian valve is an embryologic remnant of the valve directing IVC blood across the interatrial septum. Lack of the normal regression of the Eustachian valve may lead to partial or complete septation of the RA, inappropriately labeled as cor triatriatum dexter [30]. It can be best visualized on a parasternal long-axis view at the junction of IVC and RA. Although often fixed and immobile, it can be mobile and confused for a pathologic cardiac mass, or even an atrial septal defect.

A Chiari network (CN) is another embryologic remnant that is typically seen as multiple filamentous linear structures within the RA and located near the orifice of IVC. The CN is highly mobile and may be confused as a pathologic mass (e.g., vegetation or thrombi) [31].

The IVC is best visualized from subcostal views and compliance-related changes in the dimensions of IVC help estimate the RA pressure. Increased end-expiratory IVC diameter, measured proximal to the RA junction, can be secondary to the volume overload state. Furthermore, a blunted or absent respiratory variation in the IVC diameter > 50% is an excellent estimate of increased RA pressure [29, 32].

Call Out

Doppler assessment of right atrial filling is important, especially in critically ill patients. On a subcostal view, alignment of the Doppler beam with IVC flow is difficult, hence while utilizing hepatic vein flow as a surrogate due to better alignment of Doppler signal, diagnostics for various causes of elevated right atrial pressure such as severe tricuspid regurgitation, atrial fibrillation, restrictive cardiomyopathy, and pericardial constriction can be made [32].

Summary Points

- $LAVI_{max}$ measured in the biplane 2-D apical views is superior to four-chamber LA area alone or LA dimension in predicting the development of first atrial fibrillation, congestive heart failure, cerebrovascular accident, acute myocardial infarction, coronary revascularization, and cardiovascular death.

- A systematic underestimation of 2DE-acquired $LAVI_{max}$ compared to CCT and CMR is observed and is likely due to foreshortening or poor endocardial border visualization.
- Real-time 3DE is gaining popularity as the modality of choice to accurately measure cardiac chamber volumes with lower interobserver variability and higher test-retest reproducibility compared with 2DE.
- There is recent evidence suggesting that $LAVI_{min}$ may be a more important prognostic indicator using either 2DE or 3DE and current recommendations encourage the reporting of both the maximum and minimum LAVI.
- LA chamber dimensions often dilate asymmetrically with disease reiterating the importance of volume measures over dimensions.
- Accurate LAVI determination requires careful image acquisition to reduce foreshortening.
- Normal values for LA mechanics using STE are available but limited by the number of patients studied.
- Advancements in artificial intelligence with automated LA strain analysis packages continue to evolve and will likely become standard care in the future.
- LA function holds particular value in patients with HFpEF and is more sensitive than LA volume change for predicting outcomes, but requires training and expertise and there are limited standardizations.
- Doppler assessment of right atrial filling patterns is important when assessing critically ill patients.
- Hepatic vein flow is used as a surrogate marker for IVC flow due to better alignment of the Doppler cursor and offers important diagnostic estimates of right atrial pressure, severity of tricuspid regurgitation, and has unique spectral waveforms in patients with either restrictive cardiomyopathies or pericardial constriction.

Questions

1. What is the recommended optimal method for assessing the size of the left atrium with echocardiography?
   A. Visual estimation from dedicated apical four-chamber and two-chamber views
   B. Linear diameter of the LA from M-mode on the parasternal long-axis view
   C. Linear diameter of the LA from M-mode on the parasternal short-axis view
   D. Tracing the LA on dedicated transthoracic apical four-chamber and two-chamber views
   E. Tracing the LA on mid-esophageal TEE apical four-chamber and two-chamber views

   Answer: D

   The best way of estimating the LA size is by tracing the LA borders in two orthogonal views, the LA-focused apical four- and two-chamber views, and estimating the volume using the Simpson's method of disc. Option e is incorrect since TEE will rarely completely visualize the entire LA and commonly underestimates true dimensions. If the dedicated LA focus views are not obtained, the LA dimensions can be inaccurate since the LV long-axis view may foreshorten the LA [4].

2. Which of the following supports a diagnosis of intrapulmonary shunting on a 2D-TTE agitated saline bubble study?
   A. Early appearance of the saline bubbles in the LA and LV within three cardiac cycles
   B. Early appearance of the saline bubbles in the LV, but not the LA
   C. Early appearance of the saline bubbles in the LA or LV after Valsalva maneuver
   D. Late appearance of the saline bubbles in the LA or LV after five cardiac cycles
   E. Late appearance of the saline bubbles in the RA or RV after five cardiac cycles

   Answer: D

   Saline contrast study or bubble study can be used on a TTE or TEE to differentiate between intracardiac and intrapulmonary shunt. With a PFO during the agitated saline contrast study, there is an early appearance of the bubbles from right to left within three to four cardiac cycles. This can be provoked by physiological maneuvers like Valsalva or cough, which causes a transient increase in the right atrial pressures. In the case of intrapulmonary shunt, there is a late appearance of the bubble on the left heart with bubble study, usually after five to seven cardiac cycles and there is no change with the maneuvers mentioned above [24].

References

1. Ho SY, Cabrera JA, Sanchez-Quintana D. Left atrial anatomy revisited. Circ Arrhythm Electrophysiol. 2012;5(1):220–8. https://doi.org/10.1161/CIRCEP.111.962720.
2. Lang RM, Badano LP, Mor-Avi V, Afilalo J, Armstrong A, Ernande L, Flachskampf FA, Foster E, Goldstein SA, Kuznetsova T, Lancellotti P, Muraru D, Picard MH, Rietzschel ER, Rudski L, Spencer KT, Tsang W, Voigt JU. Recommendations for cardiac chamber quantification by echocardiography in adults: an update from the American Society of Echocardiography and the European Association of Cardiovascular Imaging. J Am Soc Echocardiogr. 2015;28(1):1–39.e14. https://doi.org/10.1016/j.echo.2014.10.003.
3. Mitchell C, Rahko PS, Blauwet LA, et al. Guidelines for performing a comprehensive transthoracic echocardiographic examination in adults: recommendations from the American Society of Echocardiography. J Am Soc Echocardiogr. 2019;32(1):1–64. https://doi.org/10.1016/j.echo.2018.06.004.
4. Hoit BD, Litwin SE. The new normal: how should we assess cardiac chamber sizes and proportionality across the full spectrum of body sizes with varying degrees of adiposity? J Am Soc Echocardiogr. 2021;35(2):151–3. https://doi.org/10.1016/j.echo.2021.11.013.
5. Olsen FJ, Møgelvang R, Modin D, Schnohr P, Jensen GB, Biering-Sørensen T. Association between isometric and allometric height-indexed left atrial size and atrial fibrillation. J Am Soc Echocardiogr. 2022;35(2):141–50.e4. https://doi.org/10.1016/j.echo.2021.10.010.
6. Hoit BD. Left atrial size and function: role in prognosis. J Am Coll Cardiol. 2014;63(6):493–505. https://doi.org/10.1016/j.jacc.2013.10.055.
7. Mor-Avi V, Yodwut C, Jenkins C, et al. Real-time 3D echocardiographic quantification of left atrial volume: multicenter study for validation with CMR. JACC Cardiovasc Imaging. 2012;5(8):769–77. https://doi.org/10.1016/j.jcmg.2012.05.011.
8. Shin SH, Claggett B, Inciardi RM, et al. Prognostic value of minimal left atrial volume in heart failure with preserved ejection fraction. J Am Heart Assoc. 2021;10(15):e019545. https://doi.org/10.1161/JAHA.120.019545.
9. Appleton CP, Galloway JM, Gonzalez MS, Gaballa M, Basnight MA. Estimation of left ventricular filling pressures using two-dimensional and Doppler echocardiography in adult patients with cardiac disease. Additional value of analyzing left atrial size, left atrial ejection fraction and the difference in duration of pulmonary venous and mitral flow velocity at atrial contraction. J Am Coll Cardiol. 1993;22(7):1972–82. https://doi.org/10.1016/0735-1097(93)90787-2.
10. Haji K, Huynh Q, Be KK, Wright L, Marwick TH. Interobserver agreement of left atrial strain assessment by two-dimensional speckle echocardiography. J Am Soc Echocardiogr. 2022;35(2):228–9. https://doi.org/10.1016/j.echo.2021.10.008.
11. Mochizuki A, Yuda S, Fujito T, et al. Left atrial strain assessed by three-dimensional speckle-tracking echocardiography predicts atrial fibrillation recurrence after catheter ablation in patients with paroxysmal atrial fibrillation. J Echocardiogr. 2017;15(2):79–87. https://doi.org/10.1007/s12574-017-0329-5.
12. Singh A, Carvalho Singulane C, Miyoshi T, et al. Normal values of left atrial size and function and the impact of age: results of the world Alliance societies of echocardiography study. J Am Soc Echocardiogr. 2022;35(2):154–164.e3. https://doi.org/10.1016/j.echo.2021.08.008.
13. Tsang TS, Abhayaratna WP, Barnes ME, Miyasaka Y, Gersh BJ, Bailey KR, Cha SS, Seward JB. Prediction of cardiovascular outcomes with left atrial size: is volume superior to area or diameter? J Am Coll Cardiol. 2006;47(5):1018–23. https://doi.org/10.1016/j.jacc.2005.08.077.
14. Moller JE, Hillis GS, Oh JK, Seward JB, Reeder GS, Wright RS, Park SW, Bailey KR, Pellikka PA. Left atrial volume: a powerful predictor of survival after acute myocardial infarction. Circulation. 2003;107(17):2207–12. https://doi.org/10.1161/01.CIR.0000066318.21784.43.
15. Beinart R, Boyko V, Schwammenthal E, Kuperstein R, Sagie A, Hod H, Matetzky S, Behar S, Eldar M, Feinberg MS. Long-term prognostic significance of left atrial volume in acute myocardial infarction. J Am Coll Cardiol. 2004;44(2):327–34. https://doi.org/10.1016/j.jacc.2004.03.062.
16. Tsang TS, Barnes ME, Gersh BJ, Bailey KR, Seward JB. Left atrial volume as a morphophysiologic expression of left ventricular diastolic dysfunction and relation to cardiovascular risk burden. Am J Cardiol. 2002;90(12):1284–9. https://doi.org/10.1016/s0002-9149(02)02864-3.

17. Morris DA, Takeuchi M, Krisper M, Köhncke C, Bekfani T, Carstensen T, Hassfeld S, Dorenkamp M, Otani K, Takigiku K, Izumi C, Yuda S, Sakata K, Ohte N, Tanabe K, Osmanoglou E, Kühnle Y, Düngen HD, Nakatani S, Otsuji Y, Haverkamp W, Boldt LH. Normal values and clinical relevance of left atrial myocardial function analysed by speckle-tracking echocardiography: multicentre study. Eur Heart J Cardiovasc Imaging. 2015;16(4):364–72. https://doi.org/10.1093/ehjci/jeu219.
18. Kurt M, Wang J, Torre-Amione G, Nagueh SF. Left atrial function in diastolic heart failure. Circ Cardiovasc Imaging. 2009;2(1):10–5. https://doi.org/10.1161/CIRCIMAGING.108.813071.
19. Yoon YE, Oh IY, Kim SA, Park KH, Kim SH, Park JH, Kim JE, Lee SP, Kim HK, Kim YJ, Sohn DW, Cho GY. Echocardiographic predictors of progression to persistent or permanent atrial fibrillation in patients with paroxysmal atrial fibrillation (E6P study). J Am Soc Echocardiogr. 2015;28(6):709–17. https://doi.org/10.1016/j.echo.2015.01.017.
20. Obokata M, Negishi K, Kurosawa K, Tateno R, Tange S, Arai M, Amano M, Kurabayashi M. Left atrial strain provides incremental value for embolism risk stratification over CHA_2DS_{2S}-VASc score and indicates prognostic impact in patients with atrial fibrillation. J Am Soc Echocardiogr. 2014;27(7):709–716.e4. https://doi.org/10.1016/j.echo.2014.03.010.
21. Di Salvo G, Caso P, Lo Piccolo R, Fusco A, Martiniello AR, Russo MG, D'Onofrio A, Severino S, Calabro P, Pacileo G, Mininni N, Calabro R. Atrial myocardial deformation properties predict maintenance of sinus rhythm after external cardioversion of recent-onset lone atrial fibrillation: a color Doppler myocardial imaging and transthoracic and transesophageal echocardiographic study. Circulation. 2005;112:387–95.
22. Motoki H, Dahiya A, Bhargava M, Wazni OM, Saliba WI, Marwick TH, Klein AL. Assessment of left atrial mechanics in patients with atrial fibrillation: comparison between two-dimensional speckle-based strain and velocity vector imaging. J Am Soc Echocardiogr. 2012;25(4):428–35. https://doi.org/10.1016/j.echo.2011.12.020.
23. Yang H, Marwick TH, Fukuda N, Oe H, Saito M, Thomas JD, Negishi K. Improvement in strain concordance between two major vendors after the strain standardization initiative. J Am Soc Echocardiogr. 2015;28(6):642–8.e7. https://doi.org/10.1016/j.echo.2014.12.009.
24. Goerlich E, Minhas A, Gilotra N, Barth AS, Mukherjee M, Parziale A, Wu KC, Hays AG. Left atrial function in patients with coronavirus disease 2019 and its association with incident atrial fibrillation/flutter. J Am Soc Echocardiogr. 2021;34(10):1106–9. https://doi.org/10.1016/j.echo.2021.05.015.
25. Gudmundsson GS, Smull DL, Pisani BA, Bane CD, Mendez JC, Mullen GM, Jacobs WR. Increase in atrial size in long-term survivors of heart transplant. J Am Soc Echocardiogr. 2003;16(10):1043–8. https://doi.org/10.1016/S0894-7317(03)00591-1.
26. Silvestry FE, Cohen MS, Armsby LB, et al. Guidelines for the echocardiographic assessment of atrial septal defect and patent foramen ovale: from the American Society of Echocardiography and Society for Cardiac Angiography and Interventions. J Am Soc Echocardiogr. 2015;28(8):910–58. https://doi.org/10.1016/j.echo.2015.05.015.
27. Hanley PC, Tajik AJ, Hynes JK, et al. Diagnosis and classification of atrial septal aneurysm by two-dimensional echocardiography: report of 80 consecutive cases. J Am Coll Cardiol. 1985;6(6):1370–82. https://doi.org/10.1016/s0735-1097(85)80228-x.
28. Attaran RR, Ata I, Kudithipudi V, Foster L, Sorrell VL. Protocol for optimal detection and exclusion of a patent foramen Ovale using transthoracic echocardiography with agitated saline microbubbles. Echocardiography. 2006;23:616–22. https://doi.org/10.1111/j.1540-8175.2006.00272.x.
29. Rudski LG, Lai WW, Afilalo J, et al. Guidelines for the echocardiographic assessment of the right heart in adults: a report from the American Society of Echocardiography endorsed by the European Association of Echocardiography, a registered branch of the European Society of Cardiology, and the Canadian Society of Echocardiography. J Am Soc Echocardiogr. 2010;23(7):685–788. https://doi.org/10.1016/j.echo.2010.05.010.
30. Alboliras ET, Edwards WD, Driscoll DJ, Seward JB. Cor triatriatum Dexter: two-dimensional echocardiographic diagnosis. J Am Coll Cardiol. 1987;9(2):334–7. https://doi.org/10.1016/s0735-1097(87)80385-6.
31. Peters PJ, Reinhardt S. The echocardiographic evaluation of intracardiac masses: a review. J Am Soc Echocardiogr. 2006;19(2):230–40. https://doi.org/10.1016/j.echo.2005.10.015.
32. Nagueh SF, Kopelen HA, Zoghbi WA. Relation of mean right atrial pressure to echocardiographic and Doppler parameters of right atrial and right ventricular function. Circulation. 1996;93(6):1160–9. https://doi.org/10.1161/01.cir.93.6.1160.

Left Ventricular Diastolic Function 15

Ryota Sato and Siddharth Dugar

Learning Objectives

1. Understand the physiology of diastole, including the four phases of diastole (isovolumic relaxation, early diastolic filling, diastasis, and late diastolic filling) and its mechanisms.
2. Understand how to measure parameters used to define and grade left ventricular diastolic function (E/e′, e′, tricuspid regurgitation jet peak velocity, and left atrial volume index).
3. Understand the caveats on the definition of diastolic dysfunction in critically ill patients.

Introduction

Cardiac function critically depends on diastole to provide an adequate left ventricular (LV) filling for maintenance of cardiac output and tissue perfusion. Over the last decade, it has become apparent that LV diastolic dysfunction, independent of LV systolic dysfunction, is a significant contributor to morbidity, prolonged hospital stay, and even mortality in critically ill patients [1–5]. The definition of diastolic dysfunction and the echocardiographic parameters utilized for its characterization continue to evolve. The current method of uncovering and grading diastolic dysfunction in critically ill patients is derived from the definition used in the general population. Few have questioned if the definition needs to be modified and simplified to fit the pathophysiology of critical illness where impaired relaxation may be acute/subacute with constantly changing loading conditions from fluids, inotropic agents, and mechanical ventilation [6–8]. In this chapter, we detail our current understanding of the pathophysiology of diastolic dysfunction during critical illness, elucidate parameters used to define and grade left ventricular diastolic function, and caveats to their application in critically ill patients.

Diastole

Diastole is the cardiac cycle interval between the aortic valve (AV) closure and mitral valve (MV) closure. Diastole constitutes the phase of transporting blood from one chamber (the left atrium [LA]) to another chamber (the left ventricle [LV]). This flow of blood is determined by the

Supplementary Information The online version contains supplementary material available at https://doi.org/10.1007/978-3-031-80038-2_15.

R. Sato
The Queen's Medical Center, Honolulu, HI, USA

John A. Burns School of Medicine, University of Hawai'i Manoa, Honolulu, HI, USA

S. Dugar (✉)
Department of Critical Care, Cleveland Clinic Lerner College of Medicine, Respiratory Institute, Cleveland Clinic, Cleveland, OH, USA
e-mail: dugars@ccf.org

M. J. Lanspa, A. T. Levinson (eds.), *Echocardiography and Ultrasonography in the ICU*, Respiratory Medicine, https://doi.org/10.1007/978-3-031-80038-2_15

pressure gradient between these two chambers, which in turn are determined by the characteristics of those chambers. At the end of systole, LV fibers start actively relaxing, reducing the LV pressure, and increasing the LA-LV pressure gradient, which allows the opening of the MV. During diastole, the LV, LA, and pulmonary venous system act as a single chamber allowing the blood in the pulmonary capillary bed to flow into LA and finally to LV. The diastole is partitioned into four phases: (1) Isovolumic relaxation, (2) Early diastolic filling, (3) Diastasis, and (4) Late diastolic filling. On visual assessment, the myocardium functions as a muscle-powered oscillator, seamlessly transitioning through these phases without discrete transition points. However, these four phases are essential for understanding the diastole as a hemodynamic parameter (Fig. 15.1).

Isovolumic Relaxation

Isovolumic relaxation occurs between the AV closure and MV opening. During this phase, the LV initiates relaxation to its resting unstressed length against closed MV and AV. The effect of this relaxation of the cardiac muscle fibers is a sudden drop in LV pressure. The rate of pressure decrease during the isovolumetric relaxation period directly reflects on the velocity of cardiac muscle relaxation and LV compliance. Once the LV pressure drops below the LA pressure, MV opens allowing initiation of the early diastolic filling [9].

Early Diastolic Filling

An early diastolic filling is characterized by the rapid filling of blood to the LV from LA without a significant increase in LV pressure. The relaxation of LV, which begins during isovolumic relaxation, continues in the initial phase of early diastolic filling generating the early diastolic LA-LV pressure gradient. This pressure gradient draws in the blood from LA to LV. The velocity of this blood flow is a measure of the rate of LV relaxation and, hence, compliance. Mitral inflow velocity (the flow velocity between LA and LV) during early diastolic filling measured using echocardiography is called a peak E wave velocity.

Diastasis

Diastasis is the stable phase, where the ventricular filling slows down due to the equalization of pressures between the LA and LV. During diastasis, the normal LV is composed of entirely relaxed

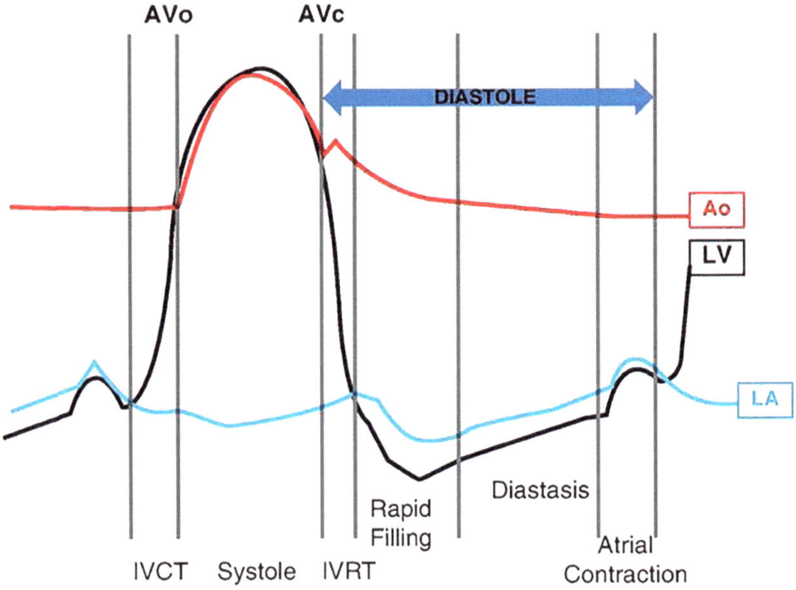

Fig. 15.1 Phases of diastole. Wiggers diagram of intra-cardiac pressures during the cardiac cycle showing simultaneous pressure tracings of the left ventricle, left atrium, and the aorta. *Ao* aorta, *AVc* aortic valve closure, *AVo* aortic valve closure, *IVCT* isovolumic contraction time, *IVRT* isovolumic relaxation time, *LA* left atrium, *LV* left ventricle

cardiomyocytes. The duration of diastasis depends on heart rate; longer at slow heart rates and shorter to completely absent at higher heart rates. The blood flow from LA to LV in diastasis may occur in a highly compliant LV, or if LA pressure is markedly elevated. However, in most normal individuals, minimal filling occurs in diastasis.

Late Diastolic Filling

The late diastolic filling is produced by atrial contraction, as LA pressure rises again from atrial contraction and exceeds LV pressure. Atrial contraction near the end of diastole contributes 20–30% to the total LV filling volume. Under normal conditions, the LV diastolic pressure increases by less than 5 mmHg. LV filling can usually be accomplished by very low filling pressures in the LA and pulmonary veins, preserving a low pulmonary capillary pressure (<12 mmHg) and a high degree of lung distensibility. Mitral inflow velocity during these phases measured using echocardiography is called a peak "A wave" velocity.

As noted, the normal diastolic function comprises LV with vigorous relaxation to pull blood from LA during early diastolic filling and high compliance, to minimize increase in the LV pressure with the flow of blood from LA. The loss of normal LV diastolic relaxation and compliance from structural and functional causes impairs LV pressure decline and filling necessitating a rise in LA and pulmonary venous pressures to maintain perfusion. This translates to an increase in pulmonary capillary pressure, an increase in lung water, and heart failure symptoms.

Unfortunately, there exists no single parameter that can encompass the pathophysiological markers of LV diastolic dysfunction namely, LV relaxation, LV and LA compliance, and filling pressure. Therefore, the assessment of diastolic function requires a comprehensive approach using a combination of several different echocardiographic parameters to assess these abnormalities (Table 15.1) [10].

Table 15.1 Parameters for the assessment of diastolic function

Mitral inflow velocity pattern		
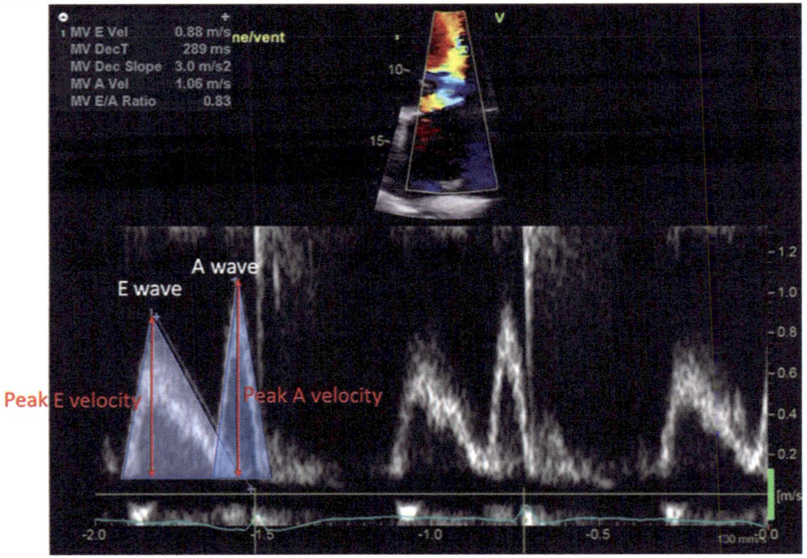	Normal E wave velocity < 50 cm/s E/A > 0.8	• Measured in A4C • Place the pulse wave Doppler at the mitral leaflet tip. • Measure peak E velocity and A velocity • Optimization of the gain and filter setting is imperative • Cannot measure it accurately in the setting of atrial fibrillation due to beat-to-beat variation • Deceleration time of E wave

Mitral annular motion velocity		
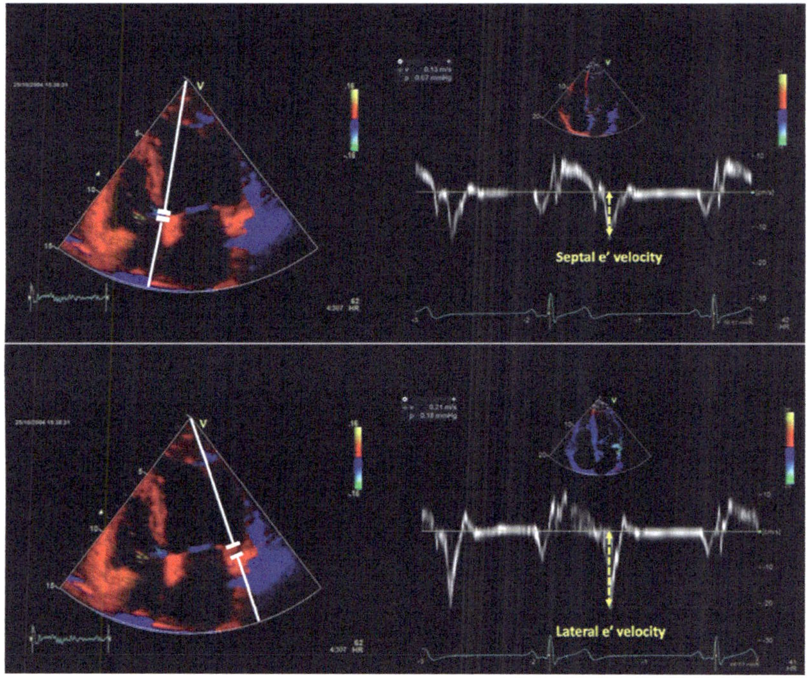	Normal Septal e′ ≥ 7 Lateral e′ ≥ 10 Average E/e′ < 10 Abnormal Septal e′ < 7 Lateral e′ < 10 Average E/e′ ≥ 10 (Average E/e′ ≥ 14 = grade 3)	• Measured in A4C • Place the tissue Doppler imaging (TDI) on the septal or lateral mitral annulus • Measure peak septal and lateral e′ tissue velocities • Positive wave is the motion toward the probe. Therefore, it represents systole (s′) • On the other hand, the subsequent negative wave represents LV relaxation during early diastolic relaxation (e′) • Ideally the measurements should be taken from both lateral and septal annulus and averaged

(continued)

Table 15.1 (continued)

Left atrial volume index		
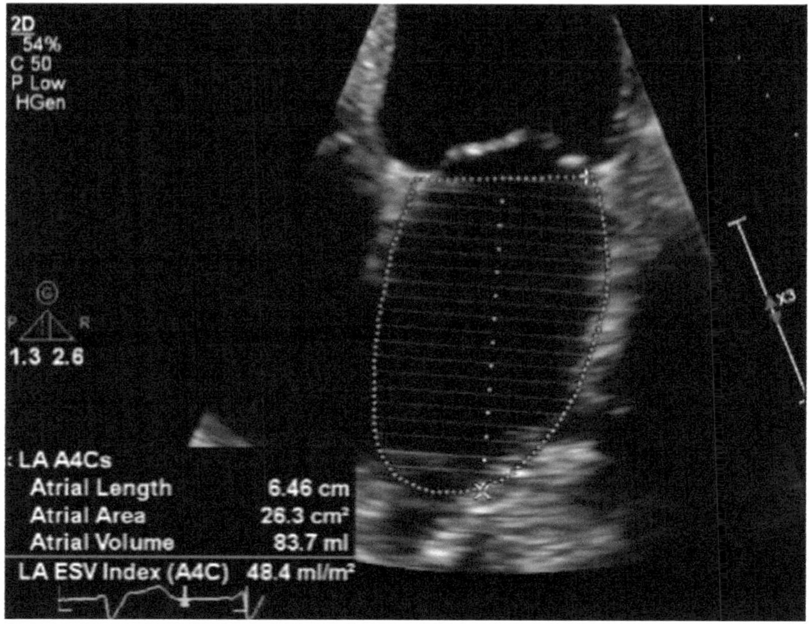	LAVI: Normal 16–34 Mildly abnormal: 35–41 Moderately abnormal: 42–48 Severely abnormal: > 48	• The measurements should be done in the end-systolic phase • Endocardium needs to be visualized for accurate measurements • The Simpson method: LA needs to be traced in apical four-chamber and two-chamber • The area-length method: The diameter from the mitral annular plane to the back wall of LA = L LA areas in A4C and A2C = A1 and A2, respectively LAV = 0.85 × A1 × A2/L • LAVI = LAV/BSA

Pulmonary venous flow		
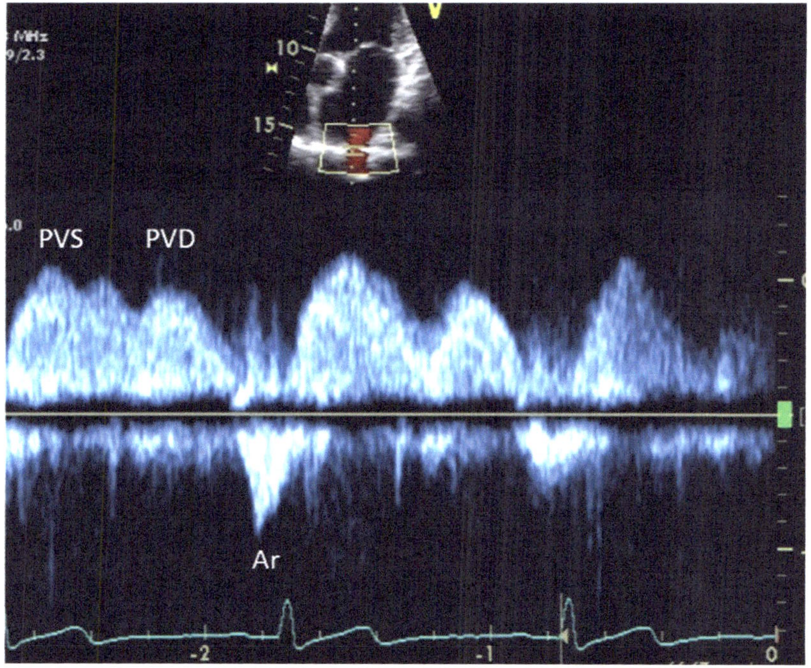	Normal S wave > D wave Diastolic dysfunction D wave > S wave	• Measured in A4C • PV flow consists of systolic wave (S), diastolic wave (D), and atrial contraction wave (Ar) • Place the pulse wave Doppler on the PV • During systole, LA cavity is expanded and the blood flows into LA from PV (toward the probe). So, the S wave is a positive wave • During diastole, LV relaxes and the blood flows into LA from PV (toward the probe). So, D wave is positive • Ar represents the regurgitation from LA to PV. So, Ar is negative wave.

(continued)

Table 15.1 (continued)

TR velocity		
RV inflow CW TR jet measurement 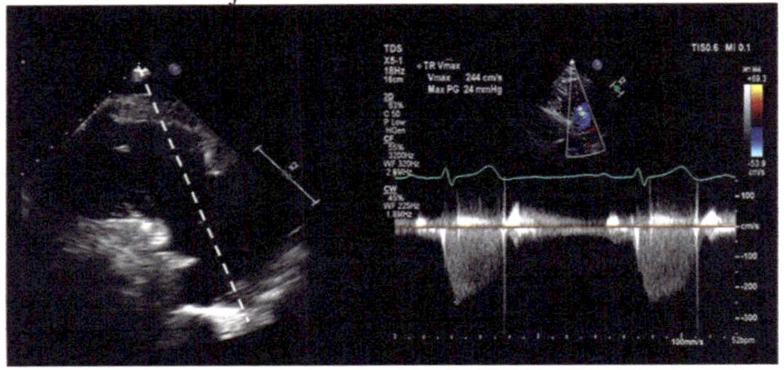	Normal ≤2.8 m/s Abnormal >2.8 m/s	• Measured from RV inflow, PSAX, A4C views • Measures the RV-RA gradient • Utilized to measure SPAP • Highest value is considered as the measurement can be underestimated if doppler not properly aligned to the blow flow
PSAX CW TR jet measurement 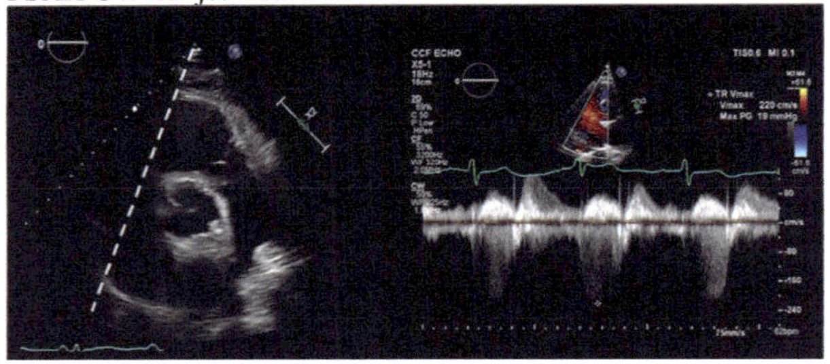		
Apical four-chamber CW TR jet measurement 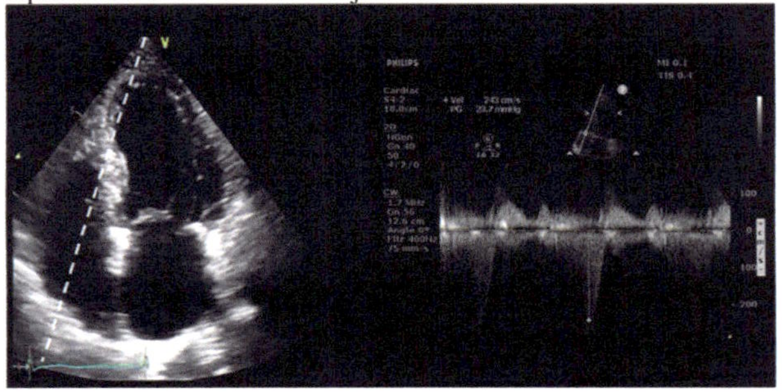		

A4C apical four-chamber view, *RV* right ventricle, *TDI* tissue Doppler imaging, *PLAX* parasternal long axis, *PSAX* parasternal short axis, *LA* left atrium, *BSA* body surface area, *LV* left ventricle, *PV* pulmonary vein, *TR* tricuspid regurgitation, *SPAP* systolic pulmonary arterial pressure

Diastolic Function Assessment

The gold standard for assessing diastolic function is the time constant (τ) of LV pressure decline during diastole. However, the measurement of τ requires an invasive pulmonary artery catheter. In a routine clinical setting, echocardiography with the Doppler technique is commonly used to assess diastolic function. The key variables currently recommended for the assessment of LV diastolic dysfunction include (1) Mitral inflow velocity pattern, (2) Mitral annular septal and lateral velocity, (3) Tricuspid regurgitation peak velocity, and (4) Left atrium volume index (Fig. 15.2).

Mitral Inflow Velocity Pattern

Mitral inflow velocity is measured using the pulse wave Doppler (PWD) in the apical four-chamber view. The sample volume (1–3 mm) is

From: Echocardiographic Evaluation of the Diastolic Function and Dysfunction

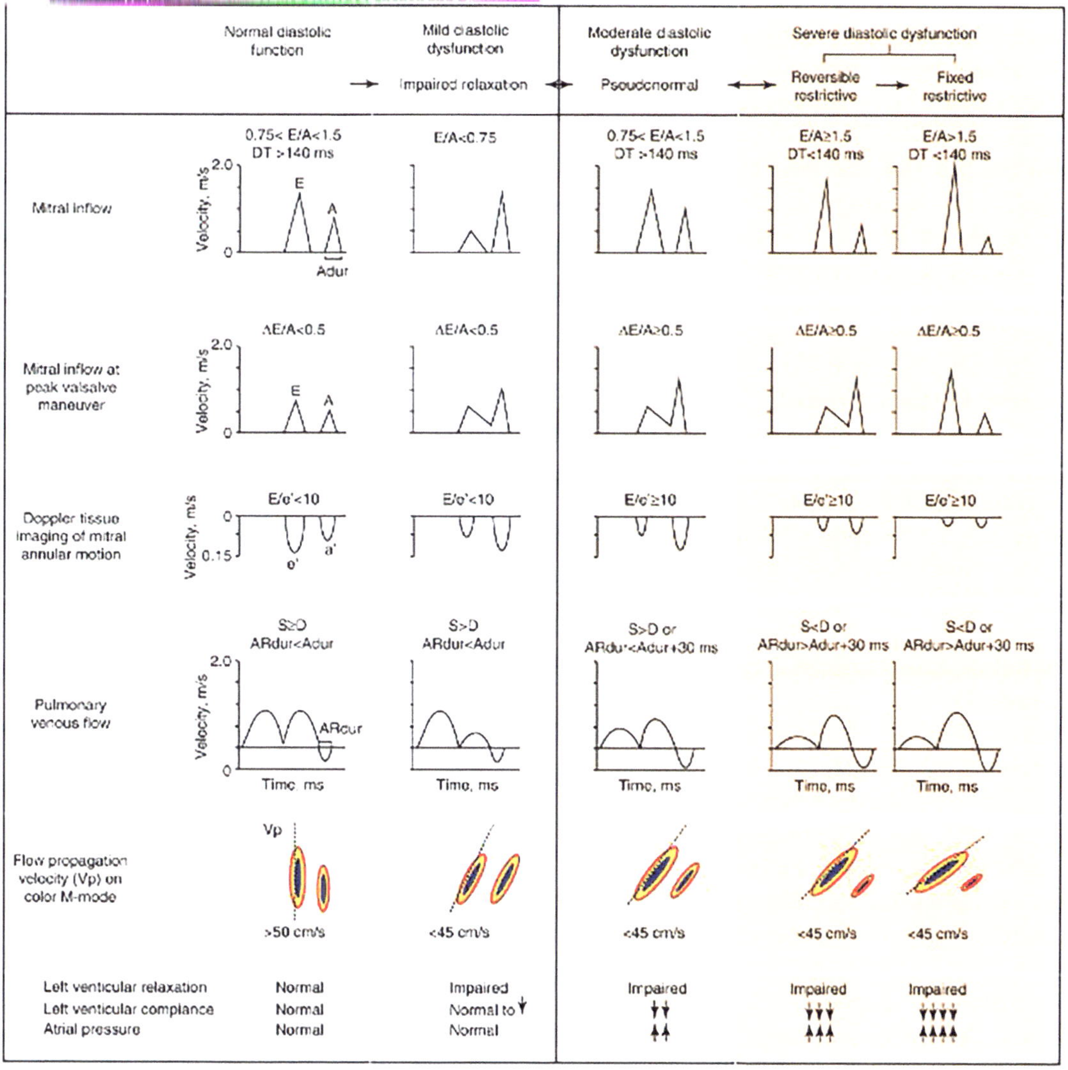

Fig. 15.2 Stages of diastolic dysfunction based on various echocardiographic parameters

placed at the mitral leaflet tip. Color flow can be used to guide the appropriate site for the placement of sample volume. Optimization of gain and filter settings is imperative to get a suitable waveform. The mitral inflow velocity pattern represents the peak velocity of blood flow from LA to LV determined by the LA-LV pressure gradient during early and late diastolic filling. Early diastolic filling velocity (E wave) is driven by the rate of LV relaxation and left-sided preload, while late diastolic filling velocity (A wave) is driven by LA contraction and LV filling pressure. In. addition to peak E and A velocity and ratio of E/A, deceleration time (DT) of E wave and isovolumic relaxation time (IVRT) can also be used to assess diastolic function. More recently, LV global longitudinal diastolic strain rate (SR) during isovolumic relaxation and early diastole has been reported to have a significant association with the time constant of LV relaxation. E/SR has been reported as a tool to estimate LV filling pressures. These novel parameters need to be validated in the ICU setting [10].

Normal Pattern (Grade 0)

The robust LV relaxation during early diastole draws a large portion of blood from LA into LV resulting in a large "E wave." The contribution of atrial kick to LV filling is relatively small generating a smaller "A wave" expressed in an E/A ratio ≥ 1.0.

LV Relaxation Abnormality Pattern (Grade 1)

As either the rate or the vigor of LV relaxation gets impaired, the reduction in LV pressure during early diastolic dysfunction declines, diminishing the LA-LV pressure gradient. The resultant "E wave" is attenuated. IVRT and DT get elongated due to prolonged relaxation. In addition, since more blood will remain in LA, the amount of blood entering LV from LA during atrial kick augments "A wave." The E/A ratio in these cases will be <0.8. It is worth noting that elderly individuals can have this pattern without myocardial pathology as a part of the aging process.

Pseudonormalization Pattern (Grade 2)

When LV compliance is impaired in addition to relaxation, LVEDP increases.

The increase in LA afterload in the setting of normal LA pressure attenuates the LV-LA gradient reducing blood flow from LA. The compensatory mechanism to maintain cardiac output leads to an increase in LA pressure to overcome the increase in afterload. The elevated LA pressure resets the LA-LV gradient, albeit at higher filling pressures restoring the large "E wave" and smaller "A wave," hence this pattern is called "pseudo-normal." As LV compliance is impaired, LV filling pressure rises quickly during early diastolic filling leading to early equalization of LV-LA pressure. This is observed in the echocardiographic waveform shortening of DT in comparison to the normal pattern. Thus, the pattern of relaxation and compliance abnormality as described using the E/A ratio is >0.8.

Restrictive Pattern (Grade 3)

Further impairment of LV compliance leads to a further increase in LA pressure and augmentation of E wave. The LV diastolic pressure in poorly compliant increases exponentially in early diastolic filling with minimal blood flow from LA to LV with atrial contraction demonstrated with further shortening of DT and attenuated A wave with E/A ≥ 2.

Mitral inflow velocity pattern has limitations. It is age-dependent. Also, the U-shaped relation with LV diastolic function as described above makes it difficult to differentiate normal diastolic function from pseudonormalization pattern. Therefore, the American Society of Echocardiography (ASE) recommends using the E/A ratio in conjunction with myocardial relaxation parameters [10].

Mitral Annular Motion Velocity

Mitral annular myocardial velocity is measured in apical four-chamber view using tissue Doppler imaging (TDI). The use of TDI differs instead of the standard Doppler eliminates the high pass filter and uses low gain amplification to exclude blood flow and measure myocardial tissue velocity. The sample volume of pulsed wave (PW) Doppler is placed on the septal and lateral mitral annulus at the level of the insertion of the mitral leaflets. These parameters measure the peak velocity of the longitudinal displacement of the septal and lateral LV basal wall as it relaxes and fills in diastole. The sample volume of PW should be adjusted to 5–10 mm to elucidate the complete excursion of the mitral annulus. In routine Apical four-chamber view, the recording displays movement toward the probe in systole and away from the probe during diastole. Systolic wave (s′) presents as a positive wave, followed by early diastolic wave (e′) and atrial systolic wave (a′), which present as negative waves. The Early diastolic annular velocity has been referenced as Ea, Em, E′, or e′, whereas late diastolic velocity is referred to as Aa, Am, A′, or a′. Measurements should ideally be taken from both the septal and lateral annulus, and then averaged to improve accuracy and reproducibility. These regional measurements of e′ at annulus are used as a surrogate for global LV relaxation. Hence, localized abnormalities affecting annulus motion such as mitral annular diseases or basal regional wall motion abnormalities will limit its utility in assessing diastolic dysfunction. A visual assessment of global myocardial activity may aid if these regional measurements can be utilized as representative of the global myocardial relaxation (Videos 15.1 and 15.2).

In patients with diastolic dysfunction, the intensity of relaxation gets progressively impaired and is displayed as attenuated e′ velocity. In the diastolic dysfunction definition, the cutoffs for impaired relaxation are <7 cm/s for septal and <10 cm/s for ateral e′. Since the E wave reflects the early diastolic mitral inflow velocity, which is determined by LV filling pressure and the strength of LV relaxation measured as e′, the ratio of E and e′ can be used as an indicator of LV filling pressure. In general, E/e′ > 14, which corresponds to an LAP of 18 is considered elevated.

$$\text{Estimated Left Atrial Pressure}(\text{LAP}) = \frac{E}{e'} + 4$$

Left Atrial Volume Index (LAVI)

The impaired LV relaxation and LV compliance increase LA afterload reducing the LV filling at normal LA pressure and hence, reducing stroke volume. In the early phase of diastolic dysfunction, LA contraction increases to surpass this reduction of stroke volume. With the progression of diastolic dysfunction, this compensatory mechanism fails to maintain cardiac output. LA remodeling ensues with chamber dilation to increase LA filling pressure to overcome the increased afterload. Therefore, left atrial volume (LAV) has been known to be associated with both the severity and chronicity of diastolic dysfunction, as well as increased risks of death, cardiovascular events, and stroke [11, 12]. LAV can be measured with the Simpson method or the Area-length method in the end-systolic phase. In the Simpson method, LA needs to be traced in apical 4 and 2 chambers. In the Area-length method, the diameter from the mitral annular plane to the back wall of LA (L) and LA areas in apical 4 and 2 chambers (A1 and A2, respectively) are used to calculate LAV with the following formula: $\text{LAV} = 0.85 \times A1 \times A2 \div L$. The echocardiographic planes should be adjusted to ensure that the maximal area of the left atrium is captured without foreshortening. LAVI, the value of LA volume divided by body surface area, is recommended as a parameter to determine the presence of diastolic dysfunction. If LAVI is >34 mL/m^2, it is considered moderately dilated LA.

Tricuspid Regurgitation (TR) Jet Peak Velocity

The measurement of TR jet velocity can provide an estimate of pulmonary systolic arterial pressure (PASP) when combined with right atrial pressure, which can be measured by a central venous catheter or estimated by the inferior vena cava measurement. An elevated PSAP can support the presence of chronic elevated LA pressure from impaired LV relaxation and decreased LV compliance. Therefore, the presence of TR can reflect the presence of diastolic dysfunction. TR jet velocity can be measured at RV inflow view, parasternal short-axis view at aortic valve level, or apical four-chamber view with continuous wave Doppler. The color flow Doppler can be used to guide the placement of continuous wave Doppler. The highest recorded velocity from all acquired views is usually reported. In case of a weak TR jet signal, agitated saline can be used to improve the delineation of the TR jet [13]. There is also a study describing that the mixture of 10% blood-10% air-80% saline further improves the delineation of TR [14]. TR jet velocity of >2.8 m/s is considered abnormal and associated with elevated right-sided pressures.

Pulmonary Vein Flow

The increase in LA pressure due to impaired LV relaxation and elevated LV filling pressure in diastolic dysfunction impedes the flow from the pulmonary venous system into LA. Hence, the pulmonary venous flow waveform pattern has been used to facilitate the diagnosis of diastolic dysfunction. Pulmonary vein (PV) flow consists of systolic wave (S), diastolic wave (D), and atrial contraction wave (Ar). It can be measured with PW Doppler at the pulmonary vein in the apical four-chamber view. Since this is typically measured in the apical four-chamber view in TTE, PVS and PVD reflect the blood flow coming into LA from PV during systole and diastole respectively, while PVAr reflects the regurgitant blood from LA to PV during atrial contraction. The PVS wave is determined by LA relaxation and compliance, while the PVD wave is determined by LV relaxation and compliance, hence, PVD follows a similar pattern to the E wave. In other words, in normal cardiac function, the pulmonary venous flow to LA is predominantly systolic with peak pulmonary vein systolic flow velocity/with peak pulmonary vein diastolic flow velocity (S/D) ratio > 1. With diastolic dysfunction with impaired LV relaxation and elevated LA filling pressure, the flow from the pulmonary vein to LA predominately occurs in diastole. An S/D ratio < 1 in the presence of impaired LV relaxation is highly suggestive of elevated LAP.

Diastolic Dysfunction Definition Over Years

ASE Recommendation 2009

ASE guidelines 2009 defined the presence of diastolic dysfunction based on mitral annulus e′ and LAVI [15]. The severity was graded based on E/A, DT, and E/e′. In this guideline, diastolic dysfunction is diagnosed if

1. Septal e′ < 8 cm/s
2. Lateral e′ < 10 cm/s
3. LAVI ≥ 34 mL/m²

The severity of diastolic dysfunction is graded as.

Parameter	Grade 1	Grade 2	Grade 3
E/A ratio	<0.8	0.8–1.5	≥2
DT (ms)	>200	160–200	<160
Average E/e′	≤8	9–12	≥13
PVAr-A	<30	≥30	≥30
Valsalva ΔE/A	<0.5	≥0.5	≥0.5

ASE Recommendation 2016

ASE guidelines 2016 defined the presence of diastolic dysfunction based using E/e′, e′, TR jet velocity, and LAVI [10]. The severity was graded based on E/A.

In this guideline, diastolic dysfunction is diagnosed if more than 50% of the following criteria are positive.

1. Septal e′ < 7 cm/s
2. Lateral e′ < 10 cm/s
3. LAVI ≥ 34 mL/m²
   with addition of
4. TR velocity > 2.8 m/s.

E/A ≤ 0.8 and E ≤ 50 cm/s are considered Grade 1. If E/A ≤ 0.8 and E > 50 cm/s or E/A 0.8–2.0, then, there are three criteria to be evaluated. If more than two of the following three criteria are positive, then, it is considered Grade 2 (1, Average E/e′ > 14; 2, TR velocity > 2.8 m/s; 3, LAVI >34 mL/m^2). If only 1 or 0 out of these three criteria is positive, it is considered Grade 1. If E/A ≥ 2.0, then this is considered Grade 3.

Comparison of ASE 2009 and 2016

In 2016, the diastolic dysfunction was simplified by minimizing the parameters required to grade the severity of diastolic dysfunction. Sanchis et al. evaluated LV diastolic function initially based on ASE 2009 guidelines followed by ASE 2016 guidelines. ASE 2016 guidelines were able to classify patients more accurately according to brain natriuretic peptide levels, the diagnosis of heart failure, and cardiovascular outcomes. In this study, most patients diagnosed with grade 1 diastolic dysfunction based on ASE 2009 guidelines were reclassified as normal diastolic function based on ASE 2016 guidelines [16]. Other studies also reported that the prevalence of diastolic function significantly decreased when using ASE 2016 guidelines as opposed to ASE 2009 guidelines [17, 18]. These findings support that ASE 2016 guidelines seem to be able to diagnose only the advanced cases in the general population.

On the other hand, Clancy et al. reported that the prevalence of diastolic dysfunction was significantly higher when using ASE 2016 compared to ASE 2009 in patients with severe sepsis and septic shock [19]. Similarly, Lanspa et al. reported that ASE 2016 guidelines categorized more sepsis and septic shock patients to have diastolic dysfunction than ASE 2009 guidelines [7]. In critically ill patients, DT and LAVI appear to be less relevant given that these parameters represent chronic changes rather than acute changes. This might explain the reason why the diagnostic characteristics of ASE 2009 and 2016 guidelines differ between relatively stable patients and critically ill patients. While ASE 2016 guidelines' grading system predicted elevated LVEDP and a poor prognosis more accurately than that of ASE 2009 in stable cardiac patients [20], it is still unclear whether the grading of diastolic dysfunction correlates with the prognosis in the critically ill population [5, 7].

Caveats on the Use of ASE Recommendations in the ICU

Caveats on the use of ASE recommendations in the ICU also need to be mentioned. ASE 2016 recommends using E/e′, e′, LAVI, and TR jet velocity. Among these parameters, LAVI and TR jet velocity may be less reliable in the critical care setting. For instance, LA dilatation is likely to reflect chronically elevated LA pressure. The acute nature of impaired LV relaxation during critical illness may not result in LA dilation. In addition, LA volume is affected by loading conditions, which can change rapidly in the critical care setting. TR jet sometimes could be difficult to assess accurately in the critical care setting due to suboptimal positioning, positive pressure ventilation, etc. Furthermore, peak TR jet velocity can occur or alter acutely by positive pressure ventilation, positive end-expiratory pressure, and fluid loading limiting its utility as a surrogate of chronically elevated left-sided filling pressure [21]. While E/e′ is also affected by several conditions, E/e′ may suffer less than other parameters from the confounding influence enhancing its utility in the assessment of elevated filling pressure along with the use of e′ as parameters of LV relaxation [22].

Conditions That Require Caution in the Assessment of Diastolic Dysfunction

1. Arrhythmias such as atrial fibrillation will result in loss of atrial kick and absence of A wave velocity. In addition, the RR interval may vary affecting the accurate assessment of Mitral inflow velocity pattern and LV relaxation limiting the utility of these parameters in the assessment of diastolic dysfunction (Fig. 15.3).
2. Valvular pathologies such as mitral stenosis and regurgitation affect mitral inflow velocity due to increased volume or pressure from valvular disease instead of LV and LA relaxation

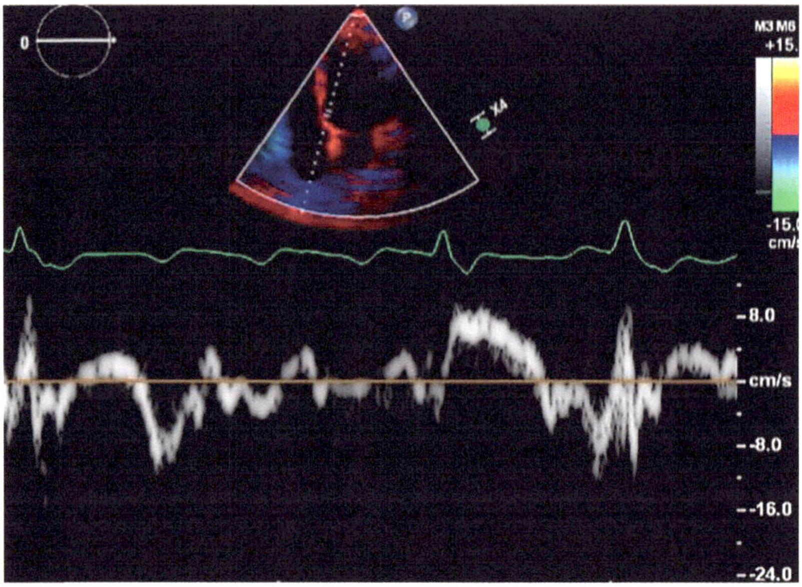

Fig. 15.3 Diastolic function assessment in presence of arrhythmia

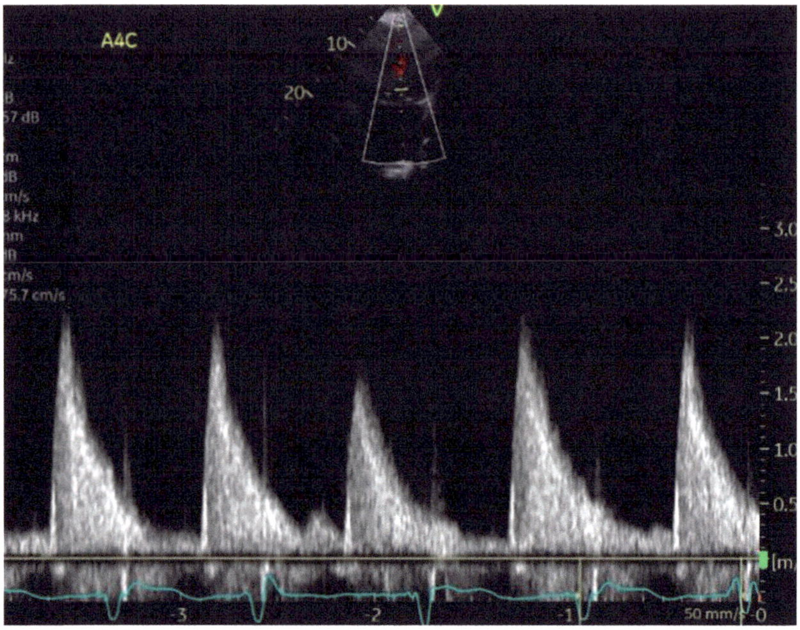

Fig. 15.4 Diastolic function assessment in presence of mitral valve pathology

properties. Therefore, if patients have any of these, mitral inflow velocity may not be reflective of the LA-LV pressure gradient and hence cannot be used to assess diastolic function. These pathologies may also result in dilation of the left atrium limiting the utility of LA dilation as criteria for diastolic dysfunction (Fig. 15.4).

3. Hypertrophic cardiomyopathy, severely reduced LV systolic function, and regional wall motion abnormality may regionally affect mitral annular motion velocity limiting the utility of these parameters as surrogates of global LV relaxation. Therefore, in such patients, comprehensive assessments including other parameters are required to assess the presence and severity of diastolic dysfunction.
4. Mitral or Aortic valve repair or replacement and mitral annulus calcification may also impair mitral annular motion and invalidate the

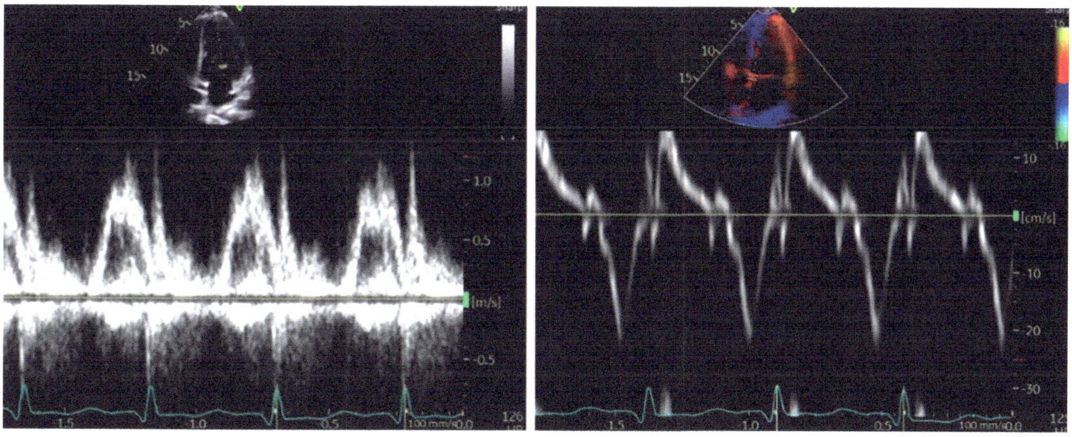

Fig. 15.5 Diastolic function assessment in presence of tachycardia

mitral inflow measurements. Therefore, in such patients, comprehensive assessments including other parameters are required to assess the presence and severity of diastolic dysfunction.

5. Age: Aging is associated with increased LV stiffness and slowing of myocardial relaxation resulting in a decrease in E/A ratio and e′ values and resembling diastolic dysfunction. Hence age-appropriate normative values should be utilized for the detection and grading of diastolic dysfunction.
6. Pericardial effusion/Constrictive pericarditis: Due to external restriction of LV relaxation, the filling pressure will be elevated despite normal myocardial tissue relaxation and compliance.
7. Tachycardia: Tachycardia may lead to the fusion of the E and A waves, resulting in an inaccurate assessment of peak E and A wave velocities (Fig. 15.5).
8. Acute cor pulmonale: The paradoxical septal motion from interventricular dependence will impair LV relaxation assessment, especially septal e′ velocity measurement.

Diastolic Function in the ICU

The prevalence of LV diastolic dysfunction is reported between 40.4% and 84%. Therefore, it is important for critical care practitioners to know the clinical situations where diastolic dysfunction could play a role in critically ill patients. These situations include estimation of filling pressure to facilitate fluid management, acute respiratory distress syndrome (ARDS), sepsis, and liberation from mechanical ventilation.

Estimation of Pulmonary Artery Occlusion Pressure

E/e′ has been evaluated as a surrogate to noninvasively estimate PAOP, especially in heart failure populations. Although transesophageal echocardiogram (TEE) appears to have a better predictive value of PAOP than transthoracic echocardiogram (TTE) [23, 24], the access to TEE in the general/medical ICU may be limited. While several estimation formulas are known [e.g., Nagueh formula: PAOP = 1.24 (E/e′) + 1.9] [25], these formulas have not been validated in the ICU population. In mechanically ventilated critically ill patients, Doppler TTE indices were highly specific but not sensitive to estimate PAOP [26]. In this study, lateral E/e′ > 15 was predictive of PAOP ≥18 mmHg with a sensitivity of 25% and specificity of 95%, whereas lateral E/e′ < 7 was predictive of PAOP <18 mmHg with a sensitivity of 32% and specificity of 81%. A more recent study suggested that simple Doppler measurements such as lateral e′ or E/A ratio provide a similar level of diagnostic performance of PAOP compared to the definition of diastolic function by the guidelines [27].

Diastolic Function and ARDS

There is no direct evidence showing the relationship between diastolic dysfunction and the prognosis of ARDS. On the other hand, in patients with ARDS, high PAOP and BNP are known to be associated with higher mortality [28–30]. In the FACTT trial, conservative fluid management improved lung function and shortened the duration of mechanical ventilation and ICU stay in patients with acute lung injury [31]. Given this evidence, it may be important to use E/e′ to guide the loading condition and diuretic therapy.

Diastolic Function and Sepsis

Diastolic dysfunction is commonly seen in septic patients and a meta-analysis reported that 48% of septic patients had diastolic dysfunction diagnosed by TDI. Diastolic dysfunction was also associated with higher mortality [3, 32] while systolic dysfunction is less common and deemed not to be associated with higher mortality in septic patients [33]. Especially a meta-analysis emphasizes the close correlation between lateral e′ < 10 cm/s and E/e′ > 14 with increased mortality. Given that e′ is partially influenced by volume loading, these values may suggest volume overload, which is known to be associated with higher mortality [34].

Diastolic Function and Liberation from Mechanical Ventilation

As many patients with diastolic dysfunction could have an exacerbation of diastolic dysfunction during exercise, a spontaneous breathing trial (SBT) could trigger heart failure symptoms. Lamia et al. first described the combination of E/A > 0.95 and E/e′ > 8.5 with TTE predicted the weaning-induced PAOP elevation [35]. Similarly, several studies showed that higher E/e′ was seen in patients who failed to wean compared with those who succeeded [36, 37]. Moschietto et al. reported that patients who succeeded in the weaning maintained the same E/e′ level with SBT while the patients who failed to wean had the elevation of E/e′, suggestive of an increase in left ventricular filling pressures [38]. Therefore, knowing diastolic dysfunction before SBT may be helpful in identifying high-risk patients for cardiogenic weaning failure.

Summary Points

- Diastole consists of four phases (isovolumic relaxation, early diastolic filling, diastasis, and late diastolic filling).
- The current American Society of Echocardiography guidelines define the presence of diastolic dysfunction based using E/e′. e′, tricuspid regurgitation (TR) jet velocity, and left atrial volume index (LAVI). Then, the severity is graded based on E/A.
- It may not be possible to reliably assess diastolic function in some situations. These situations include tachycardia, arrhythmia such as atrial fibrillation, and valvular diseases, especially mitral valve pathology. In addition, it is also important to note that aging, hypertrophic cardiomyopathy, pericardial effusion, and acute cor pulmonale will affect the measurements of diastolic function.
- Diastolic dysfunction is known to be associated with unfavorable outcomes in critically ill patients such as ARDS or sepsis.

References

1. Landesberg G, Gilon D, Meroz Y, Georgieva M, Levin PD, Goodman S, et al. Diastolic dysfunction and mortality in severe sepsis and septic shock. Eur Heart J. 2012;33(7):895–903.
2. Roche-Campo F, Bedet A, Vivier E, Brochard L, Mekontso DA. Cardiac function during weaning failure: the role of diastolic dysfunction. Ann Intensive Care. 2018;8(1):2.
3. Sanfilippo F, Corredor C, Fletcher N, Landesberg G, Benedetto U, Foex P, et al. Diastolic dysfunction and mortality in septic patients: a systematic review and meta-analysis. Intensive Care Med. 2015;41(6):1004–13.
4. Papanikolaou J, Makris D, Mpaka M, Palli E, Zygoulis P, Zakynthinos E. New insights into the

mechanisms involved in B-type natriuretic peptide elevation and its prognostic value in septic patients. Crit Care. 2014;18(3):R94.
5. Brown SM, Pittman JE, Hirshberg EL, Jones JP, Lanspa MJ, Kuttler KG, et al. Diastolic dysfunction and mortality in early severe sepsis and septic shock: a prospective, observational echocardiography study. Crit Ultrasound J. 2012;4(1):8.
6. Greenstein YY, Mayo PH. Evaluation of left ventricular diastolic function by the intensivist. Chest. 2018;153(3):723–32.
7. Lanspa MJ, Olsen TD, Wilson EL, Leguyader ML, Hirshberg EL, Anderson JL, et al. A simplified definition of diastolic function in sepsis, compared against standard definitions. J Intensive Care. 2019;7:14.
8. Sanfilippo F, Scolletta S, Morelli A, Vieillard-Baron A. Practical approach to diastolic dysfunction in light of the new guidelines and clinical applications in the operating room and in the intensive care. Ann Intensive Care. 2018;8(1):100.
9. Lang RM, Badano LP, Mor-Avi V, Afilalo J, Armstrong A, Ernande L, et al. Recommendations for cardiac chamber quantification by echocardiography in adults: an update from the American Society of Echocardiography and the European Association of Cardiovascular Imaging. J Am Soc Echocardiogr. 2015;28(1):1–39.e14.
10. Nagueh SF, Smiseth OA, Appleton CP, Byrd BF, Dokainish H, Edvardsen T, et al. Recommendations for the evaluation of left ventricular diastolic function by echocardiography: an update from the American Society of Echocardiography and the European Association of Cardiovascular Imaging. J Am Soc Echocardiogr. 2016;29(4):277–314.
11. Tsang TS, Barnes ME, Gersh BJ, Bailey KR, Seward JB. Left atrial volume as a morphophysiologic expression of left ventricular diastolic dysfunction and relation to cardiovascular risk burden. Am J Cardiol. 2002;90(12):1284–9.
12. Tsang TS, Gersh BJ, Appleton CP, Tajik AJ, Barnes ME, Bailey KR, et al. Left ventricular diastolic dysfunction as a predictor of the first diagnosed nonvalvular atrial fibrillation in 840 elderly men and women. J Am Coll Cardiol. 2002;40(9):1636–44.
13. Waggoner AD, Barzilai B, Pérez JE. Saline contrast enhancement of tricuspid regurgitant jets detected by Doppler color flow imaging. Am J Cardiol. 1990;65(20):1368–71.
14. Jeon D-S, Luo H, Iwami T, Miyamoto T, Brasch AV, Mirocha J, et al. The usefulness of a 10% air-10% blood-80% saline mixture for contrast echocardiography: Doppler measurement of pulmonary artery systolic pressure. J Am Coll Cardiol. 2002;39(1):124–9.
15. Baumgartner H, Hung J, Bermejo J, Chambers JB, Evangelista A, Griffin BP, et al. Echocardiographic assessment of valve stenosis: EAE/ASE recommendations for clinical practice. J Am Soc Echocardiogr. 2009;22(1):1–23; quiz 101–2.
16. Sanchis L, Andrea R, Falces C, Poyatos S, Vidal B, Sitges M. Differential clinical implications of current recommendations for the evaluation of left ventricular diastolic function by echocardiography. J Am Soc Echocardiogr. 2018;31(11):1203–8.
17. Huttin O, Fraser AG, Coiro S, Bozec E, Selton-Suty C, Lamiral Z, et al. Impact of changes in consensus diagnostic recommendations on the echocardiographic prevalence of diastolic dysfunction. J Am Coll Cardiol. 2017;69(25):3119–21.
18. Almeida JG, Fontes-Carvalho R, Sampaio F, Ribeiro J, Bettencourt P, Flachskampf FA, et al. Impact of the 2016 ASE/EACVI recommendations on the prevalence of diastolic dysfunction in the general population. Eur Heart J Cardiovasc Imaging. 2018;19(4):380–6.
19. Clancy DJ, Scully T, Slama M, Huang S, McLean AS, Orde SR. Application of updated guidelines on diastolic dysfunction in patients with severe sepsis and septic shock. Ann Intensive Care. 2017;7(1):121.
20. Sato K, Grant ADM, Negishi K, Cremer PC, Negishi T, Kumar A, et al. Reliability of updated left ventricular diastolic function recommendations in predicting elevated left ventricular filling pressure and prognosis. Am Heart J. 2017;189:28–39.
21. Dalla K, Bech-Hanssen O, Ricksten SE. General anesthesia and positive pressure ventilation suppress left and right ventricular myocardial shortening in patients without myocardial disease—a strain echocardiography study. Cardiovasc Ultrasound. 2019;17(1):16.
22. Sanfilippo F, Murabito P, Oliveri F, Astuto M. The value of E/e′ ratio in critically ill patients should not be underestimated. Echocardiography. 2021;38(1):155–6.
23. Combes A, Arnoult F, Trouillet JL. Tissue Doppler imaging estimation of pulmonary artery occlusion pressure in ICU patients. Intensive Care Med. 2004;30(1):75–81.
24. Vignon P, AitHssain A, François B, Preux PM, Pichon N, Clavel M, et al. Echocardiographic assessment of pulmonary artery occlusion pressure in ventilated patients: a transoesophageal study. Crit Care. 2008;12(1):R18.
25. Nagueh SF, Middleton KJ, Kopelen HA, Zoghbi WA, Quiñones MA. Doppler tissue imaging: a noninvasive technique for evaluation of left ventricular relaxation and estimation of filling pressures. J Am Coll Cardiol. 1997;30(6):1527–33.
26. Mercado P, Maizel J, Marc J, Beyls C, Zerbib Y, Zogheib E, et al. Doppler echocardiographic indices are specific but not sensitive to predict pulmonary artery occlusion pressure in critically ill patients under mechanical ventilation. Crit Care Med. 2021;49(1):e1–e10.
27. Brault C, Marc J, Mercado P, Diouf M, Tribouilloy C, Zerbib Y, et al. Estimation of pulmonary artery occlusion pressure using Doppler echocardiography in mechanically ventilated patients. Crit Care Med. 2020;48(10):e943–e50.
28. Ferguson ND, Meade MO, Hallett DC, Stewart TE. High values of the pulmonary artery wedge

pressure in patients with acute lung injury and acute respiratory distress syndrome. Intensive Care Med. 2002;28(8):1073–7.
29. Lai CC, Sung MI, Ho CH, Liu HH, Chen CM, Chiang SR, et al. The prognostic value of N-terminal proB-type natriuretic peptide in patients with acute respiratory distress syndrome. Sci Rep. 2017;7:44784.
30. Karmpaliotis D, Kirtane AJ, Ruisi CP, Polonsky T, Malhotra A, Talmor D, et al. Diagnostic and prognostic utility of brain natriuretic peptide in subjects admitted to the ICU with hypoxic respiratory failure due to noncardiogenic and cardiogenic pulmonary edema. Chest. 2007;131(4):964–71.
31. Wiedemann HP, Wheeler AP, Bernard GR, Thompson BT, Hayden D, deBoisblanc B, et al. Comparison of two fluid-management strategies in acute lung injury. N Engl J Med. 2006;354(24):2564–75.
32. Sanfilippo F, Corredor C, Arcadipane A, Landesberg G, Vieillard-Baron A, Cecconi M, et al. Tissue Doppler assessment of diastolic function and relationship with mortality in critically ill septic patients: a systematic review and meta-analysis. Br J Anaesth. 2017;119(4):583–94.
33. Sanfilippo F, Huang S, Messina A, Franchi F, Oliveri F, Vieillard-Baron A, et al. Systolic dysfunction as evaluated by tissue Doppler imaging echocardiography and mortality in septic patients: a systematic review and meta-analysis. J Crit Care. 2021;62:256–64.
34. Kelm DJ, Perrin JT, Cartin-Ceba R, Gajic O, Schenck L, Kennedy CC. Fluid overload in patients with severe sepsis and septic shock treated with early goal-directed therapy is associated with increased acute need for fluid-related medical interventions and hospital death. Shock. 2015;43(1):68–73.
35. Lamia B, Maizel J, Ochagavia A, Chemla D, Osman D, Richard C, et al. Echocardiographic diagnosis of pulmonary artery occlusion pressure elevation during weaning from mechanical ventilation. Crit Care Med. 2009;37(5):1696–701.
36. Caille V, Amiel JB, Charron C, Belliard G, Vieillard-Baron A, Vignon P. Echocardiography: a help in the weaning process. Crit Care. 2010;14(3):R120.
37. Papanikolaou J, Makris D, Saranteas T, Karakitsos D, Zintzaras E, Karabinis A, et al. New insights into weaning from mechanical ventilation: left ventricular diastolic dysfunction is a key player. Intensive Care Med. 2011;37(12):1976–85.
38. Moschietto S, Doyen D, Grech L, Dellamonica J, Hyvernat H, Bernardin G. Transthoracic echocardiography with Doppler tissue imaging predicts weaning failure from mechanical ventilation: evolution of the left ventricle relaxation rate during a spontaneous breathing trial is the key factor in weaning outcome. Crit Care. 2012;16(3):R81.

Cardiomyopathies

16

John C. Klick and Rachel Carlson

Learning Objectives

1. Review how bedside echocardiography can identify and help manage patients in the ICU with cardiomyopathies.
2. Describe the various cardiomyopathies specific echocardiographic diagnostic criteria.
3. Discuss stress-induced cardiomyopathy.

Cardiomyopathy is defined as a disease of the myocardium. The term encompasses a variety of myocardial disorders where the heart muscle is structurally and functionally abnormal in the absence of coronary artery disease, hypertension, valvular disease, or congenital disorder adequate to explain the anomalies. These disorders are frequently genetic in origin. This chapter will discuss the echocardiographic identification of the major subtypes of cardiomyopathy [1].

Supplementary Information The online version contains supplementary material available at https://doi.org/10.1007/978-3-031-80038-2_16.

J. C. Klick (✉)
Department of Anesthesiology, University of Vermont Medical Center, UVM Larner College of Medicine, Burlington, VT, USA

R. Carlson
Department of Anesthesiology, Tufts University Medical Center, Boston, MA, USA
e-mail: rcarlson@tuftsmedicalcenter.org

The World Health Organization (WHO) in 1980 defined cardiomyopathies as "heart disease of unknown cause." This was to distinguish cardiomyopathies from cardiac dysfunction due to known pathologies such as myocardial ischemia, hypertension, or valvulopathies [2]. However, in clinical practice, the terms "ischemic cardiomyopathy" and "hypertensive cardiomyopathy" remain common parlance.

In 1995, the WHO/International Society and Federation of Cardiology (ISFC) Task Force on the Definition and Classification of Cardiomyopathies expanded the classification according to anatomy and physiology, defining them as "diseases of the myocardium associated with cardiac dysfunction." The following types were outlined, each with multiple different causes: dilated cardiomyopathy (DCM), Hypertrophic cardiomyopathy (HCM), Restrictive cardiomyopathy (RCM), Arrhythmogenic right ventricular cardiomyopathy/dysplasia (ARVC/D), and unclassified cardiomyopathies. This classification system did include ischemic, valvular, and hypertensive diseases among the causes [3].

A statement from the American Heart Association (AHA) in 2006 proposed a contemporary definition and classification of cardiomyopathies. An expert consensus panel proposed that "cardiomyopathies are a heterogeneous group of diseases of the myocardium associated with mechanical and/or electrical

M. J. Lanspa, A. T. Levinson (eds.), *Echocardiography and Ultrasonography in the ICU*, Respiratory Medicine, https://doi.org/10.1007/978-3-031-80038-2_16

dysfunction that usually (but not invariably) exhibit inappropriate ventricular hypertrophy or dilation and are due to a variety of causes that frequently are genetic. Cardiomyopathies either are confined to the heart or are a part of generalized systemic disorders, often leading to cardiovascular death or progressive heart failure-related disability" [4].

In 2008, the European Society of Cardiology (ESC) presented an update to the WHO/ISFC classification. They defined cardiomyopathy as "a myocardial disorder in which the heart muscle is structurally and functionally abnormal in the absence of coronary artery disease, hypertension, valvular disease, and congenital heart disease sufficient to explain the observed myocardial abnormality." This classification emphasizes the distinction between familial/genetic and nonfamilial/nongenetic causes of cardiomyopathy and excludes heart disease secondary to valvular, ischemic, or congenital disorders. It also differs from the AHA definition by excluding ion channelopathies [5].

In 2013, the World Heart Federation (WHF) endorsed and published the MOGE(s) classification as a phenotype-genotype-based nomenclature for cardiomyopathies. It is inspired by the TNM staging of malignancy and excludes ion channelopathies [6]. The system incorporates five aspects: the morphofunctional notation (M), organ involvement (O), genetic inheritance (G), etiology (specific gene mutation (E)), and an optional functional status (S) [6]. By incorporating five aspects, the nomenclature system attempts to classify cardiomyopathy based on etiology and highlight the complex genetics for increasing specificity in registry data. However, this system has not been widely accepted into clinical practice and the applicability remains to be defined [7]. The remainder of this chapter is focused on discussing cardiomyopathy from the descriptive phenotypes commonly encountered in the clinical setting.

Dilated Cardiomyopathy

Dilated cardiomyopathy is a disease of the myocardium involving left ventricular dilation and systolic dysfunction. This dysfunction must be in the absence of abnormal loading conditions including hypertension, valve disease, or coronary artery disease, which lead to pathologic dilation [8]. Dilated cardiomyopathy is the most common cardiomyopathy, with a variable etiology that may include viral infection, toxins, parasites, alcohol, peripartum, or autoimmune disease. Up to 25% of idiopathic cases have a genetic basis and these patients may have pathologic dilation that precedes systolic dysfunction [9].

Clinically, patients present with symptoms of heart failure. The approach to echocardiography involves assessment of cardiac structures from standard TTE windows [10, 11]. **Diagnostic criteria include evidence of left ventricular systolic dysfunction with EF < 45%, and/or fractional shortening < 25% in association with left ventricular end-diastolic dimension > 112% corrected for age and BSA.** In addition to diagnostic criteria, echocardiography can offer information on the severity and sequelae of dilated cardiomyopathy. When present, right ventricular fractional area of change (FAC < 35) indicates RV dysfunction and is predictive of a worse long-term prognosis [10, 12]. It is common for valvular pathology to occur in the setting of dilated cardiomyopathy [13]. Right ventricular systolic pressures can be derived from tricuspid regurgitation Doppler velocities and left atrial and ventricular end-diastolic pressures can be estimated from mitral and aortic regurgitant Doppler velocities respectively [14]. Left ventricular thrombus in the setting of poorly functioning chambers can be identified with the assistance of contrast [10]. Echocardiography rarely alludes to the specific cause; thus patient history, family history, and imaging all contribute to the determination of cardiomyopathy etiology (i.e., infectious, alcoholic, peripartum) (see Figs. 16.1 and 16.2).

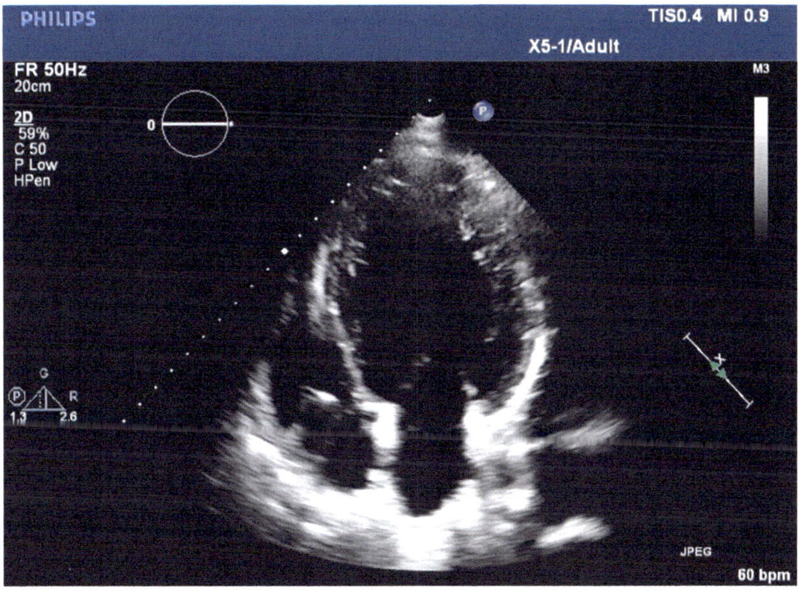

Fig. 16.1 Apical four-chamber view of a patient with dilated cardiomyopathy (see Video 16.1)

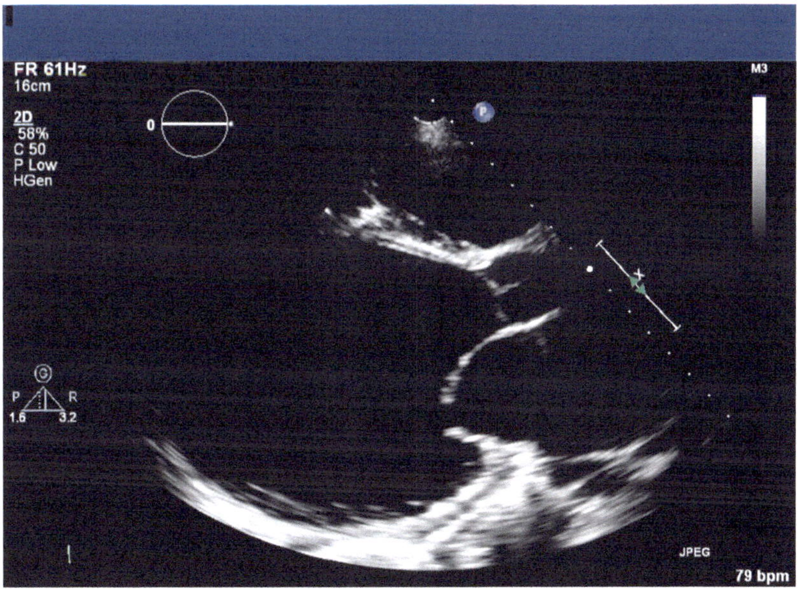

Fig. 16.2 Parasternal long-axis view of a patient with dilated cardiomyopathy secondary to methamphetamine (see Video 16.2)

Additional techniques including, evaluation with 3D echocardiography, TDI-derived strain imaging, and 2D-derived speckle-tracking strain analysis, may help assess ventricular dysfunction. Treatment remains supportive. ICD placement and cardiac resynchronization therapy are commonly used for suitable patients at risk for life-threatening arrhythmias [15, 16].

Hypertrophic Cardiomyopathy

Hypertrophic cardiomyopathy is a heterogeneous disease that develops from protein mutations in the cardiac sarcomere resulting in left ventricular hypertrophy with disorganized myocardial architecture in the absence of hypertension or valvular disease [17]. Asymmetric hypertrophy of the septum and anterior wall is the most common variant; however, there are variations including apical hypertrophy and mid-ventricular hypertrophy [18]. Diagnostic criteria include [19–21]:

- Unexplained maximal wall thickness > 15 mm in any myocardial segment or
- Septal/posterior wall thickness ratio > 1.3 in normotensive patients or
- Septal/posterior wall thickness ratio > 1.5 in hypertensive patients

Systolic function generally remains preserved as remodeling occurs; however, the diastolic left ventricular function gradually is impaired due to decreased compliance [17]. The presence of septal hypertrophy narrows the left ventricular outflow tract (LVOT) and may lead to systolic anterior motion (SAM) of the mitral valve and ultimately LVOT obstruction [22]. Up to two-thirds of patients display dynamic outflow tract obstruction with evidence of a gradient >30 mmHg. About 25% of patients experience a resting gradient, while the remainder require changes in volume and contractility to provoke a gradient indicating outflow tract obstruction [21].

Clinically, patients present with angina, dyspnea, exercise intolerance, or syncope. The approach to echocardiography involves the assessment of cardiac structures from standard TTE windows. It is important to assess interventricular septal width in diastole for asymmetric septal hypertrophy. Parasternal long- and short-axis views assess left ventricular wall thickness from the mitral, papillary, and apical levels, allowing evaluation of segmental hypertrophy [19, 21]. Systolic function is qualitatively and quantitatively normal to supranormal early in the disease process but may be reduced in the end stages. Evaluation of the mitral valve in apical four-chamber and apical five-chamber views allows determination of structure and function. Systolic anterior motion is considered mild if contact between the anterior mitral leaflet and the septum is <10% in systole and severe if >30% in systole [21]. In obstructive hypertrophic cardiomyopathy with SAM, a mitral regurgitation jet is usually present and is posteriorly directed [23]. The apical three- and five-chamber views allow for the evaluation of LVOT dynamic flow gradient. Continuous wave Doppler will often demonstrate a dagger-like profile with a peak velocity of 5 m/s or a gradient of 100 mmHg in the setting of left ventricular outflow tract obstruction. Wall thickness > 3 mm or a left ventricular outflow gradient >30 mmHg are independent predictors of sudden cardiac death [22] (see Figs. 16.3 and 16.4).

Evolving imaging techniques include using tissue Doppler imaging, one-dimensional strain imaging, and two-dimensional speckle tracking. These have shown evidence of longitudinal strain, twists, and torsion changes which can be subtle and emerge early in the disease course for hypertrophic cardiomyopathy [24–26]. This is particularly useful in assessing early disease in family members and identifying patients who may be at higher risk of developing the phenotype of hypertrophic cardiomyopathy.

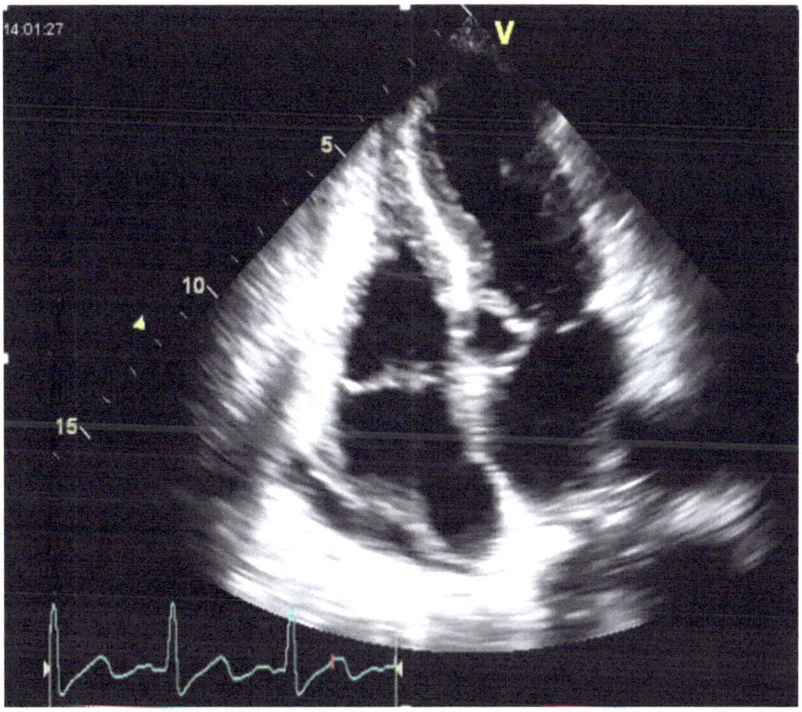

Fig. 16.3 Hypertrophic cardiomyopathy apical four-chamber demonstrating SAM (see Video 16.3)

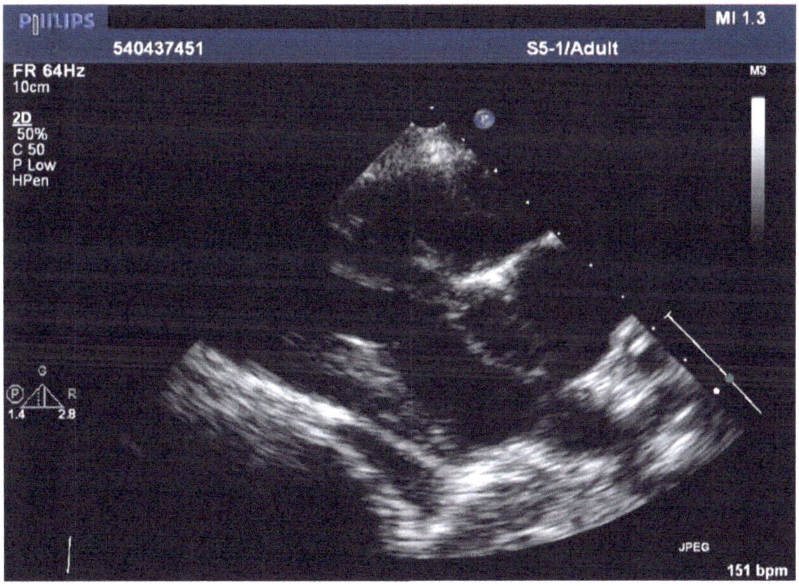

Fig. 16.4 Hypertrophic cardiomyopathy parasternal long-axis view (see Video 16.4)

Restrictive Cardiomyopathies

Restrictive Cardiomyopathy is a cardiac muscle disease characterized by increased stiffness, elevated end-diastolic pressure, and ultimately diastolic dysfunction of one or both ventricles [27]. Despite abnormal diastolic filling, the systolic function of the ventricles remains preserved. Idiopathic restrictive cardiomyopathy is uncommon, however restrictive physiology can be seen in constrictive pericarditis, and infiltrative processes including amyloidosis, hemochromatosis, sarcoidosis, and metabolic disorders [27]. It is important to identify the restrictive physiology, and thoroughly assess for its etiology to determine opportunities for intervention [28].

Clinically, patients present with evidence of heart failure including dyspnea, edema, and elevated jugular venous pressure. Infiltrative processes can disrupt the conduction system resulting in AV conduction delay/block, atrial fibrillation, or atrial arrhythmias [27]. The approach to echocardiography involves looking at the structure and both systolic and diastolic functions. Specific attention is paid to diastolic function. On initial exam, normal ventricular size and wall thickness are common with biatrial enlargement [27]. Left ventricular systolic function is typically preserved. Doppler echocardiography reveals diastolic filling abnormalities. Increased mitral E velocity, increased ratio of mitral early to late filling (E/A ratio > 2), and shortened deceleration time (<150 ms) are commonly seen [28]. Tissue Doppler is significant for decreased early mitral annular velocity (E′) [14] (see Figs. 16.5 and 16.6).

Limitations to defining restrictive cardiomyopathy involve challenges in evaluating diastolic dysfunction. Accurate Doppler evaluation of diastolic function relies on normal sinus rhythm, normal PR interval, and varies with the amount of valvular regurgitation and the phase of respiration [28–30]. The diastolic filling pattern also changes with disease progression. In early disease, the LV inflow curve shows reduced E velocity and increased A velocity, and the pulmonary vein flow curve has reduced diastolic filling and normal systolic filling. As the restrictive process progresses, there is increased E velocity, rapid early diastolic deceleration of the LV inflow, and the A velocity is reduced due to increased diastolic pressure and reduced atrial contraction. There is normal pulmonary venous inflow in diastole with decreased systolic filling. During atrial contraction, the increased resistance to left ventricular filling allows atrial flow reversal in the lower pulmonary veins. In late disease, there is increased E velocity, decreased A velocity, and steep early diastolic deceleration. Over time, end-stage restrictive cardiomyopathy can lead to biventricular enlargement and transition to echocardiographic features of a dilated cardiomyopathy [31] (see Fig. 16.7).

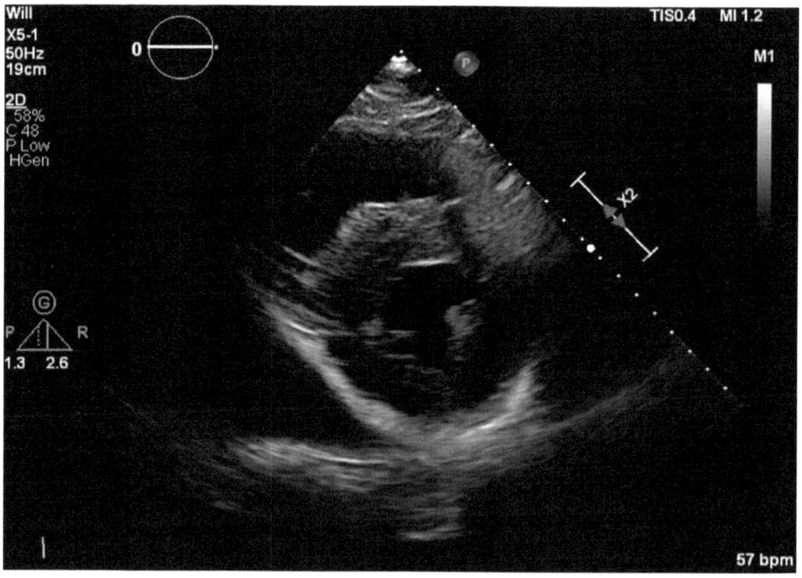

Fig. 16.5 Parasternal short-axis of a patient with restrictive cardiomyopathy secondary to amyloidosis (see Video 16.5)

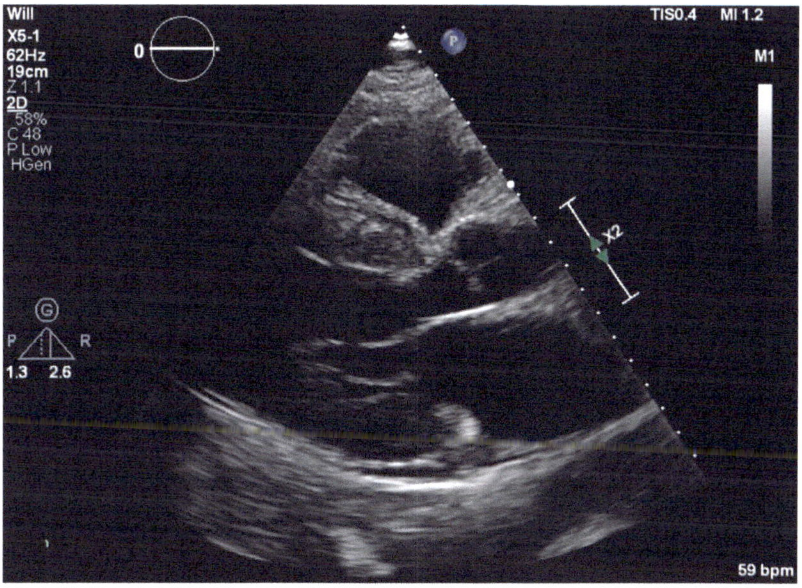

Fig. 16.6 Parasternal long-axis view of a patient with restrictive cardiomyopathy secondary to amyloidosis (see Video 16.6)

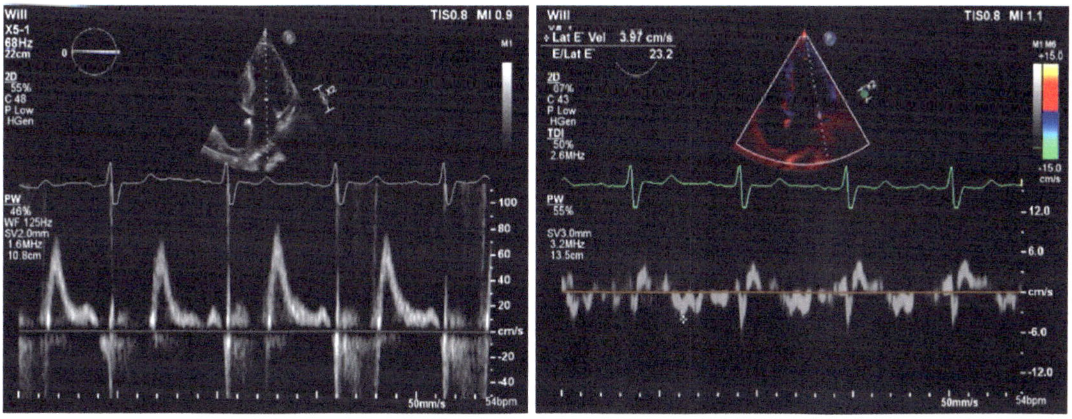

Fig. 16.7 Mitral inflow Doppler tracing and tissue Doppler tracing from a patient with restrictive cardiomyopathy demonstrating restrictive diastology

Arrhythmogenic Right Ventricular Cardiomyopathy/Dysplasia (ARVC/D)

Arrhythmogenic right ventricular cardiomyopathy/dysplasia (ARVC/D) is characterized by progressive fibrofatty replacement of the right ventricular myocardium resulting in right ventricular dilation and dysfunction [32]. ARVC/D is genetically inherited and remains the second most common cause of sudden cardiac death in patients <35 years old [33]. The right ventricular structural changes result in electrical instability and the development of ventricular arrhythmias. Adrenergic stimulation and catecholamine release associated with exercise are particularly stimulating for inducing ventricular arrhythmias [34].

Patients present with nonspecific symptoms including chest pain, syncope, and right heart failure. Sudden death by ventricular arrhythmia may be the presenting symptom with a diagnosis of ARVC/D postmortem [34]. A 1994 International Task Force created criteria for the clinical diagnosis of ARVC/D with revision in 2010. These criteria classify structural, histological, electrocardiographic, arrhythmic, and genetic features with major and minor criteria based on the specificity of diagnosis [35, 36]. The full criteria for diagnosis of ARVC/D can be referred to by Marcus et al. and is beyond the scope of this chapter [36]. Further focus will be on the specific structural components identified by echocardiography.

For patients with ventricular arrhythmia and/or undifferentiated heart failure, TTE assessment can be used to assess for ARVC/D. Updated 2010 criteria for the echocardiography structural assessment include [36]:

Major

- Regional RV akinesia, dyskinesia, or aneurysm and
- (One of the following measured at end-diastole)
  - PLAX RVOT >32 mm
  - PSAX RVOT >36 mm
  - Fractional area change ≤33%

Minor criteria include

- Regional RV akinesia or dyskinesia and
- (One of the following measured at end-diastole)
  - PLAX RVOT ≥29 to <32 mm or
  - PSAX RVOT ≥32 to <36 mm
  - Or fractional area change >33% to <40% (see Fig. 16.8)

Of note, only the echocardiography findings are summarized in the review above. Full diagnostic criteria for ARVC/D rely on echocardiography, tissue characterization of myocardium, repolarization/depolarization/conduction abnormalities, arrhythmia, and family history, requiring major and minor criteria from each category. Please refer to Marcus et al. for a more detailed description of diagnostic criteria [36].

Beyond these criteria, tricuspid annular plane systolic excursion (TAPSE), doppler tissue imaging (DTI)-derived tricuspid lateral annular systolic velocity (S′-wave), RV index of myocardial perfor-

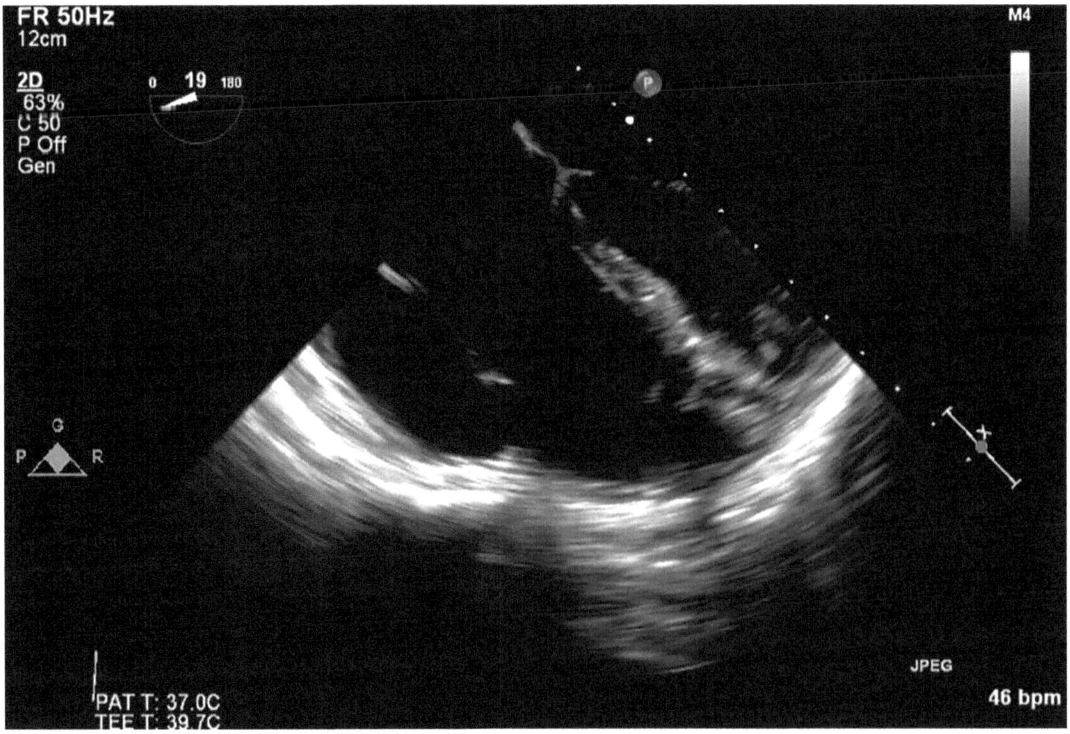

Fig. 16.8 Mid-esophageal four-chamber view of a patient with arrhythmogenic RV dysplasia (see Video 16.7)

mance (RIMP), and fractional area change (FAC) can be helpful to define the systolic and diastolic function of the right ventricle [37–39]. TAPSE <17 mm indicates right ventricular systolic dysfunction focused on right ventricular longitudinal function. RV wall thinning, aneurysm formation, outflow tract dilation, and trabecular disarray are inconsistently present [14]. While echocardiographic findings do not establish a diagnosis for ARVC/D, when right ventricular dysfunction is observed and is consistent with these parameters, ARVC/D remains an important etiology to consider. Treatment includes beta blockers, avoidance of catecholamine surges (exercise, stress, iatrogenic), and consideration of ICD placement for those at risk of life-threatening arrhythmias [34].

Stress-Induced Cardiomyopathy

Takotsubo Cardiomyopathy

Initially described in 1990, stress cardiomyopathy or "Takotsubo Syndrome," is characterized by transient ventricular systolic and diastolic dysfunction with gradual recovery in the weeks and months following diagnosis [40, 41]. Takotsubo refers to a Japanese octopus trap, which resembles the apical ballooning shape of the heart when affected by the most common variant of stress cardiomyopathy [41]. Over 90% of cases are diagnosed in postmenopausal women, and a majority experience intense emotional (close death, assault, violence) or physical (illness, surgery, trauma, stroke, or central nervous system disorder) discomfort prior to presentation [41–43]. Patients present with chest pain, shortness of breath, or evidence of cardiogenic shock, particularly in the setting of neurogenic or other acute illness [43]. Revised criteria by the Mayo Clinic are widely used for the diagnosis of stress cardiomyopathy and include [44, 45]:

(a) Transient dyskinesis, hypokinesis, or akinesis with abnormalities in regional wall motion of the left ventricular wall extending beyond epicardial vascular distribution usually in the presence of a stress trigger
(b) Absence of CAD on angiography
(c) New ECG ST-segment elevation or T wave inversions
(d) Elevation in cardiac troponin
(e) Absence of pheochromocytoma or myocarditis

Transthoracic echocardiography provides visualization of left ventricular function on presentation and allows monitoring of the ventricular recovery from the transient dysfunction. During acute illness, myocardial wall motion abnormalities exist beyond any specific coronary artery distribution [42, 46]. The classic Takotsubo Cardiomyopathy definition of "apical ballooning" involves apical hypokinesis with preserved/hyperkinetic basal segment wall motion [47]. Two additional patterns of dysfunction involve mid-ventricular and/or basal wall motion abnormalities [48, 49]. While atypical, they can occur. Diastolic dysfunction is evident with increased E/e′ ratio and has been found to be an independent predictor of heart failure and in-hospital mortality [50]. Two-dimensional strain imaging depicts decreased longitudinal strain values from base to apex in stress cardiomyopathy. Contrast echocardiography also allows for improved visualization of endocardial borders and evaluation of thrombus formation [44]. Left ventricular outflow tract obstruction (LVOTO), acute mitral regurgitation, and ventricular thrombus with distal embolization are all sequelae of cardiac dysfunction and can be periodically reevaluated throughout the course of illness by echocardiography [47] (see Fig. 16.9).

Stress cardiomyopathy is notable for the rapid recovery of LVEF; however, there is increased evidence that some degree of dysfunction remains despite supposed "normalization" of function. Months after ejection fraction recovery, patients may endorse ongoing heart failure symptoms as well as evidence of dysfunction on strain imaging with reduced global longitudinal strain, apical circumferential strain, left ventricular twist, and untwist [51, 52]. With increased evidence of cardiac dysfunction, despite recovered ejection fraction, the long-term prognosis and follow-up for these patients continue to evolve [43, 53].

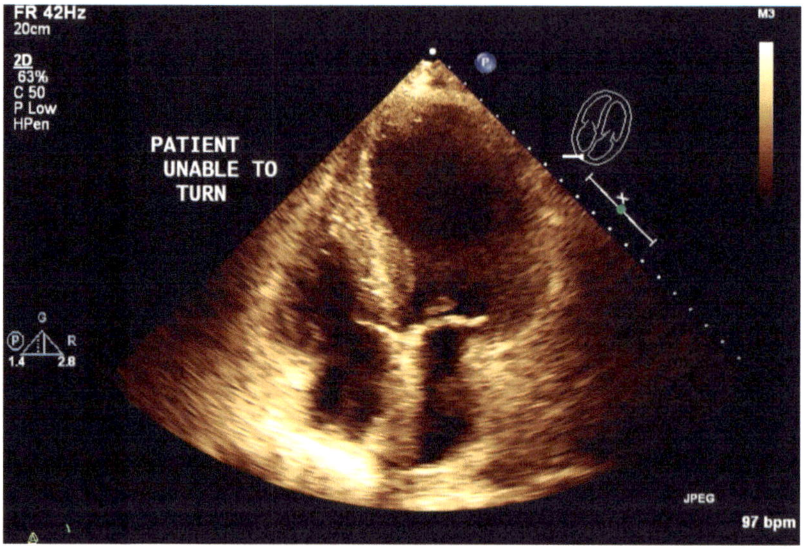

Fig. 16.9 Apical four-chamber view of a patient with Takotsubo cardiomyopathy (see Video 16.8)

Neurogenic Stress Cardiomyopathy

Cardiac abnormalities can be observed in patients who experience a severe grade subarachnoid hemorrhage, traumatic brain injury, stroke, or central nervous system infection and are considered a Neurogenic Stress Cardiomyopathy (NSC). One hypothesis attributes etiology to massive catecholamine release and has been compared to the stress response involved with Takotsubo Cardiomyopathy. NSC can be asymptomatic or have symptoms of heart failure, pulmonary edema, hypotension, or arrhythmia. Echocardiography is significant for left ventricular dysfunction with wall motion abnormalities of apical, basal, and mid-ventricular walls without correlation with coronary artery distribution, similar to Takotsubo cardiomyopathy. NSC is more likely to be associated with severe SAH and predicts cerebral vasospasm. Further research is necessary to determine outcome associations with NSC. Treatment remains supportive [54, 55].

Cirrhotic Cardiomyopathy

There has long been observation of hemodynamic changes in patients with end-stage liver disease [56, 57]. Initially attributed to alcohol use, cirrhotic cardiomyopathy is now identified as cardiac dysfunction in patients with end-stage liver disease of any source [58, 59]. The complex pathophysiology of cirrhosis, including hepatocellular dysfunction, portal hypertension, and portosystemic shunting, results in increased production of vasodilators and resistance to vasoconstrictors [60]. This delicate balance between the distribution of preload and afterload results in hyperdynamic cardiac function, low systemic vascular resistance, and an overall high cardiac output. Cardiac dysfunction for many patients is only uncovered during episodes of stress, including infection, surgery, or TIPS procedures, and can have a significant impact on morbidity and mortality [59].

Diagnostic criteria for Cirrhotic Cardiomyopathy were developed in 2005 during the World Congress of Gastroenterology in Montreal [60]. While the guidelines classified the diagnosis based on impaired contractility, systolic dysfunction, and electromechanical abnormalities, challenges emerged with identifying systolic dysfunction for patients in a hyperdynamic state [61]. A new set of guidelines were established in 2019 by the Cirrhotic Cardiomyopathy Consortium to use updated techniques to assess cardiac function including strain imaging and tissue Doppler [61, 62]. Systolic function analysis should utilize strain imaging to assess circumferential, longitudinal, radial, and transverse strain [62]. Assessment of Diastolic dysfunction utilizes 2016 ASE/EACVI guidelines [63].

2019 Cirrhotic Cardiomyopathy Consortium Criteria for diagnosis of Cirrhotic cardiomyopathy includes [61]:

- Systolic dysfunction (Any of the following)
  - LV ejection fraction <50%
  - Absolute GLS <18%
- ≥3 of the following
  - Septal mitral annular early diastolic velocity (e′) velocity < 7 cm/s
  - Mitral inflow early diastolic velocity (E) to e′ (E/e′)ratio ≥ 15
  - Left Atrial Volume Index (LAVI) >34 mL/m^2
  - Tricuspid regurgitation (TR) velocity >2.8 m/s

Cardiac dysfunction has been reported in up to 50% of patients with cirrhosis [64]. In the critical care setting, it is important to acknowledge the potential for cardiac dysfunction in cirrhotic patients and its potential contribution to an individual patient's hemodynamic instability.

Noncompaction Cardiomyopathy

Noncompaction cardiomyopathy, or left ventricular noncompaction cardiomyopathy, is characterized by excessive trabeculations of the left ventricle, intertrabecular recesses, and a bilayered myocardium with a compact epicardial layer and a thickened endocardial noncompacted layer [65]. An autosomal dominant genetic pattern is associated with the failure of the myocardium to "compact" during embryologic development resulting in a bilayer appearance [66]. Patients with noncompaction cardiomyopathy present with evidence of heart failure and are at risk of mural thrombus formation in the deep intertrabecular recesses. The risk is particularly increased in those with reduced EF or atrial fibrillation [66, 67]. Patients are also at risk of conduction abnormalities including ventricular arrhythmias associated with sudden cardiac death.

Left ventricular noncompaction cardiomyopathy is classified by the European Society of Cardiology as an unclassified Familial Cardiomyopathy and by the American Heart Association as a genetic cardiomyopathy [68, 69]. There are several proposed echocardiographic criteria for the diagnosis of noncompaction cardiomyopathy without a unified diagnostic consensus [70]. Multiple sources agree on the presence of apical trabeculations, deep intertrabecular recesses, and identification of a two-layered myocardium with a compact epicardial, and a noncompacted trabeculated endocardium as elements of this disorder [71, 72]. A ratio of noncompacted to compacted myocardium of >2:1 is considered diagnostic [14]. The left ventricular apex is most affected by trabeculations with right ventricular and biventricular involvement possible and sparing of the basal level of the ventricles [66]. Contrast echocardiography, speckle tracking, and tissue Doppler offer additional modalities which may provide important information regarding myocardial function. However, further study is required to establish the diagnostic validity of these techniques (see Fig. 16.10).

Septic Cardiomyopathy

Septic cardiomyopathy is broadly identified as acute cardiac dysfunction in the setting of systemic infection and inflammation [73]. Common characteristics include reduced left ventricular contractility, left ventricular dilatation, and reduced response to volume infusion. However, a consensus definition with diagnostic criteria does not exist [73, 74]. In 1980, septic cardiomyopathy was initially described as an acute decrease in left ventricular ejection fraction with dilation during sepsis [73, 75]. Echocardiographic characteristics include decreased LV ejection fraction which is reversible and normalizes in days, normal or low left ventricular filling pressure [75]. About 2/3 of patients have RV dysfunction on evaluation with RV fractional area change (FAC) with tricuspid annular plane systolic excursion (TAPSE), and

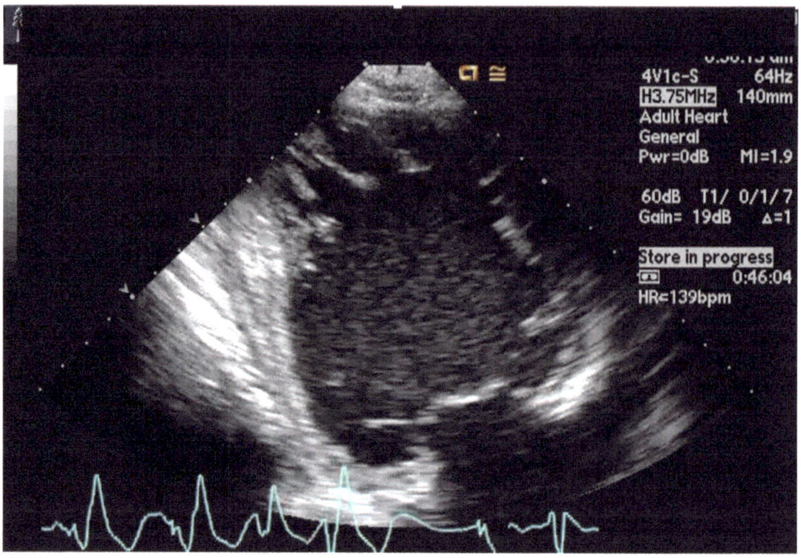

Fig. 16.10 Apical two-chamber view of a patient with noncompaction cardiomyopathy (see Video 16.9)

tricuspid annular tissue Doppler imaging (TDI, and RV wall TDI). LV Diastolic dysfunction is common and septal relaxation on TDI strongly predicted mortality in multiple studies [76, 77]. Alterations in preload and afterload during sepsis have a significant impact on LVEF, introducing concern EF may not be a reliable measure of cardiac function in a disease state known for significant alterations in systemic vascular resistance [73, 78, 79].

Speckle-tracking echocardiography has been shown to be more sensitive in sepsis in identifying LV dysfunction. Global longitudinal strain is less susceptible to alterations in preload and afterload [79–81]. While Speckle-tracking echocardiography offers potential for improved evaluation of cardiac dysfunction, the modality has not undergone evaluation with larger, randomized trials [74]. Despite unclear diagnostic criteria of septic cardiomyopathy, treatment remains focused on the treatment of the underlying infection with supportive management of hemodynamics, including inotropic support, as the inflammatory state improves [73].

Summary Points

- *Cardiomyopathy* refers to intrinsic disease of the myocardium in the absence of coronary artery disease, hypertension, valvular or congenital disease.
- Patients in the intensive care unit may present with various forms of cardiomyopathy and their sequelae.
- Bedside echocardiography is a powerful tool to identify and help manage patients in the ICU with cardiomyopathies.
- Dilated cardiomyopathy diagnostic criteria include evidence of left ventricular systolic dysfunction with EF <45%, and/or fractional shortening <25% in association with left ventricular end-diastolic dimension >112% corrected for age and BSA.
- Hypertrophic cardiomyopathy manifests left ventricular hypertrophy with disorganized myocardial architecture in the absence of hypertension or valvular disease. Up to two-thirds of patients display dynamic outflow tract obstruction with evidence of a gradient >30 mmHg.
- Restrictive Cardiomyopathy is a cardiac muscle disease characterized by increased stiffness, elevated end-diastolic pressure, and ultimately diastolic dysfunction of one or both ventricles. Despite abnormal diastolic filling, the systolic function of the ventricles remains preserved.
- Arrhythmogenic right ventricular cardiomyopathy is characterized by progressive fibrofatty replacement of the right ventricular myocardium resulting in right ventricular dilation and dysfunction.

- Stress-induced cardiomyopathy manifests as transient dyskinesis, hypokinesis, or akinesis with abnormalities in regional wall motion of the left ventricular wall extending beyond epicardial vascular distribution usually in the presence of a stress trigger.
- Cardiac dysfunction has been reported in up to 50% of patients with cirrhosis and can be identified using echocardiography.
- Noncompaction cardiomyopathy is characterized by excessive trabeculations of the left ventricle, intertrabecular recesses, and a bilayered myocardium with a compact epicardial layer and a thickened endocardial noncompacted layer.
- Septic cardiomyopathy is acute cardiac dysfunction in the setting of systemic infection and inflammation. Echocardiography is essential to its identification

Questions

1. A 55-year-old male with a history of hypertension and hypertrophic cardiomyopathy is admitted to the ICU with severe pneumonia secondary to COVID-19. The ICU team decides to intubate him for his progressive respiratory failure. After the administration of propofol sedation, he becomes tachycardic and profoundly hypotensive. The airway is secured and a bedside POCUS echocardiogram is performed. What would you expect the continuous wave Doppler profile across the aortic valve to show?
   A. Late-peaking dagger-shaped appearance
   B. Early systolic peak with a triangular shape to the velocity curve
   C. Rounded curve with a mid-systolic peak

   Answer: A

   A late-peaking dagger-shaped appearance to the continuous wave Doppler profile across the LVOT and the aortic valve is characteristic of dynamic LV outflow tract obstruction, as in SAM. An early systolic peak with a triangular shape to the CWD profile is characteristic of mild aortic valve obstruction, while a rounded curve with a mid-systolic peak is characteristic of severe aortic valve stenosis.

2. A 65-year-old female is admitted to the ICU from the ED after experiencing a "thunderclap" headache and loss of consciousness. She is diagnosed with a ruptured ACOM aneurysm and goes to neuro-IR for coiling of her ruptured aneurysm. Postprocedure she develops diffuse ST depressions on ECG and becomes profoundly hemodynamically unstable. Her troponin level is significantly elevated and your resident calls a STEMI activation. You perform a bedside TTE and note that the basal and mid-levels of the LV are hyperdynamic but the apex is dyskinetic and "ballooning" circumferentially. There does not appear to be any LVOT obstruction. What is the next most appropriate course of action?
   A. Immediate transfer to the cath lab for left heart catheterization
   B. Inotropic support
   C. Emergent CT surgery consults for emergent CABG
   D. Emergent ECMO consult

   Answer: B

   This patient is experiencing a stress-induced or Takotsubo Cardiomyopathy. This is a consequence of a massive catecholamine surge in the setting of an acute neurologic insult. The LV wall motion abnormality does not fit any one coronary distribution, hence there is no role for emergent coronary revascularization. Provided there is no echocardiographic evidence of dynamic LVOT obstruction, the patient should receive inotropic support. Mechanical circulatory support should be initiated only if the patient is refractory to inotropic pharmacologic support.

References

1. McKenna WJ, Maron BJ, Thiene G. Classification, epidemiology, and global burden of cardiomyopathies. Circ Res. 2017;121(7):722.
2. Report of the WHO/ISFC task force on the definition and classification of cardiomyopathies. Br Heart J. 1980;44(6):672–30.
3. Richardson P, McKenna W, Bristow M, Maisch B, Mautner B, O'Connell J, Olsen E, Thiene G, Goodwin

J, Gyarfas I, Martin I, Nordet P. Report of the 1995 World Health Organization/International Society and Federation of Cardiology Task Force on the Definition and Classification of cardiomyopathies. Circulation. 1996;93(5):841.
4. Maron BJ, Towbin JA, Thiene G, Antzelevitch C, Corrado D, Arnett D, Moss AJ, Seidman CE, Young JB, American Heart Association, Council on Clinical Cardiology, Heart Failure and Transplantation Committee, Quality of Care and Outcomes Research and Functional Genomics and Translational Biology Interdisciplinary Working Groups, Council on Epidemiology and Prevention. Contemporary definitions and classification of the cardiomyopathies: an American Heart Association Scientific Statement from the Council on Clinical Cardiology, Heart Failure and Transplantation Committee; Quality of Care and Outcomes Research and Functional Genomics and Translational Biology Interdisciplinary Working Groups; and Council on Epidemiology and Prevention. Circulation. 2006;113(14):1807.
5. Elliott P, Andersson B, Arbustini E, Bilinska Z, Cecchi F, Charron P, Dubourg O, Kühl U, Maisch B, McKenna WJ, Monserrat L, Pankuweit S, Rapezzi C, Seferovic P, Tavazzi L. Keren AClassification of the cardiomyopathies: a position statement from the European Society Of Cardiology Working Group on Myocardial and Pericardial Diseases. Eur Heart J. 2008;29(2):270.
6. Arbustini E, Narula N, Dec GW, Reddy KS, Greenberg B, Kushwaha S, Marwick T, Pinney S, Bellazzi R, Favalli V, Kramer C, Roberts R, Zoghbi WA, Bonow R, Tavazzi L, Fuster V, Narula J. The MOGE(S) classification for a phenotype-genotype nomenclature of cardiomyopathy: endorsed by the World Heart Federation. J Am Coll Cardiol. 2013;62(22):2046–72.
7. Elliott PM. Classification of cardiomyopathies: evolution or revolution? J Am Coll Cardiol. 2013;62(22):2073–4.
8. Kopecky SL, Gersh BJ. Dilated cardiomyopathy and myocarditis: natural history, etiology, clinical manifestations, and management. Curr Problems Cardiol. 1987;12(10):574–647.
9. Hershberger RE, Lindenfeld J, Mestroni L, Seidman CE, Taylor MR, Towbin JA. Genetic evaluation of cardiomyopathy—a Heart Failure Society of America practice guideline. J Cardiac Failure. 2009;15(2):83–97.
10. Mathew T, Williams L, Navaratnam G, Rana B, Wheeler R, Collins K, Harkness A, Jones R, Knight D, O'Gallagher K, Oxborough D. Diagnosis and assessment of dilated cardiomyopathy: a guideline protocol from the British Society of Echocardiography. Echo Res Pract. 2017;4(2):G1.
11. Thomas DE, Wheeler R, Yousef ZR, Masani ND. The role of echocardiography in guiding management in dilated cardiomyopathy. Eur J Echocardiogr. 2009;10(8):iii15–21.
12. La Vecchia L, Paccanaro M, Bonanno C, Varotto L, Ometto R, Vincenzi M. Left ventricular versus biventricular dysfunction in idiopathic dilated cardiomyopathy. Am J Cardiol. 1999;83(1):120–2.
13. Donal E, De Place C, Kervio G, Bauer F, Gervais R, Leclercq C, Mabo P, Daubert JC. Mitral regurgitation in dilated cardiomyopathy: value of both regional left ventricular contractility and dyssynchrony. Eur J Echocardiogr. 2009;10(1):133–8.
14. Wood MJ, Picard MH. Utility of echocardiography in the evaluation of individuals with cardiomyopathy. Heart. 2004;90(6):707–12.
15. Kapetanakis S, Kearney MT, Siva A, Gall N, Cooklin M, Monaghan MJ. Real-time three-dimensional echocardiography: a novel technique to quantify global left ventricular mechanical dyssynchrony. Circulation. 2005;112(7):992–1000.
16. Suffoletto MS, Dohi K, Cannesson M, Saba S, Gorcsan J III. Novel speckle-tracking radial strain from routine black-and-white echocardiographic images to quantify dyssynchrony and predict response to cardiac resynchronization therapy. Circulation. 2006;113(7):960–8.
17. Maron BJ. Hypertrophic cardiomyopathy: a systematic review. JAMA. 2002;287(10):1308–20.
18. Sherrid MV, Arabadjian M. Echocardiography to individualize treatment for hypertrophic cardiomyopathy. Progr Cardiovasc Dis. 2012;54(6):461–76.
19. Gersh BJ, Maron BJ, Bonow RO, Dearani JA, Fifer MA, Link MS, Naidu SS, Nishimura RA, Ommen SR, Rakowski H, Seidman CE. 2011 ACCF/AHA guideline for the diagnosis and treatment of hypertrophic cardiomyopathy: a report of the American College of Cardiology Foundation/American Heart Association Task Force on practice guidelines developed in collaboration with the American Association for Thoracic Surgery, American Society of echocardiography, American Society of nuclear Cardiology, Heart Failure Society of America, Heart Rhythm Society, Society for Cardiovascular Angiography and Interventions, and Society of Thoracic Surgeons. J Am Coll Cardiol. 2011;58(25):e212–60.
20. Afonso LC, Bernal J, Bax JJ, Abraham TP. Echocardiography in hypertrophic cardiomyopathy: the role of conventional and emerging technologies. JACC Cardiovasc Imaging. 2008;1(6):787–800.
21. Williams LK, Frenneaux MP, Steeds RP. Echocardiography in hypertrophic cardiomyopathy diagnosis, prognosis, and role in management. Eur J Echocardiogr. 2009;10(8):iii9–14.
22. Maron MS, Olivotto I, Zenovich AG, Link MS, Pandian NG, Kuvin JT, Nistri S, Cecchi F, Udelson JE, Maron BJ. Hypertrophic cardiomyopathy is predominantly a disease of left ventricular outflow tract obstruction. Circulation. 2006;114(21):2232–9.
23. Losi MA, Nistri S, Galderisi M, Betocchi S, Cecchi F, Olivotto I, Ballo P, Buralli S, D'Andrea A, D'Errico A, Mele D. Echocardiography in patients with hypertrophic cardiomyopathy: usefulness of old and new techniques in the diagnosis and pathophysiological assessment. Cardiovasc Ultrasound. 2010;8(1):1–9.

24. Nagueh SF, Bachinski LL, Meyer D, Hill R, Zoghbi WA, Tam JW, Quiñones MA, Roberts R, Marian AJ. Tissue Doppler imaging consistently detects myocardial abnormalities in patients with hypertrophic cardiomyopathy and provides a novel means for an early diagnosis before and independently of hypertrophy. Circulation. 2001;104(2):128–30.
25. Carasso S, Yang H, Woo A, Vannan MA, Jamorski M, Wigle ED, Rakowski H. Systolic myocardial mechanics in hypertrophic cardiomyopathy: novel concepts and implications for clinical status. J Am Soc Echocardiogr. 2008;21(6):675–83.
26. Caselli S, Pelliccia A, Maron M, Santini D, Puccio D, Marcantonio A, Pandian NG, De Castro S. Differentiation of hypertrophic cardiomyopathy from other forms of left ventricular hypertrophy by means of three-dimensional echocardiography. Am J Cardiol. 2008;102(5):616–20.
27. Kushwaha SS, Fallon JT, Fuster V. Restrictive cardiomyopathy. N Engl J Med. 1997;336(4):267–76.
28. Ammash NM, Seward JB, Bailey KR, Edwards WD, Tajik AJ. Clinical profile and outcome of idiopathic restrictive cardiomyopathy. Circulation. 2000;101(21):2490–6.
29. Appleton CP, Hatle LK, Popp RL. Relation of transmitral flow velocity patterns to left ventricular diastolic function: new insights from a combined hemodynamic and Doppler echocardiographic study. J Am Coll Cardiol. 1988;12(2):426–40.
30. Nishimura RA, Abel MD, Hatle LK, Tajik AJ. Relation of pulmonary vein to mitral flow velocities by transesophageal Doppler echocardiography. Effect of different loading conditions. Circulation. 1990;81(5):1488–97.
31. Rajagopalan N, Garcia MJ, Rodriguez L, Murray RD, Apperson-Hansen C, Stugaard M, Thomas JD, Klein AL. Comparison of new Doppler echocardiographic methods to differentiate constrictive pericardial heart disease and restrictive cardiomyopathy. Am J Cardiol. 2001;87(1):86–94.
32. Marcus FI, Fontaine GH, Guiraudon G, Frank R, Laurenceau JL, Malergue C, Grosgogeat Y. Right ventricular dysplasia: a report of 24 adult cases. Circulation. 1982;65(2):384–98.
33. Li KH, Bazoukis G, Liu T, Li G, Wu WK, Wong SH, Wong WT, Chan YS, Wong MC, Wassilew K, Vassiliou VS. Arrhythmogenic right ventricular cardiomyopathy/dysplasia (ARVC/D) in clinical practice. J Arrhythm. 2018;34(1):11–22.
34. Gemayel C, Pelliccia A, Thompson PD. Arrhythmogenic right ventricular cardiomyopathy. J Am Coll Cardiol. 2001;38(7):1773–81.
35. McKenna WJ, Thiene G, Nava A, Fontaliran F, Blomstrom-Lundqvist C, Fontaine G, Camerini F. Diagnosis of arrhythmogenic right ventricular dysplasia/cardiomyopathy. Task Force of the Working Group Myocardial and Pericardial Disease of the European Society of Cardiology and of the Scientific Council on Cardiomyopathies of the International Society and Federation of Cardiology. Br Heart J. 1994;71(3):215.
36. Marcus FI, McKenna WJ, Sherrill D, Basso C, Bauce B, Bluemke DA, Calkins H, Corrado D, Cox MG, Daubert JP, Fontaine G. Diagnosis of arrhythmogenic right ventricular cardiomyopathy/dysplasia: proposed modification of the task force criteria. Circulation. 2010;121(13):1533–41.
37. Yoerger DM, Marcus F, Sherrill D, Calkins H, Towbin JA, Zareba W, Picard MH, Multidisciplinary Study of Right Ventricular Dysplasia Investigators. Echocardiographic findings in patients meeting task force criteria for arrhythmogenic right ventricular dysplasia: new insights from the multidisciplinary study of right ventricular dysplasia. J Am Coll Cardiol. 2005;45(6):860–5.
38. Lindström L, Wilkenshoff UM, Larsson H, Wranne B. Echocardiographic assessment of arrhythmogenic right ventricular cardiomyopathy. Heart. 2001;86(1):31–8.
39. Smolarek D, Gruchała M, Sobiczewski W. Echocardiographic evaluation of right ventricular systolic function: the traditional and innovative approach. Cardiol J. 2017;24(5):563–72.
40. Sato HT. Tako-tsubo-like left ventricular dysfunction due to multivessel coronary spasm. In: Clinical aspects of myocardial injury: from ischemia to heart failure. Kagakuhyouronsha; 1990. p. 56–64.
41. Medina de Chazal H, Del Buono MG, Keyser-Marcus L, Ma L, Moeller FG, Berrocal D, Abbate A. Stress cardiomyopathy diagnosis and treatment: JACC state-of-the-art review. J Am Coll Cardiol. 2018;72(16):1955–71.
42. Lyon AR, Bossone E, Schneider B, Sechtem U, Citro R, Underwood SR, Sheppard MN, Figtree GA, Parodi G, Akashi YJ, Ruschitzka F. Current state of knowledge on Takotsubo syndrome: a position statement from the Taskforce on Takotsubo Syndrome of the Heart Failure Association of the European Society of Cardiology. Eur J Heart Failure. 2016;18(1):8–27.
43. Templin C, Ghadri JR, Diekmann J, Napp LC, Bataiosu DR, Jaguszewski M, Cammann VL, Sarcon A, Geyer V, Neumann CA, Seifert B. Clinical features and outcomes of takotsubo (stress) cardiomyopathy. N Engl J Med. 2015;373(10):929–38.
44. Ghadri JR, Wittstein IS, Prasad A, Sharkey S, Dote K, Akashi YJ, Cammann VL, Crea F, Galiuto L, Desmet W, Yoshida T. International expert consensus document on Takotsubo syndrome (part I): clinical characteristics, diagnostic criteria, and pathophysiology. Eur Heart J. 2018;39(22):2032–46.
45. Ghadri JR, Wittstein IS, Prasad A, Sharkey S, Dote K, Akashi YJ, Cammann VL, Crea F, Galiuto L, Desmet W, Yoshida T. International expert consensus document on Takotsubo syndrome (part II): diagnostic workup, outcome, and management. Eur Heart J. 2018;39(22):2047–62.
46. Citro R, Lyon AR, Meimoun P, Omerovic E, Redfors B, Buck T, Lerakis S, Parodi G, Silverio A, Eitel I, Schneider B. Standard and advanced echocardiog-

raphy in takotsubo (stress) cardiomyopathy: clinical and prognostic implications. J Am Soc Echocardiogr. 2015;28(1):57–74.
47. Izumo M, Akashi YJ. Role of echocardiography for takotsubo cardiomyopathy: clinical and prognostic implications. Cardiovasc Diagn Ther. 2018;8(1):90.
48. Mansencal N, Abbou N, N'Guetta R, Pillière R, El Mahmoud R, Dubourg O. Apical-sparing variant of Tako-Tsubo cardiomyopathy: prevalence and characteristics. Arch Cardiovasc Dis. 2010;103(2):75–9.
49. Haghi D, Papavassiliu T, Flüchter S, Kaden JJ, Pörner T, Borggrefe M, Suselbeck T. Variant form of the acute apical ballooning syndrome (takotsubo cardiomyopathy): observations on a novel entity. Heart. 2006;92(3):392–4.
50. Citro R, Rigo F, D'Andrea A, Ciampi Q, Parodi G, Provenza G, Piccolo R, Mirra M, Zito C, Giudice R, Patella MM. Echocardiographic correlates of acute heart failure, cardiogenic shock, and in-hospital mortality in tako-tsubo cardiomyopathy. JACC Cardiovasc Imaging. 2014;7(2):119–29.
51. Schwarz K, Ahearn T, Srinivasan J, Neil CJ, Scally C, Rudd A, Jagpal B, Frenneaux MP, Pislaru C, Horowitz JD, Dawson DK. Alterations in cardiac deformation, timing of contraction and relaxation, and early myocardial fibrosis accompany the apparent recovery of acute stress-induced (takotsubo) cardiomyopathy: an end to the concept of transience. J Am Soc Echocardiogr. 2017;30(8):745–55.
52. Scally C, Rudd A, Mezincescu A, Wilson H, Srivanasan J, Horgan G, Broadhurst P, Newby DE, Henning A, Dawson DK. Persistent long-term structural, functional, and metabolic changes after stress-induced (Takotsubo) cardiomyopathy. Circulation. 2018;137(10):1039–48.
53. Redfors B, Vedad R, Angerås O, Råmunddal T, Petursson P, Haraldsson I, Ali A, Dworeck C, Odenstedt J, Ioaness D, Libungan B. Mortality in takotsubo syndrome is similar to mortality in myocardial infarction—a report from the SWEDEHEART registry. Int J Cardiol. 2015;185:282–9.
54. Aronow WS. Neurogenic stress cardiomyopathy associated with subarachnoid hemorrhage. Future Cardiol. 2015;11(1):77–87.
55. Mazzeo AT, Micalizzi A, Mascia L, Scicolone A, Siracusano L. Brain–heart crosstalk: the many faces of stress-related cardiomyopathy syndromes in anaesthesia and intensive care. Br J Anaesth. 2014;112(5):803–15.
56. Kowalski HJ, Abelmann WH. The cardiac output at rest in Laennec's cirrhosis. J Clin Investig. 1953;32(10):1025–33.
57. Møller S, Henriksen JH. Cirrhotic cardiomyopathy. J Hepatol. 2010;53(1):179–90.
58. Lee SS. Cardiac abnormalities in liver cirrhosis. Western J Med. 1989;151(5):530.
59. Wiese S, Hove JD, Bendtsen F, Møller S. Cirrhotic cardiomyopathy: pathogenesis and clinical relevance. Nat Rev Gastroenterol Hepatol. 2014;11(3):177–86.
60. Møller S, Henriksen J. Cardiovascular complications of cirrhosis. Postgr Med J. 2009;85(999):44–54.
61. Izzy M, Van Wagner LB, Lin G, Altieri M, Findlay JY, Oh JK, Watt KD, Lee SS, Cirrhotic Cardiomyopathy Consortium. Redefining cirrhotic cardiomyopathy for the modern era. Hepatology. 2020;71(1):334–45.
62. Sampaio F, Pimenta J, Bettencourt N, Fontes-Carvalho R, Silva AP, Valente J, Bettencourt P, Fraga J, Gama V. Systolic and diastolic dysfunction in cirrhosis: a tissue-Doppler and speckle tracking echocardiography study. Liver Int. 2013;33(8):1158–65.
63. Nagueh SF, Appleton CP, Gillebert TC, Marino PN, Oh JK, Smiseth OA, Waggoner AD, Flachskampf FA, Pellikka PA, Evangelisa A. Recommendations for the evaluation of left ventricular diastolic function by echocardiography. Eur J Echocardiogr. 2009;10(2):165–93.
64. Nazar A, Guevara M, Sitges M, Terra C, Solà E, Guigou C, Arroyo V, Ginès P. LEFT ventricular function assessed by echocardiography in cirrhosis: relationship to systemic hemodynamics and renal dysfunction. J Hepatol. 2013;58(1):51–7.
65. Jenni R, Oechslin E, Schneider J, Jost CA, Kaufmann PA. Echocardiographic and pathoanatomical characteristics of isolated left ventricular non-compaction: a step towards classification as a distinct cardiomyopathy. Heart. 2001;86(6):666–71
66. Wengrofsky P, Armenia C, Oleszak F, Kupferstein E, Rednam C, Mitre CA, McFarlane SI. Left ventricular trabeculation and noncompaction cardiomyopathy: a review. EC Clin Exp Anat. 2019;2(6):267.
67. Hotta VT, Tendolo SC, Rodrigues AC, Fernandes F, Nastari L, Mady C. Limitations in the diagnosis of noncompaction cardiomyopathy by echocardiography. Arquivos brasileiros de cardiologia. 2017;109:483–8.
68. Maron BJ, Towbin JA, Thiene G, Antzelevitch C, Corrado D, Arnett D, Moss AJ, Seidman CE, Young JB. Contemporary definitions and classification of the cardiomyopathies: an American Heart Association Scientific Statement from the Council on Clinical Cardiology, Heart Failure and Transplantation Committee; Quality of Care and Outcomes Research and Functional Genomics and Translational Biology Interdisciplinary Working Groups; and Council on Epidemiology and Prevention. Circulation. 2006;113(14):1807–16.
69. Elliott P, Andersson B, Arbustini E, Bilinska Z, Cecchi F, Charron P, Dubourg O, Kühl U, Maisch B, McKenna WJ, Monserrat L. Classification of the cardiomyopathies: a position statement from the European Society Of Cardiology Working Group on Myocardial and Pericardial Diseases. Eur Heart J. 2008;29(2):270–6.
70. Chebrolu LH, Mehta AM, Nanda NC. Noncompaction cardiomyopathy: the role of advanced multimodality imaging techniques in diagnosis and assessment. Echocardiography. 2017;34(2):279–89.
71. Chin TK, Perloff JK, Williams RG, Jue K, Mohrmann R. Isolated noncompaction of left ventricular

myocardium. A study of eight cases. Circulation. 1990;82(2):507–13.
72. Stöllberger C, Finsterer J. Left ventricular hypertrabeculation/noncompaction. J Am Soc Echocardiogr. 2004;17(1):91–100.
73. Beesley SJ, Weber G, Sarge T, Nikravan S, Grissom CK, Lanspa MJ, Shahul S, Brown SM. Septic cardiomyopathy. Crit care Med. 2018;46(4):625–34.
74. Martin L, Derwall M, Al Zoubi S, Zechendorf E, Reuter DA, Thiemermann C, Schuerholz T. The septic heart: current understanding of molecular mechanisms and clinical implications. Chest. 2019;155(2):427–37.
75. Vieillard-Baron A. Septic cardiomyopathy. Ann Intensive Care. 2011;1(1):1–7.
76. Landesberg G, Gilon D, Meroz Y, Georgieva M, Levin PD, Goodman S, Avidan A, Beeri R, Weissman C, Jaffe AS, Sprung CL. Diastolic dysfunction and mortality in severe sepsis and septic shock. Eur Heart J. 2012;33(7):895–903.
77. L'Heureux M, Sternberg M, Brath L, Turlington J, Kashiouris MG. Sepsis-induced cardiomyopathy: a comprehensive review. Curr Cardiol Rep. 2020;22(5):1–2.
78. Berrios RA, O'Horo JC, Velagapudi V, Pulido JN. Correlation of left ventricular systolic dysfunction determined by low ejection fraction and 30-day mortality in patients with severe sepsis and septic shock: a systematic review and meta-analysis. J Crit Care. 2014;29(4):495–9.
79. Dalla K, Hallman C, Bech-Hanssen O, Haney M, Ricksten SE. Strain echocardiography identifies impaired longitudinal systolic function in patients with septic shock and preserved ejection fraction. Cardiovasc Ultrasound. 2015;13(1):1.
80. Lanspa MJ, Pittman JE, Hirshberg EL, Wilson EL, Olsen T, Brown SM, Grissom CK. Association of left ventricular longitudinal strain with central venous oxygen saturation and serum lactate in patients with early severe sepsis and septic shock. Crit Care. 2015;19(1):1–9.
81. Stanton T, Leano R, Marwick TH. Prediction of all-cause mortality from global longitudinal speckle strain: comparison with ejection fraction and wall motion scoring. Circ Cardiovasc Imaging. 2009;2(5):356–64.

Aortic Stenosis

17

Connor O'Brien and Christopher F. Barnett

Abbreviations

AoV	Aortic valve
AoV VTI	Aortic valve velocity time integral
AS	Aortic stenosis
AVA	Aortic valve area
CW	Continuous wave
DI	Dimensionless index
LVOT	Left ventricular outflow tract
LVOT VTI	Left ventricular outflow tract velocity time integral
LVOTd	Left ventricular outflow tract diameter
PLAX	Parasternal long axis
PSAX	Parasternal short axis
PW	Pulse wave
SV	Stroke volume

Learning Objectives

1. Learn to identify and grade aortic stenosis
2. Learn the methods for grading aortic stenosis
3. Understand the pitfalls for grading aortic stenosis
4. Learn how to identify aortic stenosis in low flow states

C. O'Brien (✉) · C. F. Barnett
Division of Cardiology and Critical Care Cardiology Section, Department of Medicine, University of California-San Francisco School of Medicine, CA, USA
e-mail: connor.obrien@ucsf.edu

Introduction

Aortic stenosis (AS) is most commonly caused by restricted opening of the aortic valve (AoV) leaflets. Identification and quantification of AS can be helpful to understand patient hemodynamics. AS creates an obstruction to outflow between the left ventricle and aorta. As a consequence, left ventricular stroke volume (SV) is reduced and left ventricular systolic and diastolic pressures are elevated so that myocardial oxygen demand is increased while, simultaneously, coronary perfusion and myocardial oxygen delivery are reduced.

Using ultrasound to identify and quantify AS requires an understanding of AoV anatomy, anatomic variants, ultrasound physics as applied to the measurement of valvular gradients, and hemodynamic states that can introduce error into the assessment.

Anatomy of the Aortic Valve

The AoV is composed of three thin leaflets with semilunar attachments arising from a fibrous annulus (Fig. 17.1a) [1]. The coronary arteries originate in the sinuses of Valsalva just inferior to the sinotubular junction. The names of the aortic valve leaflets and sinuses correspond to the coronary artery that originates from each. The aortic root is composed of the aortic annulus, sinuses of

M. J. Lanspa, A. T. Levinson (eds.), *Echocardiography and Ultrasonography in the ICU*, Respiratory Medicine, https://doi.org/10.1007/978-3-031-80038-2_17

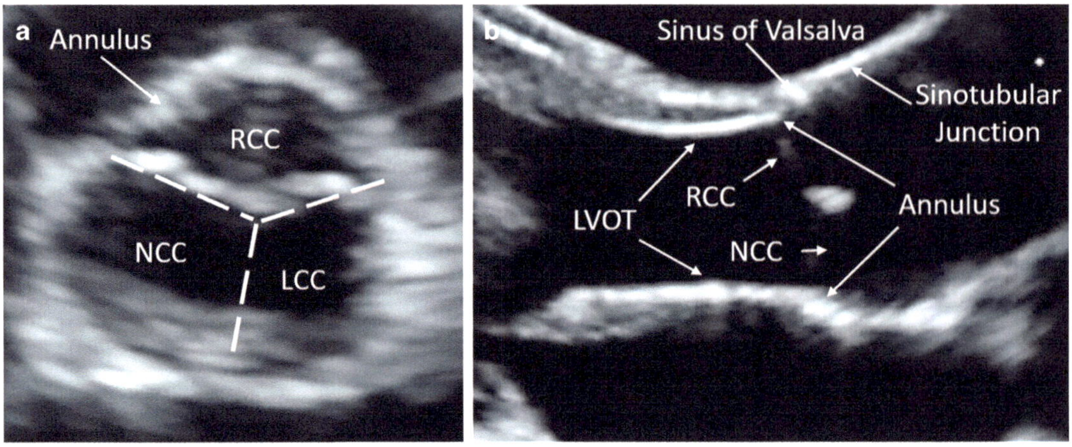

Fig. 17.1 Native AoV anatomy. (**a**) Trileaflet AoV visualized in PSAX by TTE. In this view, the annulus is a thin, echo bright circular structure. Three, thin leaflets can be seen inserting in the annulus. The dotted line demarcates leaflet edges. (**b**) AoV in PLAX illustrates the relationship between the aortic valve leaflets and annulus with the Sinuses of Valsalva and the sinotubular junction. *LCC* left coronary cusp, *NCC* noncoronary cusp, *RCC* right coronary cusp, *LVOT* left ventricular outflow tract

Valsalva, coronary ostia, and proximal ascending aorta (Fig. 17.1b).

How to Image the Aortic Valve with Ultrasound

The AoV is best viewed in parasternal long axis (PLAX) (Fig. 17.1b) and short views by transthoracic echocardiography (TTE) (Fig. 17.1a). Parasternal views offer the shortest transducer to valve distance and thus the greatest valvular resolution. Excursion of the right coronary and noncoronary cusps is best seen in PLAX (Fig. 17.2a). AS leads to restricted excursion of the cusps, which can be first identified in the PLAX (Fig. 17.2b). In this view, the cause of leaflet restriction and direction of flow acceleration can also be assessed (Fig. 17.2c, d). Rotating to parasternal short axis (PSAX) shows all three leaflets of the AoV en face and can help delineate structural causes of stenosis.

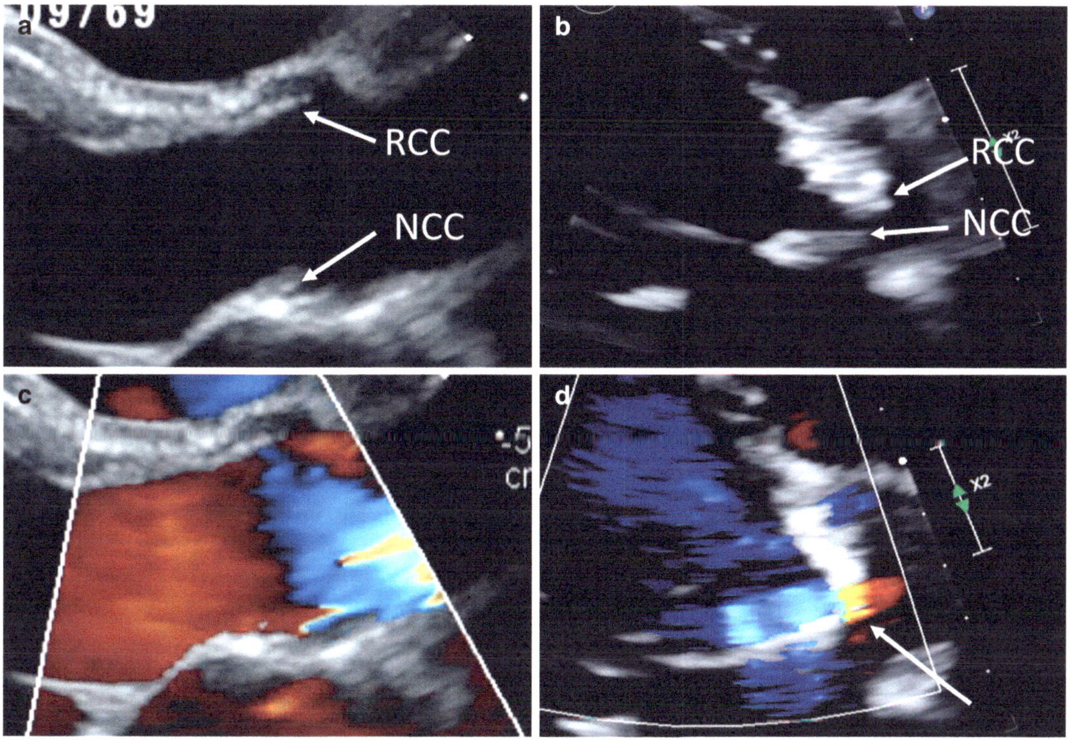

Fig. 17.2 (**a**) Normal, trileaflet AoV shown in PLAX. Thin leaflets achieve full excursion nearly opposing the wall of the aortic root. (**b**) Sclerotic aortic valve with limited leaflet opening. (**c**) Normal, trileaflet AoV during in peak systole showing laminar flow across the aortic valve. (**d**) Sclerotic aortic valve during peak systole showing nonlaminar flow acceleration across the sclerotic valve orifice. *NCC* non-coronary cusp, *RCC* right coronary cusp

Causes of Aortic Stenosis

Bicuspid AoV is the most common congenital cause of AS. Bicuspid AoV disease can be further divided into true bileaflet (Fig. 17.3a) or cusp fusion in a trileaflet valve (Fig. 17.3b) [2]. True bileaflet disease is caused by developmental abnormalities in endocardial cushion migration [3]. The resultant valve is composed of two, generally equally sized leaflets with a single commissure.

Bicuspid AoV can also be caused by leaflet fusion in a trileaflet valve. Similarly, this is caused by errors in embryological development. Fusion can occur along any fissure but is most common between the right and left coronary leaflets (~80%).

Recognizing any bicuspid AoV disease is particularly important because it is associated with other important cardiac malformations, congenital syndromes, abnormalities of aortic tissue that predispose to aneurysm and dissection.

Calcific disease of the AoV is the most common cause of AoV stenosis [4]. Stenosis is generally mediated by calcification on the aortic side of the AoV (Fig. 17.4a) but can also be subvalvular. Calcification leads to leaflet fusion and restricts leaflet excursion during systole (Fig. 17.4b). Flow acceleration can be identified through the restricted orifice (Fig. 17.4c).

Rheumatic disease and endocarditis are less common causes of aortic stenosis [2]. Rheumatic disease drives calcification and valvular sclerosis along the leaflet edges, leading to fusion of the leaflet edges commonly creating a triangular opening in the center of the AoV. Aortic insufficiency is a common feature of rheumatic AoV disease. Rheumatic aortic stenosis rarely occurs in isolation and should be suspected if rheumatic disease is seen on the mitral valve. Bulky endo-

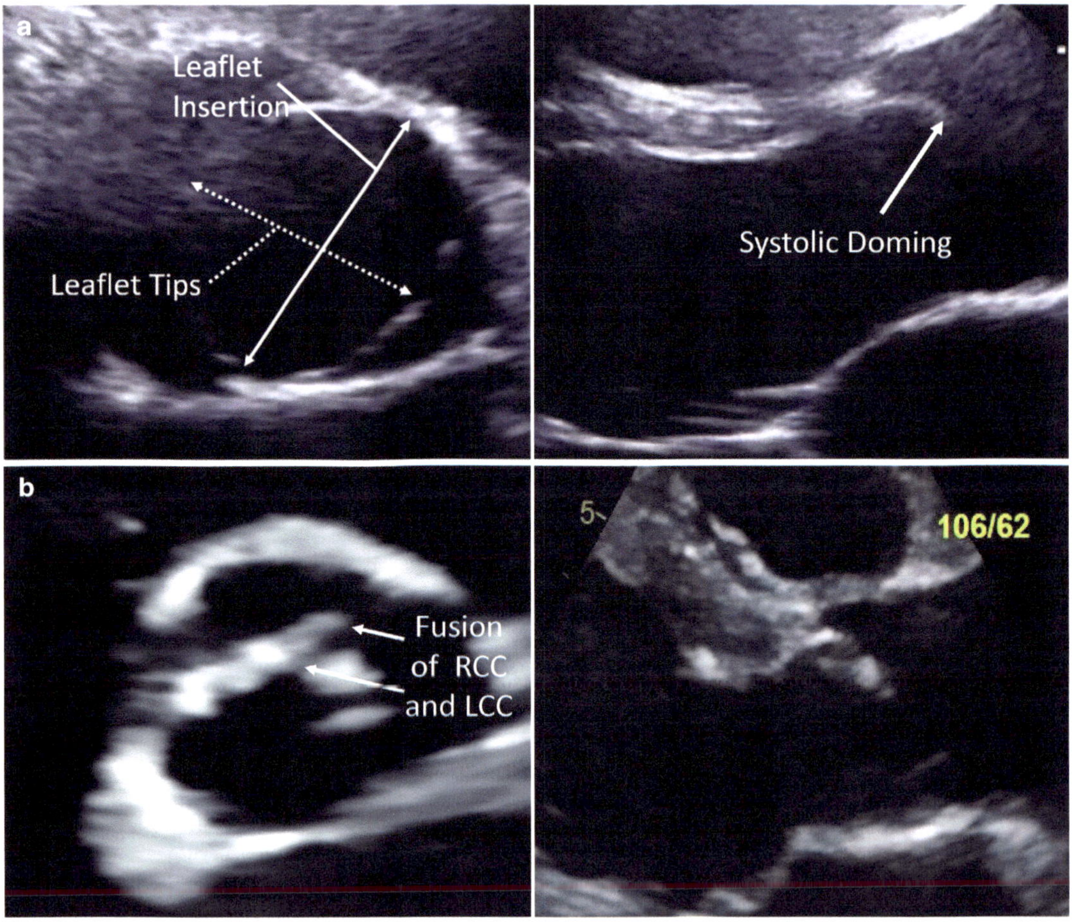

Fig. 17.3 Bicuspid AoV anatomy. (**a**) True bileaflet aortic valve. Left panel, the aortic annulus develops as an ellipse rather than circular shape. The solid, bidirectional arrow highlights the plane between the leaflets. The dotted, bidirectional arrow identifies the peak excursion along the mid-line of the valve. Right panel, shows systolic doming. (**b**) Left panel, shows leaflet fusion of the LCC and RCC. Right panel, image taken in peak systole illustrating restricted leaflet mobility. As seen here, turbulent flow can lead to sclerosis of the free edges of involved leaflets. *LCC* left coronary cusp, *RCC* right coronary cusp

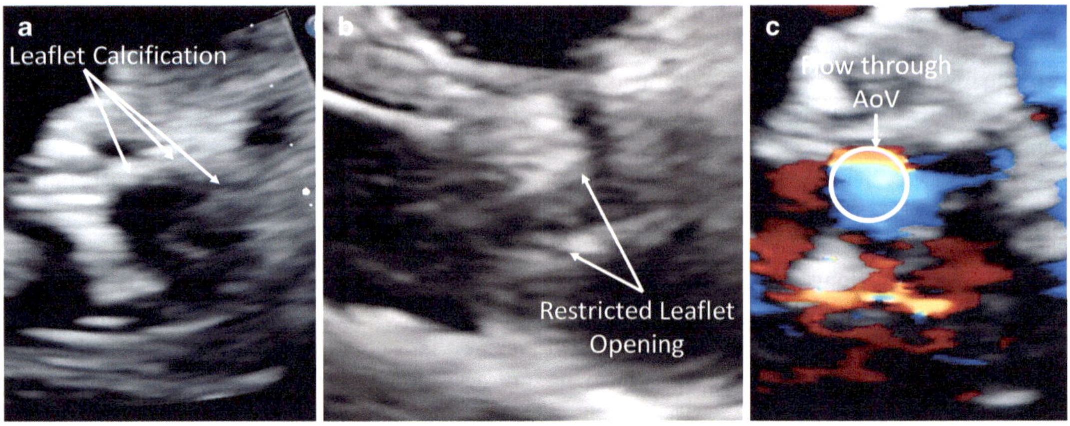

Fig. 17.4 Sclerotic AoV disease. (**a**) Sclerotic AoV in PLAX showing echo bright calcification involving the leaflet tips and annulus. (**b**) Sclerosis can be seen here tethering leaflets to both the annulus as well as each other restricting leaflet excursion. (**c**) Doppler image demonstrating flow acceleration through stenotic AoV orifice

carditis can lead to mechanical restriction of leaflet motion, and post-infectious inflammation can lead to leaflet fusion as well.

Identifying and Assessing Severity of Aortic Stenosis

Anatomic Evaluation

Bicuspid valves can be identified by recognizing distinctive echocardiographic features [5]. True bicuspid leaflets attach to the aortic annulus forming a semi-circular leaflet base. The semi-circular base creates tension along the free edge of the valve preventing full excursion giving a classic domed appearance in systole in PLAX (Fig. 17.3a). In PSAX, true bicuspid valves should have a single commissure and two equally sized leaflets. Leaflets may or may not be calcified depending on patient age and presence of other mediators of valvular sclerosis. Leaflet fusion is best described in PSAX (Fig. 17.3b). The fused leaflets will move together generally creating flow acceleration away from the leaflets. The fusion between leaflets commonly appears thickened and hyperechoic due to calcification, sclerosis, or redundant leaflet tissue.

Prosthetic valves may also become stenotic; however, identification of prosthetic valve stenosis is more complex. All prosthetic valves have transvalvular pressure gradients greater than native valves. Normative values are specific to the type and size of the prosthetic valve. Additionally, valve size and patient body surface area must be considered as patient prosthesis mismatch (typically caused by a prosthetic valve too small for the patient) can cause flow acceleration that mimics stenosis but unrelated to leaflet dysfunction.

Supravalvular and subvalvular aortic stenosis are congenital conditions commonly identified at birth or during childhood. Supravalvular stenosis is caused by a narrowing around the level of the sinotubular junction and should be expected when flow acceleration is seen above the level of the valve. Subvalvular stenosis is more common and is caused by a subaortic membrane that grows in the LVOT. There are multiple subtypes of subvalvular stenosis including discrete thin membranes, thick fibromuscular ridge, and fibrous ingrowth creating a tunnel within the LVOT [6].

Lastly, care must always be taken to distinguish AS from flow obstruction either due to cavitary obstruction or systolic anterior motion of the mitral valve. Outflow obstruction is associated with an abrupt loss of doppler signal during systole giving a classic "dagger shape" to continuous wave (CW) doppler while AS usually gives a classic dome with a mid-systolic peak (Fig. 17.5). The doppler pattern is critically evaluated as to not misconstrue out flow obstruction for AS.

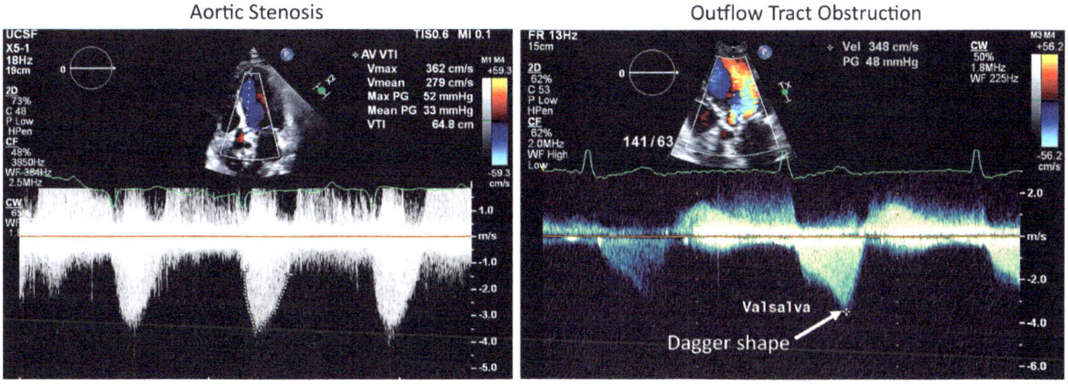

Fig. 17.5 Continuous wave doppler through the AoV. Left pane, showing a doppler pattern for AS. Right pain, showing the dagger pattern created by left ventricular outflow tract obstruction

Hemodynamic Evaluation

There are multiple complimentary approaches to assessing AS severity. The most commonly utilized measurements are the estimated aortic valve area combined with the peak blood flow velocity and mean transvalvular pressure gradient.

1. Estimated Aortic Valve Area (AVA): AVA has been shown to be a highly sensitive and specific estimate of AS, which has also been shown to predictive of outcome [7–9]. AVA can be estimated using the continuity equation (Fig. 17.6a). The continuity equation utilizes the conservation of mass principle, which assumes flow through the LVOT must be equal to flow through the AoV. To estimate SV in the LVOT, the diameter of the LVOT (LVOTd) must be measured in the PLAX in peak systole within 5 mm of aortic cusp insertion (Fig. 17.6b). Measuring inner edge to inner edge in mid-systole is recommended. Using the LVOTd, the cross-sectional area (CSA) of the LVOT can be estimated.

$$CSA_{LVOT} = \pi \left(D/2\right)^2$$

Using pulse wave (PW) doppler in either the 5-chamber (Fig. 17.6c) or 3-chamber view, a LVOT velocity time integral (VTI) must be measured. The PW signal must be measured above the level of the cusps, which can be determined by an absence of high-density doppler signal at the end of systole and diastole. In the same view, a CW doppler of

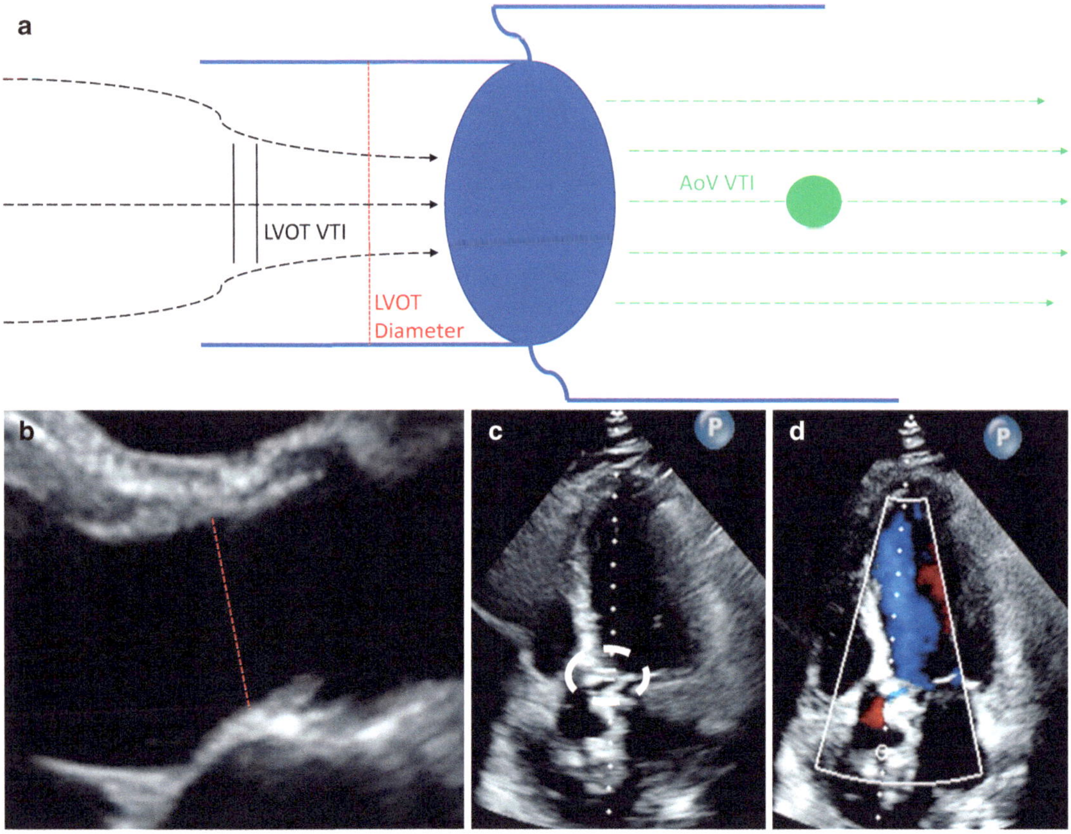

Fig. 17.6 Calculating AVA and gradients. (**a**) Diagram of the continuity equation showing points of measurement to execute the continuity equation solving for AVA. (**b**) AoV in PLAX during peak systole. Red dotted line demonstrates proper sampling for measuring LVOTd using edge-to-edge technique. (**c**) Apical four-chamber view, dotted circle shows proper PW doppler sampling position for measuring LVOT VTI. (**d**) Apical four-chamber view showing proper doppler sampling of the AoV using CW doppler. Peak and mean AoV gradients are estimated using CW doppler

the LVOT, AoV, and aortic root is taken and an aortic VTI measured (Fig. 17.6c). Values are then entered into the continuity equation to solve for AVA

$$VTI_{LVOT} \times CSA_{LVOT} = VTI_{AoV} \times AVA$$

A common pitfall of the AVA estimate is the over- or underestimation of the LVOTd. Given this contributes to continuity equation through a squared value even a small error of 1–2 mm can lead to a significant change in estimated AVA.

2. Peak Velocity and Pressure Gradients: By sampling CW doppler over the AoV, a VTI_{AoV} can be measured and traced to estimate peak velocity, peak gradient, and mean gradient over the Aov. Measurements should be acquired in multiple views to ensure maximal gradients are obtained and that signal from concomitant mitral regurgitation (MR) is not bleeding into the doppler signal. Using a PEDOF probe from the suprasternal notch can help ensure exclusion of MR. Peak and mean gradients measured by echocardiography have been shown to correlate with invasive gradients [7, 9–11]. Peak pressure gradient can be estimated applying the peak velocity in the Bernoulli equation:

$$\text{Pressure gradient} = 4 \times \text{Velocity}^2 \left(\text{m}/\text{s}\right)$$

While peak gradients measured by echocardiography and catheterization correlate, vascular compliance has been shown to significantly influence pressure transmission between the LV and aorta, which makes peak pressures prone to overestimating aortic stenosis [12, 13]. In Fig. 17.7a, the pressure transmission delay between the ventricle and aorta is demonstrated by the green dotted line. This highlights an important limitation in echocardiography. As AS becomes more severe, the delay in pressure transmission between the left ventricle and aorta becomes pronounced. In early systole LV pressure and AoV flow peak while aortic pressure remains low, illustrated in Fig. 17.7 by the red dotted line. This describes why the peak gradient measured by echo is greater than the peak-to-peak gradient reported in catheterization.

Pressure recovery is another important concept that carries particular relevance in the estimation of aortic stenosis in the setting of critical illness. During systole, there is a loss of kinetic energy as blood moves over the leaflet tips of the AoV leading to a drop in pressure immediately above the valve. The pressure rapidly recovers in the ascending aorta. Given spectral doppler only measures the greatest flow over the sampled vector, there is no opportunity to factor in pressure

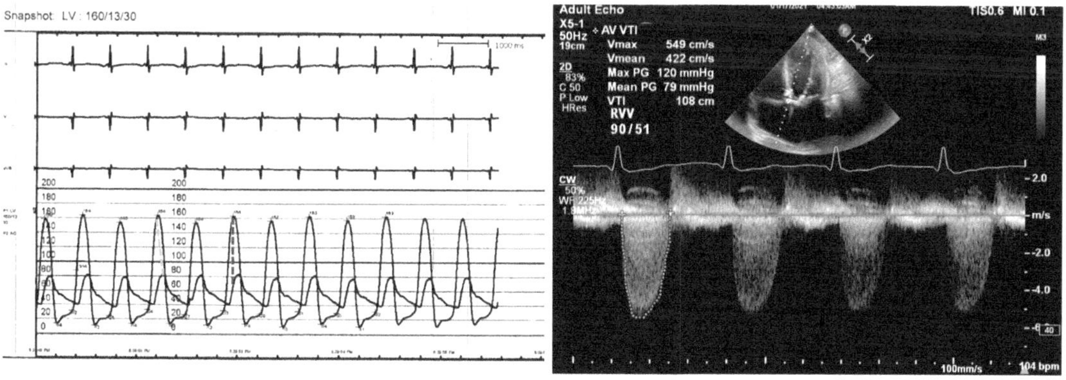

Fig. 17.7 Comparison of AoV gradients sampled by catheterization compared to echocardiography. Both samples recorded from the same patient. Left, simultaneous pressure sampling from the ascending aorta and left ventricle. Green line shows peak-to-peak estimate of peak gradient while red line shows the timing of where peak gradient is estimated by echo emphasizing how peak LV pressure is achieved before peak aortic pressure leading to an overestimation of the peak gradient shown on the right

recovery, leading to an overestimation of the gradient between the LV and true aortic pressure, which is captured on invasive measurements. Pressure recovery is affected by vascular size and tone [14], but is likely only significant when ascending aorta diameter is <30 mm [15].

Mean gradient demonstrates better correlation with invasive gradients across a diversity of hemodynamic states [16]. Mean gradient is calculated by averaging instantaneous gradients throughout the ejection period, which can be performed automatically by most clinical echocardiography software.

Given peak velocity and peak gradient track well and mean gradient is less prone to overestimation of gradient across hemodynamic states, peak velocity and mean gradient are most commonly reported in hemodynamic assessments. AS is considered severe when mean gradients measure ≥40 mmHg and peak velocity is ≥4 m/s.

3. Planimetry: Two-dimensional and three-dimensional planimetry are useful and commonly underutilized tools for assessing AS. Planimetry is the process of measuring the minimum orifice of the AoV (Fig. 17.8a). Transesophageal echocardiography (TEE) is

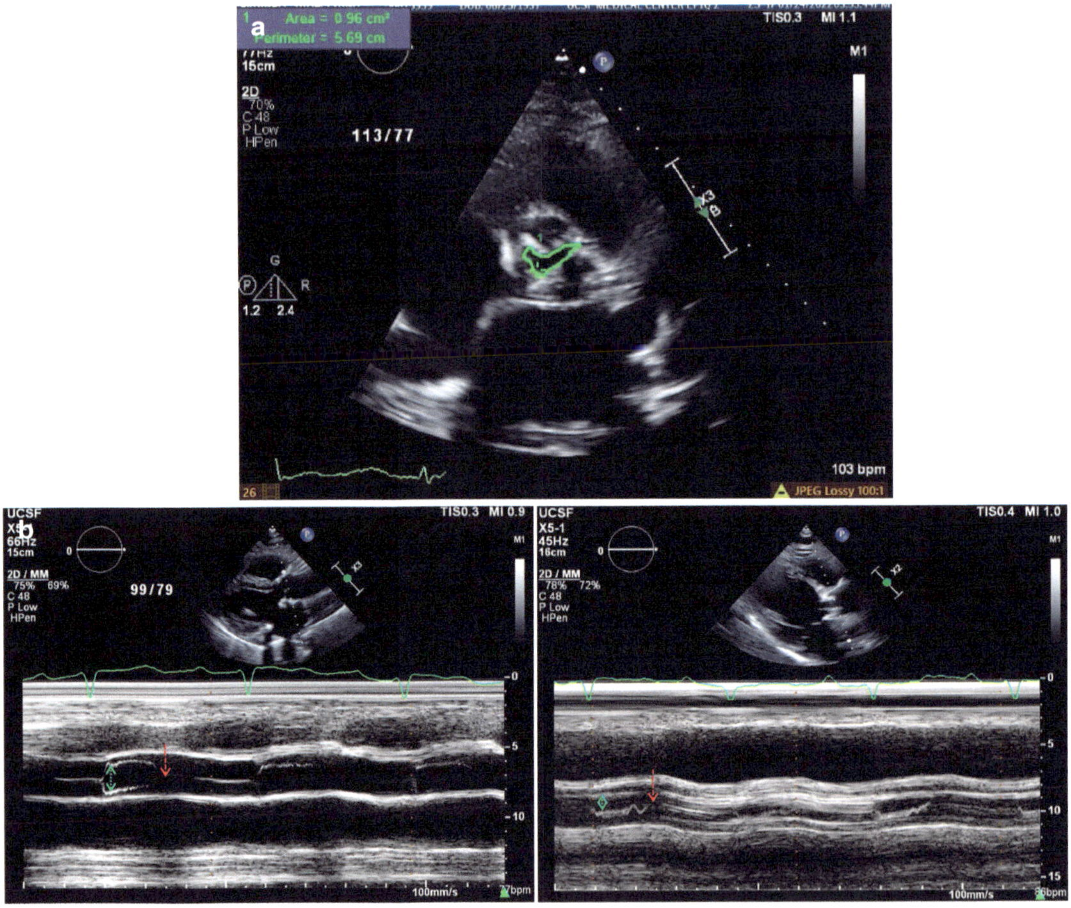

Fig. 17.8 Manual measurement of AVA. (**a**) AoV visualized in peak systole in the mid-esophageal view by TEE. Green dotted line shows proper technique for using planimetry to directly measure AVA. (**b**) M-mode sampling of the AoV in peak systole. Left panel shows sampling of a normal, trileaflet AoV. Right panel shows sampling of a sclerotic AoV with significant stenosis. Green arrows show peak valve opening. Red arrows show valvular closure in early diastole

the gold standard technique given optimal AoV resolution. In the mid-esophageal window, an enface view of the AoV can be obtained at ~45° [17]. The TEE probe can then be withdrawn or advanced to the level of the smallest orifice of the AoV during peak systole. Using TTE, measurements can be made using the PSAX at the level of the aorta, but poor resolution in this view often limits accuracy.

Depending on the etiology of stenosis, sclerosis and calcification can make tracing the orifice of the AoV challenging. Color flow, 3D echocardiography, and X-plane are useful methods for identifying the leaflet tips and orifice.

4. M-mode: M-mode can be useful for estimating valve orifice. In the PLAX, the view of the AoV leaflet tips is optimized. Color flow can help identify the point of peak flow. An M-mode sample is taken with the sample vector set at 90° to the leaflet tips during peak systole. The maximal aortic cusp separation (MACS) can then be measured. Figure 17.8b shows an example of M-mode sampling from a normal trileaflet AoV. Figure 17.8c shows an example of calcific AS with reduced MACS.

   M-mode can support an assessment of AoV composition. As is shown in Fig. 17.8b, calcified leaflets will appear echo bright, and leaflet tips will not contact the aorta in peak systole. MACS can be used as a screening study for AS, but is inadequate in isolate for making the diagnosis. MACS <8 mm has been shown a strong correlation with presence of severe AS [18] (Table 17.1).

Caveats and Pitfalls

Low-flow low-gradient aortic stenosis is a commonly underappreciated hemodynamic state. Evidence is growing showing these patients are prone to poor outcomes and can benefit from structural intervention [19]. Low-flow low-gradient AS is defined as AVA <1 cm^2, peak jet <4.0 m/s, and mean gradient <40 mmHg. These hemodynamic parameters are seen commonly when a patient's SV fall below 35 mL/m^2 [20]. Recognizing that this physiology is dictated by SV is an important lesson as this can be seen in common lesions such as heart failure with preserved (HFpEF), heart failure with reduced ejection fraction (HFrEF), and severe mitral regurgitation.

When interrogating the AoV in a low flow state, understanding the limitations of each calculation is essential. Estimating AVA in a low flow state can be influenced by incomplete valve opening due to a low-pressure differential across to AoV rather than intrinsic valve restriction. This can be induced by either severe cardiomyopathy or malignant hypertension. Optimization of afterload and initiation of dobutamine can increase SV. SV and AVA can be serially measured at increasing levels of inotropic support (Fig. 17.9). In pseudo-severe AS, AVA will increase and gradients will either remain unchanged or marginally increase while in true AS AVA will be unchanged and gradients will increase. The validity of dobutamine stress is best defined in HFrEF. Myocardium in HFpEF is commonly poorly responsive to dobutamine, making an absence of gradient augmentation difficult to interpret. Previously, an absence of response

Table 17.1 Grading of aortic stenosis

	AVA (cm^2)	Mean gradient (mmHg)	Peak jet velocity (m/s)	Dimensionless index	Maximal aortic cusp separation
Normal	3.0–4.0	<5	<2.5	N/A	N/A
Mild AS	>1.5 cm	<20	2.6–2.9	>0.5	N/A
Moderate AS	1.0–≤1.5	20–40	3.0–4.0	0.5–0.25	N/A
Severe AS	≤1.0	≥40	>4	<0.25	<8 mm

Grading of aortic stenosis from normal to severe

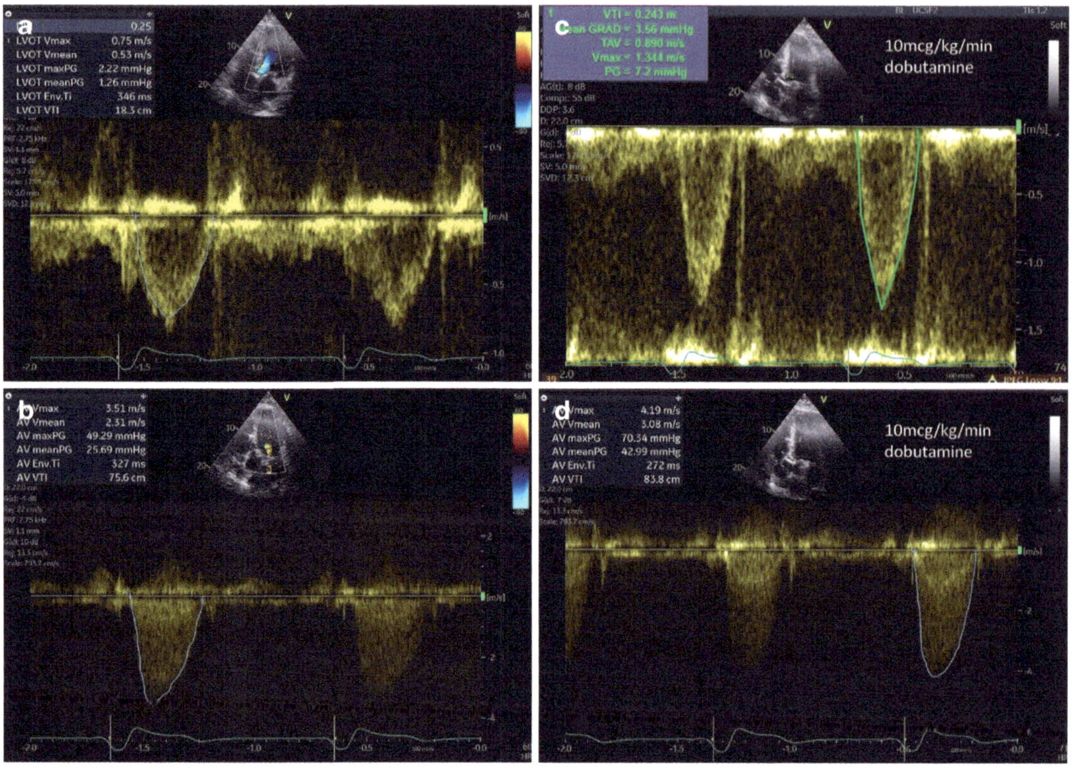

Fig. 17.9 Low-flow low-gradient aortic stenosis. (**a, b**) PW and CW Doppler, respectively, showing low SV leading to estimation of moderate AS based on mean AoV gradient. (**c, d**) PW and CW Doppler sampled after administration of dobutamine leading to a significant increase in SV estimated by LVOT VTI as well as mean gradient diagnosing severe AS

(increase in SV of ≥20%) was felt to carry a poor prognosis, but this opinion has been reconsidered [21]. Evidence now shows that valve intervention in low-flow low-gradient AS is associated with better prognosis [22].

In contrast, when AVA is found to be <1 cm^2 in the setting of a peak velocity < 4.0 m/s, mean gradient is <40 mmHg, and SV is >35 mL/m^2 outcomes appear to be more similar moderate AS [23, 24]. Given this is a rare hemodynamic scenario, measurement accuracy, especially LVOTd, should be confirmed.

Dimensionless index (DI) has emerged as a valuable tool for identifying severe AS in low flow states. Dimensionless index is a simple ratio of the peak velocity in the LVOT measured by PW doppler to the peak velocity across the AoV measured by CW doppler (V_{LVOT}: V_{AoV}). A DI < 0.25 has been shown to predict severe AS and is associated with increased mortality [25].

DI is also valuable for determining patient prosthesis mismatch and stenosis within prosthetic valves in both low and normal flow states. A DI < 0.25 is a good indicator that further screening is necessary.

Valvular calcium assessed by CT scan can be helpful in predicting the likelihood of severe AS. In men and women, a calcium score >3000 and >1600 arbitrary units (AU), respectively, make severe AS very likely while <1600 AU and <800 AU, respectively, make severe AS unlikely [26, 27].

A proposed diagnostic workflow better defining AS in the context of an AVA <1 cm^2 is outlined in Fig. 17.10.

Atrial fibrillation can also pose significant challenges in estimating gradients. Irregular rhythm leads to variable left ventricular filling and SV. Experts recommend averaging five separate measurements and using the average value for calculations [4].

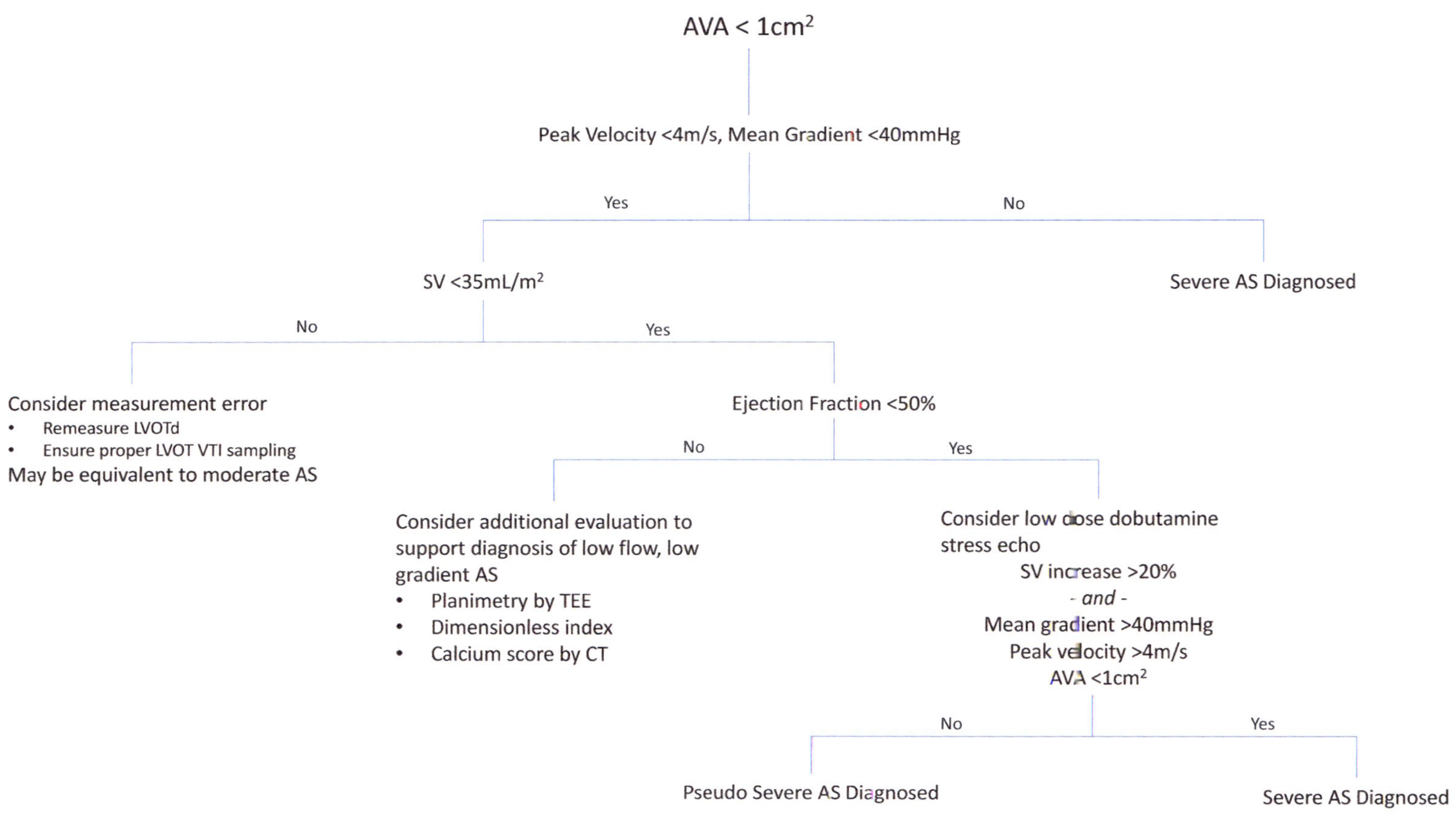

Fig. 17.10 Diagnostic approach to low-flow, low-gradient AS

Aortic regurgitation (AR) increases ventricular loading, but does not affect mean gradient or velocity assessment of AS. It should be noted, however, that moderate or greater AR associated with moderate or greater AS carry high event rates and are commonly treated like isolated severe valve disease [28].

Similarly, high flow states lead to hemodynamics achieving peak velocity > 4 m/s, mean gradient >40 mmHg, and AVA <1 cm^2. States like septic shock, shunts, anemia, and hyperthyroidism should be ruled out. These states should still be considered a state of pressure overload for the left ventricle. As high output state is reversed, aortic gradients should be re-evaluated.

Summary Points

- AS is caused by congenital or acquired leaflet restriction leading to a pressure overload state in the left ventricle.
- Severe AS is defined by an AVA <1 cm^2 combined with a mean AoV gradient >40 mmHg and evidence of flow acceleration over the AoV evidenced by a peak velocity >4 m/s.
- Low-flow, low-gradient AS requires a SV of <35 mL/m^2 and assessment must be tailored to patient physiology.
- DI can be a valuable tool for assessing the presence of severe AS across all hemodynamic states.

Acknowledgments The authors would like to thank Drs. Kirsten Tolstrup and Atif Qasim for contributing images for this chapter.

References

1. Piazza N, de Jaegere P, Schultz C, Becker AE, Serruys PW, Anderson RH. Anatomy of the aortic valvar complex and its implications for transcatheter implantation of the aortic valve. Circ Cardiovasc Interv. 2008;1:74–81.
2. Otto CM, Prendergast B. Aortic-valve stenosis—from patients at risk to severe valve obstruction. N Engl J Med. 2014;371:744–56.
3. Martin PS, Kloesel B, Norris RA, Lindsay M, Milan D, Body SC. Embryonic development of the bicuspid aortic valve. J Cardiovasc Dev Dis. 2015;2:248–72.
4. Baumgartner H, Hung J, Bermejo J, Chambers JB, Edvardsen T, Goldstein S, Lancellotti P, LeFevre M, Miller F, Otto CM. Recommendations on the echocardiographic assessment of aortic valve stenosis: a focused update from the European Association of Cardiovascular Imaging and the American society of Echocardiography. J Am Soc Echocardiogr. 2017;30:372–92.
5. Michelena HI, Della Corte A, Evangelista A, et al. International consensus statement on nomenclature and classification of the congenital bicuspid aortic valve and its aortopathy, for clinical, surgical, interventional and research purposes. J Thorac Cardiovasc Surg. 2021;162:e383–414.
6. Devabhaktuni SR, Chakfeh E, Malik AO, Pengson JA, Rana J, Ahsan CH. Subvalvular aortic stenosis: a review of current literature. Clin Cardiol. 2018;41:131–6.
7. Oh JK, Taliercio CP, Holmes DR, Reeder GS, Bailey KR, Seward JB, Tajik AJ. Prediction of the severity of aortic stenosis by Doppler aortic valve area determination: prospective Doppler-catheterization correlation in 100 patients. J Am Coll Cardiol. 1988;11:1227–34.
8. Rosenhek R, Klaar U, Schemper M, Scholten C, Heger M, Gabriel H, Binder T, Maurer G, Baumgartner H. Mild and moderate aortic stenosis: Natural history and risk stratification by echocardiography. Eur Heart J. 2004;25:199–205.
9. Otto CM, Pearlman AS, Comess KA, Reamer RP, Janko CL, Huntsman LL. Determination of the stenotic aortic valve area in adults using Doppler echocardiography. J Am Coll Cardiol. 1986;7:509–17.
10. Burwash IG, Thomas DD, Sadahiro M, Pearlman AS, Verrier ED, Thomas R, Kraft CD, Otto CM. Dependence of Gorlin formula and continuity equation valve areas on transvalvular volume flow rate in valvular aortic stenosis. Circulation. 1994;89:827–35.
11. Zhang Y, Ihlen H, Nitter-Hauge S. Estimation of the peak-to-peak pressure gradient in aortic stenosis by Doppler echocardiography. Int J Cardiol. 1986;10:197–212.
12. Panidis IP, Mintz GS, Ross J. Value and limitations of Doppler ultrasound in the evaluation of aortic stenosis: a statistical analysis of 70 consecutive patients. Am Heart J. 1986;112:150–8.
13. Kadem L, Garcia D, Durand L, Rieu R, Dumesnil J. Value and limitations of peak-to-peak gradient for evaluation of aortic stenosis. J Heart Valve Dis. 2006;15(5):609–16.
14. Giardini A, Tacy TA. Pressure recovery explains Doppler overestimation of invasive pressure gradient across segmental vascular stenosis. Echocardiography. 2010;27:21–31.
15. Baumgartner H, Stefenelli T, Niederberger J, Schima H, Maurer G. "Overestimation" of catheter gradients by Doppler ultrasound in patients with aortic stenosis: a predictable manifestation of pressure recovery. J Am Coll Cardiol. 1999;33:1655–61.
16. Bermejo J, Odreman R, Feijoo J, Mar Moreno M, Gómez-Moreno P, García-Fernández MA. Clinical efficacy of Doppler-echocardiographic indices of aor-

tic valve stenosis: a comparative test-based analysis of outcome. J Am Coll Cardiol. 2003;41:142–51.
17. Stoddard MF, Hammons RT, Longaker RA. Doppler transesophageal echocardiographic determination of aortic valve area in adults with aortic stenosis. Am Heart J. 1996;132:337–42.
18. Jayaprakash K, Dilu VP, George R. Maximal aortic valve cusp separation and severity of aortic stenosis. J Clin Diagn Res. 2017;11:OC29–32.
19. Taniguchi T, Morimoto T, Shiomi H, et al. High-Versus low-gradient severe aortic stenosis: demographics, clinical outcomes, and effects of the initial aortic valve replacement strategy on long-term prognosis. Circ Cardiovasc Interv. 2017;10:1–10.
20. Adda J, Mielot C, Giorgi R, et al. Low-Flow, low-gradient severe aortic stenosis despite normal ejection fraction is associated with severe left ventricular dysfunction as assessed by speckle-tracking echocardiography a multicenter study. Circ Cardiovasc Imaging. 2012;5:27–35.
21. Annabi MS, Clavel MA, Pibarot P. Dobutamine stress echocardiography in low-flow, low-gradient aortic stenosis: flow reserve does not matter anymore. J Am Heart Assoc. 2019;8(6):e012212. https://doi.org/10.1161/JAHA.119.012212.
22. Sato K, Sankaramangalam K, Kandregula K, et al. Contemporary outcomes in low-gradient aortic stenosis patients who underwent dobutamine stress echocardiography. J Am Heart Assoc. 2019;8(6):e011168. https://doi.org/10.1161/JAHA.118.011168.
23. Eleid MF, Sorajja P, Michelena HI, Malouf JF, Scott CG, Pellikka PA. Flow-gradient patterns in severe aortic stenosis with preserved ejection fraction: clinical characteristics and predictors of survival. Circulation. 2013;128:1781–9.
24. Mehrotra P, Jansen K, Flynn AW, Tan TC, Elmariah S, Picard MH, Hung J. Differential left ventricular remodelling and longitudinal function distinguishes low flow from normal-flow preserved ejection fraction low-gradient severe aortic stenosis. Eur Heart J. 2013;34:1906–14.
25. Altes A, Thellier N, Rusinaru D, et al. Dimensionless index in patients with low-gradient severe aortic stenosis and preserved ejection fraction. Circ Cardiovasc Imaging. 2020;13:E010925.
26. Clavel MA, Messika-Zeitoun D, Pibarot P, et al. The complex nature of discordant severe calcified aortic valve disease grading: new insights from combined Doppler echocardiographic and computed tomographic study. J Am Coll Cardiol. 2013;62:2329–38.
27. Cueff C, Serfaty JM, Cimadevilla C, et al. Measurement of aortic valve calcification using multislice computed tomography: correlation with haemodynamic severity of aortic stenosis and clinical implication for patients with low ejection fraction. Heart. 2011;97:721–6.
28. Zilberszac R, Gabriel H, Schemper M, Zahler D, Czerny M, Maurer G, Rosenhek R. Outcome of combined stenotic and regurgitant aortic valve disease. J Am Coll Cardiol. 2013;61:1489–95.

Aortic and Pulmonic Regurgitation 18

Jacqueline Sohn and Jose L. Diaz-Gomez

Learning Objectives
1. Describe the clinical significance of aortic regurgitation
2. Describe how the echocardiography assessment of aortic regurgitation can help characterize its severity, chronicity, and associated cardiac or aortic pathology
3. Review two-dimensional, color flow (CF), pulse wave (PW), and continuous wave (CW) Doppler techniques for the comprehensive assessment of patients with suspected aortic regurgitation and pulmonic regurgitation

Aortic Regurgitation

The **aortic valve** is a tri-leaflet valve composed of three semilunar cusps. The etiology of **aortic regurgitation (AR)** can be divided into two causes: either processes affecting the valve leaflets (40%) or processes affecting the aortic root (60%) (Table 18.1). AR is classified using the adapted Carpentier classification where type I (A)-(C) is due to aortic root causes, type I (D) is due to aortic cusp perforation, type II is due to cusp prolapse, and type III is due to cusp restriction (Fig. 18.1) [1]. It is also important to differentiate acute versus chronic AR because there are chronological left ventricular (LV) changes noticeable in chronic AR. In severe acute AR, the LV is not dilated, but an early mitral valve (MV) closure may be seen due to the sudden increase in LV end-diastolic pressure [2]. This can be visualized by assessing MV in M-mode. In chronic AR, LV is dilated with eccentric hypertrophy and periodic TTE helps to monitor worsening LV function and size.

AR can be quantified using various measurements. This chapter will include the Doppler findings, vena contracta (VC), jet width and area, the density of regurgitant jet, pressure half-time, and flow reversal in the aorta. An initial practical diagnostic approach is to recognize the anatomic basis for the presence of AR with 2D echocardiography, which includes bicuspid aortic valve (Fig. 18.2), incomplete closure of aortic valve cusps (>2 mm), aortic valve vegetation, or ascending aortic aneurysm. A summary of the echocardiographic criteria

Supplementary Information The online version contains supplementary material available at https://doi.org/10.1007/978-3-031-80038-2_18.

J. Sohn
Department of Anesthesiology and Critical Care Medicine, Texas Heart Institute at Baylor St. Luke's Medical Center, Houston, TX, USA
e-mail: Jacqueline.Sohn@bcm.edu

J. L. Diaz-Gomez (✉)
Department of Anesthesiology and Critical Care Medicine, Baylor College of Medicine, Texas Heart Institute at Baylor St. Luke's Medical Center, Houston, TX, USA
e-mail: Jose.Diaz-Gomez@bcm.edu

M. J. Lanspa, A. T. Levinson (eds.), *Echocardiography and Ultrasonography in the ICU*, Respiratory Medicine, https://doi.org/10.1007/978-3-031-80038-2_18

Table 18.1 Etiologies of aortic regurgitation (modified from Zoghbi et al.)

	Congenital	Acquired
Leaflet (type II)	Bicuspid, unicuspid, quadricuspid	Calcification, infective endocarditis, rheumatic disease, radiation-induced
	Ventricular septal defect	
Aortic root (type I)	Annuloaortic ectasia	Idiopathic, systemic hypertension, autoimmune diseases, aortitis (syphilitic, Takayasu's arteritis), aortic dissection, trauma
	Connective tissue diseases	

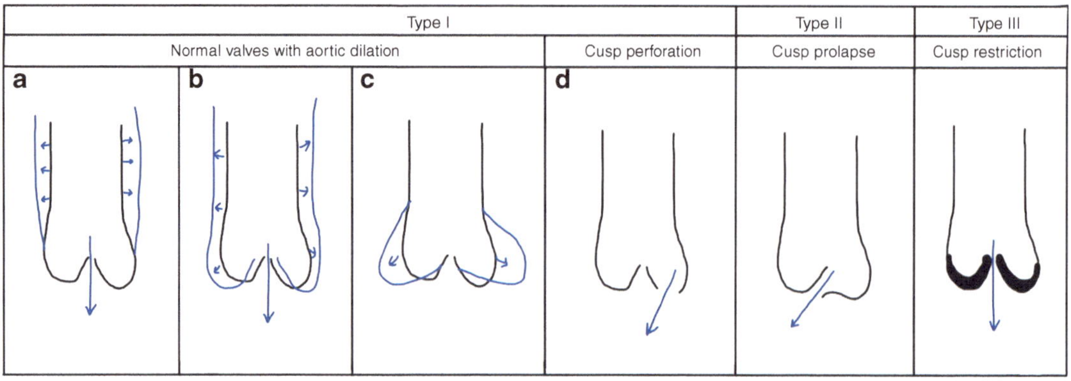

Fig. 18.1 The adaptation of the Carpentier classification for aortic regurgitation (AR). (Figure courtesy of Jacqueline Sohn, DO, Department of Anesthesiology and Critical Care at Baylor St. Luke's Medical Center—Texas Heart Institute. Permission to use obtained)

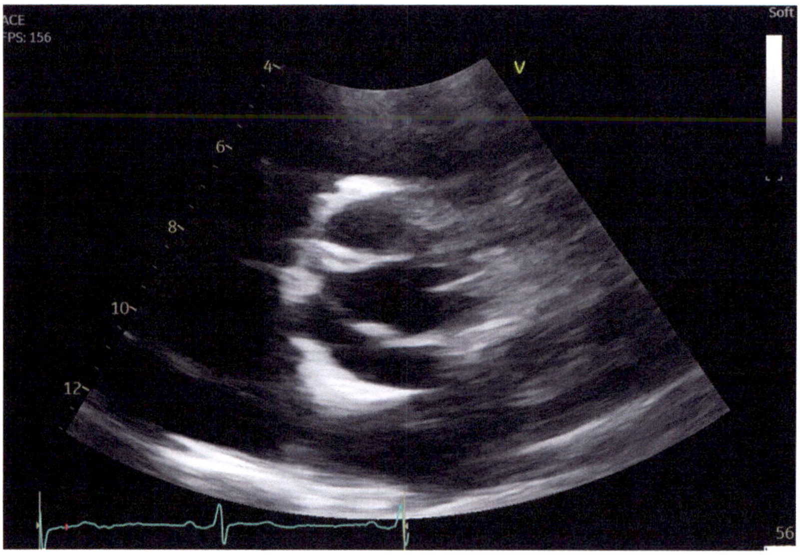

Fig. 18.2 2D-TTE image of bicuspid aortic valve. The bicuspid aortic valve must be assessed in parasternal short-axis view during systole because it may appear tricuspid when closed during diastole. The characteristic appearance of oval-shaped valve opening can be seen during systole in bicuspid aortic valve. (Figure courtesy of Department of Anesthesiology and Critical Care at Baylor St. Luke's Medical Center—Texas Heart Institute. Permission to use obtained)

Table 18.2 Summary of the echocardiographic criteria for a severe aortic regurgitation (AR) [2, 3]

Vena Contracta > 0.6 cm
Jet width/LVOT width ≥ 65%
Jet area/LVOT area ≥ 60%
Regurgitant volume ≥ 60 mL
Regurgitant fraction ≥ 50%
EROA ≥ 0.3 cm^2
Pressure half-time < 200 ms
Holodiastolic flow reversal in the abdominal aorta
Holodiastolic flow reversal in descending thoracic aorta
Abnormal or flail or wide coaptation defect
Dense regurgitant jet on CW Doppler

for a severe AR can be found at the end of the section (Table 18.2).

Doppler Findings

Doppler findings are essential in the evaluation of AR. For the evaluation of AR, color flow Doppler (CFD), pulsed wave (PW), and continuous wave (CW) Doppler are used. The PW Doppler can be used to assess the regurgitant flow in the aorta and CFD can be used to assess the signal density and the pressure half-time, which all will be discussed later in the chapter. In addition, PW Doppler can be helpful to determine increased left ventricular outflow tract (LVOT) velocity (>1.5 m/s) and velocity-time integral (>40 cm), which indicate significant AR. Furthermore, PW Doppler can determine shortened deceleration of the mitral inflow (<140 ms), increased E/A ratio, and diastolic mitral regurgitation in severe AR. In this section, we will discuss the use of the CFD.

The AR is seen in diastole with the CFD originating from the aortic valve. It is evaluated in all three views apical, parasternal long, and short axis with the apical view being the most sensitive for detection of AR (Fig. 18.3/Video 18.1) [2]. However, *the parasternal views are preferred due to the better axial resolution* [1]. There are three components to the color jet: flow convergence, VC, and jet area. The jet length of AR is not a reliable parameter because it is variable depending on the diastolic blood pressure. The AR jet usually lasts throughout diastole, but it can be brief and lower in velocity in acute AR.

Vena Contracta (VC)

Vena Contracta (VC) is defined as the narrowest portion of the regurgitant jet measured from the regurgitant orifice [1]. For AR, VC is measured in the *parasternal long-axis zoomed-in view* and measured where it is perpendicular to the color flow to obtain the most accurate VC measurement. Furthermore, to properly identify the VC, the plane should show all three components of the regurgitant jet: **flow convergence, VC, and jet area** (Fig. 18.4). The temporal and lateral resolution is also maximized by reducing the color sector size and imaging depth as narrow as possible. If the VC is measured less than 3 mm, then it is considered mild, and if it is greater than 6 mm, then it is considered severe [2]. *For intermediate values (3–6 mm), more quantitative methods are recommended.* The VC is relatively independent of flow rate and driving pressure, but it is limited by the lateral resolution of color Doppler, dynamic orifice, multiple jets, bicuspid valve, and non-circular orifice [1, 2].

Note The VC may be used in eccentric jets, and it is less dependent on technical factors.

Jet Width/Area

The **jet width** is used to assess the severity of AR. The ratio of the color jet diameter in the LVOT and the diameter of the LVOT is calculated using the parasternal long-axis view and ideally zoomed to the aortic valve. The LVOT diameter and the jet width within 1 cm of the vena contracta are measured (Fig. 18.5). *If the ratio is ≤25%, it is considered a mild AR, and if the ratio is ≥65%, then it is considered a severe AR.* Although this is an easy and fast measurement to quantify AR, it can underestimate AR in eccentric jets and overestimate it in central jets. It is also affected by the size and the measurement of the LVOT [2].

The **jet area** can be also used similarly to the jet width. The ratio of the jet area and the LVOT area can be used to assess the severity of AR. Both variables are obtained using the short-axis aortic

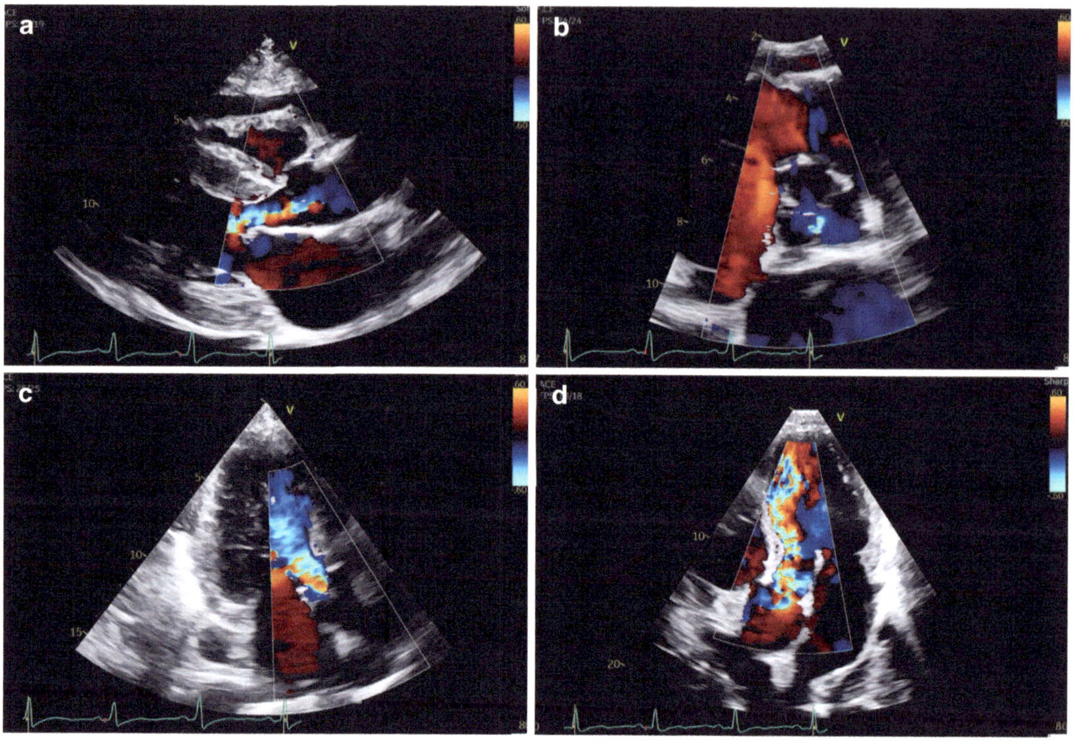

Fig. 18.3 (Video 18.1) Assessment of Aortic regurgitation in various TTE views. (**a**) Parasternal long-axis view, (**b**) parasternal short-axis view, (**c**) apical three-chamber view, (**d**) apical five-chamber view. (Figure courtesy of Department of Anesthesiology and Critical Care at Baylor St. Luke's Medical Center—Texas Heart Institute. Permission to use obtained)

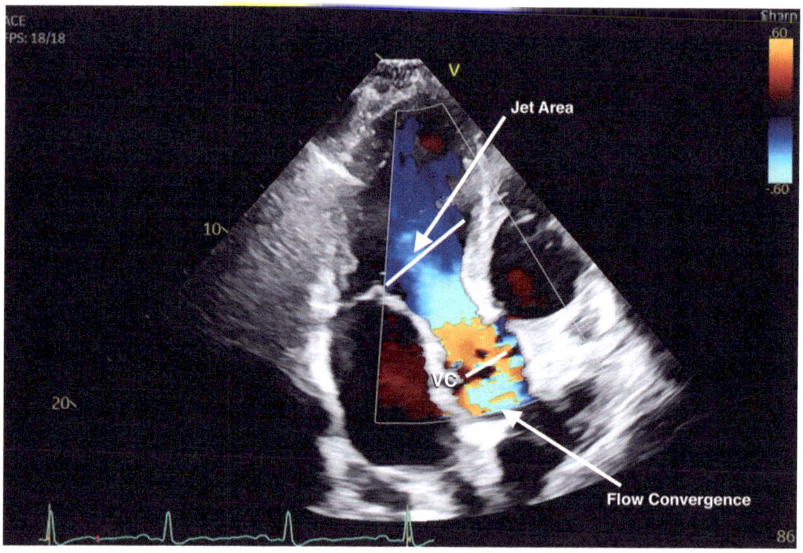

Fig. 18.4 An example of jet area, vena contracta (VC), and flow convergence. This can be also obtained in parasternal long-axis view. (Figure courtesy of Department of Anesthesiology and Critical Care at Baylor St. Luke's Medical Center—Texas Heart Institute. Permission to use obtained)

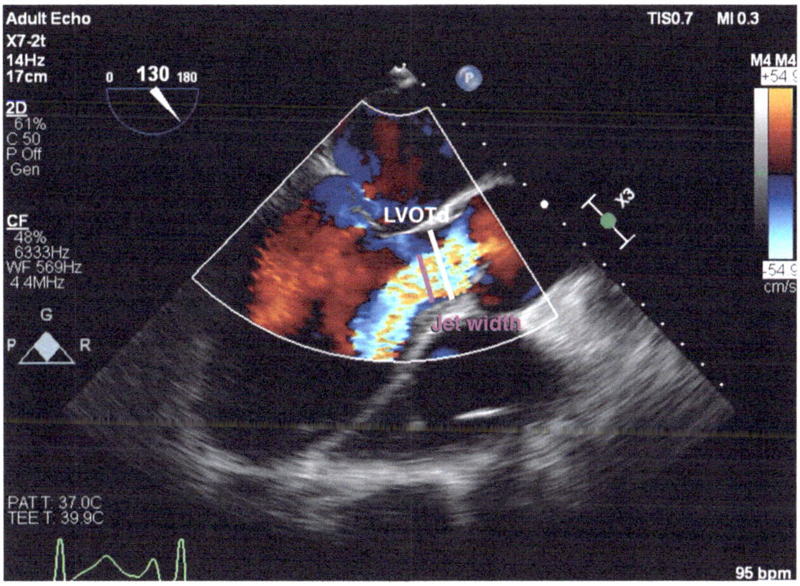

Fig. 18.5 Measurement of LVOT diameter (LVOTd) and aortic regurgitation jet width (pink) in TEE mid-esophageal long-axis view. This can also be measured in TTE parasternal long axis and apical three-chamber view. (Figure courtesy of Department of Anesthesiology and Critical Care at Baylor St. Luke's Medical Center—Texas Heart Institute. Permission to use obtained)

view and zoomed to the aortic valve. Trace the area of the aortic valve and the jet area at the narrowest point (Fig. 18.6). If the ratio is <5%, then it is considered a mild AR, and if the ratio is ≥60%, then it is considered severe. The pitfall of using jet area and LVOT area for quantifying AR is that the direction and shape of the AR jet can overestimate or underestimate the actual jet area since it is a 2D image of a 3-D structure [2].

Note The jet width may underestimate or overestimate AR in eccentric and central jets, respectively. The direction of the jet may overestimate or underestimate the jet area.

Proximal Flow Convergence

The proximal flow convergence can be obtained in both apical five-chamber and parasternal long-axis views. The aortic valve is zoomed into the view and the Nyquist limit baseline is adjusted in the direction of flow to make a better hemisphere view (Fig. 18.7) [2]. Proximal isovelocity surface area (PISA) represents the aliasing region surface area. Using the continuity equation, it is assumed that the flow through the aliasing region, PISA shell, is equal to the flow through the orifice area.

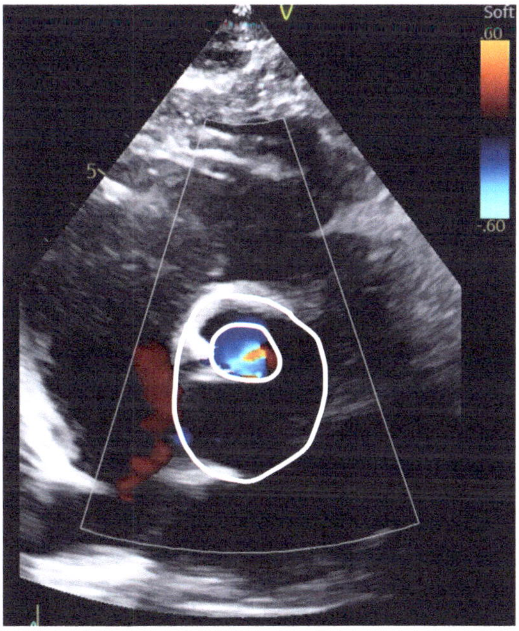

Fig. 18.6 The parasternal short-axis aortic view is obtained and trace the area of the aortic valve and the jet area at the narrowest point to measure the jet area. (Figure courtesy of Department of Anesthesiology and Critical Care at Baylor St. Luke's Medical Center—Texas Heart Institute. Permission to use obtained)

It is a rapid qualitative assessment of the aortic regurgitant jet and is used for estimated regurgitant orifice area (EROA) calculation.

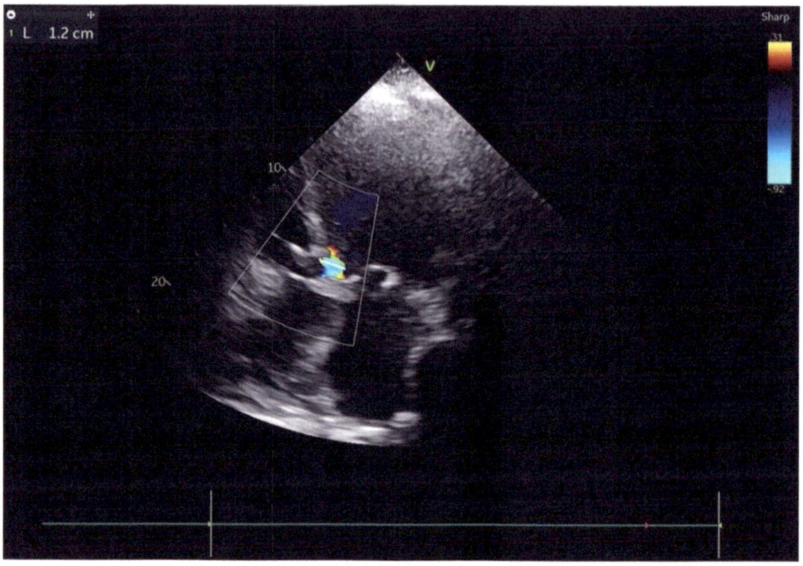

Fig. 18.7 The Proximal isovelocity surface area (PISA) can be obtained in both apical five-chamber and parasternal long-axis views. The Nyquist limit must be adjusted to obtain the hemisphere view. (Figure courtesy of Department of Anesthesiology and Critical Care at Baylor St. Luke's Medical Center—Texas Heart Institute. Permission to use obtained)

Note The proximal flow convergence is limited if non-hemispheric shape.

Regurgitant Orifice Area by PISA

Using the proximal flow convergence method, the regurgitant flow rate is calculated using the PISA radius and Nyquist limit. The equation for the regurgitant flow rate at the PISA ring is $2\pi r^2 Vn$, where the r is the PISA radius and V_n is the Nyquist limit. Then, using the continuity equation, the EROA can be calculated.

$$2\pi r^2 V_n = \text{EROA} \times V_{max} \,(\text{at the orifice})$$

$$\text{EROA}\left(\text{cm}^2\right) = \frac{2\pi r^2 V_n}{V_{max}}$$

The peak AR velocity (cm/s) is obtained using CW Doppler at the AV on the apical five-chamber view. The regurgitant orifice area (ROA, cm^2) less than 0.1 cm^2 is considered mild AR, and greater than or equal to 0.3 cm^2 is considered severe AR.

Note Small errors in the radius measurement can result in substantial errors in EROA

The *regurgitant volume* can be also calculated using the stroke volume method. EROA can be multiplied by VTI to calculate the regurgitant volume. The VTI is obtained using CW Doppler of the regurgitant jet (Fig. 18.10). Mild AR is considered regurgitant volume less than 30 mL and severe AR is considered as regurgitant volume greater than or equal to 60 mL. Another way to calculate regurgitant volume is to subtract volume across the mitral valve from the volume across the LVOT assuming that there is no mitral regurgitation.

$$\text{LVOT stroke volume} = \text{LVOT area} \times \text{LVOT VTI}$$

$$\text{MV stroke volume} = \text{MV area} \times \text{MV VTI}\left(\text{at annulus}\right)$$

$$\text{Regurgitant volume} = \text{LVOT volume} - \text{MV volume}$$

Note Requires appropriate training—accurate measurement of the mitral annulus can be challenging; if there is concomitant MR, the pulmonic stroke volume (using the right ventricle outflow tract diameter and PR VTI) is used for forward stroke volume.

Lastly, the *regurgitant fraction (RF)* is another quantitative parameter that can be calculated using the regurgitant volume. RF less than 30% is

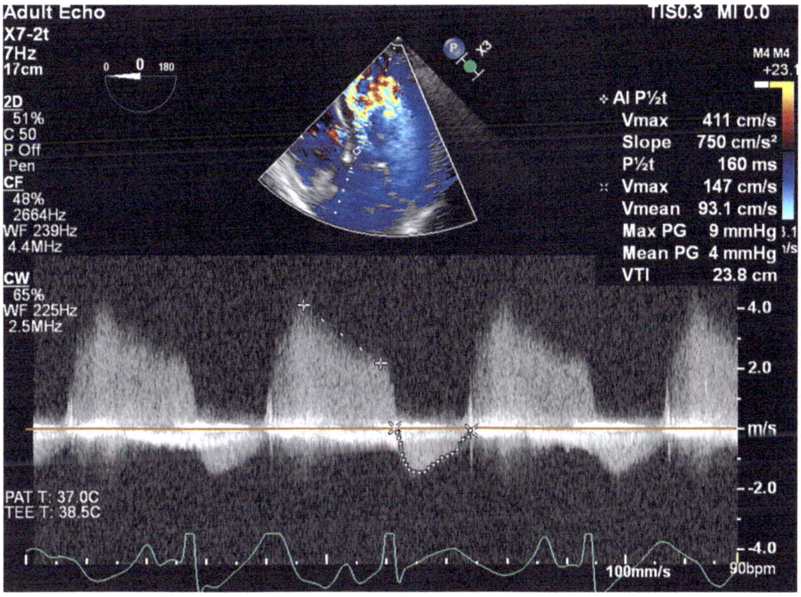

Fig. 18.8 Aortic regurgitation (AR) viewed using continuous wave (CW) Doppler. The density of the CW Doppler signal correlates with the AR volume. It suggests severe AR, if the density of the regurgitant flow is similar to the antegrade flow as shown in the figure. (Figure courtesy of Department of Anesthesiology and Critical Care at Baylor St. Luke's Medical Center—Texas Heart Institute. Permission to use obtained)

considered mild, and RF greater than or equal to 50% is considered severe AR.

$$RF(\%) = \frac{\text{Regurgitant Volume}}{\text{LVOT Stroke Volume}} * 100$$

The Density of Regurgitant Jet

A qualitative assessment of the AR jet can be performed using CFD. The CFD can be imaged in various standard views including apical five-chamber (A5CH), apical three-chamber (A3CH) or apical long-axis, and parasternal long-axis view (Fig. 18.3/Video 18.1). The signal intensity correlates to the number of red blood cells contributing to the regurgitant flow [2, 3]. The denser the CW Doppler signal, the greater the AR volume. If the density of the regurgitant flow is similar to the antegrade flow, this suggests severe AR (Fig. 18.8).

Pressure Half-Time (PHT)

Another semi-quantitative method to assess AR jet is the measurement of the jet deceleration rate or pressure half-time (PHT). It is measured using the CW Doppler at the apical window. Eccentric jet can be also measured from the parasternal window [2]. There should be a complete spectral envelop to measure the PHT. PHT is the time it takes for the peak pressure to drop to half of its value [3] (Fig. 18.9). It is a sign of pressure relation between the aorta and the left ventricle. The PHT is more accurate in acute AR than chronic AR because LV remodeling and change in diastolic pressure will affect the pressure half-time and will not reliably reflect the severity of AR. As the severity of AR increases, the aortic diastolic pressure decreases, and the LV end-diastolic pressure increases. Thus, in acute AR where the remodeling has not occurred yet, the late diastolic jet velocity is reduced and the PHT is shortened.

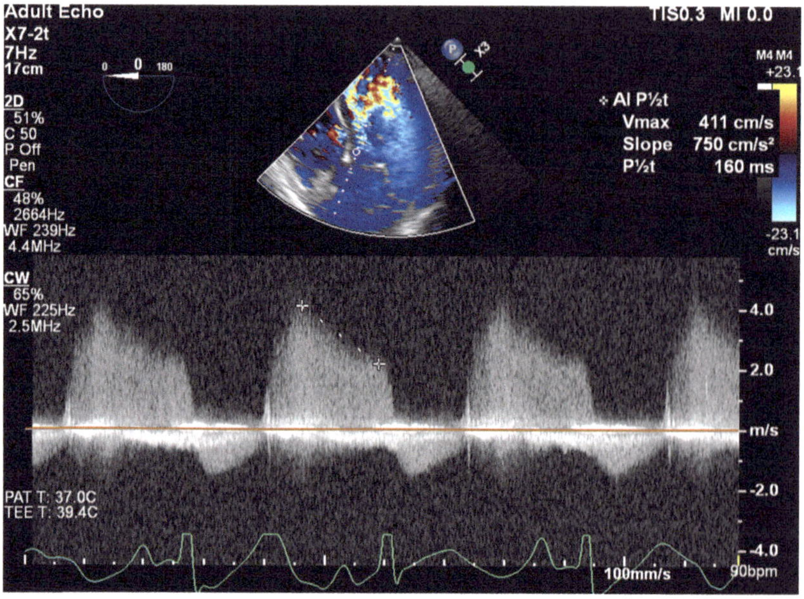

Fig. 18.9 Pressure half-time (PHT) measured using the CW Doppler. If PHT < 200 ms, it suggests severe AR. (Figure courtesy of Department of Anesthesiology and Critical Care at Baylor St. Luke's Medical Center—Texas Heart Institute. Permission to use obtained)

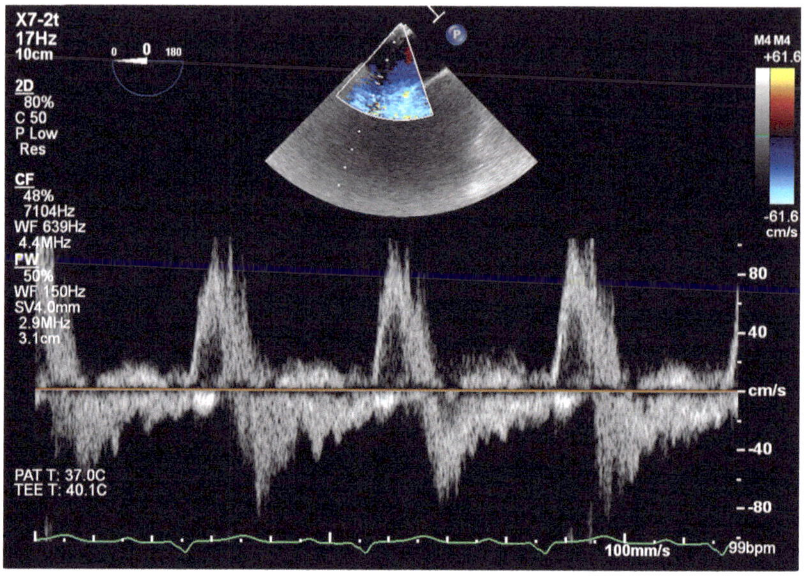

Fig. 18.10 Holodiastolic reversal seen in the descending aorta suggesting severe AR. (Figure courtesy of Department of Anesthesiology and Critical Care at Baylor St. Luke's Medical Center—Texas Heart Institute. Permission to use obtained)

On the other hand, chronic LV adaptation to AR will normalize the PHT [1, 3]. *PHT greater than 500 ms is considered mild AR and less than 200 ms meets the criteria for severe AR* [3].

Flow Reversal in the Aorta

Recognition of Holodiastolic flow reversal with PW in the descending aorta (an initial velocity > 0.6 m/s, VTI > 15 cm, and end-diastolic velocity > 20 cm/s) and abdominal aorta indicate severe AR [2, 3]. The abdominal aorta can be visualized in the subcostal view and the holodiastolic flow reversal in the abdominal aorta has 100% sensitivity and 97% specificity [3] (Fig. 18.10). The aortic arch can be visualized in the suprasternal view and although not as sensitive and specific as the abdominal aorta, holodiastolic flow reversal in the descending aorta suggests severe AR. Both color Doppler and PW Doppler can be used to assess the holodiastolic

Table 18.3 Other conditions that can cause holodiastolic flow reversal in the absence of AR [2]

A left-to-right shunt across a patent ductus arteriosus
Reduced compliance of the aorta in the elderly
An upper extremity arteriovenous fistula
A ruptured sinus of Valsalva
Aortic dissection with the diastolic flow into the false lumen

Table 18.4 TTE and TEE views for an integrated multiparametric assessment ensuring a comprehensive approach to PR

Anatomic structure of interest	TTE view	TEE view
Pulmonic valve/RVOT	Parasternal long-axis view	Mid-esophageal RV inflow-outflow view
		Upper esophageal aortic arch short-axis view
Pulmonic valve/RVOT inflow-outflow	Parasternal short-axis view	Trans-gastric RVOT and pulmonary artery views
	Subcostal view—short axis	

flow reversal. This has to be assessed with caution, however, because other etiologies can cause holodiastolic flow reversal in the absence of AR (Table 18.3). Furthermore, in an acute severe AR or bradycardia, there may be a flow reversal that is NOT holodiastolic due to the pressure equalization in the aorta and the LV before the end diastole [2].

Note The holodiastolic flow reversal in proximal descending aorta is less reliable in older patients given their lower aortic compliance. Also, it may be seen in other conditions—cerebral arteriovenous fistula, upper extremity dialysis fistula, ruptured sinus of Valsalva aneurysm, and congenital heart disease (patent ductus arteriosus) without severe AR.

Pulmonary Regurgitation

Initial echocardiographic assessment of pulmonary regurgitation (PR) should include information on cusp morphology anomalies (i.e., bicuspid or quadricuspid valves, hypoplasia, or even absence of pulmonary valve) and motion (doming or prolapse) with the utilization of transthoracic echocardiography. Moreover, transesophageal echocardiography (TEE) usually is performed when additional structural and functional details is needed (Table 18.4).

Trace to mild PR is a common finding reported in about 75% of the population. The **pulmonary valve (PV)** is a semilunar valve with three cusps that are thinner than the aortic valve cusps. Primary PR is commonly due to congenital disease or after balloon valvuloplasty for pulmonic stenosis. Acquired PR is rare but can be seen in patients with rheumatic heart disease, endocarditis, carcinoid valve disease, or pergolide-induced disease [2]. Secondary PR is seen in patients with elevated pulmonary artery (PA) pressure with dilated pulmonary artery and normal structured PV [1, 2]. Chronic severe PR can lead to right ventricle (RV) dilation and dysfunction. Primary PR can lead to RV dysfunction similar to the volume overload pattern of the septum [2]. However, there are many other etiologies for RV dilation and dysfunction, and therefore, it is not a specific sign of severe PR. Dilation may be localized to the RV outflow tract (RVOT), which can be seen in the Tetralogy of Fallot (TOF) repair. A summary of the echocardiographic criteria for a severe PR can be found at the end of the section (Table 18.5).

Table 18.5 Summary of the echocardiographic criteria for a severe pulmonary regurgitation (PR)

VCW/pulmonary artery annulus > 0.7
Color jet width occupies > 65% of the RVOT
Regurgitant volume ≥ 115 mL
Regurgitant fraction ≥ 40%
EROA ≥ 115 mm^2
Pressure half-time < 100 ms
PR index < 0.77
Dense regurgitant jet on CW Doppler

Note Despite the utilization same echocardiographic assessment techniques for other valvular heart disease, the specific PR severity criteria are less validated due to the limited number of patients studied with significant pulmonary regurgitation [1]. Only two pulmonic valve cusps can be visualized simultaneously unless a biplane (X-plane) modality is used.

Color Flow Doppler Findings: Jet Width, Jet Area, Jet Length, Vena Contracta

There is a paucity of validation studies for quantifying PR possibly due to difficulty visualizing PR. However, many of the qualitative and quantitative measuring methods for AR can be applied to PR. PR can be visualized using the color flow Doppler (CFD) with a diastolic jet toward the RV in the parasternal short-axis or the subcostal short-axis view (Fig. 18.11). If the color jet width occupies >65% of the RVOT, then it suggests severe PR. Furthermore, a holodiastolic jet in the main pulmonary artery and its branches, or a jet with wide origin, and longer (>10 mm), indicates pathologic PR [4].

VC is the most widely used semi-qualitative assessment of PR, but the data lack validation. It is measured in parasternal short axis or subcostal views by visualizing the flow convergence. The narrowest portion on the jet is measured in diastole immediately below the PV. Vena Contracta Width (VCW) and PV annular diameter ratio is another quantitative measurement for PR severity. However, it can underestimate PR in eccentric jets and overestimate in central jets. The ratio > 0.7 is considered a severe PR. Vena contracta relies on an assumption of a circular/elliptical regurgitant flow and only the TEE modality can modestly increase the reliability of PR estimation in those cases without circular/elliptical regurgitant flow.

Note Adequate evaluation of PR with CFD should include increasing frame rate, reducing the color sector size and image depth, and optimizing of color/gain scale including a Nyquist limit of 60 s/min. Of note, estimation of PR severity only based on CFD can be misleading because it is the pressure gradient between the PA and the RV, which determines the PR jet. Thus, whenever equalization between diastolic pulmonary and RV pressures occurs rapidly, the color jet can be brief and PR will be underestimated [5].

Pulse Wave Doppler: Regurgitant Volume, Regurgitant Fraction, Reverse Flow in Pulmonary Artery (PA)

The EROA can also be calculated using the same method as the AR. The EROA less than 20 mm^2 is considered mild, and greater than 115 mm^2 is considered severe PR. The regurgitant volume for PV can be calculated by multiplying the 3D measured VC with the VTI of the PR jet [1]. The regurgitant volume less than 15 mL is considered mild PR and greater than 115 mL is considered severe PR [2]. The peak velocity and VTI across the RVOT increase with moderate-to-severe PR. Indeed, the pulmonic systolic flow is significantly increased compared to the systemic flow. Another way to measure the regurgitant volume is to calculate the stroke volumes of RVOT and

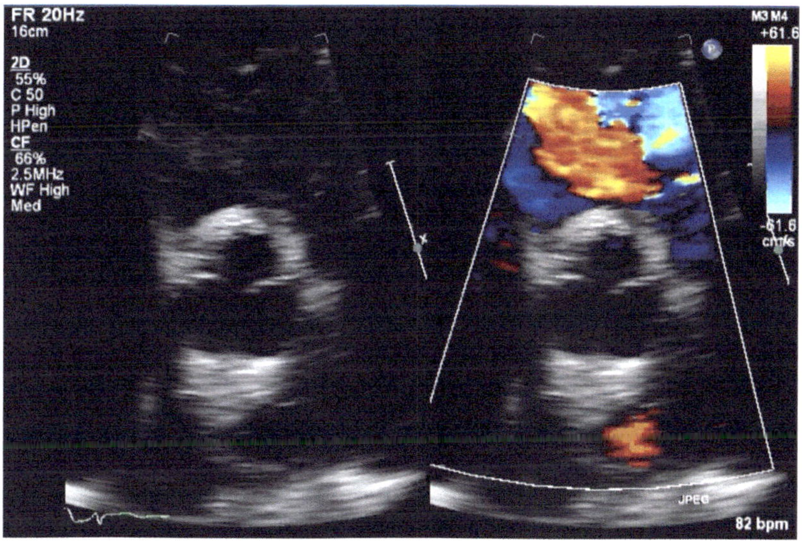

Fig. 18.11 Color flow Doppler (CFD) of severe pulmonary regurgitation (PR). (Figure courtesy of Department of Anesthesiology and Critical Care at Baylor St. Luke's Medical Center—Texas Heart Institute. Permission to use obtained)

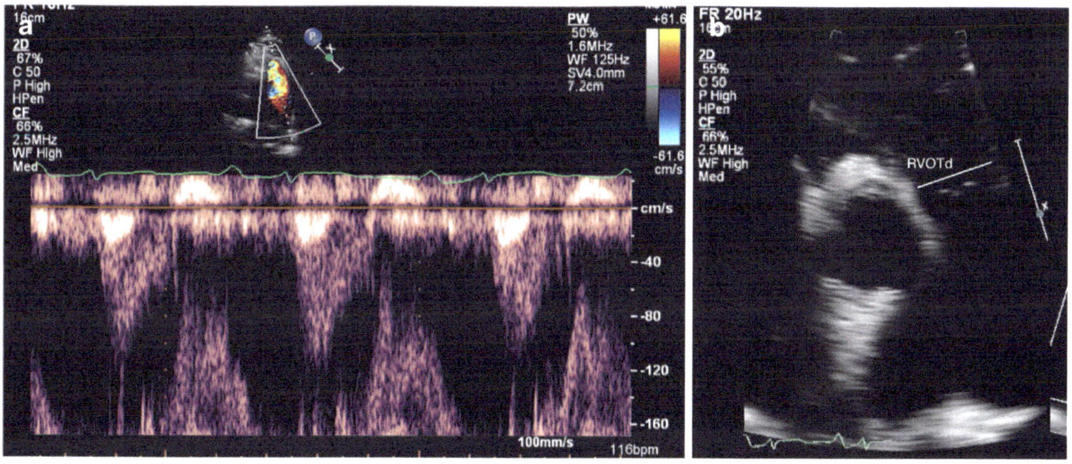

Fig. 18.12 (**a**) Pulse wave (PW) Doppler of the RVOT. (**b**) RVOT diameter measured from the parasternal short axis aortic view focused on the pulmonary valve. (Figure courtesy of Department of Anesthesiology and Critical Care at Baylor St. Luke's Medical Center—Texas Heart Institute. Permission to use obtained)

LVOT and subtract them [2] (Fig. 18.12). The RVOT diameter can be measured in the parasternal short-axis inflow-outflow view and the pulse wave Doppler at the RVOT will provide VTI measurement. This method is challenging due to the difficulties of obtaining an adequate view and measuring the RVOT diameter [2].

$$\text{RVOT stroke volume} = \text{RVOT area} \times \text{RVOT VTI}$$

The RF can also be calculated using the regurgitant volume and the RVOT stroke volume. *The RF less than 20% is mild PR and greater than 40% is considered a severe PR* [2]. Unfortunately, the cut-off values for regurgitant volume and RF are not well validated.

Continuous Wave Doppler: Jet Density, Pressure Half-Time, PR Index

Similar to the AR, the **density of the PR jet** is proportional to the number of red blood cells through the PV. This can be evaluated with CW

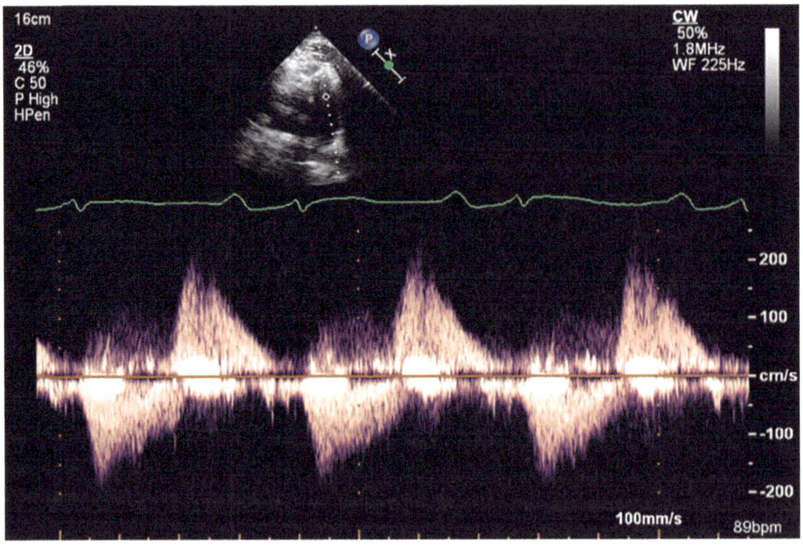

Fig. 18.13 Continuous wave (CW) Doppler of the pulmonary valve showing severe PR. Note the density of the regurgitant flow and the equalization of both inflow and outflow Doppler, which is very classic for severe PR. (Figure courtesy of Department of Anesthesiology and Critical Care at Baylor St. Luke's Medical Center—Texas Heart Institute. Permission to use obtained)

Doppler in the parasternal short-axis view and the subcostal short-axis view (Fig. 18.13). Shortened deceleration rate can be measured with the **PHT** can also be calculated using the CW Doppler and <100 ms is considered accurate (high sensitivity and specificity) for severe PR [2]. Severe PR can be suspected if there is cessation of flow before end diastole. One of the limitations of this measurement is the poor visualization and alignment of Doppler. Furthermore, RV and PA pressure differences especially due to the RV diastolic dysfunction can affect the PHT.

Lastly, the **PR index** can be calculated using the CW Doppler and it has a high diagnostic accuracy. This needs complete forward and regurgitant flow on CW Doppler, which can be challenging to obtain depending on the available window. However, this is a more advantageous measurement since it uses both PR duration and duration of diastole and accounts for the pressure differences between PA and RV [2] The disadvantage is that it does not distinguish between moderate and severe PR. The PR index less than 0.77 is considered moderate-to-severe PR [2].

$$\text{PR Index} = A / B$$

Note The main factors to determine PR severity include the size of the regurgitant orifice, the hydraulic impedance/afterload, and the right ventricular diastolic compliance, and the right ventricular diastolic filling time. Indeed, the degree of regurgitant volume depends proportionally upon the RV size and stroke volume [5]. Thus, the evaluation of RV systolic and diastolic function should be included in the PR assessment.

Key Points

- Chronic aortic regurgitation is more prevalent in older male patients, but rarely is the admission diagnosis to the intensive care unit.
- Acute aortic regurgitation is life-threatening and caused by systemic or specific structural valve disease that requires urgent surgical intervention.
- Pulmonary regurgitation is more recognized following surgical repair of congenital heart disease.
- A methodic echocardiographic approach to aortic and pulmonary regurgitations includes initial two-dimensional assessment (i.e., lack of leaflets coaptation, recognition of mobile masses) followed by CFD (regurgitant flow in diastole), PWD, and CWD to determine quantitation of regurgitant volume.

Questions

1. Which of the following echocardiographic findings is consistent with severe acute aortic regurgitation:
   A. Globular, spherical shape of the left ventricle
   B. Fluttering of the anterior mitral leaflet
   C. Late opening of the aortic valve
   D. Left atrial dilation
   E. Eccentric left ventricular hypertrophy

   Answer: B. Although fluttering of the anterior mitral leaflet has a sensitivity of 41%, yet its specificity is up to 81%, especially in grade 3 to 4+ AR. The positive predictive value is 92%. The following echocardiography findings (globular, spherical shape of the left ventricle, eccentric left ventricular hypertrophy, left atrial dilation) are findings commonly seen in chronic aortic regurgitation. Early rather than late opening of the aortic valve is seen in aortic regurgitation.
2. The following biplane TEE clip (Fig. 18.14) was obtained in a patient with suspected aortic regurgitation admitted to the ICU with acute respiratory failure. The echocardiographic finding in the mid-esophageal long-axis view is the most suggestive of:
   A. Thickened bicuspid aortic valve
   B. Rheumatic aortic valve
   C. Tricuspid aortic valve with abnormal coaptation
   D. Degenerative bicuspid aortic valve
   E. Nonbacterial thrombotic endocarditis of the aortic valve

   Answer: C. In this mid-esophageal long- and short-axis echocardiographic view, the utilization of biplane modality facilitates the recognition of lack of coaptation (short axis). A subsequent utilization of CFD in this specific area can reveal the regurgitant jet [6].
3. Which of the following echocardiographic findings is associated with severe PR and increased pulmonary vascular resistance with Spectral Doppler in a patient with repaired tetralogy of Fallot:
   A. PHT of 90 ms
   B. Narrow and short regurgitant flow with CFD
   C. Lack of late-systolic notching in RVOT PWD evaluation
   D. Lack of mid-systolic notching in RVOT PWD evaluation
   E. Atrial contraction does not induce an anterograde forward flow

   Answer: A. The pressure half-time represents the time needed for the maximum transvalvular gradient (from PA to RV in this case)

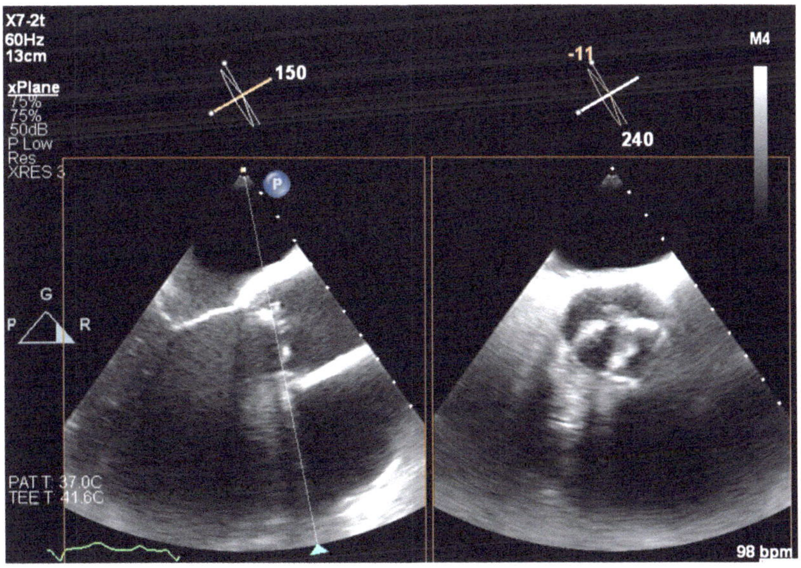

Fig. 18.14 Question 2. (Figure courtesy of Department of Anesthesiology and Critical Care at Baylor St. Luke's Medical Center—Texas Heart Institute. Permission to use obtained)

to decrease to its half value or the time interval for the peak velocity to reach 0.707 of the peak velocity value in milliseconds. The cutoff to determine significant PR has been suggested to be <100 ms [7].

References

1. Lancellotti P, Tribouilloy C, Hagendorff A, Moura L, et al. European Association of Echocardiography recommendations for the assessment of valvular regurgitation. Part 1: aortic and pulmonary regurgitation (native valve disease). Eur J Echocardiogr. 2010;11(3):223–44.
2. Zoghbi WA, Adams D, Bonow RO, Enriquez-Sarano M, et al. Recommendations for noninvasive evaluation of native valvular regurgitation. J Am Soc Echocardiogr. 2017;30(4):303–71. https://doi.org/10.1016/j.echo.2017.01.007.
3. Walpot J, Vermeiren G, Al Mafragi A, Malbrain MLNG. Comprehensive assessment of the aortic valve in critically ill patients for the non-cardiologist. Part II: chronic aortic regurgitation of the native valve. Anaesthesiol Intensive Ther. 2021;53(1):55–68. https://doi.org/10.5114/ait.2021.104892.
4. Maciel BC, Simpson IA, Valdes-Crus LM, et al. Color flow Doppler mapping studies of "physiologic" pulmonary and tricuspid regurgitation: evidence for true regurgitation as opposed to a valve closing volume. J Am Soc Echocardiogr. 1991;4:589–97.
5. Redington A. Determinants and assessment of pulmonary regurgitation in tetralogy of Fallot: practice and pitfalls. Cardiol Clin. 2006;24:631–9.
6. Grayburn PA, Smith MD, Handshoe R, Friedman BJ, DeMaria AN. Detection of aortic insufficiency by standard echocardiography, pulsed Doppler echocardiography, and auscultation. A comparison of accuracies. Ann Intern Med. 1986;104(5):599–605.
7. Silversides CK, Veldtman GR, Crossin J, Merchant N, Webb GD, McCrindle BW, et al. Pressure half-time predicts hemodynamically significant pulmonary regurgitation in adult patients with repaired tetralogy of Fallot. J Am Soc Echocardiogr. 2003;16(10):1057–62.

19 Mitral and Tricuspid Stenosis

Nicholas Levin and Christopher Kelly

Learning Objectives

1. Understand the multiple ways to obtain an estimated mitral valve area and be able to grade the severity of mitral stenosis
2. Know the consequences of long-standing mitral stenosis
3. Explain how to calculate a tricuspid valve area and know the cutoff for severe stenosis
4. Review the other echocardiographic findings indicative of hemodynamically significant tricuspid stenosis

Mitral Stenosis

The normal mitral valve area (MVA) is 4.0–5.0 cm^2. Symptoms from mitral stenosis (MS) usually occur when the valvular area is less than 2.5 cm^2; however, patients may develop symptoms prior to this cutoff during states of need for increased cardiac output such as exercise or pregnancy. Mitral valve stenosis usually becomes clinically significant at rest when the MVA is less than 1.5 cm^2. This stenosis leads to elevated transvalvular pressure gradients with subsequent left atrial pressure elevation and eventual enlargement. A further discussion regarding consequences of mitral stenosis is below. Table 19.1 lists the American Society of Echocardiography cutoffs for severity based on several criteria [1].

Etiologies

Globally, the primary etiology of mitral stenosis is rheumatic valvular disease. This predominance is largely due to the significant burden that rheumatic heart disease (RHD) continues to have in developing countries where current estimates find that it accounts for approximately >85% of the identified mitral stenosis [2]. Mitral stenosis caused by RHD has a classic appearance of the anterior leaflet of the mitral valve that is often described as a "hockey stick" as seen in Video 19.1. In developed countries, RHD carries a substantially smaller burden of disease. Other nonrheumatic causes include mitral annular calcification (MAC), radiation valvulitis, and systemic inflammatory processes such as rheumatoid arthritis and lupus. Congenital MS is exceedingly rare and accounts for approximately 1% of mitral stenosis etiologies. Congenital

Supplementary Information The online version contains supplementary material available at https://doi.org/10.1007/978-3-031-80038-2_19.

N. Levin (✉)
Stanford University, Stanford, CA, USA
e-mail: nmlevin@stanford.edu

C. Kelly
University of Utah, Salt Lake City, UT, USA
e-mail: christopher.kelly@hsc.utah.edu

M. J. Lanspa, A. T. Levinson (eds.), *Echocardiography and Ultrasonography in the ICU*, Respiratory Medicine, https://doi.org/10.1007/978-3-031-80038-2_19

Table 19.1 American Society of Echocardiography guideline cutoffs for degree of mitral stenosis based on valve area, mean gradient, and pulmonary artery pressure

	Mild	Moderate	Severe
Valve area (cm^2)	>1.5	1.0–1.5	<1.0
Mean gradient (mmHg)	<5	5–10	>10
Pulmonary artery pressure (mmHg)	<30	30–50	>50

[a] 60–80 beats/min in sinus rhythm (Circulation Volume 129, Number 23, March 3, 2014)

abnormalities include cor triatriatum, supravalvular mitral ring, double-orifice mitral valve, and parachute mitral valve. Additional functional causes of MS include cardiac masses such as myxomas or valvular vegetations such as endocarditis [3, 4].

Quantification of Mitral Valve Area

Planimetry

Direct planimetry can be utilized with 2D or 3D echocardiography imaging to calculate the anatomic mitral valve area. A short-axis view of the mitral valve during mid-diastole is obtained and the smallest orifice is then traced using the inner contours (Fig. 19.1). To optimize this measurement, biplane imaging can be used to find the optimal location and it is recommended to use the lowest gain possible to define the orifice area. In several studies, these measurements have been well validated to surgical and cardiac catheter determined areas. Calculations based on 3D echocardiography images have also been found to be more accurate than those based on 2D images as it can be difficult to ensure measurement at the true tips of the leaflets (Fig. 19.2) [5].

Continuity Equation

The continuity equation, as previously described in Chap. 17, assumes a conservation of stroke volume (SV) throughout the various chambers and valves of the heart. Diastolic stroke volume across the mitral valve is assumed to equal systolic stroke volume across the left ventricular outflow tract (LVOT). We can use this assumption to then determine the MVA utilizing measurements acquired from the LVOT. A basic formula derivation is provided below. The needed variables include the cross-sectional area and velocity time integral (VTI) of the LVOT as well as the VTI of the diastolic mitral valve inflow. An example of obtaining and measuring the mitral valve VTI is demonstrated in Fig. 19.3.

$$\mathrm{SV}\left(\mathrm{cm}^3\right) = \mathrm{Area}\left(\mathrm{cm}^2\right) \times \mathrm{VTI}(\mathrm{cm})$$

$$\mathrm{SV}_1 = \mathrm{SV}_2$$

$$\mathrm{LVOT}_{\mathrm{AREA}} \times \mathrm{LVOT}_{\mathrm{VTI}} = \mathrm{MVA} \times \mathrm{MV}_{\mathrm{VTI}}$$

$$\mathrm{MVA} = \mathrm{LVOT}_{\mathrm{AREA}} \times \frac{\mathrm{LVOT\,VTI}}{\mathrm{MV\,VTI}}$$

An important caveat to using the continuity equation to solve for the MVA is when there is concurrent aortic or mitral regurgitation. Additionally, in patients with underlying atrial fibrillation, the continuity equation should not be utilized as the primary MVA assessment [1, 6].

Pressure Half-Time

A quantitative approach using doppler measurements for MVA calculation is that of **pressure half-time (PHT)**. This approach utilizes the concept that the rate of pressure decline across a valve is related to the cross-sectional area of the valve, i.e., the smaller the cross-sectional area, the slower the decline in pressure [7]. Pressure half-time is defined as the length of time in milliseconds for the maximal early diastolic trans-mitral pressure gradient to reach one-half its value as demonstrated in Fig. 19.4. An equation was derived for calculating the MVA from the PHT [8]:

$$\mathrm{MVA}\left(\mathrm{cm}^2\right) = 220 / \mathrm{PHT}(\mathrm{ms})$$

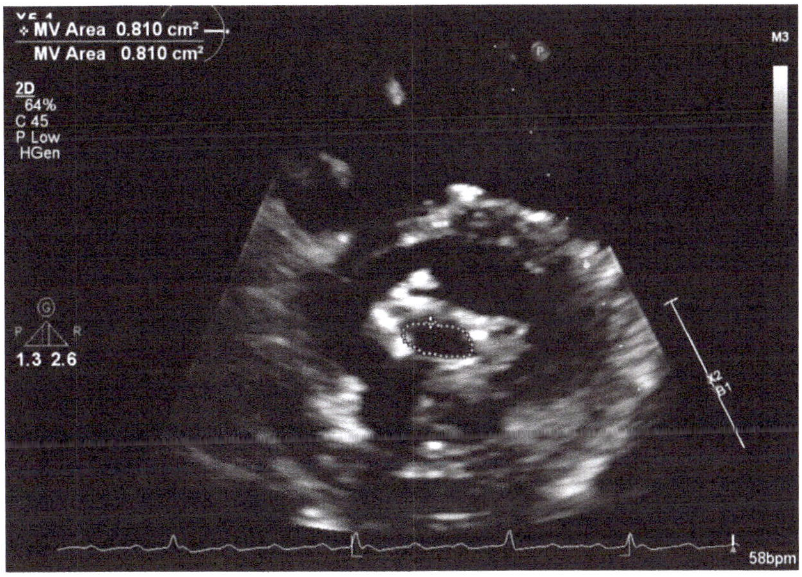

Fig. 19.1 2D parasternal short-axis view with tracing of mitral valve orifice area. (Image courtesy of University of Utah Division of Echocardiography and Perioperative Ultrasound database)

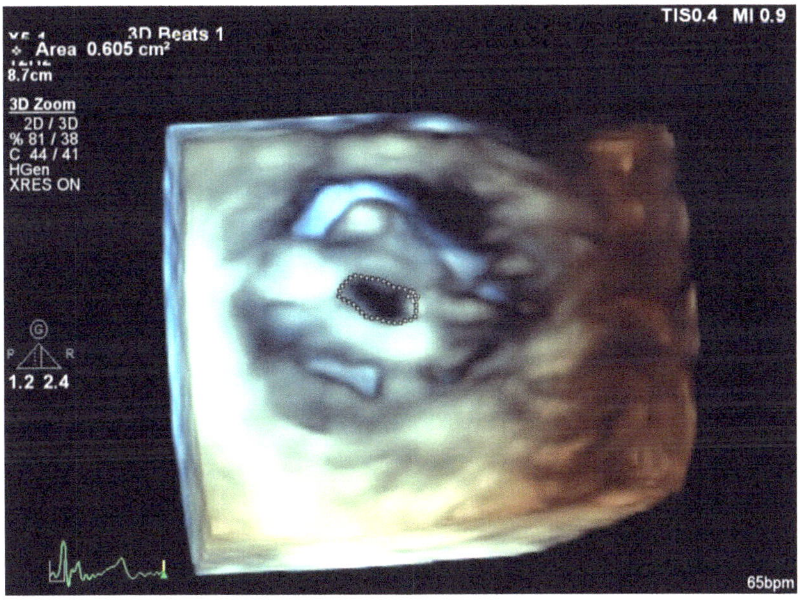

Fig. 19.2 3D parasternal short-axis view with tracing of mitral valve orifice area. Accompanying Video 19.2. (Image courtesy of University of Utah Division of Echocardiography and Perioperative Ultrasound database)

Important Considerations and Caveats [6]

Atrial fibrillation: In patients with atrial fibrillation, an average PHT should be calculated by averaging at least five cardiac cycles.

Co-existing aortic regurgitation: In patients with concomitant aortic regurgitation, transmitral filling may be affected due to retrograde filling from the aortic regurgitation or via direct impairment of mitral valve opening secondary to the retrograde aortic regurgitant jet. Special attention should be made to the aortic valve in patients with mitral stenosis in order to accurately assess the degree of mitral stenosis.

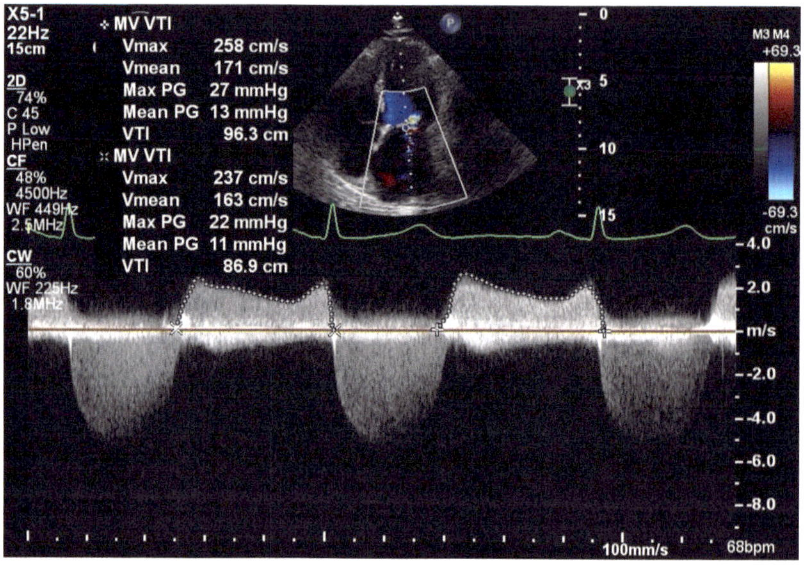

Fig. 19.3 Continuous wave Doppler through the mitral valve. Two mitral valve velocity time integral measurements are traced. (Image courtesy of University of Utah Division of Echocardiography and Perioperative Ultrasound database)

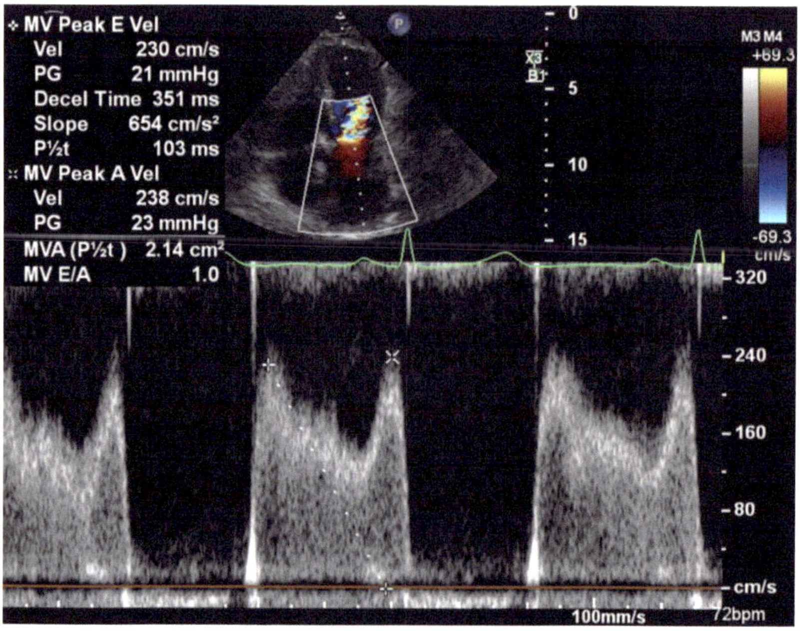

Fig. 19.4 Mitral inflow waveform demonstrating measurement location for pressure half-time (PHT) and deceleration time (DT). The mitral valve area using PHT is calculated by the formula MVA = 220/PHT which in this example would be 220/103 (in ms) = 2.14 cm^2. Alternatively, if one used the DT of 351 ms and applied it to the formula MVA = 759/DT, one would calculate the MVA as 2.16 cm^2 which is congruent with the PHT calculation. (Image courtesy of University of Utah Division of Echocardiography and Perioperative Ultrasound database)

Left ventricular Diastolic Dysfunction: Due to abnormal LV relaxation in patients with diastolic dysfunction, the PHT may be affected in either direction.

Deceleration Time

An alternative and complimentary approach for MVA using the same mitral inflow waveform as PHT is that of **deceleration time (DT)**. DT is defined as the time, in milliseconds, from peak mitral inflow E-wave velocity to the end of flow (i.e., when mitral inflow velocity = 0 cm/s) as shown in Fig. 19.5. A formula was derived to convert DT to MVA:

$$\mathrm{MVA}\left(\mathrm{cm}^2\right) = 759 / \mathrm{DT}\left(\mathrm{ms}\right)$$

The relationship between PHT and DT is demonstrated in the conversion formula:

$$\mathrm{PHT}\left(\mathrm{ms}\right) = 0.29 \times \mathrm{DT}\left(\mathrm{ms}\right)$$

Often times if mitral inflow waveform definition allows, both PHT and DT are obtained. Figure 19.4 demonstrates an example of obtaining both measurements.

Qualification of Mitral Valve Stenosis Severity

There are three categories of assessment to determine mitral valve stenosis severity as defined by the American Society of Echocardiography and shown in Table 19.1. This chapter has already covered the several ways for obtaining a mitral valve area, and additional chapters have shown how to obtain an estimated pulmonary artery pressure. We will therefore focus on the third and final severity assessment, that of mean transmitral pressure gradient.

Mean Pressure Gradient

A pressure gradient is the difference in pressure of two chambers at any one time across a valve and can be expressed as both the maximum pressure gradient and the mean pressure gradient. For qualification of mitral valve stenosis severity, the mean pressure gradient is utilized. The more stenotic the mitral valve is, the higher the mean pressure gradient will be. Pulsed or continuous wave doppler through the mitral valve can be utilized. A parallel

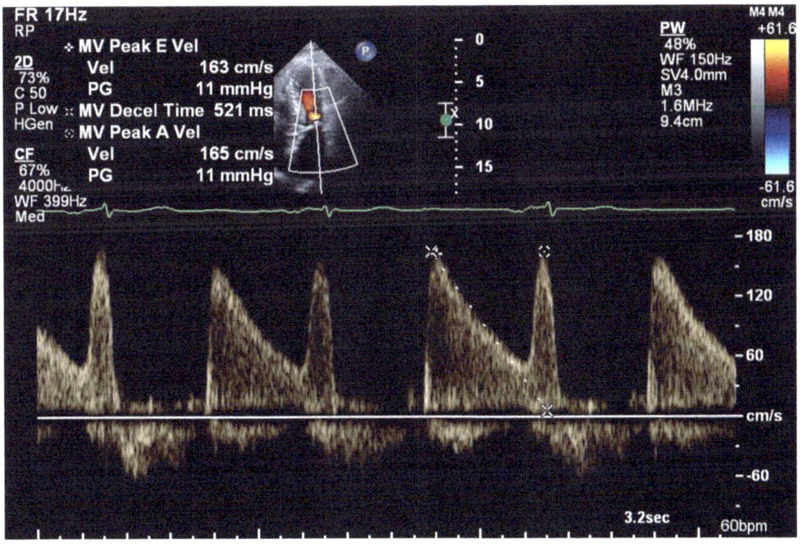

Fig. 19.5 Mitral inflow waveform demonstrating how to obtain a deceleration time. Using this value, the estimated MVA for this patient would be 759 divided by 521 ms resulting in a MVA of 1.46 cm^2. (Image courtesy of University of Utah Division of Echocardiography and Perioperative Ultrasound database)

intercept angle with regard to direction of blood flow is needed to ensure accurate velocity measurements and subsequently accurate pressure gradient calculations. It is therefore possible to have eccentric jets that makes obtaining true parallel flow assessment difficult. An example of obtaining the maximum and mean mitral valve pressure gradients is shown in Figure 19.3 [1, 4, 9].

Consequences of Long-Standing Mitral Stenosis

The consequences of mitral stenosis follow a predictable pattern of increasing left atrial pressure. Due to decreased left ventricular filling, left atrial pressure increases over time causing enlargement of the left atrium. This in turn comes with increased risk of atrial fibrillation secondary to increased atrium distension which has inherent risks with relation to thromboembolic disease due to left atrial thrombi. The increased left atrial pressure over time leads to an increase in pulmonary pressures. This in turn may lead to the cascade of right ventricular dilation, resultant tricuspid insufficiency, and ultimately right ventricular failure [1, 3].

Tricuspid Stenosis

A normal tricuspid is composed of three leaflets, the septal, anterior, and posterior. Normal tricuspid valve area (TVA) is 7–9 cm^2 with a mean gradient across the valve of less than 2 mmHg. Hemodynamically significant tricuspid stenosis typically occurs with the valve area is less than 1 cm^2. As the valve becomes increasingly stenosed, patients often present with sequela of increased venous congestion including fatigue, edema, and congestive hepatopathy. Without other valve involvement, patients rarely present with symptoms of dyspnea [1].

Etiology

Among all of the valvular stenosis, tricuspid valve stenosis is the least common and is overall extremely rare. Primary etiologies are rheumatic heart disease (RHD), carcinoid syndrome, autoimmune, metastatic processes, and complications from valvular prosthesis. Most often, tricuspid stenosis is combined with another valvular pathology. This can involve another valve (e.g., RHD will almost always have concurrent mitral stenosis) or a combined pathology with the tricuspid valve (e.g., in carcinoid syndrome there is almost always concurrent tricuspid regurgitation). Additionally, large valvular vegetations such as myxomas on the tricuspid valve can cause a relative valvular stenosis [1, 10].

Planimetry

Quantification of the tricuspid valve area can be measured by direct visualization by utilizing 3D echocardiography but the practice is neither validated nor widely utilized [1].

Continuity Equation

The continuity equation can be utilized to estimate the tricuspid valve area. Similar to the approach in mitral stenosis assessment, continuous wave doppler can be used to calculate the VTI across the tricuspid inflow. Pulmonic or aortic valve cross-sectional area and VTI measurements can then be used to complete the continuity equation where the tricuspid valve area can be calculated. Greater than mild concurrent tricuspid regurgitation presents a significant caveat to using the continuity equation and can cause underestimation of the calculated valve area. Tricuspid valve stenosis is considered severe when the valve area is less than 1 cm^2. Additionally, during this acquisition of measurements, an inflow VTI >60 cm is indicative of hemodynamically significant tricuspid stenosis (Table 19.2) [1].

Pressure Gradients

From a low parasternal right ventricular inflow view or from a RV-focused apical 4-chamber view,

Table 19.2 European Association of Echocardiography/American Society of Echocardiography Recommendations on findings indicative of hemodynamically significant tricuspid stenosis [1]

Findings of severe tricuspid stenosis	
Mean pressure gradient	≥5 mmHg
Inflow VTI	>60 cm
PHT	≥190 ms
Valve area by continuity equation	≤1 cm^2

measurements can be acquired across the tricuspid valve. As the RV inflow velocities are affected by respiration, all measurements taken should be averaged across the respiration cycle or be recorded at end-respiration. By utilizing continuous wave doppler, the pressure gradient is calculated by utilizing the simplified Bernoulli equation as previously described. A mean pressure gradient greater than 5 mmHg is considered severe tricuspid stenosis.

Pressure Half-Time

Evolving Evidence

Similar to the mitral valve, CWD can be used to measure a pressure half-time to grade tricuspid valve area and stenosis. However, given the difference between right and left heart atrio-ventricular compliance and also because of the often-concurrent tricuspid valve regurgitation, this method has significantly more variability and there are far fewer validation studies of the tricuspid valve compared to the mitral valve. Current consensus has agreed that the tricuspid valve area can be calculated by equation below:

$$\text{TVA}\left(\text{cm}^2\right) = 190 / \text{PHT}\left(\text{ms}\right)$$

Consequences

As tricuspid stenosis becomes increasingly severe, patients develop increasing right atrial pressures and venous congestion. Other echocardiographic findings supportive of this pathophysiology include an enlarged right atrium and dilated inferior vena cava. Symptomology wise, this often manifests as hepatic congestion with ascites, peripheral edema, and elevated liver enzymes as generally seen in right heart failure patients [11]. As tricuspid valve stenosis usually has concurrent left heart valvular disease, patients often have respiratory symptoms, however, if isolated tricuspid pathology, there should be an absence of respiratory complaints [12].

Summary Points

- The most common etiology of mitral stenosis and tricuspid stenosis globally is rheumatic valvular disease.
- There are several ways to obtain an estimated mitral valve area including direct 2-D or 3-D planimetry, continuity equation calculation, or via pressure half-time/deceleration time.
- The severity of stenosis is based on valvular area, mean pressure gradients, and pulmonary artery pressures.
- Tricuspid stenosis is rarely an isolated pathology.
- There are a few ways to obtain a tricuspid valve area but these come with limitations and decisions about interventions often include the patient's symptomology.

Questions

1. If you measure a PHT of 240 ms across the mitral valve, what is the calculated MVA and what severity of the stenosis does the patient have?
   (A) 0.92 cm^2, severe
   (B) 3.45 cm^2, moderate
   (C) 0.64 cm^2, severe
   (D) 0.92 cm^2, moderate

   Answer: A. 0.92 cm^2, severe. Mitral valve area is calculated by 220 (ms cm^2)/Pressure half-time (ms). 220/240 = 0.92 cm^2. A mitral valve area < 1 cm^2 is severe.
2. Which of the following is not a validated approach to obtain the MVA?
   (A) Planimetry
   (B) Continuity Eq.

(C) Pressure Half-Time
(D) Pressure Gradient

Answer: D. Pressure Gradient. Pressure gradient can offer insights into the severity of stenosis, but is insufficient to calculate mitral valve area. The other choices all offer quantitative methods to calculate mitral valve area.

3. Which of the following measurements is consistent with severe tricuspid valve stenosis?
(A) PHT of 170 ms
(B) Mean pressure gradient of 8 mmHg
(C) Tricuspid valve area of 1.2 cm^2
(D) Inflow VTI of 40 cm

Answer: B. Mean pressure gradient of 8 mmHg. A is incorrect because a pressure half-time of 170 would result in a TV area of 1.24 cm^2, and the time is lower than the threshold for severe stenosis, 190 ms. The threshold for severe stenosis is TV area of 1 cm^2. The inflow VTI is consistent with severe tricuspid stenosis when it equals or exceeds 60 cm.

References

1. Baumgartner H, Hung J, Bermejo J, Chambers JB, Evangelista A, Griffin BP, et al. Echocardiographic assessment of valve stenosis: EAE/ASE recommendations for clinical practice. Eur J Echocardiogr. 2009;10(1):1–25.
2. Iung B, Baron G, Butchart EG, et al. A prospective survey of patients with valvular heart disease in Europe: the Euro Heart Survey on valvular heart disease. Eur Heart J. 2003;24(13):1231–43. https://doi.org/10.1016/S0195-668X(03)00201-X.
3. Lang RM, Goldstein SA, Kronzon I, Khandheria B, Saric M, Mor-Avi V. 108-Rheumatic mitral stenosis. In: ASE's comprehensive echocardiography. Philadelphia: Elsevier; 2022.
4. Harb SC, Griffin BP. Mitral valve disease: a comprehensive review. Curr Cardiol Rep. 2017;19(8):73.
5. Silbiger J. Advances in rheumatic mitral stenosis: echocardiographic, pathophysiologic, and hemodynamic considerations. J Am Soc Echocardiogr. 2021;34(7):709–722.e1.
6. Lang R, Goldstein S, Kronzon I, Khandheria B, Saric M, Mor-Avi V. 109-Quantification of mitral stenosis. In: ASE's comprehensive echocardiography. Philadelphia: Elsevier; 2022.
7. Libanoff AJ, Rodbard S. Atrioventricular pressure half-time. Measure of mitral valve orifice area. Circulation. 1968;38(1):144–50. https://doi.org/10.1161/01.cir.38.1.144.
8. Hatle L, Angelsen B. Doppler ultrasound in cardiology: physical principles and clinical applications, 118. Philadelphia: Lea and Febiger; 1985.
9. Teirstein PS, Yock PG, Popp RL. The accuracy of Doppler ultrasound measurement of pressure gradients across irregular, dual, and tunnel like obstructions to blood flow. Circulation. 1985;72(3):577–84. https://doi.org/10.1161/01.CIR.72.3.577.
10. Roberts W, Ko J. Some observations on mitral and aortic valve disease. Baylor Univ Med Center Proc. 2008;21(3):282–99.
11. Coffey S, Rayner J, Newton J, Prendergast BD. Right-sided valve disease. Int J Clin Pract. 2014;68(10):1221–6. https://doi.org/10.1111/ijcp.12485.
12. Stapleton JF. Natural history of chronic valvular disease. Cardiovasc Clin. 1986;16(2):105–47.

20 Mitral and Tricuspid Regurgitation

Maxwell Hockstein and Karuna Puttur Rajkumar

Learning Objectives
1. Describe primary and secondary causes of mitral and tricuspid regurgitations
2. Review the use of Doppler to detect regurgitant jets
3. Discuss echocardiographic tools to characterize regurgitant jets
4. Analyze quantitative methods to grade the severity of regurgitant lesions

Causes

Mitral and tricuspid regurgitation are conditions in which there is incomplete coaptation of the valve leaflets, leading to retrograde flow of blood from the ventricle to the atrium. The clinical consequence of tricuspid regurgitation is reflected by venous congestion and the clinical consequence of mitral regurgitation is pulmonary congestion. Etiologies are classified into primary (organic) or secondary (functional) causes [1, 2]. Primary (organic) causes are etiologies which represent defects of the leaflets whereas secondary (functional) causes are etiologies which involve annular dilatation.

Primary Causes

- Valve Prolapse:
  - Mitral Valve Prolapse (MVP): In MVP, the mitral valve leaflets bulge back into the left atrium during contraction. This can lead to improper valve closure and regurgitation [3].
  - Tricuspid Valve Prolapse: Similar to MVP, tricuspid valve prolapse involves the tricuspid valve leaflets bulging back into the right atrium during contraction [2, 4].
- Valve Degeneration: Over time, the valves of the heart can degenerate due to aging, wear and tear, or other factors such as fibroelastic deficiency and myxomatous degeneration (Barlow's disease). This degeneration can affect the proper functioning of the valves and result in regurgitation [4].
- Rheumatic Heart Disease: Long-term inflammation and scarring associated with rheumatic disease can also lead to functional mitral and tricuspid regurgitation.
- Infective Endocarditis: Bacterial or fungal infections of the heart valves (endocarditis) can damage the valves, leading to regurgitation [2].
- Congenital Heart Defects: Congenital malformations of the mitral or tricuspid valve apparatus such as isolated cleft of the anterior mitral valve, mitral valve prolapse associated with Marfan's or Ehler-Danlos syndromes,

The original version of the chapter has been revised. A correction to this chapter can be found at https://doi.org/10.1007/978-3-031-80038-2_73

M. Hockstein (✉)
MedStar Washington Hospital Center, Washington, DC, USA

K. Puttur Rajkumar
Wake Forest Baptist Health, Winston-Salem, NC, USA

M. J. Lanspa, A. T. Levinson (eds.), *Echocardiography and Ultrasonography in the ICU*, Respiratory Medicine, https://doi.org/10.1007/978-3-031-80038-2_20

Table 20.1 Metrics for severe tricuspid and mitral valve regurgitation

	Tricuspid regurgitation	Mitral regurgitation
Jet area	>10 cm^2 [8]	>50% LA size [9]
Vena contracta	>0.7 cm	
Jet density	Equal to inflow component, early peak, triangular [8, 10]	
Effective regurgitant orifice area	>0.4 cm^2	
Regurgitant volume	>45 mL [8]	≥60 mL [11]
Regurgitant fraction	Not defined	>0.5

double orifice mitral valve, arcade mitral valve (thickened or absent chordae), and Ebstein's anomaly of tricuspid valve can lead to regurgitation [5, 6].

- Connective Tissue Disorders: Conditions that affect connective tissues, such as Marfan syndrome or Ehlers-Danlos syndrome, can lead to abnormalities in the heart valves [1, 2].
- Trauma: Physical trauma to the chest or heart externally can cause either mitral or tricuspid regurgitation [1, 2].
- Iatrogenesis: Procedures such as pulmonary artery catheters and pacemaker leads can cause damage or restrict the valve leaflets leading to tricuspid regurgitation.
- Tumors: Tumors within the heart such as left atrial myomas and carcinoid tumors though rare, affect valve function and can lead to both stenosis and regurgitation.

Secondary Causes

- Ischemic heart disease: Ischemia can cause papillary muscle rupture and/or ventricular dysfunction leading to enlargement of the ventricles, annular dilatation, and displacement of the valve leaflets resulting in incomplete coaptation of the leaflets during systole causing regurgitation.
- Dilated Cardiomyopathy: Enlargement of the heart chambers, often associated with dilated cardiomyopathy, causes insufficient coaptation of the valve leaflets leading to regurgitation [7].
- Hypertension: Chronic hypertension can lead to changes in the structure of the heart, including the valves, and contribute to regurgitation [7]. Mitral annular dilation from chronic systemic hypertension and remodeling of the left ventricle and result in mitral valve insufficiency and pulmonary hypertension and elevated right ventricular pressures can similarly lead to mitral regurgitation.

A summary of jet area metrics for mitral and tricuspid valvular regurgitation is found in Table 20.1.

Jet Area

Often the first indication of the presence of valvular insufficiency is an appreciable regurgitant jet seen with color Doppler. When color Doppler is applied over a valve with regurgitant flow, the regurgitant jet will have the color spectrum "opposite" that of antegrade flow. It should be noted that the size of a jet area does not translate into the severity of retrograde flow, rather, it simply highlights the *distribution* of regurgitant velocities [10]. In other words, a generous jet area does not imply a high regurgitant volume [10, 12]. Additionally, the area of a regurgitant jet should be contextualized to the size of the chamber in which the regurgitation occurs. The definition of jet area is the area of the regurgitant jet divided by the total chamber size. For example, mitral regurgitation jet area = mitral regurgitation jet size/left atrial size. An example of a jet area is seen in Fig. 20.1. Large atrial sizes likely indicate chronic regurgitation.

Regurgitant jets can be categorized as either central or eccentric depending on its relationship to the valve annulus. Central jets are often from a functional etiology, where the valve annulus is dilated as opposed to organic etiologies which create eccentric jets because of structural injury to the leaflets.

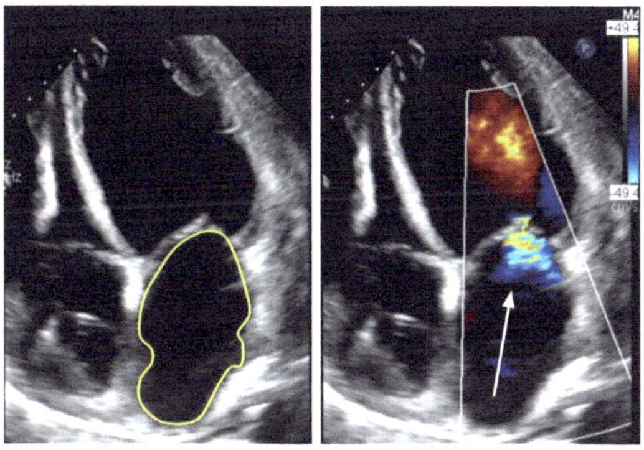

Fig. 20.1 Right-hand panel: highlighted in yellow is the LA area. Left-hand panel: arrow demonstrates the jet area

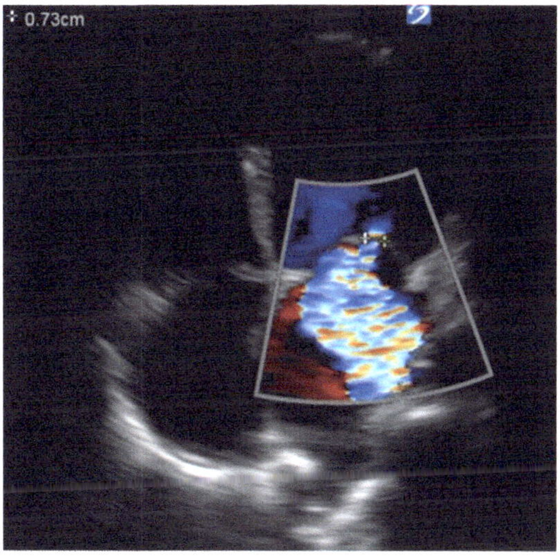

Fig. 20.2 Vena contracta measurement in mitral regurgitation

Several factors may accentuate a jet area. First, high driving pressures from the left ventricle to the left atrium may increase the jet area. Second, when multiple jets are present, the jet area often overestimates regurgitant severity [13]. Third, central, often high-velocity jets often recruit blood ("entrain") from the chamber which may augment the jet area. Once a regurgitant jet has been identified, the next step should be defining the regurgitation severity by quantitative metrics.

Vena Contracta

The vena contracta (VC), seen in Fig. 20.2, is defined as the narrowest point of the highest velocity regurgitant jet at the flow convergence region between the ventricle and atrium [1, 12, 14]. The width or diameter of the regurgitant jet is measured at this narrowest point. Vena contracta measured by either transthoracic or transesophageal echocardiography is usually reliable if the jet is symmetrical [1, 12]. A width greater than 0.7 cm is indicative of severe regurgitation. However, the vena contracta width is not a reliable measure of severity with multiple jets and may vary under dynamic changes and different afterload conditions and additional parameters are required to quantify the severity of the regurgitation [1, 12].

Jet Density

When performing continuous wave Doppler (CWD) through a valvular apparatus with regurgitant flow, there will be a regurgitant velocity jet whose density is proportional to erythrocyte density and severity [14, 15]. To maximize the signal, place the CWD through the VC as seen in Fig. 20.3 [12]. The more severe the regurgitation, higher velocities will occur in early systole, and as pressures between chambers equilibrate quickly, the CWD morphology will appear more triangular than parabolic. One caveat to the triangular appearance of the CWD with severe regurgitation is that prosthetic valves often have a similar morphology. For tricuspid valve regurgitation, jets can be best appreciated in the parasternal long right ventricular inflow view or an apical 4-chamber view. For mitral valve regurgitation, jets are best appreciated in the apical 4-chamber view. While it is possible to identify mitral regurgitation in parasternal views, the ultrasound beam is not parallel to regurgitant flow.

Tricuspid CWD provides rapid insight regarding right-heart hemodynamics. By way of the modified Bernoulli equation, right ventricular

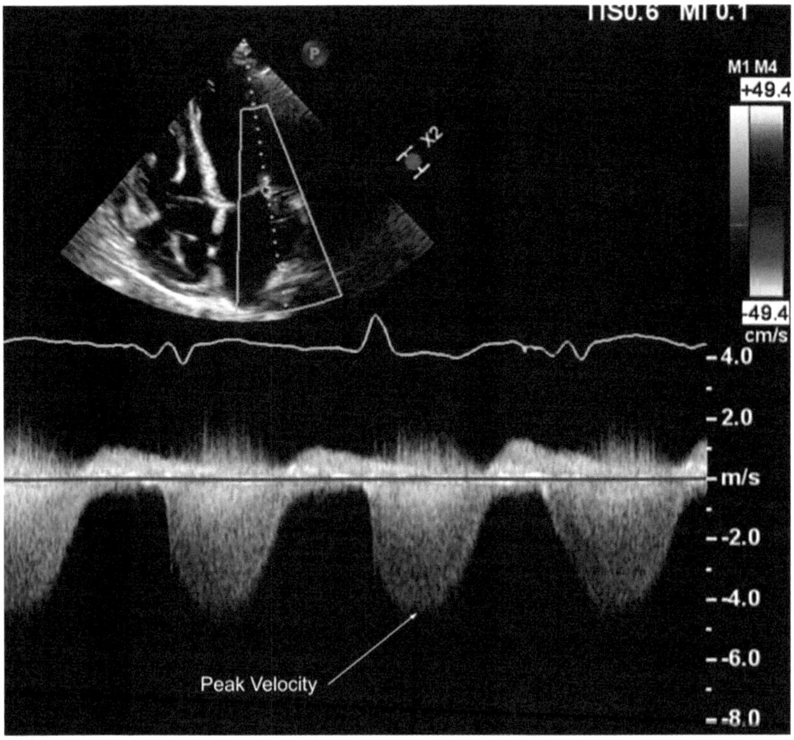

Fig. 20.3 Continuous wave Doppler (CWD) through the mitral valve

systolic pressure (RVSP), can be estimated by adding the right atrial pressure to the tricuspid valve gradient: $RVSP = 4V^2_{TR_{max}} + RAP$. Assuming there is no gradient across the pulmonic valve, RVSP equals pulmonary artery systolic pressure (PASP). Although values greater than 60 mmHg are more likely to reflect chronic pulmonary hypertension (PH), the relationship between echocardiogram-derived PASP and right heart catheterization PASP in known PH is often unreliable [16].

Pressure Half-Time

Although originally studied in mitral stenosis, pressure half-time is a marker of regurgitation severity [17]. A pressure half-time (PHT) is defined as the amount of takes that it takes for a peak pressure gradient to decrease by 50%. Commonly used in the assessment of mitral stenosis and aortic insufficiency severity, PHT is also used to estimate mitral valve area. PHT is not commonly used in the assessment of tricuspid and/or mitral regurgitation.

Proximal Isovelocity Surface Area, Effective Regurgitant Orifice Area, Regurgitant Volume, and Regurgitant Fraction

The severity of clinical consequence is proportional to the degrees of regurgitant flow. Several quantitative methods exist to grade the severity of regurgitant lesions. The proximal isovelocity surface area (PISA) method is predicated on principles of fluid dynamics which makes several assumptions, most notably a constant, laminar flow before entering the orifice. PISA is used to calculate volumetrics when quantifying regurgitation, such as effective regurgitant surface area (EROA) and regurgitant fraction (RF). PISA also assumes that as blood nears the orifice, that there is an acceleration of blood which peaks at the narrowest portion of the orifice [18]. Using color

Doppler, speeds of blood cells can be mapped in the immediate area around the valve. Conceptually, this flow acceleration can be modeled by a series of concentric spheres of blood moving at increasing velocities until reaching the center.

PISA leverages one of the artifacts of color Doppler, aliasing. Aliasing occurs when observed velocities exceed that of the set Nyquist limit. The first step to measuring PISA is to identify the aliasing velocity and to measure the PISA radius on the ventricular side of the valve as seen in Fig. 20.4 [18]. The aliasing velocity can be identified in the regurgitant jet where there is an abrupt reversal in velocities (turning from blue to red, for example) near the VC. At the point where the color transition is located is exactly the Nyquist limit and therefore the velocity of the blood at that radius [15]. It is understood that the surface area of a sphere is $4\pi r^2$, and therefore, the surface area of a hemisphere, excluding the flat base, is $2\pi r^2$. Therefore, the hemispheric area, the PISA = $2\pi r^2$.

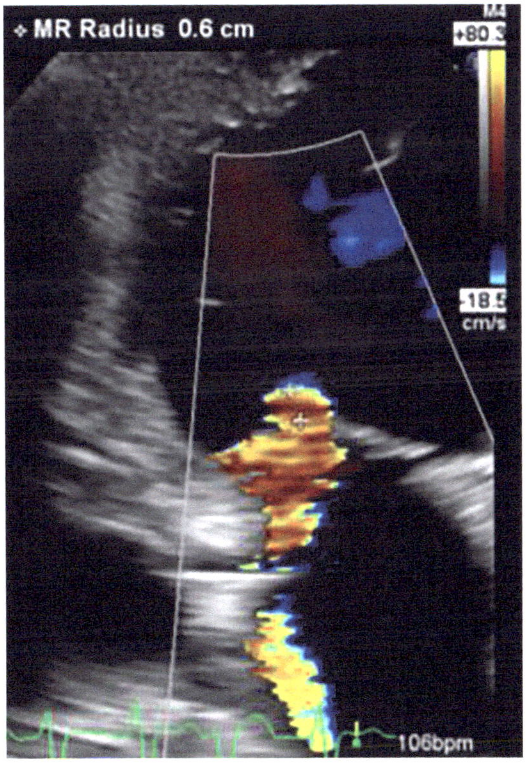

Fig. 20.4 Proximal isovelocity surface area (PISA) radius in mitral valve regurgitation

In fluid dynamics, flow is defined as an amount of fluid passing a particular point per unit time. As such, flow can be expressed as the cross-sectional area of the orifice times the velocity of the fluid ($Q = A \times V$). It is also understood that the continuity equation holds across a valve: $A_1 \times V_1 = A_2 \times V_2$. The continuity equation yields insight into the area of the regurgitant orifice, the EROA. If EROA is considered as A_1, V_1 then represents the maximum velocity of the blood traversing the regurgitant orifice. V_1 can be obtained by measuring the maximum regurgitant velocity on continuous wave Doppler through the valve (Fig. 20.3). Both A_2 and V_2 are known: $2\pi r^2$ and the Nyquist limit, respectively. Therefore, EROA = ($2\pi r^2$ × Nyquist Limit) ÷ V_{max}. It should be noted that for non-holosystolic MR, this method overestimates its severity [19].

One of the assumptions of PISA is that the regurgitant orifice occurs on a flat surface (i.e., 180°). With progressive leaflet distortion, a correction factor is applied to the EROA equation by multiplying the EROA by the ventricular side angle of the leaflets divided by 180: EROA × (∢/180).

The total volume of blood that regurgitates through the valve is known as Regurgitant Volume (RV) [11]. RV may be deduced by PISA and velocity-time-integrals (VTI) techniques. Analogous to calculation of LV stroke volume, RV = EROA × VTI. Consequently, regurgitant fraction (RF) is defined as the ratio of retrograde flow to total valvular flow (antegrade plus retrograde flow). In other words, RF = RV/SV.

Summary Points

- Primary (organic) causes are etiologies which represent defects of the leaflets whereas secondary (functional) causes are etiologies which involve annular dilatation.
- When color Doppler is applied over a valve with regurgitant flow, the size of a jet area does not translate into the severity of retrograde flow but shows the *distribution* of regurgitant velocities.

- Vena contracta width is a key parameter used in the assessment of valvular regurgitation. It represents the narrowest portion of the regurgitant jet and is measured by color Doppler flow mapping
- The proximal isovelocity surface area (PISA) is used to calculate volumetrics when quantifying regurgitation utilizing the color Doppler artifact aliasing

Questions

1. A 62-year-old man presents with complaints of exertional dyspnea and fatigue. Cardiac examination reveals a holosystolic murmur heard best at the apex, radiating to the axilla. Echocardiography demonstrates a regurgitant jet originating from the mitral valve. Which of the following parameters is commonly used to assess the severity of mitral regurgitation and is measured at the narrowest point of the regurgitant flow?
   A. Vena contracta width
   B. Ejection fraction
   C. Aortic valve area
   D. Left atrial size
   Answer: A vena contracta width Explanation: Vena contracta width is a key parameter used in the assessment of valvular regurgitation. It represents the narrowest portion of the regurgitant jet and is measured in the color Doppler flow mapping. In the context of mitral regurgitation, a wider vena contracta is indicative of more severe regurgitation. The other options are not specifically used to assess the severity of mitral regurgitation based on vena contracta.
2. Which of the following metrics is unable to reliably indicate valvular severity?
   A. EROA
   B. RF
   C. Jet area
   D. Vena contracta
   Answer: C Jet Area Explanation: Color Doppler is able to identify presence or absence of valvular regurgitation and identify the range of velocities of the regurgitation, however, does not indicate the severity of a regurgitant lesion.
3. Which of the following echocardiographic artifacts is utilized to gauge severity of mitral regurgitation?
   A. Mirroring
   B. Aliasing
   C. Shadowing
   D. Stitching
   Answer: B Aliasing Explanation: Aliasing occurs when observed velocities are outside of the preset Nyquist limits. Identification of the aliasing velocity is integral into the PISA method to determine regurgitant lesion severity.

References

1. Chan KMJ. Functional mitral and tricuspid regurgitation: pathophysiology, assessment and treatment. Springer; 2016.
2. Dal-Bianco JP, Beaudoin J, Handschumacher MD, Levine RA. Basic mechanisms of mitral regurgitation. Can J Cardiol. 2014;30(9):971–81.
3. Spartalis M, Tzatzaki E, Spartalis E, et al. Mitral valve prolapse: an underestimated cause of sudden cardiac death—a current review of the literature. J Thorac Dis. 2017;9(12):5390–8.
4. Apostolidou E, Maslow AD, Poppas A. Primary mitral valve regurgitation: update and review. Glob Cardiol Sci Pract. 2017;2017(1):e201703.
5. Nalawade D, Borikar N, Bawaskar P, Chaurasia A. Anomalous papillary muscle insertion as a cause of mitral regurgitation: multimodality imaging-based diagnosis. Circ Cardiovasc Imaging. 2020;13(12):e010592.
6. Ginghină C, Vlădaia A, Ghiorghiu I, Serban M, Popescu BA, Jurcuţ R. Echocardiography in congenital mitral valve regurgitation—the liaison between cardiologist and surgeon. J Med Life. 2009;2(4):407–13.
7. Asgar AW, Mack MJ, Stone GW. Secondary mitral regurgitation in heart failure: pathophysiology, prognosis, and therapeutic considerations. J Am Coll Cardiol. 2015;65(12):1231–48.
8. Hahn RT. State-of-the-Art review of echocardiographic imaging in the evaluation and treatment of functional tricuspid regurgitation. Circ Cardiovasc Imaging. 2016;9(12):e005332. https://doi.org/10.1161/CIRCIMAGING.116.005332.
9. Zoghbi WA, Adams D, Bonow RO, et al. Recommendations for noninvasive evaluation of native valvular regurgitation: a report from the American Society of Echocardiography Developed in Collaboration with the Society for Cardiovascular Magnetic Resonance. J Am Soc Echocardiogr. 2017;30(4):303–71.

10. Grayburn PA, Weissman NJ, Zamorano JL. Quantitation of mitral regurgitation. Circulation. 2012;126(16):2005–17. https://doi.org/10.1161/CIRCULATIONAHA.112.121590.
11. Otto CM. Textbook of clinical echocardiography. Elsevier; 2018.
12. American Society of Echocardiography. ASE's comprehensive echocardiography. Elsevier; 2021.
13. Lin BA, Forouhar AS, Pahlevan NM, et al. Color Doppler jet area overestimates regurgitant volume when multiple jets are present. J Am Soc Echocardiogr. 2010;23(9):993–1000.
14. Zoghbi WA, Enriquez-Sarano M, Foster E, et al. American Society of Echocardiography: recommendations for evaluation of the severity of native valvular regurgitation with two-dimensional and Doppler echocardiography: a report from the American Society of Echocardiography's Nomenclature and Standards Committee and The Task Force on Valvular Regurgitation, developed in conjunction with the American College of Cardiology Echocardiography Committee, The Cardiac Imaging Committee, Council on Clinical Cardiology, The American Heart Association, and the European Society of Cardiology Working Group on Echocardiography, represented by. Eur J Echocardiogr. 2003;4(4):237–61.
15. Armstrong WF, Ryan T, Feigenbaum H. Feigenbaum's echocardiography. Wolters Kluwer; 2019.
16. Fisher MR, Forfia PR, Chamera E, et al. Accuracy of Doppler echocardiography in the hemodynamic assessment of pulmonary hypertension. Am J Respir Crit Care Med. 2009;179(7):615–21.
17. Holen J, Simonsen S. Determination of pressure gradient in mitral stenosis with Doppler echocardiography. Heart. 1979;41(5):529–35.
18. Lambert AS. Proximal isovelocity surface area should be routinely measured in evaluating mitral regurgitation: a core review. Anesth Analg. 2007;105(4):940–3.
19. Grayburn PA, Thomas JD. Basic principles of the echocardiographic evaluation of mitral regurgitation. JACC Cardiovasc Imaging. 2021;14(4):843–53.

21 Calculation of Intracardiac Pressures Using Doppler Flow

Courtney Bennett

Learning Objectives

1. Describe the principle of conservation of energy and the Bernoulli equation.
2. Understand how the Bernoulli equation can be simplified and applied to measure pressure gradients between two chambers in the heart.
3. Understand the limitations of the Bernoulli equation.
4. Know how to calculate intracardiac pressures using the measured pressure gradient and a known pressure of one cardiac chamber.

The Bernoulli Equation

The assessment of intracardiac pressures and valve stenoses by echocardiography has been validated using ultrasound Doppler signals and applying the **Bernoulli principle**, which states that in the streamline flow of fluid, the sum of all forms of energy along that path is equal (Fig. 21.1) [1–3]. This concept is also described as the conservation of energy.

Bernoulli Equation

$$P1 - P2 = \frac{1}{2}\rho\left(v2^2 - v1^2\right) + \rho\int_1^2 \frac{d\vec{v}}{dt} \times \underset{ds}{\rightarrow} + R\left(\underset{v}{\rightarrow}\right)$$

Pressure decrease = convective acceleration + flow acceleration + viscous friction.

The Bernoulli equation may be modified by assuming that the contribution from both flow acceleration and viscosity are negligible in clinical applications. The upstream velocity ($v1^2$) of blood flow is also negligible and may be excluded in most settings. Finally, the mass density of blood (ρ) of convective acceleration is a constant and equal to approximately 4. Applying these assumptions, the *simplified Bernoulli* equation can be used to estimate pressure gradients between the chambers of the heart.

Simplified Bernoulli Equation

$$P1 - P2 = 4\left(v2^2\right)$$

In the presence of valvular regurgitation or an intracardiac shunt, the peak velocity of that blood flow is proportional to the difference in pressure between the two cardiac chambers (see Fig. 21.2) [4]. If the pressure of one chamber is known, such as jugular venous pressure as right atrial pressure or the systemic blood pressure, then intracardiac pressures may be derived.

There are limitations to the application of the Bernoulli equation that are important to recognize in clinical practice. For example, if there are lesions in series, such as in the clinical scenario of concomitant left ventricular outflow tract obstruction and aortic valve stenosis, then the upstream velocity ($v1^2$) is no longer negligible

C. Bennett (✉)
Mayo Clinic College of Medicine and Science, Rochester, MN, USA
e-mail: Bennett.Courtney@mayo.edu

M. J. Lanspa, A. T. Levinson (eds.), *Echocardiography and Ultrasonography in the ICU*, Respiratory Medicine, https://doi.org/10.1007/978-3-031-80038-2_21

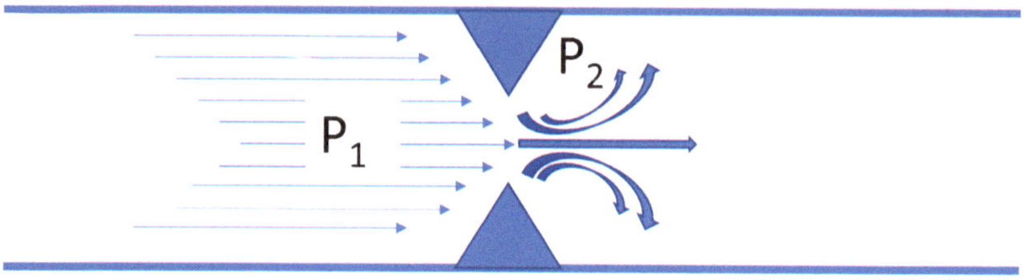

Fig. 21.1 The Bernoulli principle: The change in pressure across an orifice can be calculated by applying the concept of the conservation of energy using the Bernoulli equation

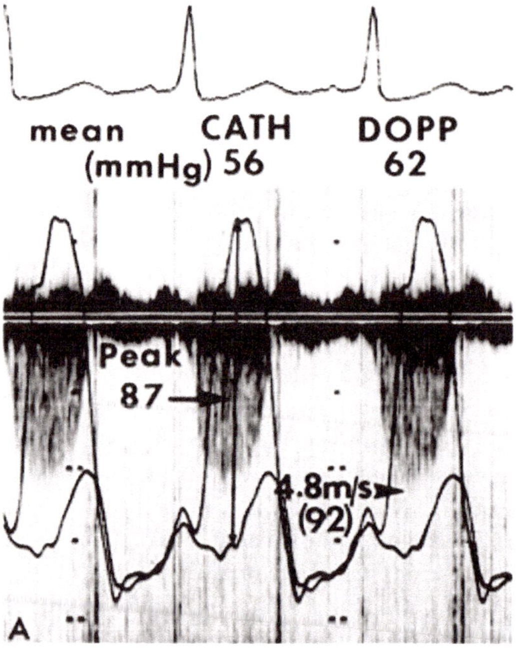

Fig. 21.2 This image shows simultaneous catheter measurements of the LA (via a transeptal approach) and LV and continuous-wave Doppler of mitral regurgitation by echocardiography. The peak gradient between the LA and LV by catheter is 87 mmHg (black arrow). The peak gradient by echocardiography using the peak velocity of 4.8 m/s (black arrowhead) is 92 mmHg. This demonstrates that the pressure difference between 2 cardiac chambers by peak catheter measurement is very similar to the calculated difference by Doppler of the regurgitant signal (Reproduced with permission from Nishimura RA, Tajik AJ). Determination of left-sided pressure gradients by utilizing Doppler aortic and mitral regurgitant signals: validation by simultaneous dual catheter and Doppler studies. J Am Coll Cardiol. 1988;11(2):317–21)

and must be applied to the equation to avoid overestimation of the downstream pressure gradient [5]. However, it is not always feasible to differentiate the velocities at each level, and therefore, hemodynamic catheterization may be necessary for workup. The other cause of increased upstream velocity may occur in the setting of increased blood flow, such as anemia or pregnancy, and needs to be taken into consideration as well. An external factor contributing to the limitations of the equation includes the accuracy of the Doppler signal, which may be faint, incomplete, or subject to poor Doppler alignment. When calculating the right ventricular systolic pressure (RVSP), there are potential errors incurred when estimating the right atrial pressure [6].

Intracardiac Pressures

Left Atrial Pressure

The left atrial pressure (LAP) may be estimated using the mitral regurgitant velocity, which occurs during systole, and the known systolic blood pressure (SBP) because the systolic blood pressure equals the left ventricular systolic pressure (LVSP) in patients *without left ventricular outflow tract obstruction*. In other words, we can use the known SBP and the calculated pressure difference between the LA and LV to solve for the LAP. It can be arranged as follows:

$$\text{LAP} = \text{SBP} - 4\left(vMR^2\right)$$

If an intraatrial shunt is present, then the maximum velocity across that shunt may be used to calculate the LAP with the addition of the right atrial pressure (RAP).

$$\text{LAP} = 4\left(vIAS^2\right) + \text{RAP}$$

Left Ventricular End-Diastolic Pressure

The left ventricular end-diastolic pressure (LVEDP) may be calculated applying the same principle as with LAP using the *end-diastolic* aortic regurgitant velocity during diastole. The aortic regurgitant velocity represents the pressure gradient between the left ventricle and the aorta. In this scenario, the calculated pressure difference between the aorta and LV is subtracted from the known aortic pressure or diastolic blood pressure (DBP) to solve for the LVEDP. It can be arranged as follows:

$$\text{LVEDP} = \text{DBP} - 4\left(vAR^2\right)$$

In addition to the above methods, diastolic tissue Doppler metrics and mitral inflow patterns can be applied to evaluate left ventricular filling pressure. The mitral inflow velocity to mitral tissue Doppler velocity ratio (E/e') has demonstrated correlation with the end-diastolic filling pressure measured by left heart catheterization.

Right Ventricular Systolic Pressure

RVSP, which occurs during systole, and the right atrial pressure. The RAP is also estimated and therefore a potential cause of error in the estimated RVSP. The calculated pressure difference between the RA and RV and the estimated RAP are added to solve for the RVSP and are arranged as follows:

$$\text{RVSP} = 4\left(vTR^2\right) + \text{RAP}$$

If there is a ventricular septal defect present, then the maximum velocity across that defect between the LV and RV plus the RAP can also be used to calculate the RVSP:

$$\text{RVSP} = 4\left(vVSD^2\right) + \text{RAP}$$

In the absence of pulmonary valve stenosis or other causes of right ventricular outflow tract obstruction, the RVSP equals the pulmonary artery systolic pressure. This can be used in the evaluation of pulmonary hypertension. Pulmonary regurgitation represents the pressure gradient between the pulmonary artery and right ventricle during diastole. Using the *end-diastolic* pulmonary regurgitant velocity with the addition of the RAP, the pulmonary artery end-diastolic pressure (PAEDP) can be calculated as follows:

$$\text{PAEDP} = 4\left(vPR^2\right) + \text{RAP}$$

Case

Doppler-derived intracardiac pressures correlate well with pressures obtained by catheterization in the laboratory. We can noninvasively assess patient hemodynamics by applying the principles discussed in this chapter.

A 70-year-old male with advanced cardiac amyloidosis and severely reduced left ventricular systolic function presents with severe shortness of breath. His blood pressure at the time of the exam is 104/68 mmHg. His echocardiogram reveals moderate tricuspid regurgitation (Fig. 21.3a) and a peak tricuspid regurgitant velocity of 2.3 m/s (Fig. 21.3b). A subcostal 4-chamber view focused on the intraatrial septum with color Doppler demonstrates left-to-right flow across a patent foramen ovale with a peak velocity of 2.0 m/s across the septum (Fig. 21.3c, d). A subcostal view of the inferior vena cava demonstrates a diameter of 29 mm and does not collapse. The interpreter estimates a RAP of 15 mmHg based on these findings. Using the equations reviewed in this chapter, we can calculate both the LAP and RVSP here:

$$\text{LAP} = 4\left(2.0^2\right) + 15 = 31\,\text{mmHg}$$

$$\text{RVSP} = 4\left(2.3^2\right) + 15 = 36\,\text{mmHg}$$

Based on these findings, the provider increased the patient's diuretic regimen and afterload reduction therapy with significant improvement in his symptoms.

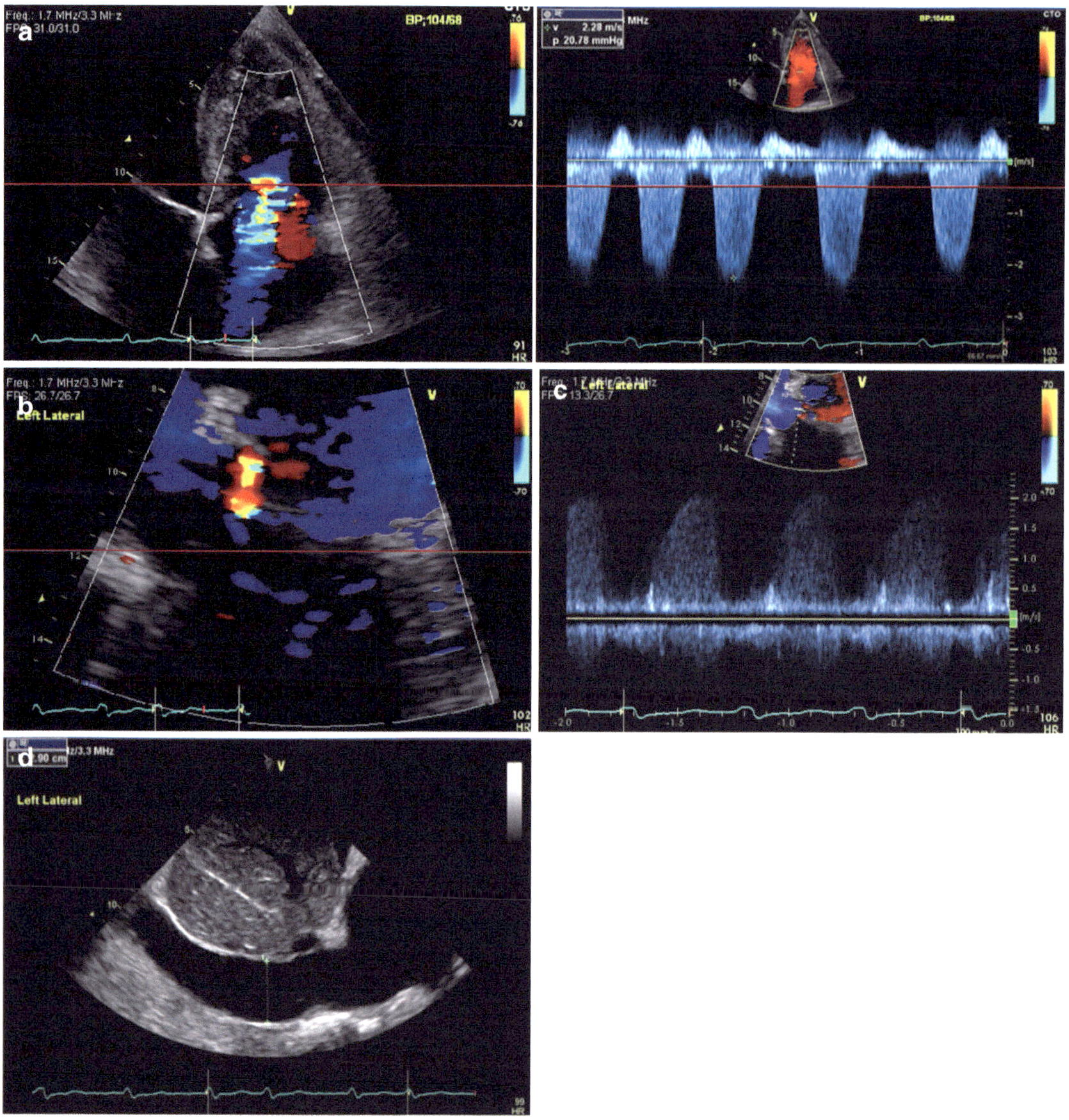

Fig. 21.3 The apical 4-chamber view focused on the right ventricle with color Doppler demonstrating moderate tricuspid regurgitation (**a**). The peak TR velocity is 2.3 m/s (**b**). A PFO is seen with left-to-right flow by color Doppler (**c**) with a peak Doppler velocity of 2.0 m/s (**d**). The IVC is dilated with <50% collapse correlating with an estimated RAP of 10–20 mmHg

Summary Points

- The assessment of intracardiac pressures and valve stenoses by echocardiography has utilized ultrasound Doppler signals.
- Calculations apply the **Bernoulli principle**, which states that in the streamline flow of fluid, the sum of all forms of energy along that path are equal.
- Intracardiac pressures are obtained using the measured pressure gradient and a known pressure of one cardiac chamber.

References

1. Hatle L. Noninvasive measurements of intracardiac blood flow velocities with Doppler ultrasound. Acta Med Scand. 1987;221(2):133–6.
2. Yock PG, Popp RL. Noninvasive evaluation of intracardiac pressures using Doppler ultrasound: a case study of panvalvular regurgitation. Clin Cardiol. 1985;8(11):565–71.
3. Nishimura RA, Miller FA Jr, Callahan MJ, Benassi RC, Seward JB, Tajik AJ. Doppler echocardiography: theory, instrumentation, technique, and application. Mayo Clin Proc. 1985;60(5):321–43.
4. Nishimura RA, Tajik AJ. Determination of left-sided pressure gradients by utilizing Doppler aortic and mitral regurgitant signals: validation by simultaneous dual catheter and Doppler studies. J Am Coll Cardiol. 1988;11(2):317–21.
5. Scantlebury DC, Geske JB, Nishimura RA. Limitations of Doppler echocardiography in the evaluation of serial stenoses. Circ Cardiovasc Imaging. 2013;6(5):850–2.
6. Finkelhor RS, Lewis SA, Pillai D. Limitations and strengths of doppler/echo pulmonary artery systolic pressure-right heart catheterization correlations: a systematic literature review. Echocardiography. 2015;32(1):10–8.

22 Prosthetic Valves

Gloria A. Ayuba and Vera Rigolin

Abbreviations

2D	Two-dimensional
3D	Three-dimensional
AT	Acceleration time
CW	Continuous wave Doppler
DI	Dimensionless index
EOA	Effective orifice area
PLAX	Parasternal long axis
PSAX	Parasternal short axis
PW	Pulsed wave Doppler
TEE	Transesophageal echocardiography
TTE	Transthoracic echocardiography

Supplementary Information The online version contains supplementary material available at https://doi.org/10.1007/978-3-031-80038-2_22.

G. A. Ayuba
Department of Medicine/Division of Cardiology, UT Southwestern, Dallas, USA
e-mail: gloria.ayuba@nm.org

V. Rigolin (✉)
Northwestern University Feinberg School of Medicine, Chicago, IL, USA

Department of Medicine, Bluhm Cardiovascular Institute, Northwestern University Feinberg School of Medicine, Chicago, IL, USA
e-mail: vrigolin@nm.org

General Imaging Principles

Echocardiography is the primary imaging modality used to evaluate prosthetic heart valves. A complete echocardiographic study in patients with prosthetic valves includes assessment of chamber sizes, systolic and diastolic ventricular function, and wall thickness in addition to evaluation of the prosthesis itself using 2D, Doppler, and 3D imaging techniques if available [1, 2].

Prosthetic valves have varying flow profiles depending on the valve type and size and have some degree of obstruction inherent to their design compared to normal native valves. So, it is important to obtain and report clinical information, including type and size of prosthetic valve, surgery date, blood pressure, heart rate, age, height, weight, and body surface area when available to allow for appropriate and accurate assessment and comprehensive reporting.

Consulting published guidelines and standards Data on normal hemodynamics of different prosthetic valves is critical to determining if the function of a specific prosthetic valve is normal [2].

Baseline prosthetic structure and function should be evaluated 1–3 months after the implantation to allow for normalization of hemodynamics and loading conditions [1]. This provides a baseline to which subsequent imaging may be compared for change.

Echo assessment should include evaluation of structural features such as mobility of the leaflets and/or sewing ring, interrogating for

M. J. Lanspa, A. T. Levinson (eds.), *Echocardiography and Ultrasonography in the ICU*, Respiratory Medicine, https://doi.org/10.1007/978-3-031-80038-2_22

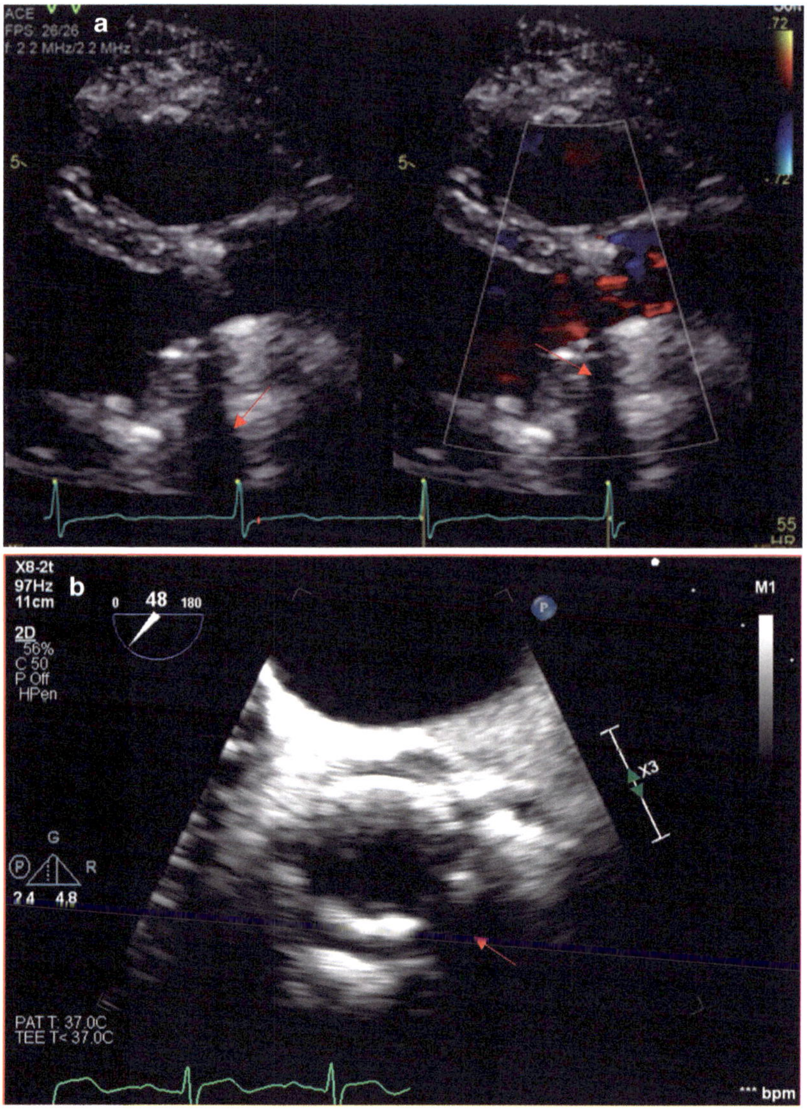

Fig. 22.1 Posterior acoustic shadow artifact (arrow) seen on TTE created by the bioprosthetic aortic valve (panel **a**). There is adequate visualization of posterior region of the prosthesis when imaged using TEE. However, note the anterior shadow artifact on the TEE image (arrow) (Panel **b**)

complications including valve thrombus, pannus in growth, vegetations, abscesses, or fistulas, and hemodynamic assessment including evaluation of peak velocity, peak/mean gradients, effective orifice area, valve regurgitation, and stroke volume.

Adequate echocardiographic evaluation using multiple windows by transthoracic echocardiography (TTE) is necessary and, if suboptimal, may require the use of transesophageal echocardiography (TEE) for better visualization given better axial resolution, particularly in the evaluation of prosthesis-associated complications such as endocarditis, thrombus or pannus ingrowth, and regurgitation, where visualization may be limited by acoustic shadowing or reverberation.

TTE and TEE can be complementary in aortic prosthetic valve assessment where shadowing and reverberations limit adequate assessment of the posterior and anterior aspects of the valve, respectively, and so assessment with both modalities may be needed for adequate visualization of the entire valve for complications such as perivalvular leaks [2] (Fig. 22.1).

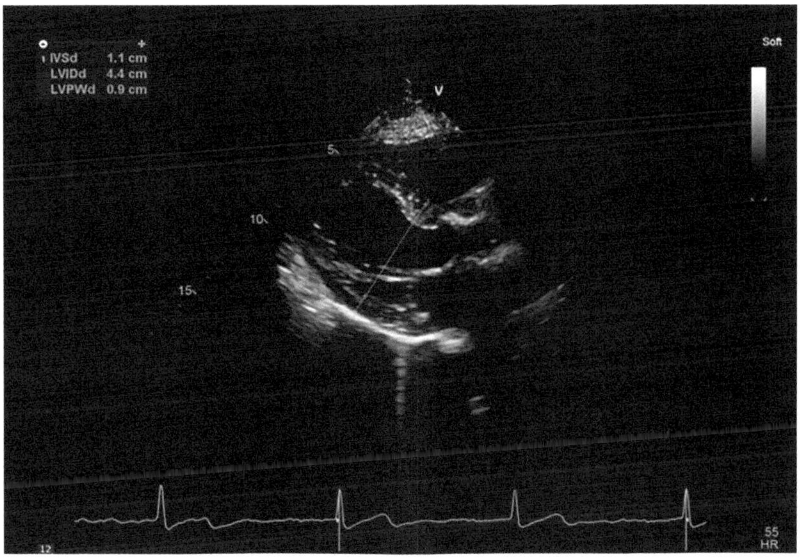

Fig. 22.2 Linear measurements in the parasternal long axis view of interventricular septal thickness, LV end diastolic internal dimension and posterior wall thickness are standard echo measurements for all patients with valvular heart disease. Although not shown in this image, LV end systolic internal dimension is also a standard measurement

2D Imaging

2D imaging assessment by TTE or TEE should include evaluation of chamber sizes, wall thickness, biventricular function (Figs. 22.2 and 22.3), prosthetic valve position, leaflet mobility, and sewing ring appearance during the entire cardiac cycle.

3D Imaging

3D Echo allows for visualization and assessment of the complex geometric shape of the heart and visualization of prosthetic valves from any perspective.

It is useful to identify the mechanisms of prosthetic dysfunction and can help localize pathology and guide transcatheter-based interventions in prosthetic valve disease. Left ventricular (LV) volumes and LV ejection fraction measurements are also more reproducible when calculated using 3D echo rather than 2D echo.

Doppler Evaluation

Doppler assessment of prosthetic valves is useful in the identification and evaluation of prosthetic valve dysfunction. Color Doppler identifies regurgitant lesions and areas of turbulent flow. Spectral Doppler (with pulsed wave (PW) and continuous wave (CW)) measures the peak velocity across the valve, peak/mean gradients, acceleration time (AT) (in the evaluation of aortic prosthesis), dimensionless index (DI), and pressure half time (of regurgitant aortic jets or stenotic mitral prostheses) and provides the data to calculate effective orifice area (EOA).

The peak velocity and gradients across a valve are determined by the valve type, valve size, and flow rate, and obtaining information on the implanted prosthesis allows appropriate contextual interpretation.

The peak gradient across prosthetic valves is calculated by the simplified Bernoulli equation [2].

Peak pressure gradient = $4 \times V^2$ [2], where V = peak velocity of jet (m/s). The mean gradient is the average gradient across the valve during systole or diastole, depending on the valve. This is obtained by averaging the instantaneous gradients over the ejection period and is usually calculated by the ultrasound system measurement package from the traced Doppler velocity curve.

Stroke volume is calculated by multiplying the velocity time integral (VTI) of the left ventricular outflow tract (LVOT) obtained with PW Doppler by the cross-sectional area (CSA) of the LVOT.

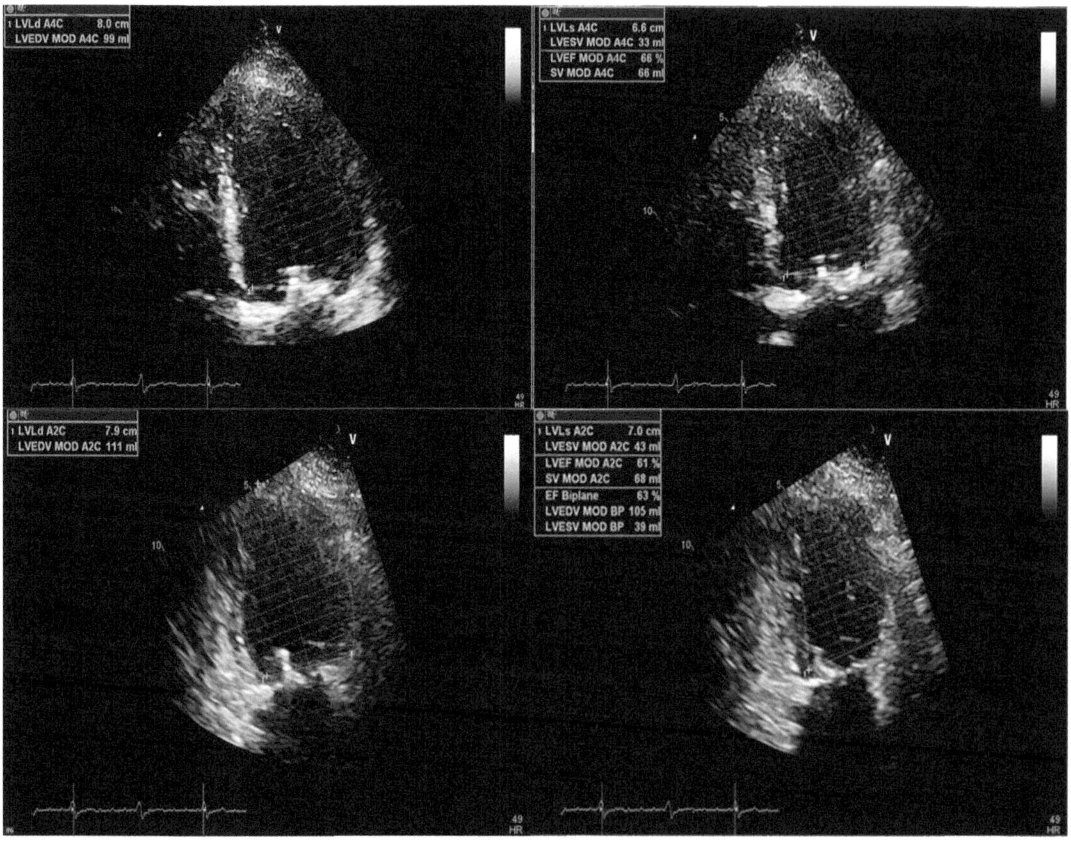

Fig. 22.3 2D LV end-diastolic and end-systolic volumes are acquired from the 4 and 2 chamber apical views. LV ejection fraction is then calculated using the Simpson's biplane method using the traced volumes

$$SV = VTI_{lvot} \times CSA_{lvot}$$

The effective orifice area (EOA) of a prosthesis is calculated using the continuity equation:

$$EOA = \text{Stroke volume} / VTIpv$$

The dimensionless index (DI) for prosthetic AV assessment is the ratio of the LVOT VTI/AV VTI, and the DI of a mitral valve prosthesis is derived from the ratio of MV VTI/LVOT VTI. Note that the continuity equation is the preferred method to calculate EOA in both AV and MV prostheses. Although pressure half-time is useful to determine the presence of prosthetic MV dysfunction, it should not be used to calculate EOA.

Role of TEE

TEE should be considered when there is suboptimal or non-diagnostic assessment of prosthetic valves by TTE, particularly when there is a concern for dysfunction. It is useful in the assessment of the etiology and mechanism of prosthetic stenosis and regurgitation and is used in transcatheter-based intervention planning and management.

TEE should be used in the assessment of complications of infective endocarditis or if there is a clinical concern for endocardial lead involvement. It may also be considered for evaluation of patients with prosthetic valves with persistent fever of unknown etiology or patients with staph aureus bacteremia without a known source to rule out infective endocarditis [1].

Overview of Types of Prosthetic Valves

Over the last six decades, prosthetic valves have been designed with the goal of having characteristics that are like native valves, including excellent durability, hemodynamics, and low thrombogenicity. At this time, no perfect valve exists, and all prosthetic valves have some inherent obstruction compared to normal native valves.

Prosthetic valves are broadly grouped into mechanical or bioprosthetic valves.

There are several makes and models of bioprosthetic valves. Some are made to be implanted surgically and can be stented or stentless. Others are implanted percutaneously (Fig. 22.4).

Mechanical valves consist of bileaflet, single tilting disc, or caged-ball valves. The latter is no longer implanted but can be seen in some patients who underwent surgery prior to 2007 (Fig. 22.5).

The choice of prosthetic types in patients is determined by several factors, including patient age, preference, valve size, expected hemodynamics, risks of long-term anticoagulation with mechanical valves, and limited durability requiring repeat interventions in the case of bioprosthetic valves.

Physiologic Regurgitation and Microcavitations

Mechanical valves have a built-in physiologic regurgitation that is important to recognize and be able to differentiate from pathologic regurgitation.

Bileaflet mechanical valves have two semilunar disks with opening angles from 75 to 90 degrees

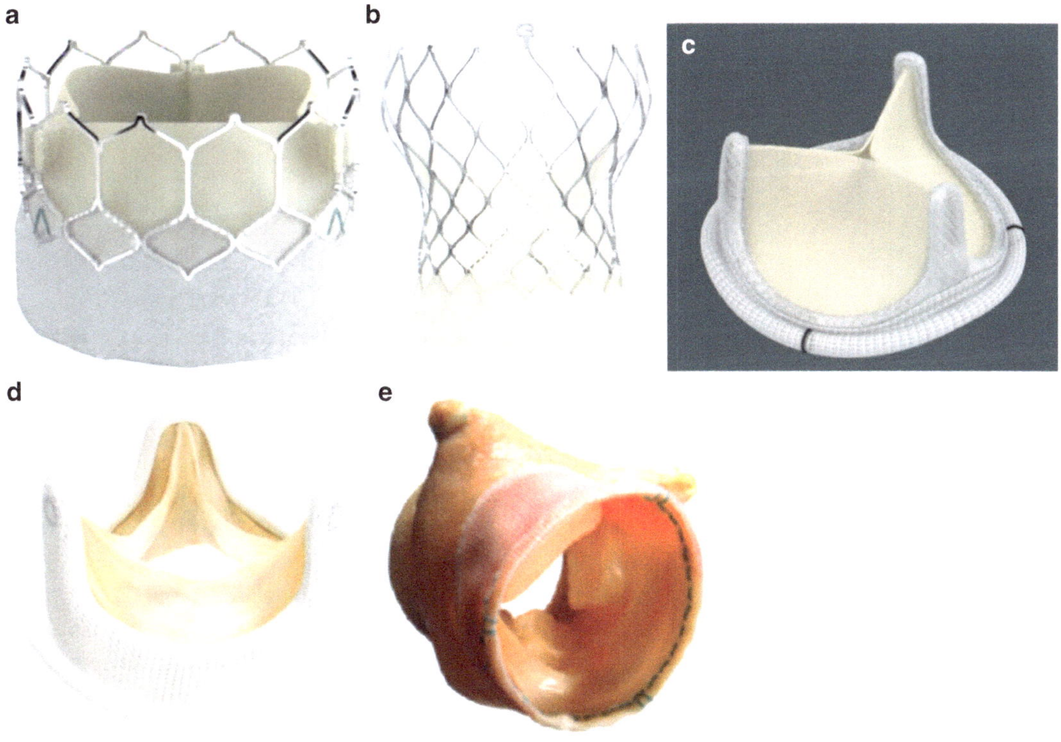

Fig. 22.4 The common types of commercially available bioprosthetic valves are shown. (**a**) Percutaneous balloon expandable bioprosthesis (Edwards Sapien); (**b**) self-expandable percutaneous bioprosthesis (Medtronic Evolut R); (**c**) stented pericardial bioprosthesis (Perimount Magna Ease); (**d**) stented porcine bioprosthesis (Medtronic Mosaic); (**e**) stentless porcine bioprosthesis (Medtronic Freestyle)

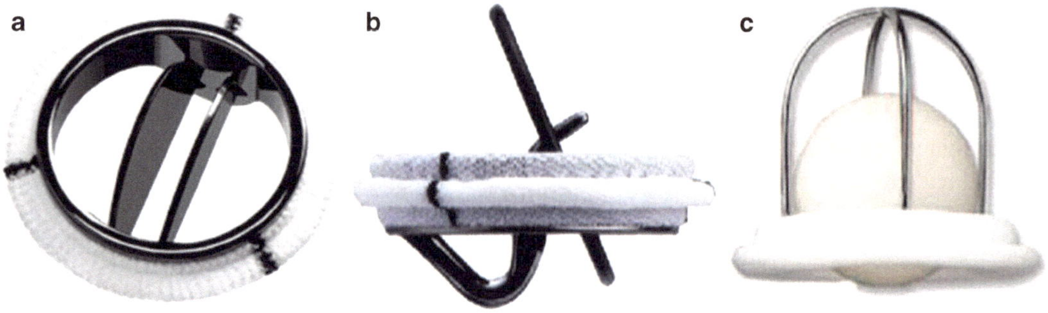

Fig. 22.5 The common types of commercially available mechanical valves are shown. (**a**) Bileaflet mechanical valve (St Jude Medical Regent); (**b**) Single leaflet mechanical valve (Medtronic Hall); (**c**) caged ball valve (Starr-Edwards)

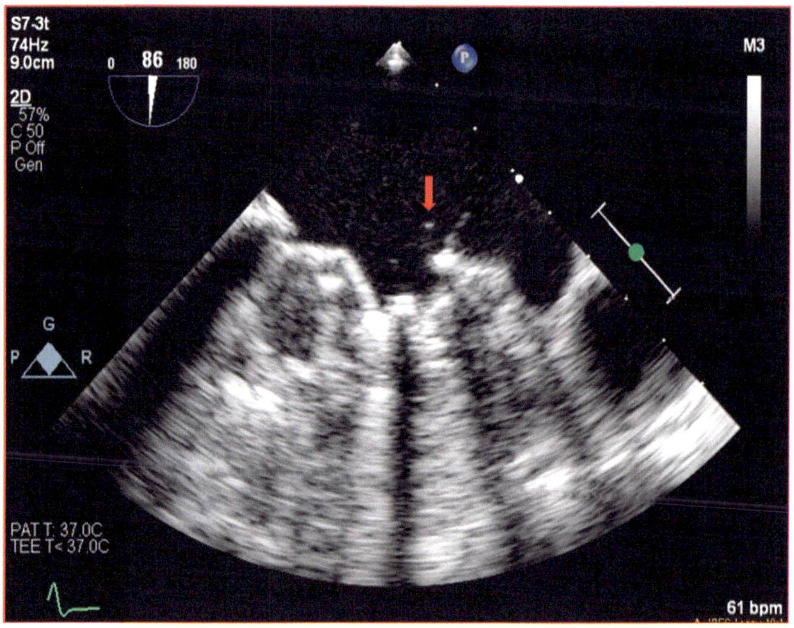

Fig. 22.6 TEE image showing microcavitations in left atrium (arrow) in patient with a mechanical bileaflet prosthetic valve in the mitral position

with three orifices noted when the valve opens and typically three built-in washing jets (physiologic regurgitation) when it closes, which is thought to prevent thrombi at sites of stasis on the valve [2, 3]. Monoleaflet valves have a single disk attached to a metal strut with an opening angle from 60 to 80 degrees with two orifices noted when it opens and a single midline built-in physiologic regurgitation when it closes [3]. The ball-shaped occluder in caged ball valves, such as the Star Edwards valve is difficult to visualize on echo, but closure of the valve, creates a small closing volume.

Microcavitations may be seen in the ventricle or atrium and appear as echo-bright bubbles that occur during the opening and closing of a mechanical valve (Figs. 22.6, 22.7 with corresponding Video 22.1). This occurs because of the vaporization of blood due to a rapid drop in pressure at the site closure of the sewing ring and prosthetic occluder [4]. These gaseous microbubbles are seen with mechanical valves and are more common in the mitral position and usually do not reflect any pathology but may be misdiagnosed as vegetation.

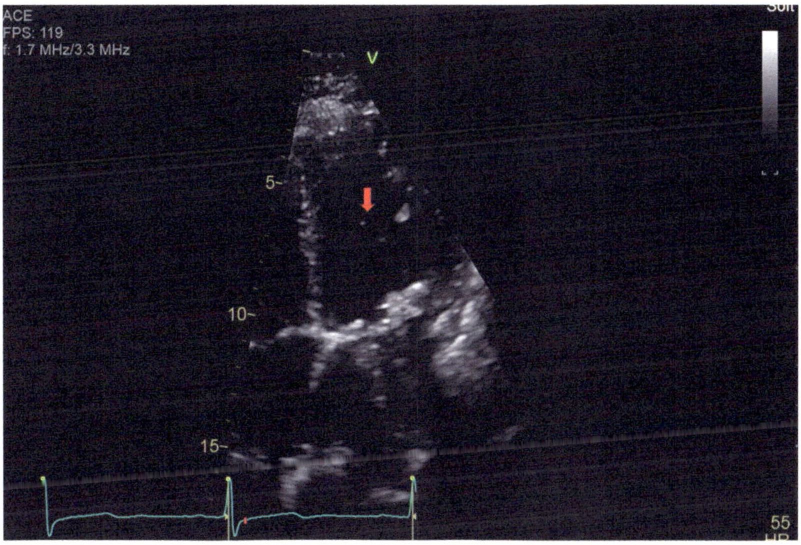

Fig. 22.7 TTE image showing microcavitations in the left ventricle (arrow) of a patient with a mechanical bileaflet prosthetic valve in the mitral position

Evaluation of Prosthetic Aortic Valves Using Echocardiography Using Illustrative Case Examples

The TTE evaluation of a patient with an AV prosthesis requires a comprehensive 2D and Doppler assessment of cardiac structure and function. The specific spectral Doppler parameters essential to assess aortic prostheses are listed in Table 22.1. Case examples will be used to illustrate how to utilize echocardiographic tools to assess prosthetic valve function.

Evaluation of Prosthetic Aortic Valves

Case 1

Patient with normal functioning bioprosthetic valve in the aortic position.

2D Evaluation

2D TTE includes a comprehensive assessment of ventricular chambers in addition to valve position and leaflet mobility. Videos 22.2 and 22.3 show that the aortic bioprosthesis appears well seated and has normal systolic leaflet excursion.

Doppler Evaluation

Color Doppler is useful to detect areas of turbulence and regurgitation. Note the laminar flow across the aortic prosthesis without turbulence or regurgitation shown in Fig. 22.8 with corresponding Video 22.4.

The first step in the hemodynamic assessment of the aortic prosthesis is measuring the diameter of the left ventricular outflow tract (LVOT). This is then followed by using CW and PW Doppler to measure peak velocity and gradients followed by calculation of the effective orifice area (EOA) and dimensionless index (DI).

The hemodynamic assessment of aortic prosthetic valve function using spectral Doppler is illustrated in Fig. 22.9.

Prosthetic Aortic Valve Dysfunction: Stenosis

Pathologic stenosis of prosthetic valves can occur due to obstructive thrombus, pannus ingrowth, malfunction of mechanical occluders, or because of degenerative processes of bioprosthetic valves over time (Figs. 22.10 and 22.11). Careful spec-

Table 22.1 Spectral Doppler parameters required for the evaluation of aortic prosthetic function

Parameter	Normal	Possible stenosis	Suggests significant stenosis
Peak velocity (m/s)	<3	3–4	>4
Mean gradient (mmHg)	<20	20–35	>35
Acceleration Time (ms)	<80	80–100	>100
Contour of jet velocity through the PrAV	Early peaking, triangular	Triangular to intermediate	Rounded
Dimensionless index (DI)	≥0.30	0.25–0.29	<0.25
Effective orifice area (EOA)	>1.2	0.8–1.2	<0.8

Adapted from Zoghbi et al. [2]

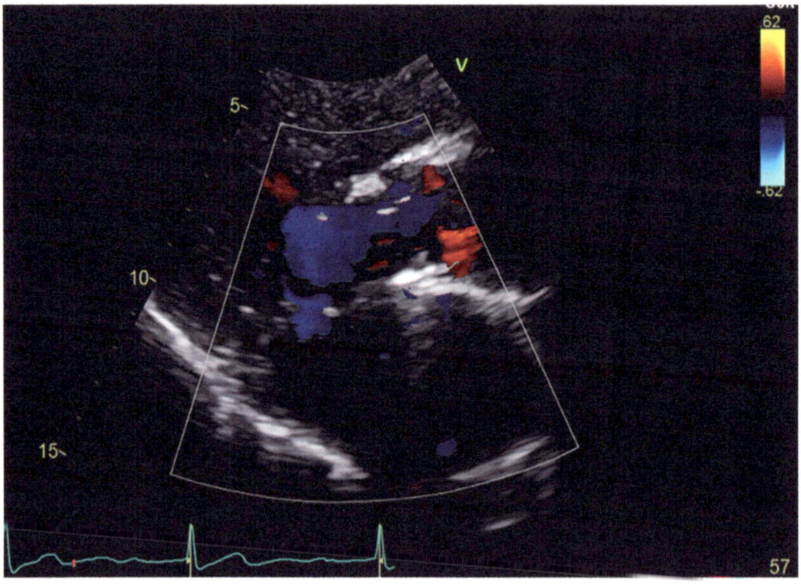

Fig. 22.8 End-systolic frame of a Color Doppler image of the aortic prosthesis showing normal laminar flow

tral Doppler evaluation can help determine the presence of stenosis (Fig. 22.12).

Case 2

85 y.o. female with aortic AV replacement 17 years prior who presented with a complaint of progressive exertional dyspnea.

2D imaging using TTE demonstrates an aortic bioprosthesis with thickened leaflets and reduced leaflet excursion (Videos 22.5 and 22.6). Spectral Doppler assessment demonstrates severe bioprosthetic AV stenosis (Fig. 22.13).

Elevated velocities and gradients across prosthetic aortic valves may not always represent pathologic obstruction. Patients may have high transvalvular gradients with a normally functioning prosthesis. This can occur in a high-flow state or when the effective orifice area is insufficient in meeting the cardiac output demand and is referred to as patient–prosthesis mismatch and may be associated with reduced short- and long-term survival [2, 5, 6].

Prosthetic Aortic Valve Dysfunction: Regurgitation

Case 3

72 y.o. male with a history of severe symptomatic aortic stenosis deemed high risk for surgical AV replacement who underwent a transcatheter aortic valve replacement (TAVR) 2 months prior. He presented with decompensated heart failure and had a TTE and TEE performed for evaluation of his AV prosthesis and paravalvular regurgitation.

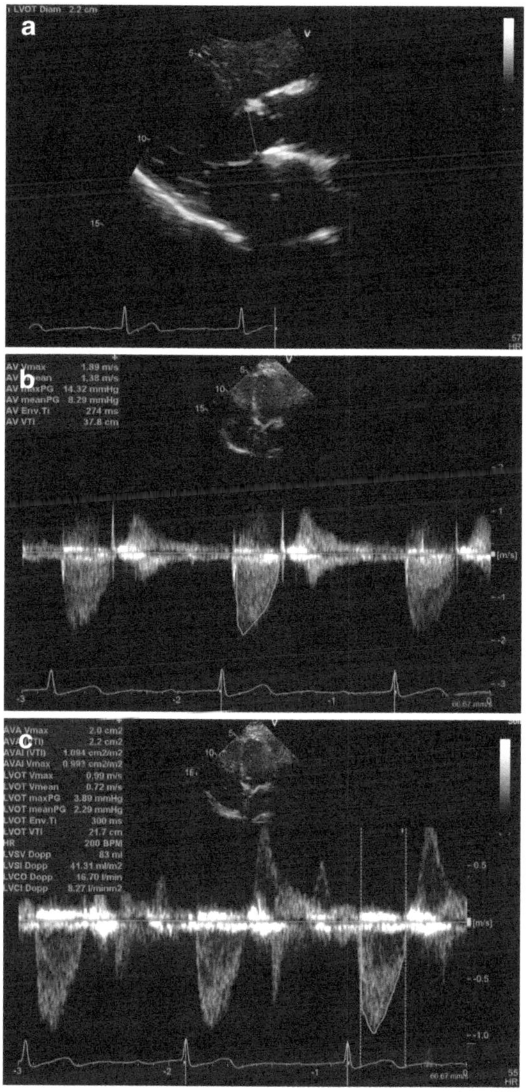

Fig. 22.9 Step by step analysis of aortic prosthetic valve function. Panel A: LVOT diameter is measured from junction of the interventricular septum and sewing ring to junction between anterior mitral leaflet and posterior sewing ring. Panel B: CW Doppler of the AV prosthesis. Panel C: PW Doppler of the LVOT

Measured variables suggest normal prosthetic valve function:

Peak velocity = 1.9 m/s; Mean gradient = 8.3 mmHg

Calculated EOA = LVOT Area × LVOT VTI ÷ AV VTI = 2.2 cm^2

Dimensionless index = LVOT VTI ÷ AV VTI = 21.7 cm ÷ 37.8 cm = 0.57

TEE color Doppler images show paravalvular regurgitation with a posterior origin surrounding a balloon-expandable percutaneous valve (Videos 22.7 and 22.8).

The presence and severity of pathologic paravalvular or transvalvular prosthetic regurgitation can be challenging to evaluate due to the difficulty visualizing color jets due to acoustic shadowing, the often serpiginous nature, and the eccentricity of paravalvular regurgitation.

Evaluation by echo should include the assessment of prosthesis position and stent/leaflet morphology in multiple views to identify the etiology or mechanism of regurgitation. Imaging should also include an adequate sweep of the prosthesis to identify the origin and location of the regurgitant jet using color Doppler. Grading the severity should include the use of color and spectral Doppler and 3D imaging assessment as recommended in published guidelines [7].

Specific parameters essential to grading the severity of aortic regurgitation following TAVR or percutaneous prosthetic valve repair are listed in Table 22.2.

Studies have shown a higher incidence of paravalvular regurgitation in transcatheter aortic valve replacement compared to surgical aortic valve replacement, and this has been shown to have an impact on clinical outcomes with an increased risk of recurrent hospitalization, cardiac death, and all-cause mortality with worsening severity [8, 9].

Evaluation of Prosthetic Mitral Valves

The TTE evaluation of a patient with an MV prosthesis requires a comprehensive 2D and Doppler assessment of cardiac structure and function. The specific spectral Doppler parameters essential to assess mitral prostheses are listed in Table 22.3.

Case 4

Patient with a history of symptomatic acute severe mitral regurgitation due to a spontaneous papillary muscle rupture who underwent an emergent MV replacement with a bioprosthetic valve.

TEE obtained intraoperatively following MV replacement shows a well-seated bioprosthetic

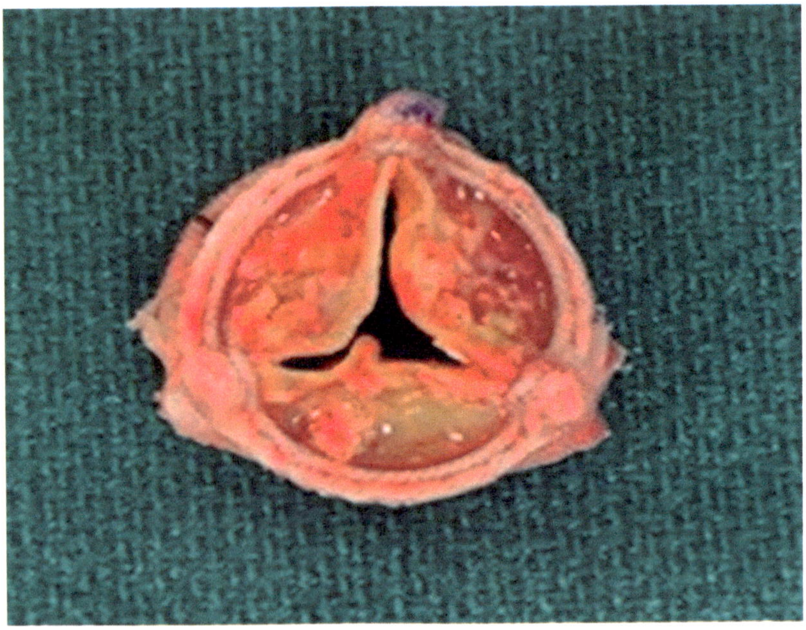

Fig. 22.10 Surgical specimen of excised degenerative calcific bioprosthetic aortic valve (Courtesy of S. Christopher Malaisrie, MD)

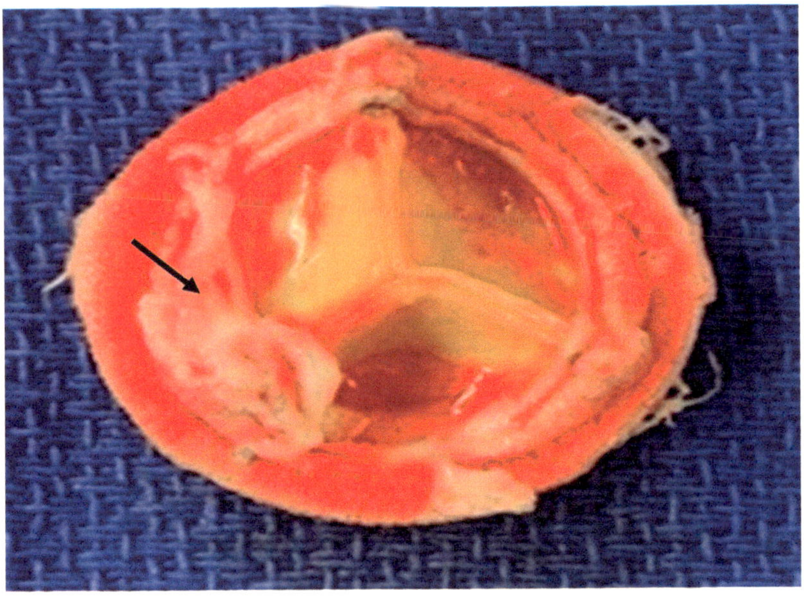

Fig. 22.11 Surgical specimen of excised bioprosthetic aortic valve with pannus ingrowth (arrow) resulting in pathologic obstruction (Courtesy of S. Christopher Malaisrie, MD)

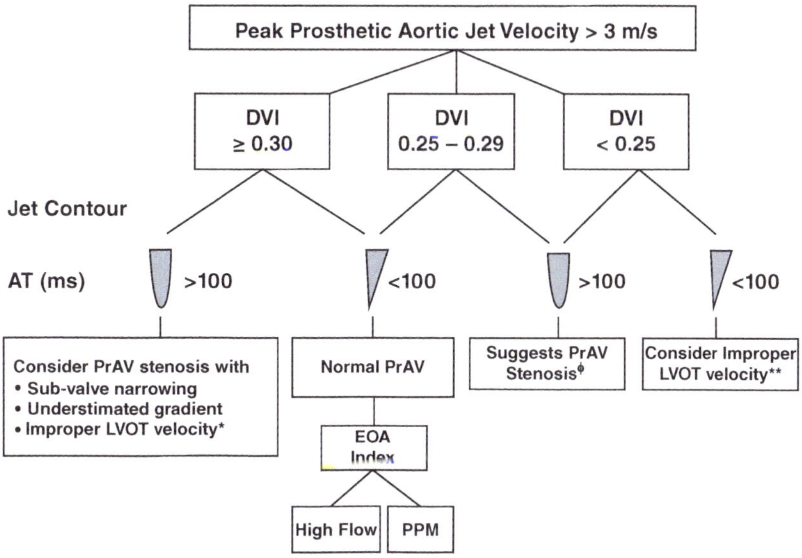

Fig. 22.12 Algorithm for evaluation of aortic valve prosthesis. Adapted with permission from Zoghbi et al. [2]

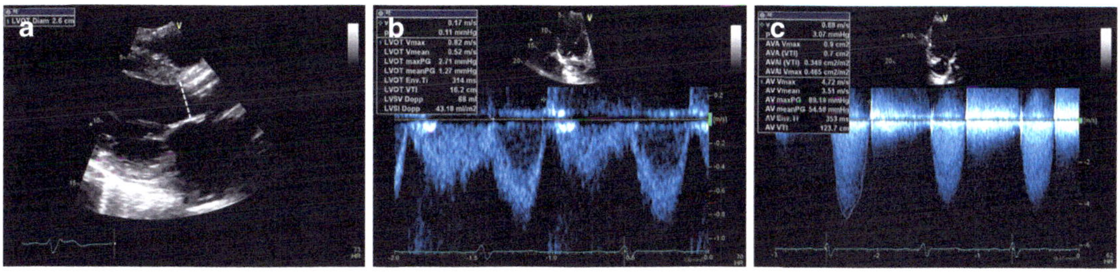

Fig. 22.13 Evaluation of parameters for prosthetic AV function assessment consistent with severe prosthetic stenosis. Panel A: Measurement of the LVOT diameter. Panel B: PW Doppler of the LVOT. Panel C: CW Doppler of the aortic valve prosthesis

Measured variable suggest severe bioprosthetic aortic stenosis

Calculated EOA = LVOT Area X LVOT VTI ÷ AV VTI = 0.7 cm^2

Dimensionless index = LVOT VTI ÷ AV VTI 16.2 cm ÷ 123.7 cm = 0.13

Mean gradient = 55 mmHg; Peak velocity = 4.72 m/s

Acceleration Time: 108 ms

Table 22.2 Doppler Parameters required for evaluation of aortic regurgitation after TAVR

	Mild AR	Moderate AR	Severe AR
Vena contracta width (cm)	<0.3	0.31–0.59	>0.6
Vena contracta area (cm^2)	<0.10	0.11–0.29	≥0.30
Circumferential extent (%)	<10	11–29	≥30%
Flow convergence	Small or absent	Intermediate	Large
PHT (ms)	>500	200–500	<200
Diastolic flow reversal in descending aorta	Absent or brief	Brief	Prominent holodiastolic flow reversal
Regurgitant volume (ml)	<30	30–59	≥60
Regurgitant fraction (%)	<30	30–49	≥50
EROA (cm^2)	<0.1	0.1–0.29	≥0.3

Adapted from Zoghbi et al. [7]

Table 22.3 Spectral Doppler parameters required for evaluation of mitral prosthetic function

	Normal	Possible stenosis	Significant stenosis
PHT (ms)	<130	130–200	>200
Peak velocity (m/s)	<1.9	1.9–2.5	>2.5
Mean gradient (mmHg)	≤5	6–10	>10
DI: VTI_{prMV}/VTI_{lvot}	<2.2	2.2–2.5	>2.5
EOA (cm^2)	≥2.0	1–2	<1

Adapted from Zoghbi et al. [2]

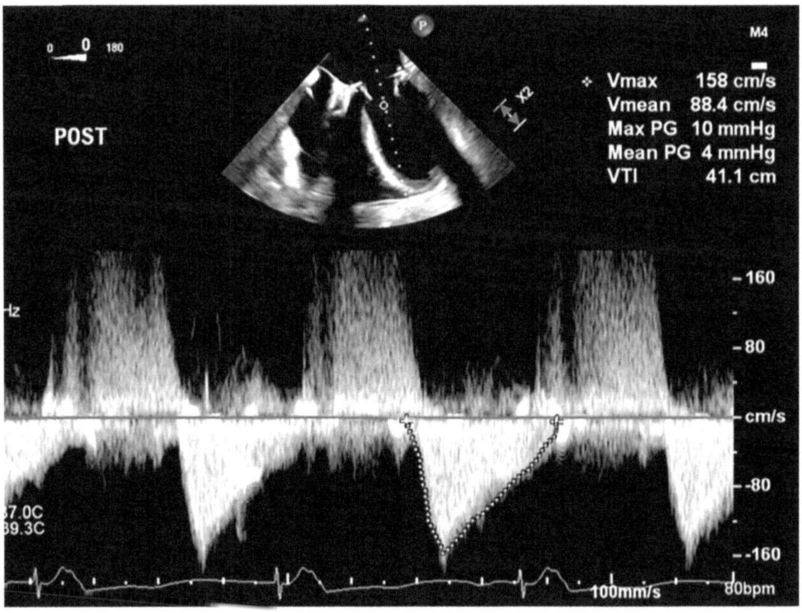

Fig. 22.14 CW Doppler assessment of a bioprosthetic mitral valve showing normal prosthetic gradient

MV with normal diastolic leaflet excursion and laminar flow across the prosthesis (Videos 22.9 and 22.10) and normal prosthetic hemodynamic assessment by spectral Doppler evaluation (Fig. 22.14) consistent with a normal functioning MV prosthesis.

Prosthetic Mitral Valve Dysfunction: Stenosis

Case 5

Patient who presented with acute decompensated heart failure. Echo demonstrated severe bioprosthetic mitral stenosis (Figs. 22.15 and 22.16 with corresponding Videos 22.11 and 22.12). The patient underwent a subsequent transcatheter valve-in-valve procedure given the elevated risk for a redo MV surgery (Fig. 22.17).

Gated CT can complement echo imaging for the evaluation of leaflets/occluder motion and visualization of potential causes of prosthetic valve dysfunction such as thrombus, vegetation, or pannus formation [2].

Prosthetic Mitral Valve Dysfunction: Regurgitation

Case 6

56 y.o. male with history of mechanical mitral valve replacement presenting with fever of 101.2 °F and chills × 3 days with positive blood cultures for staph aureus.

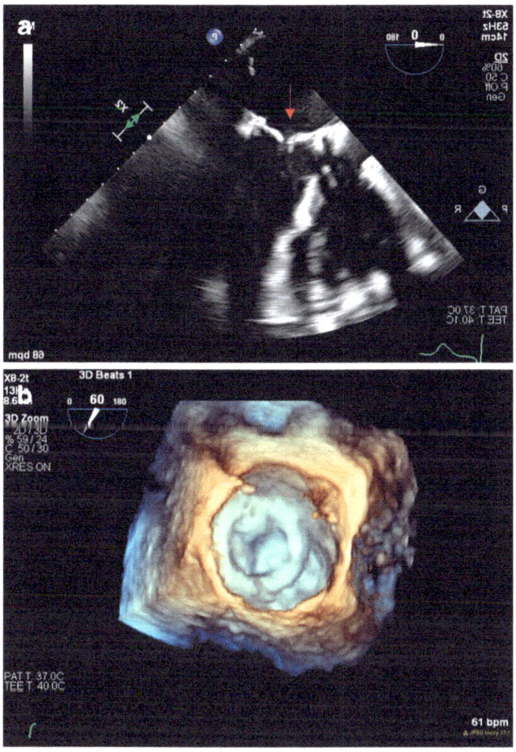

Fig. 22.15 Examples of stenotic mitral prostheses: Panel A: TEE showing a calcified stenotic bioprosthetic mitral valve with restricted leaflet opening at end diastole (arrow). Panel B: 3D image of a mitral valve prosthesis with restricted leaflet motion at end diastole

Given clinical concern for endocarditis, he underwent a TEE, which showed dehiscence of his bi-leaflet mechanical mitral valve with significant perivalvular regurgitation along the lateral aspect of the prosthetic valve (Fig. 22.18, Videos 22.13, 22.14, 22.15 and 22.16).

Evaluation of Prosthetic Pulmonic and Tricuspid Valves

Although data on right-sided prosthetic valves are limited, the same principles and concepts of prosthetic evaluation and native valve dysfunction govern their assessment.

Prosthetic Valve Endocarditis

Prosthetic valve endocarditis occurs due to microbial infection of a prosthesis and may present as vegetation characterized by an oscillating mass on the valve or supporting structures, dehiscence of the valve with new valvular regurgitation, or abscess formation. The estimated in-hospital mortality rate remains at 15–20%; thus, accurate and timely diagnosis to enable prompt and effective management is vital [10].

The modified Duke criteria is the current standard for the diagnosis of infective endocarditis and includes pathologic, imaging, and clinical findings [10–12].

Case 7

Patient with endocarditis of a bioprosthetic AV (Fig. 22.19 with corresponding Videos 22.17 and 22.18).

Prosthetic valve endocarditis has a lower incidence of vegetations compared to native valves and has a higher incidence of annular abscess and paravalvular complications, so the threshold for early TEE assessment in these patients should be low [11, 13].

Annular abscess is a life-threatening complication that requires surgical management and is associated with conduction disease resulting in heart block and a mortality rate of ≥40% [11, 13] (Fig. 22.20 with corresponding Videos 22.19, 22.20, 22.21 and 22.22).

Other indications for early surgery for patients with infective endocarditis include heart failure, persistent bacteremia, infection with highly resistant organisms, or recurrent emboli with persistent vegetations [1, 11, 13].

Recognizing normal structure and function of prosthetic valves is important to help identify the presence of dysfunction or pathology. The aortic root may be thickened in the early months (3–6 months) following aortic valve replacement due to postop hematoma and edema, which may be mistaken for an aortic root abscess. As such, corroboration with an early post-operative study is beneficial [2] (Fig. 22.21).

PET/CT is useful for evaluating patients with equivocal TEE findings and assessing complications such as annular abscess, as it is less affected by shadow artifacts that may be seen on ultrasound [2, 11].

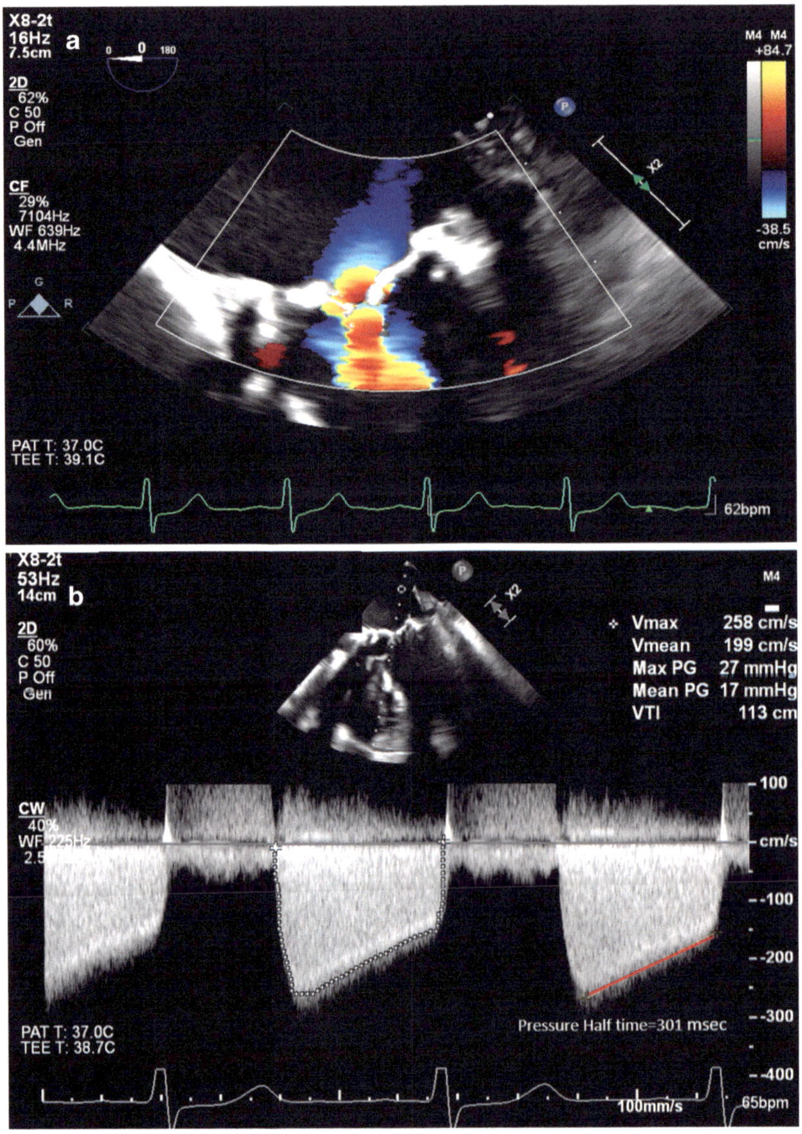

Fig. 22.16 Diastolic flow acceleration across the MV prosthesis (Panel A). Spectral Doppler of the mitral prosthesis showing a peak velocity of 2.6 m/s, a mean gradient of 17 mmHg at HR 65 bpm, VTI = 113 ms and pressure half time of 301 ms (Panel B). Not shown are the LVOT VTI = 25 cm and LVOT diameter = 2.3 cm that are used to calculate the SV of LVOT = 104 ml. The Dimensionless index: MV VTI/LVOT VTI (113 ÷ 25 = 4.5). In the absence of significant mitral and aortic regurgitation, the SV of LVOT can be used to calculate the MV EOA. EOA = SV/VTIpv = 104/113 = 0.9 cm^2. All parameters point to severe stenosis

Prosthetic Valve Thrombosis

Mechanical Valve Thrombosis

The annual rate of prosthetic valve thrombosis with mechanical valves ranges from 0.1% to 5.7% [1]. Mechanical valve thrombosis can occur acutely or subacutely, resulting in valve dysfunction, and is typically associated with subtherapeutic anticoagulation with a vitamin K antagonist (VKA). Patients may present with shortness of breath due to acute valve dysfunction or embolic phenomena.

Mechanical valves require the use of lifelong anticoagulation with a VKA at an appropriate

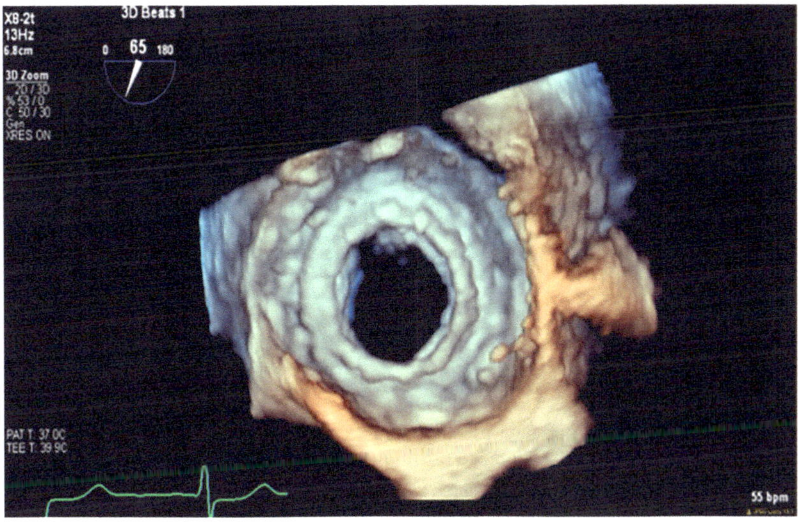

Fig. 22.17 3D image of new bioprosthetic valve within old prosthesis (valve-in-valve) with noted non-restricted pliable leaflets at end diastole

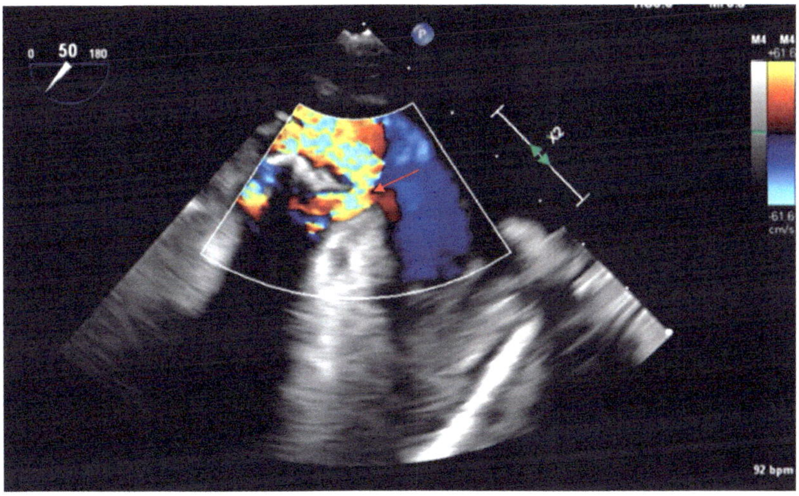

Fig. 22.18 TEE image with the arrow showing lateral periprosthetic mitral regurgitation at the site of dehiscence

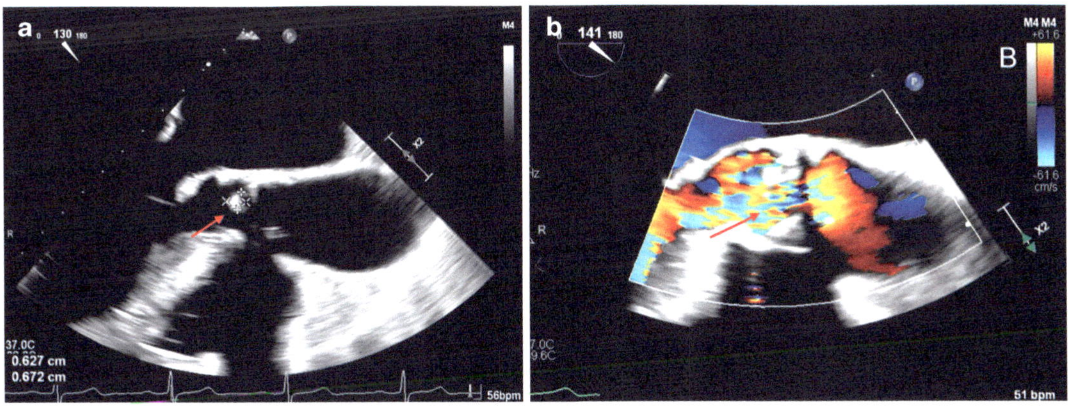

Fig. 22.19 Vegetation on a bioprosthetic AV (arrow, panel A) resulting in valve destruction and valvular regurgitation on color Doppler interrogation (arrow, panel B)

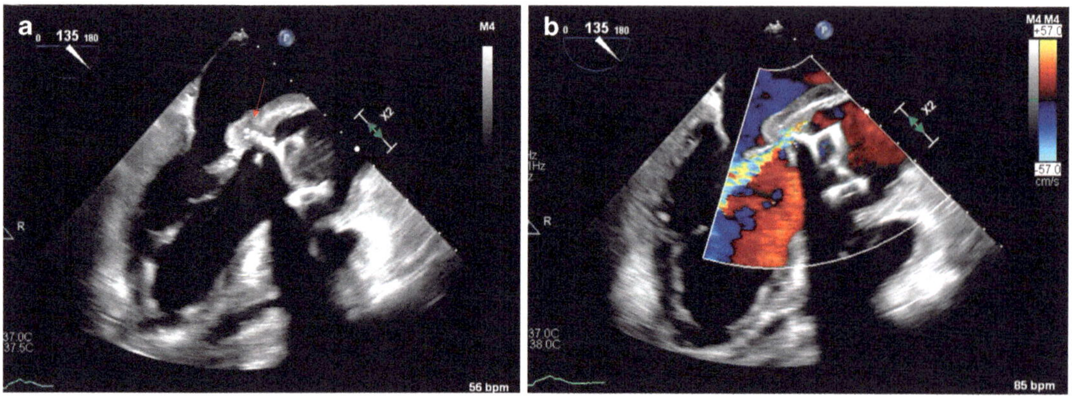

Fig. 22.20 TEE image showing prosthetic valve endocarditis in the aortic position complicated by annular abscess (arrow, panel A) and valve dehiscence resulting in posterior perivalvular regurgitation on color Doppler (panel B)

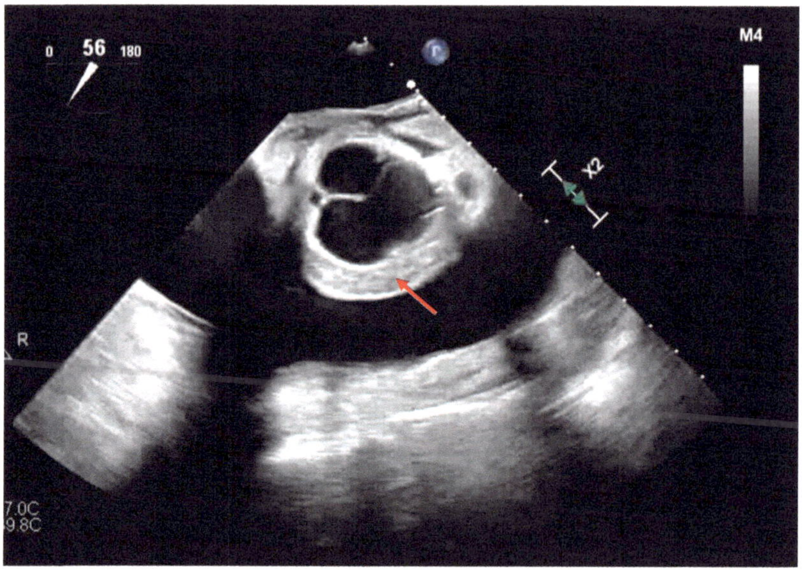

Fig. 22.21 Post op AV replacement with annular thickening due to edema (arrow)

INR goal based on valve type and position. The need for life-long anticoagulation with mechanical valves is a major consideration when electing a strategy for valve disease management [14, 15].

An INR target of 2.5 (range, 2.0–3.0) is indicated for most patients with mechanical valve prostheses in the aortic position; however, a higher target of 3.0 (range, 2.5–3.5) is recommended if patients have risk factors associated with a higher risk of thromboembolism, such as left ventricular dysfunction, atrial fibrillation, prior thromboembolism, and ball-in-cage mechanical valves [14, 15]. There is a newer generation mechanical aortic valve prosthesis that requires a lower INR target of 1.5-2.0.

By echo, mechanical prosthetic valve thrombosis is diagnosed by an abnormally elevated velocity or gradient across the prosthesis, with either limited leaflet motion or attached mobile densities consistent with thrombus.

Case 8

22 y.o. female with a history of MV replacement with a bileaflet mechanical prosthetic valve pre-

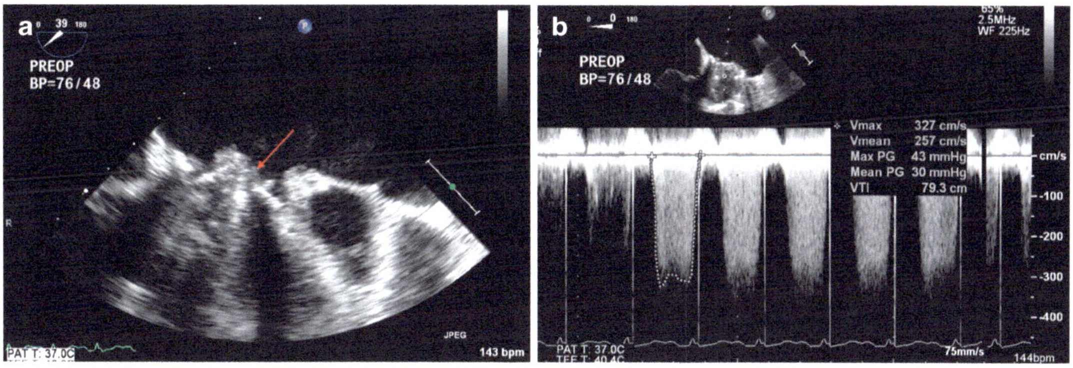

Fig. 22.22 Bileaflet mechanical valve in the mitral position with noted thrombus (arrow) and fixed lateral mechanical occluder (panel A). Spectral Doppler shows elevated gradient across MV prosthesis with mean gradient of 30 mmHg at HR of 144 bpm (panel B)

senting with cardiogenic shock following a prolonged cessation of VKA anticoagulation requiring emergent surgery. Intraoperative TEE performed showed thrombosis of the mechanical prosthetic valve (Fig. 22.22 with corresponding Video 22.23).

Bioprosthetic Valve Thrombosis

Bioprosthetic valve thrombosis, although less common compared to mechanical valves, typically occurs in the first 3 months post-implantation. However, cases of subclinical bioprosthetic valve thrombosis occurring 1 year or more post-intervention have been detected with MDCT (multidetector cardiac computed tomography) cardiac imaging and are characterized by the presence of hypoattenuating leaflet thickening and reduced leaflet motion and may represent a form of bioprosthetic dysfunction [14–16].

By echo, valve thrombosis may present as an abnormally elevated peak velocity and gradients across the prosthesis. Additional findings may include either limited leaflet motion, a fixed echogenic density on the valve leaflet, or mobile densities attached to the leaflet.

Patients with bioprosthetic valves may require anticoagulation with a VKA in the first several months after valve replacement to reduce the risk of thromboembolism until the valve is endothelialized. Most patients do not require lifelong anticoagulation unless other reasons for anticoagulation are present [15, 16].

Case 9

65 y.o. F with a history of bioprosthetic MV replacement one year prior who presented with dyspnea on exertion. TTE showed a significant increase in the MV mean gradient compared to the TTE performed 9 months prior.

She underwent a TEE that showed thrombosis of her mitral bioprosthetic valve resulting in stenosis (Fig. 22.23 with corresponding Videos 22.24 and 22.25). Pt was initiated on anticoagulation with a VKA and underwent a repeat TEE 3 months later with improvement in valve mobility and gradient noted (Fig. 22.24 with corresponding Video 22.26).

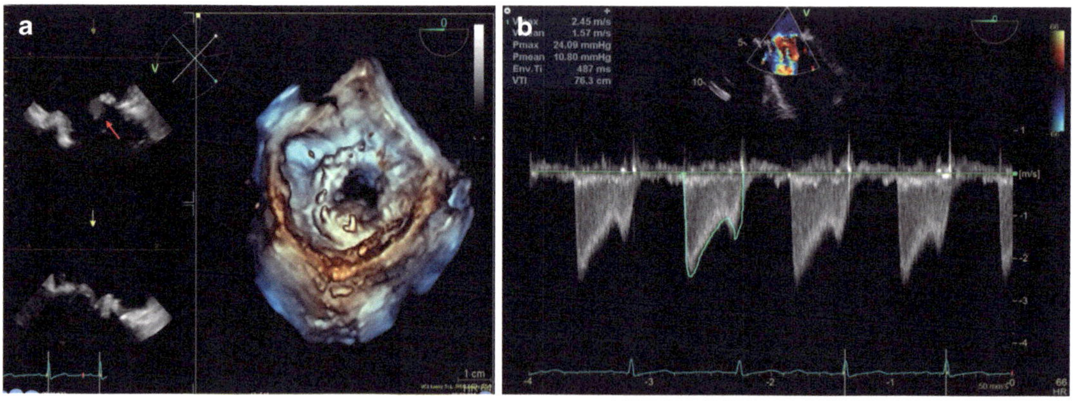

Fig. 22.23 Bioprosthetic mitral valve thrombosis with valve thickening noted (arrow, panel A) with increased mean gradient across the prosthesis measuring 11 mmHg at HR of 66 bpm (panel B)

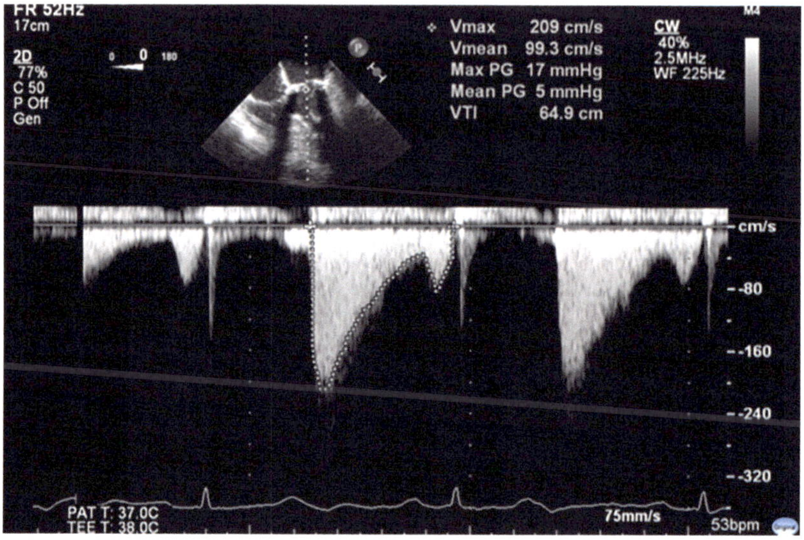

Fig. 22.24 CW Doppler of the mitral valve showing improvement of the mean gradient from 11 mmHg at HR of 66 bpm to 5 mmHg at HR of 53 bpm following 3 months of anticoagulation

Summary Points

- Echocardiography plays a key role in the assessment of prosthetic valve structure and function.
- Detailed evaluation should include two-dimentional Doppler evaluation and 3D imaging when available.
- It is important to understand the normal flow dynamics of prosthetic valve types and recognize abnormalities when present.
- Evaluation of prosthetic valve dysfunction may require transthoracic and transesophageal echocardiography and potentially other imaging modalities when ultrasound imaging is limited.

Questions

1. True or False?

   Regarding prosthetic aortic valves, an elevated gradient always represents pathologic stenosis of the prosthesis.

   Answer: False.

   Elevated gradient across an aortic prosthesis could represent prosthetic stenosis, patient prosthesis mismatch, sub valvular narrowing, high flow state or pressure recovery phenomenon. A careful and detailed evaluation should be performed to assess the etiology and mechanism of elevated gradients.

2. Patient with 21 mm bioprosthetic AV.

   Echo shows: AV velocity 3.8 m/s, mean gradient 35 mmHg, DI 0.26, triangular jet contour, AVA 1.1 cm^2, AT 76 ms, BSA 2.2 m^2, trivial aortic regurgitation. This elevated velocity likely represents what pathology?

   A. Patient with high flow state.
   B. Patient with severe prosthetic stenosis.
   C. Patient with PPM.
   D. Severe subvalvular stenosis.

   Answer: C.

   Given dimensionless index of 0.26 and short acceleration time of 76 ms, this is not consistent with severe prosthetic stenosis or severe subvalvular stenosis.

   The indexed EOA differentiates high flow from PPM with a value <0.85 cm^2/m^2 being consistent with PPM. The above patient has a calculated index EOA of 0.5 cm^2/m^2 which is consistent with severe PPM.

   (See Table 22.1 and Fig. 22.13 for reference)

3. True or False?

   Anticoagulation with a factor 10a inhibitor or VKA may be used for lifelong anticoagulation indicated for mechanical valves.

   Answer: False.

   Mechanical valves require the use of lifelong anticoagulation with a vitamin K antagonist (VKA).

   Newer anticoagulants (such as antithrombin or factor 10a inhibitors) have not been shown to be effective or safe in preventing thromboembolism associated with mechanical prosthetic valves and are currently not approved for use with mechanical prosthetic valves.

References

1. Otto CM, Nishimura RA, Bonow RO, et al. Guideline for the management of patients with Valvular Heart Disease: a report of the American College of Cardiology/American Heart Association Joint Committee on Clinical Practice Guidelines. Circulation. 2021;143:72–227.
2. Zoghbi WA, Chambers JB, Dumesnil JG, et al. Recommendations for evaluation of prosthetic valves with echocardiography and Doppler ultrasound: a report from the American Society of Echocardiography's Guidelines and Standards Committee and the Task Force on Prosthetic Valves. J Am Soc Echocardiogr. 2009;22:975–1014.
3. Pibarot P, Dumesnil JG. Prosthetic heart valves selection of the optimal prosthesis and long-term management. Circulation. 2009;119:1034–48.
4. Graf T, Reul H, Detlefs C, et al. Causes of formation of cavitation in mechanical heart valves. J Heart Valve Dis. 1994;3(1):49–64.
5. Blais C, Dumesnil JG, Baillot R, et al. Impact of valve prosthesis-patient mismatch on short-term mortality after aortic valve replacement. Circulation. 2003;108:983–8.
6. Pibarot P, Dumesnil JG. Prosthesis-patient mismatch: definition, clinical impact, and prevention. Heart. 2006;92:1022–9.
7. Zoghbi WA, Asch FM, Bruce C, et al. Guidelines for the evaluation of valvular regurgitation after percutaneous valve repair or replacement: a report from the American Society of Echocardiography. Developed in collaboration with the Society for Cardiovascular Angiography and Interventions, Japanese Society of Echocardiography, and Society for Cardiovascular Magnetic Resonance. J Am Soc Echocardiogr. 2019;32:431–75.
8. Kodali S, Pibarot P, Douglas PS, et al. Paravalvular regurgitation after transcatheter aortic valve replacement with the Edwards sapien valve in the PARTNER trial: characterizing patients and impact on outcome. Eur Heart J. 2015;36(7):449–56.
9. Makkar RR, Thourani VH, Mack MJ, et al. Five-year outcomes of transcatheter or surgical aortic-valve replacement. N Engl J Med. 2020;382:799–809.
10. Wilson W, Taubert KA, Gewitz M, et al. Prevention of Infective Endocarditis. Guidelines from the American Heart Association: a guideline from the American Heart Association Rheumatic Fever, Endocarditis, and Kawasaki Disease Committee, Council on Cardiovascular Disease in the Young, and the Council on Clinical Cardiology, Council on Cardiovascular Surgery and Anesthesia, and the Quality of Care and Outcomes Research Interdisciplinary Working Group. Circulation. 2007;116:1736–54.
11. Horstkotte D, Follath F, Gutschik F, et al. Guidelines on prevention, diagnosis and treatment of infective endocarditis executive summary: the Task Force on Infective Endocarditis of the European Society of Cardiology. Eur Heart J. 2004;3:267–76.
12. Li JS, Sexton DJ, Mick N, et al. Proposed modifications to the duke criteria for the diagnosis of infective endocarditis. Clin Infect Dis. 2000;30:633–8.
13. Piper C, Körfer R, Horstkotte D. Prosthetic valve endocarditis. Heart. 2001;85:590–3.

14. Horstkotte D, Scharf RE, Schultheiss HP. Intracardiac thrombosis: patient-related and device-related factors. J Heart Valve Dis. 1995;4:114–20.
15. Whitlock RP, Sun JC, Fremes SE, et al. Antithrombotic and thrombolytic therapy for valvular disease: Antithrombotic Therapy and Prevention of Thrombosis, 9th ed: American College of Chest Physicians Evidence-Based Clinical Practice Guidelines. Chest. 2012;141:e576S–600S.
16. Makkar RR, Blanke P, Leipsic J, et al. Subclinical leaflet thrombosis in transcatheter and surgical bioprosthetic valves: PARTNER 3 Cardiac Computed Tomography Substudy. J Am Coll Cardiol. 2020;75:3003–15.

Infective Endocarditis

23

Flora Li and Sara Nikravan

Learning Objectives

1. Discuss direct echocardiographic findings consistent with endocarditis, such as vegetations, abscesses, other perivalvular complications, and prosthetic valve dehiscence.
2. Identify normal anatomic variants on echocardiography that can be confused for vegetations.
3. Examine the indications for performing transesophageal echocardiography to aid in diagnosis.

Introduction

Infective endocarditis is a rare but life-threatening infection of the endocardial surface of the heart. The causal organism is most often bacterial, with 80% of cases of native-valve endocarditis being caused by gram-positive bacteria [1]. The in-hospital mortality for patients with endocarditis is 15–20%, with one-year mortality near 40%. Current treatments consist of a combination of prolonged antibiotic therapy and surgical management, ideally with the involvement of a multidisciplinary team including cardiology, cardiothoracic surgery, and infectious disease expertise [2]. The two main components of treatment are antibiotics and surgery. The timing and indications of surgical intervention are still not entirely clear, with some groups advocating for early surgery (within 48 h of diagnosis) and others advocating for surgery after a "cool off" period of antibiotic therapy [1–3]. Strong surgical indications include severe valvular dysfunction, heart failure, infection that is refractory to antibiotic therapy, abscess formation, and large lesions that are at high risk for embolism (Table 23.1). Patients in cardiogenic shock or with severe pulmonary edema should undergo surgery urgently [2, 3].

Although endocarditis can occur in patients with no prior cardiac issues, patients with preexisting structural abnormalities such as rheumatic or sclerotic valvular disease, congenital cardiac disease, or intracardiac prosthetic material are at higher risk of developing endocarditis. The source can be bacteremia from any source, including transient bacteremia caused by everyday occurrences such as tooth brushing and chewing. Bacteremia usually has little effect on healthy, intact cardiac endothelium. However, in the setting of endothelial damage, local inflammation and thrombus formation can promote bacterial adhesion and provide a site for bacterial colonization. Bacterial colonization leads to additional injury and inflammation, eventually

Supplementary Information The online version contains supplementary material available at https://doi.org/10.1007/978-3-031-80038-2_23.

F. Li · S. Nikravan (✉)
University of Washington, Seattle, WA, USA
e-mail: fmli@uw.edu; nikravan@uw.edu

M. J. Lanspa, A. T. Levinson (eds.), *Echocardiography and Ultrasonography in the ICU*, Respiratory Medicine, https://doi.org/10.1007/978-3-031-80038-2_23

forming a vegetation that is poorly penetrated by host neutrophils and defense molecules [4]. If left untreated, severe complications include sepsis, valvular destruction and failure, spread of infection into paravalvular structures with abscess formation, left or right ventricular failure, and emboli to systemic vessels and other organs with abscess formation and tissue infarction. This can ultimately lead to multiorgan failure and death.

Table 23.1 Indications for surgery

• Severe valvular dysfunction
• Heart failure
– Typically caused by severe valvular regurgitation or obstruction by mass
• Perivalvular complications (e.g. abscess or fistula)
• Embolic events despite appropriate antibiotic therapy
– Cerebralvascular events, provided risk of hemorrhagic conversion is low
– Other systemic embolic events: renal infarct, splenic infarct, limb ischemia
– Pulmonary embolic events: pulmonary embolism, pulmonary infarcts
• Large vegetation
– >10 mm on aortic or mitral valves
– >15 mm on tricuspid valves
• Persistent sepsis despite appropriate antibiotic therapy
• Difficult organisms
– Examples include *S. aureus, Brucella, Staphylococcus lugdunesis, Pseudomonas aeruginosa*
• Nearly all cases of prosthetic valve endocarditis

Diagnosis

Diagnosis of endocarditis can be challenging due to its variable presentation and requires utilization of clinical findings, laboratory examination using blood cultures, and echocardiography. The modified Duke criteria for diagnosis of endocarditis incorporate these findings into one system that categorizes each finding as a major or minor criterion. Under this system, the presence of two major criteria, one major criterion and three minor criteria, or five minor criteria is required for a definite diagnosis of endocarditis (Table 23.2) [5]. Although the Duke criteria were initially created for research use, subsequent studies have shown that these criteria have a high sensitivity and specificity in the clinical setting, with sensitivity reported to range from 62–76% [6–8].

Table 23.2 Modified Duke criteria

Major criteria	Minor criteria
1. One of the following on blood cultures: • Typical microorganisms (*Staphylococcus aureus*, viridans streptococci, *Streptococcus bovis*, HACEK (haemophilus, aggregatibacter, cardiobacterium, *Eikenella corrodens*, kingella) group, or community-acquired enterococci, in the absence of a primary focus • Microorganisms consistent with infective endocarditis from persistently positive blood cultures, defined as ≥2 positive cultures from blood samples drawn >12 h apart or all of 3 or a majority of ≥4 separate cultures of blood (with first and last sample drawn at least 1 h apart) • Single positive blood culture for *Coxiella burnetii* or phase I IgG antibody titer >1:800 2. Evidence of endocardial involvement • Direct echocardiographic evidence of endocarditis: vegetation, abscess, or new partial dehiscence of a prosthetic valve • New valvular regurgitation	1. Predisposing cardiac condition or intravenous drug use 2. Temperature ≥38.0 °C (100.4 °F) 3. Vascular phenomena (major arterial emboli, septic pulmonary infarcts, mycotic aneurysm, intracranial hemorrhages, conjunctival hemorrhages, Janeway lesions) 4. Immunologic phenomena (glomerulonephritis, Osler nodes, Roth spots, or rheumatoid factor) 5. Positive blood cultures that do not meet major criteria, or serologic evidence of active infection with organism consistent with infective endocarditis

Adapted from Li et al. [5]

Echocardiographic Assessment

Echocardiographic assessment plays an important role in the diagnosis of endocarditis. Of the two major criteria of the modified Duke criteria, one utilizes echocardiography heavily. The first major criterion is positive blood cultures, and the second is evidence of endocardial involvement [5, 9].

There are three echocardiographic findings that are considered direct echocardiographic findings of endocarditis: vegetations, abscesses and related perivalvular complications such as pseudoaneurysms and fistulas, and new dehiscence of a prosthetic valve (Fig. 23.1). Valvular vegetations are the classic lesion of endocarditis and are most frequently found on the low-pressure side of the valve structure. They generally present as oscillating masses that move with a motion independent of the valve. Although they are most commonly found on the valvular or subvalvular apparatus, they can also form on the endocardium, especially along the path of a turbulent regurgitant jet (Fig. 23.1a, Video 23.1) [3, 10].

Abscesses and associated perivalvular complications are the second group of major echocardiographic findings of endocarditis. Abscesses are seen on echocardiography as thickened perivalvular tissue with a heterogeneous appearance with echodense or echolucent fluid-filled areas. The fluid cavity in an abscess is not in communication with the cardiovascular lumen. Although abscesses can be associated with any location of infection, they are most common in aortic valve and prosthetic valve endocarditis (Fig. 23.1a, b, Videos 23.1 and 23.2). In contrast to abscesses, pseudoaneurysms are perivalvular cavities that do communicate with the cardiovascular lumen. They have a similar appearance to abscesses but have pulsatile flow that can be seen with color or spectral Doppler. Fistulas are complications of abscesses or pseudoaneurysms and are defined as a communication between two neighboring cardiac chambers. Flow between the two chambers should be visualized using color or spectral Doppler in order to distinguish fistulas from the other perivalvular complications.

The last major direct echocardiographic finding is new dehiscence of a prosthetic valve. Even without the other two findings, new perivalvular regurgitation in a prosthetic valve is highly suspicious for endocarditis (Fig. 23.1c, Video 23.3). Valve dehiscence and abscess formation are seen in 60% of cases of prosthetic valve endocarditis [3]. However, since perivalvular regurgitation can occur as a postoperative complication of prosthetic valve implantation, care must be taken to confirm that any regurgitation seen is new and has not been previously documented [3, 10].

In the setting of a patient with high suspicion for endocarditis, detection of new valvular regurgitation is also considered sufficient evidence for endocardial involvement. This can be diagnosed clinically (e.g., with a new murmur), but clinical findings should be confirmed with an echocardiogram. Care must be taken to ensure that any regurgitation seen is indeed new and not worsening of previously seen regurgitation. New regurgitation due to endocarditis can occur from direct destruction of the valve leaflets or subvalvular apparatus.

Echocardiographic imaging in patients with high suspicion for endocarditis can be performed using either transthoracic echocardiography (TTE) or transesophageal echocardiography (TEE) [5, 8]. TTE has a lower sensitivity than TEE (72% for TTE compared to over 90% for TEE) but is noninvasive and more widely available [3, 5, 8]. It is recommended as the initial imaging modality to use for evaluation of a suspected case of endocarditis. TEE should be used as a supplemental imaging modality to look for further cardiac complications in positive cases and as confirmation in equivocal or complicated cases [10–12] as depicted when comparing imaging from the same patient in Video 23.4 (TTE) to Video 23.5 (TEE) (Fig. 23.2). 3D TEE is an additional modality made possible by improvements in transducer technology and can provide better anatomic information than 2D TEE (Fig. 23.3, Video 23.6).

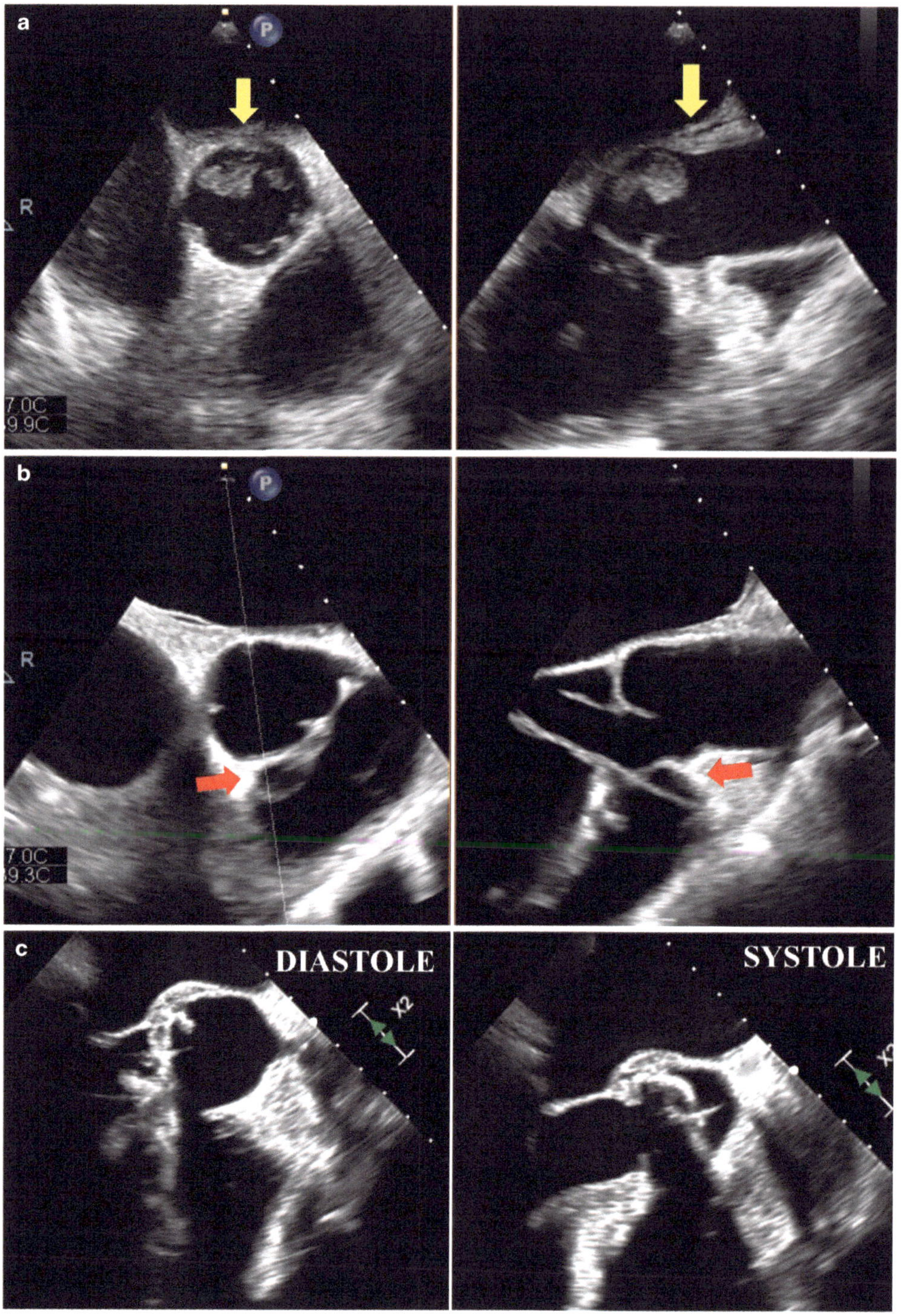

Fig. 23.1 Examples of major echocardiographic findings of endocarditisThere are three major echocardiographic findings of endocarditis: vegetation (**a**), abscess (**a** and **b**), and new valvular dehiscence (**c**). (**a**) (Video 23.1): TEE short and long axis views of a large aortic valve vegetation. Note the perivalvular thickening (yellow arrows) that is suggestive of abscess. (**b**) (Video 23.2): TEE short and long axis views of aortic valve endocarditis causing cusp destruction and abscess (red arrows). (**c**) (Video 23.3): mechanical prosthetic valve dehiscence in diastole and systole in TEE ME long axis view. Note that the lower edge of the valve annulus moves into the aortic root during systole

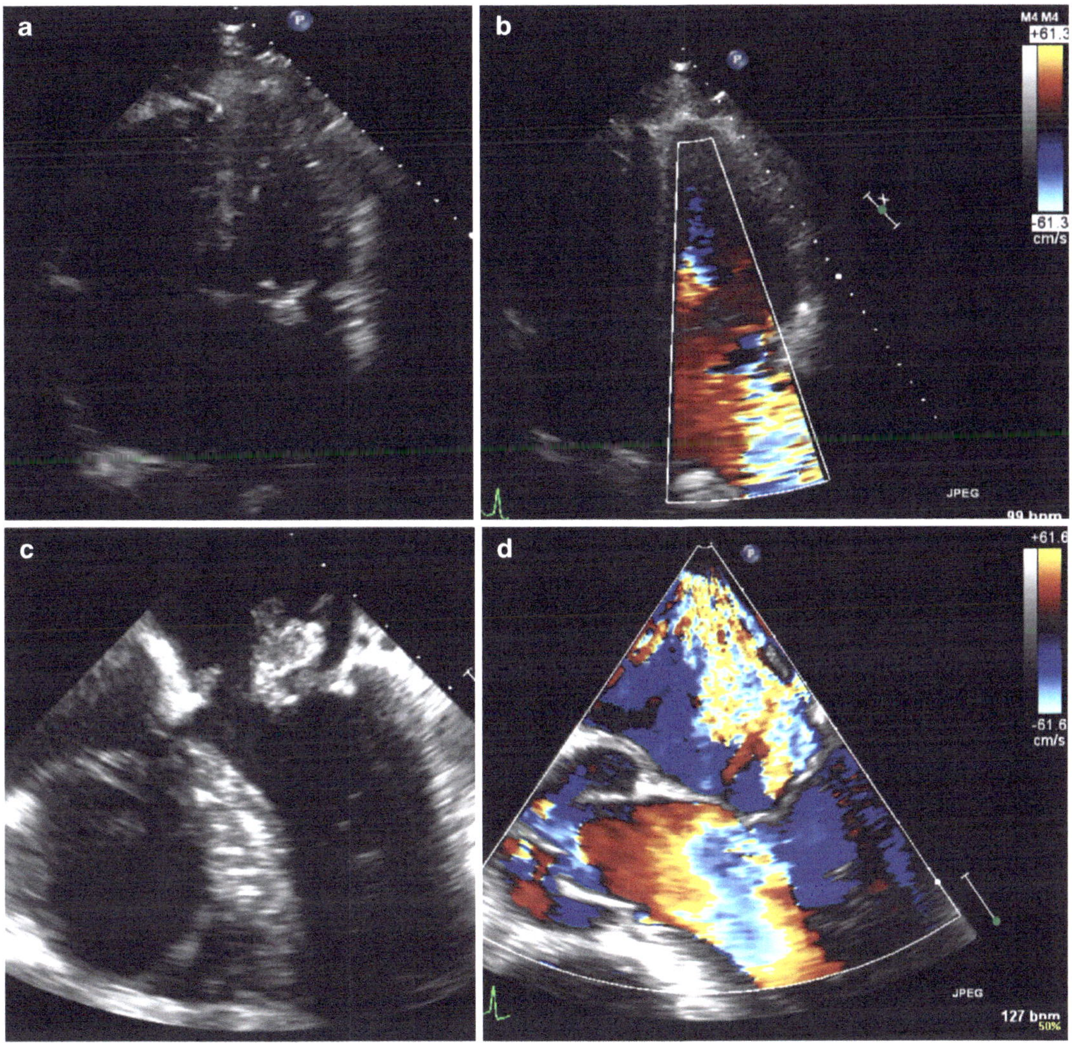

Fig. 23.2 Comparison of TTE and TEE imagingThis is a large mitral valve vegetation visualized using both TTE and TEE. Although the mass and the valvular regurgitation jet are visible in the apical 4 chamber TTE images (**a** and **b**), the analogous TEE mid-esophageal 4 chamber views (**c** and **d**) demonstrate both more clearly. Videos 23.3 and 23.4 are the clips of (**a**) and (**b**), respectively

Patients who should have supplemental TEE exams include those with prosthetic valves or intracardiac devices, patients with non-diagnostic TTE images, or patients with TTE exams that were negative but with moderate to high clinical suspicion for endocarditis. In these patient groups, TEE has significantly higher sensitivity for detecting vegetations. For example, in patients with prosthetic valves, the sensitivity of TTE decreases to 36–69% [10].

When performing echocardiographic evaluation, care must be taken to distinguish vegetations from normal anatomic variants that resemble vegetations. In the right atrium, the

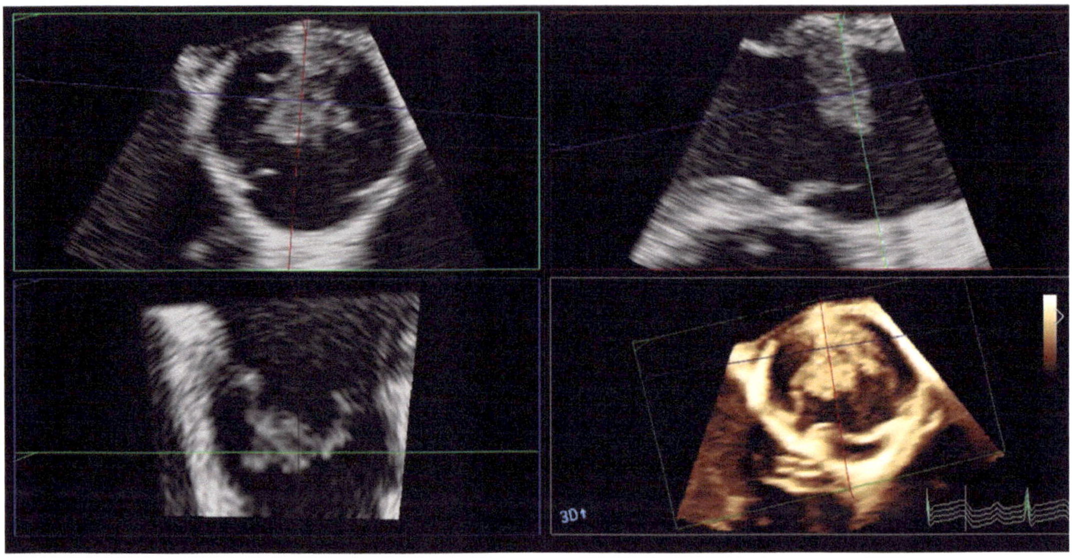

Fig. 23.3 3D rendering of the aortic valve mass from Fig. 23.1a using multiplanar reconstruction. The red, blue, and green planes show 2D cross sections at different angles. In this example, the green plane at top left shows an aortic valve short axis view, the red plane at top right shows a long axis view, and the blue plane at bottom shows a cut across the non-coronary and left coronary cusps. The 3D in the bottom right corner shows the mass at the coaptation between the non and left coronary cusps. Video 23.6 is a clip showing this view through the entire cardiac cycle

Eustachian valve, Chiari network, and crista terminalis are all normal structures that can be confused for vegetations. The Eustachian valve is an embryonic remnant located near the inferior vena cava that served to direct oxygen-rich blood from the inferior vena cava to the foramen ovale in fetuses. In adults, it is a thin structure that is attached to the junction of the inferior vena cava and the right atrium. The Chiari network is a mobile net-like structure that may be continuous with the Eustachian valve. It appears on echocardiograms as a thin, mobile structure that spans the right atrium (Fig. 23.4a, Video 23.7). The crista terminalis is a ridge of tissue running from the superior vena cava to the inferior vena cava in the right atrium.

Lambl's excrescences and fibroelastomas can be found on any valve and can be difficult to differentiate from vegetations. Lambl's excrescences are thin fibrous strands occurring at the edges of the cusps and are most often seen on the aortic valve. Unlike vegetations, they typically do not form masses and are not heterogeneous in appearance (Fig. 23.4b, Video 23.8). Cardiac fibroelastomas are bulky, often pedunculated masses that can be found on the low-pressure side of valves and on endocardial surfaces (Fig. 23.4c, Video 23.9). They can be especially difficult to distinguish from vegetations and require consideration of the whole clinical picture to determine the likelihood of endocarditis.

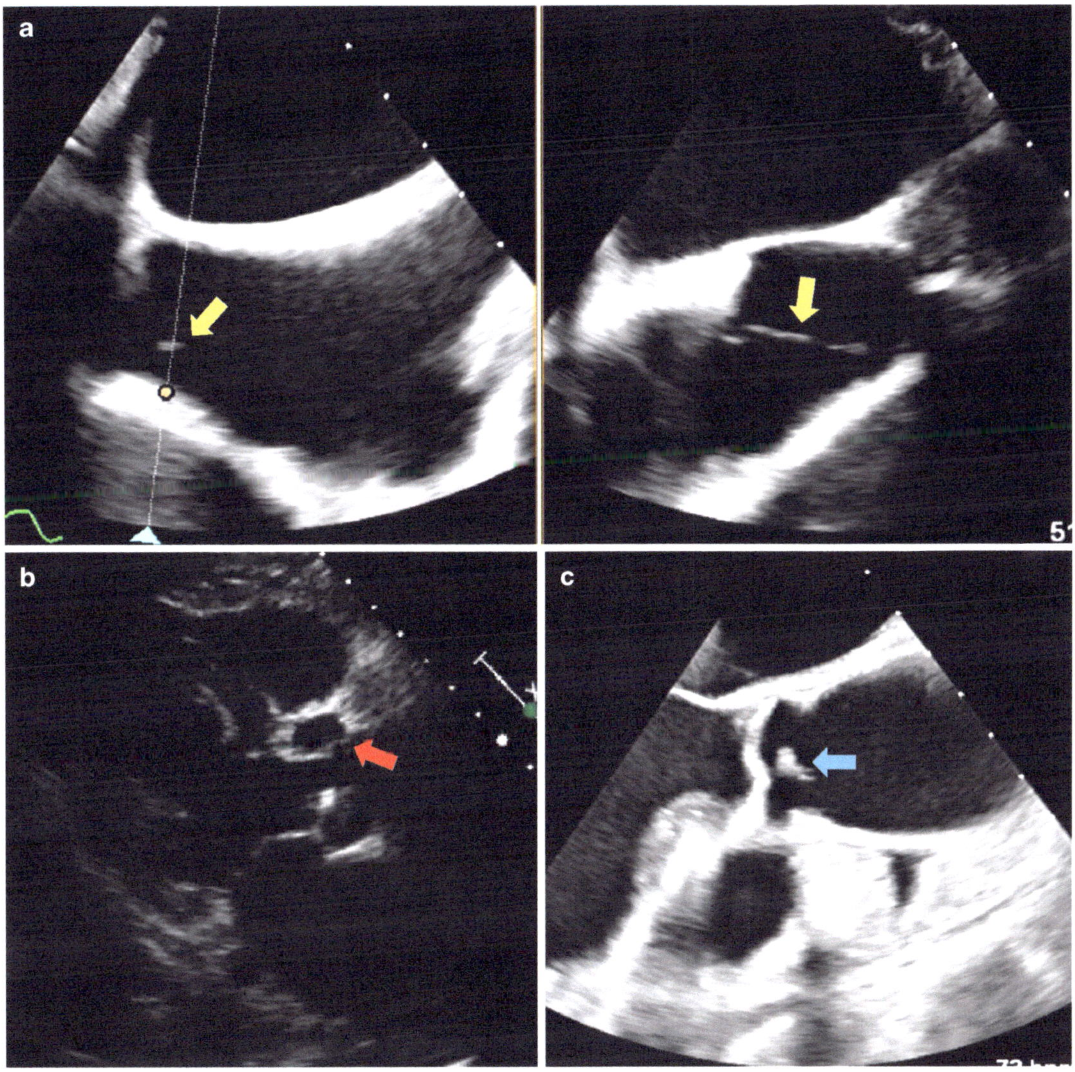

Fig. 23.4 Normal variantsExamples of normal anatomic variants that are easily confused for vegetation. (**a**) Chiari network, which appears as a filamentous structure stretching across the right atrium (yellow arrows). Seen on TEE in the midesophageal bicaval view on the left side and in the inverse 4 chamber view on the right. (**b**) Lambl's excrescence (red arrow), which appears as a thin filamentous structure on the aortic valve. Seen on TTE in the parasternal long axis view. (**c**) Fibroelastoma on the aortic valve (blue arrow), seen on TEE in the midesophageal long axis view

Left-Sided Endocarditis

Left-sided endocarditis refers to infection of the mitral valve, aortic valve, and any associated structures in the left atrium or left ventricle. It constitutes the majority of infective endocarditis cases. Patients who are at higher risk include those with structural valve abnormalities, such as severe valvular sclerosis or congenital valvular disease. The presenting symptoms may be nonspecific and include symptoms from systemic septic embolisms such as stroke, ischemic limb, renal infarcts, or splenic infarcts. Septic emboli can also seed vascular walls and form mycotic aneurysms, most commonly in the cerebral vessels. Vegetations >10 mm are an indication for urgent surgical intervention [13]. Endocarditis that is inadequately treated can lead to heart failure from severe valvular regurgitation and volume overload. Patients with baseline altered mental status, moderate to severe heart failure, endocarditis due to bacteria other than *S. viridans*, or who receive medical therapy without valve surgery have an increased six-month mortality [2]. Following diagnosis with left-sided endocarditis, the initial series of diagnostic imaging and testing should be followed by more complete imaging for systemic embolic events using modalities such as whole-body computed tomography (CT) or cerebral magnetic resonance imaging (MRI) [14].

In mitral valve endocarditis, vegetations are most commonly seen as mobile masses on the left atrial side of either leaflet. With progression of disease, valvular destruction occurs, leading to severe mitral regurgitation (Fig. 23.2, Video 23.10). Acute onset of severe mitral regurgitation may lead to dyspnea from flash pulmonary edema, volume overload of the left ventricle, and development of pulmonary hypertension. Patients with severe mitral regurgitation or heart failure require urgent surgical management. In cases with small, isolated valve lesions where mitral valve repair is feasible, valve repair instead of valve replacement may lead to better outcomes compared to valve replacement. However, this may not be an option for patients with extensive valvular destruction or perivalvular destruction. Unrepairable valves can be replaced with a bioprosthetic or mechanical prosthetic valve replacement [14, 15].

Vegetations in aortic valve endocarditis are most commonly on the left ventricular side of the valve. As with mitral valve endocarditis, aortic valve endocarditis can present with evidence of systemic emboli. Abscess formation and spread into the perivalvular space is more common in aortic valve endocarditis and can lead to complete heart block due to the proximity of the aortic valve annulus to the atrioventricular node (Fig. 23.1a, b) [16]. Perivalvular spread can involve the aorto-mitral curtain, the fibrous space that separates the aortic root from the anterior mitral leaflet, and from there spread to the mitral valve. Acute severe aortic regurgitation from valve destruction or perivalvular fistula formation causes a sudden elevation in left ventricular end-diastolic pressure. This can lead to cardiogenic shock from a sudden reduction in cardiac output, elevated left atrial pressure, and pulmonary edema. Early surgical intervention in aortic valve endocarditis improves outcomes compared to medical management alone and can prevent some of the late sequelae of aortic endocarditis. Indications for surgery are similar to those for mitral valve endocarditis [17, 18].

Right-Sided Endocarditis

Right-sided endocarditis refers to infection of the tricuspid valve, pulmonic valve, and associated right atrial and ventricular structures. It constitutes the minority of endocarditis cases and is only seen in 5–10% of all cases. Risk factors for right-sided endocarditis include intravenous drug use and the presence of venous or intracardiac hardware such as intracardiac devices and central venous catheters. Structural valve abnormalities remain a risk factor but are less common in the tricuspid and pulmonic valves. Of the common causes of right-sided endocarditis, intravenous drug use is the most common, and 2–5% of intravenous drug users develop endocarditis every year [19, 20]. With the ongoing opioid epidemic in the United States, the incidence of intravenous drug use-related endocarditis is likely to also increase. The mechanism of seeding is direct bacterial seeding from contamination of injected substances and skin flora. In addition, illicit drugs can be mixed with diluents or chemical contaminants, which cause valve thickening, prolapse, and regurgitation [19]. Successful treatment of this patient population involves not only medical and surgical management but also treatment of the underlying addiction. Addiction specialists should be engaged early in the treatment course since relapse and reinfection rates are high.

Right-sided endocarditis related to intracardiac devices is becoming more common as the number of implanted devices increases with the aging patient population. Intracardiac devices include pacemakers, implantable cardioverter defibrillators (ICD), and cardiac resynchronization therapy (CRT) devices. The risk of endocarditis rises with the complexity of the device, with ICDs being at a higher risk than pacemakers and CRT devices having the highest risk (Fig. 23.5a). Patients who have had a device replacement or revision are also at higher risk [21]. Other indwelling venous hardware that have been reported as sources for endocarditis include central lines used for inpatient care and chronic indwelling lines used for outpatient infusion therapy [22]. In addition to direct infection of the central line, a fibrin sheath may form around long-term central line catheters and remain after catheter removal, serving as a site for vegetation formation [19].

As in left-sided endocarditis, presenting symptoms are often nonspecific and consistent with bacteremia. Septic emboli from the right side of the heart cause pulmonary symptoms such as dyspnea rather than symptoms of systemic embolism, which is rare unless there is a structural abnormality allowing paradoxical embolism. Valvular destruction and severe valvular regurgitation lead to right heart volume overload and failure, which can be exacerbated by increased afterload from heavy pulmonary embolic burden. Additional evaluation with imaging should focus on detection of pulmonary complications such as pulmonary embolisms, abscesses, and infarcts [19, 20].

The tricuspid valve is involved in 90% of right-sided endocarditis (Fig. 23.5b, Video 23.11). Isolated native pulmonic valve endocarditis is rare, constituting only around 5% of cases. Although uncommon, infection of the Eustachian valve, interventricular septum, and right ventricular free wall has been reported [19]. Intravenous antibiotic therapy is the first-line treatment for right-sided endocarditis and is preferred for patients who use intravenous drugs, as the risk of reinfection is high. Patients with devices should have the device, leads, or catheters removed urgently, since those are presumed to be infected even if vegetation is not visualized on imaging. Reimplantation of new devices should be delayed until the completion of antibiotic therapy and confirmation that the infection has resolved. Indications for surgical intervention on the tricuspid valve include vegetations >20 mm, right heart failure from severe tricuspid regurgitation, persistent infection despite adequate medical therapy, perivalvular complications, and recurrent emboli. Valve repair is possible in cases with limited valve damage and has been recommended for patients who use intravenous drugs, as this reduces the amount of prosthetic material that can be later re-infected. When valve reconstruction is not possible, valve replacement is performed with either a bioprosthetic or mechanical valve. Outcomes between the two types of valves have been comparable [19, 20, 23].

Prosthetic Valve Endocarditis

Surgical and minimally invasive transcatheter prosthetic valves are increasingly common, and with that comes an increase in prosthetic valve endocarditis. Early infection after implantation is caused by direct seeding of the prosthetic material from intraoperative contamination or hematogenous spread. These infections have a mortality rate of as high as 70%. Late infection more closely resembles native valve endocarditis, since exposed prosthetic materials are protected by endothelialization. Compared to native valve endocarditis, prosthetic valve endocarditis is more difficult to diagnose and has an overall worse prognosis [3, 24]. Presenting signs and symptoms are often atypical, and imaging is often negative or indeterminate. In addition, echocardiographic assessment of prosthetic valves is challenging due to shadowing from prosthetic material and postsurgical changes that can be difficult to distinguish from endocarditis. TEE has a sensitivity of 86–94%, superior to that of TTE, and should be used for all cases of suspected prosthetic valve endocarditis. Prosthetic valve endocarditis tends to be associated with perivalvular complications such as abscess formation, conduction abnormalities, and fistulae. Vegetations are more common on mechanical valves and can be seen directly on the occluders

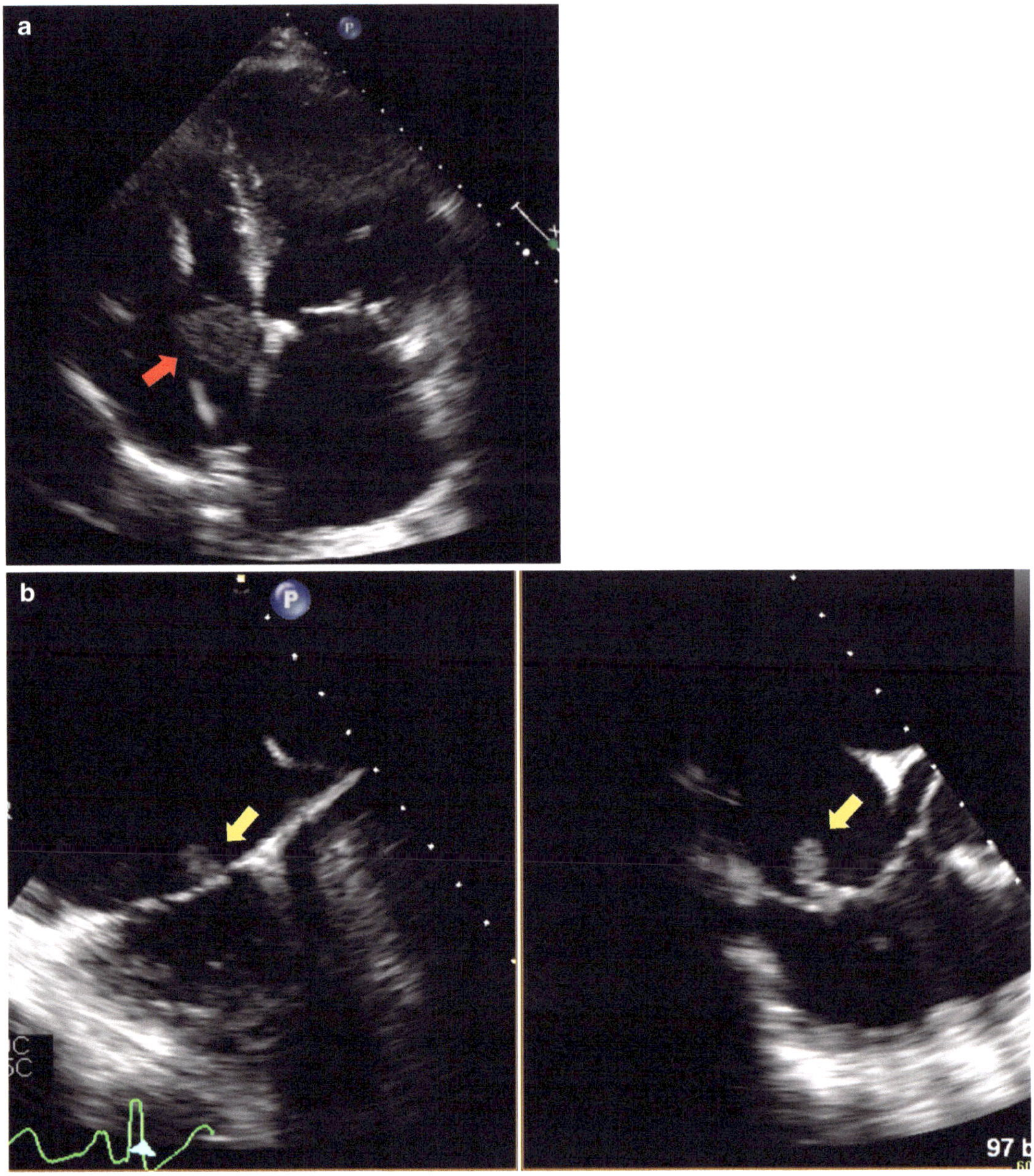

Fig. 23.5 Right sided endocarditisRight sided endocarditis can occur on native structures or on intracardiac devices, which are most often inserted into the right heart. (**a**) Large mass on a pacemaker lead (red arrow). Seen on TTE in the apical 4 chamber view. (**b**) Tricuspid mass in a patient with a history of intravenous drug use (yellow arrows). Seen in TEE midesophageal 4 chamber view on the left and RV inflow outflow view on the right

or on support material. Bioprosthetic valves present with either regurgitant or stenotic lesions, with or without visible vegetations [24]. Valve dehiscence and associated new perivalvular leak can result from the high incidence of perivalvular complications (Fig. 23.1c, Video 23.3) [3].

Prosthetic valve endocarditis often cannot be eradicated with medical therapy alone, and most cases require urgent surgical intervention [3, 24, 25]. Surgical treatment poses several challenges, such as reentry into the chest, extensive debridement and reconstruction, and poor tissue quality. Rates for reinfection are 6–15%, and up to 25% of patients require additional surgery [25].

Summary Points

- Diagnosis of endocarditis can be challenging due to its variable presentation. The modified Duke criteria incorporate clinical findings, laboratory examination using blood cultures, and echocardiography into one diagnostic system.
- Both TTE and TEE play important roles in imaging for suspected endocarditis. TTE should be used as an initial modality, with TEE as follow-up imaging in selected cases.
- Direct echocardiographic findings of endocarditis include vegetations, abscesses and related perivalvular complications such as pseudoaneurysms and fistulas, and new dehiscence of a prosthetic valve.
- Most endocarditis cases are left-sided. Right-sided endocarditis is more common in patients who use intravenous drugs and patients with intracardiac devices.
- Prosthetic valve endocarditis tends to be more challenging to diagnose and to treat, often requiring early surgical management.

Questions

1. Which of the below findings would meet criteria for diagnosis of endocarditis using the modified Duke criteria?
   A. Temperature 38.2, history of IV drug use, one positive blood culture growing Staph aureus
   B. Temperature 38.5, history of IV drug use, new-onset severe tricuspid valve regurgitation, two positive blood cultures growing Strep bovis
   C. Temperature 38.2, prior bioprosthetic AV replacement, imaging concerning for mycotic aneurysm of the ascending aorta
   D. Temperature 38.5, prior bioprosthetic AV replacement, discovery of an early diastolic decrescendo murmur

   Answer: B

   Explanation: A diagnosis of endocarditis using the modified Duke Criteria requires the presence of either two major criteria, one major and three minor criteria, or five minor criteria. Answer B depicts a patient with two major criteria: evidence of endocardial involvement with new-onset severe tricuspid valve regurgitation and two positive blood cultures growing typical microorganisms, Strep bovis being the causative organism in this case. The other choices have concerning findings but not the combination of findings that would result in a diagnosis of endocarditis using the modified Duke Criteria.
2. Direct echocardiographic findings of endocarditis include.
   A. Echocardiographic evidence of a myxomatous mitral valve in a former IV drug user
   B. Echocardiographic evidence of a perivalvular leak in a patient with a history of a prior transcatheter aortic valve replacement (TAVR) intervention.
   C. Echocardiographic evidence of an aortic root pseudoaneurysm in a patient with a prior surgical bioprosthetic aortic valve replacement
   D. Echocardiographic evidence of a bicuspid aortic valve with a newly diagnosed diastolic murmur

   Answer: C

   Explanation: Direct echocardiographic findings of endocarditis include evidence of vegetations, abscesses, and other perivalvular complications such as pseudoaneurysms and fistulas, and new dehiscence of a prosthetic valve. While a myxomatous mitral valve is a common valvular abnormality, it is defined as a degenerative valve disease causing valvular thickening, prolapse, or even flail in some cases. Despite the abnormal finding, it is not a direct echocardiographic finding of endocarditis. Similarly, although abnormal, perivalvular leaks can be seen in patients with prior history of TAVR and are not defined as direct echocardiographic findings of endocarditis. While congenital cardiac abnormalities such as a bicuspid valve may place a patient at a higher risk for developing endocarditis, a bicuspid aortic valve and associated murmurs are not direct echocardiographic findings of endocarditis. Evidence of abscesses and other perivalvular complications such as pseudoaneurysm are direct echocardiographic findings of endocarditis, making answer choice C the correct answer.

3. Prosthetic valve endocarditis…
   A. can present like native valve endocarditis
   B. can often be treated medically
   C. can easily be ruled out with negative echocardiographic imaging
   D. has a lower mortality than native valve endocarditis

   Answer: A

   Explanation: When occurring later, prosthetic valve endocarditis can present like native valve endocarditis. Unfortunately, in many cases prosthetic valve endocarditis requires more than medical treatment alone for full eradication and can be challenging to diagnose with echocardiographic imaging. For this reason, the mortality rate with prosthetic valve endocarditis is higher than that of native valve endocarditis.

References

1. Chambers HF, Bayer AS. Native-valve infective endocarditis. Solomon CG, editor. N Engl J Med. 2020;383(6):567–76.
2. Otto CM, Nishimura RA, Bonow RO, Carabello BA, Erwin JP, Gentile F, et al. ACC/AHA Guideline for the Management of Patients with Valvular Heart Disease: a report of the American College of Cardiology/American Heart Association Joint Committee on Clinical Practice Guidelines. Circulation. 2021;2020, 143(5) https://doi.org/10.1161/CIR.0000000000000923.
3. Cahill TJ, Prendergast BD. Infective endocarditis. Lancet. 2016;387(10021):882–93.
4. Lockhart PB, Brennan MT, Sasser HC, Fox PC, Paster BJ, Bahrani-Mougeot FK. Bacteremia associated with toothbrushing and dental extraction. Circulation. 2008;117(24):3118–25.
5. Li JS, Sexton DJ, Mick N, Nettles R, Fowler VG, Ryan T, et al. Proposed modifications to the Duke criteria for the diagnosis of infective endocarditis. Clin Infect Dis. 2000;30(4):633–8.
6. Prendergast BD. Diagnostic criteria and problems in infective endocarditis. Heart. 2004;90(6):611–3.
7. Topan A, Carstina D, Slavcovici A, Rancea R, Capalneanu R, Lupse M. Assesment of the Duke criteria for the diagnosis of infective endocarditis after twenty-years. An analysis of 241 cases. Med Pharm Rep. 2015;88(3):321–6.
8. Shrestha N, Shakya S, Hussain S, Pettersson G, Griffin B, Gordon S. Sensitivity and specificity of Duke criteria for diagnosis of definite infective endocarditis: a cohort study. Open Forum Infect Dis. 2017;4(Suppl. 1):S550–1.
9. Durack DT, Lukes AS, Bright DK, Duke Endocarditis Service. New criteria for diagnosis of infective endocarditis: utilization of specific echocardiographic findings. Am J Med. 1994;96(3):200–9.
10. Habib G, Badano L, Tribouilloy C, et al. Recommendations for the practice of echocardiography in infective endocarditis. Eur J Echocardiogr. 2010;11(2):202–19.
11. ACCF/ASE/AHA/ASNC/HFSA/HRS/SCAI/SCCM/SCCT/SCMR 2011 Appropriate use criteria for echocardiography. J Am Soc Echocardiogr. 2011;24(3):229–67.
12. Baddour LM, Wilson WR, Bayer AS, Fowler VG, Tleyjeh IM, Rybak MJ, et al. Infective endocarditis in adults: diagnosis, antimicrobial therapy, and management of complications: a scientific statement for healthcare professionals from the American Heart Association. Circulation. 2015;132(15):1435–86.
13. Mohananey D, Mohadjer A, Pettersson G, Navia J, Gordon S, Shrestha N, et al. Association of vegetation size with embolic risk in patients with infective endocarditis: a systematic review and meta-analysis. JAMA Intern Med. 2018;178(4):502.
14. Nappi F, Spadaccio C, Dreyfus J, Attias D, Acar C, Bando K. Mitral endocarditis: a new management framework. J Thorac Cardiovasc Surg. 2018;156(4):1486–95.
15. Rostagno C, Carone E, Stefàno PL. Role of mitral valve repair in active infective endocarditis: long term results. J Cardiothorac Surg. 2017;12(1):29.
16. Meine TJ, Nettles RE, Anderson DJ, Cabell CH, Corey GR, Sexton DJ, et al. Cardiac conduction abnormalities in endocarditis defined by the Duke criteria. Am Heart J. 2001;142(2):280–5.
17. Pettersson GB, Hussain ST. Current AATS guidelines on surgical treatment of infective endocarditis. Ann Cardiothorac Surg. 2019;8(6):630–44.
18. Gomes A, Jainandunsing JS, van Assen S, van Geel PP, Sinha B, Gelsomino S, et al. A standardized approach to treat complex aortic valve endocarditis: a case series. J Cardiothorac Surg. 2018;13(1):32.
19. Shmueli H, Thomas F, Flint N, Setia G, Janjic A, Siegel RJ. Right-sided infective endocarditis 2020: challenges and updates in diagnosis and treatment. J Am Heart Assoc. 2020;9(15) https://doi.org/10.1161/JAHA.120.017293.
20. Akinosoglou K, Apostolakis E, Marangos M, Pasvol G. Native valve right sided infective endocarditis. Eur J Intern Med. 2013;24(6):510–9.
21. Döring M, Richter S, Hindricks G. The diagnosis and treatment of pacemaker-associated infection. Dtsch Arzteblatt Int. 2018;115(26):445–52.

22. Chrissoheris MP, Libertin C, Ali RG, Ghantous A, Bekui A, Donohue T. Endocarditis complicating central venous catheter bloodstream infections: a unique form of health care associated endocarditis: endocarditis complicating CVC-BSI. Clin Cardiol. 2009;32(12):E48–54.
23. Murashita T. Surgical treatment for tricuspid valve infective endocarditis. In: Firstenberg MS, editor. Advanced concepts in endocarditis. InTech; 2018. [cited 2022 Feb 9]. Available from: http://www.intechopen.com/books/advanced-concepts-in-endocarditis/surgical-treatment-for-tricuspid-valve-infective-endocarditis.
24. Mathew JP, Nicoara A, Ayoub CM, Swaminathan M. Clinical manual and review of transesophageal echocardiography. 2019.
25. Prendergast BD, Tornos P. Surgery for infective endocarditis: who and when? Circulation. 2010;121(9):1141–52.

Cardiac Tamponade

24

Gil Allen and MaryEllen Antkowiak

Learning Objectives
1. Describe the pathophysiologic changes found in pericardial tamponade.
2. Review the echocardiographic findings of pericardial tamponade.

Pathophysiology of Pericardial Tamponade

The normal pericardium is a fibroelastic sac surrounding the heart. It is lined by smooth pericardial reflections: the outer, parietal layer, which lines the external fibrous sac, and the inner, visceral layer, which lines the epicardial surface of the heart. Under normal circumstances, this sac contains a small amount (~5–15 ml) of serous fluid [1, 2]. Under a variety of pathologic conditions, fluid can accumulate in this space, forming a pericardial effusion. Fluid will typically accumulate dependently at first in the oblique fissure, posterior to the left ventricle. As fluid accumulates, it will circumferentially surround the heart. When fluid accumulates gradually, as in chronic pericardial effusions, the pericardial sac may have time to stretch and adapt, becoming more compliant and accommodating large amounts of fluid with minimal clinical impact. In contrast, rapid accumulation of fluid in the pericardial space does not allow for adaptation in pericardial compliance, leading to the development of acute tamponade with significantly smaller volume effusions [1, 2].

Whether the accumulation of pericardial fluid occurs gradually or rapidly, cardiac tamponade occurs when pericardial pressure exceeds intracardiac pressure [1–3] (Fig. 24.1). The rise in pericardial pressure leads to impaired venous return to the right-sided cardiac chambers. As pressure increases, tamponade physiology progresses, leading to right-sided chamber collapse and reduction in cardiac output. Cardiac output is further reduced during inspiration in tamponade physiology. [1–3] While total venous return to the right-sided cardiac chambers is overall restricted in the setting of cardiac tamponade, the drop in intrathoracic pressure that accompanies inspiration still leads to increased venous return relative to that during expiration. With severe elevations of pericardial pressure, the increased volume of blood returning to the right ventricle can only be accommodated by septal bowing towards the left ventricle, leading to impaired left

Supplementary Information The online version contains supplementary material available at https://doi.org/10.1007/978-3-031-80038-2_24.

G. Allen (✉) · M. Antkowiak
Division of Pulmonary and Critical Care, Department of Medicine, University of Vermont Medical Center and Larner College of Medicine, Burlington, VT, USA
e-mail: gil.allen@uvmhealth.org; maryellen.antkowiak@uvmhealth.org

M. J. Lanspa, A. T. Levinson (eds.), *Echocardiography and Ultrasonography in the ICU*, Respiratory Medicine, https://doi.org/10.1007/978-3-031-80038-2_24

ventricular filling. This phenomenon is termed "ventricular interdependence." These physiologic alterations that occur in tamponade manifest clinical and echocardiographic findings that can be assessed to aid in the diagnosis of this life-threatening condition [4].

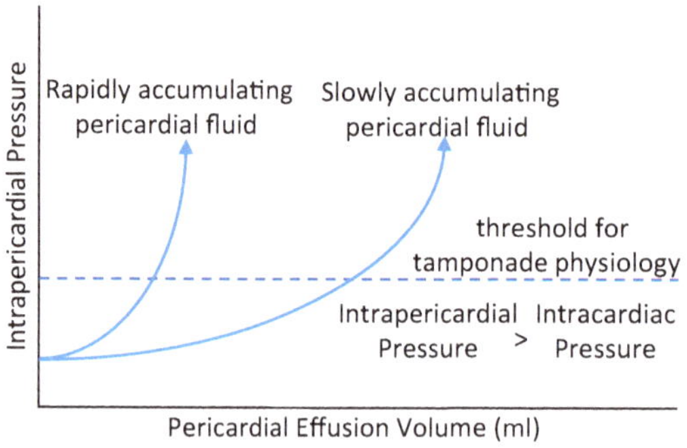

Fig. 24.1 Accumulating pericardial fluid on the horizontal axis and intrapericardial pressure on the vertical axis, demonstrating how rapidly and slowly accumulating pericardial fluid can achieve conditions of tamponade physiology (when intrapericardial pressure exceeds intracardiac pressure) at smaller and larger volumes of pericardial fluid, respectively. This is due to the pericardium having more time to stretch and accommodate volume when fluid accumulates more slowly

Clinical Criteria

Patients presenting with cardiac tamponade will present with a variety of signs and symptoms attributable to the pathologic changes that accompany increases in pericardial pressure. The majority of these are nonspecific, including dyspnea, presyncope, tachycardia, and hypotension. Chest pain, cough, and dysphagia may also be present. Advanced cases may present similarly to other forms of cardiogenic shock, with altered mental status, cold extremities, jugular venous distension, and renal failure [1, 2]. More specific findings may alert clinicians to the presence of cardiac tamponade. Heart sounds may be muffled, and patients with inflammatory pericardial effusions may exhibit a pericardial rub. Electrocardiograms may show low voltage or electrical alternans (Fig. 24.2 and Supplementary Videos 24.1 and 24.2) [1, 2]. The clinical finding most diagnostic of cardiac tamponade is *pulsus paradoxus*. Defined as a drop in systolic pressure of greater than 10 mmHg during inspiration, *pulsus paradoxus* can be detected using sphygmomanometry or via invasive arterial blood pressure

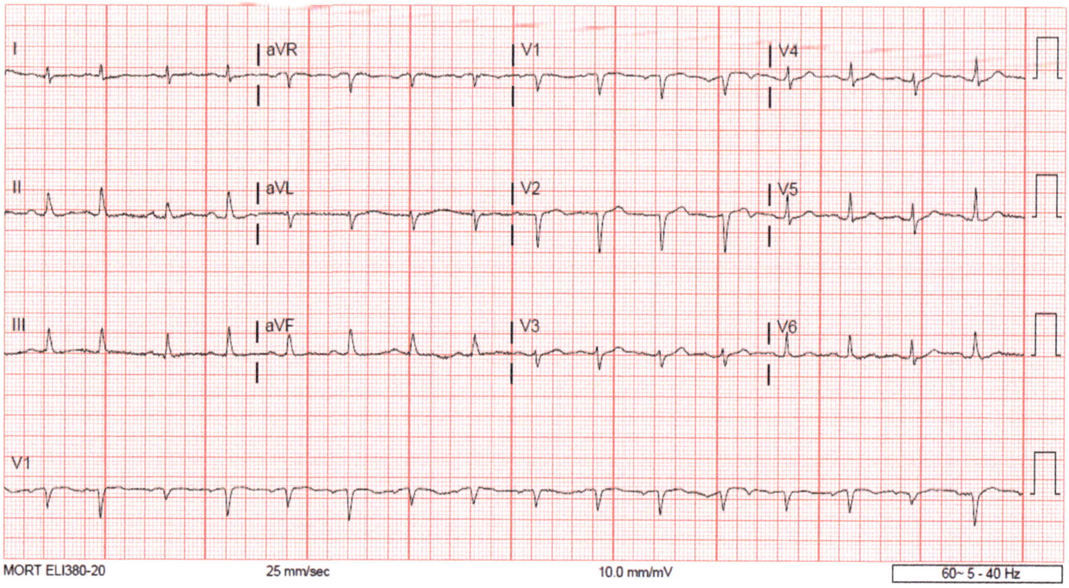

Fig. 24.2 Electrocardiogram consistent with electrical alternans, created by the shifting of the heart's electrical axis and/or variable electrical signal impedance across a variable distance of fluid to the chest wall leads while the heart rocks back and forth within the pericardial sac of fluid (see Supplementary Videos 24.1 and 24.2 for corresponding echocardiogram findings)

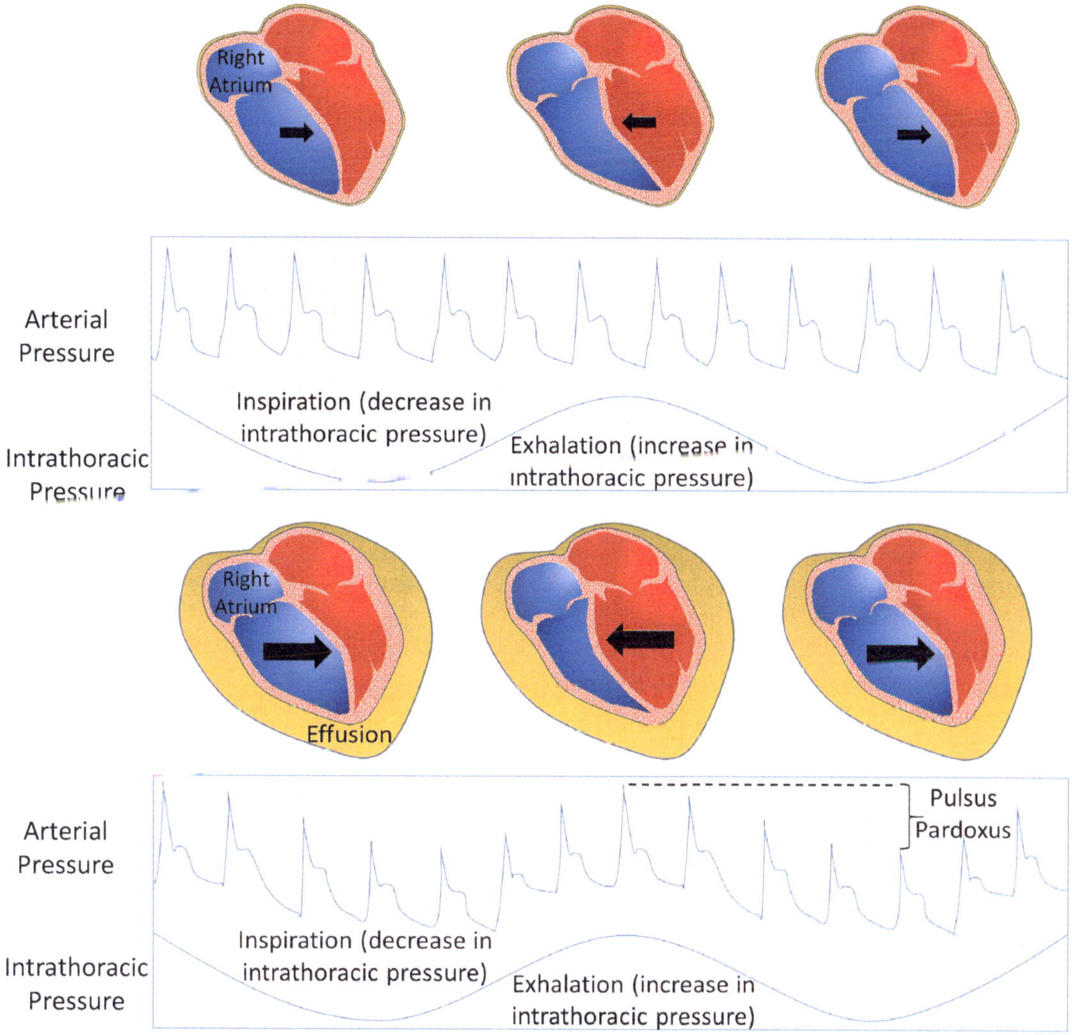

Fig. 24.3 The top section demonstrates normal and nominal ventricular interdependence under non-restrictive conditions, with negligible respirophasic variation in cardiac output and systolic blood pressure. The bottom section demonstrates the exaggerated ventricular interdependence that results from the increased restriction of accumulating pericardial effusion, resulting in respirophasic variation in both cardiac output and blood pressure (i.e., pulsus paradoxus)

monitoring [1–3]. As this drop is the result of the ventricular independence described in the previous section, it is highly suggestive of a diagnosis of cardiac tamponade in the presence of a pericardial effusion (Fig. 24.3) [4]. There are a variety of conditions that, when present, can prevent the development of pulsus paradoxus, reducing the sensitivity of this diagnostic finding [2]. Given the non-specific signs and symptoms of cardiac tamponade and the challenges encountered in evaluating pulsus paradoxus, echocardiography has become increasingly useful in the evaluation of patients presenting with pericardial effusion and concern for hemodynamic compromise. Echocardiography should be considered a supplementary tool for helping one raise or lower one's suspicion that tamponade physiology is accounting for a patient's clinical presentation, but as only some echocardiographic features of tamponade may be present in any given patient, cardiac tamponade should always be considered a clinical diagnosis.

Echocardiographic Evaluation of Pericardial Tamponade

Detection of Pericardial Effusion

The first step in the echocardiographic assessment of the patient with suspected cardiac tamponade is demonstrating the presence of pericardial effusion. Echocardiography remains the modality of choice for detecting the presence of pericardial effusion because its now wide availability at the bedside allows for rapid, noninvasive assessment [5]. Two-dimensional mode (2D mode) transthoracic echocardiography (TTE) is highly sensitive and specific for the detection of pericardial effusion. In many patients, TTE can detect effusions as small as 50 ml. Subxiphoid view is typically used in emergent cases for rapid assessment of the presence of pericardial effusion, but additional assessment in parasternal and apical views allows for a more accurate estimation of effusion size [5]. The parasternal long axis (PLAX) view should penetrate deep enough to visualize the descending aorta. Unlike pleural fluid, which will track up to but never over the descending aorta, free-flowing pericardial fluid will typically track between the descending aorta and the left atrium (Fig. 24.4 and Supplementary Videos 24.3 and 24.4). TTE also allows for the characterization of pericardial effusion, differentiating simple, free-flowing effusions from loculated or localized effusions, or those containing thrombus or other proteinaceous material [5]. It is imperative that clinicians be aware that the presence of a pericardial effusion, even when large in volume, does not imply a diagnosis of cardiac tamponade in the absence of additional supportive clinical and echocardiographic criteria. Echocardiography allows clinicians to visualize the pathophysiologic effects of increased pericardial pressure and, in many cases, correlate these with clinical exam findings.

Cardiac Chamber Collapse

Following the identification and characterization of pericardial effusion, additional assessments can be made utilizing 2D echocardiography that can alert clinicians to the development of cardiac tamponade physiology. As rising pericardial pressure exceeds intracardiac pressure, cardiac chamber collapse results. This can typically be assessed in apical and parasternal long views at various points in the car-

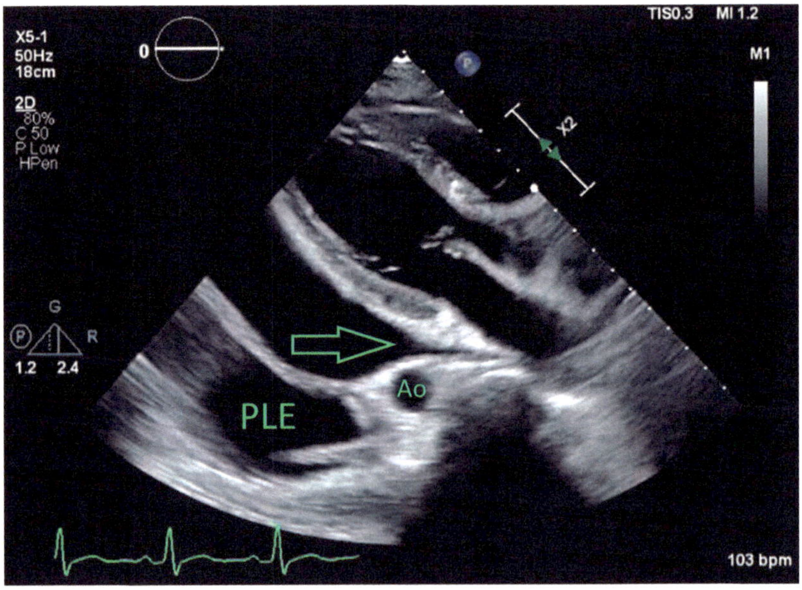

Fig. 24.4 Still shot of parasternal long axis (PLAX) view, penetrating beyond the depth of the descending aorta (Ao), demonstrating both a large pleural effusion (PLE), which terminates at the descending aorta, and a large pericardial effusion, which can be seen tracking (horizontal arrow) up and in between the descending aorta (Ao) and left atrium (see Supplementary Videos 24.3 and 24.4 for corresponding echocardiogram video clip)

diac cycle [6]. Chamber collapse will initially be evident in the right atrium, typically during early systole when intra-atrial pressure is lowest (Supplementary Videos 24.5 and 24.6). As tamponade progresses, the right atrial collapse will persist for longer periods of the cardiac cycle. The use of M-mode may aid in assessing the duration of collapse. Right atrial collapse present for greater than 1/3 of the cardiac cycle has been reported to have both a sensitivity and specificity close to 100% for the diagnosis of cardiac tamponade. [7] Left atrial collapse may also accompany right atrial collapse in the later stages of tamponade [8]. Right ventricular (RV) free wall collapse will be evident in 2D mode as tamponade progresses. In contrast to right atrial collapse, RV collapse will be observed in diastole, when intraventricular pressure is lowest. Initially, RV chamber size will be preserved in inspiration owing to increased venous return during inspiration, but as intracardial pressure rises, collapse will occur throughout the respiratory cycle [6, 9]. As observed in atrial collapse, the duration of RV free wall collapse correlates with the severity of tamponade, and the use of M-mode may aid in identifying normal RV free wall relaxation during diastole (Fig. 24.5a) or recognizing and quantifying the duration of collapse (Supplementary Videos 24.7 and 24.8; and Fig. 24.5b) [6, 9]. Although RV stroke volume will decrease as free wall collapse develops, blood pressure will remain preserved throughout the respiratory cycle, and early detection of RV free wall collapse may be an earlier indicator of tamponade than pulsus paradoxus [10]. Conversely, the absence of right-sided chamber collapse has been demonstrated to have a 90% negative predictive value for the exclusion of a diagnosis of tamponade [6]. Impaired RV filling and diastolic collapse can, in fact, manifest along a continuum, spanning from normal diastolic RV filling with a large chronic effusion (Supplementary Videos 24.9 and 24.10), intermittent RV collapse (Supplementary Videos 24.11 and 24.12), regular diastolic RV collapse (Supplementary Videos 24.13, 24.14, and 24.15), and RV filling that appears restricted throughout diastole (Supplementary Videos 24.16 and 24.17), only to be confirmed (in the same patient) by post-pericardiocentesis imaging (Supplementary Videos 24.18 and 24.19). In rare situations, chamber collapse may not be readily observed in patients with significantly elevated pericardial pressures. Severe pulmonary hypertension with accompanying right heart failure and left ventricular failure with significantly elevated left ventricular diastolic pressure, and the use of positive pressure ventilation may complicate the echocardiographic diagnosis of tamponade by blunting chamber collapse [6].

Inferior Vena Cava Plethora

As cardiac tamponade develops, increased pericardial pressure leads to increased right-sided intracardiac pressure, and venous return to the right-sided cardiac chambers becomes increasingly impaired. While this manifests clinically as jugular venous distension, impaired venous return and increased right-sided chamber pressure can be assessed echocardiographically by detection of inferior vena cava (IVC) plethora [2]. The IVC can be assessed using subxiphoid views in 2D mode. Using this view, IVC and hepatic vein distension can be detected in patients with cardiac tamponade. Plethora of the IVC is defined as an IVC diameter greater than 2 cm with less than a 50% reduction in diameter during inspiration. Assessment of variation of IVC diameter throughout the respiratory cycle is most easily assessed utilizing M-mode [6]. While IVC plethora can be seen in a variety of conditions and is not specific to tamponade, its presence in the setting of pericardial effusion and supportive clinical factors is highly suggestive of the diagnosis. Furthermore, IVC plethora has been demonstrated to be highly sensitive (>90%) for detecting cardiac tamponade, and its absence is often reassuring in helping to exclude the diagnosis [11].

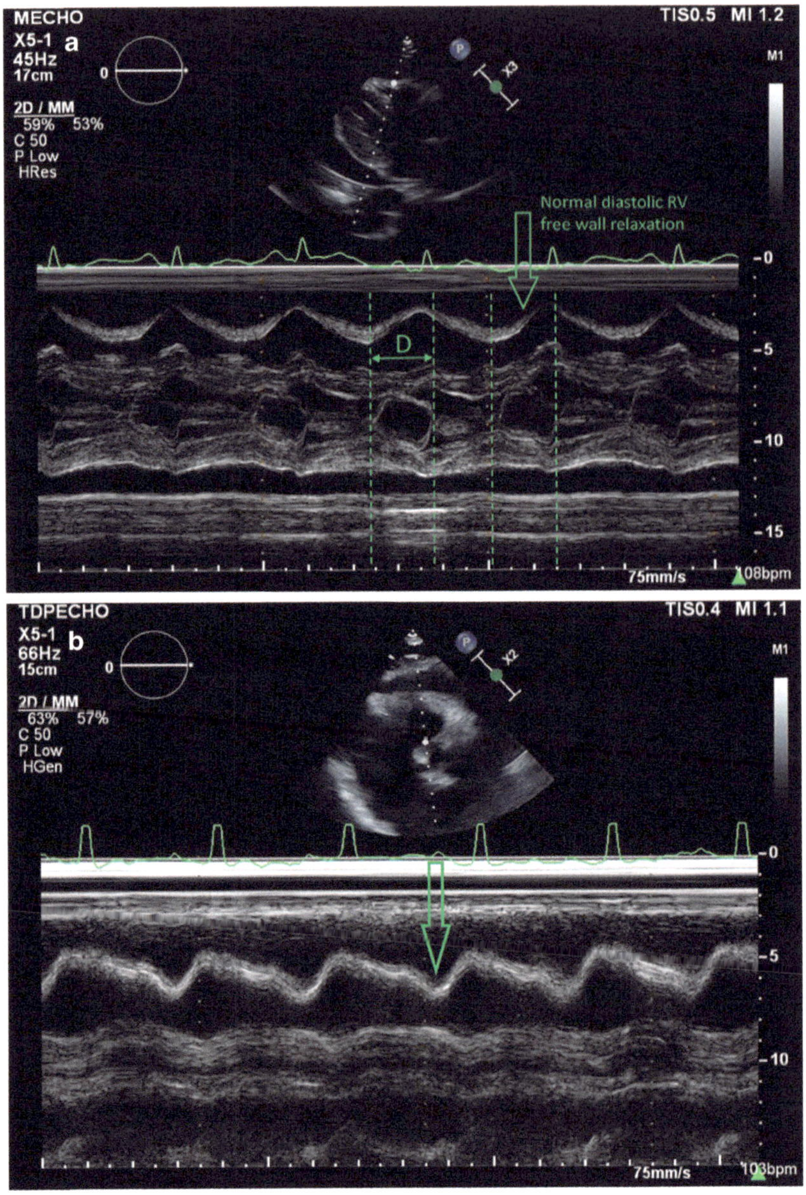

Fig. 24.5 (**a**) M-mode still from PLAX view with a slice through RV free wall, septum, and mitral leaflets. Dotted lines define the boundaries of diastole, include mitral leaflet excursion, and correspond with the ECG diastole signature. A large downward arrow demonstrates normal RV free wall relaxation and RV dilation during diastole. (**b**) M-mode still from PLAX view with a slice through RV free wall, septum, but missing the mitral leaflets. A large downward arrow corresponds with the ECG diastole signature and demonstrates depression/collapse of the RV-free wall in mid-diastole, consistent with tamponade physiology

Ventricular Interdependence and Septal Bounce

Although not typically required to support a diagnosis of cardiac tamponade, echocardiography can be used to demonstrate ventricular interdependence, the hallmark pathophysiology of the condition. Utilizing parasternal long and short-axis views in 2D echocardiography with the assistance of M-mode, ventricular size and septal positioning can be assessed throughout the respiratory cycle. In patients with increased pericardial pressure and tamponade physiology, these views will demonstrate increased RV chamber diameter, septal displacement or "bounce" towards the left ventricle, and decreased left ventricular chamber diameter during inspiration as compared with expiration [6].

Spectral Doppler Flow Variation

While pericardial effusion and tamponade physiology can be detected and characterized utilizing 2D echocardiography, in the hands of an experienced ultrasonographer, techniques utilizing spectral (pulse wave) Doppler modes can be applied to further support a diagnosis of tamponade [6]. Cardiac tamponade is associated with exaggerated variations in systemic and pulmonary venous return, resulting in exaggerated respirophasic changes in diastolic filling velocities and cardiac output [2]. These variations can be assessed clinically via assessment of pulsus paradoxus and with echocardiography using pulse wave Doppler [12]. In patients with suspected cardiac tamponade, respiratory cycle variations in right and left ventricular inflow across the mitral and tricuspid valves are commonly assessed [6, 13]. After obtaining an apical 4-chamber view, right and left ventricular inflow can be evaluated using pulse wave Doppler while positioning probe alignment across the tricuspid and mitral valves, respectively. The peak velocity of the passive ventricular filling (represented by the E wave) can then be assessed throughout the respiratory cycle [13–15]. In healthy patients without cardiac tamponade, tricuspid and mitral inflow will vary by less than 5% (Figs. 24.6 and 24.7, respectively). In patients with tamponade physiology, peak tricuspid inflow will decrease by more than 40% during expiration (Fig. 24.8), while mitral inflow will decrease by more than 25% during inspiration (Fig. 24.9) [13–15]. Spectral Doppler is less commonly used in the evaluation of cardiac tamponade to assess respirophasic changes in ventricular output in patients in normal sinus rhythm [6]. These variations are not reliable indicators of tamponade physiology in patients with irregular cardiac rhythms. Left ventricular output is best assessed using an apical five-chamber view with probe positioning over the left ventricular outflow tract. A decrease in peak left ventricular output velocity of greater than 10% during inspiration is associated with tamponade physiology (Fig. 24.10). Right ventricular outflow is best assessed by positioning a pulse wave Doppler probe across the pulmonic valve in a suprasternal or modified parasternal view. An inspiratory increase in right ventricular outflow of greater than 10% suggests cardiac tamponade [13, 15]. Alternatively, an aortic arch view from the sternal notch can also be used to corroborate these findings (Fig. 24.11). Lastly, spectral Doppler can be applied to the assessment of hepatic vein flow reversal utilizing subxiphoid windows to further support a diagnosis of cardiac tamponade [6]. In the absence of tamponade, Doppler assessment of the hepatic vein demonstrates biphasic inflow with reversal of flow during atrial contraction (Supplementary Videos 24.20 and 24.21). In tamponade, hepatic vein flow will be decreased and even reversed during diastole (Fig. 24.12). Hepatic vein flow can be challenging to assess via Doppler echocardiography in many patients, but in the presence of clear windows, the presence or absence of diastolic reversal of hepatic vein flow has been demonstrated to have a high positive and negative predictive value in the diagnosis of cardiac tamponade [6, 15].

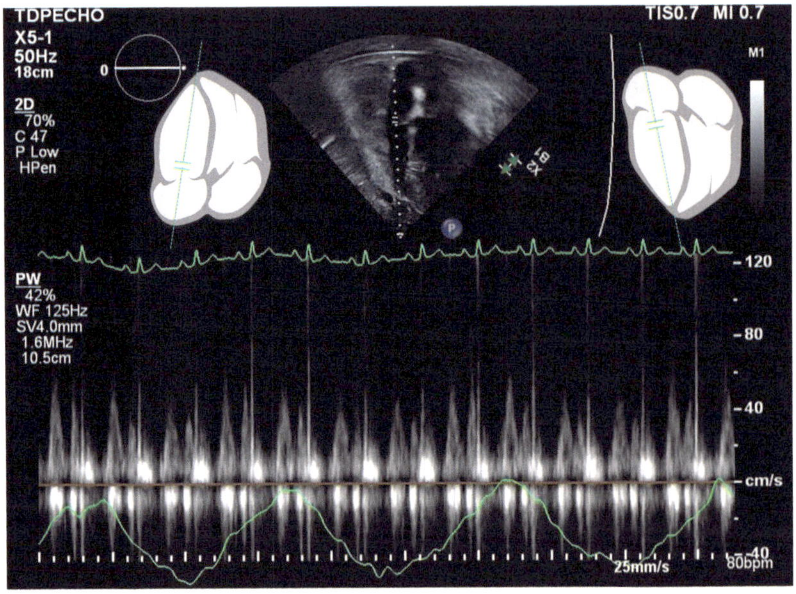

Fig. 24.6 Atria on top (Mayo) apical 4-chamber view with pulse wave Doppler indicator situated just below the leaflets of the tricuspid valve. Cartoon images on the left and right represent how standard (left) and Mayo (right) apical 4-chambers (A4C) views appear with respect to the indicator. Note the negligible variation of RV inflow velocities with inspiration (upward deflection of chest wall impedance) and exhalation (downward deflection) at the bottom of the image

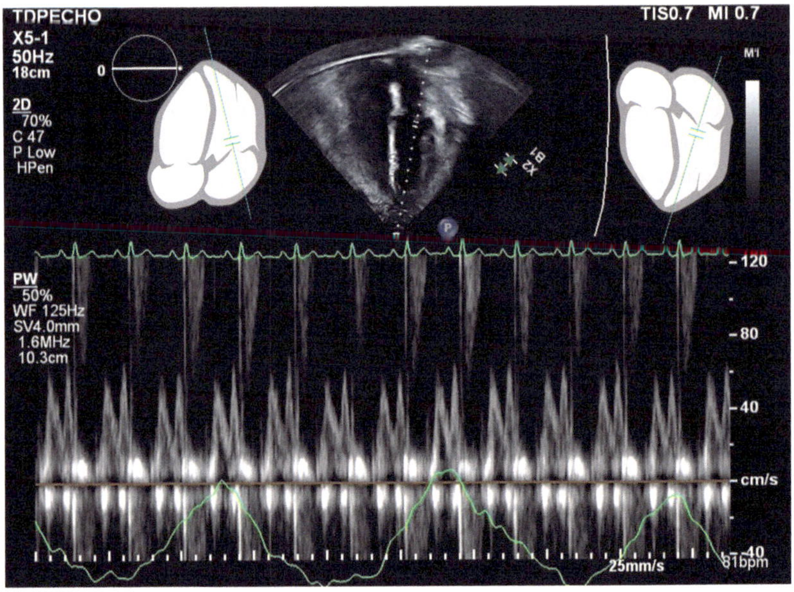

Fig. 24.7 Atria on top (Mayo) A4C view with pulse wave Doppler indicator situated just below the leaflets of the mitral valve. Similar cartoon representations of standard and Mayo A4C views are on the left and right of the echo image, respectively. Note the negligible variation of LV inflow velocities with inspiration and exhalation

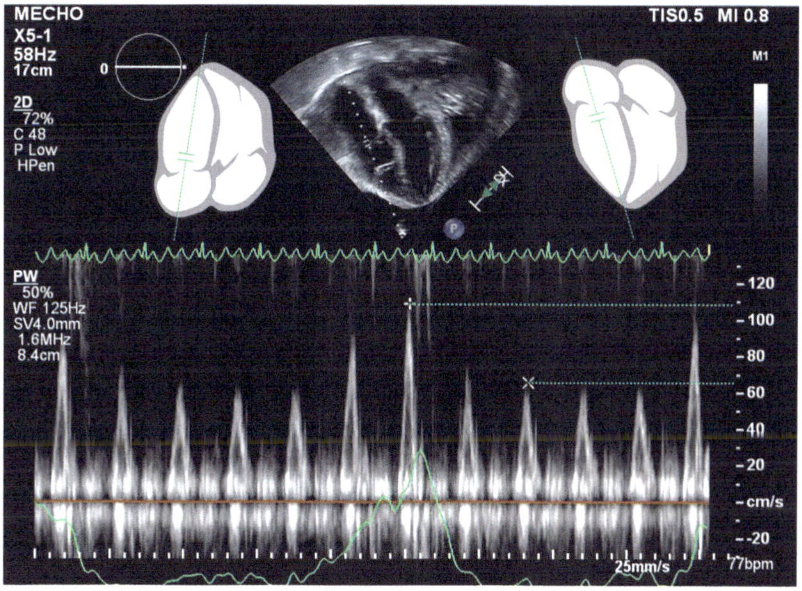

Fig. 24.8 Atria on top (Mayo) A4C view with pulse wave Doppler indicator situated just below the leaflets of the tricuspid valve. Similar cartoon representations of standard and Mayo A4C views are on the left and right, respectively. Note the significant variation of RV inflow velocities with greater velocities during augmented RV filling on inspiration, with depression during exhalation

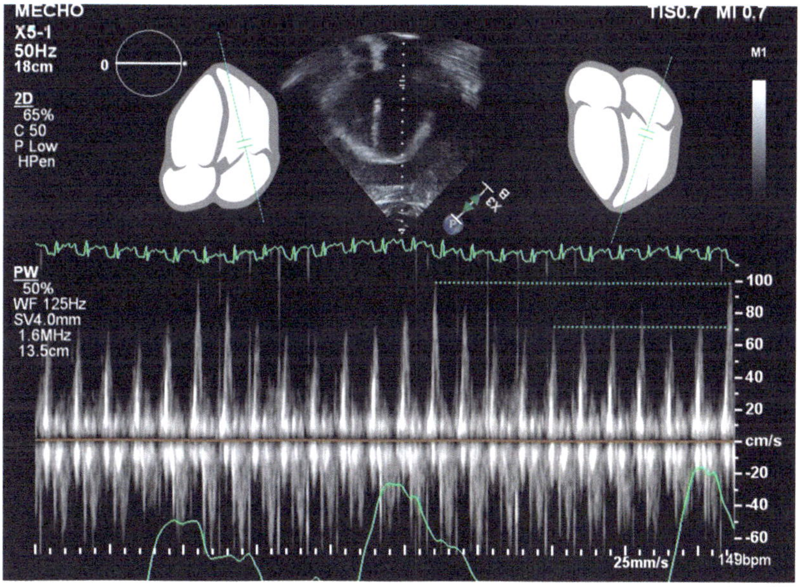

Fig. 24.9 Atria on top (Mayo) A4C view with pulse wave Doppler indicator situated just below the leaflets of the mitral valve. Similar cartoon representations of standard and Mayo A4C views are on the left and right, respectively. Note significant variation of LV inflow velocities with significantly limited inflow velocities during inspiration and augmented LV filling velocities during exhalation

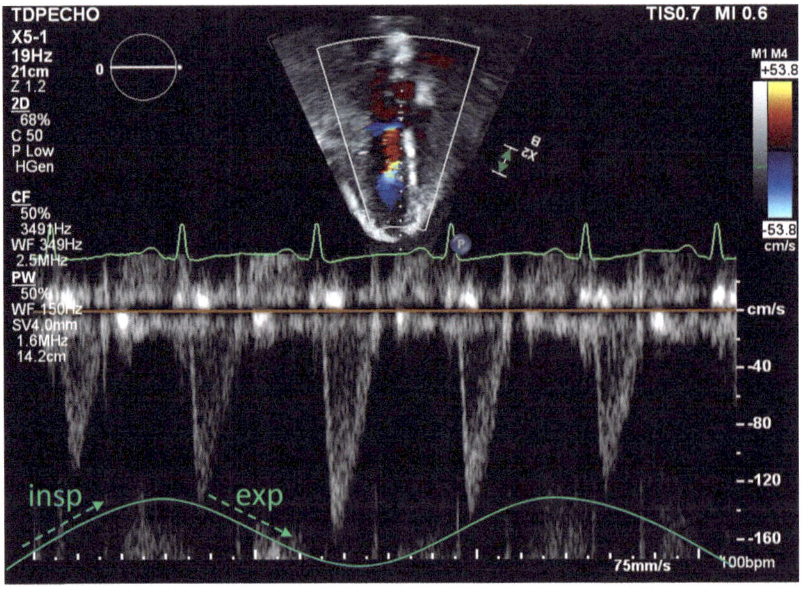

Fig. 24.10 Atria on top (Mayo) apical 5-chamber view with pulse wave Doppler indicator situated within the left ventricular outflow tract (LVOT), just behind the aortic valve. Note how peak velocities and volume time integrals (VTI) across the LVOT are augmented during exhalation (exp) when LV preload is accentuated and depressed during inspiration (insp) when RV filling is augmented and ventricular interdependence is restricting LV preload

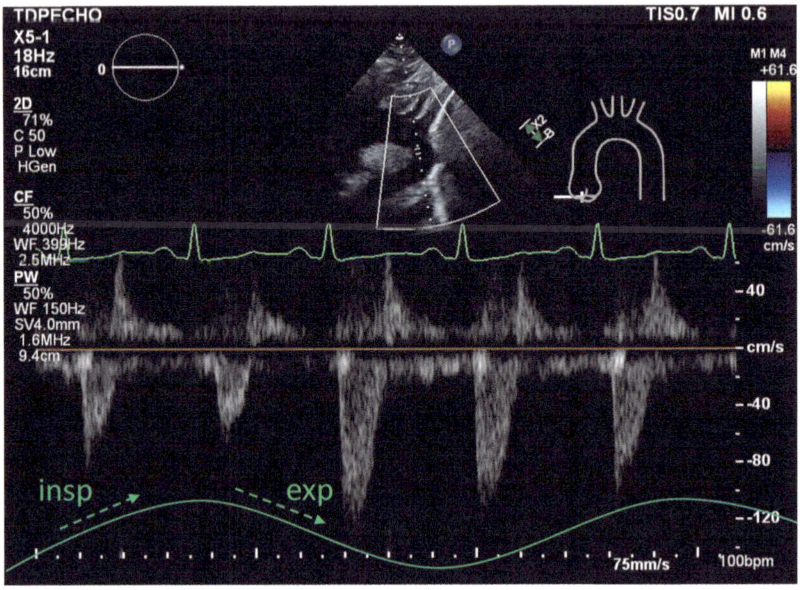

Fig. 24.11 Similar capture of aortic flow velocities and volume time integrals (VTI) in the descending aortic arch, taken from a sternal notch view, demonstrating the same respirophasic variation in VTI with stroke volume most augmented during exhalation, when ventricular interdependence is favoring LV preload

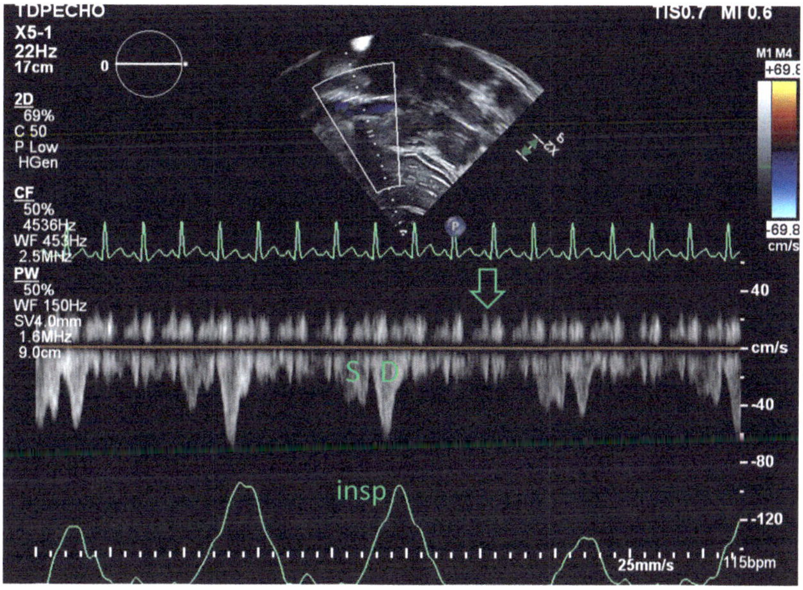

Fig. 24.12 Pulse wave Doppler measurements from the hepatic vein, feeding into the inferior vena cava. Downward augmented flow velocities labeled "S" and "D" demonstrate accelerated flow toward the atrium during systole and diastole during inspiration, when intrathoracic pressure is lowest and venous return to the heart is augmented. Note that these flow velocities are blunted during exhalation when venous return to the right heart is blunted. The downward arrow represents where one might also find augmented reversals in diastolic flow (reflux back into the IVC and hepatic vein during more extreme conditions of tamponade). Supplementary Videos 24.20 and 24.21 demonstrates IVC plethora on the right and reflux flow back into the IVC and the hepatic vein on the right

Summary Points

- Cardiac tamponade is a life-threatening yet treatable condition that can be rapidly fatal if recognition and definitive management are delayed. While ultimately a clinical diagnosis, echocardiography plays a crucial role in establishing the presence of pericardial effusion and additional findings that support clinical signs of tamponade physiology. Once a diagnosis of cardiac tamponade is established, definitive management with pericardiocentesis can be safely supported with the use of several well-described ultrasound-guided approaches. The use of ultrasound guidance in pericardiocentesis will be discussed elsewhere in this text.

References

1. Spodick DH. The normal and diseased pericardium: current concepts of pericardial physiology, diagnosis and treatment. J Am Coll Cardiol. 1983;1:240–51.
2. Spodick DH. Acute cardiac tamponade. N Engl J Med. 2003;349:684–90.
3. Reddy PS, Curtiss EI, Uretsky BF. Spectrum of hemodynamic changes in cardiac tamponade. Am J Cardiol. 1990;66:1487–91.
4. Santamore WP, Li KS, Nakamoto T, Johnston WE. Effects of increased pericardial pressure on the coupling between the ventricles. Cardiovasc Res. 1990;24:768–76.
5. Adler Y, Charron P, Imazio M, et al. 2015 ESC Guidelines for the diagnosis and management of pericardial diseases: The Task Force for the Diagnosis and Management of Pericardial Diseases of the European Society of Cardiology (ESC)Endorsed by: The European Association for Cardio-Thoracic Surgery (EACTS). Eur Heart J. 2015;36:2921–64.
6. Perez-Casares A, Cesar S, Brunet-Garcia L, Sanchez-de-Toledo J. Echocardiographic Evaluation of Pericardial Effusion and Cardiac Tamponade. Front Pediatr. 2017;5:79.
7. Gillam LD, Guyer DE, Gibson TC, King ME, Marshall JE, Weyman AE. Hydrodynamic compression of the right atrium: a new echocardiographic sign of cardiac tamponade. Circulation. 1983;68:294–301.
8. Fast J, Wielenga RP, Jansen E, Schuurmans Stekhoven JH. Abnormal wall movements of the right ventricle

and both atria in patients with pericardial effusion as indicators of cardiac tamponade. Eur Heart J. 1986;7:431–6.

9. Leimgruber PP, Klopfenstein HS, Wann LS, Brooks HL. The hemodynamic derangement associated with right ventricular diastolic collapse in cardiac tamponade: an experimental echocardiographic study. Circulation. 1983;68:612–20.
10. Singh S, Wann LS, Klopfenstein HS, Hartz A, Brooks HL. Usefulness of right ventricular diastolic collapse in diagnosing cardiac tamponade and comparison to pulsus paradoxus. Am J Cardiol. 1986;57:652–6.
11. Himelman RB, Kircher B, Rockey DC, Schiller NB. Inferior vena cava plethora with blunted respiratory response: a sensitive echocardiographic sign of cardiac tamponade. J Am Coll Cardiol. 1988;12:1470–7.
12. Merce J, Sagrista-Sauleda J, Permanyer-Miralda G, Evangelista A, Soler-Soler J. Correlation between clinical and Doppler echocardiographic findings in patients with moderate and large pericardial effusion: implications for the diagnosis of cardiac tamponade. Am Heart J. 1999;138:759–64.
13. Leeman DE, Levine MJ, Come PC. Doppler echocardiography in cardiac tamponade: exaggerated respiratory variation in transvalvular blood flow velocity integrals. J Am Coll Cardiol. 1988;11:572–8.
14. D'Cruz II, Rehman AU, Hancock HL. Quantitative Echocardiographic Assessment in Pericardial Disease. Echocardiography. 1997;14:207–14.
15. Klein AL, Cohen GI. Doppler echocardiographic assessment of constrictive pericarditis, cardiac amyloidosis, and cardiac tamponade. Cleve Clin J Med. 1992;59:278–90.

25 Ultrasound-Guided Pericardiocentesis

Lisa Rapoport and Pranjal Gupta

Learning Objectives

1. Discuss various approaches for pericardiocentesis.
2. Review ultrasound techniques for verifying needle placement prior to catheterization of the pericardial space.
3. Describe the use of ultrasound to identify post-pericardiocentesis complications.

Background

Pericardiocentesis is the aspiration of pericardial fluid from the pericardial sac. In cases with obstructive physiology, pericardiocentesis is indicated as a potentially life-saving procedure.

Echocardiography is extremely sensitive and specific for detecting pericardial effusions. Applying the physiologic concept of ventricular interdependence allows echocardiography to assess for hemodynamic significance. Furthermore, although ultimately cardiac tamponade is a clinical diagnosis, certain echocardiographic clues can point toward obstructive physiology.

L. Rapoport (✉)
Emergency and Critical Care Medicine, Kaiser Permanente Santa Clara, Santa Clara, CA, USA

Department of Emergency Medicine, Stanford University School of Medicine, Santa Clara, CA, USA

P. Gupta
Critical Care Fellow, Stanford University School of Medicine, Stanford, CA, USA
e-mail: pranjalgupta@stanford.edu

Evaluation of Pericardial Effusion on Echocardiogram

Transthoracic Echocardiogram

Point-of-care ultrasound (POCUS) can visualize the separation of the pericardium from the myocardium with high sensitivity with as little as 15–35 mL of fluid [1]. Care must be taken to differentiate a pericardial effusion from an epicardial fat pad, of which the fat pad is usually hyperechoic, granular, and moves in synchrony with the external cardiac border [2]. A pleural effusion can be confused with a pericardial effusion, but the two are differentiated via the descending thoracic aorta on parasternal long-axis view (PLAX): A pleural effusion will be adjacent or inferior to the descending aorta, while a pericardial effusion will be anterior [1]. Additionally, not all hemodynamically significant pericardial effusions need to be circumferential, as is seen in post-procedural effusions that cause obstructive physiology in a single cardiac chamber. Therefore, to best characterize a pericardial effusion, multiple different views should be obtained, as a single view can misrepresent the volume or location. Of note, the size of the effusion does not predict tamponade, but

M. J. Lanspa, A. T. Levinson (eds.), *Echocardiography and Ultrasonography in the ICU*, Respiratory Medicine, https://doi.org/10.1007/978-3-031-80038-2_25

rather the rate of accumulation of fluid and pericardial compliance [1].

When making the diagnosis of pericardial tamponade, it is important to keep the physiology in mind: tamponade is an obstructive state where the pressures outside the cardiac chambers inhibit appropriate chamber filling. Thus the most important echocardiographic signs of tamponade include the presence of a pericardial effusion, dilated inferior vena cava (IVC), and a left ventricle that has reduced end-diastolic and end-systolic dimensions with evidence of reduced cardiac output (i.e., an underfilled LV). Impaired cardiac chamber filling in turn exaggerates normal interventricular dependence during a cardiac cycle. This leads to other classic findings such as right ventricular diastolic chamber collapse, right atrial systolic collapse, and the inspiratory bulge of the interventricular septum into the left ventricle (seen bulging into the left ventricle during spontaneous inspiration and mechanical expiration). Characteristic abnormal respirophasic changes in Doppler flow velocity recordings across the mitral and tricuspid valves can also be seen and are useful findings but not necessary to make the diagnosis of tamponade (Table 25.1).

Inferior Vena Cava Plethora

A dilated or plethoric IVC with <50% respirophasic variation in diameter is correlated with elevated central venous pressure and decreased venous return, seen when pericardial pressures increase above intracardiac pressures. IVC plethora is a very sensitive sign for tamponade (95–97%) but has poor specificity (~40%) due to plethora potentially being due to a variety of other causes, such as chronic pulmonary hypertension, tricuspid regurgitation, etc. [1] M-mode can be used to track the IVC diameter across the respiratory cycle, approximately 2–3 cm from the IVC-right atrial junction. Hepatic vein dilation can also be used as a proxy for IVC plethora when the IVC is difficult to visualize [4].

Right Heart Chamber Systolic/Diastolic Collapse

Right-sided chamber collapse is a critical finding in cardiac tamponade that occurs when the pericardial pressures exceed those of the internal cardiac chambers. The right atrial collapse in systole is often considered the first sonographic sign of tamponade [5]. If the duration of right atrial collapse exceeds more than one-third of the cardiac cycle, the sensitivity and specificity of such a finding approach 100% for clinical cardiac tamponade [6]. Right ventricular collapse, usually seen in early diastole, may initially only be seen in inspiration in spontaneously breathing patients (or during expiration in mechanically ventilated patients) but may persist throughout the respiratory cycle as tamponade worsens [4]. Right heart diastolic collapse may also occur in significant hypovolemia, in which concurrently scanning for IVC plethora can be useful. Right heart diastolic collapse can be seen best in the PLAX, SX, or apical 4-chamber views (A4C). In the PLAX view, diastole corresponds with visualization of the opening of the mitral valve, and in the A4C and SX views diastole corresponds with visualization of the opening of the mitral and tricuspid valve. Keep in mind that in cases of localized tamponade, such as post-surgical tamponade, these classic findings may not be seen.

Inspiratory Bulge of the Intraventricular Septum

Spontaneous breathing causes negative intrathoracic pressure during inspiration. During spontaneous inspiration, as right heart pressures fall, RV filling is augmented, and a natural bowing of the septum towards the left ventricle is expected, given ventricular interdependence due to the shared septal wall. The opposite can be expected in mechanically ventilated patients, where bowing of the septum towards the LV occurs in mechanical expiration. RV filling pressure in turn leads to left ventricular filling variations and subsequently variations in LV stroke volume, with respect to respirophasic variations. Usually, left-sided filling changes <5% during inspiration. However, during cardiac tamponade, ventricular interdependence and thus left-sided filling changes are exaggerated. This gives rise to the phenomenon of "pulsus paradoxus." Pulsus paradoxus is generally a sign of poor specificity, seen in a variety of conditions whereby there are significant heart-lung filling pressure interactions, including COPD exacerbations and pulmonary embolism [7].

Table 25.1 Echocardiography findings of cardiac tamponade

Finding		Example
Dilated IVC	IVC dilation (>2.1 cm) with <50% reduction in diameter during inspiration. If IVC is difficult to assess, dilatation of hepatic veins is a reliable confirmatory sign	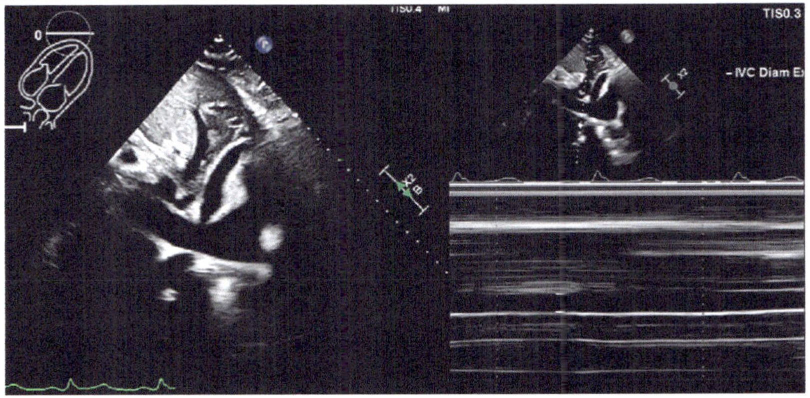 Two-dimensional subcostal view of the heart in a patient with tamponade showing a dilated IVC (2.0 cm) by 2D echocardiography—note also the dilation of the hepatic vein (HV). The image on the right shows the M-mode of the IVC throughout a spontaneous respiratory cycle and is used to calculate the inspiratory reduction in diameter
Right heart diastolic collapse	The absence of any cardiac chamber collapse has a > 90% negative predictive value for clinical cardiac tamponade [3]	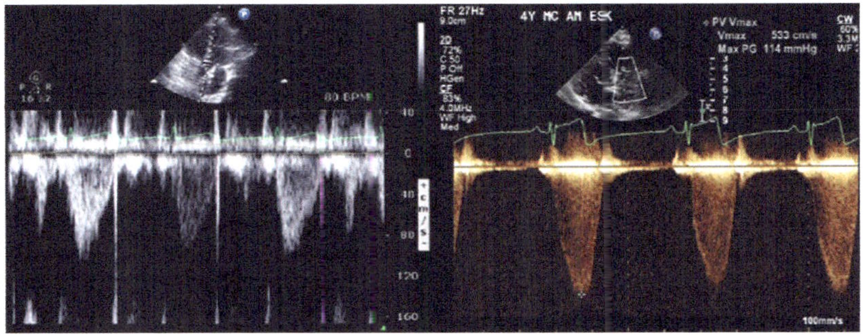 Two-dimensional subcostal view of the heart showing right atrial and RV indentation or "collapse" (small arrow). In both the right atrial and RV chambers, the indentation occurs during relaxation when their pressure is lowest and transiently falls below pericardial pressure

(continued)

Table 25.1 (continued)

Finding		Example
Inspiratory bulging of interventricular septum	Left heart filling decreases abnormally in cardiac tamponade due to ventricular interdependence, wherein an increase in filling on one side of the heart is associated with a decrease on the opposite side	An M-mode echocardiogram was obtained from a patient with pericardial effusion and cardiac tamponade. When the RV enlarges with spontaneous inspiration (insp), the LV becomes smaller (dashed arrows).The opposite changes are seen on expiration (exp)
Abnormal respiratory changes in Doppler flow velocity recordings	Generally, a decrease of 30% of mitral valve E-wave inflow velocity during inspiration is diagnostic for ultrasonographic cardiac tamponade. Similarly, an increase in roughly 40% of tricuspid valve inflow velocity during inspiration can be seen in tamponade	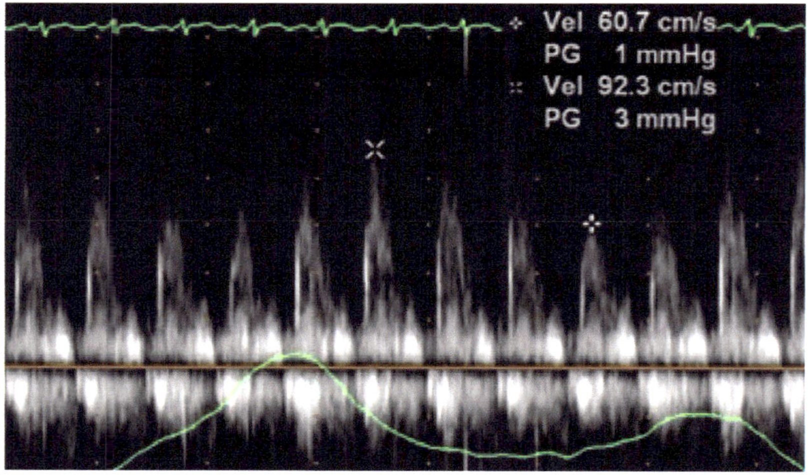 Pulse wave Doppler recording across the mitral valve of a patient in cardiac tamponade. The first beat of spontaneous inspiration should be compared to the first beat of expiration

Adapted from the American Society of Echocardiography clinical recommendations for multimodality cardiovascular imaging of patients with pericardial disease [4]

Doppler Flow Velocity Changes

Exaggerated ventricular interdependence in tamponade physiology also causes exaggerated respirophasic flows across the tricuspid and mitral valves in the pericardial tamponade. These can be evaluated via Doppler flow in ultrasonography as another tool to evaluate pericardial tamponade. Normally, changes in peak E-wave mitral velocity during spontaneous inspiration are <5% [8], but in tamponade, a decrease of 25–30% peak E-wave mitral velocity is considered diagnostic [9]. For the tricuspid valve, tamponade physiology will produce an approximately 40% increase in in-flow velocity [7]. These velocity measurements are best achieved via the A4C view when the pulse wave Doppler gate is in alignment with tricuspid and mitral valve blood flow.

Approaches to the Point-of-Care-Ultrasound (POCUS) Guided Procedure

Traditionally, pericardiocentesis is performed in a controlled, surgical setting. However, given the life-threatening nature of cardiac tamponade and the increasing use of point-of-care cardiac ultrasonography (POCUS), ultrasound-guided pericardiocentesis is an essential skill for any clinician working in an emergent setting. Multiple observational studies of ultrasound-guided pericardiocentesis report improved safety and success as compared to blind aspiration [10]. The parasternal, apical, or subxiphoid approach has all been described, but procedure selection depends on operator comfort or local expertise. Consideration should be given to the approach where the largest fluid collection is visualized on ultrasound and accessed closest to the skin surface with the safest needle trajectory. There is no clear consensus as to which approach is ideal, but some studies suggest the apical approach may be the safest. Complication rates with pericardiocentesis are reportedly lower via the parasternal or apical compared to the subxiphoid approach, as both minimize the distance from skin to fluid collection [11–13]. In addition, observational studies of pericardial effusion distribution suggest that left chest access points are often superior to the traditional subxiphoid [11, 14]. However, all three approaches (left parasternal, apical, and subxiphoid/subcostal) are described here.

- Equipment.
  - Ultrasound machine with phased-array (cardiac) and linear (vascular) probes.
  - Sterile ultrasound probe cover, sterile gown, and gloves.
  - Chlorhexidine antiseptic prep.
  - Pericardiocentesis kit, single-lumen central line kit, or a pigtail thoracostomy kit and a 6F or 8F dilator if a catheter is being left in place.
  - 18-gauge needle with sheath or 18-gauge spinal needle
  - Cardiac monitor.
  - Pulse oximetry.
  - Specimen collection tubes (for cytology and additional studies).
  - Code cart with a defibrillator.
- General Tips:
  - Systematically examine the heart and look for effusions at each imaging window (subcostal, parasternal, apical, and any additional views).
  - The optimal site contains the largest pericardial fluid that is closest to the chest wall and can be entered without puncturing an adjacent vital organ.
  - Select a target fluid layer (distance from pericardium to epicardium) of at least 1 cm to avoid cardiac puncture.
  - Real-time ultrasound visualization of the needle passage is optimal, but continuous visualization of needle tip may be difficult.
  - If available, two clinicians scrubbed in sterile attire may be superior to one, with one clinician as the designated ultrasonographer and the other clinician as the proceduralist.
  - Agitated saline injected through the pericardial catheter should create an artifact easily visualized in the pericardial space,

and this is a tenet to confirm the proper placement of the drain with any approach.
- Ultrasound can also be used to monitor for complications post-procedurally, such as pneumothorax, drain malfunction, and potentially drain malposition.
- Parasternal Approach:
Adapted from Osman et al. [15]
  - With the patient in the supine position, obtain a parasternal view using a linear probe. Patient repositioning (i.e., reverse Trendelenburg), may redistribute pericardial fluid and affect the target window.
  - Prep the skin overlying the left chest and drape the patient in a sterile manner. Place a sterile sheath over the ultrasound transducer.
  - Identify a transverse view of the sternum bone.

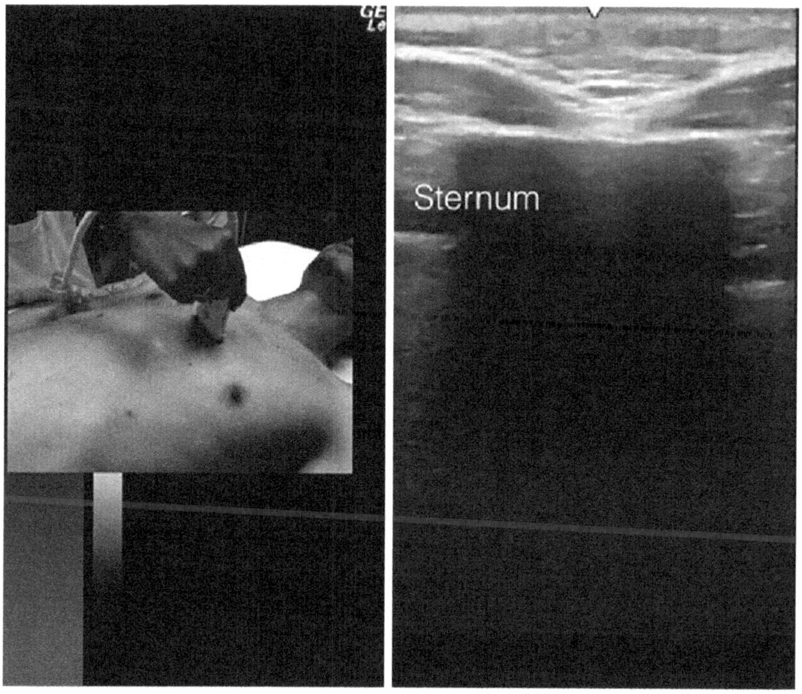

  - Move the transducer laterally to identify the internal thoracic artery vessel and pleural line (with lung sliding), just lateral to the sternum.

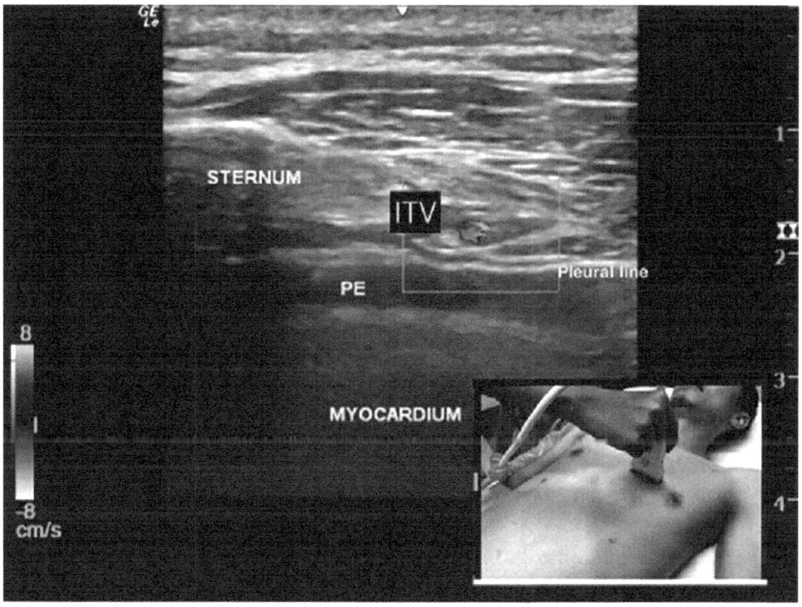

- Optimize the depth settings so that only the pericardial effusion and right ventricle are visible.
- Advance the needle tip via an in-plane medial-to-lateral approach with respect to the ultrasound probe at a 45-degree angle to penetrate the skin, intercostal muscle, and pericardial tissue until the needle tip is in the pericardial cavity. The point of needle entry should be along the superior border of the rib to prevent inadvertent injury to the intercostal vessels that run along the inferior rib border.

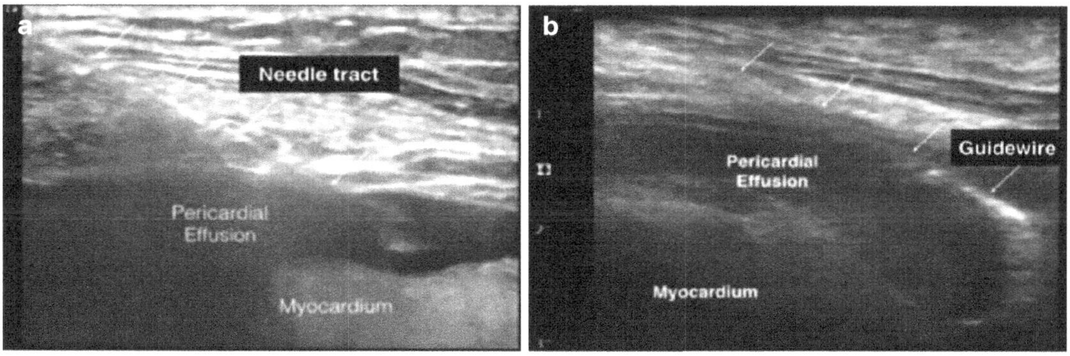

- Once within the pericardial sac, one should be able to aspirate pericardial fluid easily. Even the drainage of a small amount of fluid may have a dramatic effect on the patient's hemodynamics.
- To confirm placement, connect two 10 mL syringes via a three-way stopcock, one empty and one with 9 mL of normal saline. Rapidly agitate the saline between the two syringes with the stopcock turned off to the patient, and then open the stopcock to the patient and flush the agitated saline under continued ultrasound monitoring. This should create a "rocket flare" appearance and confirm the needle tip is in the pericardial space.

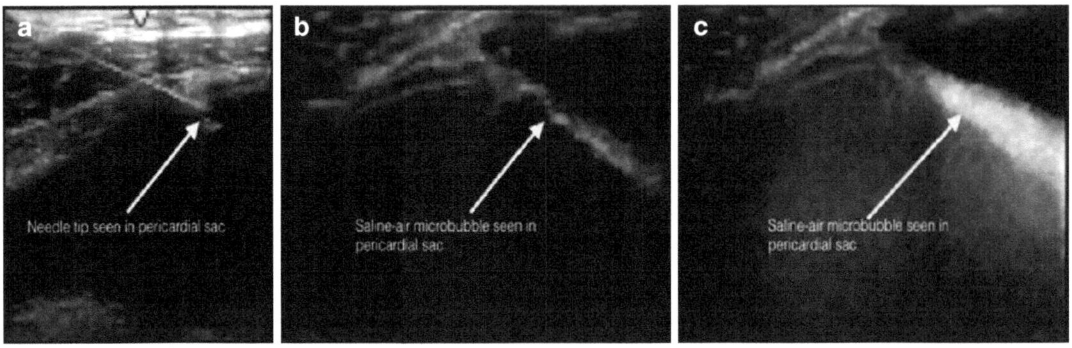

  - Agitated saline within the intracardiac areas or rapid washout of the saline may indicate an accidental myocardial puncture [16].
  - Another form of confirmation is to deploy the guidewire and visualize the guidewire within the pericardial sac under ultrasound guidance.

    Place the guide wire under real time visualization after properly confirming the placement of the needle tip as above via agitated saline. You can use the standard Seldinger technique to dilate the subcutaneous space after the needle is removed. Place a single-lumen catheter or pigtail catheter into the pericardial space.
  - After pericardial drainage, you can leave the catheter in place and then use ultrasound at serial intervals to monitor the clinical condition, effusion size, hemodynamics, and complications.
- Apical:
  - The apical approach takes advantage of a thicker left ventricle and small apical coronaries but theoretically has a higher risk of pneumothorax given the proximity to the left pleural space [17].
  - The ultrasound probe should be placed over the cardiac apex, usually found between the fifth, sixth, and seventh intercostal spaces, between the mid-clavicular and mid-axillary lines, to find the largest effusion, closest to the skin [12].
  - Prep the skin overlying the left chest and drape the patient in a sterile manner. Place a sterile sheath over the ultrasound transducer.
  - Advance the needle tip via a transverse approach with respect to the ultrasound probe at a 45-degree angle towards the right shoulder to penetrate the skin, intercostal muscle, and pericardial tissue until the needle tip is in the pericardial cavity. The point of needle entry should be along the superior border of the rib to prevent inadvertent injury to the intercostal vessels that run along the inferior rib border.
  - Follow similar steps as above regarding confirmation of needle placement and catheter placement.
- Subxiphoid Approach:
  - The subxiphoid approach is traditionally done as a blind technique but can be achieved via ultrasound guidance as well.
  - With the patient in the supine position, obtain a subxiphoid cardiac view using the phased array probe. Patient repositioning (i.e., reverse Trendelenburg), may redistribute pericardial fluid and affect the target window.
  - Prep the skin overlying the left chest and drape the patient in a sterile manner. Place a sterile sheath over the ultrasound transducer.
  - Once an appropriate pocket of fluid is identified, insert the finder needle 1 cm inferior to the left xiphocostal angle at a 30-degree angle to the skin [12]. As mentioned above, this technique can be done blind, aiming towards the left shoulder and advancing

while aspirating. If using ultrasound, a transverse out-of-plane needle approach will allow the visualization of the needle tip into the pericardial sac.
- If approaching blind and unable to aspirate fluid, attempt a redirected trajectory initially deeper posteriorly and then slowly from the patient's left to the right until aimed at the patient's right shoulder [12].

Complications

Major complications of pericardiocentesis include injury of cardiac chambers, coronary arteries, intercostal or internal thoracic vessels, abdominal viscera, pneumothorax, pneumopericardium, ventricular arrhythmias, and death. Minor complications include transient vasovagal hypotension and bradycardia, supraventricular arrhythmias, and pleuropericardial fistulas [10].

Although an immediate chest x-ray should be ordered to evaluate for pneumothorax, and if possible, an upright abdominal x-ray to evaluate for free air under the diaphragm, ultrasound can be utilized to quickly evaluate for complications at the bedside.

Some studies show bedside ultrasonography, although dependent on the skill of the operator, shows higher sensitivity and similar specificity when compared to chest radiographs in the diagnosis of pneumothorax [18–20].

Summary Points

- Pericardiocentesis is indicated for cardiac tamponade or in symptomatic pericardial effusions, clinical situations often found in intensive care units (ICU).
- Key features on bedside echocardiogram that may suggest clinical tamponade include inferior vena cava plethora, right heart collapse in diastole, bulging of the interventricular septum during inspiration, and changes in mitral and tricuspid inflow velocity on Doppler ultrasound.
- The use of ultrasound reduces complications in pericardiocentesis and may assist in identifying immediate complications.

References

1. Alerhand S, Carter JM. What echocardiographic findings suggest a pericardial effusion is causing tamponade? Am J Emerg Med. 2019;37(2):321–6. https://doi.org/10.1016/j.ajem.2018.11.004.
2. McCanny P, Colreavy F. Echocardiographic approach to cardiac tamponade in critically ill patients. J Crit Care. 2017;39:271–7. https://doi.org/10.1016/j.jcrc.2016.12.008.
3. Merce J, Sagrista-Sauleda J, Permanyer-Miralda G, Evangelista A, Soler-Soler J. Correlation between clinical and Doppler echocardiographic findings in patients with moderate and large pericardial effusion: implications for the diagnosis of cardiac tamponade. Am Heart J. 1999;138:759–64.
4. Klein AL, Abbara S, Agler DA, et al. American Society of Echocardiography clinical recommendations for multimodality cardiovascular imaging of patients with pericardial disease: endorsed by the Society for Cardiovascular Magnetic Resonance and Society of Cardiovascular Computed Tomography. J Am Soc Echocardiogr. 2013;26(9):965–1012.e15. https://doi.org/10.1016/j.echo.2013.06.023.
5. Pérez-Casares A, Cesar S, Brunet-Garcia L, Sanchez-de-Toledo J. Echocardiographic Evaluation of Pericardial Effusion and Cardiac Tamponade. Front Pediatr. 2017;5:79.
6. Gillam LD, Guyer DE, Gibson TC, King ME, Marshall JE, Weyman AE. Hydrodynamic compression of the right atrium: a new echocardiographic sign of cardiac tamponade. Circulation. 1983;68(2):294–301.
7. Hoit BD, Shaw D. The paradoxical pulse in tamponade: mechanisms and echocardiographic correlates. Echocardiography. 1994;11(5):477–87.
8. Appleton CP, Hatle LK, Popp RL. Cardiac tamponade and pericardial effusion: respiratory variation in transvalvular flow velocities studied by Doppler echocardiography. J Am Coll Cardiol. 1988;11(5):1020–30.
9. Emergency pericardiocentesis—UpToDate. [cited 2022 Jun 28]. Available from: https://www-uptodate-com.laneproxy.stanford.edu/contents/emergency-pericardiocentesis?search=emergency%20 pericardiocentesis&source=search_result&selected Title=1~70&usage_type=default&display_rank=1
10. Blanco P, Figueroa L, Menéndez MF, Berrueta B. Pericardiocentesis: ultrasound guidance is essential. Ultrasound J. 2022;14(1):9. Published 2022 Feb 14. https://doi.org/10.1186/s13089-022-00259-5.
11. Tsang TS, Enriquez-Sarano M, Freeman WK, Barnes ME, Sinak LJ, Gersh BJ, et al. Consecutive 1127 therapeutic echocardiographically guided pericardiocenteses: clinical profile, practice patterns, and outcomes spanning 21 years. Mayo Clin Proc. 2002;77:429–36.
12. Harper RJ. Pericardiocentesis. In: Roberts JR, Hedges JR, editors. Clinical procedures in emergency medicine. 5th ed. Philadelphia: W.B Saunders; 2004. p. 211–5.

13. Stolz L, Situ-LaCasse E, Acuña J, et al. What is the ideal approach for emergent pericardiocentesis using point-of-care ultrasound guidance? World J Emerg Med. 2021;12(3):169–73.
14. Cho BC, Kang SM, Kim DH, et al. Clinical and echocardiographic characteristics of pericardial effusion in patients who underwent echocardiographically guided pericardiocentesis: Yonsei Cardiovascular Center experience, 1993–2003. Yonsei Med J. 2004;45(3):462–8. https://doi.org/10.3349/ymj.2004.45.3.462.
15. Osman A, Wan Chuan T, Ab Rahman J, Via G, Tavazzi G. Ultrasound-guided pericardiocentesis: a novel parasternal approach. Eur J Emerg Med. 2018;25(5):322–7. https://doi.org/10.1097/MEJ.0000000000000471.
16. Ainsworth CD, Salehian O. Echo-guided pericardiocentesis: let the bubbles show the way. Circulation. 2011;123(4):e210–1.
17. Brown CG, Gurley HT, Hutchins GM, MacKenzie EJ, White JD. Injuries associated with percutaneous placement of transthoracic pacemakers. Ann Emerg Med. 1985;14(3):223–8.
18. Ding W, Shen Y, Yang J, He X, Zhang M. Diagnosis of pneumothorax by radiography and ultrasonography: a meta-analysis. Chest. 2011;140(4):859–66.
19. Abdalla W, Elgendy M, Abdelaziz A, Ammar M. Lung ultrasound versus chest radiography for the diagnosis of pneumothorax in critically ill patients: a prospective, single-blind study. Saudi J Anaesth. 2016;10(3):265–9.
20. Alrajab S, Youssef AM, Akkus NI, Caldito G. Pleural ultrasonography versus chest radiography for the diagnosis of pneumothorax: review of the literature and meta-analysis. Crit Care 2013;23:17(5):R208.

Pericarditis and Constriction

26

Sarah Bain and Brooks Ohlson

Learning Objectives

1. Identify the three most common etiologies of constrictive pericarditis.
2. Describe the unique pathophysiology of constrictive pericarditis in terms of increased interventricular dependence and dissociation of intrathoracic-intracardiac pressures.
3. Identify specific variables that should be included in an echocardiographic examination in the setting of suspected pericardial disease.
4. Identify the three echocardiographic principles that were found by the Mayo Clinic study to be independently associated with constrictive pericarditis.

Pro Tips

- Utilize extended clips of up to ten beats.
- Record respiration with a respirometer when assessing mitral inflow velocities, ventricular septal shift, and hepatic vein flow.

Supplementary Information The online version contains supplementary material available at https://doi.org/10.1007/978-3-031-80038-2_26.

S. Bain (✉) · B. Ohlson
Virginia Mason Franciscan Health, Seattle, WA, USA
e-mail: sarah.bain@commonspirit.org; brooks.ohlson@commonspirit.org

Causes of Constrictive Pericarditis

The epidemiology of constrictive pericarditis (CP) in the modern, developed world is nebulous. Likely owing to a relatively low prevalence [1] and changing disease burden, much of our knowledge of CP in the twenty-first century stems from single-center surgical databases. In the late 1950s, tuberculosis was estimated to represent nearly half of all cases of CP with an increasing incidence of presumed viral causes [2]. **Presently, the most common etiologies of constrictive pericarditis cited are idiopathic, post-operative, and post-radiation** [3]. While an exhaustive analysis of the causes of CP is beyond the scope of this text, any disease process that leads to inflammatory, fibrous scarring of the pericardium should be considered.

Pathophysiology

In normal circumstances, the basic mechanical functions of the pericardium promote ventricular elasticity and a low-friction structural sac for the heart [4]. Variations in ventricular filling during respiration are compensated for by pericardial stretch, minimizing the effects of ventricular interdependence. Recall that during spontaneous respiration, intrathoracic pressures influence filling pressure gradients on the left and right sides of the heart. With inspiration, negative intratho-

M. J. Lanspa, A. T. Levinson (eds.), *Echocardiography and Ultrasonography in the ICU*, Respiratory Medicine, https://doi.org/10.1007/978-3-031-80038-2_26

racic pressure promotes systemic venous return, and RV filling is enhanced. Conversely, pulmonary venous (PV) flow to the left atrium is reduced in inspiration (largely due to the intrathoracic/extrapericardial location of the pulmonary veins), with a subsequent reduction in LV end-diastolic volume. In expiration, changes to filling pressures are reversed with enhanced LV filling and reduced RV filling. A normally compliant pericardium allows for a septal shift, ventricular distensibility, and minimal impact on hemodynamics.

The fundamental pathway leading to the findings of CP results from inflammation leading to the formation of a non-compliant pericardial scar [5]. As fibrinous changes encase the heart and obliterate the normal pericardial space, diastolic function is impaired. Rather than acting as a reservoir and structural support for ventricular filling, the fibrotic and calcified pericardium forms a rigid complex with the ventricle. The rigidity of the ventricular/pericardial structure leads to an early increase in diastolic filling pressures and minimal distensibility. With this progressive impairment in ventricular relaxation, filling pressures across the cardiac chambers increase and equalize, cardiac output decreases, and venous pressure rises.

The underlying lack of ventricular compliance drives the hemodynamic changes seen with constrictive pericarditis. In general, exaggerations of ventricular interdependence and respirophasic changes in ventricular filling occur with constriction [6, 7]. During inspiration, intrapleural pressure is reduced with the expected decrease in PV inflow pressure. However, the constrictive encasement of the heart functionally limits the transmission of intrathoracic pressure changes to the heart so that left atrial pressure is less reduced than expected, resulting in a decreased pressure gradient and decreased left-sided filling. This, coupled with limited pericardial compliance, forces septal shifting from right to left (as the right-sided chambers are favored). As left-sided filling falls with inspiration, a pronounced (>10 mmHg) drop in systolic blood pressure occurs—the classic finding of pulsus paradoxus. During expiration, the reversal occurs with increased intrapleural pressure and restoration of the pressure gradient from the PVs to the left atrium. This allows left heart filling but at the expense of right heart filling due to septal shift in a fixed space.

Signs and symptoms of constrictive pericarditis are reflective of right-sided failure in the setting of normal-appearing ventricular function. Typical patients present with evidence of peripheral edema, fatigue, and dyspnea on exertion [8]. Signs of constriction include pulsus paradoxus, Kussmaul's sign (increased jugular venous distention with inspiration), a pericardial "knock" on auscultation, and a congested abdomen.

Echocardiographic Diagnosis

Clinical identification of constrictive pericarditis can be challenging (and frequently missed) as it can manifest with general symptoms of heart failure [9]. Two-dimensional and Doppler echocardiography should be utilized as an initial diagnostic tool to identify and differentiate constrictive pericarditis from other causes of heart failure, specifically restrictive cardiomyopathy, severe tricuspid regurgitation (TR), and tamponade. While some cases might require computerized tomography, MRI, cardiac catheterization, or surgical visualization for definitive diagnosis, transthoracic echocardiography is effective and noninvasive in the evaluation of patients with suspected CP.

The echocardiographic findings of CP are due to **increased ventricular interdependence** (or enhanced ventricular interaction) in a fixed space and the **dissociation of intrathoracic-intracardiac pressures** [9]. There is usually some level of ventricular dependence with a normal pericardium, but this is enhanced with a thickened sac. This noncompliant pericardial sac also insulates cardiac chambers from changes in intrathoracic pressures [9].

Evolving Evidence

In the largest, blinded study to date, 130 patients with surgically confirmed constrictive pericarditis in comparison to 36 patients with restrictive disease or severe TR was conducted by the Mayo Clinic group that evaluated the test performance of five principal echocardiographic findings in the diagnosis of CP, including (1) respiration-related ventricular septal shift, (2) variation in mitral inflow E velocity, (3) medial mitral annular velocity, (4) ratio of medial mitral annular e' to lateral e', and (5) hepatic vein expiratory diastolic reversal ratio [10].

All five varied significantly between the groups, and all but mitral inflow velocity remained significantly different in patients with atrial fibrillation or flutter.

Three of the variables were independently associated with CP: (1) ventricular septal shift, (2) medial mitral e', and (3) hepatic vein diastolic reversal ratio. The presence of septal shift in combination with either medial mitral e' ≥9 cm/s or hepatic vein diastolic reversal ratio ≥ 0.79 was sensitive (87%) and specific (91%) for a diagnosis of constrictive pericarditis [6, 10].

When pericardial disease is suspected, an echocardiographic examination should include the **2D appearance of septal motion and the IVC and Doppler interrogation of mitral inflow, the medial and lateral mitral annulus, and the hepatic veins** (9), with specific attention to ventricular septal shift, medial mitral e' velocity, and hepatic vein reversal ratio; otherwise, constrictive physiology could be overlooked. [6]

Two-Dimensional Evaluation

Septal Motion

Analysis of septal wall motion reveals two main abnormalities in patients with CP physiology, including a septal bounce and a respirophasic septal shift [9]. The septal bounce is essentially a shuddering or oscillatory motion [10] of the septal wall during diastole and is due to the difference in the diastolic pressures of the right (RV) and left ventricle (LV) (Video 26.1). It should be noted that this can look like postoperative pacing [9]. A more specific observation is the bulging of the septum towards the LV during inspiration and then towards the RV in expiration [9]. LV filling decreases during inspiration (secondary to the decreased gradient between the PVs and LV) and the septum shifts towards the LV as the RV has increased filling. The opposite then occurs during expiration. This phenomenon is due to both the dissociation of intrathoracic-intracardiac pressures and the ventricular interdependence in the fixed space caused by the noncompliant pericardium [10]. It can be observed in multiple views using 2D and M-mode.

Imaging of the IVC

Plethora or dilatation of the inferior vena cava is a common finding in CP given the expected increased venous pressure but alone does not differentiate from restrictive physiology [6].

Other 2D Findings

Assessment of the pericardial thickness can assist in making a diagnosis but 2D transthoracic echocardiography and M-mode have shown poor sensitivity and correlation to anatomic specimens. Transesophageal echocardiography has a higher specificity and sensitivity to detect thickened pericardium, but note that one in five patients with CP will have a normal pericardium, and an isolated thickened pericardium should not confirm the diagnosis [11].

Tethering of the RV free wall to the liver rather than the normal sliding motion has been observed in CP as has the **distortion in the appearance of the contour of the RV and LV** [6, 10].

Doppler Evaluation

Mitral Inflow Pulse-Wave Doppler

The dissociation of intrathoracic and intracardiac pressures that is a hallmark of CP physiology is demonstrated with pulse wave Doppler interrogation of the mitral inflow as an **inspiratory decrease in mitral E velocity** [10]. This is due to the decreased gradient between the PVs and LV during inspiration with the opposite occurring during expiration. This respiratory variation should not be observed in restrictive physiology or severe TR, as there should not be a dissociation of pressures [10]. The percent change of mitral E velocity during respiration can be calculated as follows: **[(expiratory velocity − inspiratory velocity)/expiratory velocity × 100]** and ranges from 15%–35% in constrictive physiology [6] (Fig. 26.1). While this variation can be compromised in the setting of high left atrial pressures and atrial arrhythmias [6], it can still be appreciated by utilizing extended recording clips [11].

Hepatic Vein Pulse-Wave Doppler

The phenomena of both intrathoracic and intracardiac pressure dissociation and interventricular dependence in CP are further demonstrated by the assessment of the hepatic vein flow velocities during respiration. As LV filling is increased during expiration, the septum shifts towards the right, and right-sided chamber filling decreases. Subsequently, hepatic vein forward flow is decreased with a pronounced reversal of flow during diastole. During inspiration, right heart filling increases, and the diastolic hepatic vein flow reversal becomes less prominent [6, 9, 10].

The expiratory diastolic reversal ratio (**expiratory diastolic reversal velocity/diastolic forward velocity**) can be used to quantify the respirophasic hepatic vein velocities with higher values expected in CP (Fig. 26.2). The Mayo Clinic Criteria identified that a reversal ratio of ≥0.79 was the most specific (88%) for CP (and the most specific of the five variables studied) [10].

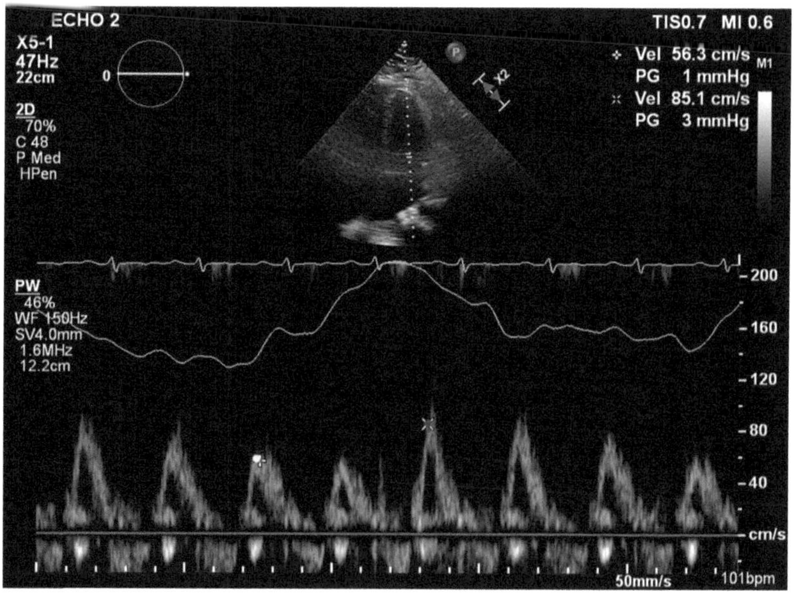

Fig. 26.1 Pulse-wave Doppler mitral inflow velocities during inspiration and expiration utilizing a respirometer. The yellow marker is the E velocity during inspiration, and the blue marker is the expiratory E velocity. There is a percent change of approximately 25% [(expiratory velocity − inspiratory velocity)/expiratory velocity × 100]

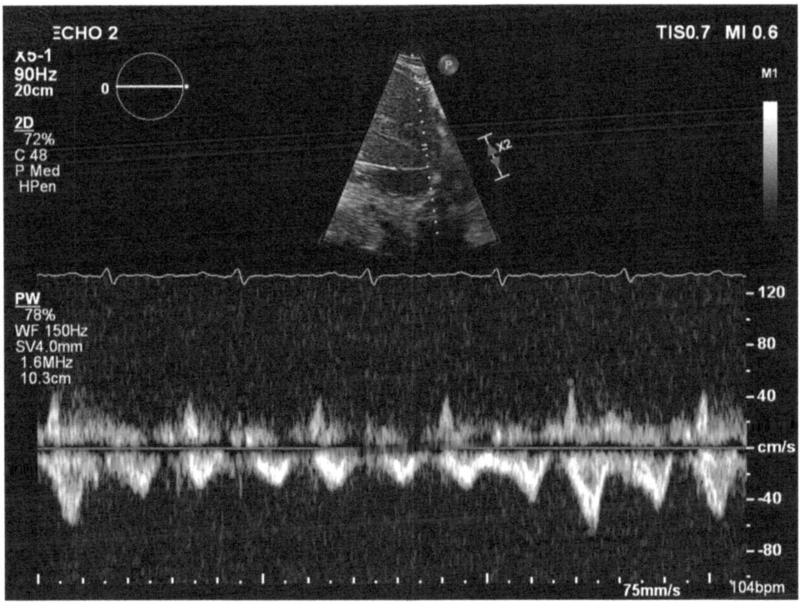

Fig. 26.2 Pulse-wave Doppler hepatic vein velocities. The red marker is the expiratory diastolic reversal velocity, and the blue marker is the diastolic forward velocity. The ratio (expiratory diastolic reversal velocity/diastolic forward velocity) is approximately 1

Tissue Doppler of the Mitral Annulus

Doppler echocardiography of the diastolic mitral annular tissue velocity (e') allows evaluation of myocardial relaxation [10]. In constrictive pericarditis (vs. restrictive myocardial disease), the myocardium is usually spared and exhibits normal to supranormal motion [6] so higher e' velocities in patients with heart failure should be a sign of constriction. It should be noted that e' velocities would be higher in primary CP vs post-operative or radiation-related cases of CP and that lateral annular e' velocities might be lower than medial e' velocities given the possibility that the lateral myocardium can be tethered to the pericardium (annulus reversus) [6, 9].

The Mayo Clinic study demonstrated that a **medial e' > 9.0 cm/s** (Fig. 26.3) was the optimal cutoff for constrictive physiology in a patient with heart failure with a sensitivity of 83% and specificity of 81% [6, 9, 10]. Note other publications and texts refer to e' > 8.0 cm/s as the limit to identify CP [12, 13].

Given that the e' velocity is preserved (or higher) in these patients, the E/e' velocity ratio will be lower than expected in the setting of higher left-sided filling pressures (annulus paradoxus) [6, 10].

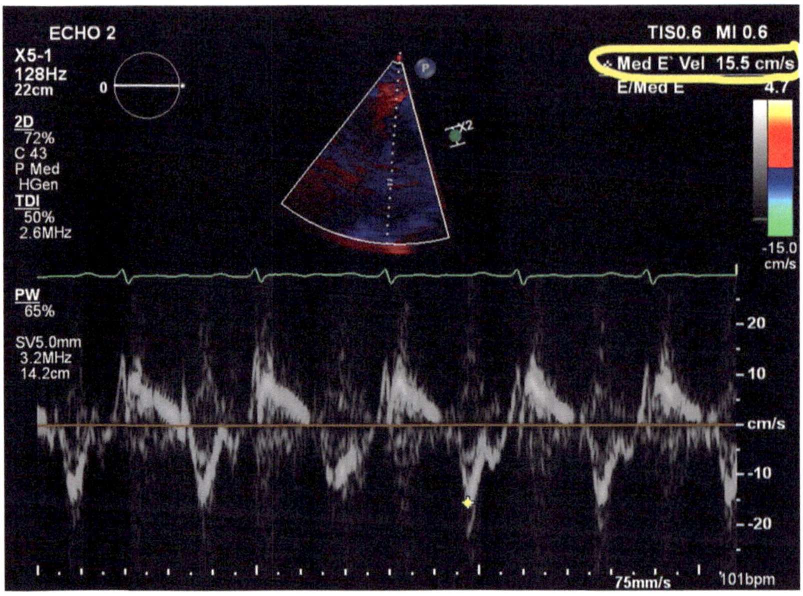

Fig. 26.3 This is an example of a pulse-wave tissue Doppler of the medial mitral annular velocity (e'). The yellow marker denotes an e' of 15.5 cm/s

Summary Points

- Previously, tuberculosis was the most common etiology of constrictive pericarditis. Now the most dominant causes are idiopathic, post-surgical, and post-radiation.
- Constrictive pericarditis is a type of diastolic heart failure with preserved systolic function in patients presenting with common right-sided heart failure symptoms like peripheral edema, fatigue, and dyspnea on exertion.
- The pathophysiology is unique from other etiologies due to the dissociation of intracardiac and intrathoracic pressures and enhanced ventricular dependence secondary to a stiff, non-compliant pericardial sac but preserved myocardial function.
- Utilization of 2D and Doppler echocardiography facilitates successful identification and diagnosis of constrictive pericarditis from other forms of diastolic heart failure.
- In patients with diastolic heart failure or suspected pericardial disease, the echocardiography exam should include specific attention to ventricular septal shift, mitral inflow velocities, mitral annular tissue velocities, hepatic vein diastolic flow reversal, and IVC appearance.
- Current evidence suggests that 3 variables (ventricular septal shift, medial mitral e', and hepatic vein expiratory diastolic reversal ratio) are independently associated with the diagnosis of constrictive pericarditis.

Questions

1. All of the following hemodynamic changes are true EXCEPT:
   A. Early, elevated diastolic filling pressures result from fibrous thickening of the pericardial-ventricular complex in constrictive pericarditis.
   B. Pulmonary venous drainage shows intrathoracic pressure dissociation in constrictive pericarditis.
   C. Septal bowing from right to left results in exaggerated systemic blood pressure decreases in constrictive pericarditis.
   D. Signs and symptoms of constrictive pericarditis are non-specific and show significant overlap with other causes of cardiac dysfunction.
   E. Patients with restrictive cardiomyopathy maintain normal intrathoracic/intracardiac pressure variability.

   Answer/Explanation: B.

The pulmonary venous system (and thus left atrial occlusion pressure) is primarily extrapericardial and remains significantly influenced by intrathoracic pressure changes while the remainder of the heart shows intrathoracic/intracardiac pressure dissociation in constrictive pericarditis. This dissociation is the result of the fibrous complex formed between the heart/pericardium. Similarly, the rigid complex causes impaired relaxation of the ventricles and early, elevated diastolic filling pressures. The right-to-left septal bowing is evidence of exaggerated interventricular dependence and reduced left-sided filling pressures, leading to a decrease in blood pressure. Constrictive pericarditis often appears as non-specific RV failure and a hallmark finding to help differentiate it from restrictive cardiomyopathy is the response to intrathoracic pressure changes.

2. Which of the following echocardiographic findings is FALSE when differentiating between constrictive pericarditis (CP)and restrictive cardiomyopathy (RCM)?
   A. There are usually enlarged right and left atria in RCM whereas patients with CP have smaller atrial size.
   B. CP is characterized by respirophasic septal bowing while there is little septal shift in RCM.
   C. Medial mitral annular tissue velocities (e') are preserved in both CP and RCM.
   D. There is minimal respiratory variation in mitral and pulmonary vein inflow in patients with RCM.

   Answer/Explanation: C.

   In restrictive myocardial disease, mitral annular motion will be inhibited (decreased e') both medially and laterally. In constrictive pericarditis (without concurrent restrictive disease), the medial mitral annular motion should be preserved or exaggerated. Lateral annular motion might be reduced due to pericardial tethering.

References

1. Mori M, Mullan CW, Bin Mahmood SU, et al. Us national trends in the management and outcomes of constrictive pericarditis: 2005-2014. Can J Cardiol. 2019;35(10):1394–9.
2. Robertson R, Arnold CR. Constrictive pericarditis with particular reference to etiology. Circulation. 1962;26:525–9.
3. George TJ, Arnaoutakis GJ, Beaty CA, Kilic A, Baumgartner WA, Conte JV. Contemporary etiologies, risk factors, and outcomes after pericardiectomy. Ann Thorac Surg. 2012;94(2):445–51.
4. Hoit BD. Anatomy and physiology of the pericardium. Cardiol Clin. 2017;35(4):481–90.
5. Kumar V, Abbas AK, Aster JC, Perkins JA, Ramzi S, Robbins, Stanley L. Robbins & Cotran pathologic basis of disease; 2021.
6. Welch TD, Oh JK. Constrictive pericarditis. Cardiol Clin. 2017;35(4):539–49.
7. Geske JB, Anavekar NS, Nishimura RA, Oh JK, Gersh BJ. Differentiation of constriction and restriction: complex cardiovascular hemodynamics. J Am Coll Cardiol. 2016;68(21):2329–47.
8. Adler Y, Charron P, Imazio M, et al. 2015 ESC guidelines for the diagnosis and management of pericardial diseases: the task force for the diagnosis and management of pericardial diseases of the European Society of Cardiology (ESC) endorsed by: the European Association for Cardio-thoracic Surgery(Eacts). Eur Heart J. 2015;36(42):2921–64.
9. Miranda WR, Oh JK. Constrictive pericarditis: a practical clinical approach. Prog Cardiovasc Dis. 2017;59(4):369–79.
10. Welch TD, Ling LH, Espinosa RE, Anavekar NS, Wiste HJ, Lahr BD, Schaff HV, Oh JK. Echocardiographic diagnosis of constrictive pericarditis: Mayo clinic criteria. Circ Cardiovasc Imaging. 2014;7(3):526–34.
11. Dal-Bianco JP, Sengupta PP, Mookadam F, Chandrasekaran K, Tajik AJ, Khandheria BK. Role of echocardiography in the diagnosis of constrictive pericarditis. J Am Soc Echocardiogr 2009;22(1):24-33; quiz 103-4.
12. Chiabrando JG, Bonaventura A, Vecchié A, Wohlford GF, Mauro AG, Jordan JH, Grizzard JD, Montecucco F, Berrocal DH, Brucato A, Imazio M, Abbate A. Management of acute and recurrent pericarditis: JACC state-of-the-art review. J Am Coll Cardiol. 2020;75(1):76–92.
13. Mathew J, Swaminathan M, Ayoub C. Clinical manual and review of transesophageal echocardiography. 2nd ed. McGraw-Hill; 2010.

Benign Masses, Normal Anatomic Variants, and Artifacts

27

Tara Brakke and Stephen Brannan

Learning Objectives

1. Assess some of the common normal anatomical variants, benign cardiac masses, and artifacts that can frequently be misinterpreted as masses or objects.
2. Describe common benign cardiac masses seen on echocardiography.
3. Review common ultrasound artifacts appearing as masses.

Introduction

Point-of-care ultrasound (POCUS), and particularly bedside echocardiographic cardiac assessment, is increasingly employed in the critical care setting to evaluate, diagnose, and guide treatment in an expanding array of hemodynamic and physiologic situations. With increasing numbers of physicians and specialties utilizing ultrasound, it is crucial to recognize and distinguish normal anatomic variants from cardiac masses, artifacts, and pathological findings. This chapter explores some of the common normal anatomical variants and benign cardiac masses and reviews some artifacts that can frequently be misinterpreted as masses or objects. We encourage the reader to verify findings in multiple windows, views, and modalities (that is, two-dimensional ultrasound, color flow Doppler, and spectral Doppler) when concerned about possible abnormalities. Wherever possible, we have included transthoracic images that reflect POCUS images, but unfortunately, some of these variants are best—or only—visualized with transesophageal echocardiography and are shown thusly herein.

Normal Anatomical Variants

Right Atrium

Crista Terminalis

The Crista Terminalis (Fig. 27.1) is a smooth, crescent-shaped ridge of myocardium located at the cavo-atrial junctions, although most often identified via imaging along the superior vena cava and right atrial junction. Anatomically this delineates the smooth right atrial muscle from the trabeculated right atrial appendage muscle. Due to its high density of adrenergic fibers, it can be an origin for atrial tachyarrhythmias and thus a target in ablation procedures.

Supplementary Information The online version contains supplementary material available at https://doi.org/10.1007/978-3-031-80038-2_27.

T. Brakke (✉) · S. Brannan
Department of Anesthesiology, University of Nebraska Medical Center, Omaha, NE, USA
e-mail: tbrakke@unmc.edu; stephen.brannan@unmc.edu

M. J. Lanspa, A. T. Levinson (eds.), *Echocardiography and Ultrasonography in the ICU*, Respiratory Medicine, https://doi.org/10.1007/978-3-031-80038-2_27

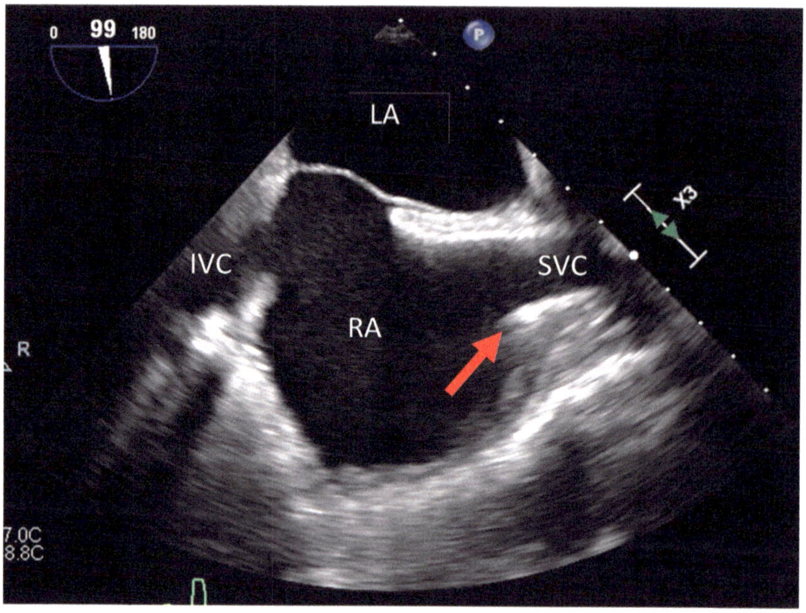

Fig. 27.1 Transesophageal midesophageal bicaval view showing the crista terminalis (red arrow) along the superior vena cava-right atrial junction and separating the trabeculated right atrial appendage wall from the smooth right atrial wall. *RA right atrium, LA left atrium, SVC superior vena cava, IVC inferior vena cava*

Eustachian Valve

The Eustachian Valve (Fig. 27.2) functions in utero to shunt oxygenated blood entering the right atrium from the inferior vena cava across the interatrial septum's fossa ovalis into the left atrium. In this way, oxygenated blood bypasses the pulmonary circulation, which at that point does not participate in gas exchange, and goes to the systemic circulation to deliver oxygen to organs and tissues. This valve does not completely regress in approximately 25% [1] of adults and appears posteriorly along the inferior vena cava as a prominent strand of tissue projecting into the right atrium. The Eustachian Valve does not cause significant blood flow disturbances when viewed with color flow Doppler. This distinguishes it from the triatriatum dexter, which is a similar-appearing thin band of tissue that traverses the entirety of the right atrium and causes flow disturbance.

Thebesian Valve

The Thebesian Valve is a thin flap of tissue covering the entrance to the coronary sinus in up to 80% of patients [2]. It can appear semilunar, fenestrated, biconcave, or bandlike and inhibit cannulation of the coronary sinus for retrograde cardioplegia or placement of a biventricular pacing wire.

Chiari Network

A Chiari Network is a remnant of sinus venosus-derived embryologic structures that appears as a thin, fenestrated, mobile, and membranous structure within the right atrium. It is distinguished from thrombus or vegetation by being visualized moving in multiple right atrial views. It is often associated with a patent foramen ovale, interatrial septal aneurysms, and paradoxical emboli.

Coronary Sinus

The coronary sinus arises from the left-sided sinus venosus, with contributory veins regressing in most adults. It runs approximately 3 cm posteriorly along the atrioventricular groove superior to the mitral valve annulus. Although it is typically less than 1 cm wide, dilation can occur due to atrial hypertension, tricuspid regurgitation, or the presence of a persistent left-sided superior vena cava.

Persistent Left Superior Vena Cava (PLSVC)

PLSVC occurs when the embryologic left-sided superior vena cava does not regress. Typically, it drains into the coronary sinus, causing the coronary sinus to dilate above 1.1 cm. It cannot be identified directly via POCUS; however, indirect suggestions are seen, such as a dilated coronary

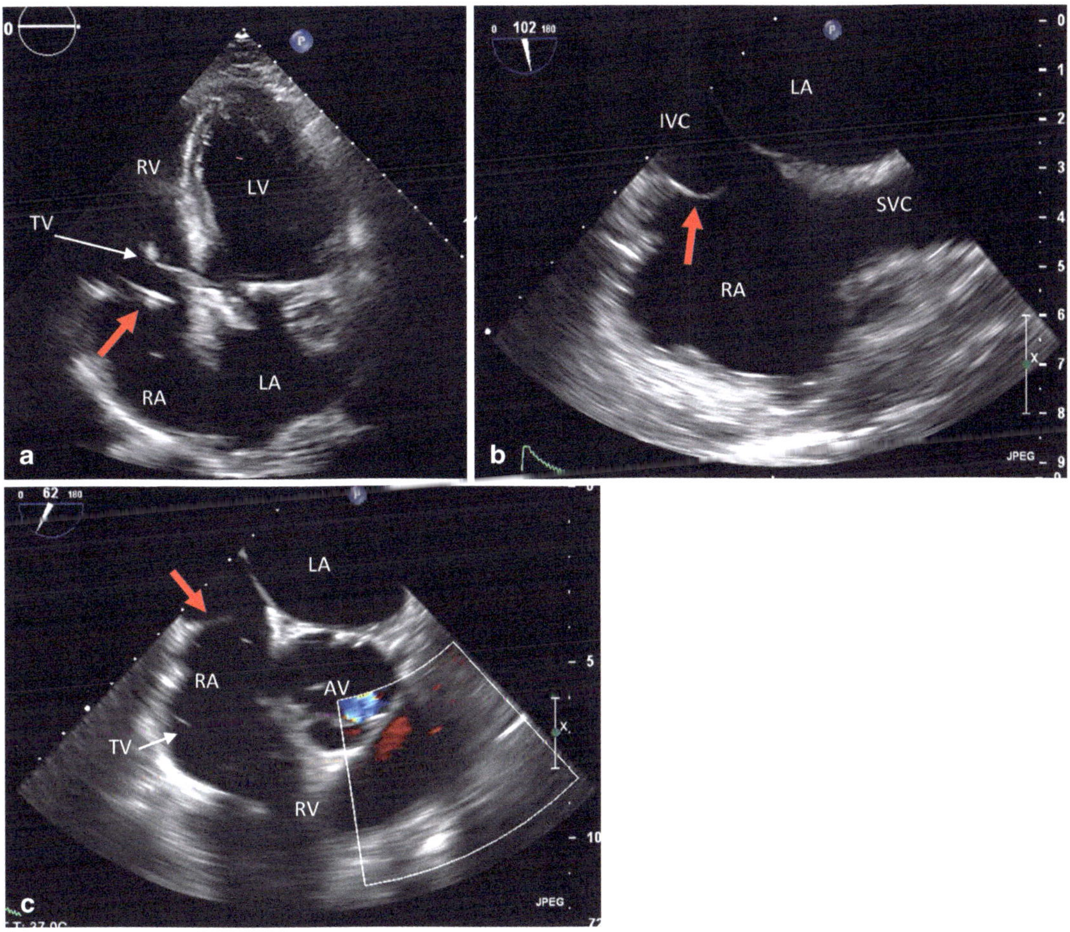

Fig. 27.2 A eustachian valve (red arrow) is noted (**a**) in a transthoracic apical four chamber view with the tricuspid valve noted by the white arrow, (**b**) in a transesophageal midesophageal bicaval view, and (**c**) in a transesophageal midesophageal right ventricle inflow and outflow view with a color flow doppler box in the right portion of the image (color flow doppler scale not pictured, tricuspid valve denoted by the white arrow). *RA right atrium, RV right ventricle, LA left atrium, LV left ventricle, TV tricuspid valve, IVC inferior vena cava, SVC superior vena cava, AV aortic valve*

sinus. A confirmatory bubble study administered via a left upper extremity peripheral IV with opacification emanating from the coronary sinus rather than the right-sided superior vena cava is confirmatory for its presence. Ineffective myocardial protection from a retrograde coronary perfusion cannula during an on-cardiopulmonary bypass open-heart procedure resulting in postoperative cardiogenic shock is also a consequence sometimes encountered in the critical care unit.

Patent Foramen Ovale (PFO)

The foramen ovale occurs in utero to shunt oxygenated blood from the highly pressurized right heart to the lower pressured left heart via a connection between the atria through the septum primum and septum secundum. With the first breaths ex utero, the left heart pressures increase above the right heart pressure from a drastic reduction in pulmonary vascular resistance as the alveoli are filled with air for the first time, causing the sep-

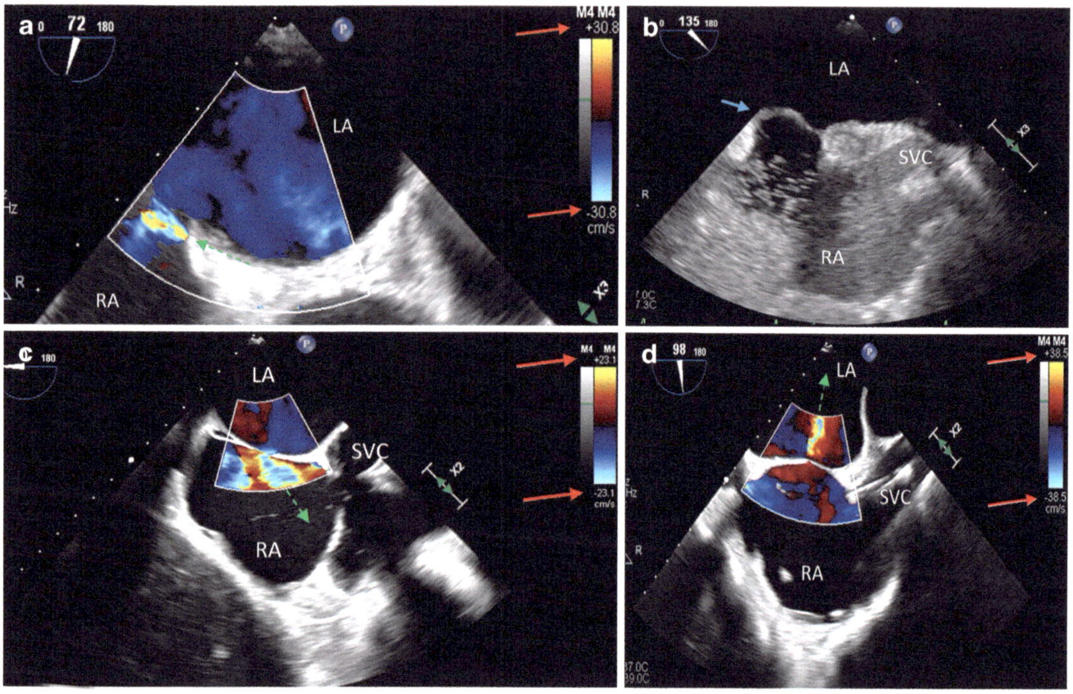

Fig. 27.3 Transesophageal midesophageal bicaval views with lowered Nyquist limits (red arrows). (**a**) Patent foramen ovale with color flow doppler showing flow parallel to the fossa ovalis (green interrupted arrow for emphasis). The fossa ovalis is the thinnest portion of the interatrial septum located between the superior and inferior limbs of the septum. This indicates flow between the two incompletely fused septae that comprise the fossa. (**b**) Representative photo from a bubble study conducted through the left upper extremity. The bubbles entered through the superior vena cava ruling out a persistent left sided superior vena cava, which in this view would enter from the coronary sinus at the left side of the screen if a persistent left sided superior vena cava was present. No bubbles appear in the left atrium within six cardiac cycles demonstrating the absence of a PFO. Importantly, note the interatrial septum (blue arrow) bowing into the left atrium with a Valsalva maneuver via the ventilator, indicating a true negative PFO test as it signifies even when the right atrial pressure is higher than left atrial pressure there is no flow across the atrial septum. (**c**) Iatrogenic PFO with left to right sided flow following placement of a left atrial appendage exclusion device. Note the flow is perpendicular to the fossa ovalis, which is characteristic for a lesion classified as an atrial septal defect, and is flowing into the right atrium (green interrupted arrow for emphasis). (**d**) Iatrogenic PFO with right to left sided flow following placement of a left atrial appendage exclusion device (green interrupted arrow for emphasis). *RA right atrium, LA left atrium, SVC superior vena cava*

tum primum to close against the septum secundum. Over time the septae fuse. In up to 25% of adults, this connection remains patent (Fig. 27.3) due to incomplete closure or incomplete fusion [3] and can increase the risk of stroke. Right-to-left shunting (Eisenmenger's physiology) can occur when the right atrial pressure exceeds the left atrial pressure, resulting in a hypoxemic shunt. One example occurs following implantation of a durable left ventricular assist device (LVAD) when right heart pressures increase secondary to pulmonary hypertension and/or right ventricular dysfunction, resulting in profound and refractory hypoxemia. Identifying and fixing a PFO is a critical component of successful durable LVAD implantation. The interatrial septum should always be evaluated by 2D and color flow Doppler. Because of the lower flow velocity in the atria, the Nyquist limit must be reduced (ideally to <30 cm/s) to help identify a PFO. Additionally, a bubble study with a Valsalva maneuver and 3D imaging provides more definitive evaluations.

Atrial Septal Aneurysm

Movement of the atrial septum at a distance of 1.5 cm or greater between the atria throughout the cardiac cycle characterizes an aneurysmal atrial septum. It is associated with a PFO and Chiari network while also increasing the risk of stroke [4]. Utilizing M-mode ultrasound modality through the septum at the point of maximum motion can more precisely visualize its full displacement, augmenting measurement accuracy.

Lipomatous Hypertrophy of the Atrial Septum

In some individuals the interatrial septum is thickened along the inferior and superior limbs while sparing the fossa ovalis, giving lipomatous hypertrophy of the atrial septum its characteristic "dumbbell-like" appearance (Fig. 27.4). The maximal thickness should be greater than 1.5 cm [5]. It occurs in 1–8% of individuals and is more common in patients who are older and obese, with a potential increased incidence in women [1].

Trabeculations and Pectinate Muscles

Muscular invaginations that form a web-like appearance are termed trabeculations. In the atria, trabeculations are referred to as pectinate muscles. Anatomically, trabeculations are found in the right and left atrial appendages but do not cross the crista terminalis into the atria proper, which separates the pectinate muscles of the appendages from the smooth wall of the atria. They are distinguished from masses and thrombi by their uniform texture and density, along with synchronous movement with the cardiac cycle. In contrast, a thrombus typically exhibits asynchrony to cardiac motion and is more common with arrhythmias and low-flow states such as atrial fibrillation and heart failure.

Left Atrium

Ligament of Marshall

Also known as the Warfarin or Coumadin® Ridge, this peninsula of atrial tissue separates the left upper pulmonary vein, and left atrial appendage (Fig. 27.5). Embryologically it is a remnant of the left common cardinal vein and fibers within it can be a focus for atrial arrhythmias.

Left Atrial Appendage

Like the right atrial appendage, the left atrial appendage (Fig. 27.5) contains trabeculated pectinate muscles. The number and shape of its lobes vary among individuals. It is a nidus for thrombus formation,

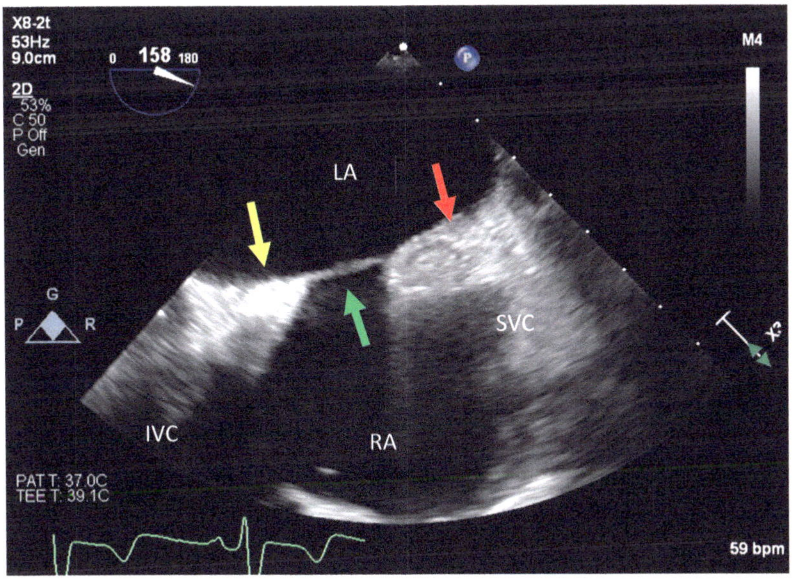

Fig. 27.4 Transesophageal midesophageal bicaval view of the interatrial septum demonstrating lipomatous hypertrophy of the superior limbus (red arrow), inferior limbus (yellow arrow), and sparing the fossa ovalis (green arrow). *LA left atrium, RA right atrium, SVC superior vena cava, IVC inferior vena cava*

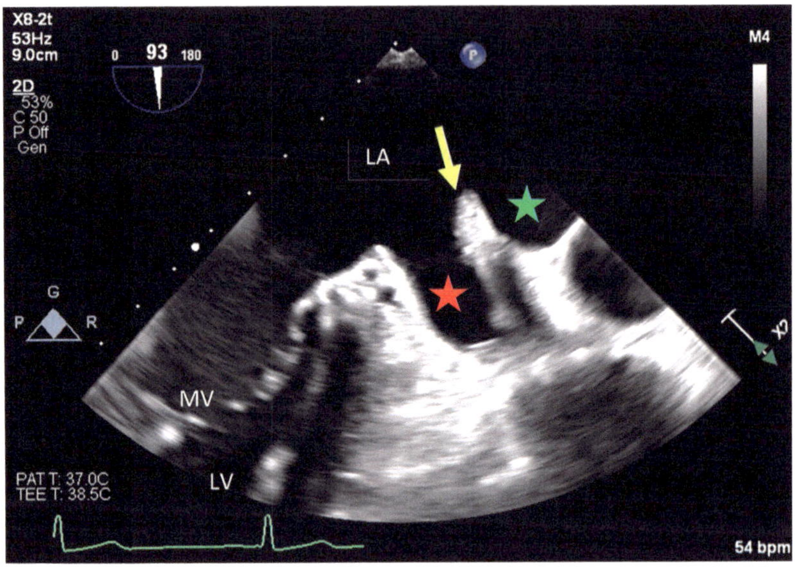

Fig. 27.5 Transesophageal midesophageal two-chamber view focusing on the left atrium, particularly the left atrial appendage (red star), left upper pulmonary vein (green star), and ligament of Marshall (yellow arrow). *LA* *left atrium*, *LV* *left ventricle*, *MV* *mitral valve*

with transesophageal echocardiography providing a better evaluation of this more posterior structure than transthoracic echocardiography. With increased use of percutaneous left atrial appendage occlusion devices and surgical exclusion during open heart procedures, the left atrial appendage may appear absent in these patients by ultrasound evaluation.

Atrial Suture Line After Cardiac Transplant

Contemporary cardiac transplant techniques normally involve anastomosing a native atrial cuff to the donor's left atrium, thus avoiding individually anastomosing the pulmonary veins and the risk of stenosis. This anastomosis is often mistaken as a pathological structure (Fig. 27.6).

Right Ventricle

Moderator Band

Also referred to as the septomarginal trabecula, the moderator band is the most prominent muscle band for most patients. Electrically, it contains Purkinje fibers that propagate cardiac depolarization laterally and basally to optimize ventricular output. Structurally, it helps limit acute dilation of the right ventricle while routing blood from the tricuspid inflow to the right ventricular outflow tract.

Left Ventricle

False Tendons

Sometimes referred to as left ventricular bands, false tendons are fibrous or fibromuscular structures in the left ventricle akin to the right ventricle's moderator band, though visually much less prominent. They are associated with murmurs and arrhythmias and may be misinterpreted as thrombi. False tendons are more commonly single, simple, and apically located [6].

Mitral Annular Calcification

Calcification of the mitral annulus (Fig. 27.7) creates hyperechoic foci associated with artifacts such as acoustic shadowing or side lobe. Either the calcification itself or the artifacts it can cause are commonly mistaken for pathological findings or foreign objects. Furthermore, the artifacts can obscure deeper structures. Because the transducer is at the apex for transthoracic imaging and the left ventricle is in the near field, left ventricular assessment is minimally affected by mitral annular calcification artifacts. However, transesophageal echocardiography ultrasound beams travel through left atrium down across the mitral valve and finally into the left ventricle in the far field so artifacts created by mitral annular calcifi-

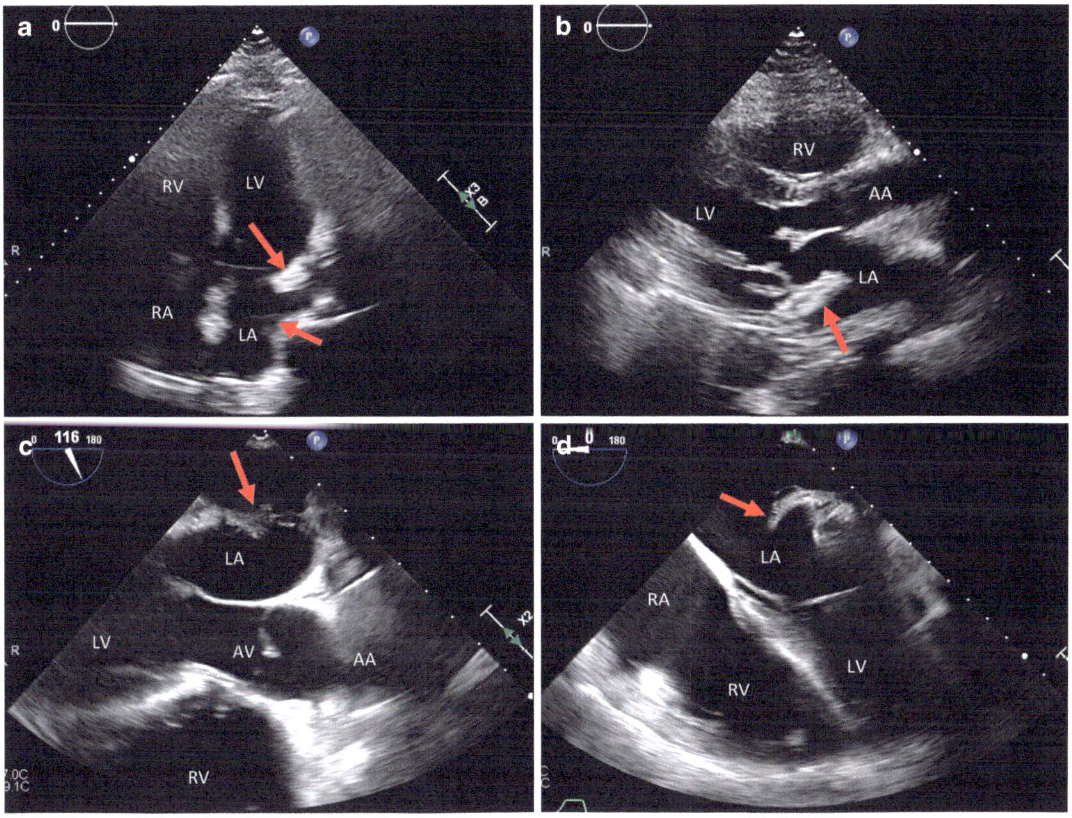

Fig. 27.6 The red arrows demonstrates atrial suture lines following cardiac transplantation in (**a**) transthoracic apical four chamber view, (**b**) transthoracic parasternal long axis view, (**c**) transesophageal midesophageal aortic valve long axis view, and (**d**) transesophageal midesophageal four chamber view. *RA right atrium, LA left atrium, RV right ventricle, LV left ventricle, AV aortic valve, AA ascending aorta*

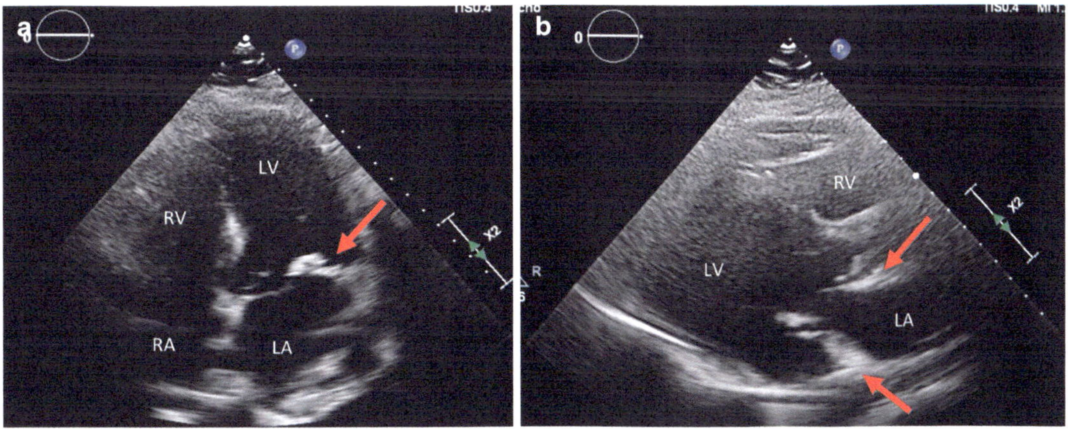

Fig. 27.7 Mitral annular calcification (red arrows) as shown in a transthoracic (**a**) apical four chamber view and (**b**) parasternal long axis view

cation project into the left ventricle which can make evaluation of systolic function and wall motion challenging.

Extracardiac Spaces

Pericardial Space

Although the pericardial space normally contains a very small amount of fluid, it usually is not well visualized. While most imagine fluid occupying the pericardial space, it is important to note additional materials such as calcium and adipose can accumulate in the space, causing constrictive or restrictive physiological effects. Commonly, pericardial fat can resemble a sizable pericardial effusion. Left-sided pericardial effusions are typically more lateral (away from the septum) and posterior near the descending aorta (Fig. 27.8a), which is consistent with how the heart lies anatomically within the chest. Right-sided pericardial effusions (Fig. 27.8b, c) usually occur more laterally (away from the septum) and superiorly near the liver. Effusions can be simple or complex, along with localized or diffusely surrounding the heart. Pericardial effusions are distinguished from pleural effusions on TTE parasternal views as occurring between the heart and the descending aorta (Fig. 27.8a), whereas pleural effusions are located beyond the descending aorta.

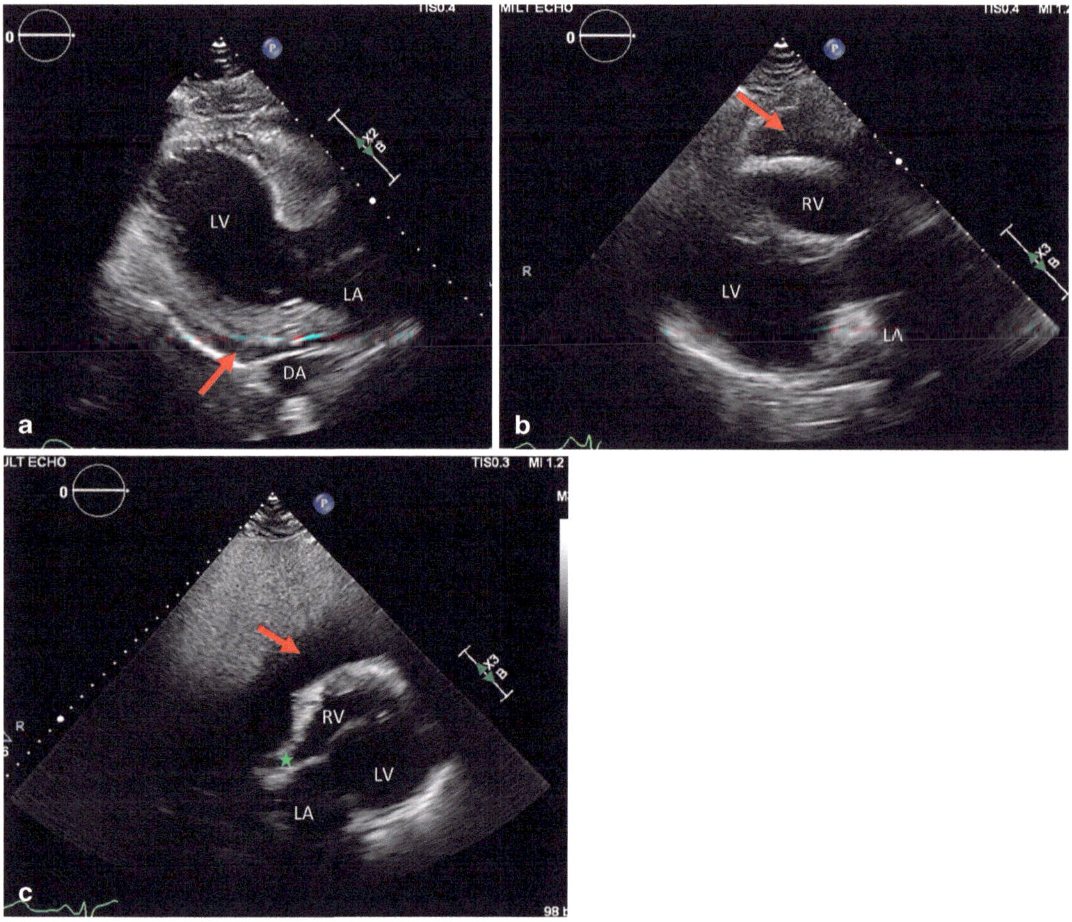

Fig. 27.8 Pericardial effusion (red arrows) viewed through several transthoracic windows. (**a**) Parasternal long axis view demonstrating the pericardial effusion between the left ventricle myocardium and the descending aorta. (**b**) Parasternal long axis view showing the pericardial effusion is concentrated more along the right ventricle in this situation. (**c**) Subcostal view illustrating the pericardial effusion with tamponade physiology, as the right atrium is almost completely collapsed (green star). *LA left atrium, LV left ventricle, RV right ventricle, DA descending aorta*

Sinuses

The transverse sinus is a reflection of the pericardium located at the confluence of the posterior aspect of the ascending aorta, anterior left atrium, and posterior pulmonary artery. More simply, it is a space where the great vessels leave the heart. Meanwhile, the oblique sinus is a reflection of the pericardium located posteriorly to the entry of the four pulmonary veins into the left atrium. Normally, neither pericardial sinus should contain any blood or fluid.

Exogenous Devices

When performing cardiac POCUS, it is imperative to keep in mind any exogenous devices. Pacemaker wires, pulmonary arterial catheters, central venous catheters, mechanical support devices or cannulas, percutaneous left atrial appendage exclusion devices, and percutaneous atrial septal closure devices are examples of some benign objects that may appear in a standard cardiac ultrasound examination. Correlating expected device location to the view and any prior radiographic studies can help confirm the proper location or raise concern for improper placement, which may or may not contribute to physiological perturbations.

Benign Masses

Myxoma

Cardiac myxomas are the most common benign cardiac tumors (27% overall) and most frequently located in the left atrium (75% of the time) [7]. These masses are often pedunculated, attached to an endocardial surface via a stalk, and composed of mucopolysaccharides, giving them a friable characteristic. The most serious consequences of myxomas are obstructed intracardiac blood flow and embolization of tumor materials.

Fibroelastomas

Fibroelastomas (Fig. 27.9) are small, solitary, pedunculated, or sessile-shaped benign tumors found on cardiac valves away from lines of closures. They are associated with thromboembolic events, although their management from an anticoagulation and surgical removal standpoint remains controversial.

Lambl's Excrescences

A specific type of fiberoelastoma, Lambl's excrescences are smaller and thinner filiform structures usually arising from the line of valve closure. However, they most commonly arise from the aortic surface of the aortic valve. Like other fibroelastomas, they are associated with but not necessarily proven to cause strokes, and their medical and surgical management is debated.

Nodule of Arantius

These nodules are located in the center of the free edges of most aortic valve cusps, likely arising from chronic wear and tear. They can become calcified and appear as a mass contributing to valvular regurgitation.

Common Artifacts Appearing as Masses

Reverberations

Recall that ultrasound transducers send out a signal and measure the time it takes for the signal to return. The duration between sending and receiving is converted to a distance on the display screen. When the transducer sends out a primary ultrasound beam, it hits a reflector and then travels back to the transducer. When the beam encounters a second strong reflector, the beam reflects back away from the transducer towards the initial reflector and then back to either the secondary reflector again (the cycle repeats) or back to the transducer. Because the beam reflected from a secondary strong reflector takes longer to return to the transducer than the primary beam, the machine believes the initial target is further from the transducer than it actually is located. Thus, the machine displays a copy of the target deeper or more distal to the actual target location on the screen. This copy is a reverberation artifact. Depending on the number of cycles the beam travels between the target and the secondary strong reflector, multiple copies can appear on the screen, with each one deeper to the target. Examples include A-lines on lung ultrasound and mitral annular calcification on cardiac ultrasound.

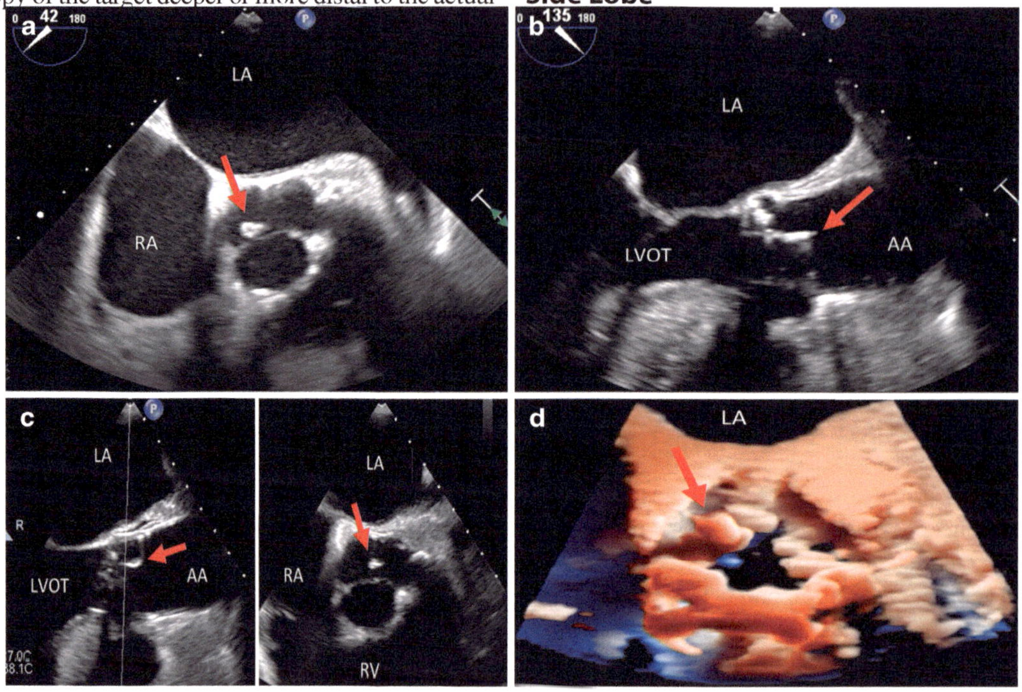

Fig. 27.9 Transesophageal views of an aortic valve fibroelastoma (red arrows). (**a**) Midesophageal aortic valve short axis view. (**b**) Midesophageal aortic valve long axis view. (**c**) Midesophageal biplane view of the aortic valve long axis. In this view the mass appears to originate near the midpoint of the commissure rather than centrally along the line of closure and has a pedunculated appearance. These suggest fibroelastoma over a Lambl's excrescence, the latter of which typically has a thinner and more fibrinous look. (**d**) Three-dimentional aortic valve short axis view with the fibroelastoma

Mirror Image

These artifacts occur when an ultrasound beam bounces once off a strong reflector, back to the target, and then to the transducer. It creates a single copy of the target twice as far as its true location from the transducer. It is essentially a "single copy reverberation." They can also occur in color flow Doppler.

Side Lobe

All artifacts occur because they violate an assumption about ultrasound wave behavior. In the case of side lobe artifacts, the transducer produces more than a single beam, and the extra beams do not travel parallel to the primary beam. The lateral edges of the transducer generate extraneous beams that diverge and travel in a non-parallel direction compared to the primary beam. When these extraneous beams hit a target and reflect back to the transducer, the machine assumes the location they arrive at on the transducer was their origination point and displays the target correspondingly on the screen. However, these extra beams originated elsewhere, contacted a reflector in a non-parallel pathway as the primary beam, and then traveled back to the transducer at a non-parallel angle. Therefore, the machine displays a copy/copies of the target at a uniform distance from the transducer but along a curvilinear line from the actual target's location, otherwise known as side lobe artifacts. Side lobe artifacts appear to disrupt blood flow when viewed in 2D or B mode, but the use of color flow Doppler or spectral Doppler fails to demonstrate a disruption. An example would be a calcified aortic valve annulus appearing as a dissection flap in the ascending aorta.

Acoustic Shadowing

Some tissues or materials have high acoustic impedance, meaning they prevent an ultrasound beam from travelling further. Because the beam cannot penetrate beyond the object, it is unable to contact distal targets and display them on the screen. Thus, the machine displays an echolucent "shadow" deeper/distal to the high acoustic impedance object. For example, in midesophageal transesophageal views, a mechanical mitral valve often casts a shadow over the left ventricular walls, making it impossible to assess for systolic function and wall motion abnormalities. Other common causes include other types of prosthetic valves, patches, implants, and heavily calcified structures.

Conclusion

Point of care Cardiac ultrasound is used more prevalently for critically ill patients in the intensive care unit setting by an increased number of providers. Accurately distinguishing among normal anatomical variants, benign masses, and artifacts is paramount to a proper diagnosis of physiological etiologies of hemodynamic instability and employment of subsequent treatment modalities. This chapter has covered a number of these commonly mistaken structures and findings. Whenever in doubt, we recommend always evaluating the suspected target in multiple windows, views, and modalities.

Summary Points

- Every physician performing echocardiographic assessment of the heart needs to distinguish between normal anatomical variants and pathological findings by becoming familiar with common variants that cause confusion and reconfirming suspicions with multiple views and modalities.
- Benign cardiac masses such as myxomas and fibroelastomas are found incidentally on cardiac ultrasounds and may or may not require medical or surgical attention.
- Several ultrasound artifacts like reverberation, side lobe, and acoustic shadowing can hamper the full evaluation of the heart in a particular view and falsely create abnormal appearing structures.

Questions

1. A 72-year-old male with a past medical history of diabetes mellitus type 2, hypertension, hyperlipidemia, and chronic obstructive pulmonary disease presents to the emergency room after experiencing new-onset left facial droop and slurred speech thirty minutes prior to arrival at the hospital. Which of the following normal anatomic variants is this patient most likely to show on echocardiographic imaging:
   A. Patent foramen ovale.
   B. Chiari network.
   C. Left atrial appendage.
   D. Atrial septal aneurysm.
   E. Crista terminalis.
   F. A, B, and C.
   G. A, B, and D.
   H. A and B.

   Answer 1:

   G— A patent foramen ovale, Chiari network, and atrial septal aneurysm are all associated with an increased risk of stroke, which is the clinical diagnosis for this patient. The crista terminalis (E) separates the pectinate muscles of the right atrial appendage from the smooth wall of the right atrium and is most commonly visualized at the junction of the superior vena cava and right atrium on transesophageal echocardiography in the midesophageal bicaval view. The left atrial appendage (C) is a normal structure that should be found in every patient, except for those who have undergone surgical or percutaneous left atrial appendage exclusion. It is a nidus for thrombus in low-flow states, such as atrial arrhythmias like atrial fibrillation and heart failure. This patient did not endorse any history of dysrhythmias, palpitations, heart failure, or other risk factors for having a thrombus in the left atrial appendage. Therefore, a patent foramen ovale, Chiari network, and atrial septal aneurysm are more likely in this patient.

2. A 64-year-old female with normal heart function, coronary artery disease, and severe aortic valve insufficiency is admitted on veno-arterial extracorporeal membrane oxygenation support to the cardiovascular intensive care unit following combined coronary artery bypass grafting and aortic valve replacement for failure to separate from cardiopulmonary bypass due to cardiogenic shock. Which of the following could have prevented this from occurring?
   A. Perform a 3D assessment of the aortic valve.
   B. Insert a pulmonary arterial catheter for added monitoring under TEE guidance.
   C. Perform a bubble study through a left upper extremity peripheral IV.
   D. Confirm the arterial cannula placement on TEE.

   Answer 2:

   C—While undergoing a combined on-pump coronary artery bypass grafting and aortic valve replacement surgery, the heart is arrested by administering cardioplegia either antegrade (into the aortic root so that it goes down the coronary arteries) or retrograde (through a cannula placed into the coronary sinus). Antegrade flow down the coronary arteries is dependent upon sufficient pressurization of the root between the aortic cross-clamp and a competent aortic valve. In this case, the patient has severe aortic valve insufficiency, which results in antegrade cardioplegia leaking into the left ventricle rather than going down the coronary arteries. Therefore, the surgeon placed a retrograde cardioplegia line in the coronary sinus to frequently dose the cardioplegia.

   In patients with a persistent left superior vena cava (PLSVC), primarily left upper extremity venous blood drains into the coronary sinus directly and eventually into the right atrium. This results in the coronary sinus usually being dilated greater than 1 cm and should clue echocardiographers into its possible existence. Conversely, when administering retrograde cardioplegia through a coronary sinus catheter, the retrograde cardioplegia travels backward into the systemic circulation rather than to the myocardium for myocardial protection. Therefore, this patient had a PLSVC with frequent administration of retrograde cardioplegia resulting in no cardioprotection. Diagnosing PLSVC involves conducting a bubble study through a left upper extremity PIV and observing opacification of the coronary sinus rather than the right-sided superior vena cava. Had this been done before the institution of cardiopulmonary bypass, a different myocardial protection plan could have preserved this patient's heart function on pump.

   Performing a 3D assessment of the aortic valve (A) can further evaluate the patient's aortic insufficiency and would prompt the use of retrograde cardioplegia. It would still require evaluation for a PLSVC. Placing a pulmonary arterial catheter under TEE guidance (B) can be a useful monitor in some situations, but for this patient, it would not have improved myocardial protection. Confirming arterial cannula placement (D) would not have improved this patient's myocardial protection.

3. What is the most common location to find a myxoma?
   A. Left atrium.
   B. Right atrium.
   C. Left ventricle.
   D. Right ventricle.

   Answer 3:

   The most common location for a cardiac myxoma, which is the most common benign cardiac tumor, is the left atrium (A) in approximately 75% of patients. The other locations can be home to myxomas but are less frequent than the left atrium.

References

1. Sidebotham D, Merry A, Legget M, Wright G. Practical perioperative transoesophageal echocardiography. 3rd ed. New York City, NY: Oxford University Press; 2018.
2. Pejković B, Krajnc I, Anderhuber F, Kosutić D. Anatomical variations of the coronary sinus ostium area of the human heart. J Int Med Res. 2008;36(2):314–21.
3. Otto C. Textbook of clinical echocardiography. 6th ed. Philadelphia, PA: Elsevier; 2018.
4. Mas JL, Arquizan C, Lamy C, Zuber M, Cabanes L, Derumeaux G, et al. Recurrent cerebrovascular events associated with patent foramen ovale, atrial septal aneurysm, or both. N Engl J Med. 2002;3(11):93.
5. Mattioli AV, Aquilina M, Oldani A, Longhini C, Mattioli G. Atrial septal aneurysm as a cardioembolic source in adult patients with stroke and normal carotid arteries. A multicentre study. Eur Heart J. 2001;22(3):261–8.
6. Ahmad ZS, Koshy C, Koshy GA. Echocardiographic study of left ventricular false tendons. J Indian Acad Echocardiogr Cardiovasc Imaging. 2019;3(3):150–5.
7. Swaminathan M, Mathew J, Nicoara A, Ayoub C. Clinical manual and review of transesophageal echocardiography. 3rd ed. New York City, NY: McGraw Hill; 2019.

28 Left Ventricular Thrombus Part 1

Donald R. Maberry and Babar Fiza

Learning Objectives

1. Discuss the pathophysiology of LV thrombus.
2. Examine the utility of using contrast enhancement to improve the echocardiographic diagnosis of LV thrombus.
3. Review echocardiographic techniques for reducing erroneous findings of LV thrombus.

Introduction

Left ventricular thrombus (LVT) is a potentially fatal complication of anterior myocardial infarction and dilated cardiomyopathies. Prompt and accurate diagnosis of LVT is crucial as the presence of LVT can significantly impact both acute and long-term management strategies. The diagnosis of LVT can be challenging to establish with point-of-care ultrasound but can be achieved with meticulous imaging techniques and a thorough understanding of the echocardiographic characteristics of LVT. This chapter details the epidemiology, pathophysiology, and role of point-of-care echocardiography in diagnosing LVT. Additionally, we discuss the diagnostic limitations of ultrasonography and the role of contrast-enhanced echocardiography in the LVT diagnostic algorithms.

Etiology

Epidemiology and Pathophysiology

Left ventricular thrombus was a common complication of myocardial infarction before the widespread use of PCI treatments [1]. Early studies using 2D echocardiography alone to diagnose LVT reported an incidence of 4–17% in all cases of myocardial infarction and 10–34% for anterior myocardial infarctions [1, 2]. In contrast, contemporary studies using cardiac magnetic resonance (CMR) report an overall incidence of LVT of 5.4% and 7–15% of anterior MIs [3].

The formation of left ventricular thrombi occurs because of Virchow's triad, which consists of three factors: hypercoagulability, stasis, and endothelial injury [3]. During a myocardial infarction, subendothelial ischemia leads to tissue damage and localized inflammatory changes that activate platelets and the coagulation cascade. Simultaneously, the decrease in cardiac blood flow leads to areas of myocardial dyskinesis

Supplementary Information The online version contains supplementary material available at https://doi.org/10.1007/978-3-031-80038-2_28.

D. R. Maberry · B. Fiza (✉)
Division of Critical Care Medicine, Department of Anesthesiology, Emory School of Medicine, Atlanta, GA, USA
e-mail: donald.reed.maberry@emory.edu; babar.fiza@emory.edu

M. J. Lanspa, A. T. Levinson (eds.), *Echocardiography and Ultrasonography in the ICU*, Respiratory Medicine, https://doi.org/10.1007/978-3-031-80038-2_28

and potentially aneurysm or pseudoaneurysm formation. Myocardial dyskinesis and myocardial architectural distortion alter blood flow through the left ventricle and lead to areas of relative blood stasis. The severity of blood stasis increases as the left ventricle ejection fraction decreases. Finally, acute coronary syndrome is associated with a hypercoagulable state, specifically with increased levels of von Willebrand factor, prothrombin, and fibrinopeptide-A that can persist for months after the MI [3, 4]. This pathophysiology demonstrates two important phenomena about left ventricular thrombus. First, approximately 90% of thrombi form in the first 2 weeks after myocardial infarction [3]. Although the risk of developing an LVT decreases with time, one study using cardiac MRI found an additional 6% of patients with a new LV thrombus at 4 months [5]. Second, myocardial dyskinesis and decreased ejection fraction are major risk factors for developing LV thrombus after myocardial infarction. Interestingly, other pathologic states with decreased ejection fraction and myocardial dyskinesis, such as takotsubo, have an LVT incidence of only 1–2%, despite low rates of anticoagulation [6]. It is theorized that the delayed formation of thrombi after MI and the relative lack of thrombi in Takotsubo demonstrate the importance of the persistent hypercoagulable state following an acute MI [6].

Biostatistics and Risk Factors

Multiple modalities are available for diagnosing a left ventricular thrombus: standard echocardiography, contrast-enhanced echocardiography, and cardiac MRI. Understanding the indications and limitations of each of these tools is vital for making a prompt diagnosis of LVT. A traditional non-contrast transthoracic echocardiogram (TTE) has a sensitivity of 24–33%, specificity of 95%, a positive predictive value (PPV) of 57%, and a negative predictive value (NPV) of 85% for diagnosing LVT [7, 8]. Interestingly, when evaluation for LVT is listed as the specific indication for a TTE, the sensitivity and PPV of echocardiography increase to 60% and 75%, respectively [9]. The use of contrast-enhanced echocardiography improves the diagnostic yield, with a sensitivity of 61%, specificity of 99%, a PPV of 93%, and an NPH of 91% [6]. When LV thrombus was the specified indication and performed on very high-risk patients (anterior MI and reduced ejection fraction), the sensitivity was 94.7% and the specificity was 98.5% [10]. In comparison, delayed enhancement cardiac MRI has a sensitivity of 88% and a specificity of 99% [11].

There are several well-known risk factors for LVT that should be taken into consideration when choosing a diagnostic modality. The primary risk factor for developing an LVT is an acute anterior myocardial infarction. Other important risk factors include LV ejection fraction <40%, large infarct size, severe apical dyskinesis, LV aneurysm, LV pseudoaneurysm, and dilated cardiomyopathy [3, 11]. Of note, the risk of LV thrombus in non-anterior MI increases as the necrosis progresses towards the posterolateral wall [3]. Given the limited sensitivity of echocardiography to diagnose an LV thrombus, any patient at high risk for LVT should be referred for a contrast-enhanced echocardiogram or a delayed enhancement cardiac MRI [12].

Diagnosis

Definition and Differential Diagnosis

A left ventricular thrombus is a ventricular cavity mass that appears adjacent to a dyskinetic segment of the myocardium with margins that are distinct from the blood and the endocardium. To make the diagnosis, the mass in question should be present for the entire cardiac cycle and be visible in at least two views [10]. Finally, the thrombus should be clearly distinguishable from the chordae tendineae, papillary muscles, and myocardial trabeculae [9]. An LVT can be further characterized by its location, shape, mobility, and chronicity. Most LV thrombi occur in the LV apex, but they can occur at any location throughout the left ventricle [11, 13].

An LV thrombus can be categorized based on the thrombus characteristics. A protruding thrombus is any thrombus that projects directly into the ventricular cavity and has multiple surfaces that interface with the bloodstream (Fig. 28.1; Video 28.1). This is contrasted with a mural thrombus, which is flat, parallel to the endocardium, and has only one surface that contacts the bloodstream (Fig. 28.2; Videos 28.2 and 28.3). A mobile thrombus is any LVT that moves independently from the myocardium. Finally, a thrombus can be described by its chronicity. An acute thrombus consists primarily of platelets and clotting cascade proteins. As the clot ages, fibroblasts create a collagen matrix, forming a stronger, more organized clot [14]. Generally, acute LV thrombi are irregular, protruding, highly mobile, and commonly have an echo-lucent core (Fig. 28.3; Video 28.4). In contrast, chronic thrombi are less mobile and more likely to have a mural appearance [15]. Although beyond the scope of this text, echocardiography can be used to measure the elastic deformation of an LV thrombus as a marker for thrombus chronicity [14].

The size, shape, and mobility of the LVT are of diagnostic and clinical significance. The sensitivity of echocardiography to detect an LV thrombus is variable. The likelihood of a false-negative echocardiogram is higher for small thrombi, nonapical thrombi, and mural thrombi [9]. Clinically, acute thrombi, large thrombi, protruding thrombi, and highly mobile thrombi are at higher risk of embolization [15]. Other risk factors for embolization include increasing age, a history of congestive heart failure, and an adjacent hyperdynamic myocardial segment [15].

The differential diagnosis for an LVT is broad and includes both normal and pathologic entities. False tendons, trabeculae, and misplaced papillary muscles are common normal variants that can be mistaken for LVT [15]. Potentially pathologic causes of an LV mass include left ventricular fibroma, myxoma, papillary fibroelastoma, Lamble excrescence, metastatic cancer, primary cardiac neoplasm, and cardiac hamartoma. Melanoma commonly metastasizes to the pericardium and myocardium. Primary cardiac tumors are rare and are usually a primary sarcoma or lymphoma. LVT is strongly associated with myocardial dyskinesis; if there are no adjacent areas of dyskinesis, you should seriously consider another diagnosis [13, 15, 16]. Uncommon causes of LVT in the setting of normal LV function include eosinophilic endocarditis, antiphospholipid syndrome, protein C deficiency, myeloproliferative disorders, and cardiac trauma [15].

Echocardiography Technique

When evaluating a patient for LVT, the initial echocardiogram examination should consist of parasternal long, parasternal short, and apical 2, 3, and 4 chamber windows [9]. The standard apical windows may miss small LV thrombi, and

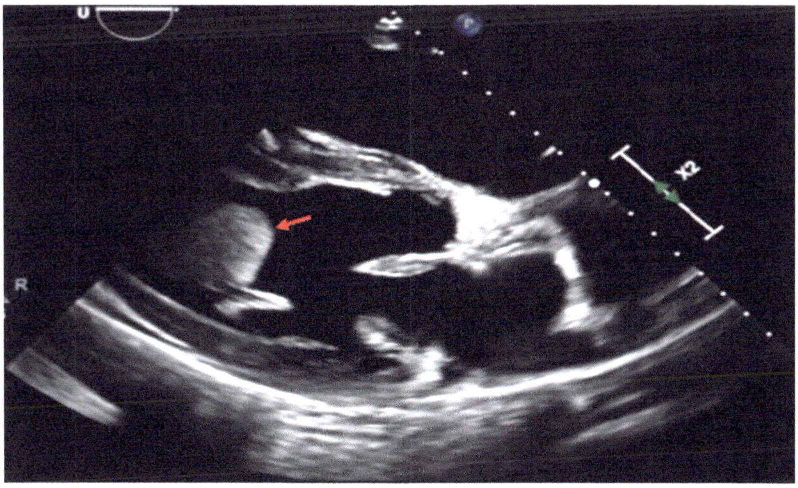

Fig. 28.1 A large, protruding, and mobile thrombus (red arrow) is visualized within the left ventricle on the parasternal long-axis view

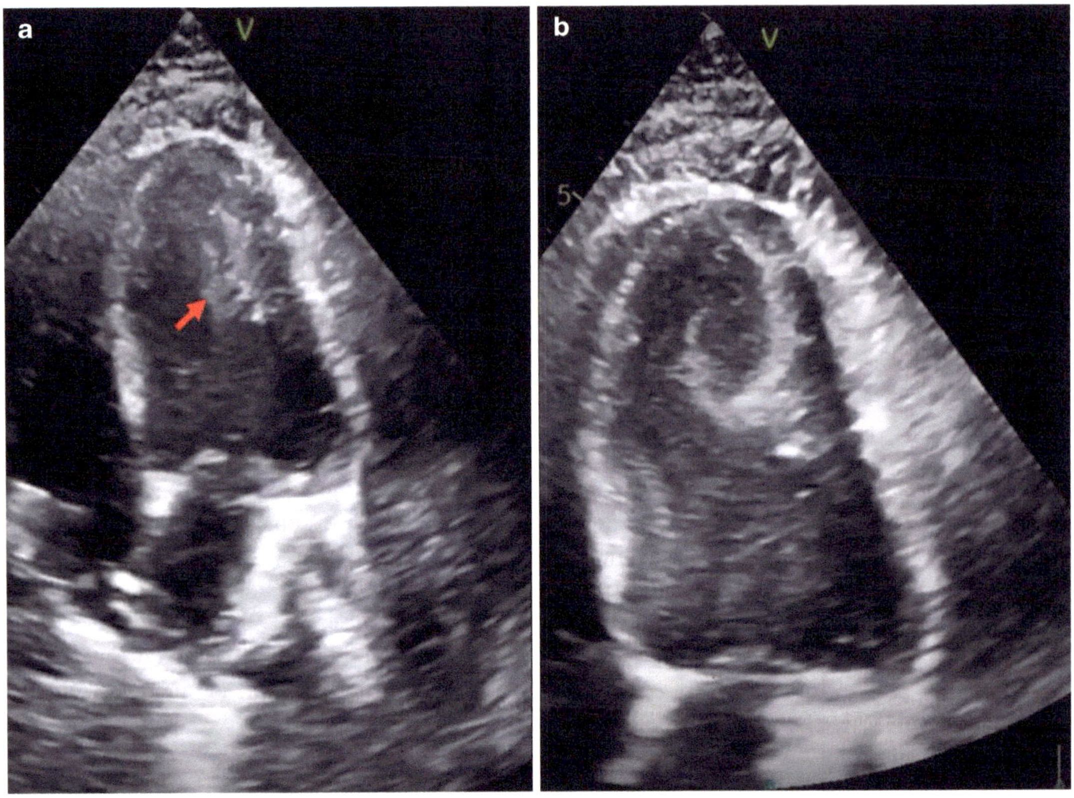

Fig. 28.2 (**a**) A mural thrombus is visualized in the apical four-chamber view (red arrow), adherent to the left ventricular apex and apical lateral wall. (**b**) A zoomed-in view highlights the mural thrombus and spontaneous echo contrast (smoke) within the left ventricle

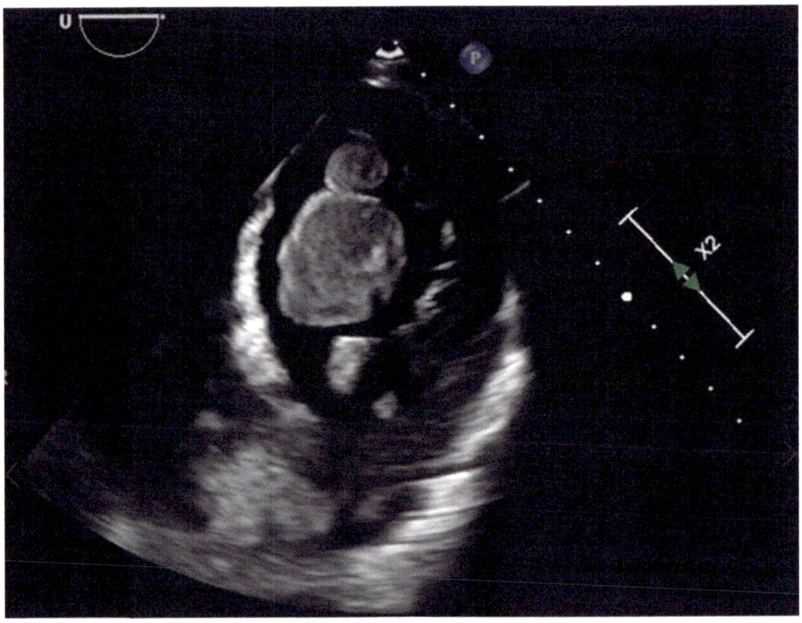

Fig. 28.3 Multiple protruding and mobile left ventricular thrombi are visualized in this off-axis apical two-chamber view. The largest thrombus demonstrates a hypoechoic center relative to its echogenic margins, suggestive of an acute thrombus

obtaining off-axis or tangential apical views can increase the diagnostic yield (Fig. 28.3; Video 28.4) [13]. Using probes with different frequencies, varying the gain settings, and adjusting the depth of field can reduce the risk of false positive studies [5]. You can also consider measuring Doppler flow patterns in the LV cavity, as both apical flow stasis and apical swirling are linked to LVT formation [15]. LV cavity Doppler flow is also useful for differentiating between an apical thrombus and common mimics such as a false tendon or a myocardial trabeculae. A false tendon is a fibrous band, like a chordae tendinea, that stretches across the LV cavity but does not connect with the mitral valve. Both false tendons and trabeculae create an echogenic line on ultrasound that mimics the edge of an apical thrombus. When color Doppler is placed over a false tendon or trabeculae, it will show flow on both sides of the line, confirming the presence of a false tendon or trabeculae. An apical thrombus will not have an internal Doppler signal [13]. Similarly, it is important to be aware of near-field clutter artifacts and reverberation artifacts, as both artifacts mimic an apical thrombus but will move with probe repositioning [13]. Finally, the diagnosis of LVT is dependent upon clear delineation of the LV endocardial border. If the endocardial border cannot be clearly defined, the patient should be considered for contrast-enhanced echocardiography or cardiac MRI [15].

Contrast-Enhanced Echocardiography

The clear delineation of the endocardial border is a key component in diagnosing LVT and a primary limitation of the traditional non-contrast echocardiography. The use of ultrasound contrast to opacify the left ventricle cavity to improve endocardial delineation significantly increases the sensitivity and positive predictive value of echocardiography for diagnosing LVT. As such, LV thrombus is listed as a primary indication for the use of ultrasound contrast in the American Society of Echocardiography Guidelines [17]. Ultrasound contrast is a solution of microbubbles made up of a lipid, protein, or polymer shell filled with a perfluorocarbon or sulfur hexafluoride gas. These microbubbles undergo volumetric oscillations when they are exposed to sound waves and reverberate at a frequency that can be detected by vendor-specific detection modalities, allowing for improved visualization of the endocardial border [18].

When using ultrasound contrast agents, it is important to make the following considerations. First, the machine should be set to a low mechanical index, approximately 02–0.5; the exact level will be determined by the type of contrast used. The contrast infusion rate should be optimized so that the LV opacification is uniform throughout. If the contrast agent is infused too rapidly, it can lead to signal attenuation and poor study quality. If the contrast agent is infused too slowly, or if the mechanical index is too high, it can lead to a swirling artifact or a loss of apical opacification. When used properly, contrast-enhanced echocardiography reduces the number of studies deemed uninterpretable, increases visualization of the LV segments, improves the ability to detect wall motion abnormalities, and increases the detection of LV thrombi (Figs. 28.4 and 28.5) [19]. Finally, ultrasound contrast is associated with back pain and transient headache, but serious reactions are rare, and it is considered safe for use in pulmonary hypertension and critically ill patients [16].

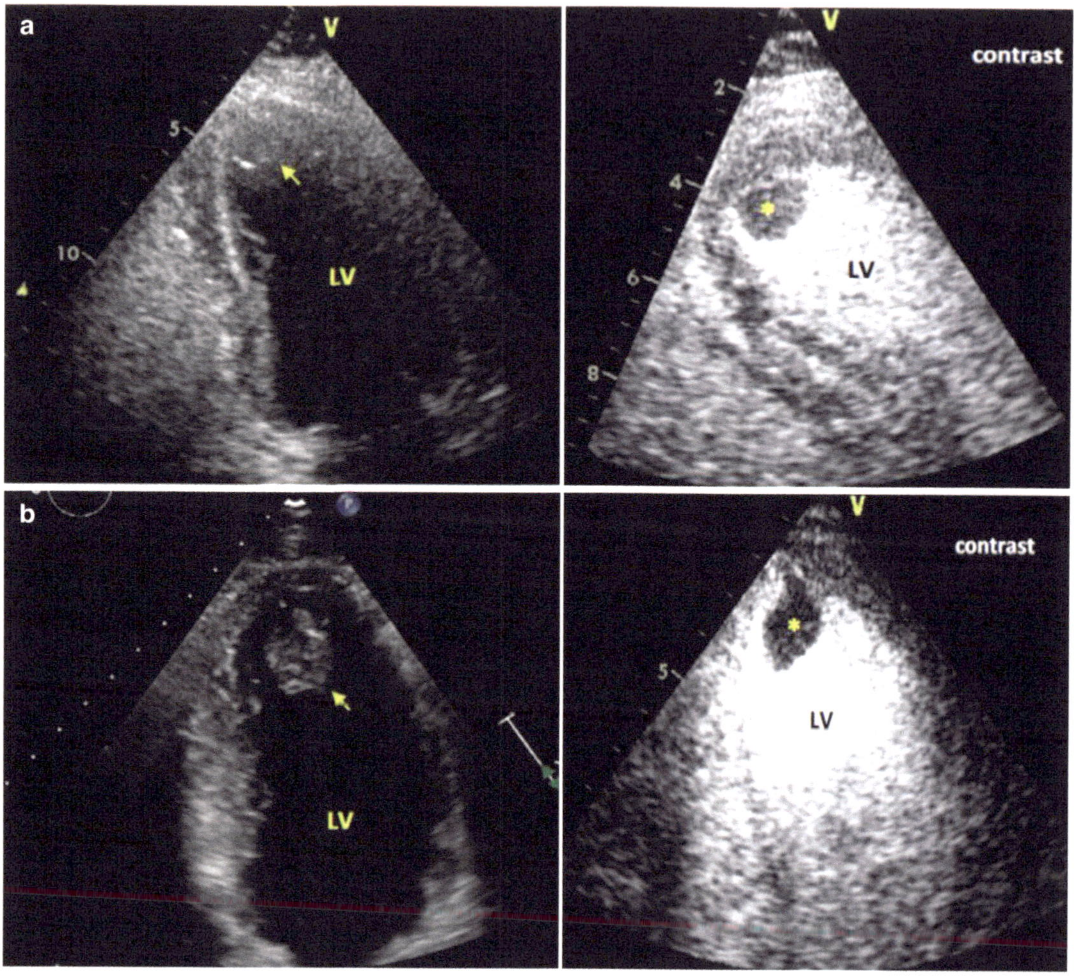

Fig. 28.4 Two examples of apical thrombi are demonstrated before and after ultrasound contrast enhancement. (**a**) A hyperechoic region is noted near the apex (yellow arrow); however, poor endocardial border definition limits diagnostic confidence. Following contrast administration, a protruding left ventricular thrombus is clearly delineated (yellow asterisk). (**b**) A large apical thrombus is visualized both before (yellow arrow) and after (yellow asterisk) contrast enhancement, with contrast markedly improving thrombus visualization and endocardial border definition.

Image adapted from Barbieri A, Mantovani F, Bursi F, Faggiano A, Boriani G, Faggiano P. Optimal Use of Echocardiography in Management of Thrombosis After Anterior Myocardial Infarction. Echocardiography. 2020;37(8):1287–1295

Permission Granted from John Wiley and Sons and Copyright Clearance Center

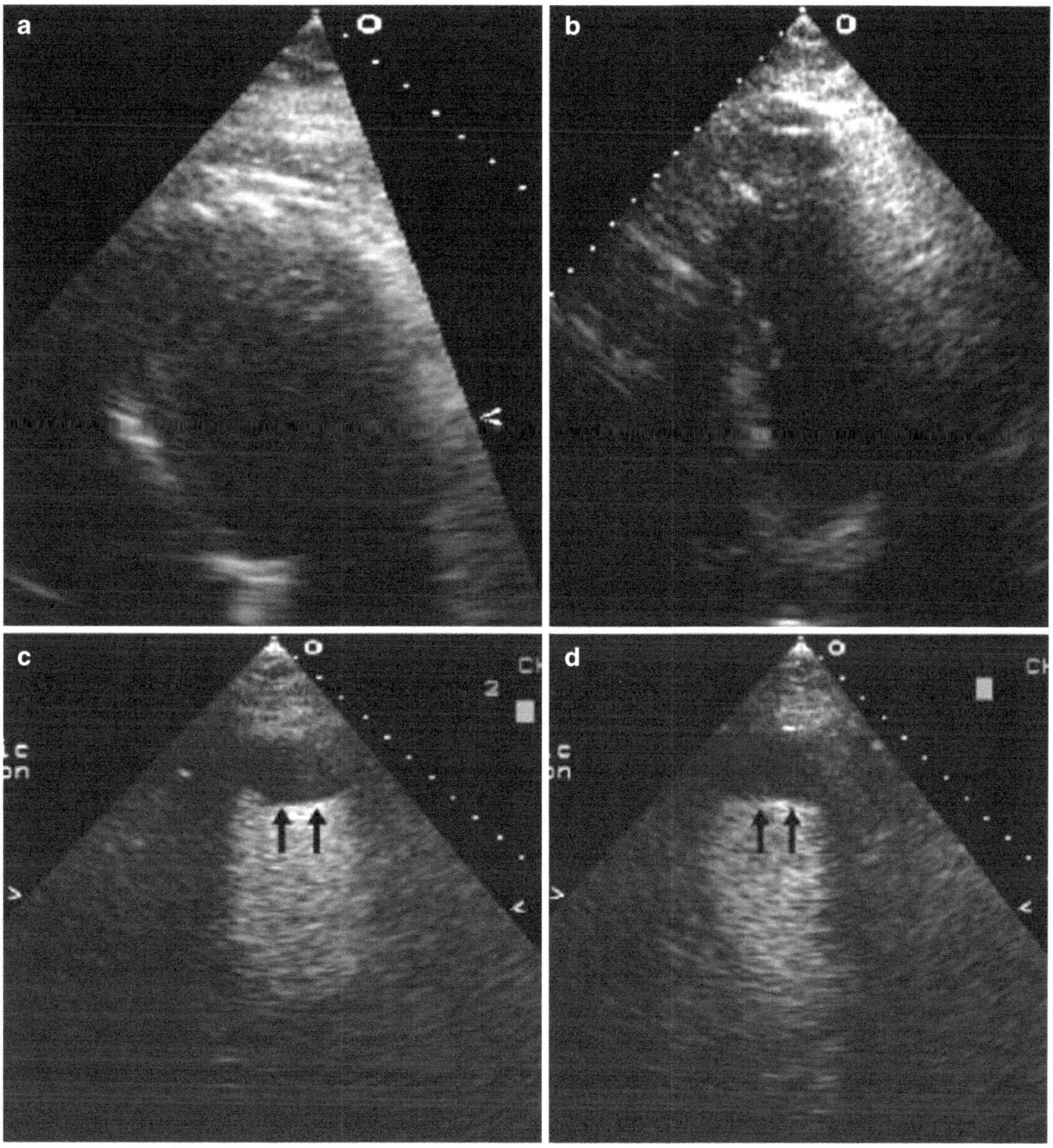

Fig. 28.5 Visualization of Apical Thrombi Before and After Ultrasound Contrast Enhancement. Panels (**a**) and (**c**) show an apical two-chamber view acquired before and after contrast administration, respectively. In panel (**a**), the endocardial border at the apex is poorly defined, limiting diagnostic clarity. Contrast enhancement in panel (**c**) reveals a well-delineated apical thrombus. Panels (**b**) and (**d**) depict an apical three-chamber view before and after contrast. While no thrombus is identified in panel (**b**) due to suboptimal visualization, panel (**d**) demonstrates improved endocardial border definition and confirms the presence of an apical thrombus following contrast administration

Image adapted from: Srichai MB, Junor C, Rodriguez LL, Stillman AE, Grimm RA, Lieber ML, et al. Imaging and pathological characteristics of left ventricular thrombus: a comparison of contrast-enhanced magnetic resonance imaging, transthoracic echocardiography, and transesophageal echocardiography with surgical or pathological validation. American Heart Journal. 2006;152(1):75–84

Permission Granted from Elsevier Publishing

Clinical Implications

Patients with an LV thrombus are at increased risk of cardioembolic events and require anticoagulation and repeat imaging to evaluate for thrombus resolution [8]. When the diagnosis of LVT is made, the patient should be started on anticoagulation with warfarin and a heparin bridge. Direct-acting oral anticoagulants (DOACs) can be used, but a recent retrospective study found that patients treated with DOACs had a higher incidence of stroke after 1 year [20]. The rate of LVT-related cardioembolic events is approximately 5.5% and can be as low as 3% in patients who are therapeutic on warfarin more than 50% of the time [20]. It is important to recognize that the risk of a cardioembolic event is highest during the first 2 weeks after thrombus formation and then gradually decreases over the next 3 months [20].

Delayed enhancement Cardiac MRI is considered the diagnostic standard, but it has limited availability, limited ability to perform serial exams, increased cost, and may not be tolerated by the patient. The diagnosis of LV thrombus can be made on point-of-care (POC) ultrasound if a ventricular cavity mass with distinct margins is seen adjacent to a dyskinetic segment of the myocardium. It is important to understand the limitations of point-of-care ultrasound in making this diagnosis. It is crucial that high-risk patients with a negative POC ultrasound are referred for additional testing with contrast-enhanced echocardiography or a cardiac MRI. It is also reasonable to consider repeat contrast-enhanced echocardiography in 2 weeks for high-risk patients with a negative initial scan [20].In patients with an LVT on their initial study, a repeat echocardiogram may be performed in 2–4 weeks to assess for resolution of the thrombus, as 62.3% of patients may have total resolution of the thrombus with a median time to resolution of 103 days [21]. This has important therapeutic implications, as patients with thrombus resolution can discontinue their anticoagulation while patients with persistent LVT remain at a higher risk of complications [20].

Summary Points

- Left ventricular thrombus (LVT) affects 5.4% of all MIs and 7–15% of anterior MIs [3].
- LV thrombus should also be considered in patients with severe apical dyskinesis, LV aneurysm, LV pseudoaneurysm, and dilated cardiomyopathy [3, 11].
- Patients with LVT are at increased risk of cardioembolic events and require anticoagulation and further imaging to monitor for thrombus resolution [21].
- Traditional transthoracic echocardiograms have a sensitivity of 24–33% and specificity of 95% [7, 8].
- Specifying LVT as the indication for the study increases the sensitivity [9].
- Contrast-enhanced echocardiography improves delineation of the endocardial border and increases the sensitivity to 61% and specificity of 99% [6].
- The likelihood of a false-negative echocardiogram is higher for small thrombi, non-apical thrombi, and mural thrombi [9].
- Obtaining off-axis or tangential apical views, using probes with different frequencies, varying the gain settings, and adjusting the depth of field can reduce the risk of false positive studies [5, 13].
- LV cavity Doppler flow is useful for differentiating between an apical thrombus and common mimics such as a false tendon or a myocardial trabecula [13].
- Contrast-enhanced echocardiography should be considered in all high-risk patients and in any study where the endocardial border is not clearly defined [17].

Questions

1. Which of the following ultrasound modalities can be used to differentiate between a left ventricular thrombus and similarly appearing non-pathologic conditions such as a false tendon or a trabecula?
   A. Pulse wave Doppler.
   B. Continuous wave Doppler.

C. **Color Doppler.**
D. M-mode.

Explanation: LV cavity Doppler flow is useful for differentiating between an apical thrombus and common mimics such as a false tendon or a myocardial trabecula. A false tendon is a fibrous band, like a chordae tendinea, that stretches across the LV cavity. Both false tendons and trabeculae create an echogenic line on ultrasound that mimics the edge of a ventricular thrombus. When color Doppler is placed over a false tendon or trabeculae, it will show flow on both sides of the line, confirming the presence of a false tendon or trabeculae. An apical thrombus will not have an internal Doppler signal [13]. Pulse wave Doppler allows you to measure low velocities in a small, gated area. Continuous wave Doppler can measure both the direction and the velocity of flow along a given path but cannot determine the exact location [22]. M-mode allows you to visualize motion and timing in a selected region [23].

2. You are caring for a 55-year-old man with acute heart failure after an anterior myocardial infarction. He is now 7 days out from PCI and has been progressing as expected. You are completing your morning exam when you notice that his right leg is cold and no longer has a palpable dorsalis pedis pulse. You perform a bedside echocardiogram and notice a moderately reduced ejection fraction with anterior wall dyskinesis but do not visualize an LV thrombus. Which of the following scenarios is most likely to result in a false-negative echocardiogram for LV thrombus?
   A. A left ventricle apex thrombus of any size.
   B. A large mural thrombus.
   C. A small apical thrombus.
   D. **A small, non-apical, mural thrombus.**
   E. A small, non-apical, protruding thrombus.

Explanation: In a study by Weinsaft et al. (2011) comparing echocardiography and delayed enhancement cardiac MRI in 243 patients, they found that small thrombi and mural thrombi were the most likely to be missed on transthoracic echocardiography. In this study, the positive predictive value was also related to the image quality of the echocardiogram [9]. A second study by Weinsaft et al. published in 2009 found that non-apical thrombi were less likely to be detected [7].

References

1. Kalra A, Jang I-K. Prevalence of early left ventricular thrombus after primary coronary intervention for acute myocardial infarction. J Thromb Thrombolysis. 2000;10(2):133–6. https://doi.org/10.1023/a:1018710425817.
2. Asinger RW, Mikell FL, Elsperger J, Hodges M. Incidence of left-ventricular thrombosis after acute transmural myocardial infarction. N Engl J Med. 1981;305(6):297–302. https://doi.org/10.1056/nejm198108063050601.
3. Delewi R, Zijlstra F, Piek JJ. Left ventricular thrombus formation after acute myocardial infarction. Heart. 2012;98(23):1743–9. https://doi.org/10.1136/heartjnl-2012-301962.
4. Merlini PA, Bauer KA, Oltrona L, et al. Persistent activation of coagulation mechanism in unstable angina and myocardial infarction. Circulation. 1994;90(1):61–8. https://doi.org/10.1161/01.cir.90.1.61.
5. Delewi R, Nijveldt R, Hirsch A, et al. Left ventricular thrombus formation after acute myocardial infarction as assessed by cardiovascular magnetic resonance imaging. Eur J Radiol. 2012;81(12):3900–4. https://doi.org/10.1016/j.ejrad.2012.06.029.
6. Templin C, Ghadri JR, Diekmann J, et al. Clinical features and outcomes of Takotsubo (stress) cardiomyopathy. N Engl J Med. 2015;373(10):929–38. https://doi.org/10.1056/nejmoa1406761.
7. Weinsaft JW, Kim RJ, Ross M, et al. Contrast-enhanced anatomic imaging as compared to contrast-enhanced tissue characterization for detection of left ventricular thrombus. JACC: Cardiovasc. Imaging. 2009;2(8):969–79. https://doi.org/10.1016/j.jcmg.2009.03.017.
8. Barbieri A, Mantovani F, Bursi F, Faggiano A, Boriani G, Faggiano P. Optimal use of echocardiography in management of thrombosis after anterior myocardial infarction. Echocardiography. 2020;37(8):1287–95. https://doi.org/10.1111/echo.14808.
9. Weinsaft JW, Kim HW, Crowley AL, et al. LV thrombus detection by routine echocardiography. Cardiovasc Imaging. 2011;4(7):702–12. https://doi.org/10.1016/j.jcmg.2011.03.017.
10. Meurin P, Brandao Carreira V, Dumaine R, et al. Incidence, diagnostic methods, and evolution of left ventricular thrombus in patients with anterior myocardial infarction and low left ventricular ejection fraction: a prospective multicenter study. Am Heart J. 2015;170(2):256–62. https://doi.org/10.1016/j.ahj.2015.04.029.

11. Srichai MB, Junor C, Rodriguez LL, et al. Clinical, imaging, and pathological characteristics of left ventricular thrombus: a comparison of contrast-enhanced magnetic resonance imaging, transthoracic echocardiography, and transesophageal echocardiography with surgical or pathological validation. Am Heart J. 2006;152(1):75–84. https://doi.org/10.1016/j.ahj.2005.08.021.
12. Weinsaft JW, Kim J, Medicherla CB, et al. Echocardiographic algorithm for post–myocardial infarction LV thrombus. JACC: Cardiovasc. Imaging. 2016;9(5):505–15. https://doi.org/10.1016/j.jcmg.2015.06.017.
13. Armstrong WF, Ryan T. Feigenbaum's echocardiography: Ebook without multimedia. 8th ed. Wolters Kluwer Health; 2018. Accessed December 7, 2021. https://search-ebscohost-com.proxy.library.emory.edu/login.aspx?direct=true&db=e000xna&AN=2356848&site=ehost-live&scope=site
14. Niemann M, Gaudron PD, Bijnens B, et al. Differentiation between fresh and old left ventricular thrombi by deformation imaging. Circ: Cardiovasc. Imaging. 2012;5(5):667–75. https://doi.org/10.1161/circimaging.112.974964.
15. Lang RM. ASE's comprehensive echocardiography. 3rd ed. Elsevier; 2022. Accessed 12/14/2021. https://www-clinicalkey-com.proxy.library.emory.edu/#!/browse/book/3-s2.0-C20160019678
16. Oh JK, Kane GC. The echo manual: Ebook without multimedia. 4th ed. Wolters Kluwer Health; 2018. Accessed December 8, 2021. https://search-ebscohost-com.proxy.library.emory.edu/login.aspx?direct=true&db=e000xna&AN=2356924&site=ehost-live&scope=site
17. Porter TR, Mulvagh SL, Abdelmoneim SS, et al. Clinical applications of ultrasonic enhancing agents in echocardiography: 2018 American Society of Echocardiography Guidelines Update. J Am Soc Echocardiogr. 2018;31(3):241–74. https://doi.org/10.1016/j.echo.2017.11.013.
18. Abdelmoneim SS, Pellikka PA, Mulvagh SL. Contrast echocardiography for assessment of left ventricular thrombi. J Ultrasound Med. 2014;33(8):1337–44. https://doi.org/10.7863/ultra.33.8.1337.
19. Kurt M, Shaikh KA, Peterson L, et al. Impact of contrast echocardiography on evaluation of ventricular function and clinical management in a large prospective cohort. J Am College Cardiol. 2009;53(9):802–10. https://doi.org/10.1016/j.jacc.2009.01.005.
20. Robinson AA, Trankle CR, Eubanks G, et al. Off-label use of direct oral anticoagulants compared with warfarin for left ventricular thrombi. JAMA Cardiol. 2020;5(6):685. https://doi.org/10.1001/jamacardio.2020.0652.
21. Lattuca B, Bouziri N, Kerneis M, et al. Antithrombotic therapy for patients with left ventricular mural thrombus. J Am College Cardiol. 2020;75(14):1676–85. https://doi.org/10.1016/j.jacc.2020.01.057.
22. Narasimhan M, Koenig SJ, Mayo PH. Advanced echocardiography for the critical care physician: Part 1. Chest. 2014;145(1):129–34.
23. Prada G, Vicillard-Baron A, Martin AK, Hernandez A, Mookadam F, Ramakrishna H, et al. Echocardiographic applications of M-mode ultrasonography in anesthesiology and critical care. J Cardiothorac Vasc Anesth. 2019;33(6):1559–83.

Left Ventricular Thrombus Part 2

29

John L. Maurer and Matthew E. Prekker

Learning Objectives

1. Identify risk factors for LV thrombus formation.
2. Recognize the sonographic features of an LV thrombus.
3. Know the utility of ultrasound-enhancing agents and the limits of imaging modalities for the diagnosis of LV thrombus.
4. Understand the clinical implications and treatment of an LV thrombus.

In: "Echocardiography and Ultrasonography in the ICU: A Comprehensive Text" Eds. Michael Lanspa, MD, MS, and Andrew Levinson, MD, MPH

Supplementary Information The online version contains supplementary material available at https://doi.org/10.1007/978-3-031-80038-2_29.

J. L. Maurer
Department of Critical Care, University of Minnesota Physicians, Minneapolis, MN, USA
e-mail: Jmaurer10@umphysicians.umn.edu

M. E. Prekker (✉)
Department of Medicine, Division of Pulmonary, Allergy, and Critical Care Medicine, Hennepin County Medical Center, Minneapolis, MN, USA
e-mail: Matthew.prekker@hcmed.org

LV Thrombus Formation: Pathophysiology and Clinical Context

LV thrombosis most commonly occurs within the LV apex (Figures/Videos 29.1, 29.2, 29.3 and 29.4) where there is blood stasis in the setting of acute myocardial infarction (AMI) or heart failure with reduced ejection fraction (HFrEF). In the case of AMI, most LV thrombi are diagnosed within 2 weeks of the inciting event and commonly within the first 72 h [1]. In the era of percutaneous coronary intervention (PCI), the reported incidence of LV thrombus-complicating AMI has declined to 1.6–4% [2–4]. However, incidence estimates are influenced by diagnostic modality and screening intervals. For example, studies utilizing gadolinium-enhanced cardiac magnetic resonance imaging (CMR) have reported an LV thrombus incidence of 8–15% following AMI [5, 6].

The pathophysiology of LV thrombosis is driven by Virchows triad (circulatory stasis, endothelial injury, and hypercoagulability). In the setting of AMI, regional LV akinesia or dyskinesia may lead to blood stasis [7]. Transmural or endocardial injury contributes to LV thrombus formation by exposing blood to a damaged endothelial surface. Patients with acute coronary syndrome (ACS) may exhibit an increased basal level activation of the coagulation system following clinical ACS resolution which may predispose to late thrombosis [8].

M. J. Lanspa, A. T. Levinson (eds.), *Echocardiography and Ultrasonography in the ICU*, Respiratory Medicine, https://doi.org/10.1007/978-3-031-80038-2_29

The published literature over several decades highlights a number of clinical risk factors for the diagnosis of LV thrombus: anterior AMI, large AMI size, the magnitude of cardiac enzyme elevation, LV regional akinesis or dyskinesis including the presence of an LV aneurysm, and incident HFrEF. According to a 2019 retrospective analysis using two-dimensional echocardiography, the common precipitants of LV thrombus were heart failure (69% of cases) followed by AMI (26%) [9]. Moreover, dilated cardiomyopathy, independent of AMI, is an established risk factor for LV thrombus formation [10]. Thus, heart failure has likely supplanted AMI as the most common disease associated with LV thrombosis.

LV Thrombus Recognition: Sonographic Features

The typical sonographic appearance of an LV thrombus is an echodense mass adherent to the endocardium with distinct margins (Figs. 29.1a and 29.2a/Videos 29.1 and 29.3) and, in some instances, independent motion. LV thrombus formation typically occurs in regions of stagnant or slow blood flow such as adjacent to segmental wall motion abnormalities, LV aneurysm or pseudoaneurysm, and in the setting of diffuse LV dysfunction [11, 12]. Thus, these cardiac pathologies often provide indirect evidence to an ultrasonographer that an LV thrombus may be present.

Pro-Tips: Sonography for LV Thrombus Detection

1. The apex is best visualized with the patient in the left lateral decubitus position which promotes the leftward shift of the heart from beneath the high attenuation tissue of the sternum.
2. The transducer is placed near the point of maximal impulse (PMI) or the shortest distance between the chest wall and the cardiac apex to maximize resolution.
3. Multiple apical views should be sought as the LV may appear foreshortened if the transducer is not placed at the true apex.
4. Decreasing depth to better visualize the apex favorably affects the pulse repetition frequency and increases the framerate of the desired image, potentially improving image resolution [11].
5. Near-field gain should be reduced to mitigate near-field artifact. This type of artifact may mimic the appearance of an LV thrombus and result in false positive findings [11].
6. Near-field resolution of apical structures may be enhanced by using high-frequency transducers (5–7.5 MHz).
7. The presence of "spontaneous echo contrast," or smoke-like swirling of hyperechoic speckles in the LV cavity, is thought to represent low-velocity blood flow and indicates greater risk of thrombosis [12].
8. Doppler analysis of apical flow patterns with identification of apical flow stasis or continuous swirling of flow around the apex may also indicate greater risk for apical thrombosis [13].

There are three distinct morphologic features of LV thrombus: (1) **mural** thrombus—thin clot oriented parallel to the endocardium with a concave free margin and a single surface exposed to blood; (2) **protruding** thrombus—convex extension from the endocardium with multiple surfaces exposed to blood (Figs. 29.1a-c and 29.3; Videos 29.1 and 29.2); and (3) **mobile** thrombus—extension from the endocardium with independent motion of part or all of the thrombus (Figs. 29.2a-c; Videos 29.3 and 29.4). Multiple features may co-exist in a single thrombus. In all three thrombus morphologies, a discrete interface between clotted and non-clotted blood is typically observed given differences in their acoustic impedance. Thrombus chronicity also contributes to sonographic appearance: mature thrombi may

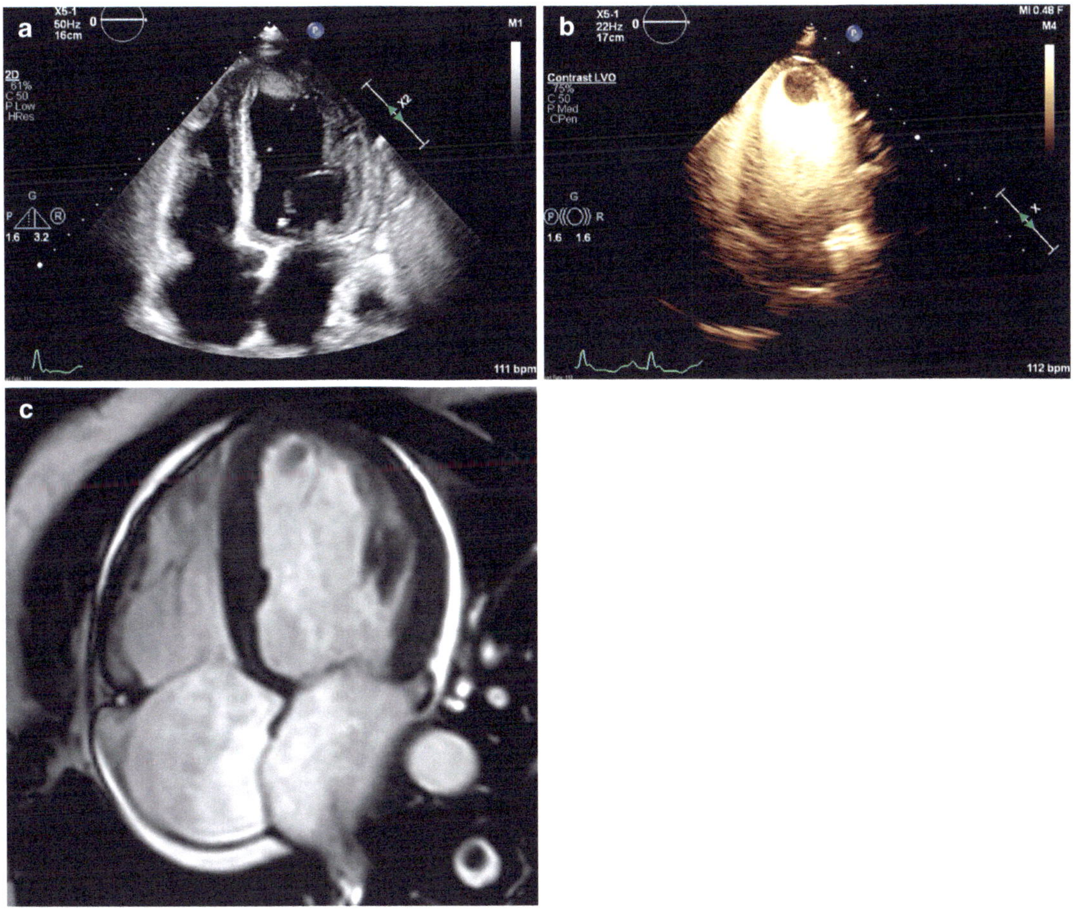

Fig. 29.1 (**a**) Transthoracic echocardiography (TTE): apical four chamber view depicting biventricular, apical, protruding thrombi. (**b**) Contrast-enhanced TTE in the same patient: apical four chamber view depicting biventricular, apical, protruding thrombi. Note: the left ventricular opacification (LVO) technique using an ultrasound-enhancing agent (UEA) renders the blood in the left ventricular cavity hyperechoic but does not penetrate or opacify the avascular thrombi. The right ventricle may be more difficult to see in contrast enhanced images. (**c**) Non-contrast cardiac magnetic resonance (CMR) imaging in the same patient: this horizontal long axis (HLA) view utilizing steady-state free precession demonstrates biventricular, apical, protruding thrombi

appear hyperechoic, while immature thrombi may be relatively hypoechoic and difficult to distinguish from blood. Larger thrombi may exhibit heterogeneous echodensity. In many cases, the acoustic properties of thrombus and myocardium are similar making this diagnosis challenging; a mural thrombus can be nearly indistinguishable from the adjacent myocardium.

An LV thrombus must be distinguished from the normal intraventricular anatomy such as papillary muscles, muscular trabeculae, chordal structures, endocardium, and other intraventricular masses. Thrombus mimics may be identified in part by, (1) an intracavitary location that would be atypical for LV thrombus (e.g., the base of the heart), (2) the absence of pathology associated with an LV thrombus such as segmental hypokinesis or akinesis, LV aneurysm, or diffuse LV dysfunction, or (3) the absence of variation in sonographic appearance of a suspicious structure over time (LV thrombi tend to change in appearance with serial imaging).

Sonographic artifacts may also mimic an LV thrombus. An anatomic structure exhibits an immutable position within the LV cavity whereas an artifact changes position or disappears with

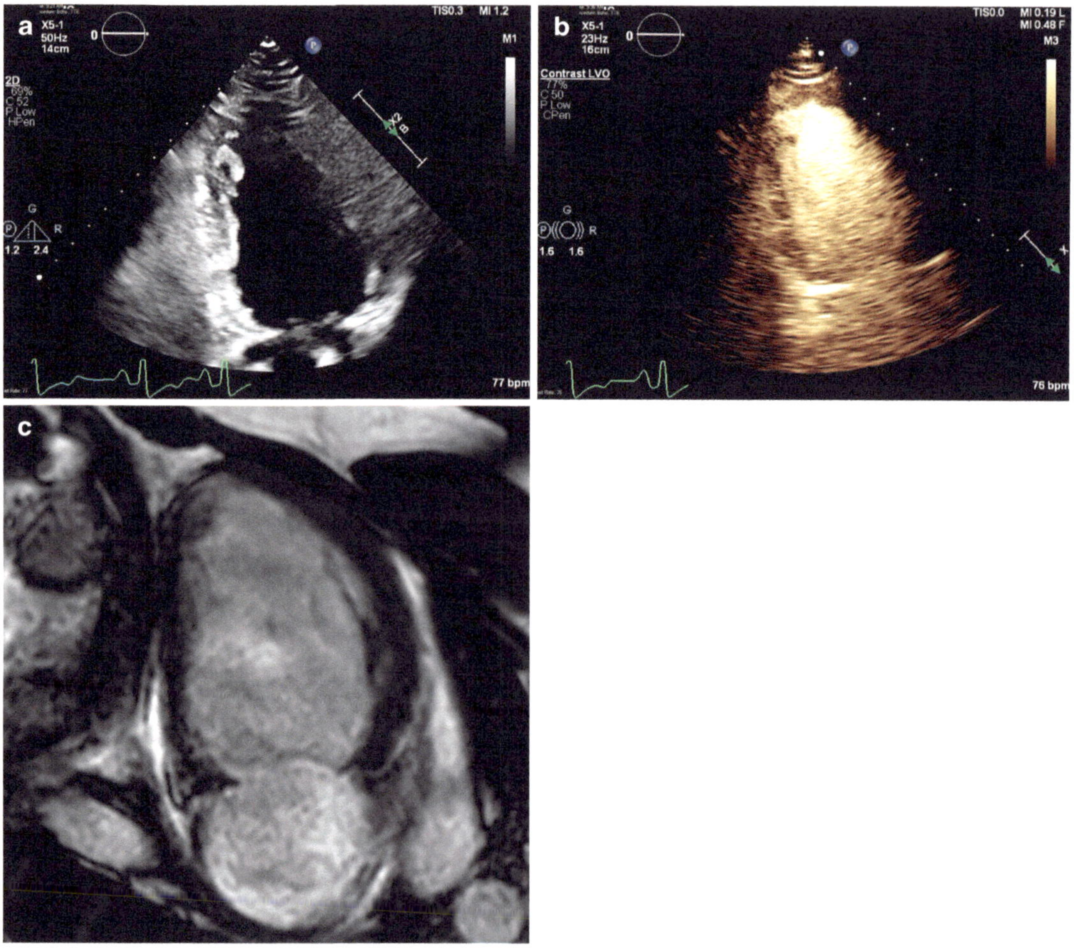

Fig. 29.2 (**a**) Transthoracic echocardiography (TTE): apical two chamber view depicting a left ventricular mobile thrombus adherent to the apical inferior wall. Note the irregular endocardial border and hyperechoic structure (thrombus). (**b**) Contrast-enhanced TTE: apical two chamber view depicting the same left ventricular mobile thrombus located on the apical inferior wall. (**c**) Non-contrast cardiac magnetic resonance (CMR) imaging of the same patient: vertical long axis view depicting the left ventricular, apical inferior, mobile thrombus (dark grey)

changes in orientation. Therefore, spurious structures should be interrogated with multiple orthogonal views in order to exclude artifacts. The use of color flow Doppler to evaluate for flow across an area of interest may further distinguish artifacts from structures that warrant additional interrogation.

Thus, features that favor the diagnosis of LV thrombus include apical location, adjacent position relative to hypokinetic or akinetic myocardium such as LV aneurysm, the presence of diffuse LV dysfunction, "spontaneous echo contrast," acoustic differentiation from underlying myocardium, distinct thrombus margins, free-motion of the intracavity thrombus margin, static position within the LV cavity on multiple views, and variation in appearance on serial examinations. However, the diagnosis is not straightforward in a substantial number of cases, and serial echocardiography, the application of UEAs or "echo contrast," or CMR will be necessary to optimize diagnostic accuracy (Fig. 29.4a-c; Videos 29.5 and 29.6).

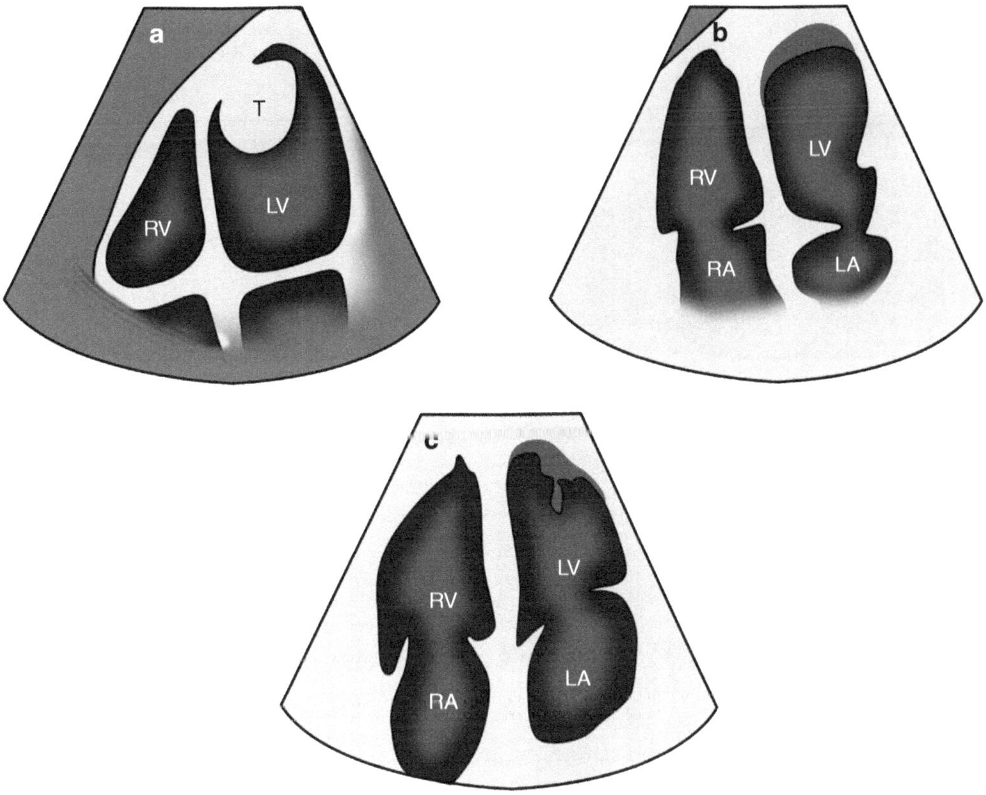

Fig. 29.3 There are three distinct morphologies of LV thrombi, a protruding thrombus (**a**), a mural thrombus (**b**), and a mobile thrombus (**c**). Multiple morphologies may co-exist in a single thrombus

Advanced Diagnosis: Ultrasound Enhancing Agents (UEAs) and Cardiac Magnetic Resonance Imaging (CMR)

Standard two-dimensional echocardiography for the evaluation of LV thrombus has a specificity of 96–98% and a sensitivity of 23–35%, while the addition of UEA use has been shown to increase sensitivity to 61–64% without compromising specificity [6, 14, 15]. The American Society of Echocardiography recommends that "ultrasound enhancement should be used in patients in whom LV thrombus cannot be ruled in or out with non-contrast echocardiography" [16].

For the purpose of cardiac imaging, three UEAs are available currently: Optison, Definity (Luminity in Europe), and Lumason (SonoVue outside the United States). These commercially produced, gas-filled microbubble agents are designed to survive transpulmonary passage and exhibit compressibility, or the capacity to oscillate, creating a visually sharp interface between blood and tissue. At low mechanical index (MI) and power output, microbubbles exhibit a nonlinear oscillation pattern that generates acoustic signals distinct from that of tissue. The backscattered acoustic signals appear as opacification (so-called "enhancement") on ultrasound. In the absence of LV thrombus, UEA-facilitated **left-ventricular opacification (LVO)** will demonstrate a smooth LV endocardial border, following the ventricular contour in an uninterrupted fashion. In the presence of LV thrombus, UEA-facilitated LVO may reveal an irregular endocardial border (Fig. 29.2b/Video 29.4). Moreover, the use of UEAs at low MI with multipulse cancellation techniques improves visualization of the blood-endocardial boundary and facilitates real-time visualization of wall motion

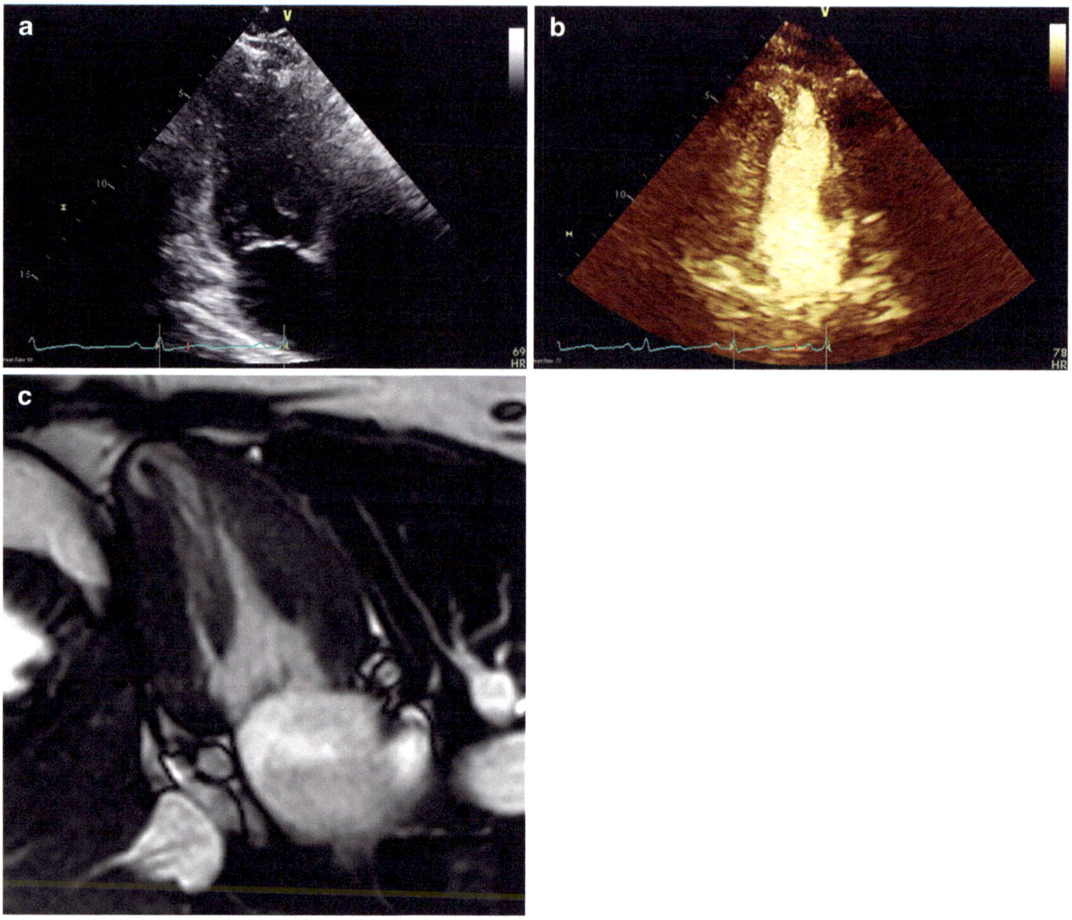

Fig. 29.4 (**a**) Transthoracic echocardiography (TTE): apical two chamber view depicting prominent trabeculation mimicking a thrombus in the setting of adjacent wall-motion hypokinesis. (**b**) Contrast enhanced TTE: apical two chamber view depicting the same prominent trabeculation mimicking a thrombus in the setting of an adjacent hypokinetic myocardial segment. (**c**) Non-contrast cardiac magnetic resonance (CMR) imaging: vertical long axis view depicting prominent trabeculation mimicking a thrombus in the setting of an adjacent hypokinetic myocardial segment

so that the characteristic LV thrombus milieu may be detected [16, 17]. The utilization of UEA LVO also mitigates apical reverberation artifacts.

The compressibility and resonant properties of microbubbles relative to tissue can be exploited by different imaging techniques to enhance the endocardial border, define intra-cavitary structures, and evaluate for perfusion of cardiac structures. For example, the use of intermittent imaging with destruction/reperfusion at high MI may facilitate visualization of a perfusion defect in the adjacent myocardium as a substrate for thrombus formation and differentiate avascular thrombus from vascularized cardiac tissue [16, 17].

Pro-Tips: Use of Ultrasound Enhancing Agents (UEAs)

1. Ensure that your ultrasound equipment is compatible with UEAs by contacting your equipment representative.
2. You may have to adjust the power output or mechanical index within the range of 0.2–0.5 until visualization is most favorable.
3. Position the focus of the ultrasound beam at the bottom of the imaging sector in order to optimize near-field visualization.

(continued)

4. There are at least three methods to deliver UEAs: bolus with or without dilution or infusion. UEA boluses, sometimes diluted in saline, are satisfactory for LVO studies. The agent must be activated and prepared according to manufacturer recommendations and delivery method.
5. UEA bolus injection is performed slowly in order to achieve homogenous opacification, which facilitates clear visualization of the endocardium and wall thickening with minimization of basal attenuation and apical artifact (Fig. 29.5a, b).
6. LVO may persist for several minutes. Repeat bolus dosing may be necessary.

Multiple studies have demonstrated the superiority of gadolinium-enhanced CMR over transthoracic echocardiography with UEA. Thus, if echocardiography shows a suspicious intracavitary structure, but diagnostic uncertainty remains, then gadolinium-enhanced CMR should be considered in centers experienced with image acquisition and interpretation using this modality. Transesophageal echocardiography (TEE) is not recommended for the evaluation of LV thrombus. There is an unfavorable distance between an ultrasound probe positioned in the esophagus and the LV apex which leads to apical foreshortening and poor visualization at the most common locus of LV thrombi.

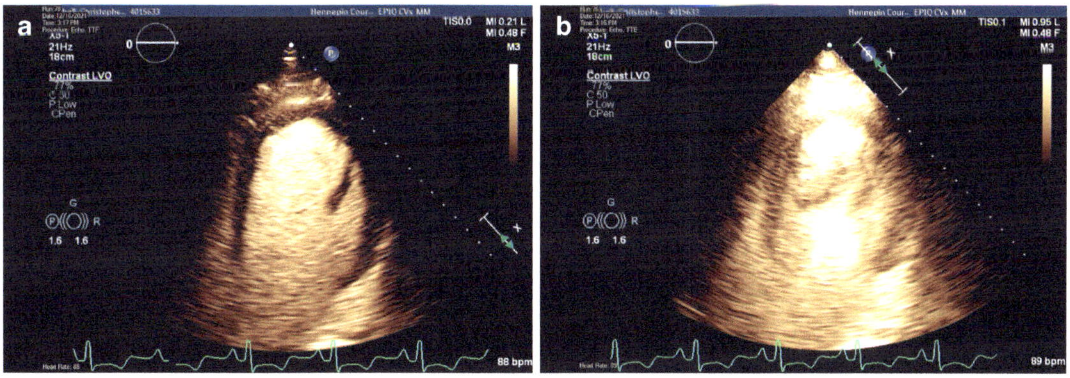

Fig. 29.5 (**a**) Contrast enhanced transthoracic echocardiography using proper UEA technique: apical two chamber view. Note the homogenous LV opacification and focus positioned at the bottom of the imaging sector with optimal visualization of a papillary muscle. (**b**) Contrast enhanced transthoracic echocardiography using poor UEA technique: apical two chamber view. Suboptimal visualization of an LV structure is the result of positioning the focus at the top, rather than at the bottom, of the imaging sector. Contrast swirling is observed

Clinical Implications and Treatment of LV Thrombus

The natural history of an LV thrombus is unpredictable and may entail regression with or without therapy, partial regression, change in morphology, or calcification. The most feared complication of LV thrombus is embolization. In the absence of therapeutic anticoagulation, the risk of LV thrombus embolization has historically ranged from 13% to 22% [2, 18]. Embolization risk is greater among protruding and mobile thrombi. After 3 months, the risk of systemic embolization may be lower as the thrombus matures and incorporates into LV wall segments. A 2020 observational study evaluating the prognosis of patients treated with anticoagulation for a confirmed LV thrombus identified an overall incidence of major adverse cardiac events of 37% [18]. Over a median follow-up period of 632 days in this study, mortality was 19%, stroke was diagnosed in 13%, and major bleeding occurred in 13% [18].

Systemic anticoagulation reduces the risk of LV thrombus embolization. Professional society guidelines for the management of STEMI complicated by LV thrombus, including the American College of Cardiology/American Heart Association (ACC/AHA) and the European Society of Cardiology (ESC), recommend anticoagulation therapy for at least 3–6 months duration [19, 20]. The American Heart Association/American Stroke Association (AHA/ASA) guidelines for the secondary prevention of ischemic stroke recommend anticoagulation therapy for at least 3 months duration for patients with LV thrombus who are diagnosed with stroke or transient ischemic attack [21]. Professional societies unanimously agree that screening for an LV thrombus should be pursued in the setting of frequently coexistent pathology. However, the optimal timing for screening, imaging frequency, and duration of follow-up imaging in the setting of an identified LV thrombus all remain controversial.

Evolving Evidence: The Choice of Anticoagulant to Treat LV Thrombus

Historically, guidelines have recommended vitamin K antagonists (VKAs) for the treatment or prevention of LV thrombus [19, 21]. Heparins are often used until the target INR is achieved. The efficacy of direct oral anticoagulants (DOACs) in LV thrombus treatment could perhaps be extrapolated from experience treating atrial fibrillation (AF) and venous thromboembolism (VTE). Accordingly, the use of DOACs to treat LV thrombi has increased, and the literature now contains reports of thrombus regression with apixaban, rivaroxaban, and dabigatran. However, in a 2020 retrospective cohort study, DOAC treatment was associated with a higher risk of systemic embolization in patients with an LV thrombus compared with warfarin use [22]. We recommend that the risks and benefits of DOAC use in patients with LV thrombus be weighed on a case-by-case basis.

The combination of anticoagulation therapy and dual antiplatelet therapy (DAPT), so-called "triple therapy," increases the risk of bleeding two- to threefold compared to anticoagulation therapy alone. There are no randomized clinical trials comparing "double therapy" (oral anticoagulation plus a single antiplatelet agent) with "triple therapy" in acute coronary syndrome (ACS) patients with LV thrombus. However, data gleaned from studies comparing double versus triple therapy for patients with ACS and other conditions suggest that double therapy is associated with reduced bleeding risk and potentially similar efficacy compared with triple therapy [23, 24]. Future clinical research should clarify the role of DOAC therapy for patients with LV thrombus as well as compare the benefits and harms of double vs triple therapy for ACS patients with LV thrombus who require platelet inhibition after PCI.

Summary Points

- The typical sonographic appearance of an LV thrombus is an echodense mass adherent to the endocardium with distinct margins and, in some instances, a motion that is independent of other cardiac structures.
- The majority of LV thrombi form in the LV apex, often in conjunction with an LV apical aneurysm.
- Careful echocardiographic evaluation with multiple apical views should be performed if the diagnosis of an LV thrombus is suspected.
- There are three common morphologic variants of LV thrombus (mural, protruding, and mobile), but a single thrombus may exhibit more than one of these features.
- Utilization of an ultrasound enhancing agent (UEA), with appropriate mechanical index or power output adjustments, improves the sensitivity of transthoracic echocardiography for the diagnosis of LV thrombus.
- Left-ventricular opacification (LVO) using UEAs improves visualization of the blood-endocardial boundary and facilitates: (1) LV thrombus diagnosis and (2) evaluation of abnormalities in wall motion.
- Systemic anticoagulation reduces the risk of LV thrombus embolization and treatment is generally prescribed for at least 3–6 months.

Questions

1. A 40-year-old woman presents 2 weeks after childbirth for progressive dyspnea, peripheral edema, and new onset right-sided weakness. She is admitted to the intensive care unit for acute hypoxemic respiratory failure requiring mechanical ventilation. Head imaging demonstrated an acute ischemic stroke. While performing bedside echocardiography you estimate an ejection fraction of <30% and are concerned that an LV thrombus may be present. Which of the following maneuvers would be may assist in the diagnosis of an LV thrombus?
   A. Place the patient in the left lateral decubitus position and the transducer at the point of.
   B. maximal impulse.
   C. Avoid foreshortening of the left ventricular apex and obtain multiple orthogonal views.
   D. Slowly administer an IV bolus of ultrasound contrast while pursuing left ventricular apical views.
   E. All of the above.

   Answer D

   Peripartum cardiomyopathy (PPCM) is a well-established risk factor for LV thrombus, especially in the setting of an ejection fraction of <35%. In the setting of concurrent heart failure and stroke symptoms, evaluation for an LV thrombus is critical. Standard two-dimensional echocardiography for the evaluation of LV thrombus has a specificity of 96–98% and a sensitivity of 23–35%, while the addition of UEA use has been shown to increase sensitivity to 61–64% without compromising specificity [6, 14, 15]. The American Society of Echocardiography recommends that "ultrasound enhancement should be used in patients in whom LV thrombus cannot be ruled in or out with noncontrast echocardiography" [16]. Time-gain compensation (TGC) should be adjusted such that near-field gain is reduced in order to mitigate near-field artifacts and false positive evaluation. Decreasing depth to better visualize the apex favorably affects the pulse repetition frequency (PRF) and increases the frame rate of the desired image. Depth of field settings of 7–9 cm may be most favorable.

2. A 55-year-old man with a history of ischemic heart disease is admitted from a clinic for further evaluation of fatigue, cough, dyspnea, and severe peripheral eosinophilia. After admission, he exhibits a complete heart block with a ventricular escape rhythm prompting transfer to the intensive care unit. Bedside echocardiography with the use of an ultrasound-enhancing agent demonstrates reduced LV function and a mobile echodense mass adherent to the apical endocardium. Which of the following statements is false?

A. Embolization risk is greater among protruding thrombi and especially mobile thrombi.
B. A true intra-cavitary structure should exhibit an immutable position within the LV cavity whereas an artifact will change position or disappear with changes in orientation.
C. In patients with heart disease, the administration of UEAs may be poorly tolerated evidenced by studies that have demonstrated a greater risk of adverse events with the application of perflutren compared with placebo.
D. In the absence of absolute contraindications, anticoagulation therapy should be instituted for a minimum of 3 months duration and guided by follow-up imaging.

Answer C

This patient most likely has Hypereosinophilic syndrome (HES) complicated by cardiac disease. Hypereosinophilic myocarditis is associated with heterogeneous mechanisms. A large body of published clinical data, evaluating the application of UEAs under conditions of stress and coronary artery disease, has established the safety of UEAs. Accordingly, the FDA has approved three agents for cardiac indications after extensive safety evaluations, including direct comparisons with placebo, that showed no significant difference in total or specific adverse events [16, 25].

Acknowledgments Special thank you to the following for their generous contributions to this chapter: Dr. Michelle Carlson, MD, FACC; Melissa Madsen, cardiac sonographer; and Dr. Laura Hubbard, PharmD.

References

1. Funke Küpper AJ, Verheugt FWA, Peels CH, Galema TW, Roos JP. Left ventricular thrombus incidence and behavior studied by serial two-dimensional echocardiography in acute anterior myocardial infarction: left ventricular wall motion, systemic embolism and oral anticoagulation. J Am College Cardiol. 1989;13:1514–20.
2. Robinson AA, Jain A, Gentry M, McNamara RL. Left ventricular thrombi after STEMI in the primary PCI era: a systematic review and meta-analysis. Int J Cardiol. 2016;221:554–9.
3. Gianstefani S, Douiri A, Delithanasis I, Rogers T, Sen A, Kalra S, Charangwa L, Reiken J, Monaghan M, MacCarthy P. Incidence and predictors of early left ventricular thrombus after ST-elevation myocardial infarction in the contemporary era of primary percutaneous coronary intervention. Am J Cardiol. 2014;113:1111–6.
4. Mao TF, Bajwa A, Muskula P, Coggins TR, Kennedy K, Magalski A, Skolnick DG, Main ML. Incidence of left ventricular thrombus in patients with acute ST-segment elevation myocardial infarction treated with percutaneous coronary intervention. Am J Cardiol. 2018;121:27–31.
5. Delewi R, Nijveldt R, Hirsch A, Marcu CB, Robbers L, Hassell MECJ, de Bruin RHA, Vleugels J, van der Laan AM, Bouma BJ. Left ventricular thrombus formation after acute myocardial infarction as assessed by cardiovascular magnetic resonance imaging. Eur J Radiol. 2012;81:3900–4.
6. Weinsaft JW, Kim J, Medicherla CB, Ma CL, Codella NCF, Kukar N, Alaref S, Kim RJ, Devereux RB. Echocardiographic algorithm for post–myocardial infarction LV thrombus. JACC: Cardiovasc Imaging. 2016;9:505–15.
7. Stein B, Fuster V. Antithrombotic therapy in acute myocardial infarction: prevention of venous, left ventricular and coronary artery thromboembolism. Am J Cardiol. 1989;64:33B–40B.
8. Merlini PA, Bauer KA, Oltrona L, Ardissino D, Cattaneo M, Belli C, Mannucci PM, Rosenberg RD. Persistent activation of coagulation mechanism in unstable angina and myocardial infarction. Circulation. 1994;90:61–8.
9. McCarthy CP, Murphy S, Venkateswaran RV, Singh A, Chang LL, Joice MG, Rivero JM, Vaduganathan M, Januzzi JL, Bhatt DL. Left ventricular thrombus. J Am College Cardiol. 2019;73:2007–9.
10. Falk RH, Foster E, Coats MH. Ventricular thrombi and thromboembolism in dilated cardiomyopathy: a prospective follow-up study. Am Heart J. 1992;123:136–42.
11. Asinger RW, Mikell FL, Elsperger J, Hodges M. Incidence of left-ventricular thrombosis after acute transmural myocardial infarction. N Engl J Med. 1981;305:297–302.
12. Asinger RW, Mikell FL, Sharma B, Hodges M. Observations on detecting left ventricular thrombus with two dimensional echocardiography: emphasis on avoidance of false positive diagnoses. Am J Cardiol. 1981;47:145–56.
13. Delemarre BJ, Visser CA, Bot H, Dunning AJ. Prediction of apical thrombus formation in acute myocardial infarction based on left ventricular spatial flow pattern. J Am College Cardiol. 1990;15:355–60.

14. Srichai MB, Junor C, Rodriguez LL, Stillman AE, Grimm RA, Lieber ML, Weaver JA, Smedira NG, White RD. Clinical, imaging, and pathological characteristics of left ventricular thrombus: a comparison of contrast-enhanced magnetic resonance imaging, transthoracic echocardiography, and transesophageal echocardiography with surgical or pathological validation. Am Heart J. 2006;152:75–84.
15. Weinsaft JW, Kim RJ, Ross M, Krauser D, Manoushagian S, LaBounty TM, Cham MD, Min JK, Healy K, Wang Y. Contrast-enhanced anatomic imaging as compared to contrast-enhanced tissue characterization for detection of left ventricular thrombus. JACC: Cardiovasc Imaging. 2009;2:969–79.
16. Porter TR, Mulvagh SL, Abdelmoneim SS, Becher H, Belcik JT, Bierig M, Choy J, Gaibazzi N, Gillam LD, Janardhanan R. Clinical applications of ultrasonic enhancing agents in echocardiography. 2018 American Society of Echocardiography Guidelines Update. J Am Soc of Echocardiogr. 2018;31:241–74.
17. Kaufmann BA, Wei K, Lindner JR. Contrast echocardiography. Curr Problems Cardiol. 2007;32:51–96.
18. Lattuca B, Bouziri N, Kerneis M, Portal J-J, Zhou J, Hauguel-Moreau M, Mameri A, Zeitouni M, Guedeney P, Hammoudi N. Antithrombotic therapy for patients with left ventricular mural thrombus. J Am College Cardiol. 2020;75:1676–85.
19. O'Gara PT, Kushner FG, Aschcim DD, Casey DE, Chung MK, de Lemos JA, Ettinger SM, Fang JC, Fesmire FM. 2013 ACCF/AHA guideline for the management of ST-elevation myocardial infarction. Circulation. 2013;127:362–425.
20. Ibanez B, James S, Agewall S, Antunes MJ, Bucciarelli-Ducci C, Bueno H, Caforio ALP, Crea F, Goudevenos JA, Halvorsen S. 2017 ESC Guidelines for the management of acute myocardial infarction in patients presenting with ST-segment elevation. Kardiol Pol. 2018;76:229–313.
21. Kleindorfer DO, Towfighi A, Chaturvedi S, Cockroft KM, Gutierrez J, Lombardi-Hill D, Kamel H, Kernan WN, Kittner SJ, Leira EC. 2021 Guideline for the prevention of stroke in patients with stroke and transient ischemic attack: a guideline from the American Heart Association/American Stroke Association. Stroke. 2021;52:364–467.
22. Robinson AA, Trankle CR, Eubanks G, Schumann C, Thompson P, Wallace RL, Gottiparthi S, Ruth B, Kramer CM, Salerno M. Off-label use of direct oral anticoagulants compared with Warfarin for left ventricular thrombi. JAMA Cardiol. 2020;5:685.
23. Dewilde WJ, Oirbans T, Verheugt FW, Kelder JC, De Smet BJ, Herrman J-P, Adriaenssens T, Vrolix M, Heestermans AA, Vis MM. Use of clopidogrel with or without aspirin in patients taking oral anticoagulant therapy and undergoing percutaneous coronary intervention: an open-label, randomised, controlled trial. Lancet. 2013;381:1107–15.
24. Gibson CM, Mehran R, Bode C, Halperin J, Verheugt FW, Wildgoose P, Birmingham M, Ianus J, Burton P, van Eickels M. Prevention of bleeding in patients with atrial fibrillation undergoing PCI. N Engl J Med. 2016;375:2423–34.
25. Kitzman DW, Goldman ME, Gillam LD, Cohen JL, Aurigemma GP, Gottdiener JS. Efficacy and safety of the novel ultrasound contrast agent perflutren (definity) in patients with suboptimal baseline left ventricular echocardiographic image: a list of participating investigators appears in the Appendix. Am J Cardiol. 2000;86:669–74.
26. Stratton JR, Resnick AD. Increased embolic risk in patients with left ventricular thrombi. Circulation. 1987;75:1004–11.
27. Visser CA, Kan G, Meltzer RS, Dunning AJ, Roelandt J. Embolic potential of left ventricular thrombus after myocardial infarction: a two-dimensional echocardiographic study of 119 patients. J Am College Cardiol. 1985;5:1276–80.

Left Atrial Thrombus

30

Megan H. Hicks and Manender Kumar Singla

Etiology

Left atrial (LA) thrombus is typically the result of blood stasis in the left atrium. The most common site of thrombosis in the LA is the left atrial appendage (LAA), but the formation of floating and ball thrombus in the LA can occur [1, 2]. The complex anatomy and histologic features of the LAA as an embryologic remnant predispose it to thrombogenicity, which is exacerbated in the presence of the hypercoagulable state associated with atrial fibrillation (AF) [3].

The majority of LAAs are multilobar, with 80% of patients having two or more lobes, leading to differential blood flow and predisposition to stasis [3, 4]. There are four common morphologies that have been demonstrated to follow genetic and regional patterns [2]. The chicken wing is the most common shape, found in nearly half of patients, alongside cactus, windsock, and cauliflower shapes [3, 4]. The muscle bundles and pectinate muscles that speckle the myocardial surface also predispose the LAA to harbor thrombus [3].

M. H. Hicks (✉)
Wake Forest University School of Medicine, Winston-Salem, NC, USA
e-mail: mhhicks@wakehealth.edu

M. K. Singla
Fortis Hospital, Ludhiana, India

Virchow described three factors responsible for the pathogenesis of LA thrombus formation (Virchow's triad): (1) Wall injury via endothelial or endocardial damage; (2) blood stasis via sluggish or turbulent flow due to atypical hemodynamics; and (3) increased coagulability [2, 5]. Collectively, this triad results in the formation of activated platelet aggregates and leukocyte- or fibrinogen-mediated erythrocyte aggregates which present on echocardiography as spontaneous dense echocardiographic contrast (SEC) or "smoke." [3, 6] These aggregates can progress to thickened, slow-moving blood called "sludge" and eventually thrombus.

The most frequent cause of LAA thrombus formation is AF. Nearly 15% of patients with acute AF, defined as a duration of less than 3 days, have LAA thrombi [4]. Thrombogenesis occurs through a hyperactive clotting cascade driven by inflammation and oxidative stress [3]. Multiple cytokines and inflammatory markers known to be involved in coagulation are found to be elevated in patients with atrial fibrillation, including C-reactive protein, interleukin 6, tumor necrosis factor-alpha, D-dimer, fibrinogen, prothrombin, lipoprotein a, platelet factor-4, and von Willebrand factor [2, 3]. Thrombus can develop even in therapeutically anticoagulated AF patients [4, 7].

Although the mechanism of clot formation is multifactorial, local factors such as size, morphology, and function of the LAA can play a role.

M. J. Lanspa, A. T. Levinson (eds.), *Echocardiography and Ultrasonography in the ICU*, Respiratory Medicine, https://doi.org/10.1007/978-3-031-80038-2_30

Increasing numbers of LAA lobes are associated with an increased risk of LA SEC and LAA thrombus [2, 8, 9]. As such, the non-chicken wing shapes of LAA, especially the cauliflower type, are associated with a three-fold higher stroke risk [2, 10, 11]. Stroke and thromboembolism risk also correlate with an LAA volume greater than 34 mL [3]. Reduced LAA blood flow velocities, smaller LAA ostium size, a shorter distance from ostium to the first bend of the LAA, as well as shorter lengths of LAA, are associated with a greater risk of thrombus formation and thromboembolism [3].

Mitral stenosis (MS) is another important risk factor for thrombus formation due to left atrial stasis, portending a 17-fold increased risk in patients with MS and AF [2, 12]. In contrast, mitral regurgitation may be somewhat protective due to high-velocity left atrial washing [2]. Left ventricular dysfunction has been associated with a decrease in LAA emptying velocity, which presumably increases stasis [3]. LAA dysfunction is also common in dilated cardiomyopathy, even in sinus rhythm, with LAA thrombosis noted in many of these patients [13]. LAA dysfunction in the absence of AF has been commonly observed in patients with hypertrophic obstructive cardiomyopathy.

Diagnosis

While cardiac computed tomography and intracardiac echocardiography have emerged as effective alternative imaging modalities, TEE remains a mainstay of left atrial evaluation [10, 11, 14]. TEE has been reported to have a sensitivity and specificity approaching 100% and 99%, respectively, with an estimated 86% positive predictive value and 100% negative predictive value [3, 15].

The left atrium is visualized abutting the TEE probe in all mid-esophageal views, with the LAA best visualized in the mid-esophageal two-chamber and aortic valve short-axis views [16]. It is seen in the long axis abutting the Coumadin (lateral) ridge, which separates the LAA from the more superior and posterior left upper pulmonary vein (Fig. 30.1). Of the multiple classic morphologies of the LAA, the windsock is the easiest to fully examine, while the fan/broccoli and C/chicken wing morphologies present more challenges due to more extensive lobar architectures [2, 11].

Thrombi may appear as both mobile or immobile hyperechoic tissue, usually acoustically different from the abutting endocardium [11]. To effectively exclude thrombus, the LAA must be examined in multiple planes. Simultaneous orthogonal (X-plane) imaging is often useful to

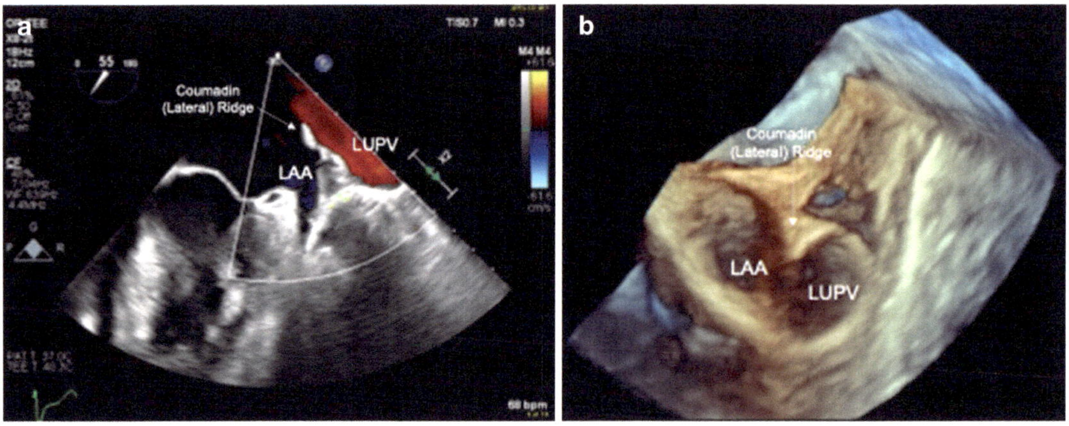

Fig. 30.1 (**a**) Midesophageal aortic valve short axis view. (**b**) 3D view. *LAA* left atrial appendage, *LUPV* left upper pulmonary vein

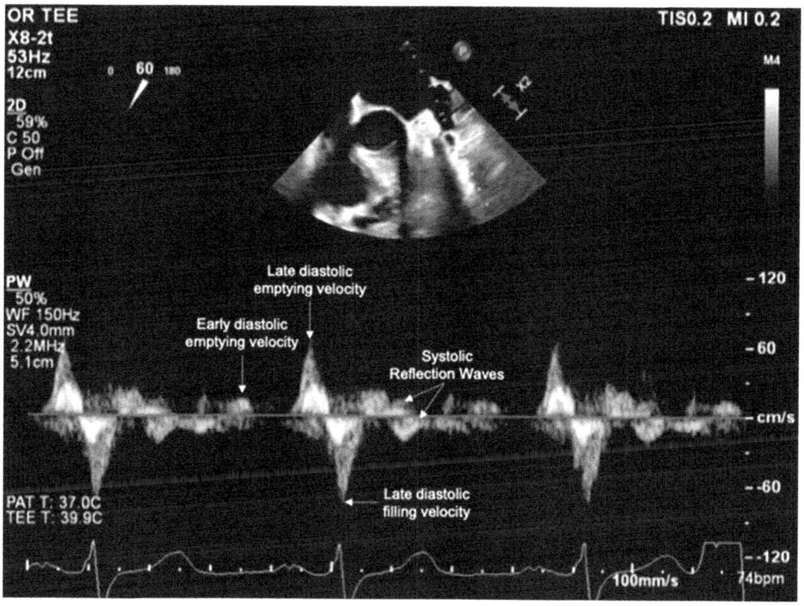

Fig. 30.2 Normal quadriphasic LAA velocity waveform

distinguish artifact or pectinate muscle from thrombus. Both color flow Doppler and injectable ultrasound contrast with or without power Doppler imaging may be useful adjuncts to exclude or confirm thrombus by revealing defects in color or contrast; this is particularly helpful when confounding SEC is also noted [11, 17, 18].

LAA function is frequently estimated using the LAA flow velocity, though its utility is limited in certain populations [2, 19]. Pulsed Doppler of the LAA in normal sinus rhythm demonstrates a quadriphasic pattern consisting of pairs of early and late ventricular diastolic waves that represent emptying and filling [19] (Fig. 30.2). The dominant late diastolic emptying wave is usually referenced as a surrogate of LAA ejection, with the peak velocity having been correlated with the risk for LAA stasis and thus thrombus formation [19]. Normal peak velocities range from 50 to 64 cm/s [20]. In patients with atrial fibrillation, the LAA waveform adopts a more sawtooth pattern with variable amplitude, and mean LAA flow velocities may better represent function [13].

SEC is common at velocities below 20 cm/s and is an independent risk factor for thrombus regardless of anticoagulation and CHA_2DS_2-VASc score [9, 11, 18]. Thrombus is less likely at velocities above 40 cm/s with a negative predictive value of 99–100% at LAA velocities greater than 55 cm/s [9, 21, 22]. The velocity should be obtained at either the level of the LAA orifice or within the first third of the visualized depth, as velocity expectedly decreases as flow reaches the LAA apex [13, 23].

The LAA filling velocity does decrease with age and is highly variable in the setting of arrhythmia [19]. Other methods of assessment of LAA function include tissue Doppler imaging of the LAA wall, with a velocity <10 cm/s being highly specific for SEC [19].

As catheter-based LAA occlusion has become more frequent, 3D evaluation of the LAA has been deployed more often. Processing of 3D data sets allows the LAA to be aligned in three axes to provide reliable dimensions, improved functional assessment, and enhanced visualization and differentiation of thrombus from endocardial tissue [11, 24] (Fig. 30.3).

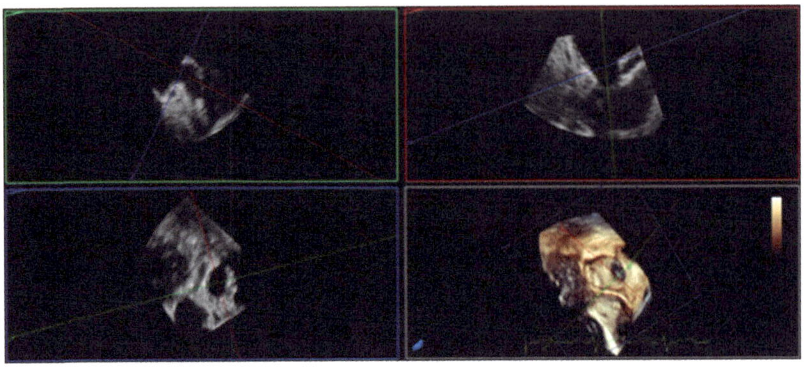

Fig. 30.3 3-D evaluation of the LAA orifice

Clinical Implications

LAA thromboembolism is the leading cause of morbidity and mortality in patients with atrial fibrillation [2]. LA and LAA thrombi are some of the very important causes of ischemic stroke [3]. Approximately 20% of strokes are thought to be cardioembolic, with the majority of these in patients with atrial fibrillation. The source of 75% of those is the left atrial appendage [13, 25]. Over 90% of thromboembolic strokes in nonvalvular atrial fibrillation are due to LAA thrombus [3, 26]. The incidence of stroke is much higher when atrial fibrillation is due to mitral stenosis [3]. Stroke risk can be estimated using validated scoring systems based on comorbidities like the $CHADS_2$ and CHA_2DS_2-VASc [3].

The presence of LAA thrombus on preoperative imaging prevents performing cardioversion to restore sinus rhythm [27]. This thus perpetuates low cardiac output states through loss of the atrial kick, which contributes up to 30% of left ventricular filling [27, 28]. Although the mechanism is not clear, transiently worsened LAA ejection and increased SEC can occur after spontaneous, pharmacological, or electrical cardioversion from AF or atrial flutter [18]. Paradoxically depressed LAA flow velocities have also been noted after transcatheter radiofrequency or surgical ablation [18]. This can itself predispose to the formation of thromboembolism. This LAA stunning is known to improve within 7–30 days after cardioversion [18].

Apart from the cerebral circulation, thrombus dislodgement from the LA can cause occlusive vascular symptoms in arterial branches to limbs, the mesentery, and other distant organs. Echocardiographic and CT imaging of the LAA is becoming increasingly important in ruling out thrombus prior to cardioversion or ablative procedures as well as in anatomic assessment and procedural guidance for minimally invasive LAA occlusion procedures.

Questions

1. Which of the following patients is LEAST likely to be diagnosed with a left atrial appendage thrombus?
   A. 54-year-old female with atrial fibrillation, 1+ spontaneous echo contrast, LAA peak velocity 40 cm/s
   B. 80-year-old male with ischemic cardiomyopathy, no spontaneous echo contrast, LAA peak velocity 28 cm/s
   C. 60-year-old female with restrictive diastolic dysfunction, no spontaneous echo contrast, LAA peak velocity 62 cm/s
   D. 74-year-old male with severe mitral stenosis, 2+ spontaneous echo contrast, LAA peak velocity 18 cm/s

   Answer: C

   Explanation: A left atrial appendage peak emptying velocity greater than 55 cm/s is associated with a negative predictive value of nearly 100%, meaning that there is almost zero chance of the patient having an LAA thrombus. While patients with a velocity >40 cm/s are less likely to develop a thrombus, spontaneous echo contrast is an independent risk factor for developing left atrial appendage thrombus. A velocity <40 cm/s, particularly those less than 20 cm/s suggests a high risk for thrombus formation.

2. Which of the following letters represents the appropriate waveform from which to measure the left atrial appendage peak emptying velocity?

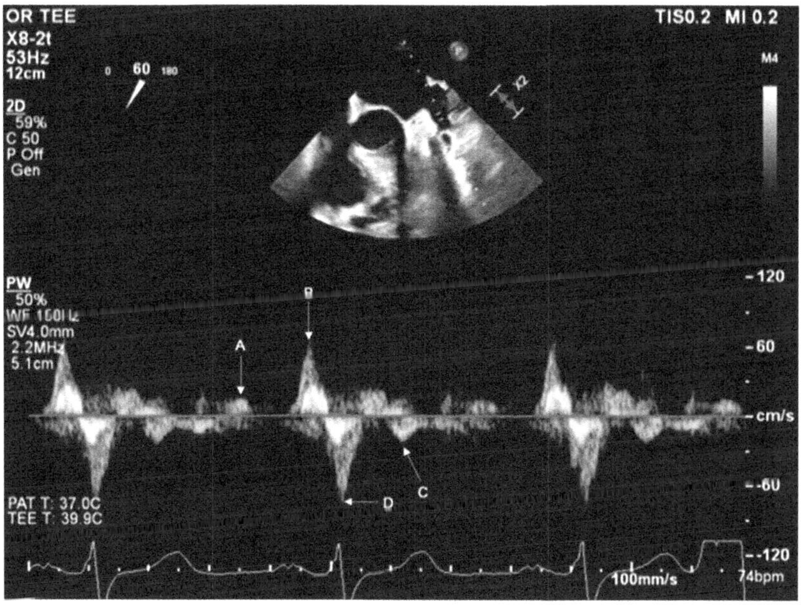

A. A
B. B
C. C
D. D

Answer: B

Explanation: The large diastolic upstroke above the axis indicates flow out of the left atrial appendage toward the probe and thus corresponds with the emptying of the LAA. The peak velocity, measured at the apex of this inflection, will represent the LAA peak emptying velocity.

References

1. Omoto T, Aoki A, Maruta K, Masuda T, Hirono M. Left atrial thrombus in a patient without mitral valve disease or atrial fibrillation. J Cardiol Cases. 2016;14(4):115–8.
2. Cresti A, Camara O. Left atrial thrombus—are all atria and appendages equal? Intervent Cardiol Clin. 2022;11:121–34.
3. Kanmanthareddy A, Reddy YM, Vallakati A, Earnest MB, Nath J, Ferrell R, Dawn B, Lakkireddy D. Embryology and anatomy of the left atrial appendage: why does thrombus form? Interv Cardiol Clin. 2014;3(2):191–202.
4. Beigel R, Wunderlich NC, Ho SY, et al. The left atrial appendage: anatomy, function, and noninvasive evaluation. JACC Cardiovasc Imaging. 2014;7(12):1251–65.
5. Watson T, Shantsila E, Lip GY. Mechanisms of thrombogenesis in atrial fibrillation: Virchow's triad revisited. Lancet. 2009;373(9658):155–66.
6. Pathan F, Hecht H, Narula J, Marwick TH. Roles of transesophageal echocardiography and cardiac computed tomography for evaluation of left atrial thrombus and associated pathology: a review and critical analysis. JACC Cardiovasc Imaging. 2018;11(4):616–27.
7. Erickson M, Yadav H, Sneij E, Austin J, Manyam H. Incidence of left atrial appendage thrombus despite 3 weeks of anticoagulation and the need for precardioversion echocardiography. Ann Noninvasive Electrocardiol. 2022;27(5):e12989.
8. Wang F, Zhu M, Wang X, et al. Predictive value of left atrial appendage lobes on left atrial thrombus or spontaneous echo contrast in patients with nonvalvular atrial fibrillation. BMC Cardiovasc Disord. 2018;18:153.

9. Fatkin D, Kelly RP, Feneley MP. Relations between left atrial appendage blood flow velocity, spontaneous echocardiographic contrast and thromboembolic risk in vivo. JACC. 1994;23(4):961–9.
10. Smiseth OA, Baron T, Marino PN, Marwick TH, Flachskampf FA. Imaging of the left atrium: pathophysiology insights and clinical utility. Eur Heart J. 2022;23:2–13.
11. Abdelmoneim SS, Mulvagh SL. Techniques to improve left atrial appendage imaging. J Atr Fibrillation. 2014;7(1):85–94.
12. Al-Saady NM, Obel OA, Camm AJ. Left atrial appendage: structure, function, and role in thromboembolism. Heart. 1999;82(5):547–54.
13. Agmon Y, Khandheria BK, Gentile F, Seward JB. Echocardiographic assessment of the left atrial appendage. JACC. 1999;34(7):1867–77.
14. Ge J, Chen T, Chuanzhen M, Maduray K, Zhong J. Can intracardiac echocardiography completely replace transesophageal echocardiography to guide left atrial appendate closure? The comparisons of intracardiac echocardiography with transesophageal echocardiography. J Card Surg. 2022;37:2766–75.
15. Manning WJ, Silverman DI, Gordon SP, et al. Cardioversion from atrial fibrillation without prolonged anticoagulation with use of transesophageal echocardiography to exclude the presence of atrial thrombi. N Engl J Med. 1993;328:750–5.
16. Shanewise JS, Cheung AT, Aronson S, et al. ASE/SCA guidelines for performing a comprehensive intraoperative multiplane transesophageal echocardiography examination: recommendations of the Society of Echocardiography Council for Intraoperative Echocardiography and the Society of Cardiovascular Anesthesiologists Task Force for Certification in Perioperative Transesophageal Echocardiography. J Am Soc Echocardiogr. 1999;12:884–900.
17. Hamper UM, DeJong MR, Caskey CI, Sleth S. Power Doppler imaging: clinical experience and correlation with color Doppler US and other imaging modailities. Radiographics. 1997;17(2):499–513.
18. Bansal M, Kasliwal RR. Echocardiography for left atrial appendage structure and function. Indian Heart J. 2012;64(5):469–75.
19. Ito T, Suwa M. Assessment of left atrial appendage function by echocardiography. Heart Fail Rev. 2023;28(5):1177–87.
20. Donal E, Yanada H, Leclercq C, Herpin D. The left atrial appendage, a small, blind-ended structure. Chest. 2005;128(3):1853–62.
21. Herring N, Page SP, Ahmed M, et al. The prevalence of low left atrial appendage emptying velocity and thrombus in patients undergoing catheter ablation for atrial fibrillation on uninterrupted peri-procedural warfarin therapy. J Atr Fibrillation. 2013;5(6):761.
22. Handke M, Harloff A, Hetzel A, et al. Left atrial appendage flow velocity as a quantitative surrogate parameter for thromboembolic risk: determinants and relationship to spontaneous echocontrast and thrombus formation—a transesophageal echocardiographic study in 500 patients with cerebral ischemia. J Am Soc Echocardiogr. 2005;18(12):1366–72.
23. Goldberg TH, Gordon SC, Spevack DM, Gordon GM. Disparities in emptying velocity within the left atrial appendage. Eur J Echocardiogr. 2010;11(3):290–5.
24. Nucifora G, Faletra F, Regoli F, et al. Evaluation of the left atrial appendage with real-time 3-dimensional transesophageal echocardiography. Circ Cardiovasc Imaging. 2011;4:514–23.
25. Dudzińska-Szczerba K, Kulakowski P, Michalowska I, Baran J. Association between left atrial appendage morphology and function and the risk of ischaemic stroke in patients with atrial fibrillation. Arrhythm Electrophysiol Rev. 2022 Apr;11:e09.
26. Wang D, Forbes TJ, Lee JC, Eng MH. Echocardiographic imaging for left atrial appendage occlusion. Intervent Cardiol Clin. 2018;7:219–28.
27. Hautmann M, Zacher M, Fuchs S, et al. Left atrial appendage thrombus formation, potential of resolution and association with prognosis in a large real-world cohort. Sci Rep. 2023;13:889.
28. Namana V, Gupta SS, Sabharwal N, Hollander G. Clinical significance of atrial kick. QJM. 2018;111(8):569–70.

Right-Sided Thrombus

31

Karim El-Kersh and Bilal Athar Jalil

Learning Objectives

1. Identify the causes of right-sided thrombi (RST).
2. Know the different echocardiographic patterns of RST.
3. Understand different treatments for RST.

Introduction

Intra-cardiac thrombi include both left- and right-sided thrombi (RST). While left-sided thrombi, such as those in the left atrial appendage and the left ventricle, are not uncommon, RSTs are exceedingly rare yet carry a high mortality [1]. The broad categories of RST include true thrombi and tumor thrombi. This chapter discusses the etiology, diagnosis, echocardiographic appearance, and clinical implications of right-sided thrombi. Pulmonary embolism and right-heart dysfunction are discussed in a separate chapter.

Supplementary Information The online version contains supplementary material available at https://doi.org/10.1007/978-3-031-80038-2_31.

K. El-Kersh
Division of Pulmonary, Critical Care, and Sleep Medicine, Department of Medicine, University of Arizona College of Medicine, Phoenix, AZ, USA
e-mail: Karimelkersh@arizona.edu

B. A. Jalil (✉)
Divisions of Cardiovascular Critical Care and Advanced Heart Failure, Heart and Vascular Institute, West Virginia University, Morgantown, WV, USA
e-mail: bilal.jalil@wvumedicine.org

Etiology

There are two broad categories of RST: true thrombi and tumor thrombi. True thrombi can be further subdivided into thrombi-in-transit, which represent embolized thrombi from peripheral veins that get trapped en route within the right heart, and those associated with devices such as central venous catheters and implantable cardiovascular leads.

Mobile RSTs are diagnosed in about 4%–18% of patients with acute pulmonary embolism (PE), with the higher incidence being reported in critically ill patients [2, 3]. The increased utilization of echocardiography in the risk stratification of PE patients has led to an increased detection of RST; however, the true incidence remains unknown. Mobile RST typically represents embolized thrombi from a more peripheral vein that temporarily lodges in the right atrium or right ventricle and is considered life-threatening [4]. Several predisposing factors are implicated in the temporary entrapment of mobile thrombi in the right heart. These may include the presence of a prominent Eustachian valve, a low cardiac output state, tricuspid regurgitation, and pulmonary hypertension [5].

M. J. Lanspa, A. T. Levinson (eds.), *Echocardiography and Ultrasonography in the ICU*, Respiratory Medicine, https://doi.org/10.1007/978-3-031-80038-2_31

The other group of true thrombi are those associated with the presence of indwelling central venous catheters or cardiovascular device leads. The presence of a foreign body can be an inciting factor for thrombi formation, which is usually seen in the right atrium. Right atrial thrombi (RAT) have been documented in end-stage renal disease patients with indwelling hemodialysis catheters with an incidence of 5.4% [6]. They have also been reported in patients with central venous catheters and pulmonary artery catheters in autopsy studies with an incidence between 29–33% [7]. Mobile thrombi on implantable cardiovascular device leads have been documented as high as 30% [8]. These catheter- and device-related thrombi are harder to recognize using transthoracic echocardiography (TTE), and since patients with RAT are asymptomatic, the incidence of RAT is likely underestimated [9].

"Tumor thrombi" is a misnomer, as these are not true thrombi but rather represent venous extension of tumors from the inferior vena cava to the right atrium. These can be seen in advanced-stage hepatocellular and renal cell carcinomas and are often considered poor prognostic indicators [10, 11].

Diagnosis

RSTs are usually diagnosed by TTE initially, and they can be occasionally noted in contrast to chest computed tomography (CT) studies aimed to assess for an acute PE. Thrombi are seen as hyperechoic densities within the right atrium, right ventricle, or the right ventricular outflow tract. Their appearance is characterized by their shape (serpiginous or globular) and motion (mobile or immobile), and they are usually classified into three types based on their echocardiographic appearance. Type A thrombi are usually seen in patients with acute PE and deep vein thrombosis and are highly mobile and serpiginous in morphology. Type B thrombi are nonmobile and may arise from an in-situ thrombosis related to cardiac structural abnormalities or the presence of foreign bodies. Type C thrombi are highly mobile and appear globular and multilobular, similar in appearance to right atrial myxomas [12]. The types of thrombi are depicted in Fig. 31.1a–c and Videos 31.1, 31.2, and 31.3.

The best views to evaluate for RST are those that best delineate the right atrium, the right ventricle, and the right ventricular outflow tract. The apical 4-chamber view (Fig. 31.2 and Video 31.4) and the subcostal 4-chamber views (Fig. 31.1c and Video 31.3) visualize the right-heart chambers well. Additionally, the subcostal view of the inferior vena cava can identify tumor thrombi traversing through the inferior vena cava into the right atrium (Fig. 31.3 and Video 31.5). Right-ventricular inflow views may be used to better visualize the right heart chambers and to help differentiate a freely mobile thrombus from vegetation attached to tricuspid valve leaflets (Fig. 31.4 and Video 31.6). The parasternal short- and long-axis views can be used to identify RST and to assess the right ventricular outflow tract (Fig. 31.5a, b and Videos 31.7 and 31.8).

With the increasing use of TTE in PE risk stratification, the detection of RST is expected to increase. The sensitivity of TTE could be reduced due to poor acoustic windows, normal anatomic variants such as the presence of a prominent Eustachian valve, Chiari network, crista terminalis, false chordae tendineae, and the presence of congenital heart disease [13]. Contrast echocardiography may be of additional value in delineating the presence of thrombi that are not well visualized on non-contrast-enhanced images and may help to differentiate thrombi from tumors (Fig. 31.6a, b and Videos 31.9 and 31.10).

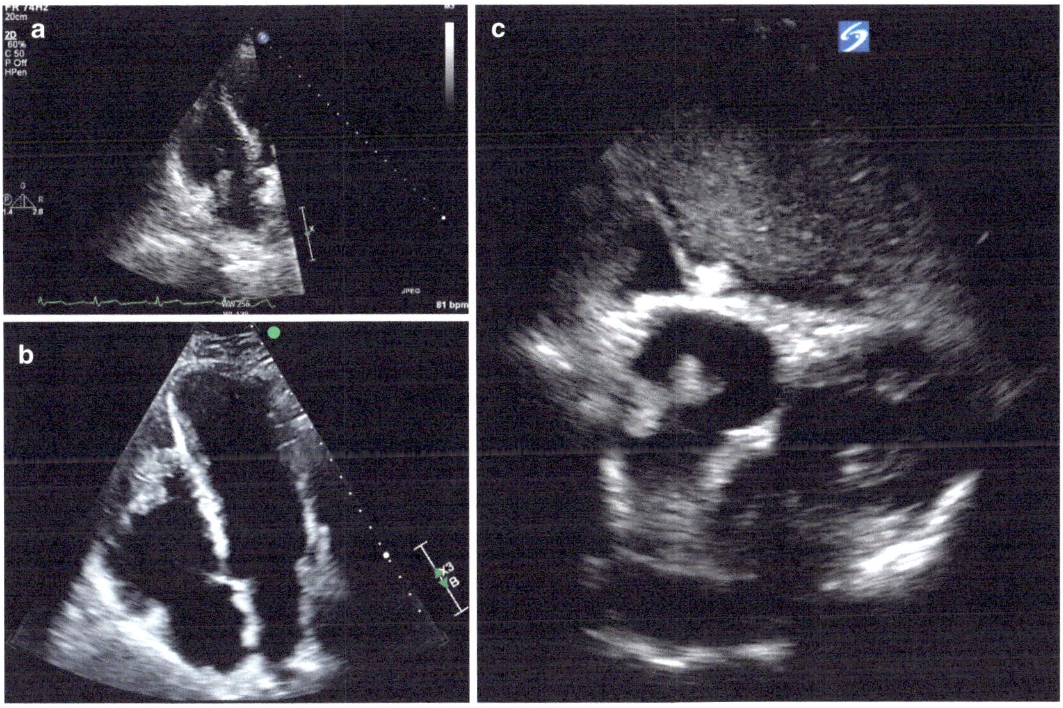

Fig. 31.1 A depiction of the types of thrombi. (**a**) A truncated apical 4-chamber view focusing on the right ventricle showing a type A mobile thrombus in the right atrium with a serpiginous appearance. (**b**) Apical 4 chamber view showing a type B non-mobile thrombus in the right ventricle adherent to the interatrial septum. (**c**) Subcostal view showing a type C multilobulated thrombus in the right atrium

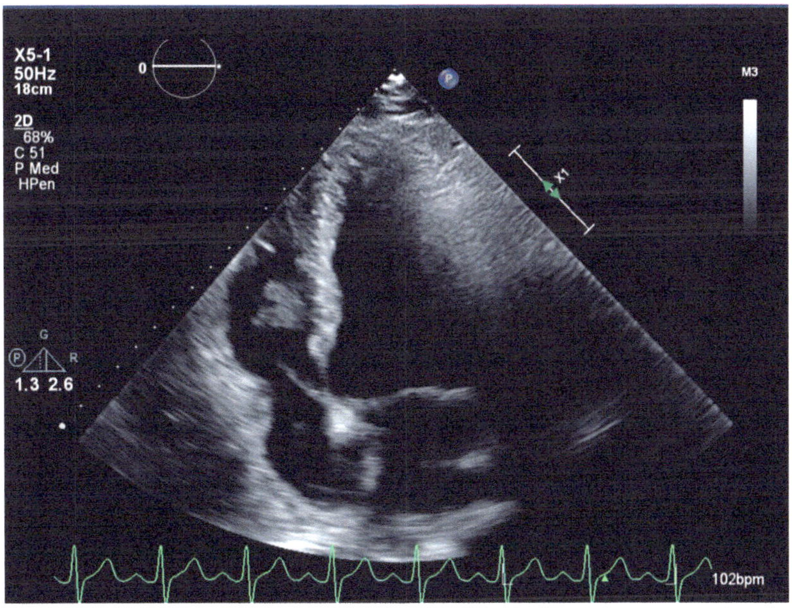

Fig. 31.2 Apical 4 chamber view showing a mobile thrombus in the right ventricle

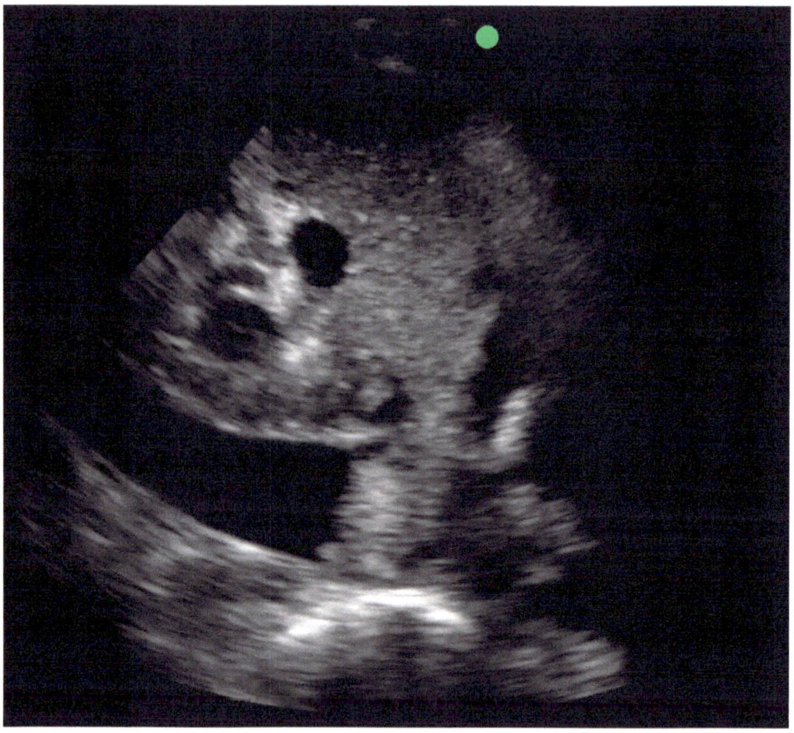

Fig. 31.3 A subcostal view of the inferior vena cava showing tumor thrombus within the hepatic vein and extending into the inferior vena cava and the right atrium

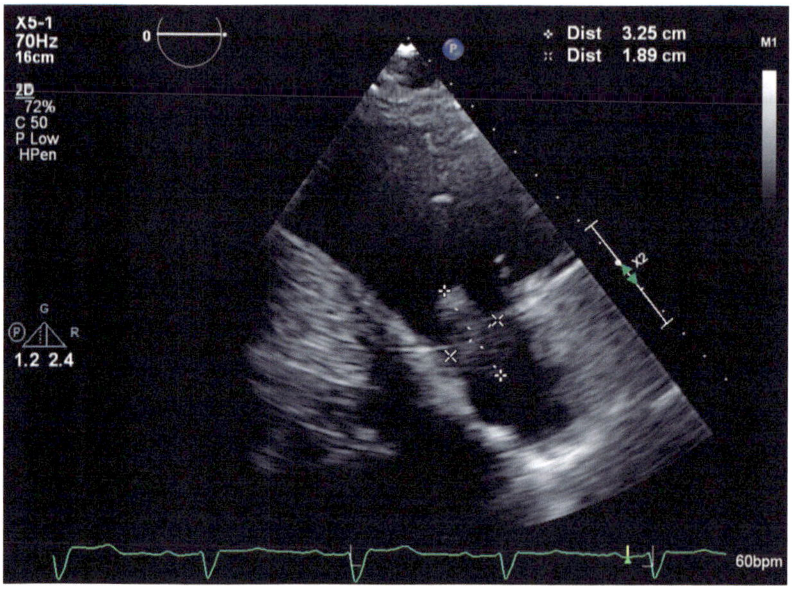

Fig. 31.4 A right-ventricular inflow view showing a mobile globular appearing thrombus in the right atrium with to-and-fro motion traversing the tricuspid valve

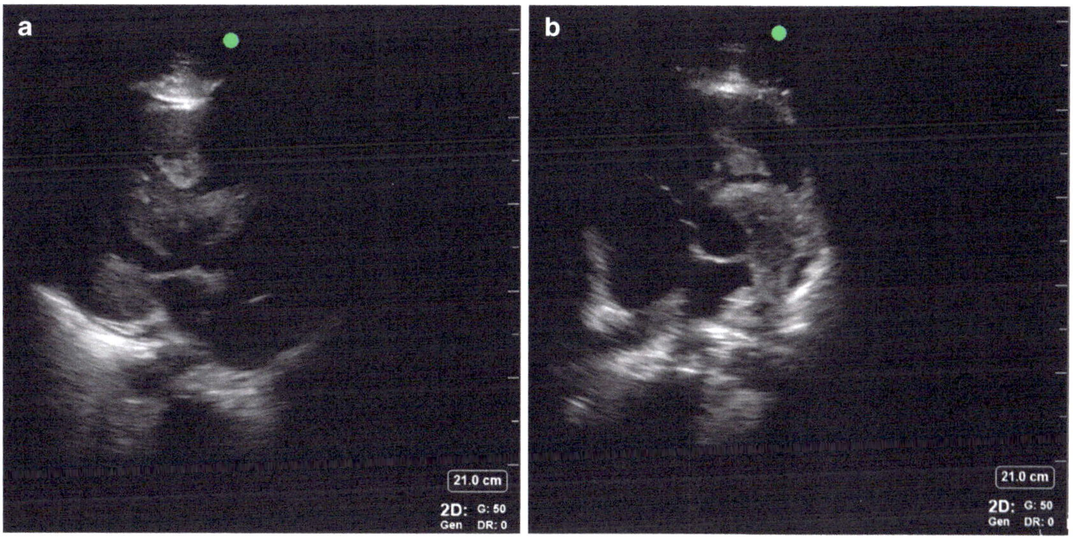

Fig. 31.5 A right ventricular outflow tract thrombus seen in a patient during cardiac arrest. (**a**) A parasternal long-axis view showing a mobile thrombus in the right ventricular outflow tract. (**b**) A parasternal short-axis view at the level of the aortic valve showing the same thrombus in the right ventricular outflow tract with associated thrombus in the proximal main and right pulmonary artery

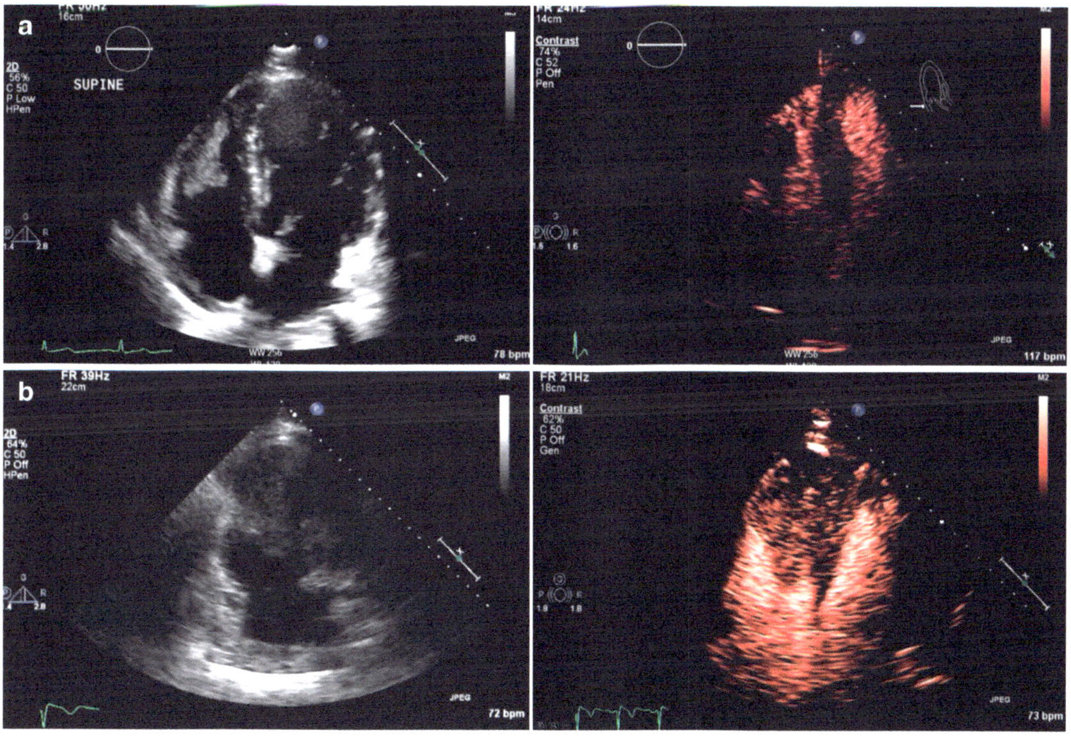

Fig. 31.6 Apical 4-chamber views showing a side-by-side comparison between the difference in contrast enhancement in true thombus and a mass. (**a**) A right-ventricular thrombus with contrast-ehanced images showing a filling defect within the right ventricle. (**b**) A right-ventricular malignant mass showing contrast uptake and enhancement of the mass

In contrast echocardiography, thrombi show no enhancement as they are avascular, while malignant tumors show enhancement due to abnormal neovascularization and high vascularity, and myxomas show partial enhancement due to poor blood supply [14]. The adjunctive use of 3-dimensional echocardiographic imaging may permit better visualization of thrombi and allow their volumetric measurements, similar to its use in intracardiac masses [15].

Transesophageal echocardiography (TEE) has distinct advantages of higher-resolution imaging and confers superior sensitivity in the right-heart chambers' surveillance and thrombi detection [16]. An added benefit of using TEE in RST is the ability to detect small thrombi that are beyond the resolution of TTE and accurately determine their morphology and size (Fig. 31.7 and Video 31.11). The use of cardiac magnetic resonance (CMR) imaging has also been reported to detect RST and may be a valuable alternative in patients with a high suspicion of RST who cannot undergo TEE imaging [12]. Some clots are very small and may be better delineated on CMR as seen in Fig. 31.8 and Video 31.12.

A careful review of contrast chest computed tomography (CT) images may also be helpful in evaluating patients with RST. Contrasted chest CTs may show filling defects within the right heart chambers as shown in Fig. 31.9. This may help strengthen the suspicion of a thrombus seen initially on TTE or vice versa. Additionally, computed tomography imaging of the abdomen in the case of tumor thrombus associated with renal cell carcinoma and magnetic resonance imaging of the liver in patients with hepatocellular carcinoma may be useful in confirming a suspected tumor thrombus seen on echocardiography.

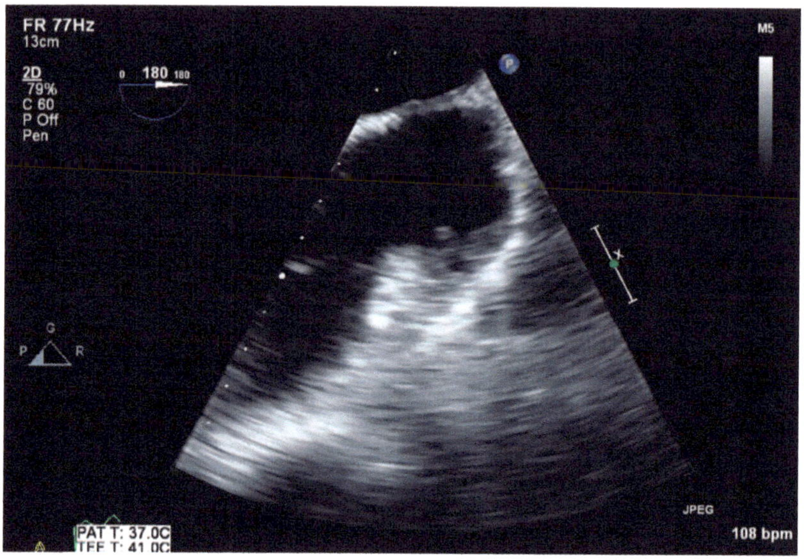

Fig. 31.7 Transesophageal echocardiogram of the right atrial appendage showing a mobile thrombus

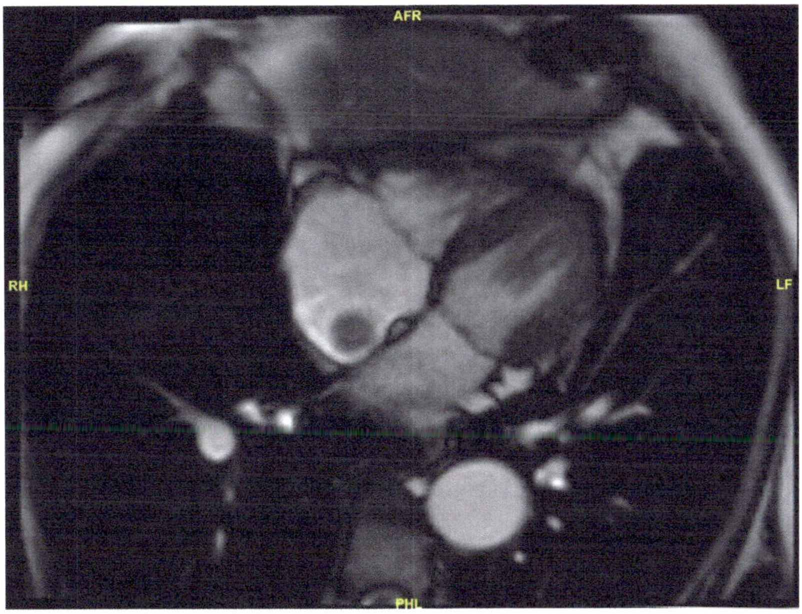

Fig. 31.8 Cardiac magnetic resonance image showing a small globular appearing right atrial thrombus

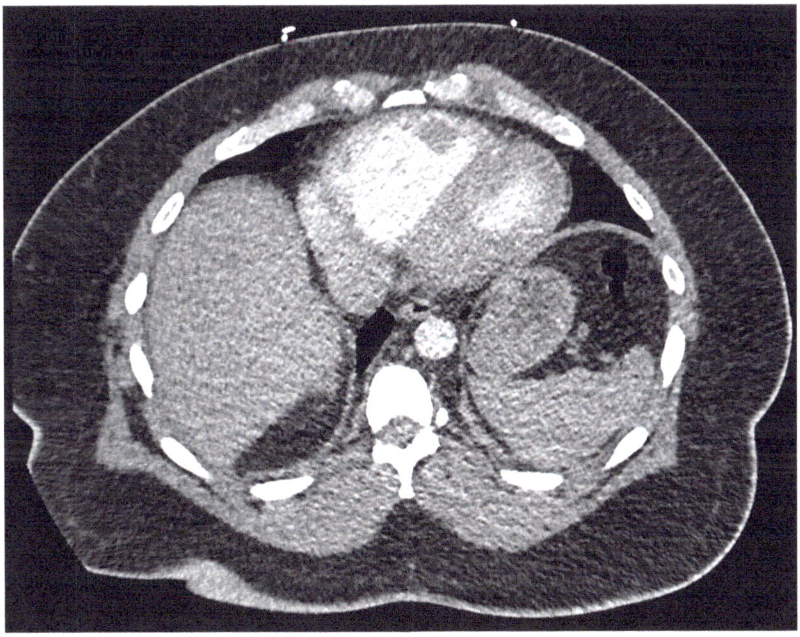

Fig. 31.9 Computer tomography image of the chest with contrast showing a filling defect in the apex of the right ventricle

Clinical Implications

In patients with RST on echocardiography without documented PE, it is imperative to evaluate these patients for the presence of concurrent PE. Mobile RSTs are associated with an increased mortality in the setting of acute PE, especially in the presence of right ventricular dysfunction [17, 18]. Despite the noted higher mortality, the current guidelines don't include the presence or absence of RST in the formal PE risk assessment, which mainly utilizes hemodynamic instability, clinical parameters of severity or comorbidities, right ventricular dysfunction, and elevated cardiac biomarkers such as troponins in early risk assessment [4]. It is difficult to differentiate tumors, tumor thrombi, and true thrombi based on their sonographic appearance; it is important to consider contrast-enhanced echocardiography and the use of multimodality imaging, including TEE and CMR, to better differentiate the findings on TTE.

There is a risk of RST causing hemodynamic instability; initial triage should include an individualized approach to consider monitoring these patients who may be at a higher risk of hemodynamic collapse in the intensive care unit. Multidisciplinary Pulmonary Embolism Response Teams (PERT) can be a valuable resource in triage and treatment decision-making. Treatment decisions can be affected by several factors, including the center's experience, bleeding risk, size and location of the thrombus, overall clot burden, right ventricular dysfunction, and presence of patent foramen ovale [20]. Besides anticoagulation, systemic thrombolysis, catheter-directed therapy including catheter embolectomies such as AngioVac systems, and surgical embolectomy can be considered in the treatment of mobile RST [20]. Thrombus-in-transit across a PFO represents a unique challenge. Despite limited evidence, in this situation, surgical embolectomy can be considered due to the risk of stroke and intracranial hemorrhage with other therapeutic modalities [19].

Evolving Evidence

Due to the lack of prospective randomized trials that evaluate different treatment modalities of mobile RST, there is no consensus on optimal management strategy and an individualized treatment approach should be considered in each case.

Summary Points

- RST can be associated with pulmonary embolism (thrombus-in-transit) or catheters/devices.
- The echocardiographic appearance of RST can be grouped into three patterns (type A, type B, and type C).
- Mobile RSTs are associated with increased mortality in the setting of acute pulmonary embolism.
- Individualized treatment approaches should be considered in patients with mobile RST.
- Multidisciplinary PERT can be a valuable resource in management.

Questions

1. A 45-year-old female without known prior medical problems, presented to the emergency room after a syncopal episode. She was hypoxic, requiring oxygen at 6 L/min via nasal cannula, had sinus tachycardia with a heart rate of 145/min, a respiratory rate of 28/min, and her blood pressure was 87/36 mmHg. She was given a bolus of 500 ml lactated Ringer's solution without improvement in her blood pressure, and she was subsequently started on a norepinephrine infusion. A contrast chest computed tomography showed a saddle pulmonary embolism, and she was started on a heparin infusion. An emergent echocardiogram showed severe right ventricular dilation with severely depressed right ventricular function. An incidental note was made of a highly mobile serpiginous density in the right atrium concerning a clot-in-transit. What is the next best step in the management of this patient?
   A. Continue anticoagulation with heparin and repeat serial echocardiograms to evaluate the right atrial density.
   B. Switch intravenous heparin to subcutaneous low-molecular-weight heparin.
   C. Review the thrombolytics contraindication checklist and treat the patient with systemic thrombolytics in the absence of contraindications.
   D. Review the thrombolytics contraindication checklist and prepare the patient for catheter-directed thrombolysis in the absence of contraindications.

   Answer: C

   Explanation: The patient has a high-risk acute pulmonary embolism evidenced by hemodynamic instability and significant right ventricular dysfunction. Furthermore, she has a right atrial thrombus-in-transit. In the absence of contraindication, systemic thrombolysis is the treatment of choice in this case (answer C). Anticoagulation alone (answers A and B) or catheter-directed thrombolysis (answer D) is not the treatment of choice in high-risk pulmonary embolism complicated with thrombus-in-transit in the absence of contraindication for systemic thrombolysis.

2. A 65-year-old male with COVID-19 infection was admitted to the ICU and was intubated for progressive acute hypoxic respiratory failure. Over the course of this ICU stay, his oxygen requirement gradually improved. His Fio2 and positive end-expiratory pressure were weaned gradually in anticipation of extubation. You were alerted about a sudden worsening in the patient's oxygen requirement and the development of circulatory failure, necessitating the initiation of vasopressors. A point-of-care ultrasound showed bilateral lung sliding, preserved left ventricular ejection fraction without regional wall motion abnormalities, dilated inferior vena cava at 2.3 cm without respiratory variations, and a mobile density in the right ventricular outflow tract. Soon after, the patient became pulseless with asystole on the cardiac monitor, and cardiopulmonary resuscitation was initiated. What is the most likely cause of the patient's cardiac arrest?
   A. Acute pulmonary embolism
   B. Anterior wall myocardial infarction
   C. Tension pneumothorax
   D. Hypovolemic shock

   Answer: A

   Explanation: The sudden deterioration in oxygenation and hemodynamics in the presence of a mobile density in the right ventricular outflow tract on point-of-care ultrasound is highly suggestive of acute pulmonary embolism (answer A) as the cause of cardiac arrest. Tension pneumothorax (answer C) is less likely in the presence of bilateral lung sliding on ultrasound lung examination. Anterior wall myocardial infarction (answer B) is less likely in the absence of regional wall motion abnormalities. The dilation of the inferior vena cava without respiratory variations argues against hypovolemia (answer D).

References

1. Rose PS, Punjabi NM, Pearse DB. Treatment of right heart thromboemboli. Chest. 2002;121(3):806–14.
2. Torbicki A, Galie N, Covezzoli A, Rossi E, De Rosa M, Goldhaber SZ, et al. Right heart thrombi in pulmonary embolism: results from the international cooperative pulmonary embolism registry. J Am Coll Cardiol. 2003;41(12):2245–51.
3. Casazza F, Bongarzoni A, Centonze F, Morpurgo M. Prevalence and prognostic significance of right-sided cardiac mobile thrombi in acute massive pulmonary embolism. Am J Cardiol. 1997;79(10):1433–5.
4. Konstantinides SV, Meyer G, Becattini C, Bueno H, Geersing GJ, Harjola VP, et al. 2019 ESC guidelines for the diagnosis and management of acute pulmonary embolism developed in collaboration with the European Respiratory Society (ERS). Eur Heart J. 2020;41(4):543–603.
5. Ferrari E, Benhamou M, Berthier F, Baudouy M. Mobile thrombi of the right heart in pulmonary embolism: delayed disappearance after thrombolytic treatment. Chest. 2005;127(3):1051–3.
6. Shah A, Murray M, Nzerue C. Right atrial thrombi complicating use of central venous catheters in hemodialysis. Int J Artif Organs. 2004;27(9):772–8.
7. Ducatman BS, McMichan JC, Edwards WD. Catheter-induced lesions of the right side of the heart. A one-year prospective study of 141 autopsies. JAMA. 1985;253(6):791–5.
8. Supple GE, Ren JF, Zado ES, Marchlinski FE. Mobile thrombus on device leads in patients undergoing ablation: identification, incidence, location, and association with increased pulmonary artery systolic pressure. Circulation. 2011;124(7):772–8.
9. van Laecke S, Dhondt A, de Sutter J, Vanholder R. Right atrial thrombus in an asymptomatic hemodialysis patient with malfunctioning catheter and patent foramen ovale. Hemodial Int. 2005;9(3):236–40.
10. Wang Y, Yuan L, Ge RL, Sun Y, Wei G. Survival benefit of surgical treatment for hepatocellular carcinoma with inferior vena cava/right atrium tumor thrombus: results of a retrospective cohort study. Ann Surg Oncol. 2013;20(3):914–22.
11. Chiappini B, Savini C, Marinelli G, Suarez SM, Di Eusanio M, Fiorani V, et al. Cavoatrial tumor thrombus: single-stage surgical approach with profound hypothermia and circulatory arrest, including a review of the literature. J Thorac Cardiovasc Surg. 2002;124(4):684–8.
12. Tsang BK, Platts DG, Javorsky G, Brown MR. Right ventricular thrombus detection and multimodality

imaging using contrast echocardiography and cardiac magnetic resonance imaging. Heart Lung Circ. 2012;21(3):185–8.
13. Horner SM, Bell JA, Swanton RH. Infected right atrial thrombus—an important but rare complication of central venous lines. Eur Heart J. 1993;14(1):138–40.
14. Mansencal N, Revault-d'Allonnes L, Pelage JP, Farcot JC, Lacombe P, Dubourg O. Usefulness of contrast echocardiography for assessment of intracardiac masses. Arch Cardiovasc Dis. 2009;102(3):177–83.
15. Zaragoza-Macias E, Chen MA, Gill EA. Real time three-dimensional echocardiography evaluation of intracardiac masses. Echocardiography. 2012;29(2):207–19.
16. Cohen GI, Klein AL, Chan KL, Stewart WJ, Salcedo EE. Transesophageal echocardiographic diagnosis of right-sided cardiac masses in patients with central lines. Am J Cardiol. 1992;70(9):925–9.
17. Barrios D, Rosa-Salazar V, Morillo R, Nieto R, Fernandez S, Zamorano JL, et al. Prognostic significance of right heart thrombi in patients with acute symptomatic pulmonary embolism: systematic review and meta-analysis. Chest. 2017;151(2):409–16.
18. Koc M, Kostrubiec M, Elikowski W, Meneveau N, Lankeit M, Grifoni S, et al. Outcome of patients with right heart thrombi: the right heart thrombi European registry. Eur Respir J. 2016;47(3):869–75.
19. Rivera-Lebron B, McDaniel M, Ahrar K, Alrifai A, Dudzinski DM, Fanola C, et al. Diagnosis, treatment and follow up of acute pulmonary embolism: consensus practice from the PERT consortium. Clin Appl Thromb Hemost. 2019;25:1076029619853037.
20. Carroll BJ, Larnard EA, Pinto DS, Giri J, Secemsky EA. Percutaneous Management of High-Risk Pulmonary Embolism. Circ Cardiovasc Interv. 2023;16(2):e012166. https://doi.org/10.1161/CIRCINTERVENTIONS.122.012166. Epub 2023 Feb 6. PMID: 36744463.

Diagnosing Acute Aortic Syndromes with Ultrasound

32

Meghan Snuckel and Andrew T. Levinson

Learning Objectives

1. Review aortic pathology relevant to critically ill patients.
2. Describe image acquisition of the aorta via transthoracic and transabdominal views.
3. Examine the diagnostic accuracy of TTE and TEE for detecting acute aortic pathology.
4. Evaluate the evidence for the use of POCUS in the rapid diagnosis of aortic syndromes.

Introduction

Imaging of the aorta with ultrasound can be critical in the rapid triage of the patient who presents with back, abdominal, or chest pain and hypotension or shock. Acute aortic syndromes and emergencies in critically ill or injured patients include ruptured abdominal aortic aneurysm, traumatic aortic injury, aortic dissection, and aortic intraluminal thrombus. Acute aortic syndromes can either be spontaneous or traumatic and are often difficult to diagnose. Delayed diagnosis and misdiagnosis of acute aortic syndromes contribute to significant morbidity and mortality [1–3].

Risk factors for acute aortic pathology include a history of connective tissue disease, family history, aortic valve disease, hypertension, known prior aortic aneurysm, hyperlipidemia, COPD, smoking history, and prior aortic endovascular procedures or previous aortic surgeries [4]. Presenting symptoms of acute aortic pathology can be non-specific and include chest pain, back pain, abdominal pain, syncope, and focal neurological deficits. Confounding the diagnosis is the fact that a significant percentage of patients with acute aortic pathology may not have significant symptoms. Exam findings may include diastolic murmurs, pulse deficit, and hypotension [2].

Aortic pathology can be detected and characterized by various radiographic modalities, including chest radiography, contrast-enhanced computed tomography (CT), trans-thoracic echocardiogram (TTE), trans-abdominal ultrasound, trans-esophageal echocardiography (TEE), magnetic resonance imaging (MRI), and angiography. In trauma, a positive Focused Assessment with Sonography for Trauma (FAST) exam showing free fluid in the abdomen may be an indication for surgery in an unstable patient.

Supplementary Information The online version contains supplementary material available at https://doi.org/10.1007/978-3-031-80038-2_32.

M. Snuckel · A. T. Levinson (✉)
Division of Pulmonary, Critical Care, and Sleep Medicine, The Warren Alpert Medical School, Brown University, Providence, RI, USA
e-mail: andrew_levinson@brown.edu

M. J. Lanspa, A. T. Levinson (eds.), *Echocardiography and Ultrasonography in the ICU*, Respiratory Medicine, https://doi.org/10.1007/978-3-031-80038-2_32

Aortic Dissection

An aortic dissection results from a disruption in the medial layer of the aorta, often in the setting of an aortic intimal tear. Ultrasound findings consistent with possible aortic dissection include pericardial effusions, intimal flaps, or an aortic outflow track diameter measuring more than 35 mm [5] (Videos 32.8, 32.9, 32.10, and 32.11).

DeBakey and Stanford are two different classification systems to describe the location of aortic dissections that are used. DeBakey type I includes the ascending aorta, arch, and descending thoracic aorta. Debakey type II, in contrast, is limited to the ascending aorta, while Debakey type III includes the descending aorta distal to the left subclavian artery origin. Stanford classification type A includes the ascending aorta, while type B does not involve the ascending aorta. Most Stanford type B dissections are distal to the left subclavian artery but may include the arch involvement without involving the ascending aorta [2]. Stanford type A dissections are mostly managed surgically, while Stanford type B dissections involving the descending aorta are usually managed medically [3, 6].

Abdominal Aortic Aneurysm

An abdominal aortic aneurysm is defined as any focal dilation along the abdominal aorta. The aneurysm can be anywhere from an incidental finding requiring incremental radiographic monitoring to emergent surgery. When evaluating aortic size with ultrasound, the accepted standard is to measure the inner-to-inner maximum anterior-posterior aortic diameter [4].

At the level of the infrarenal aorta, an abdominal aortic aneurysm is considered to be present when the inner-to-inner diameter exceeds 3.0 cm [3]. Surgery and/or endovascular repair should be considered for symptomatic or quickly expanding. Aneurysms >4 cm and poorly controlled diastolic blood pressure are risk factors for rupture [3] (Video 32.5, 32.6, and 32.7).

Aortic Thrombus

Multiple etiologies of acute aortic clot (Video 32.6) have been described, including secondary to aortic dissection, AAA, atrial fibrillation, and other factors predisposing to hypercoagulability [7]. Treatment may include systemic anticoagulation, anti-thrombotic therapy, maximal medical therapy, and/or surgery.

Image Acquisition

Images of the aorta can be obtained by transthoracic and transabdominal views and by TEE. To visualize the aorta, standard TTE views and abdominal ultrasound are recommended.

For the thoracic aorta, transthoracic image acquisition refers to the subcoastal views sections in Chap. 5: transthoracic echocardiography views and windows. For TEE, see Chap. 9: TEE views. Transthoracic views often allow imaging of the ascending aorta and aortic arch, descending thoracic aorta, and the origins of the right brachiocephalic, left common carotid, and left subclavian arteries. It is recommended that particular attention be placed on the parasternal and apical and subcostal views with the patient supine and/or in the left lateral decubital position [2].

It has also been described in the literature that in patients with pneumonia and/or consolidation patterns, the thoracic descending aorta and even occasionally the aortic arch can be well visualized with TTE, positioning the probe on the left lateral and posterior chest wall [8].

Abdominal aorta image acquisition and views are well described in the literature [9]. For abdominal views (Videos 32.1, 32.2, and 32.3), the proximal (Image 32.1), mid (Images 32.2 and 32.3), and distal abdominal aorta (Images 32.4 and 32.5) should be visualized and measured both in transverse and longitudinal views. The aorta is visualized deep into the IVC. If there is any confusion about whether the IVC or aorta is being visualized, compression and the use of Doppler signaling may be helpful.

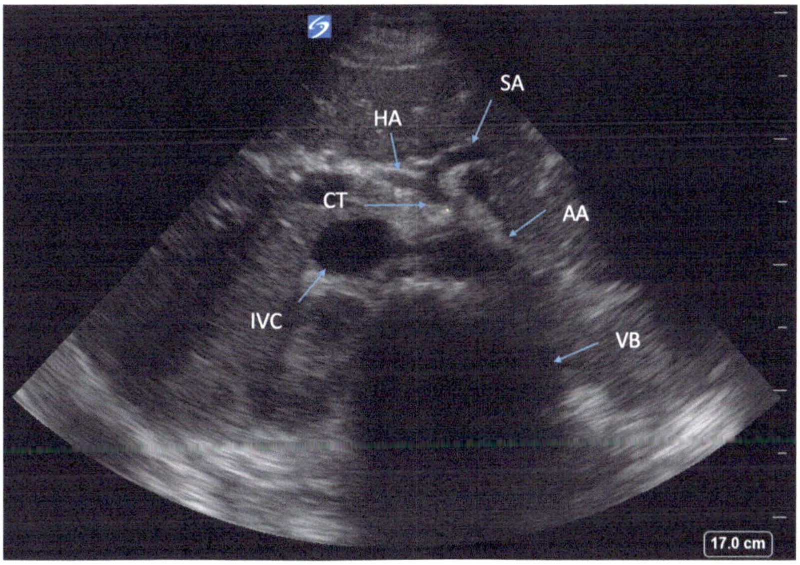

Image 32.1 Transverse axis, proximal aorta, "seagull sign". *AA* abdominal aorta, *SA* splenic artery, *HA* hepatic artery, *CT* celiac trunk, *IVC* inferior vena cava, *VB* vertebral body

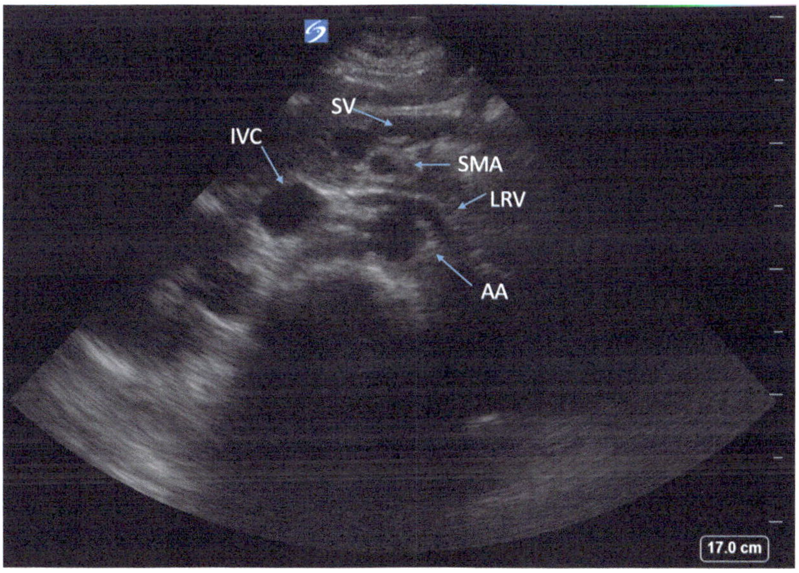

Image 32.2 Transverse axis, mid abdominal aorta. *AA* abdominal aorta, *LRV* left renal vein, *IVC* Inferior vena cava, *SV* splenic vein, *SMA* superior mesenteric artery

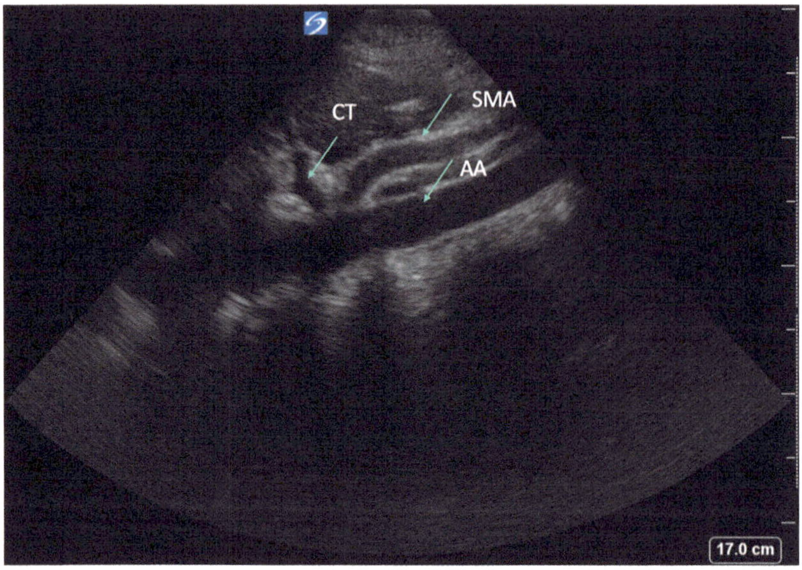

Image 32.3 Longitudinal view, proximal and mid abdominal aorta with branching of the celiac and superior mesenteric artery. *CT* celiac trunk, *SMA* superior mesenteric artery

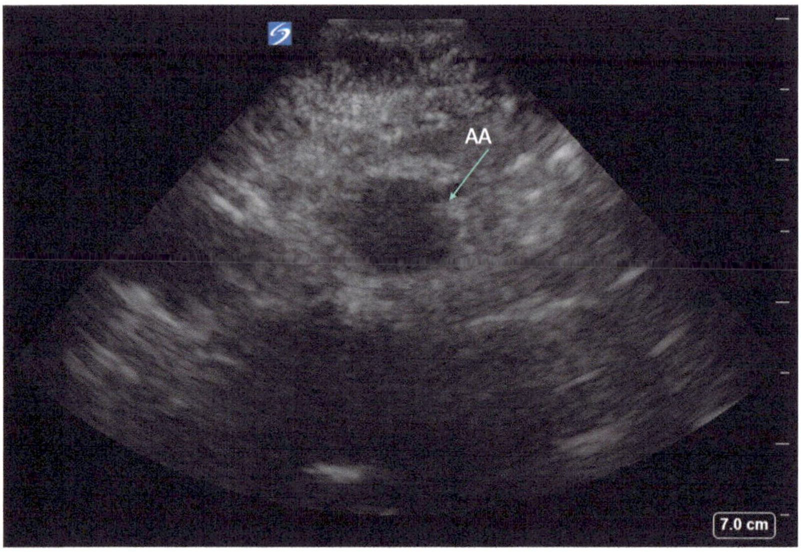

Image 32.4 Transverse view, distal abdominal aorta. *AA* Abdominal aorta

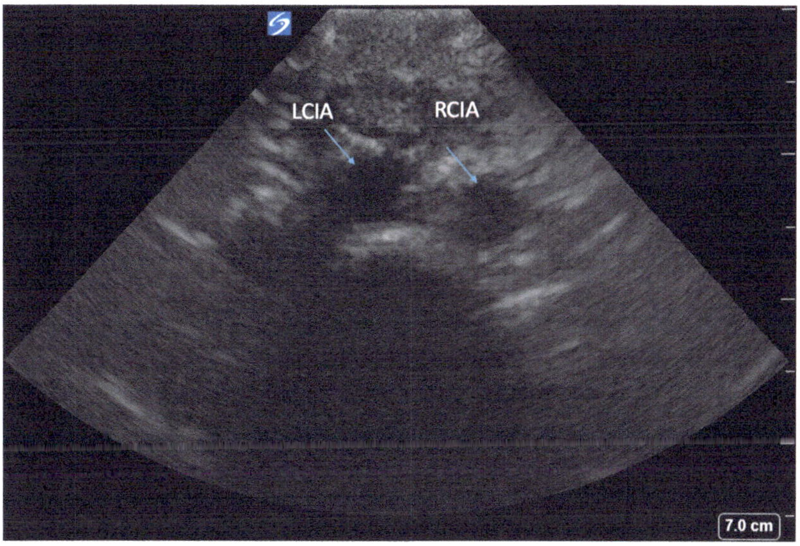

Image 32.5 Transverse view, distal abdominal aorta, branching of the common iliac arteries. *LCIA* left common iliac artery, *RCIA* right common iliac artery

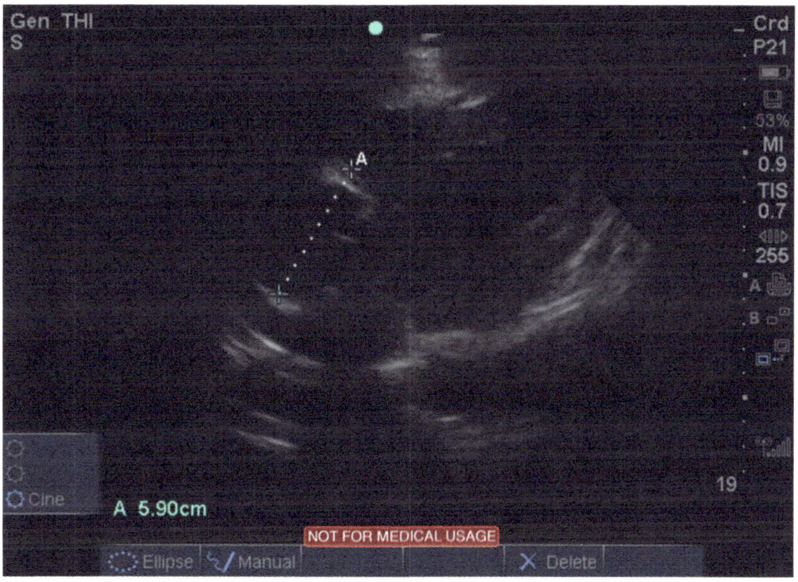

Image 32.6 Abdominal aortic aneurysm. Courtesy Dr. Kristin Dwyer

TEE artifacts are discussed extensively in Chap. 10, Artifacts and Pitfalls in TEE. Thoracic aortic dissection can be well visualized with TEE (Videos 32.8, 32.9, and 32.11).

Specific POCUS findings for the diagnosis of acute aortic syndromes include the visualization of an intraluminal aortic flap (Videos 32.4 and 32.9), an intramural aortic clot (video 32.6), and a visible aortic ulcer. Indirect findings may include aortic dilatation at any level >4 cm (Image 32.6, Videos 32.5 and 32.6), pericardial effusion and/or tamponade, and aortic regurgitation [2, 10].

Pitfalls

The aorta is visualized deep into the IVC. If there is any confusion about whether the IVC or aorta is being visualized, compression and the use of Doppler signaling may be helpful.

The TEE often provides very limited visualization of the aortic arch and cannot diagnose pathology there. Suprasternal TTE can be performed in addition to TEE to possibly better evaluate aortic arch pathology.

Some ultrasound artifacts can mimic aortic dissection. For example, on TTE, a side-lobe artifact from a central venous catheter in the innominate vein and/or SVC can mimic dissection.

Evidence for the Use of POCUS in the Rapid Diagnosis of Aortic Syndromes

Diagnostic accuracy of POCUS for acute aortic processes can be useful but cannot exclude the absence of pathology in symptomatic patients. For patients with a high pretest probability of an acute aortic process but a negative POCUS exam, formal imaging is suggested, such as CTA.

TTE has been estimated to have a *sensitivity* of 88–91%, but CTA, MRA, and TEE all have sensitivities >95% for both types of aortic dissection. Formal cardiology-performed TTE has a sensitivity >95% for type A aortic dissection. POCUS in the literature has a sensitivity between 80% and 90% for type A aortic dissection and 70% for type B aortic dissection [5].

One recent point-of-care ultrasound (POCUS) protocol prospective study combining transthoracic echocardiography (TTE) and ultrasound imaging of the abdominal aorta found a sensitivity of 93.2% (95% CI 81.3–98.6), specificity of 90.9 (95% CI 89.2–92.5), positive predictive values of 26.3%, and a negative predictive value of 99.7% [5]. The prospective multicenter study enrolled 1324 patients who presented to emergency departments and compared the protocolized TTE and abdominal aorta scans to the findings from a CT angiogram utilizing a dissection protocol [6].

Regarding abdominal aortic pathology, transesophageal echocardiography (TEE) has been well described for some time in the critical care literature as a very rapid and sensitive tool for diagnosing aortic injury. Diagnostic accuracy is quite high in diagnosing acute dissection, compared to the gold standard of angiography, MRI, or CT angiography [11–13].

With basic training, both physicians and students have been shown to have high diagnostic accuracy at measuring the aorta and detecting aortic dissection rapidly using trans-thoracic and trans-abdominal ultrasound [14–16].

Specifically for thoracic acute aortic syndromes, it is not recommended by most experts as a stand-alone test. If acute findings are noted, they can be extremely helpful given ease of use, cost, lack of radiation, and timeliness. However, if they are not diagnostic and there is a moderate to high pre-test probability, additional tests that have higher diagnostic accuracy, especially for descending thoracic aortic processes, should be performed, such as computed tomography (CT), magnetic resonance imaging (MRI), and/or transesophageal echocardiography (TEE) [2].

TTE has not been recognized as a useful modality for the assessment and/or diagnosis of diseases of the descending thoracic aorta. This is because standard TTE windows usually do not offer good visualization due to the larger distance from the anterior chest to the descending thoracic aorta and because of lung artifacts. One recent small single-center study, however, suggested that, compared to contrast-enhanced CT as the gold standard, a posterior para-vertebral approach for TTE with the patient in a lateral decubitus position has significantly increased sensitivity (compared to standard anterior TTE views) for detecting acute aortic pathology in the descending thoracic aorta [17].

Summary Points

- Transesophageal echocardiography (TEE) has been well described for some time in the critical care literature as a very rapid and sensitive tool for diagnosing aortic injury.
- TTE and Transabdominal point-of-care ultrasound have been shown to have high diagnos-

tic accuracy in measuring the aorta and detecting aortic dissection rapidly using transthoracic and transabdominal ultrasound.

- TTE should not be used as a stand-alone test for acute thoracic aortic pathology. If acute findings are noted, they can be extremely helpful given timeliness and ease of use while waiting for a gold-standard test; however, if they are not diagnostic, additional tests that have higher diagnostic accuracy, especially for descending thoracic aortic processes, should be performed.

References

1. Azhar B, Patel SR, Holt PJ, Hinchliffe RJ, Thompson MM, Karthikesalingam A. Misdiagnosis of ruptured abdominal aortic aneurysm: systematic review and meta-analysis. J Endovasc Ther. 2014;21:568–75.
2. Morello F, Santoro M, Fargion AT, Grifoni S, Nazerian P. Diagnosis and management of acute aortic syndromes in the emergency department. Intern Emerg Med. 2021;16:171–81.
3. Chinthamuneedi M. Diseases of the aorta in the critically ill. Crit Care Resusc. 2000;2:117–24.
4. Abdominal aortic aneurysm: diagnosis and management. NICE; 2020. Accessed 3 Jan 2024.
5. Gibbons RC, Smith D, Feig R, Mulflur M, Costantino TG. The sonographic protocol for the emergent evaluation of aortic dissections (SPEED protocol): a multicenter, prospective, observational study. Acad Emerg Med. 2024;31:112–8.
6. Gibbons RC, Singh G, Donuru A, Young M. Abdominal Aortic Aneurysm Imaging. StatPearls. Treasure Island (FL) ineligible companies. Disclosure: Gagandeep Singh declares no relevant financial relationships with ineligible companies. Disclosure: Achala Donuru declares no relevant financial relationships with ineligible companies. Disclosure: Michael Young declares no relevant financial relationships with ineligible companies. 2024.
7. Boivin Z, Mensel E, She T. Role of POCUS in assessing an acute aortic thrombus. POCUS J. 2023;8:129–31.
8. Barbry T, Bouhemad B, Leleu K, de Castro V, Remerand F, Rouby JJ. Transthoracic ultrasound approach of thoracic aorta in critically ill patients with lung consolidation. J Crit Care. 2006;21:203–8.
9. Hartrich M, Eilbert W. An approach to point-of-care ultrasound evaluation of the abdominal aorta. J Vis Exp. 2023.
10. Hansen MS, Nogareda GJ, Hutchison SJ. Frequency of and inappropriate treatment of misdiagnosis of acute aortic dissection. Am J Cardiol. 2007;99:852–6.
11. Khalil A, Helmy T, Porembka DT. Aortic pathology: aortic trauma, debris, dissection, and aneurysm. Crit Care Med. 2007;35:S392–400.
12. Porembka DT. Importance of transesophageal echocardiography in the critically ill and injured patient. Crit Care Med. 2007;35:S414–30.
13. Shiga T, Wajima Z, Apfel CC, Inoue T, Ohe Y. Diagnostic accuracy of transesophageal echocardiography, helical computed tomography, and magnetic resonance imaging for suspected thoracic aortic dissection: systematic review and meta-analysis. Arch Intern Med. 2006;166:1350–6.
14. Jaynstein D, Baeten R, Bafuma P, et al. Point-of-care ultrasound assessment of the abdominal aorta by physician assistant students: a pilot study. Emerg Radiol. 2021;28:245–50.
15. Pare JR, Liu R, Moore CL, et al. Emergency physician focused cardiac ultrasound improves diagnosis of ascending aortic dissection. Am J Emerg Med. 2016;34:486–92.
16. Nazerian P, Vanni S, Morello F, et al. Diagnostic performance of focused cardiac ultrasound performed by emergency physicians for the assessment of ascending aorta dilation and aneurysm. Acad Emerg Med. 2015;22:536–41.
17. Yamaguchi S, Murakami H, Kudo T, et al. Usefulness of the echocardiographic paravertebral approach for the diagnosis of descending thoracic aortic dissection. J Echocardiogr. 2017;15:127–34.

Adult Congenital Heart Disease

33

Erik Su and Saul Flores

Learning Objectives

1. Understand the most common congenital heart defects
2. Recognize diagnostic echocardiographic targets for patients with suspected congenital heart defects
3. Correlate congenital lesions with echocardiographic findings

Summary Points

- Identification of congenital heart defects requires an excellent working knowledge of normal cardiac anatomy and function, as well as advanced qualitative and quantitative skills in echocardiography.
- As point-of-care ultrasound (POCUS) becomes increasingly used in initial hemodynamic assessment, the recognition of congenital abnormalities and their physiological sequelae is important for optimal evaluation and management of critically ill patients.

This chapter is intended for clinicians experienced in focused cardiac ultrasound or critical care echocardiography optimally with a level of verified and mentored experience examining patients in acute hemodynamic instability with structurally normal hearts. A necessary skill in assessing patients with cardiac morphology skills is sweeping (also fanning or tilting) the beam of an ultrasound toward and away from the operator along a direction perpendicular to the plane of the view. As an operator performs this while visualizing the heart, different sections of the heart are visible and a slow sweep can identify structures outside of traditional view planes. This is instrumental for identifying structures such as coronary arteries in the parasternal short axis view at the aortic valve level, and the coronary sinus in the apical four-chamber view. With color Doppler, it may be used to survey for atrial and septal defects from the subcostal four-chamber window.

The exhaustive views used to comprehensively phenotype a heart with dysmorphology often exceed 100 images in echocardiography labs and are unfortunately too extensive for this discussion. Rather traditional views used in critical care echocardiography are mentioned with accompanying caveats for assisting readers in discussing these patients for timely cardiac referral and consultation.

Within congenital heart disease, defects are often classified into three, sometimes four categories based on physiology in infancy:

1. Problems causing increased pulmonary blood flow (Qp > Qs)

E. Su (✉) · S. Flores
Adult Congenital Heart Disease ICU, Division of Critical Care Medicine in the Department of Pediatrics, Baylor College of Medicine at Texas Children's Hospital, Houston, TX, USA
e-mail: saul.flores2@bcm.edu

M. J. Lanspa, A. T. Levinson (eds.), *Echocardiography and Ultrasonography in the ICU*, Respiratory Medicine, https://doi.org/10.1007/978-3-031-80038-2_33

   (a) Septal defects, Patent Ductus Arteriosus, Anomalous Pulmonary Veins
2. Problems causing too little pulmonary blood flow (Qp < Qs)
   (a) Tetralogy of Fallot with Major Aorto-Pulmonary Collateral Arteries (MAPCAs), Ebstein's Malformation, Pulmonary Stenosis
3. Obstruction to systemic blood flow
   (a) Aortic Stenosis, Coarctation of the Aorta
4. Cardiomyopathy (discussed in Chapter IIc)
   (a) Congenitally Corrected Transposition of the Great Arteries (L-TGA)

Recognizing the long-term sequelae of CHD as clues that will help you seek timely consultation is crucial when a patient with known or unknown CHD presents to your care.

Within this chapter, unless otherwise noted, apical and subcostal views appear in the pediatric convention where the probe is at the bottom of the screen and structures distal to it appear at the top of the screen.

Problems Causing Increased Pulmonary Blood Flow

These lesions proceed toward Eisenmenger's syndrome, due to a left to right shunt. Depending on location of the shunt, the excess volume load to the heart initially leads to left heart dilatation and insufficiency, and increased left atrial (LA) pressure. Increasing pulmonary vascular pressures lead to progressive right heart dilatation and insufficiency. Increasing pulmonary vascular pressures over time can reverse shunt physiology as well. In congenital heart disease of this type that persists into adult ages, patients may manifest progressive left heart failure and potential biventricular failure with pulmonary hypertension.

Patent Ductus Arteriosus (PDA)

PDA occurs in 1 per 2000 live infant births and occurs when the ductus arteriosus, which serves a left-to-right shunt in the normal fetal circulation, fails to close more than 48 h after birth [1].

In terms of physiology and presentation, PDA is a risk factor for endarteritis and a major cause of morbidity and mortality in untreated PDA. This is irrespective of the size of the shunt. Vegetations appear on the pulmonary side of the PDA, and embolization typically travels to the lungs as opposed to the systemic vasculature. Patients with a large shunt will demonstrate a wide pulse pressure. The majority of patients may be asymptomatic with a machine-like continuous murmur in the left upper chest, others may have significant congestive heart failure in the case of increasing longstanding shunt. Pathological PDA is usually diagnosed in childhood and if untreated over a lifetime, the persistent left to right shunt causes volume overload of the heart. Variability in the degree of the shunt leads to heterogeneous presentations along a spectrum congestive heart failure (CHF) as well as secondary pulmonary hypertension (PHTN). Patients may present with impaired exercise tolerance, syncope, and palpitations depending on the degree of heart failure.

Findings on the image of the patient may demonstrate dilation of the left heart chambers with some level of compromised function, and potentially mitral valve regurgitation (Fig. 33.1). ECG may demonstrate left atrial dilatation and left ventricular strain depending on the degree of CHF. Targets of diagnostic echocardiography include identifying the location of the PDA and its flow direction, and a detailed functional assessment of the right and left heart. The PDA is visualized using dedicated ductal views modified from parasternal long and short axis views at the level of the pulmonary arteries. The pressure gradient across the PDA is used for determining right ventricular systolic pressure. Architecture and size of the PDA is relevant in its procedural management. Diastolic runoff through the PDA can result in reversal of aortic flow in the descending abdominal aorta during diastole.

In critical care echocardiography, recognizing left heart dilatation and function, and valvular competence are essential. Assessing right heart dilatation and function, and right ventricular systolic pressures are also important. The PDA

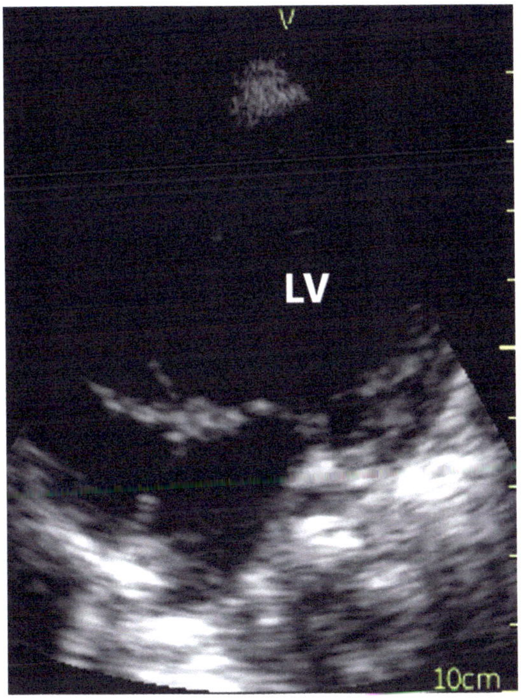

Fig. 33.1 Apical four-Chamber view of 6-month-old with untreated PDA and subsequent left heart failure. Image is shown in traditional echocardiography convention with probe at the top of the screen and objects distal to the probe at the bottom of the screen. LV: left ventricle

views are challenging in adults and difficult to render even if the windows are obtainable due to thoracic ossification and air artifact.

Atrial Septal Defect (ASD)/Patent Foramen Ovale (PFO) (Unrepaired/Repaired)

ASDs arise from various causes but comprise roughly 1–2 per 1000 of live births. ASDs appear in a variety of forms:

- Primum ASDs appear immediately above the atrioventricular (AV) valves due to a failure of the septum primum in fetal embryology. They may be associated with other ventricular septal and AV valve malformation issues
- Secundum ASDs arise from failure of the septum secundum and occur in the middle of the septum
- Coronary sinus ASDs occur in the vicinity of the coronary sinus when the sinus is unroofed and exposed to the left atrium
- Sinus venosus ASDs occur at the posterior margin of the atrial septum where either the superior or inferior vena cava insert in a way that overrides the septum and are commonly associated with anomalous pulmonary venous return
- Iatrogenic leakage around prior instrumentation

The degree of pathology imaged is influenced by the size of the defect and evolves from complications left-to-right shunting physiology. Closure is indicated in many situations given the risk of paradoxical emboli causing a cerebrovascular accident, though ASDs may also aid in decompressing the right heart as a “pop-off” in pulmonary hypertension.

Diagnostic imaging targets include a detailed functional assessment of the left and right heart comparing function and size. A defect may or may not be visible. Defects of the atrial septum are not readily assessed in apical views where the septum can be parallel to the beam and dropout of signal in the fossa ovalis, where a secundum ASD would appear. Subcostal (Fig. 33.2) and parasternal (Fig. 33.3) views are helpful sweeping through the entire septum. Defects are sometimes associated with anomalous pulmonary vein return though the sites where the veins connect can vary greatly. Targets for critical care echocardiography include assessment of left and right heart function, with right heart failure a possibility. A cardiology consultation is recommended for identification of an ASD, but techniques that may identify them include performing:

- A subcostal sweep through the septum in the long and short axis with and without color Doppler.
- A parasternal sweep in the short axis with and without color Doppler.
- Agitated saline (Bubble) study.
- An evaluation of left and right heart function.
- Areas around ASD device closures, presence of patch repair and noteworthy artifacts.

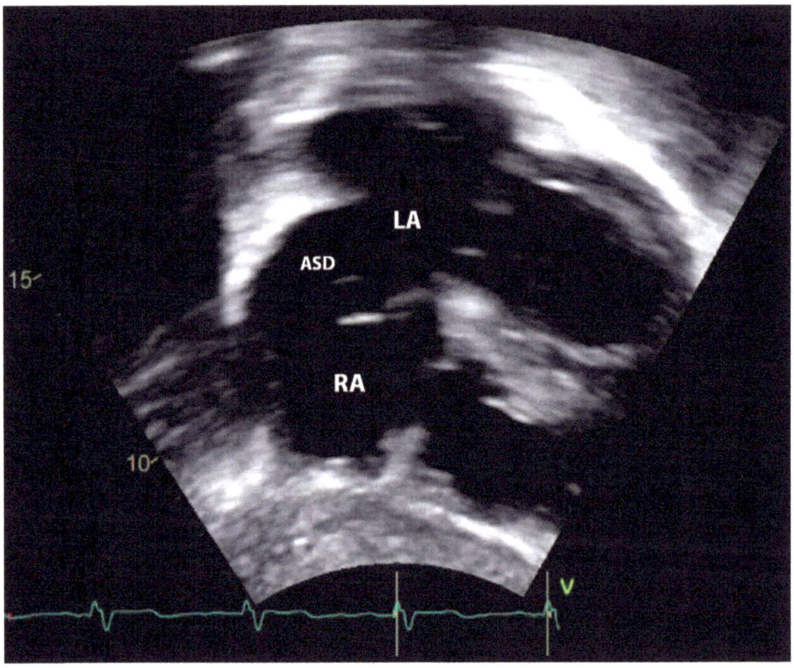

Fig. 33.2 Subcostal long axis view of 17-year-old male with previously undiagnosed secundum ASD. LA (Left Atrium), RA (Right Atrium), and ASD (Atrial Septal Defect)

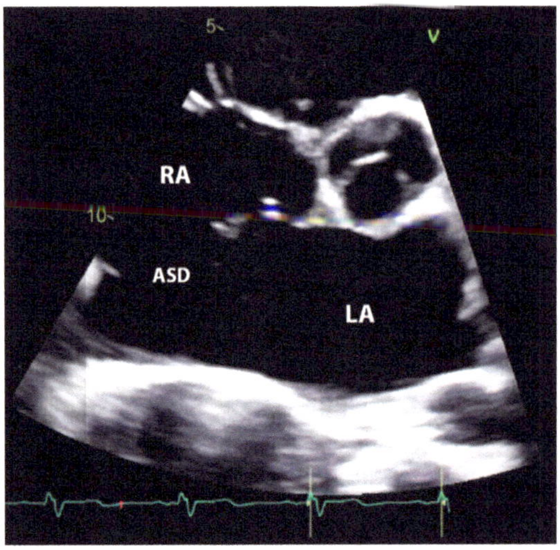

Fig. 33.3 Parasternal short axis view of 17-year-old male with previously undiagnosed secundum ASD. LA (Left Atrium), RA (Right Atrium), and ASD (Atrial Septal Defect)

Targets to note include that partial anomalous pulmonary vein return (PAPVR) can result in a continuous right-to-left shunt across an ASD independent of pulmonary hypertension. Additionally, a large coronary sinus seen in an apical view can also reflect PAPVR, as well as a left-sided SVC.

Ventricular Septal Defects (VSDs) and Atrioventricular Septal Defect (AVSD)

Ventricular septal defects (VSDs) are common in children but only comprise 10% of CHD in adults as some close through development.

There are multiple types of VSDs (Fig. 33.4), due to the conformation of the interventricular septum as a delta shaped structure curved to the contour of the left ventricle (LV) comprised of differing tissue types. Consequently defects can occur each of the five areas of the septum

- Infundibular Type 1 VSDs occur just beneath the semilunar valves and can cause prolapse of the left aortic valve cusp, resulting in aortic insufficiency.
- Membranous Type 2 VSDs are the most common VSDs in adults and occur inferior to the crista supraventricular is adjacent to the infundibular septum and therefore, are less proximate to the aortic valve but border the septal leaflet of the tricuspid valve.
- Inlet Type 3 VSDs (also known as AV canal type) are located below the AV valves but are

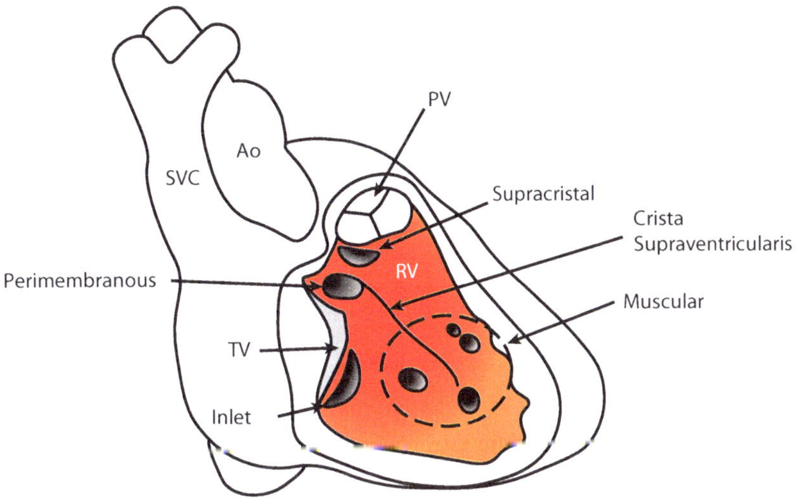

Fig. 33.4 Types of ventricular septal defects (VSDs)

not typically associated with valvular insufficiency unless the defect is an atrioventricular septal defect.

- Muscular Type 4 VSDs may appear in multiples in the muscular septum closer to the papillary muscle level of the septum.
- A Gerbode defect is a rare VSD of the atrioventricular septum that occurs in the small area of ventricular septum above the tricuspid valve and base of the right ventricle (RV) where a defect permits blood flow directly from the left ventricle to the right atria.
- VSDs can also occur as a complication of cardiac injury and/or complications of instrumentation.

Given the variety of VSD types, presentation, and imaging findings can vary significantly. In the setting of a symptomatic VSD, left to right shunting will vary based on the size of defect as well as the pressure gradient between the ventricles as pulmonary arterial hypertension may develop from increased flows. Ventricular size may not provide insights particularly in VSDs occurring in the outflow tract. Most membranous Type 2 and muscular Type 4 VSDs close in childhood with cardiac growth. Endocarditis is a possible presenting diagnosis in patients with small restrictive VSDs. With increased left to right shunting, left heart enlargement from volume overload can occur and in the progression of pulmonary hypertension right heart failure can ensue. In moderate defects, where Qp:Qs exceeds 1.5:1, left heart overload and pulmonary hypertension can develop. In severe defects where the area of the defect exceeds 75%, these patients often require surgery while infants and untreated will progress to pulmonary hypertension and Eisemenger complex more rapidly.

Typical complete echocardiogram targets include a detailed functional assessment of the left and right heart comparing function and size. The defect again may or may not be visible due to size, windows, and location. An agitated saline (bubble) study may help identify a VSD.

- Infundibular Type 1 VSDs are differentiable from perimembranous Type 2 VSDs in the parasternal short axis view at the level of the aortic valve. If looking at the aortic valve *en face* as a clock face, an infundibular VSD will appear on Doppler imaging as a jet from the aorta into the right ventricular outflow tract (RVOT) in the 11 o'clock to 3 o'clock range. A perimembranous VSD will appear as a jet from the aorta into the RV near the tricuspid valve at the 9 o'clock to 11 o'clock position. A sweeping motion up and down the Left Ventricular Outflow Tract (LVOT) in this view will be necessary to identify the VSD.

- Muscular Type 4 VSDs may be identifiable in apical, parasternal, or subcostal sweeps of the long-axis view anterior and posterior through the ventricular septum with color Doppler on and optimized.
- Inlet Type 3 VSDs and Gerbode defects can also be identified using apical sweeps with color Doppler.

It is important that indices of LV and/or RV dysfunction are assessed in critical care echocardiography, as well as the presence of pulmonary hypertension.

In pursuing complete diagnostic echocardiography, the following are assessed. The tricuspid valve orifice descends toward the apex as can be seen in multiple views and the RV cavity may not be visible in apical views in severe cases (Figs. 33.5 and 33.6). Due to its smaller size, the appearance of RV movement may overestimate its function. In critical care echocardiography, an operator should assess tricuspid valve regurgitation, and also right atrial enlargement, which may increase the chance of arrhythmias. Flow-related ASD enlargement and right-to-left shunting may predispose to paradoxical embolic event.

Problems Causing Decreased Pulmonary Blood Flow

A decrease in pulmonary blood flow is a consequence of obstruction of right heart outflow with a right-to-left diversion of blood flow to the systemic circulation. Examples including those below can include pulmonary stenosis. This results in early manifestations of cyanotic heart disease, and patients with untreated CHD in this category may see exercise intolerance and growth restriction over their lifespan potentially resulting in chronic end organ hypoxemia. A patient may experience renal and hepatic insufficiency as well clubbing.

Ebstein's Malformation (Unrepaired)

An Ebstein's Malformation occurs rarely in 1 in 20,000 births. It may be associated with intrapartum exposure to lithium. In this defect, the septal and posterior leaflets of the tricuspid valve are displaced toward the apex of the RV and the degree of this is variable, and the upper RV chamber is "atrialized" as the tricuspid valve (TV) orifice appears lower in the ventricle. This results in variable amounts of TV regurgitation. An ASD is commonly associated with Ebstein's malformation and commonly a source for right-to-left shunting.

Tetralogy of Fallot (TOF)

Tetralogy of Fallot occurs in 7% of CHD and the most common cyanotic heart disease to reach adulthood without repair. It is defined as four anatomic components consisting of pulmonary stenosis, VSD (Fig. 33.7), overriding aorta over the muscular interventricular septum, and RV hypertrophy. Methods for repair in childhood can include a transannular patch to widen the RV outflow, resection of obstructive trabecular structures, replacement of the outflow tract with a valved conduit, monocusp revision of the valve. Repairs may also require shunts or stenting for preservation of pulmonary blood flow pending complete repair. Later in life, pulmonary stenosis and/or insufficiency can develop with negative effects on RV function. In adults, repair is possible though pulmonary valve repair is often required. Symptoms early in life relate to inadequate pulmonary blood flow with right-to-left shunting and cyanosis. Later in life, RV failure can develop.

Typical full diagnostic echocardiography targets include a detailed functional assessment of the right heart evaluating the RV outflow tract and pulmonary arteries. Identification of the VSD in parasternal and apical views as mentioned above encompasses the membranous septum and passes under an overriding aortic orifice. Coronary artery position and aortic arch position is identified as these can be abnormal. It is also

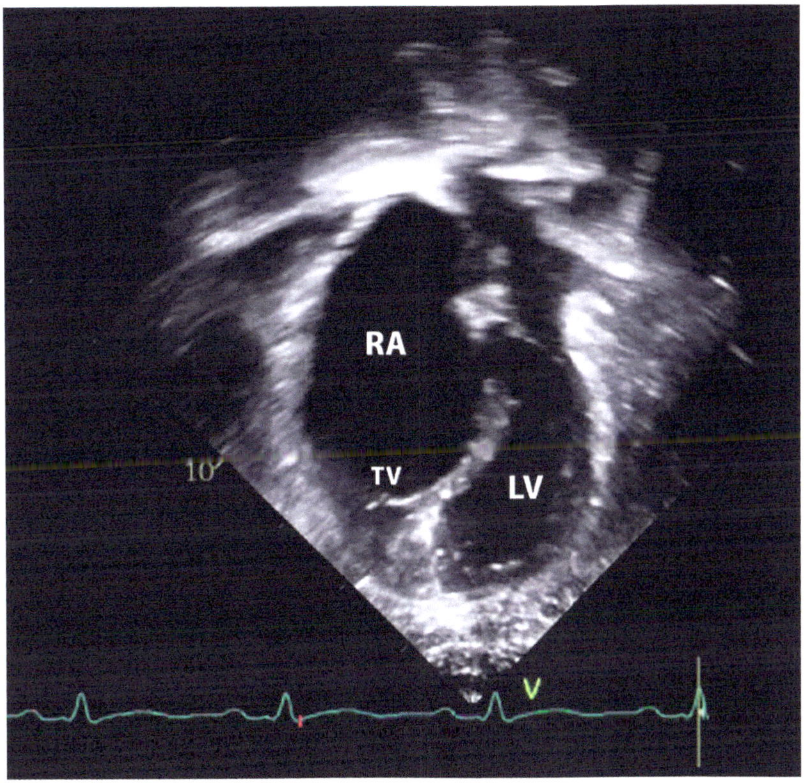

Fig. 33.5 Apical four-Chamber view of 17-year-old female with Ebstein's malformation. Note apical displacement of the tricuspid valve and large atrialized portion of the RV. Right atrium (RA), tricuspid valve (TV), and left ventricle (LV)

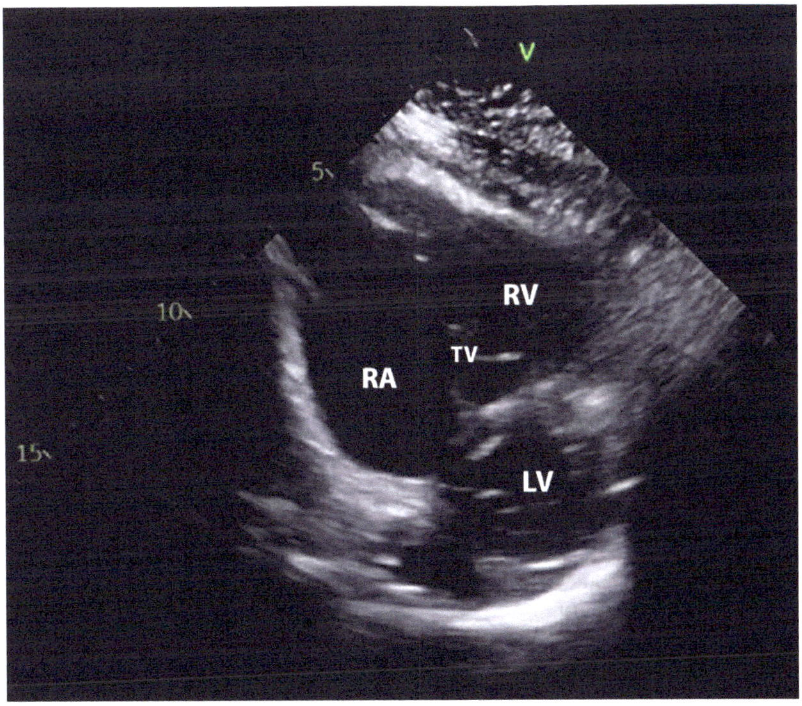

Fig. 33.6 Parasternal short axis view of 17-year-old female with Ebstein's malformation. Right atrium (RA), tricuspid valve (TV), right ventricle (RV), and left ventricle (LV)

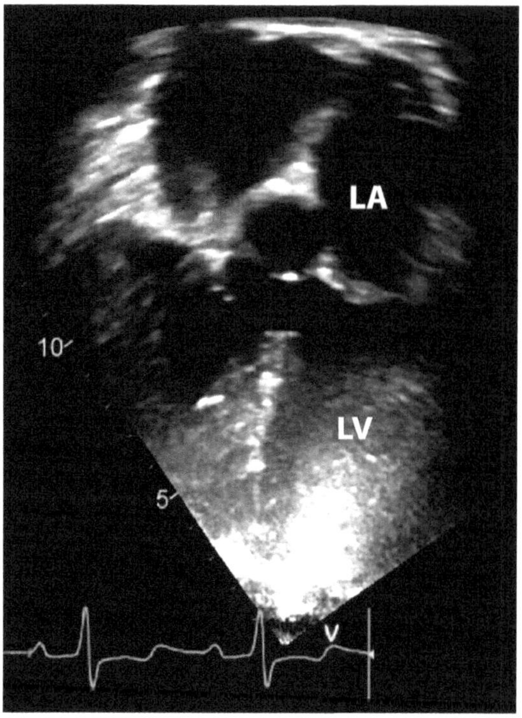

Fig. 33.7 Apical five-Chamber view of the patient with unrepaired Tetralogy of Fallot, demonstrating overriding aorta over VSD. Left atrium (LA) and left ventricle (LV)

associated with aorto-pulmonary collateralization and these large collaterals are potentially visualizable. Additionally, ASDs are possible and are evaluated for features that should be recognized in critical care echocardiography include the assessment of right ventricular function and its loading status given the nature of the abnormality.

Problems Causing Obstruction to Blood Flow

Anomalies of the left heart outflow lead to obstruction of systemic perfusion that lead to shock and heart failure. In the adult, the degree of shock is either survivably mild or progressively worsens over the lifespan.

Bicuspid Aortic Valve

At 1% of the population, this is one of the most common congenital heart defects. It may occur alone or with other defects. In patients with bicuspid aortic valve, fusion of the left and the right coronary leaflets is most common. However, fusion of the right and the noncoronary leaflets is associated with greater valve dysfunction. These patients may develop valve calcification, stenosis and/or regurgitation, subsequently resulting in root dilatation. Bicuspid aortic valve is also an independent risk factor for aortic dissection as well as endocarditis.

Typical echo targets for assessment of bicuspid aortic valve include detailed views of valve morphology. These consist of a variety of views including those in the parasternal short axis at the aortic valve level that can identify fusion of the valve leaflets (Figs. 33.8, 33.9, 33.10, and 33.11). Parasternal long axis views focusing on the aortic valve can help identify dilation of the aortic root as well as valvular insufficiency and abnormal leaflet excursion. A complete evaluation of left ventricular functional exam is indicated given the effect of aortic stenosis on afterload and regurgitation on preload. There is the potential for a Type A (DeBakey I or II) dissection involving the ascending aorta and this can potentially be evaluated using arch views..

Features that need to be recognized in critical care echocardiography include a significantly dilated aortic root and left ventricular function.

Coarctation of the Aorta

Coarctation occurs in 4% of congenital heart disease and can be repaired using a variety of techniques. These include end to end anastomosis, a subclavian flap repair using a segment of sacrificed subclavian artery to widen the coarctation site, patch angioplasty, or an interposition graft for restoring aortic patency. The physiology of

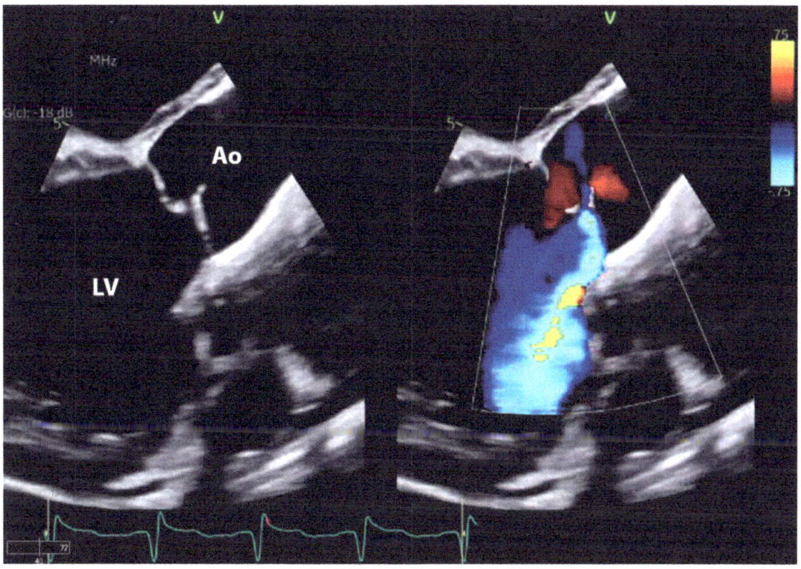

Fig. 33.8 Parasternal short axis view at the aortic valve level of a 16-year-old male demonstrating bicuspid aortic valve and fusion of the right and left aortic valve leaflets. Aorta (Ao) and left ventricle (LV)

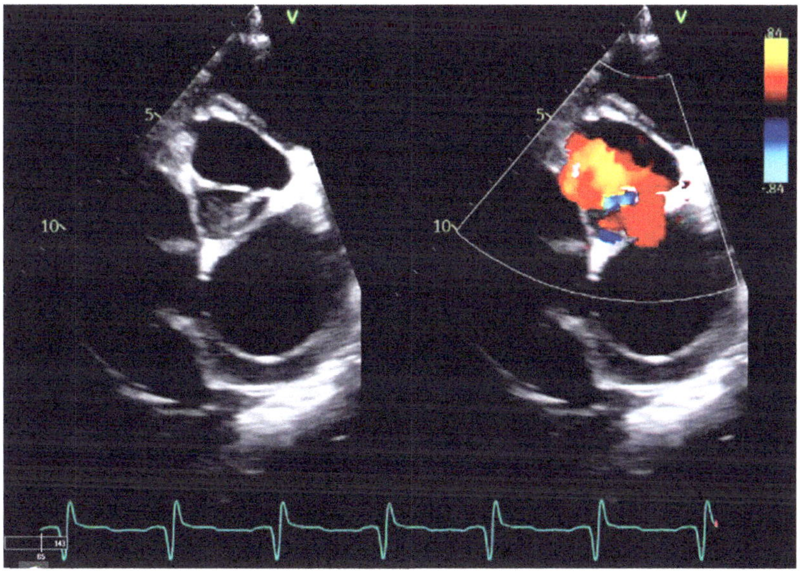

Fig. 33.9 Color Doppler of Parasternal long axis view of 16-year-old male with bicuspid aortic valve demonstrating moderate-severe aortic insufficiency

coarctation involves aortic intimal thickening and hyperplasia that obstructs the aortic lumen. Patients who do not receive repair can manifest systemic hypertension, coronary artery disease, stroke, aortic dissection, and heart failure. It is also a risk factor for endocarditis.

Typical echocardiography targets include evaluation of left ventricular function, as well as a detailed arch examination performed with high parasternal or suprasternal views to identify the coarctation. The coarctation appears in the proximal descending thoracic arch and is

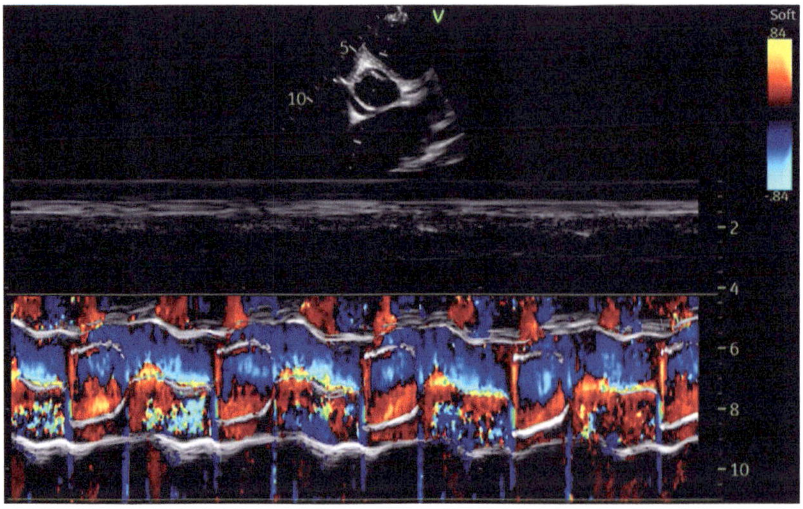

Fig. 33.10 Color Doppler M-Mode through the valve demonstrating AI during diastole

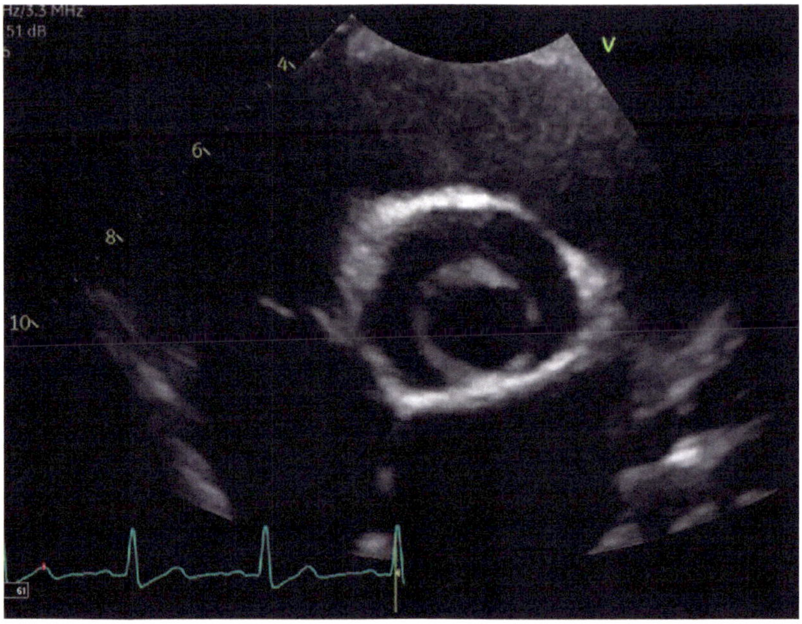

Fig. 33.11 Parasternal short axis view at the aortic valve level of a 16-year-old male demonstrating monocusp aortic valve, notice circular cross-section of annulus in systole

identified with 2D imaging and color Doppler. A stenosis pattern can be seen in aortic flow proximal to the coarctation where the peak flow increases between the area proximal (Fig. 33.12) to and the area distal (Fig. 33.13) to the coarctation. In the area proximal to the coarctation, flow in systole extends into the diastolic phase of the cardiac cycle whereas it is dampened in diastole distal to the coarctation. In the older unrepaired patient, collateralization around the coarctation can diminish coarctation gradients and magnitude of findings though heart failure is still a risk.

Features that need to be recognized include evidence of global or regional left ventricular dysfunction as well as the aortic Doppler features mentioned above. They would likely be consistent with exam findings of diminished lower extremity pulses.

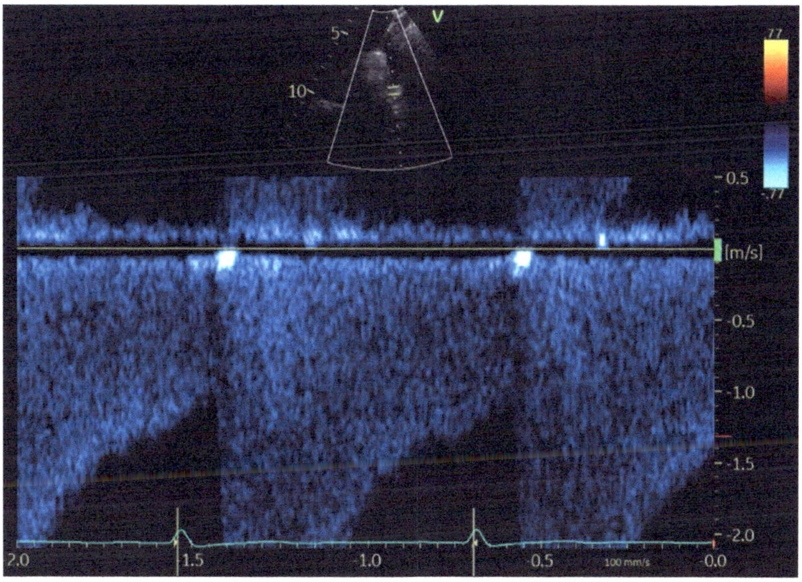

Fig. 33.12 Spectral Doppler of transverse aortic arch in a 17-year-old male with untreated coarctation of the aorta demonstrating pronounced systolic amplitude and prolongation of ejection into diastole

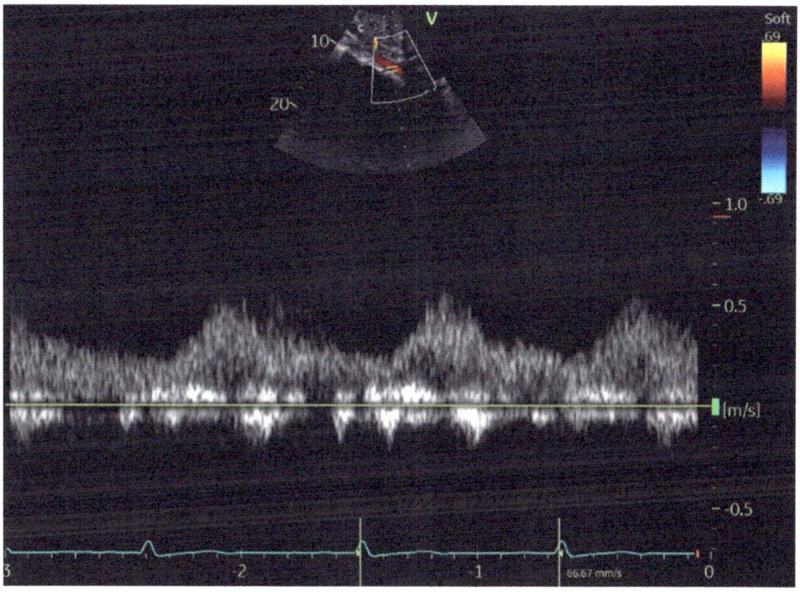

Fig. 33.13 Spectral Doppler of descending aorta in the same 17-year-old male as in Fig. 33.10 demonstrating marked dampening of systolic peak compared to previous

Summary

Identification of congenital heart defects is heavily dependent on an excellent working knowledge of normal cardiac anatomy and function, as well as advanced qualitative and quantitative skills in echocardiography. As POCUS becomes increasingly used in initial hemodynamic assessment, some recognition of congenital abnormalities and their physiological sequelae is likely appropriate for optimal evaluation and management of critically ill patients.

References

1. Wiyono SA, Witsenburg M, de Jaegere PP, Roos-Hesselink JW. Patent ductus arteriosus in adults: case report and review illustrating the spectrum of the disease. Neth Heart J. 2008;16(7–8):255–9. https://doi.org/10.1007/BF03086157. PMID: 18711613; PMCID: PMC2516289

Further Reading

Mulder BJ. Epidemiology of adult congenital heart disease: demographic variations worldwide. Neth Heart J. 2012;20(12):505–8. https://doi.org/10.1007/s12471-012-0335-1. PMID: 23225563; PMCID: PMC3515732

Gilboa SM, Devine OJ, Kucik JE, Oster ME, Riehle-Colarusso T, Nembhard WN, Xu P, Correa A, Jenkins K, Marelli AJ. Congenital heart defects in the United States: estimating the magnitude of the affected population in 2010. Circulation. 2016;134(2):101–9. https://doi.org/10.1161/CIRCULATIONAHA.115.019307. Epub 2016 Jul 5. PMID: 27382105; PMCID: PMC4942347

Part III

Ultrasonography

Effusion

34

Nicholas A. Leverone and Daniel A. Sweeney

Learning Objectives

1. Learn how to perform an ultrasound exam to identify pleural fluid in a critically ill patient
2. Learn methods to estimate pleural fluid volume with bedside ultrasound
3. Recognize and interpret sonographic characteristics of pleural fluid
4. Understand how Point-of-care ultrasound (POCUS) can inform pleural fluid management decisions including whether to place a chest tube; in the future, POCUS may prove to be useful in identifying patients who would be best served with video-assisted thoracoscopic surgery

Ultrasound Technique for Identifying Pleural Fluid

Patient and Machine Positioning

In the intensive care unit (ICU) bedside ultrasound examination for the identification and treatment of pleural effusions should be performed with the patient in a supine or semi-recumbent position (Fig. 34.1a). Machine placement is variable. Some experts advocate having both the examiner and ultrasound machine on the patient's right side so that the examiner is holding the probe in their dominant right hand and manipulating ultrasound buttons with their left hand. Alternatively, if the examiner stands on one side of the patient and places the machine on the opposite side of the patient then the patient and the machine are in the same line of sight, similar to how an interventional cardiologist performs a cardiac catheterization. While this position makes live imaging more intuitive to interpret and is optimal for ultrasound guided procedures, it does require either using two operators or the examiner must reach across the patient to manipulate ultrasound controls.

Scanning Technique

A low frequency (2–5 MHz) phased array probe (cardiac or abdominal preset) is used as this provides adequate penetration and the small footprint allows for the probe to be positioned in between ribs. The probe should be held in the horizontal orientation in the palm of the hand that is resting on the patient's bed (Fig. 34.1b). Scanning is performed along the posterior axillary line as free-flowing dependent fluid will settle in the posterior chest of a supine patient. After first identifying the liver (right side) or the spleen (left side), the probe is moved cephalad from one

N. A. Leverone · D. A. Sweeney (✉)
Division of Pulmonary, Critical Care, Sleep Medicine and Physiology, Department of Medicine, University of California, San Diego, La Jolla, CA, USA
e-mail: nleverone@health.ucsd.edu

M. J. Lanspa, A. T. Levinson (eds.), *Echocardiography and Ultrasonography in the ICU*, Respiratory Medicine, https://doi.org/10.1007/978-3-031-80038-2_34

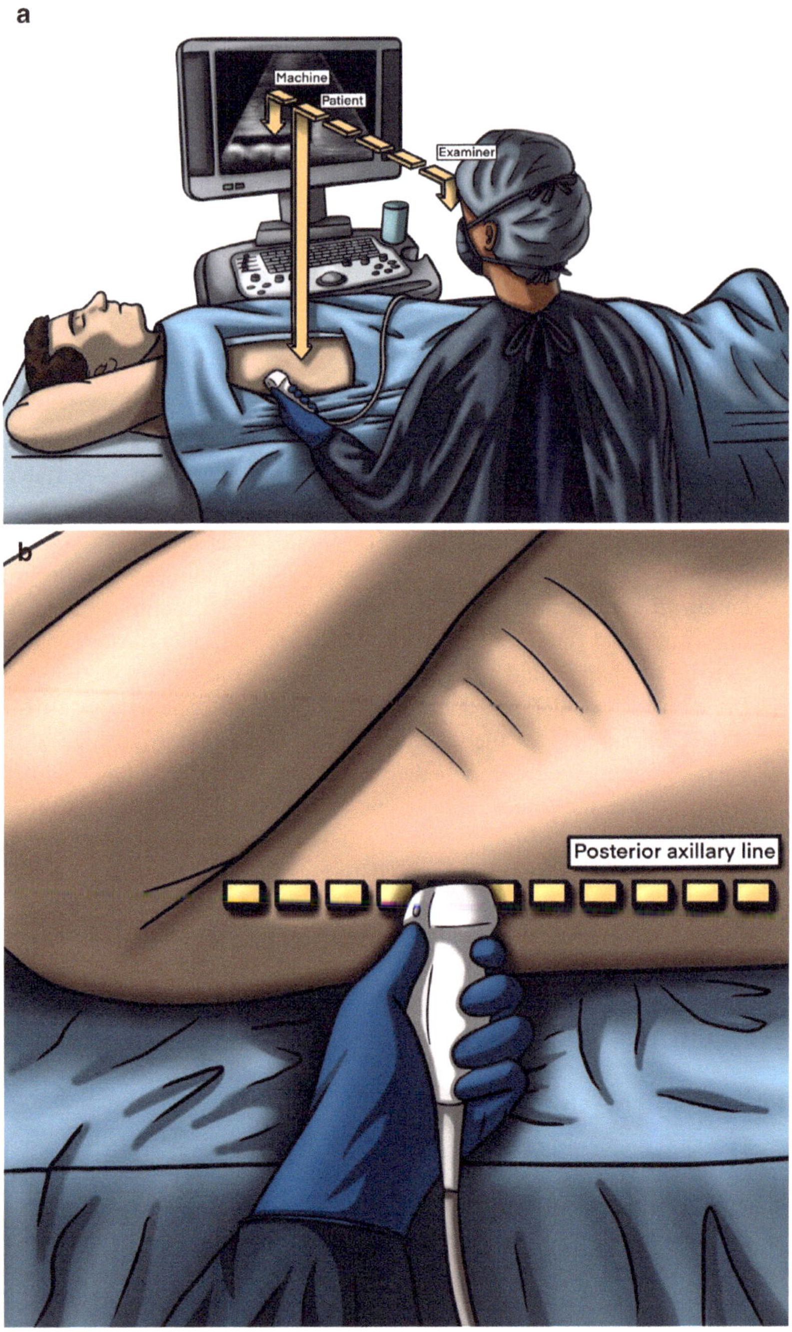

Fig. 34.1 Examiner, patient, and ultrasound machine can be positioned all along the same visual axis to prevent forcing the examiner to have to twist and turn during examination or procedure (**a**). When holding the ultrasound probe to obtain initial imaging and orientation, the probe marker should be aimed cephalad, along the posterior axillary line sliding superiorly or inferiorly to identify the diaphragm (**b**). Here you can see the dorsal aspect of the hand resting against the bed to achieve alignment with the posterior axillary line in the supine patient. Courtesy of Catherine Cichon, MD

intercostal space to another along the posterior axillary line. Within each intercostal space, the probe should be fanned anteriorly to posteriorly to fully interrogate the space.

In the absence of a pleural effusion, lung consolidation, or atelectasis at the base of the lung, the structures visualized by POCUS include: the chest wall, the dome of diaphragm, and the spine with spine shadow posterior to the liver or the spleen (Fig. 34.2). If the spine and spine shadow (referred to as “the spine sign”) are imaged cephalad to the diaphragm, this necessarily means that pathology

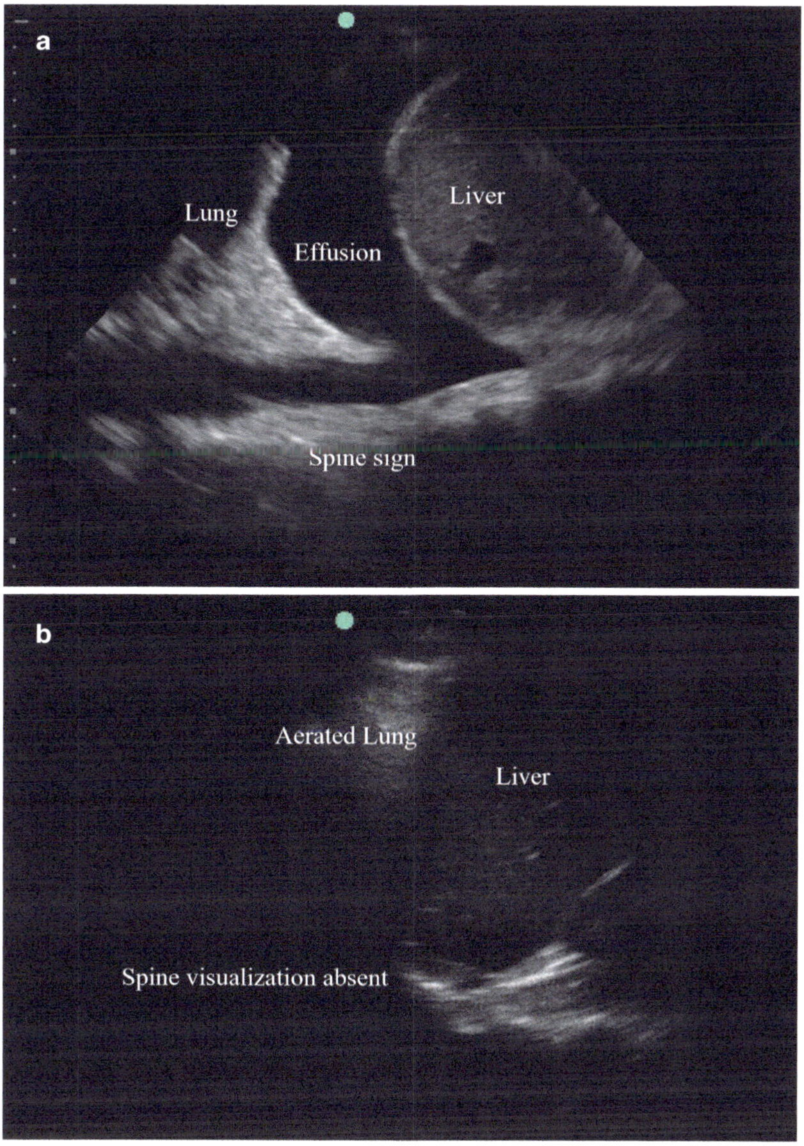

Fig. 34.2 Landmarks in the presence (**a**) and absence (**b**) of pleural effusion demonstrating visualization of spine sign in the presence of intrathoracic pathology. Consolidated lung and fluid both allow transmission of ultrasound waves, permitting visualization of deeper structures normally impossible to see through aerated lung tissue

is present in the chest cavity. This is because normally ultrasound waves do not transmit through aerated lung, preventing visualization of the underlying spine. The **spine sign** occurs when consolidation, atelectatic lung, pleural effusion, or some combination of these is present making it possible to visualize the vertebral column through the thoracic cavity. When a pleural effusion is present, then both the fluid and accompanying "drowned" lung will be visible via POCUS. In the event that the ultrasound image is saved, radiology convention dictates that the image be orientated such that the left side of the image is cephalad and the right side is caudad; if for some reason the saved image violates this convention, then simply label the picture accordingly.

Quantification of Pleural Fluid Volume Using Ultrasound

The volume of a pleural effusion has implications for clinical management in critical care. Studies have shown that the drainage of effusions greater than 500 mL result in significant improvement in patient oxygenation and respiratory mechanics, including lung compliance and end expiratory lung volume, although these benefits are likely reduced in patients with acute respiratory distress syndrome (ARDS) [1–5]. While there is no agreed upon method of using POCUS to estimate the volume of a pleural effusion in a critically ill, supine patient, a handful of approaches have been proposed [4, 6, 7]. In general, these investigators have derived formulas for estimating the volume of the effusion based upon the maximal inter-pleural distance separating the surface of the drowned lung and the chest wall, using a transverse/axial image (i.e., probe placed along posterior axillary line and oriented perpendicular to the axis of the patient similar to a chest CT image) (Fig. 34.3). In one study by Balik et al, the maximal distance ("Sep") separating drowned lung (at the lung base) from the chest wall was measured at the end of expiration in 81 mechanically ventilated patients, who subsequently underwent thoracentesis with complete drainage of their pleural effusions. The authors derived a formula to estimate the pleural effusion volume: Volume (mL) = 20 × Sep(mm) showing a positive correlation between Sep and effusion volume (R = 0.72, R^2 = 0.52; P < 0.001)) [6]. Thus, a Sep ≥ 25 mm would suggest an effusion volume of at least 500 mL. In clinical practice, however, qualitative volume assessment (i.e., small, medium, or large) of the pleural effusion with ultrasound is more commonly used.

Characterization of Pleural Fluid Based on Ultrasound Imaging

Pleural fluid ultrasound characteristics are described along a spectrum ranging from anechoic (black fluid), complex nonseptated (echogenic debris heterogenously present but without loculations), complex septated (loculations present) to complex homogeneously echogenic fluid pattern (echogenic material with brightness approaching that of soft tissue) (Fig. 34.4) [8–10].

Transudative Versus Exudative Fluid

Bedside ultrasound image characteristics of pleural fluid cannot always predict whether an effusion is a transudate or exudate. Across studies, complex homogeneous echogenic effusions are uniformly exudative and the presence of septated fluid is highly predictive for exudative fluid (positive predictive value of ≥89%) [8–11]. Unfortunately, the appearance of anechoic or complex nonseptated fluid is not reliably informative in terms of whether a pleural collection is transudative or exudative. Traditionally, anechoic fluid was thought to be highly suggestive of a transudate; however, more recent studies do not support this finding [10]. Furthermore, differences in gain and other control settings chosen by the operator, as well as advances in ultrasound image quality have made it challenging to uniformly discern between anechoic and complex nonseptated fluid. Measuring pixel intensity of pleural fluid ultrasound images is another possible tool for differentiating transudative versus exudative effusions [12, 13]. However, this technology is not yet widely available on commercial ultrasound machines.

Malignant Fluid

While it has been suggested that a swirling pattern of complex nonseptated fluid pleural fluid is suggestive of a malignant effusion in patients with an underlying diagnosis of cancer, others have identified this finding in both patients with exudative (nonmalignant) and transudative effusions [14, 15]. Instead of the ultrasound character of the fluid, more telling signs suggestive of a malignant effusion involve the pleura and include pleural thickening >1 cm, pleural nodularity, and diaphragmatic thickening >7 mm [16].

Empyema

One of the most important and time sensitive questions to answer, following identification of

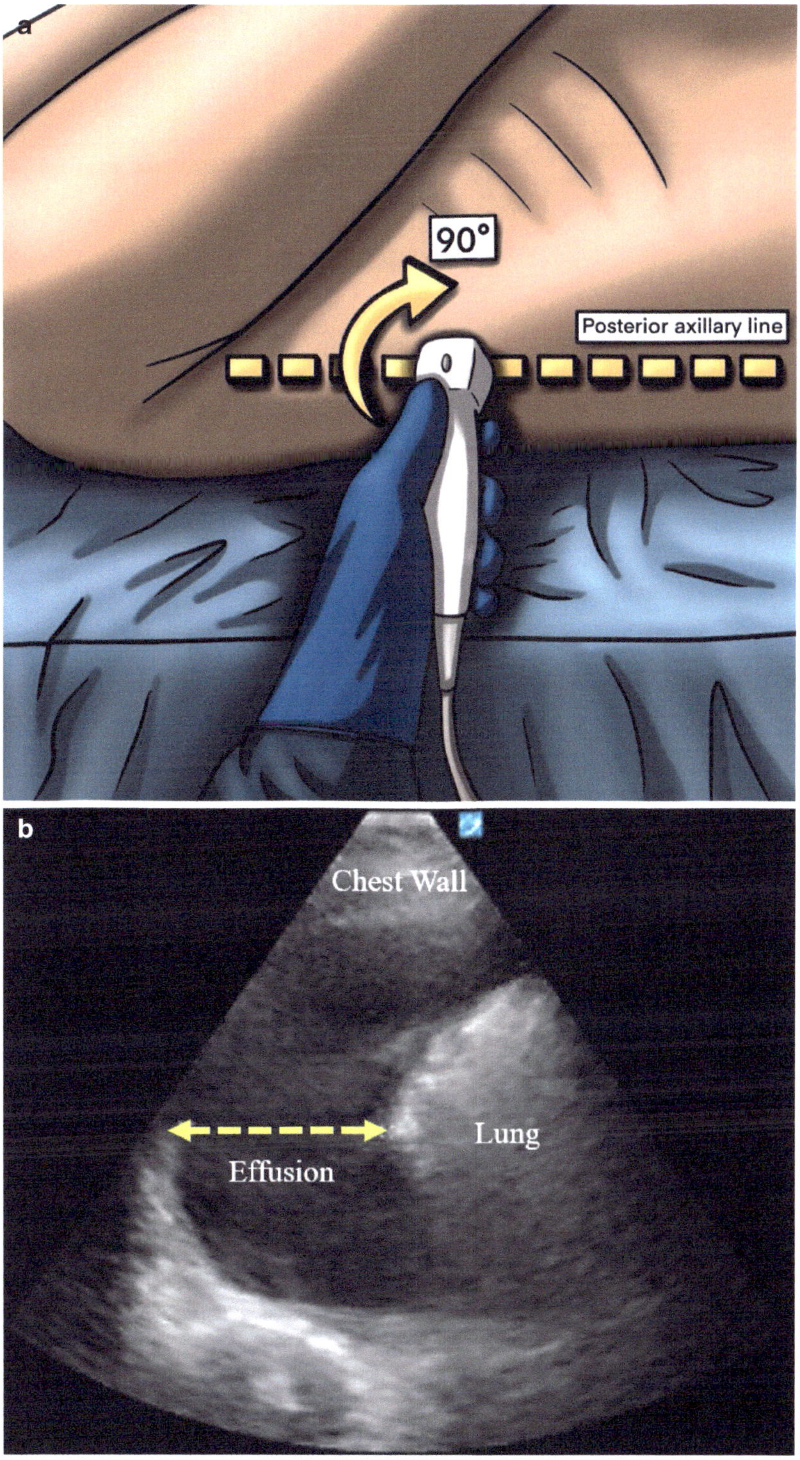

Fig. 34.3 In order to perform quantification of pleural fluid using the Balik or similar formulas, the transducer probe must be rotated 90 degrees (**a**) in order to measure the distance between the parietal and visceral pleura as visualized similar to axial CT imaging (**b**). In the case of the Balik formula, the maximal end-expiratory distance between parietal and visceral pleura (Sep) is used in the equation: pleural effusion volume (mL) = 20 × Sep (mm). Courtesy of Catherine Cichon, MD

pleural fluid, is whether or not the collection represents an empyema, as early source control with chest tube placement is crucial. In a study of 94 patients with fever and a pleural effusion, 118 diagnostic thoracentesis were performed and 15 empyemas were identified [11]. There were no

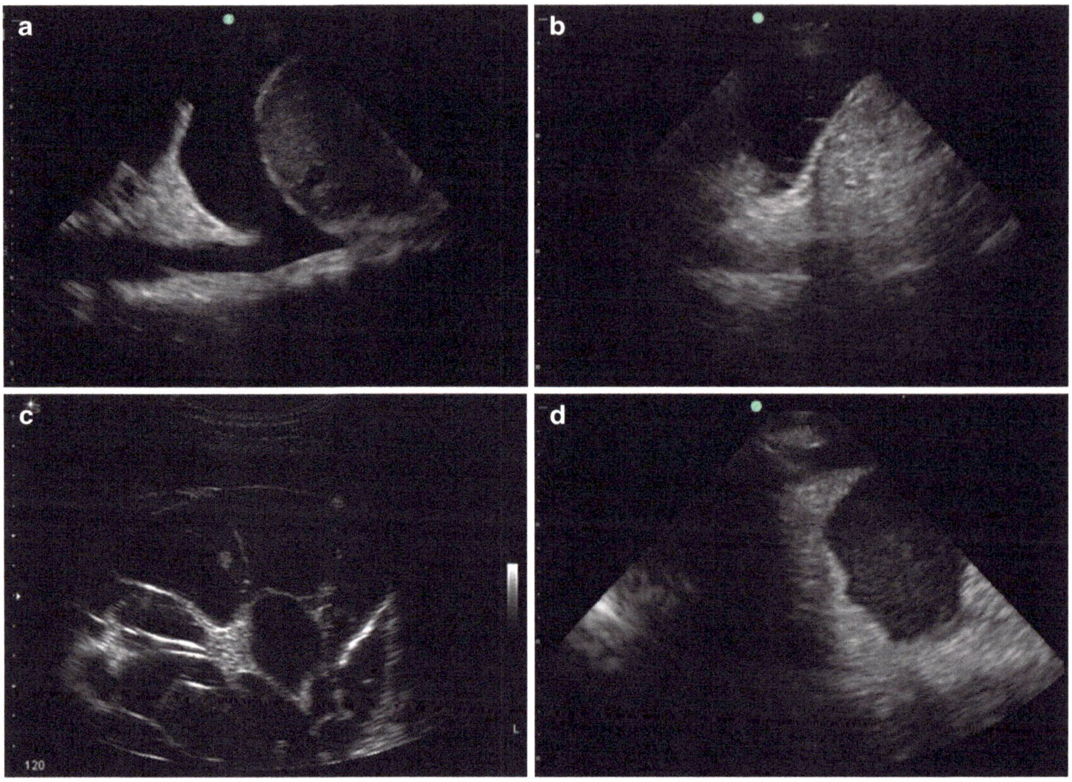

Fig. 34.4 Pleural fluid quality can be described along a spectrum based on the complexity and heterogeneity of the fluid. Here you can see examples of anechoic (**a**), complex nonseptated (**b**), complex septated (**c**), and complex homogeneously echogenic fluid (**d**). The characteristics of the visualized fluid can lend to the differential, such as anechoic fluid almost never seen in patients with empyema

empyemas in cases in which the fluid was either anechoic (0/47 cases) or complex nonseptated and relatively hypoechoic (0/36 cases). This study strongly suggests that the diagnosis of an empyema can be safely excluded in patients with anechoic fluid. Moreover, the authors demonstrated the value of serial POCUS exam to assess pleural effusion characteristics. There were three cases of empyemas in which the initial thoracentesis revealed sterile fluid, but because these patients remained febrile, a repeat thoracentesis was performed and the diagnosis of an empyema was made on a subsequent fluid sampling. In each of these cases, the ultrasound fluid characteristics became more complex or more hyperechoic between the time the initial and repeat thoracenteses were performed.

Ultrasound to Guide the Management of Pleural Effusions

POCUS should be viewed as an additional, complementary imaging tool to chest radiography (CXR) and chest computed topography (CT) in the management of pleural effusions. The volume of a pleural effusion is a factor in deciding whether to place a chest tube; likewise determining if other interventions such as diuretic therapy are effectively decreasing pleural effusion volume can also be vital information to patient management. Bedside ultrasound can answer both these, and other clinical questions in relation to the pleural space. POCUS can also rule out the presence of an empyema when anechoic fluid is present. However, this does not obviate the need for repeat

POCUS assessment of an effusion if such a patient fails to improve, as changes in ultrasound imaging can herald the development of an empyema.

Compared to free-flowing pleural effusions, there is greater uncertainty surrounding the optimal management of empyemas or complex parapneumonic effusions. Specifically, there is some controversy regarding the decision to treat these effusions with chest tube placement and intrapleural fibrinolytic therapy, or instead proceed directly to video-assisted thoracoscopic surgery (VATS) [17]. While chest tube drainage combined with intrapleural therapy is commonly used as the initial approach for the treatment of complicated pleural effusions, failure rates have been reported to occur in up to 22–32% of cases [18, 19]. However, POCUS imaging could potentially aid in determining the best initial management strategy for patients with empyemas. Loculations in the form of septations are more readily visualized using POCUS compared to CT, and the appearance of sonographic septations is predictive of the outcome of simple catheter drainage for the treatment of empyemas and complicated parapneumonic effusions [20–26]. Additionally, analysis of the pixel intensity of pleural fluid ultrasound images has been shown to correlate with the duration of the chest tube drainage, days until apyrexia, and total length of hospitalization [13]. Thus, it is possible that POCUS could have a growing role in guiding the initial treatment of loculated effusions in terms of whether to begin with medical therapy or proceed directly to VATS.

Summary Points

- Lung ultrasound is an essential tool for identifying, characterizing, and managing pleural effusions in the critically ill patient.
- Ultrasound scanning of pleural effusion and ultrasound-guided procedures can be performed safely with the critically ill patient in the supine position.
- Pleural effusions are common in the ICU and their identification can be helpful in understanding the pathology of a critically ill patient.
- Lung ultrasound is more sensitive than CXR for identifying the presence of a pleural effusion and can be used to estimate the volume of an effusion.
- Ultrasound image characteristics aid in predicting whether a fluid collection is exudative, transudative, or may represent an empyema.
- Both the estimated size and the ultrasound image characteristics of a pleural effusion can be helpful in deciding whether to perform a thoracentesis versus placing a thoracostomy tube.
- While complicated pleural fluid can be identified using bedside ultrasound this information has not yet been shown to inform the decision of whether to place a chest tube or proceed to video-assisted thoracoscopic surgery.

Pro-Tips Call Outs

POCUS imaging has been shown to be remarkably sensitive for the detection of pleural effusions and volume is easily estimated either quantitatively or qualitatively.

Recognize the importance of finding a spine shadow cephalad to the diaphragm as this unequivocally means there is pathology in the chest cavity—lung atelectasis, consolidation, or a pleural effusion.

Large effusions can be estimated using various formulas or qualitative assessment.

In one well done study, the finding of only anechoic fluid ruled out the possibility of an empyema.

Evolving Evidence

Defining the optimal management of complicated, loculated effusion has been elusive with advocates for VATS versus chest tube being the two primary options. Septations and debris can be easily identified using POCUS. Ultrasound characterization of pleural fluid has the potential to guide this initial management decision.

References

1. Chiumello D, Marino A, Cressoni M, Mietto C, Berto V, Gallazzi E, Chiurazzi C, Lazzerini M, Cadringher P, Quintel M, Gattinoni L. Pleural effusion in patients with acute lung injury: a CT scan study. Crit Care Med. 2013;41(4):935–44.

2. Goligher EC, Leis JA, Fowler RA, Pinto R, Adhikari NK, Ferguson ND. Utility and safety of draining pleural effusions in mechanically ventilated patients: a systematic review and meta-analysis. Crit Care. 2011;15(1):R46.
3. Razazi K, Thille AW, Carteaux G, Beji O, Brun-Buisson C, Brochard L, Mekontso Dessap A. Effects of pleural effusion drainage on oxygenation, respiratory mechanics, and hemodynamics in mechanically ventilated patients. Ann Am Thorac Soc. 2014;11(7):1018–24.
4. Roch A, Bojan M, Michelet P, Romain F, Bregeon F, Papazian L, Auffray JP. Usefulness of ultrasonography in predicting pleural effusions > 500 mL in patients receiving mechanical ventilation. Chest. 2005;127(1):224–32.
5. Talmor M, Hydo L, Gershenwald JG, Barie PS. Beneficial effects of chest tube drainage of pleural effusion in acute respiratory failure refractory to positive end-expiratory pressure ventilation. Surgery. 1998;123(2):137–43.
6. Balik M, Plasil P, Waldauf P, Pazout J, Fric M, Otahal M, Pachl J. Ultrasound estimation of volume of pleural fluid in mechanically ventilated patients. Intensive Care Med. 2006;32(2):318.
7. Vignon P, Chastagner C, Berkane V, Chardac E, Francois B, Normand S, Bonnivard M, Clavel M, Pichon N, Preux PM, Maubon A, Gastinne H. Quantitative assessment of pleural effusion in critically ill patients by means of ultrasonography. Crit Care Med. 2005;33(8):1757–63.
8. Evans AL, Gleeson FV. Radiology in pleural disease: state of the art. Respirology. 2004;9(3):300–12.
9. Shkolnik B, Judson MA, Austin A, Hu K, D'Souza M, Zumbrunn A, Huggins JT, Yucel R, Chopra A. Diagnostic accuracy of thoracic ultrasonography to differentiate transudative from exudative pleural effusion. Chest. 2020;158(2):692–7.
10. Yang PC, Luh KT, Chang DB, Wu HD, Yu CJ, Kuo SH. Value of sonography in determining the nature of pleural effusion: analysis of 320 cases. AJR Am J Roentgenol. 1992;159(1):29–33.
11. Tu CY, Hsu WH, Hsia TC, Chen HJ, Tsai KD, Hung CW, Shih CM. Pleural effusions in febrile medical ICU patients: chest ultrasound study. Chest. 2004;126(4):1274–80.
12. Soni NJ, Dreyfuss ZS, Ali S, Enenmoh A, Proud KC, Mader MJ, Velez MI, Smith SB, Peters JI, Restrepo MI. Pleural fluid echogenicity measured by ultrasound image pixel density to differentiate transudative vs. exudative pleural effusions. Ann Am Thorac Soc. 2022;19(5):857–60.
13. Varsamas C, Kalkanis A, Gourgoulianis KI, Malli F. The use of a novel quantitative marker of echogenicity of pleural fluid in parapneumonic pleural effusions. Can Respir J. 2020;2020:1283590.
14. Chian CF, Su WL, Soh LH, Yan HC, Perng WC, Wu CP. Echogenic swirling pattern as a predictor of malignant pleural effusions in patients with malignancies. Chest. 2004;126(1):129–34.
15. Lane AB, Petteys S, Ginn M, Nations JA. Clinical importance of echogenic swirling pleural effusions. J Ultrasound Med. 2016;35(4):843–7.
16. Qureshi NR, Rahman NM, Gleeson FV. Thoracic ultrasound in the diagnosis of malignant pleural effusion. Thorax. 2009;64(2):139–43.
17. Godfrey MS, Bramley KT, Detterbeck F. Medical and surgical management of empyema. Semin Respir Crit Care Med. 2019;40(3):361–74.
18. Kheir F, Cheng G, Rivera E, Folch A, Folch E, Fernandez-Bussy S, Keyes C, Parikh M, Channick C, Chee A, Majid A. Concurrent versus sequential intrapleural instillation of tissue plasminogen activator and deoxyribonuclease for pleural infection. J Bronchol Interv Pulmonol. 2018;25(2):125–31.
19. Khemasuwan D, Sorensen J, Griffin DC. Predictive variables for failure in administration of intrapleural tissue plasminogen activator/deoxyribonuclease in patients with complicated parapneumonic effusions/empyema. Chest. 2018;154(3):550–6.
20. Chen CH, Chen W, Chen HJ, Yu YH, Lin YC, Tu CY, Hsu WH. Transthoracic ultrasonography in predicting the outcome of small-bore catheter drainage in empyemas or complicated parapneumonic effusions. Ultrasound Med Biol. 2009;35(9):1468–74.
21. McLoud TC, Flower CD. Imaging the pleura: sonography, CT, and MR imaging. AJR Am J Roentgenol. 1991;156(6):1145–53.
22. Esmadi M, Lone N, Ahmad DS, Onofrio J, Brush RG. Multiloculated pleural effusion detected by ultrasound only in a critically-ill patient. Am J Case Rep. 2013;14:63–6.
23. Grimberg A, Shigueoka DC, Atallah AN, Ajzen S, Iared W. Diagnostic accuracy of sonography for pleural effusion: systematic review. Sao Paulo Med J. 2010;128(2):90–5.
24. Kearney SE, Davies CW, Davies RJ, Gleeson FV. Computed tomography and ultrasound in parapneumonic effusions and empyema. Clin Radiol. 2000;55(7):542–7.
25. Mattison LE, Coppage L, Alderman DF, Herlong JO, Sahn SA. Pleural effusions in the medical ICU: prevalence, causes, and clinical implications. Chest. 1997;111(4):1018–23.
26. Rothlin MA, Naf R, Amgwerd M, Candinas D, Frick T, Trentz O. Ultrasound in blunt abdominal and thoracic trauma. J Trauma. 1993;34(4):488–95.

35 Point-of-Care Ultrasound for the Diagnosis of Pneumothorax

Joel Turner

Learning Objectives

1. Pneumothorax (PTx) is a potentially life-threatening diagnosis in patients complaining of chest pain and dyspnea.
2. Undiagnosed, pneumothorax can lead to significant morbidity and mortality if not rapidly managed accordingly.
3. Current methods of diagnosis, including physical exam and chest X-ray, are insensitive in identifying pneumothoraces.
4. Lung point of care ultrasound has been used for over 15 years for the accurate and rapid bedside diagnosis of pneumothorax.
5. Lung ultrasound for the rapid diagnosis of pneumothorax has diagnostic sensitivities approaching those of CT.
6. By recognizing the presence or absence of lung sliding, B-line artefacts, lung pulse, and lung points, a trained user of POCUS can detect or rule out pneumothorax within a few minutes.

Supplementary Information The online version contains supplementary material available at https://doi.org/10.1007/978-3-031-80038-2_35.

J. Turner (✉)
Department of Emergency Medicine, Jewish General Hospital, McGill University, Montreal, QC, Canada

Introduction

Dyspnea and acute chest pain are among the most common, potentially dangerous, symptoms that physicians are faced to diagnose on a daily basis. While the differential diagnosis is extensive, there are only a handful of potential diagnoses which require rapid, accurate recognition. These include acute myocardial infarction (AMI), Pulmonary embolism (PE), acute exacerbation of chronic obstructive lung disease (AECOPD), Pneumonia, pericarditis, and of course pneumothorax.

Pneumothorax occurs when air is introduced into the pleural space. This can occur spontaneously, or following a traumatic event. In all cases, depending on the size of the pneumothorax, pain and respiratory difficulty can ensue. However, if the air within the pleural space is under positive pressure, this results in a tension pneumothorax which can quickly lead to cardiorespiratory collapse. A patient with a tension pneumothorax requires urgent recognition and management. Traditionally, the diagnosis of pneumothorax is done through the combination of auscultation and chest X-ray (CXR). Unfortunately, the literature has repeatedly shown that these modalities are very poor at ruling out pneumothorax, which can lead to significant morbidity and/or mortality. While computer tomography (CT) remains the gold standard for pneumothorax diagnosis, it is expensive, time consuming, and often not feasi-

M. J. Lanspa, A. T. Levinson (eds.), *Echocardiography and Ultrasonography in the ICU*, Respiratory Medicine, https://doi.org/10.1007/978-3-031-80038-2_35

ble or readily available. Over the past 15 years, point-of-care ultrasound (POCUS) of the lung has been shown to be significantly more accurate than exam findings and CXR at diagnosing pneumothorax. As a result of this, along with it being a rapid and safe test to perform, lung POCUS has become an essential bedside tool to timely assess the possibility of pneumothorax.

This chapter will review the current understanding of lung POCUS in the diagnosis of pneumothorax. We will review the basic concepts of lung sonography, discuss the techniques to perform lung POCUS to rule out pneumothorax, and review the findings of the normal and pathologic lung.

Background

Pneumothorax is often classified based on its etiology. A primary spontaneous pneumothorax (PSP) is defined as occurring without any precipitating event and in the absence of any known lung disease. These are relatively common, tend to occur in younger males (tall stature), with an incidence that ranges between 34 and 52 cases per 100,000 population [1, 2]. Secondary spontaneous pneumothorax (SSP) occurs as a result of underlying lung disease, and is much more common in adults and in the elderly [3]. By far, the most common cause of SSP is COPD, associated with 50–70% of all cases [3, 4]. Other causes of SSP include cystic fibrosis, lung malignancy, interstitial lung disease, and necrotizing pulmonary infection.

Trauma is probably the most common overall cause of pneumothorax. These can be caused by either blunt, or more commonly penetrating external trauma, or through iatrogenic mechanisms following an invasive procedure performed in the hospital setting [5].

Iatrogenic pneumothoraces are an important cause of pneumothorax, occurring more often in teaching vs non-teaching hospitals [6]. The most common procedure causing pneumothorax is central venous catheterization (if venous access, dialysis catheterization, transvenous pacemaker insertion), followed by thoracentesis, and mechanical ventilation-induced barotrauma. Together, these three procedures account for approximately 75% of hospital-acquired pneumothorax [7, 8].

Historically, the diagnosis of pneumothorax starts with history and physical exam, followed soon after by chest X-ray. In fact, it is still considered standard of practice to use chest radiography as the initial investigation to diagnose pneumothorax [9, 10].

Unfortunately, several studies confirm that radiography is extremely insensitive in detecting pneumothorax regardless of the cause. In multiple systematic reviews, comparing chest radiography to other diagnostic modalities in over 1000 patients, chest X-ray has a sensitivity and specificity of 52% and 99%, respectively [11–13].

Point-of-care ultrasound has several significant advantages for diagnosing pneumothorax. Literature confirms that the sensitivity and specificity of lung POCUS is substantially better than physical exam and especially chest X-ray [11, 12]. A 2020 Cochrane Review examining the accuracy of lung POCUS vs supine chest radiography for the diagnosis of pneumothorax examined 1271 patients from 9 studies [14]. The overall sensitivity and specificity of lung ultrasound was 91% (95% CI 85–94%) and 99% (95% CI 97–100%), respectively. This is compared to the sensitivity and specificity of chest radiography of 47% (95% CI 31–63%) and 100% (95% CI 97–100%) in the same studies. POCUS can be performed within minutes of patient contact, at the bedside and without any risk to move the patient to the radiology department for further imaging. It is a test that can be done rapidly in the span of less than 5 min [15], is easily reproducible in patients whose clinical status changes, and lacks the risks of significant radiation exposure.

General Principles of Lung POCUS

Almost all sonographic patterns of lung pathology, and especially for the assessment of pneumothorax, arise from the pleural line; a bright echogenic line consisting of the apposition of the parietal and visceral pleura [15–19].

For the diagnosis of pneumothorax, it is important to use a probe with high frequency, in order to maximize the resolution of structures that lie close to the skin surface. The linear array probe, generally with a frequency range of 5–12 MHz is optimal. However, the curvilinear and phased array probes can be used, albeit with slightly decreased resolution. Furthermore, lung POCUS focusses on the analysis and visualization of artefacts that are created when sound waves interact with air, water, and lung tissue. It is for this reason that filters on the ultrasound machine be turned off or a dedicated lung preset be used to enhance the visualization of these artefacts [15–17].

Technique

Because air within a Pneumothorax is non-dependent, ultrasound assessment is done by scanning the anterior chest wall of the supine chest. With the use of a high-frequency linear array probe, scanning is performed with the probe in a longitudinal orientation with the probe marker facing cephalad [18, 19] (Fig. 35.1).

In order to diagnose a pneumothorax, it has been traditionally taught to scan 2–3 successive intercostal spaces along the midclavicular line on either side [20, 21]. However, recently, it has been shown through CT mapping that the majority of traumatic pneumothoraces are located in an area between the parasternal border and the midclavicular line, and from the inferior aspect of the clavicle to the physiologic lung points (liver lung point on the right and cardiac lung point on the left) [22]. As a result, the author suggests that both lungs be scanned along two sagittal planes, parasternal and midclavicular, from the angle of

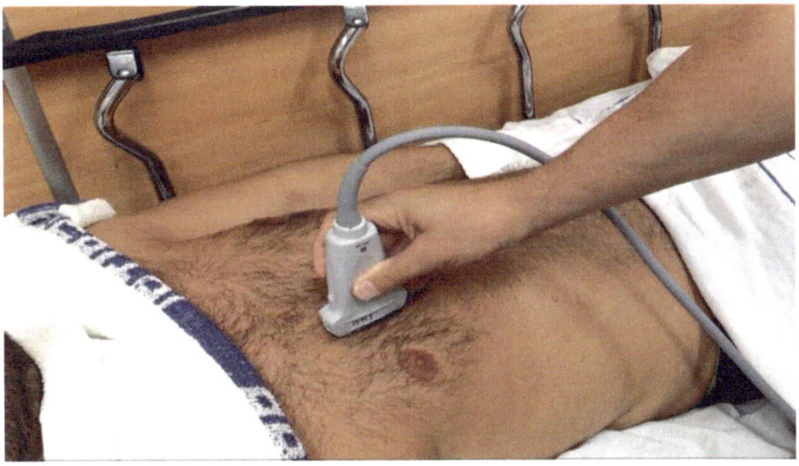

Fig. 35.1 To diagnose pneumothorax, a linear array probe is placed along the anterior chest, in a longitudinal orientation

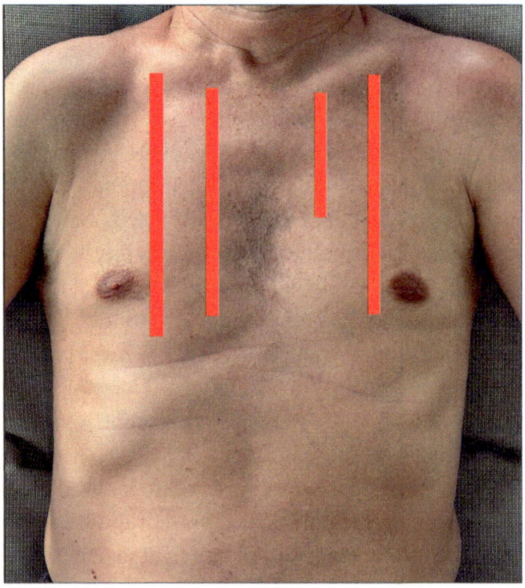

Fig. 35.2 Areas to scan on both lungs to assess for pneumothorax (red boxes)

Louie to the liver lung point (on the right) and to the cardiac lung point (on the left) (Fig. 35.2). It can be extrapolated that this technique will maximize the sensitivity and specificity of lung POCUS for the diagnosis of pneumothorax.

Normal Findings and Nomenclature of Lung at the Pleura

Once the probe is placed onto the patient's chest wall, identify the ribs with their corresponding rib shadow (Fig. 35.3). Approximately 0.5–1.0 cm deep to the ribs, you will find the more echogenic pleural line. This is the area of interest and where you must focus your eyes.

During cycles of respiration, the normal visceral and parietal pleural will slide back and forth, causing a **lung sliding** motion visualized on your screen (Video 35.1). Some characterize this shimmering effect similar to a column of ants walking along the pleural line.

You may at times identify horizontal echogenic lines equidistant and in the far field of the pleural line. These "**A-lines**" represent a reverberation artifact from the pleura and provide no meaningful information in the assessment for pneumothorax.

Another artefact to identify (if present) are **B-lines and comet tails**. These are vertical hyperechogenic reverberation artefacts that originate from the pleural line, and move along the pleural with respirations. These vertical lines only originate from the visceral pleura and is therefore, an indication of normal lung in contact with parietal pleura.

Anatomically, the anterior right lung extends from the angle of Louis of the sternum superiorly, to the pleura/liver interface inferiorly This intersection between the lung and liver capsule is called the **liver lung point** (Video 35.2). On the left anterior lung, due to the cardiac image extending into the lung, the intersection between the pleura and the pericardium produces a **cardiac lung point** (Video 35.3). Both of these liver and cardiac lung points can mimic a pneumothorax and are important to identify [18].

Findings of PTx

In 2012, Volpicelli et al. published international evidence-based recommendations for point-of-care lung ultrasound [21]. It is important to use a stepwise approach to identify the structures or artefacts that allow you to rule out or rule in a pneumothorax (Fig. 35.4).

1. **Lung sliding**: The first finding to look for is for the presence or absence of lung sliding. Once the entire anterior lung is scanned, if there is lung sliding throughout, you have ruled out PTx in that lung. While the absence of lung sliding strongly suggests the possibility of a pneumothorax, there is an important differential of other pathologies that can result in an absence of lung sliding (Table 35.1).
2. **B-lines/comet tails**: Since these artefacts only occur through the interaction of air and water within lung tissue, and only originate from the visceral pleura, the presence of either confirms the apposition of the visceral pleura against the parietal pleura, effectively ruling

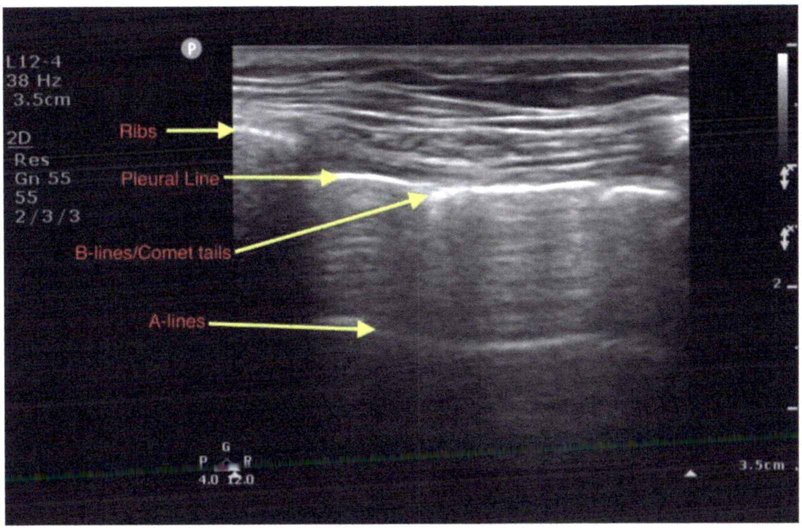

Fig. 35.3 Normal appearing lung

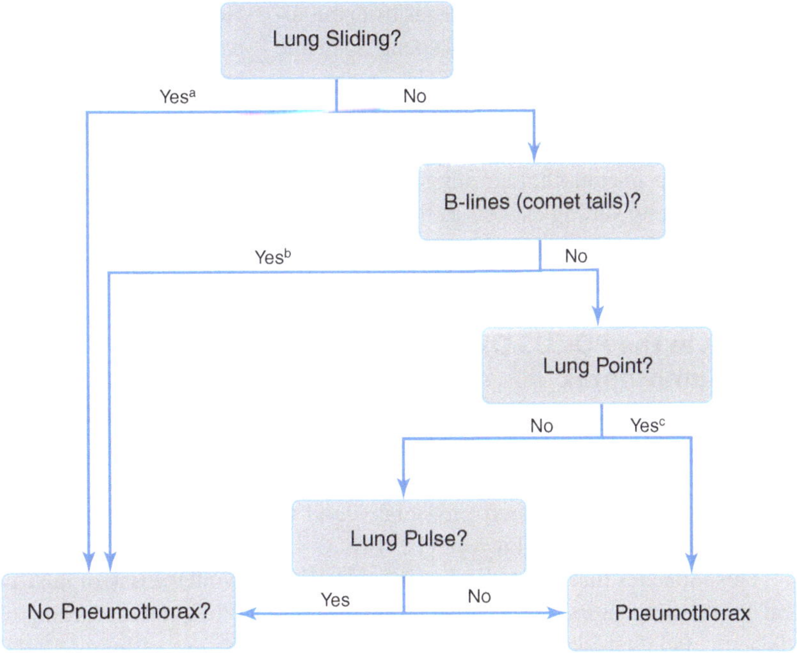

Fig. 35.4 Stepwise approach to assessing for pneumothorax

out pneumothorax in the area being scanned (Video 35.4). However, it is important to note that not all patients will exhibit comet tails or B-lines. Therefore, their absence does not suggest pneumothorax.

3. **Lung Pulse**: The lung pulse is caused by the rhythmic transmission of cardiac activity through an intact lung. Its presence therefore also rules out pneumothorax. This is an important feature found in right main stem intubations, where a lung pulse will be present in the **left lung** despite the lack of lung sliding due to the absence of ventilation on that side (Video 35.5).
4. **Lung Point**: A pneumothorax can be confirmed with the detection of a lung point. The lung point refers to the specific location where the visceral and parietal pleura separate from each other to form the pneumothorax. On the ultrasound image, a lung point will be

Table 35.1 Differential diagnosis of absent lung sliding

Pneumothorax
Significant atelectasis/consolidation
Main stem intubation
Acute respiratory distress syndrome (ARDS)
Severe fibrosis
Pleural adhesions
Apnea
Pulmonary contusion
Bullous disease

identified as a specific area alternating between a more echogenic lung sliding and an area of absent lung sliding (or movement of any kind) (Video 35.6). In emergency situations, it is suggested that the absence of both lung sliding and B-lines provides enough information for the safe diagnosis of pneumothorax, without the need to spend valuable time identifying a lung point [21].

Videos 35.7, 35.8, and 35.9 provide typical findings of a pneumothorax, suggested by both the lack of lung sliding as well as the lack of any comet tail/B-line artefacts.

Pitfalls in the POCUS Diagnosis of Pneumothorax

There is clear evidence that the level of training effects the reliability of POCUS to diagnose pneumothorax, as non-expert physicians tend to show lower accuracy for this tool [12, 14].

This indicates that the type of training is critical in ensuring proper technique (both through didactic and bedside teaching). However, this author believes this to be true of any diagnostic modality taught in medical school, residency, or post residency training. In cases of missed pneumothorax, it is not the ultrasound that is necessarily at fault, but the user's ability to generate and interpret images. For example, using the absence of lung sliding as the sole criteria to confirm a pneumothorax, without considering alternate diagnoses or using additional criteria (B-lines, lung pulse) is a clear cause of decreased accuracy. In addition, a common pit-fall is to look for lung-sliding in only one or two chest locations, rather than in multiple locations.

Case reports have reported missed pneumothorax based on atypical locations of located lung collapse [23]. These case reports underline the importance of careful and complete assessment of each lung using both the step-wise approach as well as the two sagittal scan approach outlined above. Confusing the liver and cardiac lung points as true lung points of a pneumothorax is also reported and proper methodology to minimize this error is of critical importance [24].

It has been previously considered that the location of the lung point can provide information with respect to the size of the pneumothorax. However, up to now, lung POCUS is not recognized as an accurate method to differentiate between small and large pneumothoraces [17].

Conclusion

Pneumothorax is a diagnosis that must be quickly and accurately made to prevent morbidity and mortality. Historical use of chest radiography has been shown to be inadequate to rule out pneumothorax, and the use of CT is neither feasible nor justified with the advent of POCUS. POCUS is a rapid, reproducible bedside tool, that can rule in and rule out pneumothorax as reliably as CT without any of the inherent risks. However, proper technique must be employed in order to avoid the risk of false negatives as outlined above. While not discarding other diagnostic modalities, the use of lung POCUS should be considered as the initial diagnostic tool for the diagnosis of pneumothorax.

Summary Points

- Pneumothorax is a diagnosis that must be considered in any patient complaining of chest pain and/or dyspnea. It is a diagnosis that must be made quickly to avoid potential morbidity and mortality.

- Chest radiography, while very specific for the diagnosis, is poorly sensitive and should not be relied upon to exclude PTx.
- Lung POCUS is both sensitive and specific for the diagnosis of pneumothorax, approaching that of computer tomography (when proper and careful technique is be used).
- Using s stepwise approach, assessing for the presence or absence of lung sliding, B-lines, lung pulse, and lung point can provide a diagnosis rapidly, accurately, and safely.
- Two sagittal scans (parasternal and midclavicular line) should be performed on both sides to maximize your accuracy.
- While POCUS is excellent for the diagnosis of pneumothorax, it should not be used to determine its size.

Evolving Evidence

There are reports of missed pneumothorax based on atypical locations of lung collapse [23]. These case reports underline the importance of careful and complete assessment of each lung using a step-wise approach and a two-two sagittal scan approach.

Pro-Tips (Call-Out)

While the absence of lung sliding strongly suggests the possibility of a pneumothorax, there is an important differential of other pathologies that can result in an absence of lung sliding.

The absence of both lung sliding and B-lines provides enough information for the safe diagnosis of pneumothorax, without the need to spend valuable time identifying a lung point.

Both lungs should be scanned along two sagittal planes, parasternal and midclavicular, from the angle of Louie to the liver lung point (on the right) and to the cardiac lung point (on the left).

Questions

1. Which two findings on POCUS effectively rule out pneumothorax on POCUS?
   A. Presence of Lung Pulse and Lung Point
   B. Absence of lung sliding and B-lines
   C. Absence of lung sliding and presence of Lung Point
   D. Presence of B-lines and lung pulse
   E. Absence of Lung sliding and Liver lung point
   Answer: A
2. All of the following can cause an absence of lung sliding in the right lung, except,
   A. Right main stem intubation
   B. Massive atelectasis
   C. Cardiac arrest
   D. Pleurodesis
   E. ARDS
3. Which of the following is correct regarding lung POCUS for the diagnosis of PTx?
   A. In an urgent situation, you should still identify the lung point in order to determine the size of the PTx
   B. Presence of lung sliding in one view is adequate to rule out PTx on that side?
   C. Absence of B-lines is diagnostic for PTx
   D. Identifying a lung point definitively rules in a PTx
   E. The liver lung point is a surrogate for a lung point on the right lung, and therefore, diagnostic of a PTx

References

1. Dotson K, Timm N, Gittelman M. Is spontaneous pneumothorax really a pediatric problem? A National Perspective. Pediatr Emerg Care. 2012;28(4):340–4.
2. Huang Y, Chang P, Wong K, Chang C, Lai J, Chen J. An age-stratified longitudinal study of primary spontaneous pneumothorax. J Adolesc Health. 2017;61(4):527–32.
3. Noppen M, De Keukeleire T. Pneumothorax. Respiration. 2008;76(2):121–7.
4. Hallifax R, Goldacre R, Landray M, Rahman N, Goldacre M. Trends in the incidence and recurrence of inpatient-treated spontaneous pneumothorax, 1968–2016. JAMA. 2018;320(14):1471.
5. Lee G.UpToDate. 2022 [online] Uptodate.com. https://www.uptodate.com/contents/pneumothorax-in-adults-epidemiology-and-etiology
6. John J, Seifi A. Incidence of iatrogenic pneumothorax in the United States in teaching vs. non-teaching hospitals from 2000 to 2012. J Crit Care. 2016;34:66–8.

7. Çelik B, Sahin E, Nadir A, Kaptanoglu M. Iatrogenic pneumothorax: etiology, incidence and risk factors. Thorac Cardiovasc Surg. 2009;57(05):286–90.
8. Loiselle A, Parish J, Wilkens J, Jaroszewski D. Managing iatrogenic pneumothorax and chest tubes. J Hosp Med. 2013;8(7):402–8.
9. Gulati M, Levy P, Mukherjee D, Amsterdam E, Bhatt D, Birtcher K, Blankstein R, Boyd J, Bullock-Palmer R, Conejo T, Diercks D, Gentile F, Greenwood J, Hess E, Hollenberg S, Jaber W, Jneid H, Joglar J, Morrow D, O'Connor R, Ross M, Shaw L. 2021 AHA/ACC/ASE/CHEST/SAEM/SCCT/SCMR Guideline for the Evaluation and Diagnosis of Chest Pain: Executive Summary: A Report of the American College of Cardiology/American Heart Association Joint Committee on Clinical Practice Guidelines. Circulation. 2021;144(22)
10. Tschopp J, Bintcliffe O, Astoul P, Canalis E, Driesen P, Janssen J, Krasnik M, Maskell N, Van Schil P, Tonia T, Waller D, Marquette C, Cardillo G. ERS task force statement: diagnosis and treatment of primary spontaneous pneumothorax. Eur Respir J. 2015;46(2):321–35.
11. Ding W, Shen Y, Yang J, He X, Zhang M. Diagnosis of pneumothorax by radiography and ultrasonography. Chest. 2011;140(4):859–66.
12. Alrajhi K, Woo M, Vaillancourt C. Test characteristics of ultrasonography for the detection of pneumothorax. Chest. 2012;141(3):703–8.
13. Ron E, Alattar Z, Hoebee S, Kang P, van Sonnenberg E. Current trends in the use of ultrasound over chest X-ray to identify pneumothoraces in ICU, trauma, and ARDS patients. J Intensive Care Med. 2021;37(1):5–11.
14. Chan K, Joo D, McRae A, Takwoingi Y, Premji Z, Lang E, Wakai A. Chest ultrasonography versus supine chest radiography for diagnosis of pneumothorax in trauma patients in the emergency department. Cochrane Database Syst Rev. 2020;2020(8)
15. Lichtenstein D, Mezière G. Relevance of lung ultrasound in the diagnosis of acute respiratory failure*: the BLUE protocol. Chest. 2008;134(1):117–25.
16. Volpicelli G. Sonographic diagnosis of pneumothorax. Intensive Care Med. 2010;37(2):224–32.
17. Gargani L, Volpicelli G. How I do it: lung ultrasound. Cardiovasc Ultrasound. 2014;12(1):1–10.
18. Socransky S, Wiss R, Hall G, Ho B, Skinner A, Turner J, Woo M, Chen R. Essentials of point-of-care ultrasound. 1st ed. Sudbury: The EDE 2 Course Inc.; 2014.
19. Turner J, Dankoff J. Thoracic ultrasound. Emerg Med Clin North Am. 2012;30(2):451–73.
20. Helland G, Gaspari R, Licciardo S, Sanseverino A, Torres U, Emhoff T, Blehar D. Comparison of four views to single-view ultrasound protocols to identify clinically significant pneumothorax. Acad Emerg Med. 2016;23(10):1170–5.
21. Volpicelli G, Elbarbary M, Blaivas M, Lichtenstein D, Mathis G, Kirkpatrick A, Melniker L, Gargani L, Noble V, Via G, Dean A, Tsung J, Soldati G, Copetti R, Bouhemad B, Reissig A, Agricola E, Rouby J, Arbelot C, Liteplo A, Sargsyan A, Silva F, Hoppmann R, Breitkreutz R, Seibel A, Neri L, Storti E, Petrovic T. International evidence-based recommendations for point-of-care lung ultrasound. Intensive Care Med. 2012;38(4):577–91.
22. Bignucolo A, Acton C, Ohle R, Socransky S. Traumatic pneumothorax mapping using computed tomography to assess optimal area to scan with POCUS. CJEM. 2020;22(5):708–11.
23. Retief J, Chopra M. Pitfalls in the ultrasonographic diagnosis of pneumothorax. J Intensive Care Soc. 2016;18(2):143–5.
24. Blanco P, Volpicelli G. Common pitfalls in point-of-care ultrasound: a practical guide for emergency and critical care physicians. Crit Ultrasound J. 2016;8(1):1–12.

Pulmonary Edema

36

Daniel Gerber and Paul K. Mohabir

Learning Objectives

1. Explore how an A-line pattern strongly correlates with dry pulmonary interstitium, low pulmonary capillary wedge pressure, and therefore, low likelihood of cardiogenic pulmonary edema.
2. Examine how B-line artifacts are nonspecific markers of subpleural interstitial thickening with a broad differential.
3. Demonstrate how a B-line predominance is characteristic of pulmonary edema, acute respiratory distress syndrome, interstitial lung diseases, pneumonia, pneumonitis, pulmonary infarcts, and pulmonary contusions.
4. Review protocols, algorithms, and scoring systems have been proposed to qualitatively determine the underlying etiology of respiratory failure.

Explanation of B-Lines

B-lines are vertical *ring-down artifacts* that form when there is an increase in subpleural alveolar or interstitial lung density disrupting normal pleural reflection. Aerated lung creates a significant shift in acoustic impedance at the pleural-air interface acting as a near total reflector. Reflection between the transducer and the pleural line generates artifactual horizontal A-lines. By contrast, interstitial thickening by fluid, inflammation, or fibrosis forms acoustic windows and surrounds alveolar air bubbles. Rather than reflecting, ultrasound waves resonate within these air-interstitium complexes creating B-lines. Characteristically, they are hyperechoic vertical artifacts that originate from the pleural line, extend the entire depth of the visual field without fading, obliterate A-lines, and move with lung sliding.

While occasional B-lines are physiologic, especially in dependent lung zones, 3 or more within a single field-of-view are considered pathological. B-lines are characteristic of pulmonary edema, yet are nonspecific and encompass a broad differential, including acute respiratory distress syndrome (ARDS), pneumonia, pneumonitis, interstitial lung diseases (ILD), pulmonary infarcts, and pulmonary contusions.

Image
B/A/Z lines

Call Out Pro-Tip
B-lines

D. Gerber · P. K. Mohabir (✉)
Stanford University School of Medicine, Stanford, CA, USA
e-mail: dgerber@stanford.edu; mohabir@stanford.edu

M. J. Lanspa, A. T. Levinson (eds.), *Echocardiography and Ultrasonography in the ICU*, Respiratory Medicine, https://doi.org/10.1007/978-3-031-80038-2_36

- Hyperechoic vertical artifacts
- Originate from the pleural line
- Extend the depth of the visual field without fading
- Obliterate horizontal A-lines
- Move with lung sliding

Call Out Pro-Tip
≥3 B-lines in a single field of view is pathological.

Cardiogenic Vs. Noncardiogenic

Pulmonary edema represents the accumulation of extravascular fluid in the pulmonary interstitium and alveolar air spaces. Any mechanism that causes pulmonary edema via increased pulmonary venous and capillary hydrostatic pressures is considered cardiogenic. Common etiologies include left ventricular systolic or diastolic dysfunction, aortic or mitral valvular disease, and atrial or ventricular arrhythmias. By contrast, noncardiogenic pulmonary edema is the result of decreased oncotic pressure or increased pulmonary capillary permeability. This broad differential includes ARDS, pneumonitis, pulmonary infarcts and contusions, transfusion-related acute lung injury (TRALI), high altitude pulmonary edema (HAPE), opiate and salicylate overdose, re-expansion pulmonary edema, and many others [1, 2].

Call Out
Pulmonary Edema
- Cardiogenic: increased pulmonary capillary hydrostatic pressure
- Noncardiogenic: increased pulmonary capillary permeability or decreased oncotic pressure

Diagnostically, the gold standard for confirming cardiogenic pulmonary edema is invasive cardiac catheterization demonstrating elevated left atrial or pulmonary capillary wedge pressure (PCWP). While lung ultrasonography to assess PCWP is an area of evolving evidence, it provides a promising method of rapidly and noninvasively identifying pulmonary edema, assessing its distribution and severity, and determining etiology.

Soldati and colleagues have outlined a succinct approach to the ultrasonographic evaluation of parenchymal lung pathology [1]. Their algorithm focuses on (1) confirming the presence of a B-line pattern, (2) determining focal versus diffuse involvement, and (3) assessing for heterogeneity. Cardiogenic pulmonary edema causes a diffuse and homogenous increase in interstitial edema with B-line predominance, yet without evidence of parenchymal lung injury [1]. While B-lines are nonspecific and correlate poorly with PCWP, their absence, A-line predominance, is highly specific for a low PCWP and essentially rules out cardiogenic edema [3]. Pathological B-lines limited to a specific lung region unilaterally imply focality, as is seen in pneumonia, atelectasis, pulmonary contusion, pulmonary infarct, or malignancy. Finally, diffuse B-line patterns are further categorized as homogenous, suggestive of cardiogenic pulmonary edema, or heterogenous with features of parenchymal lung injury. Areas of patchy lung sparing, pleural irregularities, altered lung sliding, and subpleural consolidations all suggest underlying parenchymal damage with atelectasis or fibrosis consistent with noncardiogenic pulmonary edema, ARDS, or diffuse interstitial fibrosis [4].

Quantitative and Semi-Quantitative Scores

As discussed above, lung ultrasonography is a powerful noninvasive tool to estimate pulmonary edema, or extravascular lung water (EVLW). Multiple scoring systems and protocols have been proposed to standardize this assessment, though this remains an area of evolving evidence. Semiquantitative scores rely on visual estimation of B-line predominance. Each intercostal space is scored based on the total number of B-lines present, percentage of occupied intercostal space, or presence and extent of coalescence, which occurs when numerous B-lines fuse and become indistinguishable [5, 6]. While semiquantitative scores correlate with gold-standard invasive metrics of EVLW, they are prone to operator interpretation and error. Quantitative methods employ computer-assisted analysis, reducing error and providing superior accuracy [7, 8].

Differentiating Z-Lines

Similar in appearance to B-lines, Z-lines are vertical hyperechoic artifacts that originate from the pleural line. These reverberation artifacts are thought to be generated by reflection between pleura and extra-pulmonary fascia [9, 10]. Unlike B-lines, they fade 2–4 cm beyond the pleural line, do not move in synchrony with lung sliding, and do not obliterate A-lines. Z-lines are of no apparent clinical significance and are considered artifactual.

CALL OUT
Z-lines evolving evidence:
- Hyperechoic vertical artifacts
- Originate from the pleural line
- Fade after 2–4 cm
- Do not obliterate horizontal A-lines
- Do not move with lung sliding

Lung Zones/Locations

A standard lung ultrasound examination is performed with the patient in the reclined or supine position. The transducer is placed perpendicular to the chest wall in the vertical or cranial-caudal plane with the indicator, and by convention the left side of the image, oriented toward the patient's head. Each hemithorax is divided based on anatomical landmarks and imaged according to a variety of protocols. A standard bilateral exam consists of 12 lung zones: anterior, lateral, and posterior zones demarcated by the sternum, anterior and posterior axillary lines, and thoracic spine subdivided into upper and lower halves by the clavicle, fourth rib, and diaphragm. In the critical care setting, an eight-zone approach omitting the posterior lung fields is often preferred, and is recommended by the International Liaison Committee on Lung Ultrasound [11]. The Bedside Lung Ultrasound in Emergency (BLUE) protocol further simplifies this to three standardized "BLUE-points" on each hemithorax to improve speed and reproducibility [12].

Summary Points
- Coupled with focused echocardiography, lung ultrasonography is an invaluable tool in identifying and differentiating the etiology of pulmonary edema by quantitative and semiquantitative measures of B-line predominance.
- B-lines are hyperechoic vertical artifacts that originate from the pleural line, extend the depth of the visual field without fading, obliterate horizontal A-lines, and move with lung sliding. These are nonspecific markers of increased interstitial lung density most commonly seen in the setting of pulmonary edema, ARDS, pneumonia or pneumonitis, pulmonary infarcts or contusions, and interstitial lung diseases.
- Cardiogenic pulmonary edema is the result of increased pulmonary capillary hydrostatic pressure, whereas noncardiogenic edema is the result of decreased oncotic pressure or increased vascular permeability.

Questions
1. A 65-year-old man with a history of hypertension, hyperlipidemia, aortic stenosis, and transfusion-dependent myelodysplastic syndrome presents to the emergency department with dyspnea 12 h after scheduled transfusion of two packed red blood cells. Vitals are notable for a heart rate of 85 bpm, BP 120/80 mmHg, and oxygen saturation 92% on 2 L O_2 by nasal cannula. Exam is notable for a systolic murmur and bibasilar crackles. ECG shows sinus rhythm. While awaiting the results of his labs and chest X-ray, you perform bedside lung ultrasonography which shows >3 B-lines in each lung zone. Which of the following additional sonographic findings would support a diagnosis of cardiogenic pulmonary edema?
   A. Pleural effusions
   B. Subpleural consolidations

C. Areas of lung sparing
D. Impaired pleural sliding
E. Pleural irregularities
Answer: A.

2. A previously heathy 19-year-old man presents to the emergency department with palpitations and dyspnea 2 h after smoking methamphetamines. Heart rate is 110 bpm, BP 150/90 mmHg, and oxygen saturation is 100% on room air. Exam shows an anxious young man with clear lungs, no murmurs, and no other focal findings. ECG shows sinus tachycardia. Labs, toxicology, and chest X-ray are pending. Lung ultrasonography shows hyperechoic vertical artifacts that originate from the pleural line. Which of the following additional findings confirm that these artifacts are Z-lines rather than B-lines?
A. Fade after 2–4 cm
B. Erase A-lines
C. Move with lung sliding
D. Extend the entire depth of the visual field
Answer: A.

References

1. Soldati G, Demi M, Demi L. Ultrasound patterns of pulmonary edema. Ann Transl Med. 2019;7(Suppl 1):S16. https://doi.org/10.21037/atm.2019.01.49.
2. Soldati G, Demi M. The use of lung ultrasound images for the differential diagnosis of pulmonary and cardiac interstitial pathology. J Ultrasound. 2017;20:91–6. https://doi.org/10.1007/s40477-017-0244-7.
3. Sekiguchi H, Schenck LA, Horie R, et al. Critical care ultrasonography differentiates ARDS, pulmonary edema, and other causes in the early course of acute hypoxemic respiratory failure. Chest. 2015;148:912–8. https://doi.org/10.1378/chest.15-0341.
4. Copetti R, Soldati G, Copetti P. Chest sonography: a useful tool to differentiate acute cardiogenic pulmonary edema from acute respiratory distress syndrome. Cardiovasc Ultrasound. 2008;29(6):16.
5. Gargani L. Lung ultrasound: a new tool for the cardiologist. Cardiovasc Ultrasound. 2011;9:6.
6. Mongodi S, Bouhemad B, Orlando A, Stella A, Tavazzi G, Via G, Iotti GA, Braschi A, Mojoli F. Modified lung ultrasound score for assessing and monitoring pulmonary aeration. Ultraschall Med. 2017;38(5):530–7.
7. Corradi F, Ball L, Brusasco C, Riccio AM, Baroffio M, Bovio G, Pelosi P, Brusasco V. Assessment of extravascular lung water by quantitative ultrasound and CT in isolated bovine lung. Respir Physiol Neurobiol. 2013;187(3):244–9.
8. Corradi F, Brusasco C, Vezzani A, Santori G, Manca T, Ball L, Nicolini F, Gherli T, Brusasco V. Computer-aided quantitative ultrasonography for detection of pulmonary edema in mechanically ventilated cardiac surgery patients. Chest. 2016;150(3):640–51.
9. Francisco MJN, et al. Advances in lung ultrasound. Einstein (Sao Paulo, Brazil). 2016;14(3):443–8. https://doi.org/10.1590/S1679-45082016MD3557.
10. Lee FCY. Lung ultrasound-a primary survey of the acutely dyspneic patient. J Intensive Care. 2016;4(1):57. https://doi.org/10.1186/s40560-016-0180-1.
11. Volpicelli G, Elbarbary M, Blaivas M, et al. International evidence-based recommendations for point-of-care lung ultrasound. Intensive Care Med. 2012;38:577–91. https://doi.org/10.1007/s00134-012-2513-4.
12. Lichtenstein DA, Mezière GA. Relevance of lung ultrasound in the diagnosis of acute respiratory failure: the BLUE protocol. Chest. 2008;134:117–25.

Pneumonia and Consolidation

37

Andrew Foderaro and Andrew T. Levinson

Learning Objectives

1. Compare lung ultrasound (LUS) to other imaging modalities for diagnosing pneumonia
2. Describe various ultrasound features seen in patients with pneumonia
3. Examine LUS for the diagnosis of pneumonia in the Covid-19 era

Lung ultrasound has a long history of clinical application for lung pathologies with good evidence especially in evaluating pleural effusions, pulmonary edema, and pneumothoracies [1–3]. More recently the use of point-of-care ultrasound for the investigation of pneumonia has become more common in practice. During the coronavirus disease-2019 (COVID-19) pandemic there has been opportunity for some advancement of the understanding of lung ultrasound especially in viral pneumonia. Point-of-care ultrasound for pneumonia has been especially useful clinically. It has shown improved capabilities compared to the chest x-ray which is often the preferred first imaging modality. When compared to computed tomography (CT) scan, the use of lung ultrasound (LUS) can reduce patient risk by eliminating the need for transport across the hospital to access a CT scanner, which is especially pertinent in a critically ill patient [4, 5]. Over this chapter, the focus will be on the use of lung ultrasound in the evaluation of lung consultation/pneumonia with some focus on the pandemic as a novel source of experience in this area of point-of-care ultrasound.

Ultrasound Features of Pneumonia

As discussed in more detail elsewhere, the image acquisition for LUS uses a high frequency linear probe which is placed between the ribs and is often the preferred choice for pleural or subpleural imaging. For patients with a thick chest wall, or with obesity, a lower-frequency probe can be used. As with other lung protocols, such as the BLUE-protocol, a comprehensive assessment of the lung includes the evaluation of multiple lung zones [5, 6]. This evaluation can lead to a diagnosis of lung consolidation and thus pneumonia by identifying various ultrasound findings such as lung hepatization, shred sign, and air bronchograms. Set apart from the normal pattern of healthy lung, which demonstrate an A-line pattern (Fig. 37.1; Video 37.3), and lung sliding, the identification of these findings added to the

Supplementary Information The online version contains supplementary material available at https://doi.org/10.1007/978-3-031-80038-2_37.

A. Foderaro · A. T. Levinson (✉)
Division of Pulmonary, Critical Care, and Sleep Medicine, The Warren Alpert Medical School, Brown University, Providence, RI, USA
e-mail: andrew_levinson@brown.edu

M. J. Lanspa, A. T. Levinson (eds.), *Echocardiography and Ultrasonography in the ICU*, Respiratory Medicine, https://doi.org/10.1007/978-3-031-80038-2_37

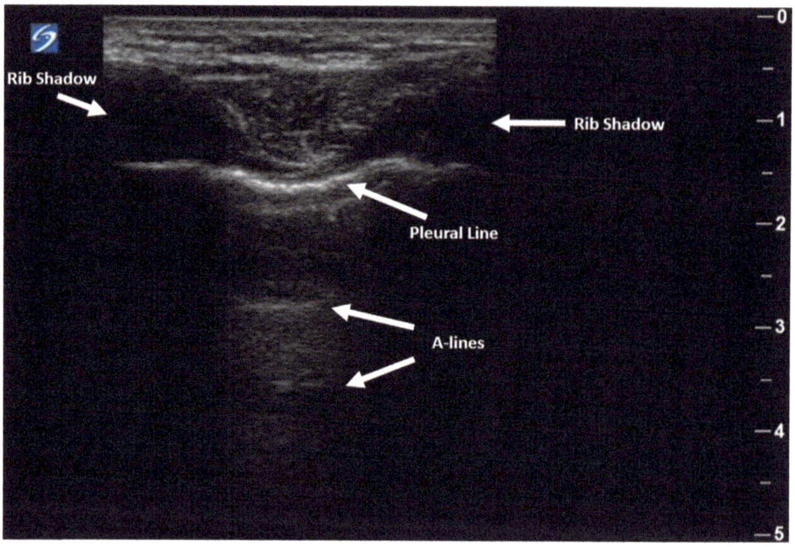

Fig. 37.1 A line pattern with lung sliding

clinical evaluation of respiratory failure help produce a more specific diagnosis of lung consolidative processes. In addition to differentiating from normal lung, the various findings aid in differentiating between causes of consolidation, including pneumonia, non-cardiogenic pulmonary edema, or acute respiratory distress syndrome (ARDS), and cardiogenic pulmonary edema (CPE).

When obtaining imaging within each lung zone, the ultrasound findings can also be used to differentiate translobar versus nontranslobar lung consolidation. **Translobar alveolar consolidation** on ultrasound is seen as sonographic lung hepatization. In a severe translobar pneumonia, the alveoli are filled with exudative inflammation, increasing acoustic impedance, which causes the image to resemble that of the liver (Fig. 37.2; Video 37.2) as opposed to the lower impedance image produced with air-filled alveoli in normal lung [7].

Nontranslobar pneumonia is signified by a differentiation of the area of consolidation and the air-filled lung within the same lobe. The ultrasound finding is an irregular line between the area of consolidated lung and the aerated lung at the pleural surface, which has some resemblance to a torn piece of paper, and thus, is referred to as the shred sign (Fig. 37.3) [8].

Air bronchograms, both dynamic and static, can be seen on lung ultrasound and are helpful in determining processes such as pneumonia and atelectasis. Sonographic air bronchograms appear as hyperechoic lines within a hypoechoic area of lung (Fig. 37.4; Video 37.5). This finding is produced as the air within the airway is highlighted by the dense and less echogenic consolidation. If the air bronchograms are moving within the image, this is referred to as **dynamic air bronchograms** and have been shown to be specific for pneumonia as compared to atelectasis [9]. Conversely, a **static air bronchogram** can be seen in both pneumonia and atelectasis.

Lung pulse is a sonographic observation of pleural line movement corresponding to heart beats. This finding is seen transmitted through consolidated lung and, in addition to dynamic air bronchograms, can be helpful in differentiating pneumonia from atelectasis [10] (Video 37.4 Lung pulse).

B-lines are vertical lines arising from the pleura and are sharply defined (Fig. 37.5; Video

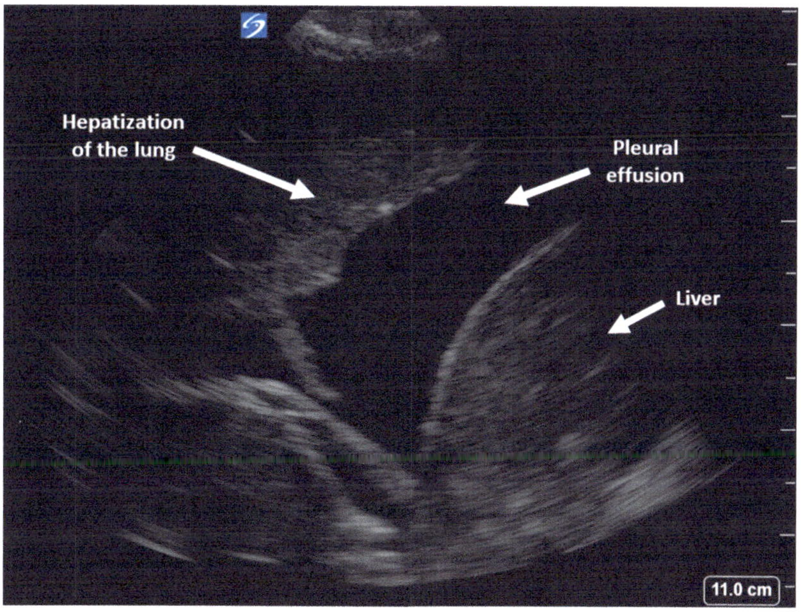

Fig. 37.2 Translobar pneumonia with lung hepatization

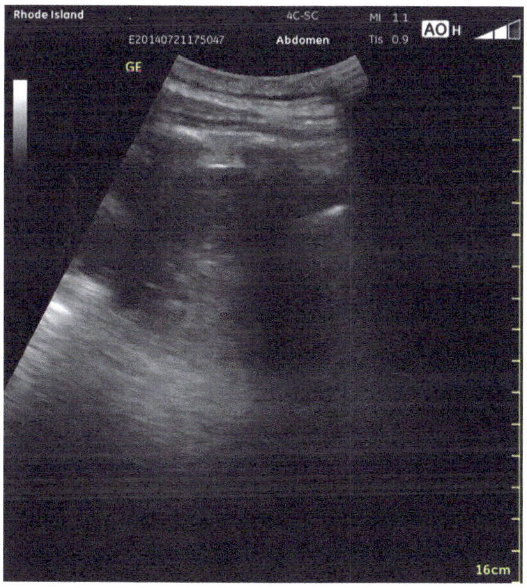

Fig. 37.3 Shred sign

37.1). This finding can be seen in numerous lung pathologies and thus needs to be interpreted with other clinical parameters. Typically, B-lines associated with pneumonia are often more focal and unilateral whereas a more diffuse identification of B-lines is more specific for CPE [11].

Pleural effusions can be easily identified using point-of-care ultrasound [12]. Light et al. in 1980 showed that 44% of patients in their cohort of 203 patients developed a parapneumonic effusion [13]. When evaluating a parapneumonic effusion associated with an infectious inflammatory pneumonia, generally they will be unilateral and demonstrate other findings such as septations [14]. Evaluation demonstrating bilateral free flowing effusions can again be helpful in differentiating pneumonia from a process such as CPE (Fig. 37.6; Videos 37.2 and 37.5).

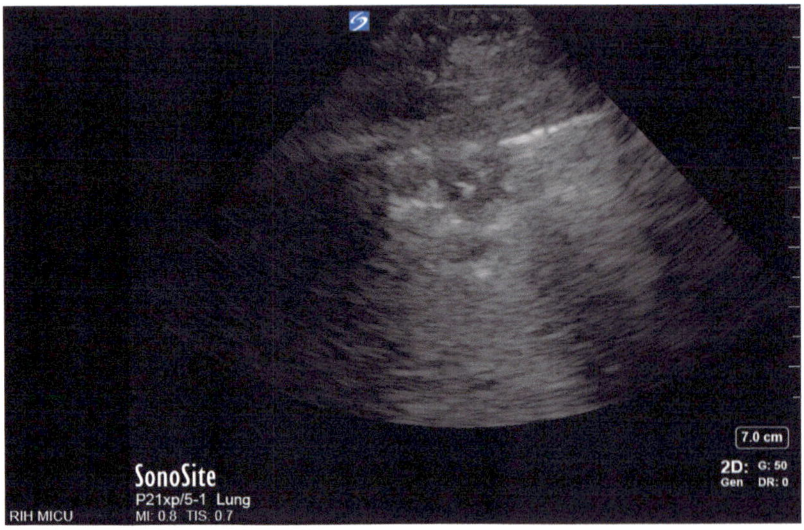

Fig. 37.4 Sonographic air bronchograms

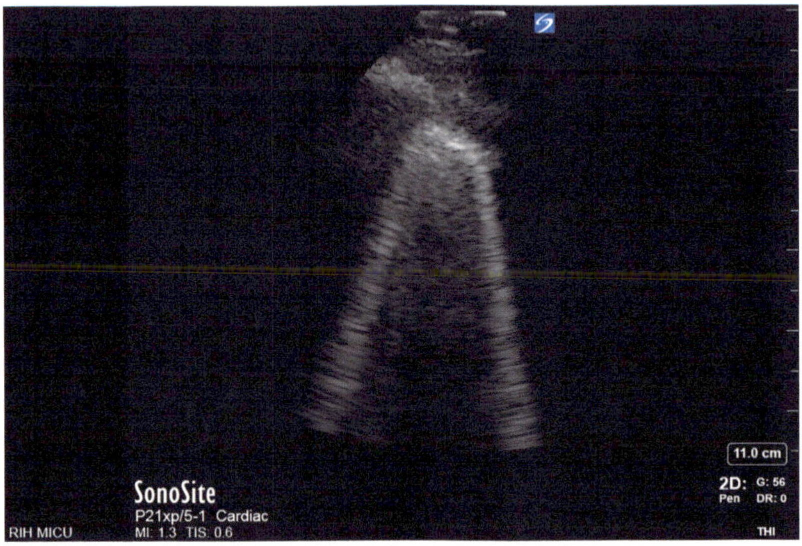

Fig. 37.5 B Lines

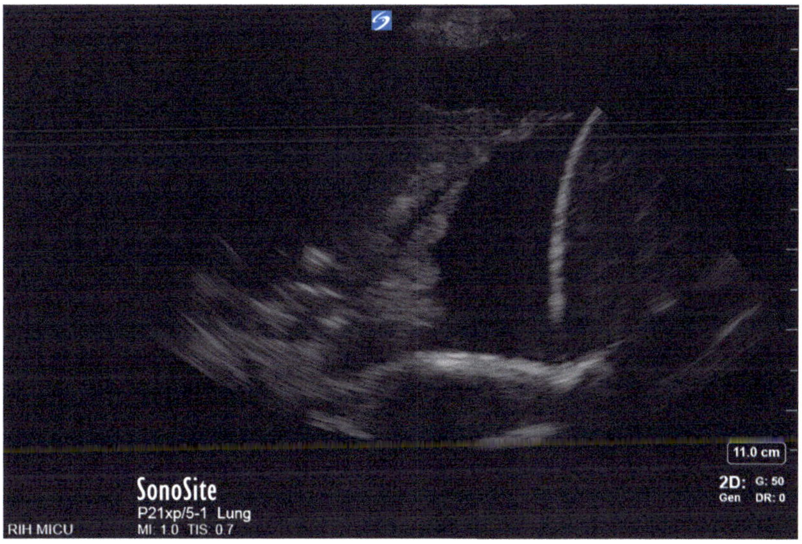

Fig. 37.6 Pleural effusion and lung consolidation

Comparing Ultrasound to Other Imaging Modalities

The diagnosis of pneumonia has often been made in real time combining clinical history, labs, and often x-ray imaging. It is quite clear that history, examination, and experience are not enough to diagnose pneumonia with any adequate sensitivity or specificity [15]. Ultrasound continues to show improved diagnostic accuracy when compared to x-ray in multiple studies, including a 2015 meta-analysis using CT as the gold standard [16]. A systematic review in 2017 showed that ultrasound, although not as sensitive as CT scan, was a clinical tool which had excellent test characteristics as well as significantly decreased cost and transport needs compared to CT scan. The 95% confidence interval for sensitivity was 80–90% and the specificity 70–90% [17]. These evidence-based findings show ultrasound to be an important addition to patient care in patients with consolidative pulmonary processes, especially in critical care settings where transportation within the hospital carries risk.

Lung Ultrasound for Pneumonia in the Era of COVID-19

Overall, the findings associated with COVID-19 have been found to be similar to what is discussed above for other forms of pneumonia but there are some unique features to the COVID-19 pandemic that make LUS especially appealing. The ability to perform LUS at the bedside is especially helpful as it removes the need for transport across the hospital and thus minimizes exposure to others.

As stated above, the findings of COVID-19 pneumonia are similar overall to the findings in non-COVID pneumonia. There have been a significant number of case series and small studies during the last 2 years and a variety of both systemic reviews and meta-analyses. Early in the pandemic, a systematic review and meta-analysis demonstrated that the CT findings of COVID-19 involved a bilateral, peripheral predominant, and heterogeneous distribution [18]. Given the wide area of involvement, a protocoled evaluation of multiple lung zones is important when using point-of-care LUS. Subsequently, Castelao et al. confirmed similar findings with LUS; however, noting a posterior and lower lobe predominance [18, 19].

Due to the heterogeneity of location in the lungs, as well as diversity of LUS findings, there were several proposals for standardization of COVID-19 LUS. Soldati et al. proposed a LUS score for evaluation scanning 14 zones with a score being produced, using many of the discussed findings for pneumonia, between 0 and 3. This score was evaluated by Gil-Rodriguez et al. in a 2022 systematic review of 66 articles with pooled population of 4687 patients, which demonstrated that a higher LUS score was associated with worse outcomes, including death and need for ICU admission.

Pit Falls of Lung Ultrasound

As with all imaging modalities, ultrasound and specifically LUS carry some downsides. As noted previously, one of the issues can be related to the high number of lung zones which need to be imaged for a complete evaluation. This brings with it a need for patient mobilization and positioning which can be difficult, especially in hospitalized patients or those who are critically ill. Another potential issue can be in relation to body habitus and obesity. In obese patients, the ultrasound waves have greater distance to travel, therefore affecting the signal-to-noise ratio, decreasing image quality and increasing the difficulty in interpretation of the images. Further investigations into techniques and creation of efficient protocols will be important to make ultrasound imaging clinically practical in heterogenous patient populations.

Summary Point

- Lung ultrasound to detect alveolar consolidation/pneumonia, although not as sensitive as CT scan, is a useful clinical tool which has excellent test characteristics.

Pro-Tips (Call-Out)

- **Lung pulse** is a sonographic observation of pleural line movement corresponding to heart beats. This finding is seen transmitted through consolidated lung and, in addition to dynamic air bronchograms, can be helpful in differentiating pneumonia from atelectasis.

Evolving Evidence (Call-Out)

- If the air bronchograms are moving within the image, this is referred to as **dynamic air bronchograms** and have been shown to be specific for pneumonia as compared to atelectasis. Conversely, a **static air bronchogram** can be seen in both pneumonia and atelectasis.

References

1. Xirouchaki N, et al. Lung ultrasound in critically ill patients: comparison with bedside chest radiography. Intensive Care Med. 2011;37(9):1488–93.
2. Hagaman JT, et al. Admission chest radiograph lacks sensitivity in the diagnosis of community-acquired pneumonia. Am J Med Sci. 2009;337(4):236–40.
3. Lichtenstein DA. Lung ultrasound in the critically ill. Ann Intensive Care. 2014;4(1):1–12.
4. Durant A, Nagdev A. Ultrasound detection of lung hepatization. West J Emerg Med. 2010;11(4):322–3.
5. Biswas A, et al. The utility of the "shred sign" in the diagnosis of acute respiratory distress syndrome resulting from multifocal pneumonia. Am J Respir Crit Care Med. 2017;195(2):e20–2.
6. Lichtenstein D, Mezière G, Seitz J. The dynamic air bronchogram: a lung ultrasound sign of alveolar consolidation ruling out atelectasis. Chest. 2009;135(6):1421–5.
7. Lichtenstein DA. Lung ultrasound in the critically ill. Ann Intensive Care. 2014;4:1.
8. Al Deeb M, Barbic S, Featherstone R, et al. Point-of-care ultrasonography for the diagnosis of acute cardiogenic pulmonary edema in patients presenting with acute dyspnea: a systematic review and meta-analysis. Acad Emerg Med. 2014;21:843–52.
9. Soni NJ, et al. Ultrasound in the diagnosis and management of pleural effusions. J Hosp Med. 2015;10(12):811–6.

10. Light RW, et al. Parapneumonic effusions. Am J Med. 1980;69(4):507–12.
11. Kearney SE, et al. Computed tomography and ultrasound in parapneumonic effusions and empyema. Clin Radiol. 2000;55(7):542–7.
12. Metlay JP, Kapoor WN, Fine MJ. Does this patient have community-acquired pneumonia? Diagnosing pneumonia by history and physical examination. JAMA. 1997;278(17):1440–5.
13. Ye X, Xiao H, Chen B, et al. Accuracy of lung ultrasonography versus chest radiography for the diagnosis of adult community-acquired pneumonia: review of the literature and meta-analysis. PLoS One. 2015;10:e0130066.
14. Llamas-Alvarez AM, Tenza-Lozano EM, Latour-Perez J. Accuracy of lung ultrasonography in the diagnosis of pneumonia in adults: systematic review and meta-analysis. Chest. 2017;151:374–82.
15. Bao C, et al. Coronavirus disease 2019 (COVID-19) CT findings: a systematic review and meta-analysis. J Am Coll Radiol. 2020;17(6):701–9.
16. Castelao J, et al. Findings and prognostic value of lung ultrasound in COVID-19 pneumonia. J Ultrasound Med. 2021;40(7):1315–24.
17. Yasukawa K, Minami T, Boulware DR, Shimada A, Fischer EA. Point-of-care lung ultrasound for COVID-19: findings and prognostic implications from 105 consecutive patients. J Intensive Care Med. 2021;36(3):334–42.
18. Soldati G, et al. Proposal for international standardization of the use of lung ultrasound for patients with COVID-19: a simple, quantitative, reproducible method. J Ultrasound Med. 2020;39(7):1413–9.
19. Gil-Rodríguez J, et al. Ultrasound findings of lung ultrasonography in COVID-19: a systematic review. Eur J Radiol. 2022;148:110156.

Diaphragm

38

Idunn Morris and Ewan Goligher

Learning Objectives

1. Use ultrasound to measure diaphragm thickness, thickening, excursion, echodensity, strain, and tissue velocity
2. Understand the caveats and limitations of each modality of assessment and know when and how to use them diagnostically and prognostically
3. Be able to synthesize information obtained from diaphragm ultrasound and apply this to a clinical context to aid decision making

I. Morris
Interdepartmental Division of Critical Care Medicine, University of Toronto, Toronto, ON, Canada

Division of Respirology, Department of Medicine, University Health Network, Toronto, ON, Canada

Department of Intensive Care Medicine, Nepean Hospital, Sydney, Australia
e-mail: idunn.morris@uhn.ca

E. Goligher (✉)
Interdepartmental Division of Critical Care Medicine, University of Toronto, Toronto, ON, Canada

Division of Respirology, Department of Medicine, University Health Network, Toronto, ON, Canada

Toronto General Hospital Research Institute, Toronto, ON, Canada
e-mail: ewan.goligher@utoronto.ca; ewan.goligher@uhn.ca

Introduction

The diaphragm is the primary muscle of ventilation. It is composed of the muscular central tendon, the crural diaphragm which inserts into the first three lumbar vertebrae, and the costal diaphragm which inserts onto rib cage and xiphoid process (Fig. 38.1). The crural diaphragm lowers the dome of the diaphragm while the costal diaphragm lowers the diaphragm dome and elevates the lower rib cage. The force generated by the action of the diaphragm is quantified as the transdiaphragmatic pressure (difference in intrathoracic and intraabdominal pressures). This force is modified by the length of the diaphragm at the onset of contraction (i.e., the length-tension relation) and by the rate of shortening during contraction (i.e. the force-velocity relationship). Transdiaphragmatic pressure can be computed from the difference in esophageal and gastric pressures measured using an esophageal catheter fitted with esophageal and gastric balloons. Obtaining these measurements requires specialized equipment and considerable time and technical expertise.

Diaphragm ultrasound is a comparatively novel technique that enables non-invasive assessment of the structure and function of the right and left hemidiaphragm. Assessment of abnormal diaphragm structure and function by ultrasound can aid clinical decision-making in both outpatients presenting with respiratory complaints and

M. J. Lanspa, A. T. Levinson (eds.), *Echocardiography and Ultrasonography in the ICU*, Respiratory Medicine, https://doi.org/10.1007/978-3-031-80038-2_38

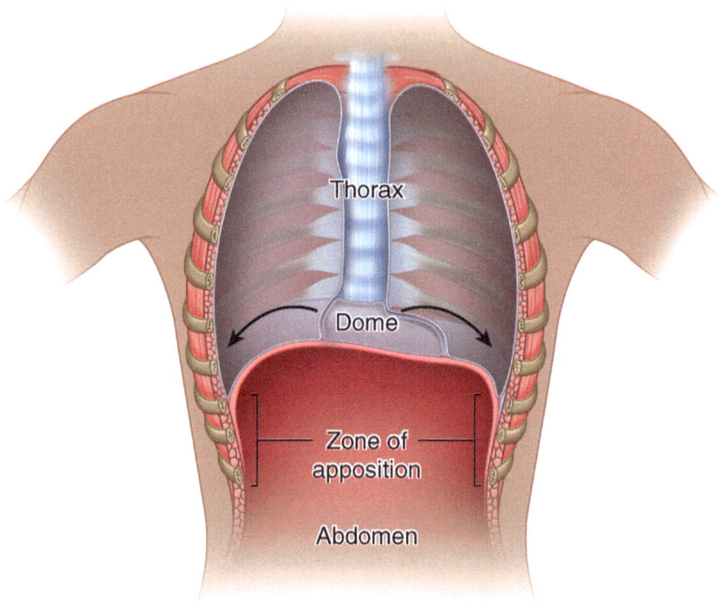

Fig. 38.1 Zone of apposition: the portion of the costal diaphragm that lies adjacent to the lower rib cage throughout the entirety of the respiratory cycle

in hospitalized and mechanically ventilated patients with acute or chronic respiratory failure.

Diaphragm Thickness and Echodensity

Measurement

Diaphragm thickness (T_{di}) is measured by visualizing the diaphragm in cross section using a high resolution (10–15 MHz) linear array transducer held perpendicular to the chest wall along the eighth, nineth, or tenth intercostal space between the mid and anterior axillary line. The relatively anechoic costal diaphragm is located between the highly echogenic pleural and peritoneal membranes. The costal diaphragm covers approximately one third of the lower rib cage (zone of apposition, Fig. 38.1). Its thickness tapers from its costal insertion to the central tendon as well as from anterior to posterior regions. Given this variability in thickness, to detect changes in diaphragm thickness over time, serial measurements should be made at exactly the same location by marking the probe position at the skin. The resting (relaxed) thickness of the muscle at end-expiration (functional residual capacity, FRC) is taken as the diaphragm thickness (Fig. 38.2). T_{di} can be measured in B mode if adequately timed to end expiration, or this can be done more easily in M mode. However, in M mode, doppler alignment is important so as to avoid overestimation of T_{di} by off-axis imaging.

Echodensity of the diaphragm can also be measured in this view in B mode. The grayscale density of pixels contained within the region of the diaphragm muscle is quantified using image analysis software (e.g., ImageJ, National Institutes of Health, Bethesda MD, https://imagej.nih.gov/ij/). Increases in echodensity in other muscles during critical illness have been shown to correlate with inflammation and necrosis [1].

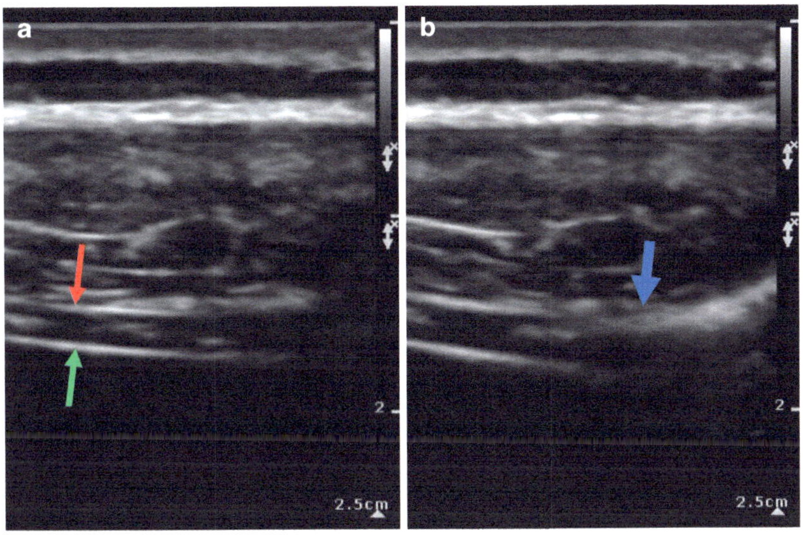

Fig. 38.2 (**a**) B mode imaging of the diaphragm in cross section at end-expiration. The relatively anechoic diaphragm lies between the highly echogenic pleural (red arrow) and peritoneal (green arrow) membranes. (**b**) During inspiration, the lung shadow (blue arrow) enters the ultrasound field. This indicates that the probe is positioned cephalad relative to the zone of apposition and should be moved down 1–2 intercostal spaces

Caveats

T_{di} measured at FRC in healthy volunteers has varied across studies but is usually slightly greater in men as compared to women and right as compared to left (see Table 38.1) [2–4]. It is also somewhat correlated with height and weight [5], is physiologically increased in association with physical training (e.g., weight-lifting) [5], and is pathologically increased in those with chronic asthma and Duchenne muscular dystrophy [6, 7]. T_{di} varies in different chronic cardiopulmonary disease states (increased, decreased, or unchanged). Isolated values of T_{di} (unless markedly abnormal, e.g., below the lower limit of normal or fifth percentile; Table 38.1) need to be interpreted with caution. Ultrasound measurement of T_{di} has been validated in autopsy studies [8] and has high intra-observer and inter-observer reproducibility (±0.2 mm) [9].

Interpretation and Evidence

Lower T_{di} measured at the outset of mechanical ventilation is strongly associated with prolonged ventilation and increased mortality [10]. This association may reflect the impact of diaphragm atrophy or it may suggest a more general lack of physiological reserve. Both increases and decreases in T_{di} over time during mechanical ventilation are associated with diaphragm dysfunction, prolonged ventilation, and poor outcomes [11]. Decreases in T_{di} over time reflect diaphragm atrophy as observed in animal models of ventilator-induced diaphragm function [12, 13]; the mechanism underlying pathological increases in T_{di} is uncertain but may reflect load-induced injury. Increases in echodensity over time during mechanical ventilation may represent muscle necrosis and/or edema. Increased echodensity is associated with fewer ventilator-free days and a trend toward increased mortality [1].

Table 38.1 Normal values taken from studies in healthy non-ventilated volunteers

Diaphragm thickness at end FRC						
Study	**Number**	**Side**	**Men**		**Women**	
			Mean ± SD (mm)	**LLN (mm)**	**Mean ± SD (mm)**	**LLN (mm)**
Boon et al. (2013) [4]	150 Supine	Right Left	3.8 ± 1.5 3.7 ± 1.7	1.7 1.6	2.7 ± 1.0 3.1 ± 1.9	1.5 1.4
Cardenas (2018) [3]	64 Semi-recumbent	Right	1.9 ± 0.3	1.3	1.8 ± 0.3	1.2
Boussuges et al. (2021) [2]	200 Seated	Right Left	2.1 ± 0.4 2.0 ± 0.4	1.3 1.3	1.9 ± 0.4 1.7 ± 0.3	1.1 1.1
Diaphragm thickening fraction expressed as %						
Study	**Number**	**Breath type**	**Mean (%)**		**LLN (%)**	
Boon et al. (2013) [4][a]	150 supine	Inspiratory capacity				
		Men (right) Men (left) Women (right) Women (left)	80 100 80 90		20 30 30 30	
Harper et al. (2013) [15][a]	150 supine	Quiet breathing				
		Right Left	20 23		18 20	
Cardenas et al. (2018) [3]	64 semi-recumbent	Inspiratory capacity				
		Men (right) Women (right)	204 170		80 82	
Boussuges et al. (2021) [2]	200 seated	Inspiratory capacity				
		Men (right) Men (left) Women (right) Women (left)	106 112 116 121		40 39 39 48	
Diaphragm excursion						
Study	**Number**	**Breath type**	**Men**		**Women**	
			Mean ± SD (cm)	**LLN (cm)**	**Mean ± SD (cm)**	**LLN (cm)**
Cardenas et al. (2018) [3]	64 semi-recumbent	Right				
		Quiet breathing Deep breathing	1.52 ± 0.43 7.79 ± 0.82	0.66 6.15	1.41 ± 0.32 6.41 ± 1.02	0.77 4.37
Boussuges et al. (2021) [2]	200 seated	Quiet breathing				
		Right Left	2.0 ± 0.5 2.2 ± 0.6	n/a	1.9 ± 0.5 1.9 ± 0.5	n/a
		Deep breathing				
		Right Left	6.0 ± 0.9 6.2 ± 0.9	n/a	5.0 ± 0.9 5.0 ± 0.7	n/a
		Voluntary sniff				
		Right Left	2.7 ± 0.7 2.8 ± 0.8	n/a	2.3 ± 0.7 2.4 ± 0.6	n/a

FRC functional residual capacity, *SD* standard deviation, *LLN* lower limit of normal, *n/a* not applicable

[a]Values of thickening ratio re-expressed as thickening fraction (%)

Diaphragm Thickening

Measurement

As the diaphragm contracts, it shortens. The resulting overlap of myofilaments causes the muscle to thicken. This contractile thickening can be quantified by ultrasound using M mode. It is imperative to keep the probe perpendicular to the muscle at the zone of apposition to avoid biasing measurements by off-axis imaging. Maximal (peak inspiratory thickness, T_{pi}) and minimal (end expiratory thickness, T_{di}) thicknesses can be measured (Fig. 38.3) and expressed as either thickening ratio (T_{pi}/T_{di}) [2, 4, 14, 15] or thickening fraction (TF_{di}, $(T_{pi}-T_{di})/T_{di}$ (×100 to express as percentage)) with the latter being more commonly used in the critical care literature. TF_{di} can be measured during tidal breathing to assess resting diaphragm contractile activity or during a maximal inspiratory maneuver (FRC to total lung capacity) to quantify maximal diaphragm thickening as a measure of diaphragm function. Measurement of maximal TF_{di} requires a vigorous inspiratory effort from a cooperative patient. In non-cooperative spontaneously ventilated patients, a maximal inspiratory effort can be obtained by transiently occluding the endotracheal tube with a one-way valve which only permits exhalation, for up to 20 s (the Marini maneuver) [16, 17]. Immediately following release of the occlusion, maximal TF_{di} can be measured from the stimulated respiratory efforts. The highest value of 3–5 maximal inspiratory efforts should be taken as the maximal TF_{di}. During passive mechanical ventilation, breaths at <50% of maximal inspiratory capacity and volumes <1.5 L (e.g., during tidal breathing) have shown to not cause inadvertent diaphragm thickening [9] and therefore, thickening that occurs during inspiration represents synergistic diaphragm contraction.

Callouts Pro–Tips

- Changes in diaphragm thickness during mechanical ventilation are associated with prolonged mechanical ventilation
- For a given level of muscular effort, the thickening and descent of the diaphragm as visualized by ultrasound is dependent on the respiratory mechanics and clinical context remains essential for interpretation

Caveats

The relationship between inspiratory thickening of the diaphragm and muscular force generation is complex. The presence of marked resistive or elastic mechanical loads may reduce shortening

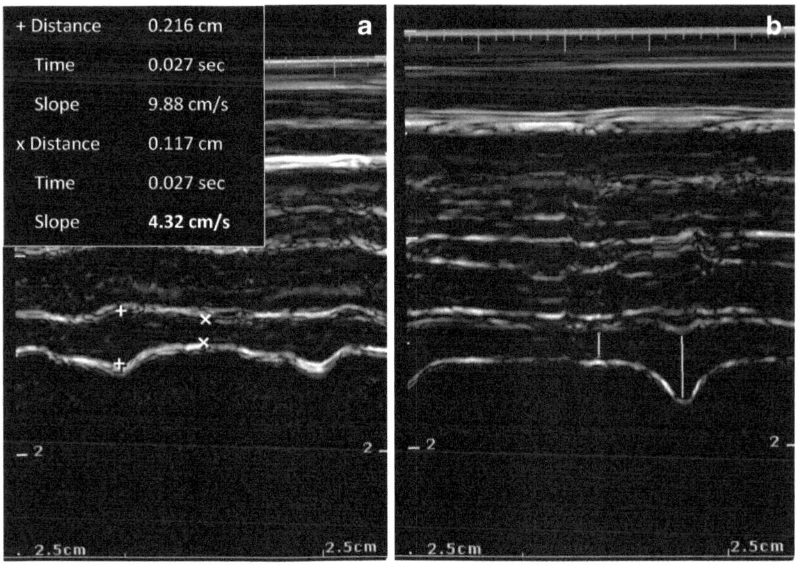

Fig. 38.3 (**a**) M mode imaging of diaphragm thickness and inspiratory thickening during tidal breathing. Measurements of thickness at end expiration (T_{di}) and inspiration (maximal thickness) allow calculation of thickening fraction or thickening ratio. (**b**) M mode imaging of diaphragm thickening during a sniff inspiratory maneuver

and thickening of the diaphragm, even as it generates very large transdiaphragmatic pressures. Additionally, when other ribcage inspiratory muscles are vigorously contracting, the diaphragm dome may be "pulled" upward, reducing diaphragmatic shortening during contraction. This reduces thickening of the muscle on ultrasound relative to force generation. Despite the complexity of this mechanical system, diaphragm thickening is a clinically useful measurement to assess for the presence and magnitude of diaphragm contractile activation [11, 18, 19]. Measurement of TF_{di} has moderately good repeatability (intra-user) and reproducibility (inter-user) noting that TF_{di} incorporates measurement errors from both T_{di} and T_{pi} [9].

Interpretation and Evidence

Maximal TF_{di} correlates with maximal inspiratory pressure [16] and a maximal TF_{di} value of <20% is diagnostic for severe diaphragm weakness [11, 20]. Tidal TF_{di} has also been shown to correlate with diaphragm strength and a value below 25% measured in patients on a pressure support mode of mechanical ventilation was found to be as effective in predicting weaning failure as diaphragm function assessed by twitch tracheal pressure obtained by supramaximal magnetic phrenic nerve stimulation [21]. During the spontaneous breathing trial (whether on pressure support or T piece), a tidal TF_{di} of >30% predicts extubation success with greater discrimination than clinical assessment by use of the rapid shallow breathing index [22]. Finally, a resting tidal TF_{di} between 15 and 30% has been shown to be associated with the shortest duration of mechanical ventilation [11] and targeting this level of diaphragm activity during invasive ventilation may protect the diaphragm from both atrophy and load-induced injury [23].

Diaphragm Excursion

Measurement

The motion and descent ("excursion") of the dome of the diaphragm can be visualized using a 2–5 MHz phased array ultrasound probe placed below the subcostal margin at the midclavicular line (Fig. 38.4). The cursor of the probe must be kept perpendicular to the dome to prevent mea-

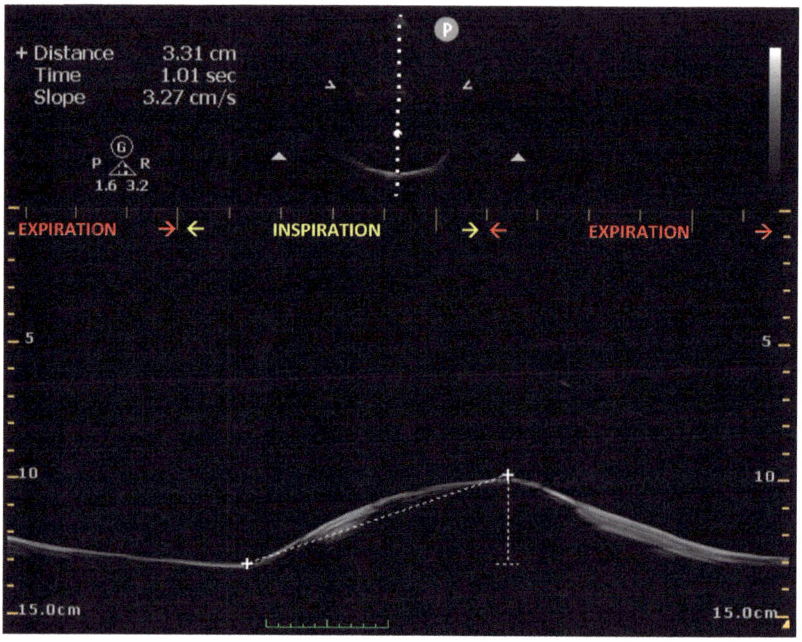

Fig. 38.4 Diaphragm excursion is measured by quantifying the maximal descent of the dome of the diaphragm on M mode (bottom image). The dome of the diaphragm can be best identified on B mode (upper image) and this is used to confirm that the ultrasound beam is approximately perpendicular to its peak

surement error from foreshortening. Excursion can be quantified in M mode during quiet breathing or during a maximal inspiratory effort. M mode tracings can also be used to assess expiratory relaxation time, a measure of muscle fatigue.

Caveats

For a given contractile force, the distance that the diaphragm dome descends will vary with changes in end-expiratory lung volume and respiratory mechanics (and as such may vary with posture [24]). In patients receiving mechanical ventilatory support, pressure and flow delivered by the ventilator inflate the chest and contribute to diaphragm excursion apart from any muscular contraction. Consequently, this measurement can only be used in ventilated patients to evaluate diaphragm function when ventilatory assistance is removed (i.e., continuous positive airway pressure, CPAP, or T-piece). Paradoxical motion of the diaphragm can sometimes be observed in patients with severe diaphragm dysfunction, unilateral phrenic nerve palsy, or in the presence of large pleural effusions that invert the diaphragm [25–27].

Interpretation and Evidence

Diaphragm excursion has excellent inter and intra-observer reproducibility with limits of agreement within approximately 10–15% of mean measurements [28]. The normal range of values for excursion has been published for a variety of diaphragmatic maneuvers including tidal breathing, sniffing, and maximal inspiration (Table 38.1). Diaphragm excursion <2.5 cm during a maximal inspiratory effort [29] and <1 cm during quiet breathing [30, 31] predicts diaphragm dysfunction. Reduced diaphragm excursion also predicts an increased duration of mechanical ventilation and hospitalization [30].

Diaphragmatic Strain and Tissue Doppler Imaging

Measurement

Diaphragmatic strain is measured by the speckle tracking technique applied to cross-sectional imaging of the diaphragm in the zone of apposition similar to the method for measuring T_{di} [32]. Strain reflects muscular deformation, theoretically a more direct assessment of contractile activation. Diaphragm motion has also been quantified by tissue doppler imaging, an echocardiographic method of assessing high-amplitude low-velocity signals of moving tissues. A 2–4 MHz phased array probe is placed subcostally between the midclavicular and anterior axillary lines, perpendicular to the mid or posterior 1/3 of the hemidiaphragm. The velocities of contraction and relaxation can be computed from the M-mode waveform, and this is correlated with transdiaphragmatic pressure [33].

Caveats

Measurement of strain by speckle tracking requires specialized ultrasound equipment and software not available on all bedside ultrasound devices. Tissue doppler measurements are generally obtained for the right hemidiaphragm as the contrast with the liver makes it easier to identify and follow the motion of the diaphragm. Tissue doppler measurements of diaphragmatic motion are unable to distinguish passive and active force generation during passive mechanical ventilation, and can only be used when inspiratory assistance is removed (i.e., CPAP or T-piece in ventilated patients or in non-ventilated patients).

Interpretation and Evidence

The utility of diaphragmatic strain measurements in the clinical setting is uncertain. Peak contraction velocity measured by tissue doppler imaging is strongly correlated with peak transdiaphragmatic pressure and pressure-time product. Maximal relaxation rate measured by tissue doppler correlates with the maximal relaxation rate of transdiaphragmatic pressure and is markedly increased in weaning failure [33]. During a spontaneous breathing trial, inspiratory peak and mean excursion velocity as well as acceleration have been found to be significantly higher in patients who subsequently went on to fail extubation (3.1 vs. 1.8 cm/s; 1.6 vs. 1.1 cm/s; 8.8 vs. 4.2 cm/s^2, respectively) [34].

Applications of Diaphragm Ultrasound and Implications for Weaning

Diaphragm ultrasound has a number of clinical applications to include diagnostic, prognostic, and procedural uses. The diagnostic applications include assisting in evaluation of diaphragm function in patients with possible neuromuscular causes of respiratory disease and guiding needle placement for diaphragm intramuscular electromyography [35]. Paradoxical diaphragm motion can identify patients with potential phrenic nerve injury, severe diaphragm dysfunction, or in the presence of pleural effusions identify those in whom drainage is likely to improve respiratory mechanics [25]. Ultrasound can also be used to assess diaphragm function in patients who are difficult to liberate from mechanical ventilation (Table 38.2). Serial measurements can detect the development of diaphragm atrophy or myotrauma and sonographic assessment of contractility might be useful to guide a diaphragm-protective ventilatory strategy from early in the course of mechanical ventilation.

Table 38.2 Diaphragm ultrasound measurements predicting prolonged mechanical ventilation

Diaphragm thickness (T_{di}) and echodensity
Lower T_{di} at outset of mechanical ventilation [10]
Increase or decrease (≥10%) in T_{di} from baseline [11]
Increasing echodensity [1]
Diaphragm thickening fraction (TF_{di}) expressed as %
Maximal TF_{di} <20% (diagnostic for severe diaphragm weakness) [20]
TF_{di} <15 or >30% (average value over first 3 days of ventilation) [11]
Tidal TF_{di} <25% during a spontaneous breathing trial [21]
Diaphragm excursion
Paradoxical movement on excursion assessment [27]
Excursion <2.5 cm during maximal inspiratory effort [29]
Excursion <1 cm during tidal breathing [30, 31]

Call-Out Evolving Evidence

- Diaphragm thickening is a useful predictor of ability to wean from mechanical ventilation and extubation success. It may also provide a therapeutic target for safe diaphragm activity

Summary Points

- The costal diaphragm can be visualized at the zone of apposition and thickness at end expiration (T_{di}) can be measured in B or M mode
- Thickening fraction (TF_{di} during tidal or maximal inspiratory breath) is generally measured in M mode to more easily identify the peak diaphragm thickness during inspiration.
- Diaphragm excursion (tidal or maximal inspiratory breath) is measured subcostally in M mode in spontaneously ventilating patients only
- Diaphragm thickness, thickening fraction, and excursion provide diagnostic and prognostically useful information in mechanically ventilated patients
- Emerging data on diaphragm echodensity, strain, and tissue doppler may provide further robust markers and thresholds to guide assessment of diaphragm function in the future

Questions

1. A 52-year-old female is 8 days post bilateral lung transplant for interstitial pulmonary fibrosis on a background of moderate pulmonary hypertension and previous ventricular septal defect repair. She was reintubated within 6 h of extubation on day 3 due to increased work of breathing and poor sputum clearance. Despite subsequent completion of antimicrobial treatment for staphylococcus aureus grown from a donor bronchoaleveolar lavage specimen and optimization of fluid status, she is slow to wean from mechanical ventilation. Her clinical examination is significant for hypoactive delirium and mild-moderate global weakness while off sedation for more than 48 h. As part of a work-up, the team requests an echocardiogram and a diaphragm ultrasound. Diaphragm excursion (right hemidiaphragm) is shown below and was performed on continuous positive airway pressure (CPAP) 8cmH_2O, FiO_2 0.4. What information if any does this give?
   A. Diaphragmatic excursion is within normal limits for tidal breathing in women. Diaphragm dysfunction (right side only assessed here) is unlikely to significantly contribute to failure to wean.
   B. Reduced diaphragm excursion is suggestive of diaphragm dysfunction. Ensure imaging is not off axis (and thereby underestimating true value) and assess other diaphragm parameters such as TF_{di}.
   C. Diaphragm excursion is excessive for normal tidal breathing suggesting the diaphragm is not the primary cause of failure to wean. If excessive efforts continue, however, under-assistance, myotrauma may lead to diaphragm dysfunction.
   D. Paradoxical diaphragm movement is suggestive of phrenic nerve injury, severe diaphragm dysfunction, or clinically significant pleural effusion, further investigation into cause is warranted.
   E. Diaphragm excursion is an unreliable assessment of diaphragm dysfunction in this scenario due to the presence of significant positive pressure from the ventilator.

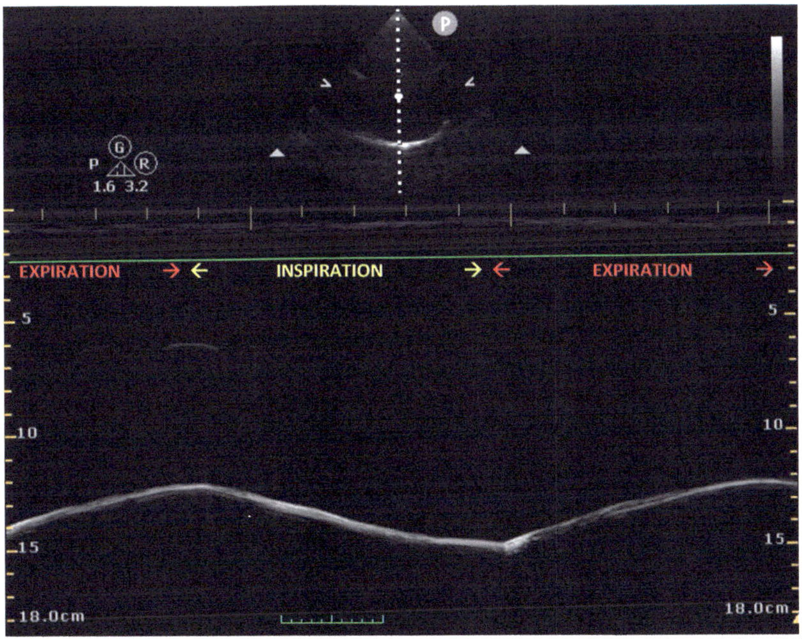

Answer: D

Explanation: M-mode image demonstrates paradoxical movement (diaphragm ascent during inspiration is demonstrated by movement of the dome AWAY from the probe).

2. A 32-year-old male with a background history of poorly controlled asthma presented 14 days earlier with a ruptured appendix. His postoperative course was complicated by intra-abdominal sepsis (requiring surgical drainage of collections and multiple washouts, as well as moderate vasopressor support), acute kidney injury (however, no renal replacement therapy indicated), and acute respiratory distress syndrome (ARDS, featuring both hypoxemic respiratory failure and significant impairment in respiratory mechanics). Despite substantial improvement in his overall clinical condition, he is intolerant to further weaning of pressure support (PEEP 6 cm H_2O, pressure support 14 cm H_2O, FiO_2 0.3). The treating team considers several potential contributing factors to include ongoing pain, hyperactive delirium necessitating intermittent sedative use, resolving ARDS, and ventilator induced diaphragm dysfunction (VIDD). The team requests a diaphragm ultrasound to assess diaphragmatic effort and function. With regards to the image below taken during tidal breathing, which of the following statements is *NOT* true?
   A. T_{di} may be lower than expected given age, gender, and asthma history, suggesting a potential for diaphragm atrophy to have occurred. However, care needs to be taken in interpreting isolated T_{di} measurements.
   B. If T_{di} is increased from the patient's baseline, this would suggest an increase in diaphragm muscle mass and would correlate well with an ability to generate higher transdiaphragmatic pressures and excludes diaphragm dysfunction.
   C. Although within normal range, given known respiratory and abdominal pathologies, TF_{di} may represent excessive force and a risk of underassistance myotrauma.
   D. Despite significant ventilatory support TF_{di} still provides valuable information about the patient's respiratory effort and diaphragm function.
   E. Normal diaphragm excursion would not prove useful in excluding diaphragm dysfunction in this scenario.

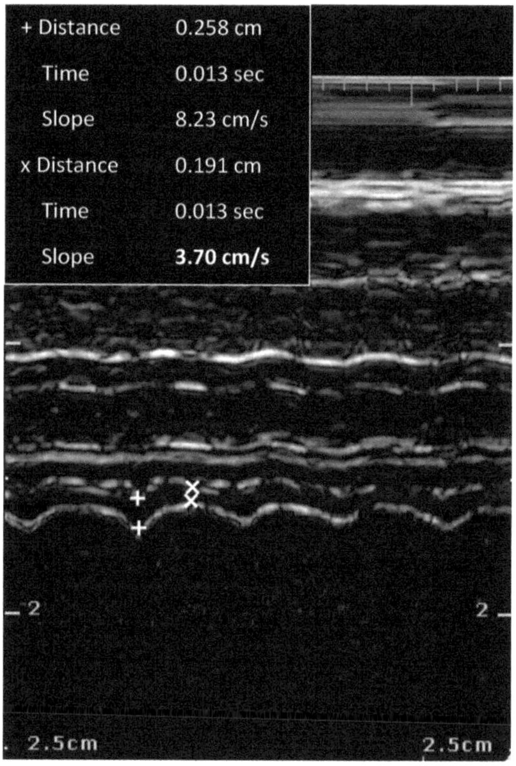

Answer: B

Explanation: Acute increases in diaphragm thickness during critical illness are often considered to be due to load-induced injury, edema, or necrosis and is associated with prolonged mechanical ventilation.

References

1. Coiffard B, Riegler S, Sklar MC, Dres M, Vorona S, Reid WD, et al. Diaphragm echodensity in mechanically ventilated patients: a description of technique and outcomes. Crit Care. 2021;25(1):64.
2. Boussuges A, Rives S, Finance J, Chaumet G, Vallée N, Risso J-J, et al. Ultrasound assessment of diaphragm thickness and thickening: reference values and limits of normality when in a seated position. Front Med. 2021;8:742703.

3. Cardenas LZ, Santana PV, Caruso P, de Carvalho CR, de Albuquerque AL. Diaphragmatic ultrasound correlates with inspiratory muscle strength and pulmonary function in healthy subjects. Ultrasound Med Biol. 2018;44(4):786–93.
4. Boon AJ, Harper CJ, Ghahfarokhi LS, Strommen JA, Watson JC, Sorenson EJ. Two-dimensional ultrasound imaging of the diaphragm: quantitative values in normal subjects. Muscle Nerve. 2013;47(6):884–9.
5. McCool FD, Benditt JO, Conomos P, Anderson L, Sherman CB Jr, FGH. Variability of diaphragm structure among healthy individuals. Am J Resp Crit Care. 2012;155(4):1323–8.
6. Bruin PFD, Ueki J, Bush A, Khan Y, Watson A, Pride NB. Diaphragm thickness and inspiratory strength in patients with Duchenne muscular dystrophy. Thorax. 1997;52(5):472.
7. de Bruin PF, Ueki J, Watson A, Pride NB. Size and strength of the respiratory and quadriceps muscles in patients with chronic asthma. European Respir J. 1997;10(1):59–64.
8. Wait JL, Nahormek PA, Yost WT, Rochester DP. Diaphragmatic thickness-lung volume relationship in vivo. J Appl Physiol. 1989;67(4):1560–8.
9. Goligher EC, Laghi F, Detsky ME, Farias P, Murray A, Brace D, et al. Measuring diaphragm thickness with ultrasound in mechanically ventilated patients: feasibility, reproducibility and validity. Intens Care Med. 2015;41(4):642–9.
10. Sklar MC, Dres M, Fan E, Rubenfeld GD, Scales DC, Herridge MS, et al. Association of low baseline diaphragm muscle mass with prolonged mechanical ventilation and mortality among critically ill adults. JAMA Netw Open. 2020;3(2):e1921520.
11. Goligher EC, Dres M, Fan E, Rubenfeld GD, Scales DC, Herridge MS, et al. Mechanical ventilation-induced diaphragm atrophy strongly impacts clinical outcomes. Am J Resp Crit Care. 2018;197(2):204–13.
12. Sassoon CSH, Caiozzo VJ, Manka A, Sieck GC. Altered diaphragm contractile properties with controlled mechanical ventilation. J Appl Physiol. 2002;92(6):2585–95.
13. Powers SK, Shanely RA, Coombes JS, Koesterer TJ, McKenzie M, Gammeren DV, et al. Mechanical ventilation results in progressive contractile dysfunction in the diaphragm. J Appl Physiol. 2002;92(5):1851–8.
14. Ueki J, Bruin PFD, Pride NB. In vivo assessment of diaphragm contraction by ultrasound in normal subjects. Thorax. 1995;50(11):1157–61.
15. Harper CJ, Shahgholi L, Cieslak K, Hellyer NJ, Strommen JA, Boon AJ. Variability in diaphragm motion during normal breathing, assessed with B-mode ultrasound. J Orthop Sports Phys Ther. 2013;43(12):927–31.
16. Marini JJ, Smith TC, Lamb V. Estimation of inspiratory muscle strength in mechanically ventilated patients: the measurement of maximal inspiratory pressure. J Crit Care. 1986;1(1):32–8.
17. Truwit JD, Marini JJ. Validation of a technique to assess maximal inspiratory pressure in poorly cooperative patients. Chest. 1992;102(4):1216–9.
18. Cohn D, Benditt JO, Eveloff S, McCool FD. Diaphragm thickening during inspiration. J Appl Physiol. 1997;83(1):291–6.
19. Vivier E, Dessap AM, Dimassi S, Vargas F, Lyazidi A, Thille AW, et al. Diaphragm ultrasonography to estimate the work of breathing during non-invasive ventilation. Intens Care Med. 2012;38(5):796–803.
20. Gottesman E, McCool FD. Ultrasound evaluation of the paralyzed diaphragm. Am J Resp Crit Care. 1997;155(5):1570–4.
21. Dres M, Goligher EC, Dubé B-P, Morawiec E, Dangers L, Reuter D, et al. Diaphragm function and weaning from mechanical ventilation: an ultrasound and phrenic nerve stimulation clinical study. Ann Intensive Care. 2018;8(1):53.
22. DiNino E, Gartman EJ, Sethi JM, McCool FD. Diaphragm ultrasound as a predictor of successful extubation from mechanical ventilation. Thorax. 2014;69(5):431.
23. Goligher EC, Jonkman AH, Dianti J, Vaporidi K, Beitler JR, Patel BK, et al. Clinical strategies for implementing lung and diaphragm-protective ventilation: avoiding insufficient and excessive effort. Intens Care Med [Internet]. 2020;46(12):2314–26. https://doi.org/10.1007/s00134-020-06288-9.
24. Chen CF, Lien IN, Wu MC. Respiratory function in patients with spinal cord injuries: effects of posture. Spinal Cord. 1990;28(2):81–6.
25. Cooper JC, Elliott ST. Pleural effusions, diaphragm inversion, and paradox: new observations using sonography. AJR Am J Roentgenol. 1995;164(2):510.
26. Goligher EC, Ferguson ND. Utility of draining pleural effusions in mechanically ventilated patients. Curr Opin Pulm Med. 2012;18(4):359–65.
27. Nason LK, Walker CM, McNeeley MF, Burivong W, Fligner CL, Godwin JD. Imaging of the diaphragm: anatomy and function. Radiographics. 2012;32(2):E51–70.
28. Boussuges A, Gole Y, Blanc P. Diaphragmatic motion studied by M-mode ultrasonography methods, reproducibility, and normal values. Chest. 2009;135(2):391–400.
29. Lerolle N, Guérot E, Dimassi S, Zegdi R, Faisy C, Fagon J-Y, et al. Ultrasonographic diagnostic criterion for severe diaphragmatic dysfunction after cardiac surgery. Chest. 2009;135(2):401–7.
30. Kim WY, Suh HJ, Hong S-B, Koh Y, Lim C-M. Diaphragm dysfunction assessed by ultrasonography: influence on weaning from mechanical ventilation*. Crit Care Med. 2011;39(12):2627–30.
31. Farghaly S, Hasan AA. Diaphragm ultrasound as a new method to predict extubation outcome in mechanically ventilated patients. Aust Crit Care. 2017;30(1):37–43.

32. Orde SR, Boon AJ, Firth DG, Villarraga HR, Sekiguchi H. Diaphragm assessment by two dimensional speckle tracking imaging in normal subjects. BMC Anesthesiol. 2016;16(1):43.
33. Soilemezi E, Savvidou S, Sotiriou P, Smyrniotis D, Tsagourias M, Matamis D. Tissue Doppler imaging of the diaphragm in healthy subjects and critically ill patients. Am J Resp Crit Care. 2020;202(7):1005–12.
34. Cammarota G, Boniolo E, Santangelo E, Vita ND, Verdina F, Crudo S, et al. Diaphragmatic kinetics assessment by tissue Doppler imaging and extubation outcome. Respir Care. 2021;66(6):983–93.
35. Boon AJ, Oney-Marlow TM, Murthy NS, Harper CM, McNamara TR, Smith J. Accuracy of electromyography needle placement in cadavers: non-guided vs. ultrasound guided. Muscle Nerve. 2011;44(1):45–9.

Thoracentesis and Thoracostomy Procedural Guidance

39

Tahir Ahmad and Jen-Ting Chen

Learning Objectives

1. Learn the technique, required equipment, and patient positioning needed for successful ultrasound (U/S)-guided thoracentesis and tube thoracostomy.
2. Understand the principles of manometry and its uses.
3. Familiarize with the procedural complications of thoracentesis and tube thoracostomy.
4. Understand the indications for confirmatory chest X-ray after thoracentesis, its evidence, and limitations.
5. Understand the benefits and utility of ultrasound in subpleural mass biopsies.

Introduction

Thoracentesis and tube thoracostomy are important procedures utilized for the diagnosis and treatment of pleural effusions, empyema, pneumothoracies, and systemic diseases. Ultrasound plays a significant role in the diagnosis and characterization of pleural pathology, as well as the planning for these two diagnostic and therapeutic procedures, and as such will be the first step in performing these procedures. The ultrasound diagnosis and characterization of fluid collections and pneumothoracies have been described elsewhere in this section.

Thoracentesis Technique

For thoracentesis, ultrasound should be utilized to assess two things: to image the location of the largest pocket of fluid for the procedural approach, and to interrogate the site of the procedure for vascular structures and adjacent lung that can lead to complications. Ideally, one would use the phased array probe to look for the largest pocket of fluid, and then utilize the linear probe to assess the subcutaneous and cutaneous tissues for vascular structures. In general, the approach will be to insert the needle or catheter used for the thoracentesis as close to the superior aspect of the identified rib space as possible to avoid the intercostal artery, which runs along the inferior rib border.

Prior to the procedure, obtain adequate equipment necessary for thoracentesis: sterile drape, chlorhexidine antiseptic, needles of various sizes—a 22 or 25 gauge needle for anesthetic and

Supplementary Information The online version contains supplementary material available at https://doi.org/10.1007/978-3-031-80038-2_39.

T. Ahmad · J.-T. Chen (✉)
Division of Critical Care Medicine, Department of Medicine, Montefiore Medical Center, Albert Einstein College of Medicine, Bronx, NY, USA
e-mail: tahmad@montefiore.org; Tina.Chen@ucsf.edu

M. J. Lanspa, A. T. Levinson (eds.), *Echocardiography and Ultrasonography in the ICU*, Respiratory Medicine, https://doi.org/10.1007/978-3-031-80038-2_39

an 18 or 20 gauge needle with a length of at least 5 cm depending on the thickness of the patient's subcutaneous tissue—a large bore IV catheter, lidocaine for anesthetic injection, at least 2 syringes (one for anesthetic injection and a second for withdrawing fluid), scalpel, one way tubing, a three-way stopcock, and a drainage bag. This is in addition to a sterile gown, gloves, mask, and cap for sterile technique (Fig. 39.1). Commercial drainage kits may be available, and one should familiarize with the equipment prior to proceeding.

Ideally, if your patient is hemodynamically stable, position them in a sitting position for thoracentesis leaning forward against a stable table for a posterior thorax approach to maximize the intercostal space and amount of fluid in the posterior gutter [1, 2] (Fig. 39.2). However, this position may not be feasible in all situations, especially in the critical care setting.

In a supine patient, raising the head of the bed or placing wedges allows fluid to drain to the base of the thorax (Fig. 39.3). The arm on the side of the procedure should be securely placed away from the procedural site, either above the head or extended. With the use of ultrasound, visualize the exact approach to the fluid pocket, which is dependent on the proximity of the surrounding organs and the diaphragm. A safe needle insertion depth of >1 cm of fluid thickness from the pleura has been cited in the literature from the 2010 British Thoracic Society Pleural Disease Guidelines [3]; however, a minimum depth of 1 cm for the performance of this procedure may not be sufficient for safety. A retrospective study by Schecthman et al. on the incidence and risk factors for pneumothorax after ultrasound guided thoracentesis found that patients who developed a pneumothorax had a smaller depth of pleural fluid at a mean of 3.37 cm [4]. While there is a paucity of literature for what fluid depth is exactly safe, this determination is best guided by clinical judgement on whether the needle can be inserted safely into a fluid pocket. Given these findings, our usual practice considers a safe fluid pocket for thoracentesis to be at least 3 cm of fluid from pleura and the surrounding structures and should not

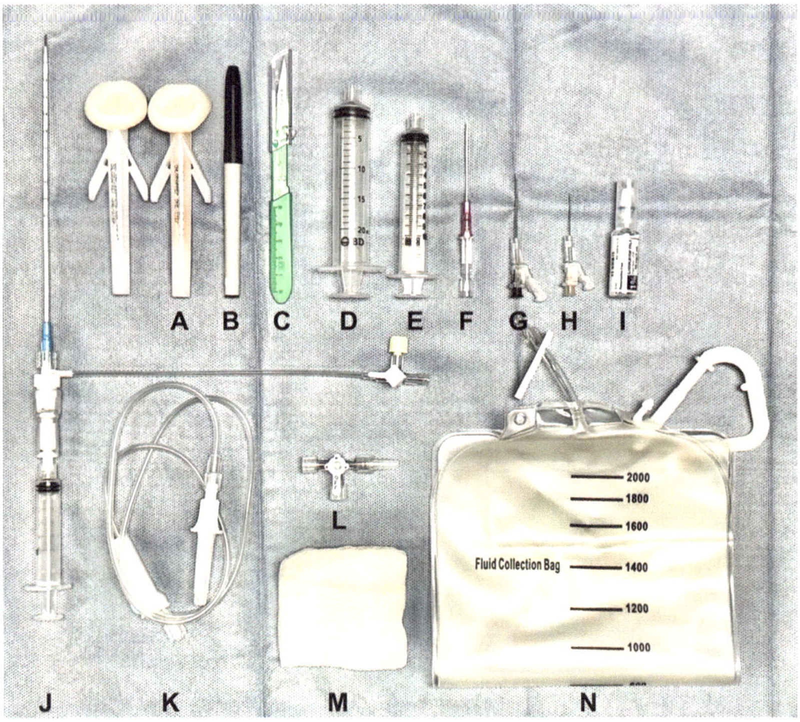

Fig. 39.1 Equipment needed for thoracentesis. (**a**) Chlorhexidine antiseptic prep, (**b**) marking pen, (**c**) 11 blade scalpel, (**d**) 20 mL syringe, (**e**) 10 mL syringe, (**f**) 20 gauge angiocatheter for drainage, (**g**) 22 gauge needle for deep lidocaine infiltration, (**h**) 25 gauge needle for superficial lidocaine infiltration, (**i**) Lidocaine 1% for anesthetization, (**j**) commercial blunt catheter-based needle with trochar, (**k**) one-way tubing, (**l**) three-way stopcock, (**m**) gauze, and (**n**) drainage bag

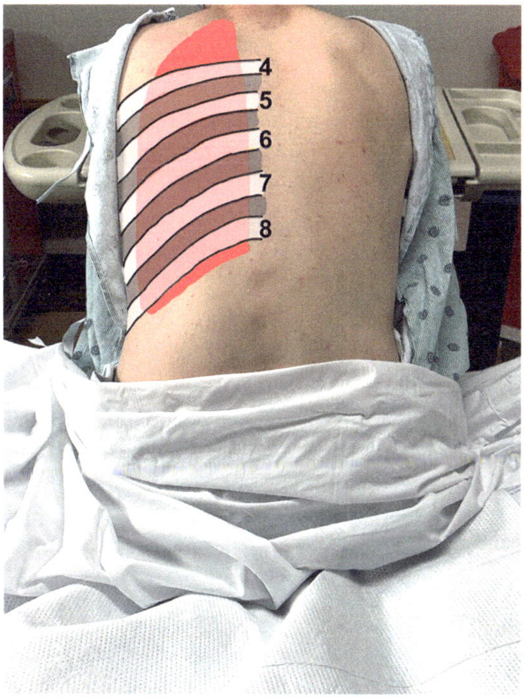

Fig. 39.2 Patient in the upright position for thoracentesis. Patient in this image is leaning forward to maximize intercostal space width. Numbered are ribs four through eight, with highlighted lung

have lung within the path of the needle, lung overlapping the diaphragm in the path of the needle, or the diaphragm within the direction of the needle.

Use ultrasound to interrogate the potential space of insertion, taking note of the pocket with the largest size of fluid, the distance your needle will need to travel exactly to enter the space, and vascular structures in the area. Mark the entry site of the needle while performing ultrasound. This should be placed approximately at the level of the superior aspect of the rib inferior to the intercostal space of interest. Whenever possible, we recommend the use of a blunt catheter-based needle (such as a specialized cavity drainage catheter) to minimize risk of lung puncture. Once the intercostal space of interest is identified, carefully mark the site of entry with a marking pen. Use sterile technique and provide local anesthetic to the surrounding rib space and pleura accordingly with 10 mL of lidocaine 1% [3]. Pay attention to whether air or pleural fluid is aspirated while anesthetizing and when performing the procedure.

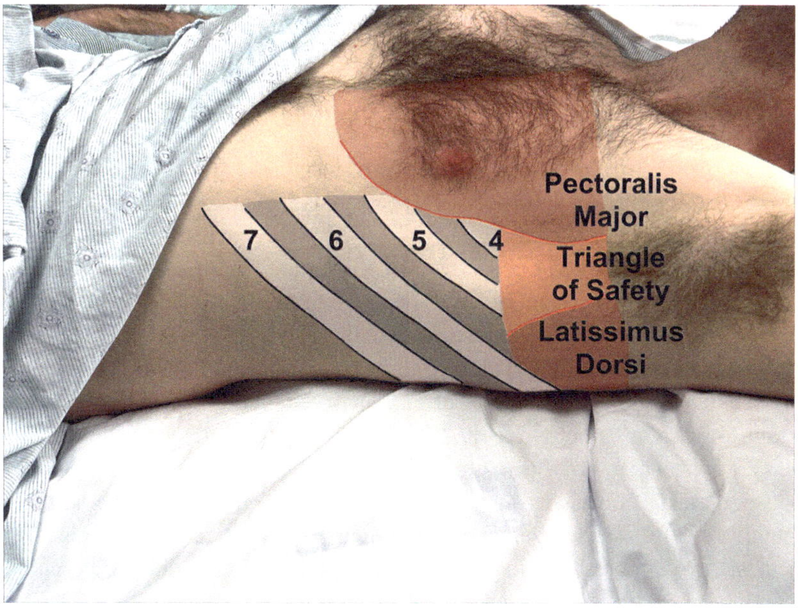

Fig. 39.3 Patient in supine position for thoracentesis. Numbered are ribs four through seven, and highlighted are the borders of the triangle of safety: pectoralis major, latissimus dorsi, and the superior border of the fifth intercostal space

Pro Tip Call-Out
In an obese patient or patient with excess skin, we recommend pulling the patient's skin taut when puncturing the skin and maintaining the same tension throughout the procedure.

For a simple diagnostic aspiration, using an 18-to-20-gauge needle with a 20 mL syringe is sufficient for the procedure). Insert the needle applying negative pressure until you enter the pleural space. Insertion can either be performed after ultrasound used to mark insertion site and then putting U/S probe down prior to cleaning site following same angle of probe used previously and maintaining same patient positionings (static technique). Alternatively, the ultrasound probe can be used dynamically using a sterile probe cover in real time (dynamic technique). It is our opinion that needle insertion should be done under real-time ultrasound guidance with a sterile probe cover with the probe angled adjacent to the needle to demonstrate its movement, or immediately before the procedure [3]. Direct ultrasound guidance increases the chances of aspirating fluid both successfully and safely. There is limited evidence that with a pleural effusion with 3 cm or greater depth below the pleural line that real time technique in a skilled operator is superior to the static technique (Mayo chest 2004).

Pro Tip Call-Out
Adjust the angle of your ultrasound probe during thoracentesis to keep your needle always visualized while advancing.

Remove the needle or catheter during exhalation to avoid entrapment of air. When using a large bore catheter-based system, you will need to make a small incision of the cutaneous tissue horizontal to the rib at the site of entry prior to insertion of the catheter-needle system to allow easy advancement of the catheter over needle system. Basic fluid assessment to determine the nature of effusion includes pH, lactate dehydrogenase, protein, gram stain microscopy, culture, cytology, as well as cell count with differential. Additional studies can be sent as needed where there is clinical suspicion. The procedure should stop if the patient has chest discomfort or persistent coughing, when no more fluid can be aspirated, or if 1.5 L of fluid has been removed [1, 5]. The procedure should stop after 1.5 L of volume is removed due to an increased risk of pneumothoracies and re-expansion pulmonary.

Tube Thoracostomy Technique

Tube thoracostomy, or chest tube placement, is performed to drain a pleural fluid collection, and to treat pneumothoracies. It is generally performed in the fifth intercostal space, mid-axillary line using landmarks within a space called the triangle of safety (Fig. 39.3). The triangle of safety is defined by the lateral border of pectoralis major, the lateral border of latissimus dorsi, and the superior border of the fifth intercostal space (nipple line).

Landmark based approaches have a considerable risk of complications, such as subdiaphragmatic tube placement, organ injury, bleeding from injury to a vessel, and infection. These risks can be mitigated by ultrasound. A prospective randomized study on trauma patients in the emergency department found that ultrasound identified thoracostomy insertion sites above the diaphragm 97% of the time [6]. Gray et al., in a prospective study, found that almost 20% of potential thoracostomy sites assessed by landmarks either were below the diaphragm or crossed the diaphragm when the fifth intercostal space was evaluated by ultrasound [7]. Tube thoracostomy can be performed either with seldinger technique or direct manual surgical chest tube. Both methods require localization of pleural space devoid of lung sliding or the presence of a lung point. The patient is positioned in a semi-recumbent position at 30° elevation and with the ipsilateral arm secured away from the procedural field. Providing proper analgesia and anxiolysis help with the success of the procedure. Both anterior and lateral approaches can be utilized under ultrasound guidance for tube thoracostomy provided adequate ultrasound guidance and diagnosis of pneumothorax in the rib space of interest. We recommend the use of ultrasound to identify the safest fluid pocket, as well as identifying the largest air pocket, determined by the area with the largest number of contiguous rib spaces without lung sliding.

For this procedure, you will need a chest tray, antiseptic, sterile drapes, gown, gloves, mask, cap, lidocaine, sutures, scalpel, gauze, and tape. A drainage system with a water seal to prevent air entry into the thoracic cavity is necessary and allows for safe suction [8]. Commercial tube thoracostomy kits may also be available. The following procedural guidance will describe the use of a commercial tube thoracostomy kit that uses seldinger technique to insert a chest tube. Prep your patient prior to the procedure with antiseptic and maintain universal precautions. Identify thoracostomy site and anesthetize liberally with lidocaine 1% in the tissue and pleural space. Use ultrasound to guide the insertion of the needle into the pleural space while aspirating by placing the probe adjacent to the needle insertion site for visualization. Confirmation of entrance into the pleural space can be confirmed by aspiration of pleural fluid if treating a pleural collection, and evacuation of air for a pneumothorax. A small amount of sterile saline within the syringe can facilitate visualization of air. Once the needle is in place, use seldinger technique to deploy the chest tube. Additionally, prior to chest tube deployment, the guidewire can be visualized under ultrasound guidance for confirmation of entry into the pleural space (Video 39.1) (Fig. 39.4).

A size 10–14 Fr chest tube suffices for treatment of simple pneumothoracies, drainage of pleural fluid, parapneumonic effusions, and empyema [3]. In our practice, we opt for larger diameter chest tubes for proteinaceous or thick pleural fluid to minimize resistance to flow. Parapneumonic effusions and empyema will require intrapleural tPA/DNase instillation via the chest tube [9]. Secure the chest tube to the skin with #0–#1 silk suture, dress it with gauze and tape, while attaching it to the drainage system. Confirm chest tube placement by repeating lung ultrasound to visualize the catheter within pleural fluid or presence of lung sliding. The gold standard however remains radiograph for confirmation. For the blunt insertion of chest tubes (also known as a surgical chest tube), ultrasound should be utilized similarly in assessing an appropriate insertion site as described above. An incision will need to be made to accommodate the index finger and chest tube at the same time, within which a Kelly clamp or index finger will be used to bluntly dissect a path angled superiorly, followed by the entrance of the pleural space with the tip of the Kelly clamp [10]. Once the tip of the clamp is within the pleural space (signified by a pop), insert your index finger alongside the chest tube within the pleural space and guide the chest tube into the pleural space, ensure the side ports are within the thoracic cavity, and immediately connect it to the drainage system afterwards. Secure the chest tube with suture and cover the chest tube site with gauze and tape.

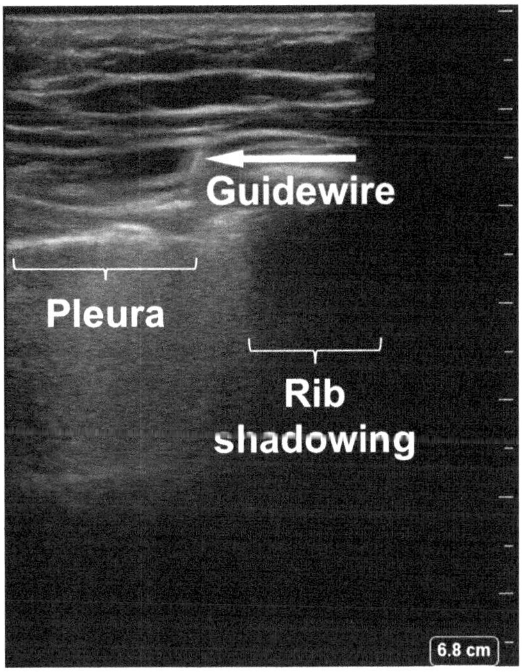

Fig. 39.4 Guidewire confirmation within pneumothorax using ultrasound. In this image, brackets highlight the pleura and rib shadowing, and an arrow highlights the guidewire. Still image is from the associated video highlighting ultrasound findings in a patient undergoing chest tube placement for treatment of a pneumothorax

Manometry

Manometry can be used as a safeguard to monitor pleural pressures to help prevent complications of thoracentesis such as pulmonary edema, chest discomfort, and breathlessness, especially in those with non-expanding lungs due to trapped lung. Pressures lower than −20 cm H_2O are cited as excessively negative based on early research models, where pressures greater than this had the lowest incidence of complications [11]. These complications are more likely to occur in those with lung entrapment or trapped lung. Manometry can be performed in various ways by connecting the pleural catheter to either a digital manometer, a hemodynamic transducer with an ICU monitor, or a column manometer. Your choice of monitor is attached to the pleural catheter and measurements can be taken in intervals after removing aliquots of fluid. Measurements are taken during expiration. Pleural elastance can be calculated by taking an initial pleural pressure measurement, subtracting the final pleural pressure measurement after completing thoracentesis, and dividing it by the amount of fluid removed (calculated in H_2O/L).

$$\text{PEL} = \frac{(\text{Opening pressure} - \text{Closing pressure})}{\text{Volume removed}}$$

While manometry can assist in mitigating complications, it is not commonly performed, and often symptoms during thoracentesis are used to guide the clinician's removal of fluid. A 2019 randomized single blinded study on the utilization of manometry during large volume thoracentesis to prevent related complications demonstrated that its utilization did not lead to a statistically significant reduction in procedure related chest discomfort [12]. There were some limitations to the study, such as most patients had 1 L of fluid or less removed (60%), with fewer patients having more than 1.2 L of fluid removed, which questions whether the study findings are generalizable to those patients who have large volume thoracentesis performed [13].

Procedural Complications

Complications during performance of thoracentesis and tube thoracostomy can occur. These complications include pneumothorax, bleeding, re-expansion pulmonary edema [5], as well as pain, and procedure failure. Pneumothorax has a higher incidence of occurrence when thoracentesis is performed without ultrasound guidance [14]. Bleeding can manifest as puncture site bleeding, intercostal blood vessel injuries resulting in hemothorax, and chest wall hematoma. Use of ultrasound to identify vasculature prior to procedure can assist in reducing the risk of bleeding. Finally, re-expansion pulmonary edema, while uncommon, can occur after thoracentesis, and manifests as hypoxemia and new infiltrates on chest X-ray within 24 h of thoracentesis, usually within in the re-expanded lung.

The Need for Chest X-Ray After Thoracentesis

Some proceduralists may obtain a chest X-ray post procedurally after a thoracentesis to confirm the absence of a pneumothorax. Early literature has suggested that thoracentesis had a considerable rate of pneumothorax ranging from 5.2% to as high as 26% [14]. However, ultrasound guided thoracentesis has shown to have significantly reduced this risk. A 1997 retrospective review of ultrasound guided thoracentesis by Gervais et al. found that out of 434 patients who underwent thoracentesis (342 spontaneously breathing, 92 intubated), only 10 patients developed a pneumothorax (6 in intubated patients, and 4 in spontaneously breathing patients) [15]. In another retrospective study of ultrasound guided thoracentesis by Cavanna et al. in 2014, among 445 patients with malignant pleural effusions who underwent thoracentesis with and without ultrasound, pneumothorax occurred in less than 1% of those guided with ultrasound (3/310), and in 8.89% of those without ultrasound guidance

(12/135) [14]. Tube thoracostomy was required in three patients only, and only in those who had thoracentesis performed without ultrasound. Pneumothorax can occur due to several reasons, such as introduction of air during procedure into the pleural cavity, direct lung puncture, and failure for the lung to expand after removal of fluid, known as pneumothorax ex vacuo. Pneumothorax ex vacuo does not require treatment with a chest tube. A review of the available literature suggests obtaining a repeat chest radiograph after thoracentesis if the patient had multiple attempts, if there was aspiration of air, if they are on a mechanical ventilator, if large volume thoracentesis was performed, or if they have advanced lung disease [16]. The decision to obtain a chest radiograph should be guided by patient symptoms and clinical suspicion. Ultrasound should also be utilized to check for post-procedural pneumothorax after a thoracentesis and be used to assess for residual pleural effusion in lieu of chest X-ray and has the benefit of preventing additional radiation exposure. Outside of the above, obtaining routine chest radiography to rule out pneumothorax after a thoracentesis is not required [3]. Obtaining a chest radiograph after tube thoracostomy is a usual practice and should be performed post procedurally.

Subpleural Mass Biopsy

Ultrasound has been shown to be safe and effective in ultrasound-guided needle biopsies of subpleural masses. A retrospective study by Mychajlowycz et al. found that ultrasound and CT guidance for subpleural biopsies have similar safety and diagnostic adequacy but with the benefit of shorter procedure times and wait times when done under ultrasound guidance [17]. The lesions biopsied in this study were noted to be larger than those biopsied by CT, with an average axial diameter of 4.8 cm (±2.6) compared to lesions biopsied via CT with an average axial diameter of 3.2 cm (±1.9), and additionally demonstrated equivalent sampling adequacy and similar rate of pneumothoracies. Biopsies were performed with a semi-automatic 18-gauge needle with a Menghini type tip. Furthermore, a prospective analysis on the diagnostic accuracy of ultrasound guided subpleural mass biopsies by Sperandeo et al. found that ultrasound guided biopsies were 93% accurate with 0.79% rate of pneumothorax, demonstrating that ultrasound guidance is both safe and effective compared to CT guidance [18]. Diagnostic accuracy in this study however depended on the size of the subpleural mass, with masses greater than 5.0 cm and smaller than 2.0 cm having a higher rate of non-statistically significant non-diagnostic biopsies compared to masses with sizes between 2.0 cm and 5.0 cm.

Conclusion

Thoracentesis and tube thoracostomy are critical procedures for clinicians to perform precisely and safely. The use of ultrasound has allowed for intensivists to mitigate the risk of pneumothorax and organ injury. In addition, ultrasound can be used to confirm lung re-expansion after chest tube placement for pneumothorax and to re-assess the pleural space after fluid drainage, helping to reduce the need for chest X-ray. Ultrasound is used to interrogate the site of procedure for findings that ensure safety, such as, largest area with absence of lung sliding, and largest fluid pocket for pneumothoracies and pleural effusions, respectively. Symptom monitoring during therapeutic thoracentesis is largely used over manometry. Finally, ultrasound is safe and effective in obtaining subpleural biopsies, with the added benefit of shorter wait times for the procedure.

Summary Points

- Use ultrasound to interrogate the site of the procedure to identify vital structures, vasculature, and to plan the approach for thoracentesis and tube thoracostomy for pneumothorax and pleural fluid drainage.

- Use direct ultrasound guidance whenever possible to increase safety, success, and to help prevent complications.
- Manometry is not used commonly during pleural fluid drainage but can be an additional safeguard. Pleural drainage should be stopped upon the patient experiencing chest discomfort.
- Routine chest X-ray is not needed after thoracentesis, unless air has been aspirated, multiple attempts were made, the patient is on a mechanical ventilator, or if the patient becomes symptomatic. Use ultrasound to check for pneumothorax after thoracentesis instead.
- Ultrasound is safe for subpleural mass biopsies, has similar yield to CT guided biopsies, and has benefits of shorter procedure and wait times.

Questions

1. A 40-year-old man with type 1 diabetes mellitus (DM1), hypertension, and interstitial lung disease (ILD) is admitted to the ICU for respiratory failure due to influenza A and Diabetic Ketoacidosis (DKA). Bedsides, ultrasound performed demonstrates a moderate left sided pleural effusion adjacent to consolidated lung with air bronchograms. Which of the following after performing bedside thoracentesis would necessitate performing a portable chest X-ray?
   A. Mechanical ventilation
   B. History of interstitial lung disease
   C. Multiple attempts during thoracentesis
   D. Aspiration of free air during the procedure
   E. All of the above
   Answer: E
2. Which of the following statements is true regarding the use of ultrasound in performing thoracentesis and tube thoracostomy?
   A. Tube thoracostomy under ultrasound guidance does not lead to fewer subdiaphragmatic chest tubes.
   B. The incidence of pneumothorax is the same after thoracentesis and tube thoracostomy with and without ultrasound guidance.
   C. Landmark based tube thoracostomy placement leads to the same incidence of iatrogenic injury when compared to ultrasound guided placement.
   D. Ultrasound-guided thoracentesis has a lower incidence of post-procedural pneumothorax.
   Answer: D

References

1. Kalanjeri S, Pastores SM. Thoracentesis. In: Oropello JM, Pastores SM, Kvetan V, editors. Critical care. McGraw-Hill Education.
2. Kollef MH, Isakow W, Burks AC, Despotovic V, Burks AC, Chen AC. Thoracentesis. The Washington manual of critical care. 3rd ed. Wolters Kluwer; 2018. p. 695–700. Chapter 81
3. Havelock T, Teoh R, Fau-Laws D, Laws D, Fau-Gleeson F, Gleeson F. Pleural procedures and thoracic ultrasound: British Thoracic Society Pleural Disease Guideline 2010. (1468–3296 (Electronic)).
4. Shechtman L, Shrem M, Kleinbaum Y, Bornstein G, Gilad L, Grossman C. Incidence and risk factors of pneumothorax following pre-procedural ultrasound-guided thoracentesis. J Thorac Dis. 2020;12(3):942–8. https://doi.org/10.21037/jtd.2019.12.39.
5. Cantey EP, Walter JM, Corbridge T, Barsuk JH. Complications of thoracentesis: incidence, risk factors, and strategies for prevention. Curr Opin Pulm Med. 2016;22(4):378–85. https://doi.org/10.1097/MCP.0000000000000285.
6. Taylor LA, Stenberg R, Tozer J, et al. Novel approach to ultrasound-guided thoracostomy. J Ultrasound Med. 2022;41(3):743–7. https://doi.org/10.1002/jum.15759.
7. Gray EJ, Cranford JA, Betcher JA, et al. Sonogram of safety: ultrasound outperforms the fifth intercostal space landmark for tube thoracostomy site selection. J Clin Ultrasound. 2020;48(6):303–6. https://doi.org/10.1002/jcu.22851.
8. Zisis C, Tsirgogianni K, Lazaridis G, et al. Chest drainage systems in use. Ann Transl Med. 2015;3(3):43. https://doi.org/10.3978/j.issn.2305-5839.2015.02.09.
9. Rahman NM, Maskell NA, West A, et al. Intrapleural use of tissue plasminogen activator and DNase in pleural infection. N Engl J Med. 2011;365(6):518–26. https://doi.org/10.1056/NEJMoa1012740.
10. Watson GAHB. E12: chest tube placement, care, and removal. In: Texbook of critical care. 7th ed. Elsevier; 2016.
11. Light RW, Jenkinson SG, Minh VD, George RB. Observations on pleural fluid pressures as fluid is withdrawn during thoracentesis. Am Rev Respir Dis. 1980;121(5):799–804. https://doi.org/10.1164/arrd.1980.121.5.799.

12. Lentz RJ, Lerner AD, Pannu JK, et al. Routine monitoring with pleural manometry during therapeutic large-volume thoracentesis to prevent pleural-pressure-related complications: a multicentre, single-blind randomised controlled trial. Lancet Respir Med. 2019;7(5):447–55. https://doi.org/10.1016/s2213-2600(18)30421-1.
13. Krenke R, Grabczak EM. Pleural manometry and thoracentesis—is the issue resolved? Lancet Respir Med. 2019;7(5):374–6. https://doi.org/10.1016/s2213-2600(19)30033-5.
14. Cavanna L, Mordenti P, Bertè R, et al. Ultrasound guidance reduces pneumothorax rate and improves safety of thoracentesis in malignant pleural effusion: report on 445 consecutive patients with advanced cancer. World J Surg Oncol. 2014;12(1):139. https://doi.org/10.1186/1477-7819-12-139.
15. Gervais DA, Petersein A, Lee MJ, Hahn PF, Saini S, Mueller PR. US-guided thoracentesis: requirement for postprocedure chest radiography in patients who receive mechanical ventilation versus patients who breathe spontaneously. Radiology. 1997;204(2):503–6. https://doi.org/10.1148/radiology.204.2.9240544.
16. Mirrakhimov AE, Barbaryan A, Ayach T, Canepa Escaro F, Talari G, Gray A. Is chest radiography routinely needed after thoracentesis? Cleve Clin J Med. 2019;86(6):371–3. https://doi.org/10.3949/ccjm.86a.17058.
17. Mychajlowycz M, Alabousi A, Mironov O. Ultrasound- versus CT-guided subpleural lung and pleural biopsy: an analysis of wait times, procedure time, safety, and diagnostic adequacy. Can Assoc Radiol J. 2021;72(4):883–9. https://doi.org/10.1177/0846537120939073.
18. Sperandeo M, Maiello E, Graziano P, et al. Effectiveness and safety of transthoracic ultrasound in guiding percutaneous needle biopsy in the lung and comparison vs. CT scan in assessing morphology of subpleural consolidations. Diagnostics (Basel). 2021;11(9):1641. https://doi.org/10.3390/diagnostics11091641.

Ultrasound During Intubation

40

Youyou Duanmu and Erin J. Liang

Learning Objectives

1. Recognize sonographic findings of tracheal and esophageal anatomy
2. Identify sonographic findings of tracheal intubation and esophageal intubation

Anatomy and Technique

Ultrasound has been proposed as an adjunct for visualizing and confirming endotracheal intubation in the acute care setting in conjunction with video laryngoscopy, capnography, lung auscultation, and chest X-ray. The high-frequency linear probe is most commonly used to visualize airway anatomy under ultrasonography, the curvilinear probe can be used in patients with greater neck soft tissue depth. Place the probe above the suprasternal notch in the transverse plane with the indicator to the patient's right. Identify the proximal wall of the trachea and the esophagus. When viewed under ultrasonography the trachea is a midline, curved hyperechoic structure with posterior shadowing. The esophageal is located posterior and lateral, most often to the patient's left, of the trachea and appears as a smaller oblong structure. Move the probe laterally if unable to identify the esophagus as it may be underlying the trachea shadow. The carotid arteries will also appear lateral to the trachea. Do not mistake the carotid artery for the esophagus, the carotid artery will be a more lateral, round-walled, hypoechoic and pulsating structure [1, 2] (Fig. 40.1).

For real-time assessment of endotracheal tube (ETT) placement, the trachea and esophagus should be identified prior to intubation and dynamic monitoring of the trachea and esophagus should continue as the endotracheal tube is being advanced during intubation. Successful tracheal intubation will result in increased mucosal air artifact and shadowing of the trachea as the tube enters. The sonographer should simultaneously assess for signs of esophageal intubation. If an esophageal intubation occurs, a second round structure with a hyperechoic anterior rim and hypoechoic shadowing appears just lateral and behind the trachea, almost appearing as if there is a second trachea ("double-tract" sign) [3].

Static ultrasonography can also be used to confirm endotracheal tube placement after intubation has already occurred. Ultrasound following successful tracheal intubation will show a single, midline air-mucosal interface with shadowing representing the trachea with ETT in place. Conversely if esophageal intubation has

Y. Duanmu (✉)
Department of Emergency Medicine, Stanford University School of Medicine, Palo Alto, CA, USA
e-mail: yduanmu@stanford.edu

E. J. Liang
Department of Emergency Medicine, Kaiser Permanente San Diego, San Diego, CA, USA

M. J. Lanspa, A. T. Levinson (eds.), *Echocardiography and Ultrasonography in the ICU*, Respiratory Medicine, https://doi.org/10.1007/978-3-031-80038-2_40

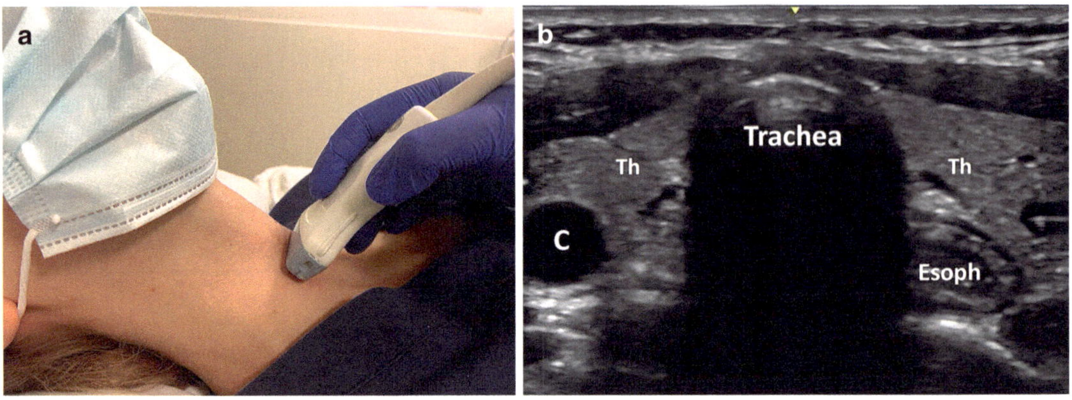

Fig. 40.1 (**a**) The linear ultrasound transducer is placed 1–2 cm above the suprasternal notch in the transverse orientation. (**b**) The trachea is a superficial, midline structure with a hyperechoic anterior arch with posterior shadowing and flanked by the thyroid gland (Th). The esophagus (Esoph) is a muscular-walled ovoid structure slightly lateral and posterior to the trachea. The carotid arteries (**c**) may be visible lateral to the trachea and esophagus

occurred, two rounded air-filled artifacts or the "double-tract" sign is seen. A gentle side-to-side rotation of the ETT while visualizing the above structures on ultrasound can help confirm its location by the presence of motion artifact [4].

Lung ultrasound has been utilized in many clinical settings for the detection of lung expansion with respiration, which is reflected as movement at the junction of the visceral and parietal pleura. This motion at the pleural line is lost in the presence of pneumothorax, lung scarring, pulmonary bleb, or in the absence of mechanical ventilation in intubated patients. To assess for expansion of each lung, the linear transducer is placed in the sagittal orientation between the second and third rib in the midclavicular line. Each rib is delineated by a thin anterior hyperechoic arch with dark posterior shadowing and the hyperechoic pleural line is seen between and slightly posterior to the ribs. Lung sliding movement seen at the pleural line bilaterally indicates tracheal intubation, while lack of lung sliding of one lung suggests either ipsilateral pneumothorax or mainstem bronchial intubation of the contralateral side.

Evidence

The utility of ultrasonography to confirm ETT placement was summarized in a 2020 meta-analysis of 30 studies involving over 2500 patients. The majority of studies took place in the emergency department, four were performed in the critical care setting. There were 28 prospective observational studies and two randomized controlled trials. Ultrasound showed good accuracy for differentiating between tracheal and esophageal intubation with a pooled specificity of 98.2% and a pooled specificity of 95.7% [5].

There is emerging evidence to expand the use of ultrasound for ETT confirmation and to predict the difficulty of intubation as well as intubation depth. While color doppler has been proposed as an adjunct for dynamic monitoring of ETT placement, studies comparing color doppler with B-mode ultrasound have not shown superior accuracy for visualizing tracheal vs esophageal intubation [6, 7]. Ultrasound has also been studied as a tool for predicting challenging ETT placement. Measurements such as increased distance from skin surface to the hyoid bone or epiglottis (as measured in the transverse plane), and increased hyomental distance (as measured in the sagittal plane with probe placed below the mandible) have been associated with difficult intubation [8, 9].

For assessing depth of intubation, one study showed that ultrasound to assess for anterior lung sliding had superior sensitivity (93 vs. 66%) and specificity (96 vs. 59%) for differentiating tracheal from bronchial mainstem intubation relative to lung auscultation [10]. In the pediatric population, filling the ETT balloon with saline and evaluating for its presence at the sternal notch has been proposed to aid in the assessment of intubation depth, while measuring the subglottic trachea diameter has been used to predict proper ETT size [11, 12]. Further validation may be required for these emerging airway ultrasound techniques.

Limitations

Monitoring for tracheal intubation requires identifying pertinent ultrasound anatomy prior to the procedure. The visibility of normal trachea and esophageal landmarks can vary between patients. Esophageal intubation can be difficult to identify if the esophagus is directly underlying the trachea. Therefore, it is helpful to identify the collapsed esophagus prior to intubation, and to attempt a more lateral view if it is not visible from the midline transverse probe orientation.

Summary Point

- Ultrasound shows good accuracy for differentiating between tracheal and esophageal intubation.

Question

1. What qualities distinguish the trachea from the esophagus on ultrasound?
   A. The esophagus has a posterior air shadow behind it.
   B. The trachea has a hyperechoic anterior border.
   C. The trachea is generally lateral and posterior relative to the esophagus.
   D. The esophagus may contain lines parallel to the anterior border due to reverberation.

   Answer: B

   Explanation: The trachea can be differentiated from the esophagus on ultrasound by its hyperechoic anterior border with posterior shadowing. Parallel hyperechoic lines may also be seen posterior to the trachea border reflecting reverberation artifact from the air mucosal interface of the trachea.

Conflicts of Interest The authors have no real or potential conflicts of interest related to the manuscript.

References

1. Chou EH, Dickman E, Tsou PY, et al. Ultrasonography for confirmation of endotracheal tube placement: a systematic review and meta-analysis. Resuscitation. 2015;90:97–103.
2. Das SK, Choupoo NS, Haldar R, et al. Transtracheal ultrasound for verification of endotracheal tube placement: a systematic review and meta-analysis. Can J Anesth. 2015;62(4):413–23.
3. You-Ten KE, Siddiqui N, Teoh WH, et al. Point-of-care ultrasound (POCUS) of the upper airway. Can J Anesth. 2018;65(4):473–84.
4. Gottlieb M, Nakitende D, Sundaram T, et al. Comparison of static versus dynamic ultrasound for the detection of endotracheal intubation. West J Emerg Med. 2018;19(2):412–6.
5. Sahu AK, Bhoi S, Aggarwal P, et al. Endotracheal tube placement confirmation by ultrasonography: a systematic review and meta-analysis of more than 2500 patients. J Emerg Med. 2020;59(2):254–64.
6. Gildea TH, Anderson KL, Niknam KR, et al. The utility of color doppler to confirm endotracheal tube placement: a pilot study. West J Emerg Med. 2020;21(4):870–5.
7. Gottlieb M, Holladay D, Serici A, et al. Comparison of color flow with standard ultrasound for the detection of endotracheal intubation. Am J Emerg Med. 2018;36(7):1166–9.
8. Alessandri F, Antenucci G, Piervincenzi E, et al. Ultrasound as a new tool in the assessment of airway difficulties: an observational study. Eur J Anaesthesiol. 2019;36(7):509–15.

9. Abraham S, Himarani J, Mary Nancy S, et al. Ultrasound as an assessment method in predicting difficult intubation: a prospective clinical study. J Maxillofac Oral Surg. 2018;17(4):563–9.
10. Ramsingh D, Frank E, Haughton R, et al. Auscultation versus point-of-care ultrasound to determine endotracheal versus bronchial intubation. Anesthesiology. 2016;124(5):1012–20.
11. Tessaro MO, Arroyo AC, Haines LE, et al. Inflating the endotracheal tube cuff with saline to confirm correct depth using bedside ultrasonography. Can J Emerg Med. 2015;17(1):94–8.
12. Shibasaki M, Nakajima Y, Ishii S, Shimizu F, Shime N, Sessler DI. Prediction of pediatric endotracheal tube size by ultrasonography. Anesthesiology. 2010;113(4):819–24.

Transcutaneous Laryngeal Ultrasonography: Vocal Fold Ultrasound

41

Akiva Leibowitz and Achikam Oren-Grinberg

Introduction

Multimodal ultrasound has been recognized as a potentially useful tool for noninvasively evaluating the airways and vocal folds, with the increasing availability of this tool for use by bedside clinicians since the 1980s [1–3]. B-mode ultrasound can be used to identify glottic structures and their dynamic movements, while spectral doppler can be utilized to evaluate motion and vibration. Some vocal movement disorders such as bilateral vocal cord paralysis, paradoxical vocal fold motion movement abnormalities, arytenoid dislocation, and laryngeal edema may be the underlying pathologies causing respiratory distress and stridor. Laryngeal nerve injury has been reported during thyroid, anterior cervical spine, esophageal, and mediastinal surgical procedures in the surgical patient population. The reported incidence is 2.3% among patients following cardiac and great vessel surgery [4], 3.9% following initial thyroid surgery [5], and 45.3% following radical esophagectomy [6]. Paradoxical vocal motion abnormalities occur when vocal cords close (adduct) rather than abduct when they should be opening (mostly on inspiration) and may present with inspiratory stridor and respiratory distress [7]. Hence, early identification of these abnormalities may have a role in the management of patients presenting with respiratory distress or in those developing post-extubation respiratory failure in the ICU. The mainstay for diagnosis of vocal cord motion abnormalities remains clinical exam and indirect fiberoptic laryngoscopy (IFL) [8], which may be replaced in certain instances with less invasive Transcutaneous Laryngeal Ultrasonography (TLUS). Ultrasound has been used for the identification of important laryngeal landmarks (Thyroid cartilage, cricothyroid membrane, laryngeal rings, vocal folds, arytenoid cartilage, and vascular structures) as well as delineating functionality (vocal fold movement, vocal cord palsies). The unique characteristics of the larynx, particularly the presence of air in the laryngotracheal space, encased by cartilaginous structures—present unique challenges when assessing the airway with ultrasound.

Supplementary Information The online version contains supplementary material available at https://doi.org/10.1007/978-3-031-80038-2_41.

A. Leibowitz (✉) · A. Oren-Grinberg
Department of Anesthesia, Critical Care and Pain Medicine, Harvard Medical School, Beth Israel Deaconess Medical Center, Boston, MA, USA
e-mail: aleibow1@bidmc.harvard.edu

M. J. Lanspa, A. T. Levinson (eds.), *Echocardiography and Ultrasonography in the ICU*, Respiratory Medicine, https://doi.org/10.1007/978-3-031-80038-2_41

Ultrasound Anatomy of the Vocal Cords

A standard linear high-frequency probe (6–13 MHz) may be used for the visualization of laryngeal structures. Low-frequency curvilinear probes (2–5 MHz) may be used as well, albeit with some loss of resolution. The vocal cords are composed of mucous membrane infoldings attached anteriorly at the angle on the interior surface of the thyroid cartilage and project posteriorly to the arytenoid cartilages on either side [9]. The true vocal cords overlie hypoechoic muscle, whereas the false cords contain echoic fat. The tissue air interface appears on ultrasound as a bright white line, for which anything behind it will be considered an artifact. The vocal folds are visualized by placing the transducer transversely over the thyroid cartilage, slightly tilting the probe cephalad (Fig. 41.1). A study with 24 healthy volunteers showed that the thyroid cartilage provides the best acoustic window [2], with the operator able to identify true and false vocal cords in all participants. Calcified thyroid cartilage and male gender have been associated with impaired ability to adequately visualize the vocal cords [10]. However, in individuals with calcified thyroid cartilages, the vocal cords and the arytenoid cartilages can still be seen by combining the scanning from just cranially to the superior thyroid notch angled caudally and scanning from the cricothyroid membrane in the midline and on each side with the transducer angled 30° cranially [1]. A lateral approach, with the transducer placed at a 30° angle—has been shown to improve overall vocal cord visualization rate compared to the midline approach (93.3 vs. 82.2%, p = <0.001), especially for males (75.0

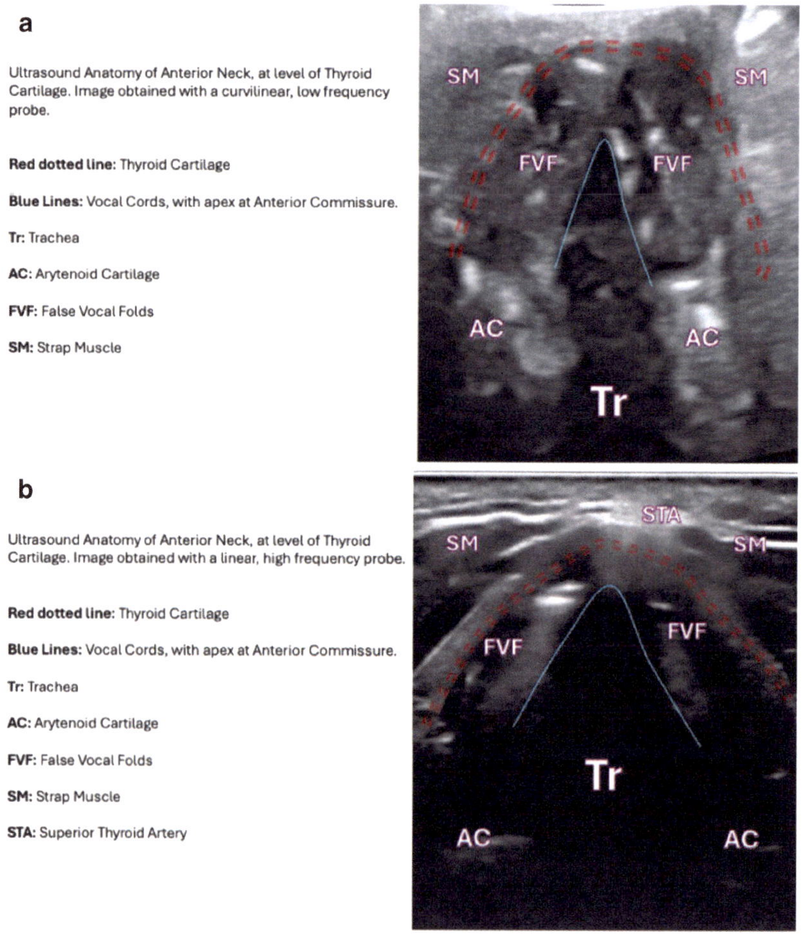

Fig. 41.1 (**a**) Ultrasound anatomy of anterior neck, at level of thyroid cartilage. Image obtained with a curvilinear, low frequency probe. (**b**) Ultrasound anatomy of anterior neck, at level of thyroid cartilage. Image obtained with a linear, high frequency probe. **Red dotted line**: Thyroid cartilage, **Blue lines**: Vocal cords, with apex at anterior commissure, **Tr**: Trachea, **AC**: Arytenoid cartilage, **FVF**: False vocal folds, **SM**: Strap muscle, **STA**: Superior thyroid artery

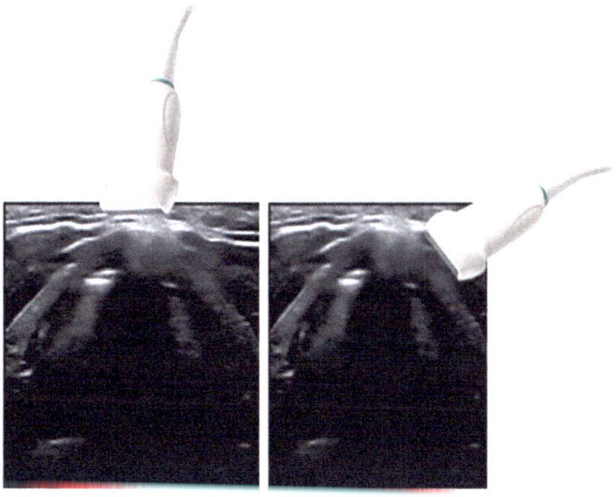

Fig. 41.2 Ultrasound probe position for imaging of vocal cords at level of thyroid cartilage. Midline (left) and 30° (right)

vs. 33.3%, $p = 0.002$) [11] (Fig. 41.2). The true vocal cords appear as two triangular hypoechoic structures (the vocalis muscles), outlined medially by the hyperechoic vocal ligaments [2]. The cords oscillate and move toward the midline during phonation, adduct during Valsalva maneuver, and abduct upon relaxation. During normal respiration, the cords open upon inspiration to allow an unobstructed flow of air (Video 41.1). When paradoxical vocal fold motion abnormality is present—the cords adduct during inspiration—leading to stridor and dyspnea. The false vocal cords lay parallel and cephalad to the true cords, are more hyperechoic in appearance, and remain relatively immobile during phonation but appear to open and close with respiration [12].

Vocal Cord Motion - B mode Ultrasound / Transcutaneous Laryngeal Ultrasonography (TLUS)
Image acquisition tips and tricks

Lowering of probe frequency
and increase gain at the time of VC scanning

Tilting of probe cephalocaudal

Sliding probe from the midline to 30 degrees

Valsalva maneuver —> TVC adducted on the midline, followed by confirmation of bilateral mobility when the TVC abduct with inspiration

Motion evaluation using passive breathing is possible, but it is more challenging and time-consuming because the TVC movement is often subtle.

Application of Doppler ultrasound CDI or PWD for assessment of movement, vibration, and airflow patterns

Vocal Fold Motion Abnormalities

All intrinsic muscles of the larynx, but the crico-arytenoid muscle, which is an abductor, are vocal cord adductors. These (aside from the tensor cricothyroid muscle) are innervated by the recurrent laryngeal nerve. Complete paralysis of the vocal cord will result in a paramedian position, which may be observed with static ultrasound of the neck. Bilateral paralysis may manifest as dyspnea and respiratory distress. Absent movement of the cords with phonation may also be observed with ultrasound [3, 13]. Since this technique was described in 1989, several studies have been carried out, evaluating the sensitivity and specificity of this approach compared to indirect fiberoptic laryngoscopy (IFL), which is considered the gold standard, with varying levels of success. The vast majority of these studies were conducted either with healthy volunteers or patients undergoing Thyroid and Parathyroid surgery [14–18]. The accuracy and reliability of Trans Cutaneous Laryngeal Ultrasonography (TLUS) for the detection of motion abnormalities depends not only on adequate visualization of the cords but also identification of real-time movement of the vocal cords and arytenoids, which may be challenging in patients in respiratory distress. Therefore, the interpretation of these studies when applied to the critical care setting should call for some caution. Several studies report the utility of B-mode TLUS either as a screening tool or when laryngoscopy is not available, for the identification of vocal cord motion abnormalities [14–18] with reported sensitivity and specificity of up to 100% and 98%, respectively [10, 14, 16–18], while other single-center studies report poorer utility with values of sensitivity and specificity only in the 40–60% range and with a positive predictive value of 73% and negative predictive value of 95% [19, 20]. This may be explained in part, by the frame rate on most ultrasound machines which is significantly lower than the vibration frequency of the cords, as well as the significant variability in the ability to accurately detect the relevant structures. Further studies which included the addition of Doppler imaging demonstrated improved accuracy. Ooi et al. demonstrated the ability to identify vocal fold palsy with color doppler imaging (CDI) based on showing airflow pattern asymmetry [21], whereas Dedjecus et al. were able to identify all motion abnormalities by applying pulsed wave doppler both in the horizontal and lateral positions [15] (Fig. 41.3). A recent meta-analysis by Kim et al. which included 17 eligible studies found that Transcutaneous laryngeal ultrasonography exhibited a pooled sensitivity of 0.91, pooled specificity of 0.97, pooled negative predictive value of 0.99, and AUC of 0.94. The SROC curve value was 0.9–1.00, suggesting excellent diagnostic accuracy. Authors concluded that given its accuracy—TLUS may be used in certain situations as an alternative to IFL [16]. Phung et al. conducted a similar meta-analysis with a more reserved conclusion with negative

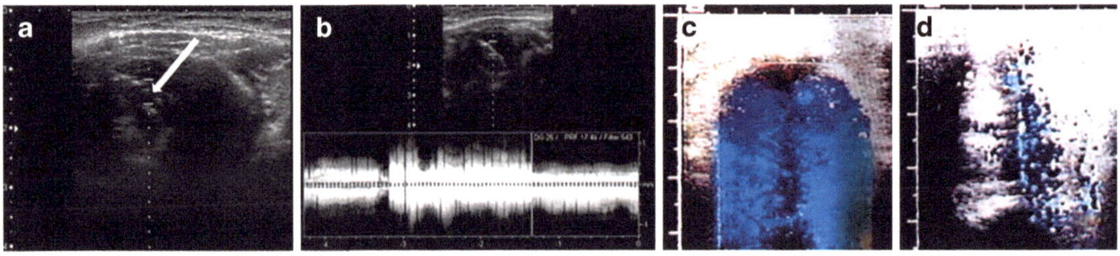

Fig. 41.3 Application of Doppler imaging for evaluation of vocal fold motion. (**a**) Placement of ultrasound probe on the lateral thyroid cartilage, with PW volume gate over the vocal cord. (**b**) Registering vocal fold displacement velocity with and without phonation (*Dedecjus M, Adamczewski Z, Brzeziński J, Lewiński A. Real-time, high-resolution ultrasonography of the vocal folds—a prospective pilot study in patients before and after thyroidectomy. Langenbeck's Arch Surg 2010;395(7):859–64.*) (**c**) Color Doppler Imaging (CDI) demonstrating normal air flow patterns over both cords. (**d**) Paralyzed right vocal cord adducted to midline, with asymmetric color triangle. (*Ooi LL, Chan HS, Soo KC. Color Doppler imaging for vocal cord palsy. Head Neck 1995 Feb;17(1):20–3*)

predictive values ranging 60–100%, given the limitations set forth by inter-user variability, older age, and male gender. They conclude that TLUS may be a good alternative in the postoperative setting in a young patient following uncomplicated surgery with a normal voice on clinical examination, to confirm recurrent laryngeal nerve integrity [22].

Paradoxical Vocal Cord Motion Disorder

Paradoxical Vocal Fold Motion Disorder (PVCMD) is a condition where the vocal folds adduct instead of abduct on inspiration. Common symptoms include stridor, wheezing, coughing, throat tightness, dyspnea, and respiratory distress. Many factors have been implied in the underlying etiology of PVCM, among them are lung factors, exercise, stressful events, psychogenic, functional-neurologic, reflux, or idiopathic [23–26]. PVCMD is not an uncommon cause of post-extubation stridor in the post-anesthesia recovery unit or the ICU [27]. Presentation may be confounded with other causes of stridor, including glottic and subglottic edema, anaphylaxis, mucous plugging, and airway obstruction. Typical inspiratory vocal closure can be visualized without airway edema or allergic features. Distinguishing PCVM from other causes of respiratory distress is paramount, as this condition can often be treated with anxiolytics and induction of a slow rhythmic pattern of breathing. Most often, when properly diagnosed and treated, respiratory distress may be resolved, obviating the need for invasive respiratory support. Several practitioners report that timely diagnosis has prevented patients from being reintubated (personal communication). Definitive diagnosis is made with IFL, which is a minimally invasive procedure, though this is not always feasible in the uncooperative patient in distress. TLUS offers a noninvasive mode of diagnosis at the bedside. Application of TLUS for PCVM has not been as extensively studied—as in vocal cord paralysis, although similar principles apply. Small-scale feasibility studies have demonstrated the potential utility of this tool [12], and preliminary data from clinical cases in the ICU are promising [28]. A standard linear high-frequency probe (6–13 MHz) is placed horizontally over the thyroid cartilage. After identifying the laryngeal structures—the opening and closing of the vocal folds are noted and correlated with inspiration and expiration. When a normal pattern is present—the cords will open on inspiration (Video 41.1). When PCVM is present, the cords will adduct and close on inspiration, with the concomitant typical inspiratory stridor sound (Video 41.2).

Summary Points

- Transcutaneous Laryngeal Ultrasonography allows visualization of important laryngeal structures, namely the thyroid cartilage, True/False vocal folds, and arytenoid cartilages and their function throughout the respiratory cycle and during phonation.
- TLUS is a noninvasive alternative to indirect flexible laryngoscopy readily available to the intensivist at the patient's bedside and can assist in diagnosing vocal fold motion abnormalities underlying respiratory distress and stridor.
- Use of TLUS may be limited by patient habitus, male gender, older age, and calcified thyroid cartilage. The application of spectral Doppler modes may increase diagnostic accuracy.

Pro-Tips

When PCVM is present, the cords will adduct and close on inspiration, with the concomitant typical inspiratory stridor sound.

Evolving Evidence

A recent meta-analysis of 17 eligible studies suggested TLUS had excellent diagnostic accuracy.

References

1. Kristensen MS. Ultrasonography in the management of the airway. Acta Anaesthesiol Scand. 2011;55(10):1155–73.
2. Singh M, Chin KJ, Chan VWS, Wong DT, Prasad GA, Yu E. Use of sonography for airway assessment. J Ultrasound Med. 2010;29(1):79–85.
3. Miles KA. Ultrasound demonstration of vocal cord movements. Br J Radiol. 1989;62(741):871–2.
4. Itagaki T, Kikura M, Sato S. Incidence and risk factors of postoperative vocal cord paralysis in 987 patients after cardiovascular surgery. Ann Thorac Surg. 2007;83(6):2147–52.
5. Bergenfelz A, Jansson S, Kristoffersson A, Mårtensson H, Reihnér E, Wallin G, et al. Complications to thyroid surgery: results as reported in a database from a multicenter audit comprising 3,660 patients. Langenbeck's Arch Surg. 2008;393(5):667–73.
6. Nishimaki T, Suzuki T, Suzuki S, Kuwabara S, Hatakeyama K. Outcomes of extended radical esophagectomy for thoracic esophageal cancer. J Am Coll Surg. 1998;186(3):306–12.
7. Malaty J, Wu V. Vocal cord dysfunction: rapid evidence review. Am Fam Physician. 2021;104(5):471–5.
8. Paul BC, Rafii B, Achlatis S, Amin MR, Branski RC. Morbidity and patient perception of flexible laryngoscopy. Ann Otol Rhinol Laryngol. 2012;121(11):708–13.
9. Saran M, Georgakopoulos B, Bordoni B. Anatomy, head and neck, larynx vocal cords. In: StatPearls [Internet], Treasure Island, FL: StatPearls Publishing; 2022. http://www.ncbi.nlm.nih.gov/books/NBK535342/.
10. Carneiro-Pla D, Miller BS, Wilhelm SM, Milas M, Gauger PG, Cohen MS, et al. Feasibility of surgeon-performed transcutaneous vocal cord ultrasonography in identifying vocal cord mobility: a multi-institutional experience. Surgery. 2014;156(6):1597–604.
11. MMH F, Lang BH-H. A prospective study comparing the midline and lateral trans-laryngeal ultrasonography approaches in vocal cord assessment before and after thyroid and neck surgeries. Am J Surg. 2022;223(4):676–80. https://www.americanjournalofsurgery.com/article/S0002-9610(21)00347-0/fulltext
12. Finnoff JT, Orbelo DM, Ekbom DC. Can ultrasound identify paradoxical vocal fold movement? A pilot study. Clin J Sport Med. 2020;30(5):e120–3.
13. Amis RJ, Gupta D, Dowdall JR, Srirajakalindini A, Folbe A. Ultrasound assessment of vocal fold paresis: a correlation case series with flexible fiberoptic laryngoscopy and adding the third dimension (3-D) to vocal fold mobility assessment. Middle East J Anaesthesiol. 2012;21(4):493–8.
14. Cheng S-P, Lee J-J, Liu T-P, Lee K-S, Liu C-L. Preoperative ultrasonography assessment of vocal cord movement during thyroid and parathyroid surgery. World J Surg. 2012;36(10):2509–15.
15. Dedecjus M, Adamczewski Z, Brzeziński J, Lewiński A. Real-time, high-resolution ultrasonography of the vocal folds—a prospective pilot study in patients before and after thyroidectomy. Langenbeck's Arch Surg. 2010;395(7):859–64.
16. Kim DH, Lee J, Seo Y, Kim SW, Hwang SH. Perioperative transcutaneous laryngeal ultrasonography to assess vocal cord function in thyroid surgery. Am J Surg. 2022;223(5):893–9.
17. Wong K-P, Lang BH-H, Ng S-H, Cheung C-Y, Chan CT-Y, Lo C-Y. A prospective, assessor-blind evaluation of surgeon-performed transcutaneous laryngeal ultrasonography in vocal cord examination before and after thyroidectomy. Surgery. 2013 Dec;154(6):1158–65.
18. Wang C-P, Chen T-C, Yang T-L, Chen C-N, Lin C-F, Lou P-J, et al. Transcutaneous ultrasound for evaluation of vocal fold movement in patients with thyroid disease. Eur J Radiol. 2012 Mar;81(3):e288–91.
19. Sidhu S, Stanton R, Shahidi S, Chu J, Chew S, Campbell P. Initial experience of vocal cord evaluation using grey-scale, real-time, B-mode ultrasound ANZ. J Surg. 2001;71(12):737–9.
20. Kandil E, Deniwar A, Noureldine SI, Hammad AY, Mohamed H, Al-Qurayshi Z, et al. Assessment of vocal fold function using transcutaneous laryngeal ultrasonography and flexible laryngoscopy. JAMA Otolaryngol Head Neck Surg. 2016;142(1):74–8.
21. Ooi LL, Chan HS, Soo KC. Color Doppler imaging for vocal cord palsy. Head Neck. 1995;17(1):20–3.
22. Phung D, Fradet L, Riffat F, Novakovic D, Elliott MS, Nguyen K, et al. Translaryngeal ultrasound in thyroid surgery: state of the art review. ANZ J Surg. 2022;92:385–9.
23. Leong P, Phyland DJ, Koh J, Baxter M, Bardin PG. Middle airway obstruction: phenotyping vocal cord dysfunction or inducible laryngeal obstructions. Lancet Respir Med. 2022 Jan;10(1):3–5.
24. Altman KW, Mirza N, Ruiz C, Sataloff RT. Paradoxical vocal fold motion: presentation and treatment options. J Voice. 2000 Mar;14(1):99–103.
25. Denipah N, Dominguez CM, Kraai EP, Kraai TL, Leos P, Braude D. Acute management of paradoxical vocal fold motion (vocal cord dysfunction). Ann Emerg Med. 2017;69(1):18–23.
26. Kenn K, Balkissoon R. Vocal cord dysfunction: what do we know? Eur Respir J. 2011;37(1):194–200.
27. Farley JD, Cheney M, Eckmann MS, Wallisch B. Paradoxical vocal fold motion disorder in the postanesthesia care unit. Anesthesiology. 2021;134(4):626–7. https://doi.org/10.1097/ALN.0000000000003683.
28. Leibowitz A, Oren-Grinberg A. Clinical application of vocal cord ultrasound. In: Advanced critical care ultrasound summit. Park City, UT: Utah Thoracic Society; 2022.

Focused Assessment of Sonography in Trauma (FAST)

42

Monica Saxena

Learning Objectives
1. Describe the components of the FAST exam
2. Review indications for the FAST exam
3. Explore the limitations of the FAST exam

Concept, Indications, and Limitations

Concept

The FAST exam is used to detect intraperitoneal fluid in the abdomen and around the heart. The exam has utility in critical care units as well as the emergency department and inpatient floors. The FAST exam was developed in the 1990s by trauma surgeons [1]. Over time, it has become an accepted protocol for patient evaluation in both acute and critical care settings [2].

Indications

In general, a FAST exam is indicated in any clinical situation in which there is a concern for intra-abdominal free fluid or for hemorrhage [3]. An extended version of the FAST exam, the E-FAST, also examines the lungs for pneumothorax [4]. There are no absolute contraindications to obtaining a FAST exam. A relative contraindication is performing a FAST exam when it delays or interferes with time-sensitive life-saving care.

Limitations

Though the FAST exam is now a standard part of the evaluation of free fluid in the hemoperitoneum and pericardial spaces, it is important to note that urine, ascites, and bowel fluid appear similarly to free fluid in ultrasound visualization [5]. A determination of whether the finding is free fluid depends on the clinical presentation. Also, the FAST exam has limited utility in evaluating for penetrating bowel or organ injury [6]. Additionally, there are limitations in detecting free fluid in mesenteric, diaphragmatic, or hollow viscus injuries. Also, in certain specific clinical presentations, free fluid detected on FAST exam is not necessarily pathologic such as identification of free fluid in patients with ventriculoperitoneal shunts and or peritoneal dialysis catheters.

Supplementary Information The online version contains supplementary material available at https://doi.org/10.1007/978-3-031-80038-2_42.

M. Saxena (✉)
Department of Emergency Medicine, Stanford School of Medicine, Stanford University, Stanford, CA, USA
e-mail: saxenam@stanford.edu

M. J. Lanspa, A. T. Levinson (eds.), *Echocardiography and Ultrasonography in the ICU*, Respiratory Medicine, https://doi.org/10.1007/978-3-031-80038-2_42

Views

There are 4 standard views in the FAST exam that are used to evaluate for the presence of intraperitoneal fluid: the hepatorenal recess, the splenorenal recess, the rectouterine (female)/retrovesical (male) space, and the pericardium [4]. The e-FAST exam includes the additional view of the lungs to evaluate for pneumothorax (Video 42.5).

The Hepatorenal Recess (Morrison's Pouch)

The interface of the liver and kidney is often referred to by the eponym of Morrison's pouch. Often this is the first view obtained in the FAST exam because it is one of the most dependent areas in the body and fluid from the peritoneal cavity is likely to collect here first before the other views. For optimal evaluation, the patient should be lying supine as fluid will collect in the most dependent areas of the body. To obtain the view, either the phased array or curvilinear probe can be used. The probe marker is aimed superiorly and the probe is angled between the 8th and 11th intercostal spaces in the mid-axillary line. The entire renal hepatic interface should be visualized (Video 42.1). In particular, the inferior liver tip and renal interface, called the paracolic gutter, should be evaluated for free fluid as fluid may initially collect here before spreading to Morrison's pouch. The hepatorenal recess should also be used to evaluate for hemothorax by looking for fluid above the diaphragm. If the depth of the ultrasound image is decreased, the spine appears as hyperechoic lines. Also, the space above the diaphragm should be evaluated for free fluid. To evaluate for fluid above the diaphragm (pleural effusion or hemothorax), the depth of splenorenal interface is decreased so that the vertebral bodies appear as hyperechoic lines at the bottom of the screen. The probe is then moved towards the patient's head and visualization of the spine below the diaphragm ("spine sign) is indicative of hemothorax or pleural effusion.

The Splenorenal Recess

The spleen kidney interface is often the second view obtained because fluid can communicate between the left and right upper quadrants. Similar to the right-sided liver and kidney interface, either the phased array or the curvilinear probe can be used to obtain the image. The probe marker is aimed superiorly and placed in the posterior axillary line. The splenorenal interface is visualized looking for any anechoic spaces indicating free fluid. Next, the subphrenic space (interface between the spleen and the diaphragm) should be examined for free fluid as this is the first place fluid often collects in the left thorax (Video 42.2). Finally, the left paracolic gutter at the inferior tip of the spleen should also be evaluated for any free fluid.

The Pericardial Space

Depending on the indication for fast exam, in some instances, the pericardial space is the first view obtained, for example, if there is concern for cardiac tamponade. The phased array probe is used to obtain the image. The probe marker is aimed towards the patient's right side. The probe is placed inferior and to the right of the patient's xiphoid process aiming the probe towards the patient's left shoulder. The edges of the pericardium should be evaluated for any pathologic free fluid presenting as a pericardial effusion (Video 42.3). When assessing the pericardium for fluid, the depth of the image should be set to at least 20 cm to fully evaluate the borders of the heart for any free fluid.

The Pelvis

The common location of free fluid in the pelvis is different between females and males, though the image is obtained in the same way. Similar to the right and left thorax, either the curvilinear or phased array probe can be used to obtain the proper view. The probe marker should be pointing towards the patient's right and the probe should be placed in the abdominal midline above the pubic symphysis and the borders of the bladder should be fully visualized (Video 42.4). The bladder should also be visualized with the probe marker pointed towards the patient's head, sweeping the probe from left to right to fully view the entire bladder. In females, the uterus will be visualized superior to the bladder (or on the right side of the screen) and free fluid, if present, will commonly collect posterior to the uterus (Pouch of Doulas) first before collecting between the bladder and uterus. In males, free fluid often collects in the retrovesical pouch which is a potential anatomic space between the bladder and the prostate which lies directly posterior (inferior on the ultrasound screen) to the bladder.

Pathologic Findings

As noted, free fluid in a FAST exam is pathologic in the following areas:

Pericardial Fluid
Morrison's pouch: The liver and kidney interface in the right thorax

Right paracolic gutter: The space between the inferior liver tip and the right kidney

Below the diaphragm: If vertebral bodies are visualized below the diaphragm ("spine sign"), this indicates free fluid

Splenorenal recess: The spleen and kidney interface in the left thorax

Subphrenic space: The space between the diaphragm and the spleen

Left paracolic gutter: The space between the inferior tip of the spleen and the left kidney

Pouch of Douglas: Posterior to the uterus

Retrovesical pouch: The space between the bladder and prostate

Evolving Evidence (Call-Out)
An extended version of the FAST exam, the E-FAST also examines the lungs for pneumothorax

Pro-Tips: (Call-Out)

- In males, free fluid often collects in the retrovesical pouch which is a potential anatomic space between the bladder and the prostate which lies directly posterior to the bladder

Summary Points

- In critical care settings, the FAST exam has multiple applications.
- Specific indications include massive ascites, ruptured viscus, spontaneous intra-abdominal bleeding and intraperitoneal rupture of an AAA.
- The FAST exam is also useful in evaluating undifferentiated hypotension or shock.
- Outside the critical care settings, the FAST exam is part of standard practice when evaluating trauma patients who present with blunt or thoracoabdominal trauma.
- The FAST exam is also useful to evaluate for ruptured ectopic pregnancy.

References

1. Rozycki GS, Ochsner MG, Jaffin JH, Champion HR. Prospective evaluation of surgeons' use of ultrasound in the evaluation of trauma patients. J Trauma. 1993;34:516–27.
2. Balmert N, Espinosa J, Arafeh M-O, Costello J, Markle S. Integration of bedside ultrasound into the ICU—a review of indications, techniques and interventions. J Emerg Crit Care Med. 2018;2:17.
3. Dawson M, Mallin M. Introduction to bedside ultrasound volumes 1 and 2. Lexington, KY: Emergency Ultrasound Solutions; 2012.
4. Chapter 5. Trauma ultrasound: The FAST exam. In: Reichman EF, editor. Emergency medicine procedures. 2nd ed. McGraw Hill; 2013. https://accessemergencymedicine.mhmedical.com/content.aspx?bookid=683&sectionid=45343641. Accessed 23 January 2022.
5. Chapter 5. Trauma ultrasound: the FAST exam. In: Reichman EF, editor. Emergency medicine procedures. 2nd ed. The McGraw-Hill Companies; 2013. https://accessemergencymedicine.mhmedical.com/content.aspx?bookid=683&sectionid=45343641. Accessed 22 June 2024.
6. Quinn AC, Sinert R. What is the utility of the focused assessment with sonography in trauma (FAST) exam in penetrating torso trauma? Injury. 2011;42(5):482–7. https://doi.org/10.1016/j.injury.2010.07.249.

43 Renal and Bladder Ultrasonography for the Intensivist

David N. Suwondo and Cristiana Baloescu

Learning Objectives

1. Review the utility of using point-of-care ultrasound to diagnose hydronephrosis and urinary retention
2. Discuss the limitations of point-of-care ultrasound for diagnosing hydronephrosis

Indications and Limitations

Indications

The incidence of acute kidney injury (AKI) among patients admitted to the intensive care unit (ICU) is rising, and a recent international study found that AKI occurs in 57% of patients admitted to ICUs worldwide [1]. The American College of Radiology (ACR) Appropriateness Criteria for Renal Failure recommend renal ultrasound for the initial evaluation of unspecified AKI [2]. Although point-of-care renal ultrasound is not generally used to diagnose prerenal or intrinsic causes of AKI, it can rapidly detect post-renal etiologies through the presence of hydronephrosis. The overall rate of hydronephrosis among patients with AKI is low, ranging from 5 to 10% [3, 4], but it represents a reversible cause of AKI, for which early intervention is crucial, given the clear association between AKI and increased mortality risk among ICU patients [1, 5]. Point-of-care ultrasound (POCUS) of the bladder can also be used to accurately measure bladder volume and assess bladder catheterization. Urinary catheter use has been reported in 61% of ICU patients in the United States, compared to 20% of non-ICU patients [6]. POCUS can be used to identify malposition of the catheter balloon or tip, visualize catheter obstruction, or detect the presence of echogenic bladder debris or clots. Among patients with abdominal pain or urinary tract infection (UTI), POCUS of the kidneys and bladder may be used to diagnose an obstructing renal stone. This is especially useful for patients unable to travel for CT scan. In patients with urinary tract infections causing severe sepsis or septic shock, identification of a suspected obstructing stone may change management and prompt urgent procedural intervention.

Limitations

In the absence of prior imaging or other information, the degree of hydronephrosis seen on ultrasound does not necessarily correlate with either the acuity or the degree of urinary obstruction [7, 8]. The ureters are not easily imaged on transabdominal ultrasound due to overlying bowel gas, and an obstructing ureteral stone may not be directly visualized or measured. Moreover,

D. N. Suwondo (✉) · C. Baloescu
Department of Emergency Medicine, Yale University School of Medicine, New Haven, CT, USA
e-mail: david.suwondo@yale.edu; cristiana.baloescu@yale.edu

M. J. Lanspa, A. T. Levinson (eds.), *Echocardiography and Ultrasonography in the ICU*, Respiratory Medicine, https://doi.org/10.1007/978-3-031-80038-2_43

hydronephrosis may be caused by other less common etiologies, such as malignancy, pregnancy, ureteral reflux, or diabetes [9]. Hydronephrosis may not be immediately apparent despite acute urinary obstruction in patients who are intravascularly depleted or who have significantly decreased renal function until after the patient is adequately fluid resuscitated, potentially leading to a false negative study [7, 8]. Ultrasound evaluation of the bladder is significantly limited by an under-distended or empty bladder.

Anatomy and Imaging Technique

Anatomy of the Kidneys

The kidneys are located retroperitoneally, at the level of the T12–L3 vertebrae on the right and the L1–L4 vertebrae on the left [10]. The kidneys range from 9 to 12 cm in length, 4 to 6 cm in width, and 2.5 to 3.5 cm in the anterior-posterior dimension [7, 9, 10]. Each kidney is encapsulated by a well-defined and smooth hyperechoic border consisting of a fibrous capsule, perinephric fat, and renal fascia (Gerota's fascia) [7, 8]. Within this capsule lies the renal parenchyma, composed of the renal cortex peripherally and the renal medulla (containing the renal pyramids and papillae) centrally. At the center of the kidney lies the renal sinus, which consists of the renal calyces and pelvis, renal vessels, and peripelvic fat [10]. The renal sinus appears hyperechoic on ultrasound due to the presence of peripelvic fat along with the collapsed, nondistended calyces and pelvis (Fig. 43.1b). The renal cortex is slightly less echogenic than the liver or spleen, and the renal medullary pyramids are hypoechoic to the renal cortex [7–9]. Chronic kidney disease (CKD) is associated with decreased kidney size and decreased renal cortical thickness on ultrasound (Fig. 43.1c), and both measurements have been found to correlate with estimated glomerular filtration rate [11]. Both AKI and CKD are associated with increased renal echogenicity on ultrasound, although this finding by itself is neither sensitive nor specific [2].

Imaging the Kidneys

A curvilinear low-frequency transducer is typically used to image the kidneys and bladder while the patient is in a supine position. The kidneys are first imaged in the coronal plane, which provides a long-axis view of the kidney. In this plane, the kidney appears bean-shaped (Fig. 43.1a). To image the right kidney, the transducer is placed coronally in the anterior or mid-axillary line, superior to the subcostal margin, with the probe indicator oriented towards the patient's head. The transducer is fanned posteriorly towards the patient's back to view the kidney, using the liver as an acoustic window. To center the kidney on screen, the operator may need to slide the transducer superiorly or inferiorly by one or two intercostal spaces. Rotating the transducer in an oblique fashion to better align the imaging plane parallel to the intercostal space prevents structures of interest from being obscured by shadowing from overlying ribs. In thin patients, using the phased-array transducer may be helpful, as the entire footprint of the transducer can be placed in one intercostal space without rib interference. The left kidney is more difficult to image than the right, due to the smaller acoustic window provided by the spleen and the presence of air in the stomach; the left kidney is often found more superior and posterior than the right kidney. The transducer is placed coronally in the left posterior axillary line, one or two intercostal spaces higher than on the right, with the probe indicator oriented towards the patient's head. Each kidney should be scanned in long axis all the way through from anterior surface to posterior surface by fanning the transducer. After obtaining images along the long axis of the kidney, the transducer is rotated 90 degrees with the probe indicator oriented towards the anterior or posterior aspect of the patient to obtain short axis views of the kidney in a transverse plane. In this plane, the kidney appears circular (Fig. 43.1d). The operator should scan the kidney from superior pole to inferior pole by fanning the transducer.

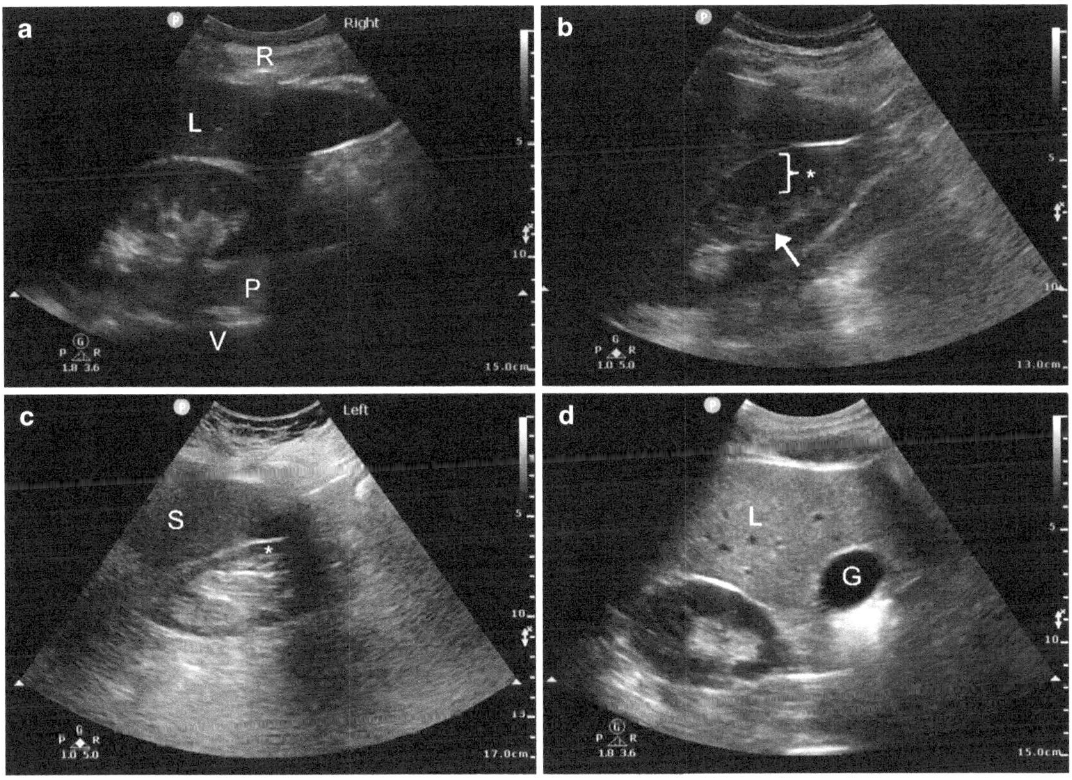

Fig. 43.1 (**a**) Normal right kidney in long axis, showing relationships with liver *(L)*, psoas muscle (*P*), and vertebrae (*V*), and acoustic shadowing from a rib (*R*), (**b**) Normal kidney in long axis, highlighting hypoechoic renal parenchyma *(asterisk)* surrounding hyperechoic renal sinus (*arrow*), (**c**) Left kidney in long axis, showing relationship with spleen (*S*), with abnormal thinning of the renal cortex (*asterisk*), which may be seen in chronic kidney disease, (**d**) Normal right kidney in short axis (transverse plane), showing relationships with liver (*L*) and gallbladder (*G*). Suwondo DN and Baloescu C. Renal and Bladder Ultrasonography for the Intensivist. In: Lanspa MJ and Levinson AT, editors. Echocardiography and Ultrasonography in the ICU: A Comprehensive Text. Springer; *in preparation*, 2022

Imaging the Bladder

The bladder, when empty or under-distended, is located entirely in the pelvis behind the pubic symphysis [12] and may be difficult to identify or evaluate on ultrasound. When distended, the bladder extends superiorly into the abdomen [12] and is easily identifiable. The bladder is imaged in two planes: transverse and sagittal. To obtain a transverse view of the bladder, the transducer is placed in the midline suprapubic region, with the probe indicator pointed towards the patient's right side. From here, the transducer is fanned inferiorly towards the patient's feet and the sound beam is directed behind the pubic symphysis into the pelvis to locate the bladder, which appears as a well-circumscribed round or rectangular anechoic structure with posterior acoustic enhancement and with smooth hyperechoic walls. The bladder wall ranges from 3 to 6 mm in thickness and varies with the degree of bladder distension. Bladder wall thickening is a nonspecific finding due to under-distension, cystitis, elevated intravesical pressures secondary to obstruction or neurogenic bladder, or malignancy [9, 13]. The operator should fan the transducer from superior to inferior to fully image the bladder in transverse view. To obtain a sagittal view of the bladder, the transducer is rotated into a sagittal plane in the midline suprapubic region, with the probe indicator pointed towards the patient's head. From here, the transducer is tilted inferiorly using a rocking hand maneuver and the sound beam is directed into the pelvis. In the sagittal plane, the bladder is scanned from edge-to-edge by fanning the transducer left and right. In males, the prostate is located in the midline at the posterior-inferior aspect of the bladder and can often be seen on the transverse view, particularly when enlarged (Fig. 43.2c). In females, the cer-

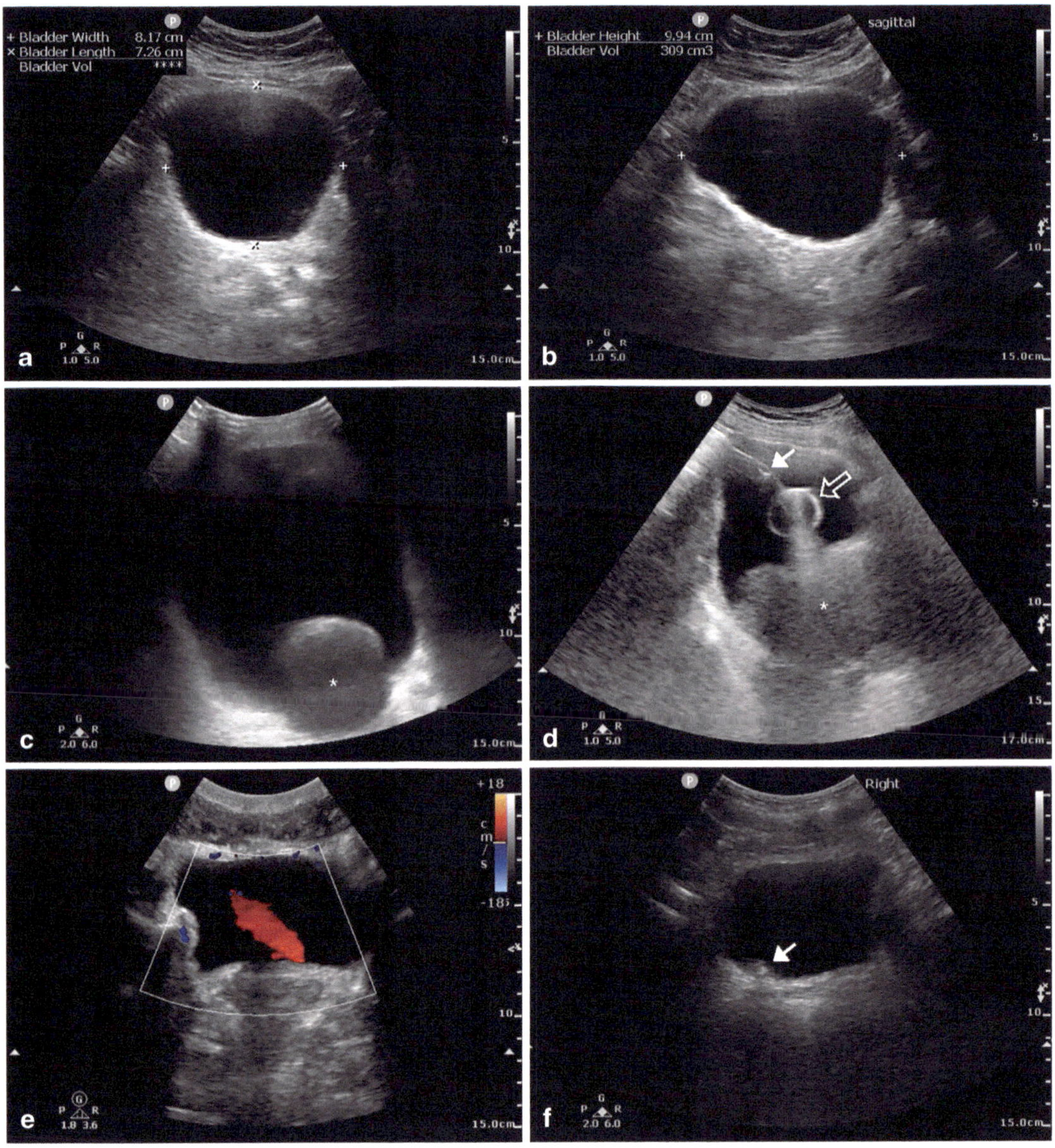

Fig. 43.2 (**a**) Normal bladder in transverse plane, from which two of the three measurements needed to calculate bladder volume can be obtained, (**b**) Normal bladder in sagittal plane, from which the third measurement can be obtained and the bladder volume calculated, (**c**) Transverse view of a severely distended bladder in a patient with urinary retention due to an enlarged prostate (*asterisk*), with more than 1 L of urine in the bladder, (**d**) Sagittal view of a bladder after placement of a urinary catheter, showing an enlarged prostate (*asterisk*) at the base of the bladder, the opening at the tip of the catheter (*thin arrow*), and the inflated catheter balloon (*block arrow*) properly located within the lumen of the bladder, (**e**) Transverse view of bladder with color-flow Doppler showing left ureteral jet, confirming patency of left ureter, (**f**) Transverse view of bladder showing hyperechoic stone (*arrow*) at right ureterovesical junction (UVJ) with acoustic shadowing. Suwondo DN and Baloescu C. Renal and Bladder Ultrasonography for the Intensivist. In: Lanspa MJ and Levinson AT, editors. Echocardiography and Ultrasonography in the ICU: A Comprehensive Text. Springer; *in preparation*, 2022

vix is located posterior to the bladder and the anteverted uterus is located superior to the bladder, and best visualized on the sagittal view. The presence of intraperitoneal free fluid in the pelvis is typically identified as irregularly shaped, uncontained anechoic areas tracking between the bladder wall and surrounding structures such as bowel. This is unlike urine in the bladder, which is also anechoic but well-circumscribed and fully encapsulated in a spherical or cuboid shape.

Bladder Ultrasound

Point-of-care bladder ultrasound can be used by the intensivist to accurately measure bladder volume, diagnose acute urinary retention, troubleshoot malfunctioning urinary catheters, and assess ureteral patency via the presence of ureteral jets.

Bladder Volume

Although bladder volume is commonly estimated using commercial handheld bladder scanning devices, these devices may have decreased accuracy when compared to POCUS-based measurements, particularly in patients with morbid obesity or ascites [14, 15]. Using POCUS, the intensivist can quickly and accurately identify a urine-filled bladder based on anatomic landmarks and appearance, which may help differentiate the bladder from other potential abdominopelvic fluid-containing pathologies such as ascites, distended fluid-filled loops of bowel, an abdominal aortic aneurysm, or adnexal cysts. To calculate bladder volume, the maximal length and width of the bladder lumen are measured in the transverse plane (Fig. 43.2a), and the maximal height of the bladder lumen is measured in the sagittal plane (Fig. 43.2b), yielding three orthogonal measurements. Most ultrasound machines will automatically calculate a bladder volume from these three measurements, although a variety of formulas for manually calculating the volume have been described, the simplest of which is L*W*H*0.75 [7, 16]. As ultrasound vendors have introduced artificial intelligence algorithms into their machines, some devices may have an automatic feature which calculates bladder volume without need for manual scanning in different planes.

Urinary Catheters

POCUS can also help the intensivist identify and troubleshoot problems with urinary catheters. In catheterized patients who develop anuria, suprapubic pain, or hematuria, POCUS can be used to identify signs of urinary catheter obstruction or malposition and to differentiate catheter obstruction from true anuria. An inflated Foley balloon typically appears as a perfectly spherical structure comprising a thin hyperechoic border with anechoic contents (Fig. 43.2d) near the tip of the catheter [13]. A distended bladder on ultrasound despite the presence of a urinary catheter suggests catheter obstruction or malposition. POCUS can also reveal hyperechoic debris or clot layering in dependent areas of the bladder, or a Foley balloon inappropriately positioned within the prostatic urethra. In both non-catheterized and catheterized patients with decreased output or hematuria, the presence of a large clot burden filling the bladder may dissuade blindly performing brisk bladder irrigation.

Ureteral Stones and Jets

In patients with known or suspected ureteral stones, POCUS can help confirm ureteral patency by visualizing the presence of ureteral "jets" at the ureterovesical junction (UVJ) using color-flow Doppler. On a transverse view of the bladder with color-flow Doppler applied, jets appear as intermittent streams of color flow originating from the posterior wall of the bladder at the left or right UVJ and angled towards the center of the bladder lumen (Fig. 43.2e). Jets represent expulsion of urine from the ureter into the bladder during ureteral peristalsis, and depending on hydration status, may be seen one or more times per minute, each lasting up to a second [7, 8]. The presence of bilateral jets makes complete ureteral obstruction unlikely, while their unilateral absence can suggest ureteral obstruction. Although ultrasound is generally insensitive for the detection of ureteral stones, sufficiently large UVJ stones may be identified on ultrasound as an echogenic focus which may exhibit posterior acoustic shadowing on B-mode imaging (Fig. 43.2f) or a "twinkling" artifact on color-flow Doppler, which manifests as a rapidly alternating or shifting color signal behind the stone surface and which has been reported to have a 78% positive predictive value for the presence of nephrolithiasis on unenhanced CT [17]. Large ureteropelvic junction (UPJ) stones may also be visible on ultrasound at the proximal ureter.

Hydronephrosis

Grading of Hydronephrosis

Hydronephrosis in adults is typically graded as mild, moderate, or severe [7–9]. Mild hydronephrosis involves mild dilation or "splaying" of the renal pelvis, without significant distortion of the calyces (Fig. 43.3a). Moderate hydronephrosis involves significant renal pelvic dilation that extends into the calyceal system, causing enlargement and blunting of the calyces; this results in a characteristic multipronged broccoli-like or claw-like appearance (Fig. 43.3b), which spares the renal cortex. In severe hydronephrosis, the calyceal dilation results in thinning of the renal parenchyma (Fig. 43.3c). Severe hydronephrosis with cortical atrophy may represent chronic rather than acute etiology [18]. Among ED patients with suspected renal colic, the finding of moderate or severe hydronephrosis on POCUS has a pooled specificity of 94% for the presence of a renal stone on CT [19]. POCUS may also reveal the presence of other non-obstructing renal stones, which may appear as echogenic foci with acoustic shadowing. In a critically ill ICU patient with urosepsis, the finding of unilateral hydronephrosis on POCUS suggests the presence of an infected obstructing stone and may prompt urgent procedural intervention. In a patient with a renal transplant, isolated hydronephrosis of the transplanted kidney without bladder distension can suggest edema or obstruction at the ureteral anastomosis site [9].

Pitfalls

When evaluating for hydronephrosis in patients with unilateral symptoms, it may be helpful to first scan the unaffected contralateral kidney to obtain a set of baseline images against which to compare the renal collecting system of the affected side, particularly when the degree of hydronephrosis is mild. Prominent renal vasculature, particularly the veins at the level of the hilum, can be misidentified as hydronephrosis on grayscale imaging; applying color-flow Doppler can rapidly differentiate the renal pelvis from surrounding vasculature (Fig. 43.3e). A renal cyst, particularly a parapelvic cyst, may also be misidentified as hydronephrosis; however, cysts are fully circumscribed with a smooth rounded shape, may exhibit posterior acoustic enhancement, and are not associated with dilation of the renal pelvis or surrounding calyces (Fig. 43.3d). Hydronephrosis, by comparison, manifests as renal pelvic dilation that extends into all the calyces.

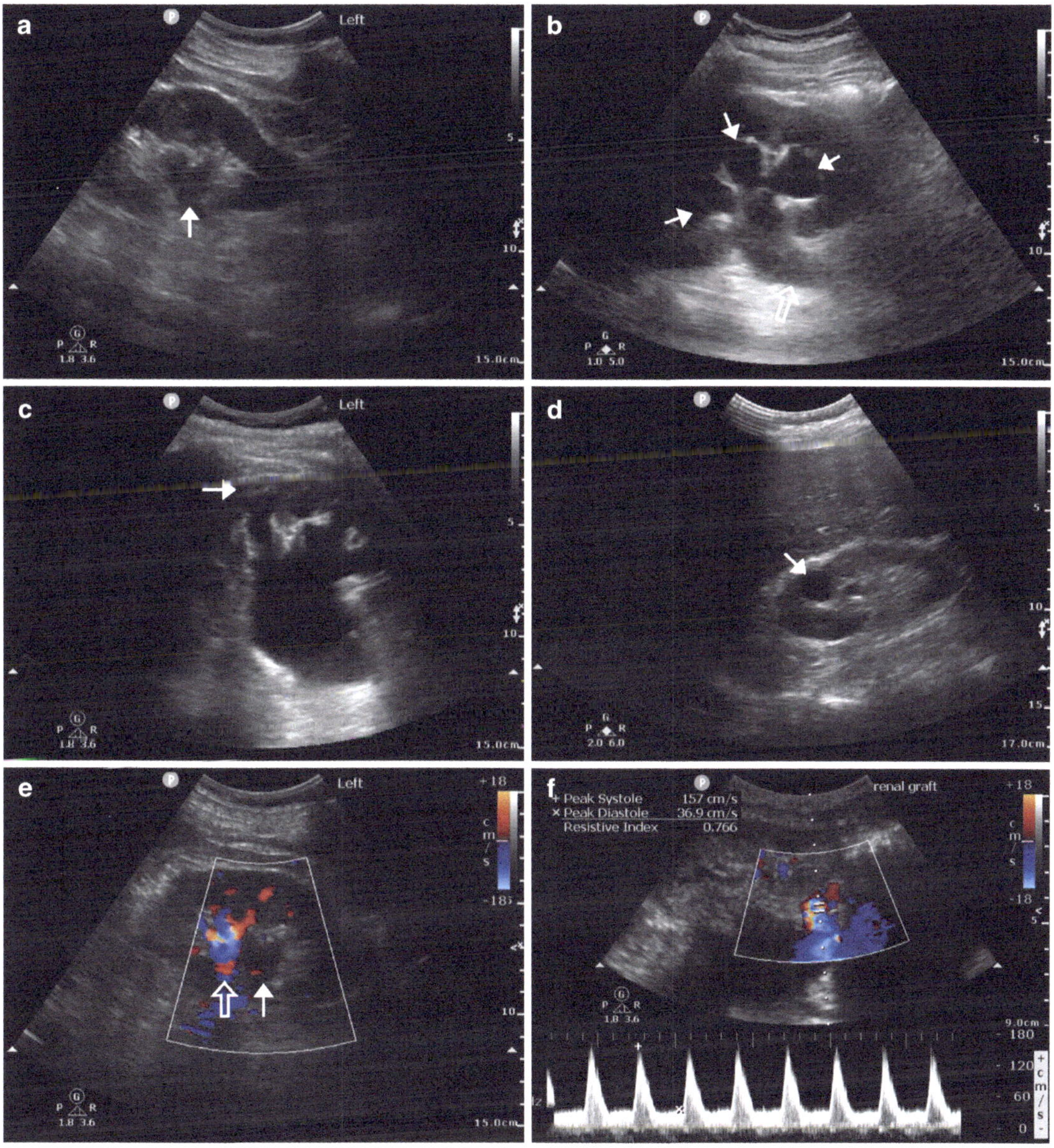

Fig. 43.3 (**a**) Mild hydronephrosis, with splaying of the renal pelvis (*arrow*), (**b**) Moderate hydronephrosis, which extends into the calyces (*arrows*), and hydroureter (*block arrow*), (**c**) Severe hydronephrosis, with thinning of the renal cortex (*arrow*), (**d**) Simple renal cyst (*arrow*), which may be mistaken for hydronephrosis, (**e**) Color-flow Doppler can be used to differentiate the renal blood vessels (*block arrow*) from mild hydronephrosis (*arrow*), (**f**) Pulsed-wave spectral Doppler of a transplanted kidney. Angle-corrected pulsed-wave spectral Doppler can be used to measure the peak systolic velocity in the main renal artery, and can be used to calculate the resistive index (RI) in the renal parenchymal arteries. Suwondo DN and Baloescu C. Renal and Bladder Ultrasonography for the Intensivist. In: Lanspa MJ and Levinson AT, editors. Echocardiography and Ultrasonography in the ICU: A Comprehensive Text. Springer; *in preparation*, 2022

Renal Blood Flow

Renal duplex Doppler ultrasound is typically used in the evaluation of renal transplants and in cases where renal artery stenosis or renal vein thrombosis is suspected. An elevated peak systolic velocity of >285 cm/s on angle-corrected spectral Doppler in the main renal artery and a delayed acceleration time of >0.1 s from end-diastole to peak-systole in the renal parenchymal arteries suggest renal artery stenosis [2, 9, 20]. The resistive index (RI), calculated from the peak systolic velocity (PSV) and end diastolic velocity (EDV) as (PSV-EDV)/PSV, is normally 0.58 ± 0.10 (Fig. 43.3f) [20]. A clinically significant elevated RI is typically >0.80. This may predict persistent AKI in critically ill patients [21], but is nonspecific as to the cause of AKI [2, 8, 9] and represents an area of evolving evidence.

Along with flow pattern assessment of the hepatic and portal veins, Doppler of the renal vein plays a role in the Venous Excess UltraSound (VExUS) score that was developed as an attempt to detect early congestion and avoid end-organ damage. (Details are discussed in Chap. 54) Intrarenal venous Doppler demonstrates a steady monophasic flow beneath the baseline in normal circumstances. It is considered abnormal if discontinuous flow patterns are seen in systolic and diastolic phases, or in the diastolic phase alone [22]. This topic is also an emerging area of evolving evidence.

Summary Points

- Post-renal AKI can be readily diagnosed using POCUS of the kidneys and bladder
- POCUS of the bladder can be used to more accurately measure bladder volume and to troubleshoot problems with urinary catheters
- POCUS of the kidneys can be used to identify hydronephrosis, particularly moderate or severe hydronephrosis
- Mild hydronephrosis involves mild dilation or splaying of the renal pelvis
- Moderate hydronephrosis involves significant dilation of the renal pelvis and extends to the calyces, producing a characteristic multi-pronged claw-like appearance
- Severe hydronephrosis results in thinning of the renal cortex
- The presence of bilateral ureteral jets on color-flow Doppler of the bladder suggests ureteral patency
- Spectral Doppler can be used to evaluate for renal artery stenosis and venous congestion

Pro-Tip (Call-Out)

To calculate bladder volume, the maximal length and width of the bladder lumen are measured in the transverse plane and the maximal height of the bladder lumen is measured in the sagittal plane, yielding three orthogonal measurements.

Emerging Evidence (Call-Out)

Among ED patients with suspected renal colic, the finding of moderate or severe hydronephrosis on POCUS has high (>90%) specificity for the presence of a renal stone on CT.

Questions

1. On point-of-care ultrasound of the right kidney, you note a dilated anechoic structure at the renal pelvis which appears to branch into three dilated rounded structures. The thickness of the surrounding renal cortex appears similar to the contralateral side. On color-flow Doppler, there is no flow within the structure. How would you grade this finding?
   A. Normal finding.
   B. Mild hydronephrosis.
   C. Moderate hydronephrosis.
   D. Severe hydronephrosis.

   Answer: (C) Moderate hydronephrosis. Mild hydronephrosis is primarily limited to the renal pelvis. This patient has moderate hydronephrosis, which extends into the calyceal system. Severe hydronephrosis involves thinning of the renal cortex.
2. You suspect a complete obstruction of the right ureter. Which of the following findings, if present, most suggests patency of the right ureter?

A. The presence of only mild right hydronephrosis, rather than moderate or severe hydronephrosis.
B. The presence of a ureteral jet originating from the right ureterovesical junction on color-flow Doppler of the bladder.
C. A resistive index of 0.60 in the right renal artery on pulsed-wave spectral Doppler.
D. A distended bladder with a bladder volume of 550 cc.

Answer: (B) Ureteral jet. Recall that the degree of hydronephrosis does not necessarily correspond to the acuity or severity of obstruction and may appear falsely minor in hypovolemic patients until adequate fluid resuscitation.

References

1. Hoste EA, Bagshaw SM, Bellomo R, Cely CM, Colman R, Cruz DN, et al. Epidemiology of acute kidney injury in critically ill patients: the multinational AKI-EPI study. Intensive Care Med. 2015;41(8):1411–23. https://doi.org/10.1007/s00134-015-3934-7.
2. Wong-You-Cheong JJ, Nikolaidis P, Khatri G, Dogra VS, Ganeshan D, Goldfarb S, et al. ACR Appropriateness Criteria® renal failure. J Am Coll Radiol. 2021;18(5S):S174–S88. https://doi.org/10.1016/j.jacr.2021.02.019.
3. Podoll A, Walther C, Finkel K. Clinical utility of gray scale renal ultrasound in acute kidney injury. BMC Nephrol. 2013;14:188. https://doi.org/10.1186/1471-2369-14-188.
4. Gamss R, Stein MW, Rispoli JM, Cohen HW, Roberts JH, Koenigsberg M, et al. What is the appropriate use of renal sonography in an inner-city population with new-onset acute kidney injury? J Ultrasound Med. 2015;34(9):1639–44. https://doi.org/10.7863/ultra.15.14.04026.
5. Srisawat N, Sileanu FE, Murugan R, Bellomod R, Calzavacca P, Cartin-Ceba R, et al. Variation in risk and mortality of acute kidney injury in critically ill patients: a multicenter study. Am J Nephrol. 2015;41(1):81–8. https://doi.org/10.1159/000371748.
6. Greene MT, Fakih MG, Fowler KE, Meddings J, Ratz D, Safdar N, et al. Regional variation in urinary catheter use and catheter-associated urinary tract infection: results from a national collaborative. Infect Control Hosp Epidemiol. 2014;35(Suppl 3):S99–S106. https://doi.org/10.1086/677825.
7. Hwang JQ, Poffenberger CM. Chapter 10. Renal and urinary system ultrasound. In: Carmody KA, Moore CL, Feller-Kopman D, editors. Handbook of critical care and emergency ultrasound. New York, NY: The McGraw-Hill Companies; 2011.
8. Sheynkin YR. Ultrasound evaluation of the renal system and the bladder. In: Levitov AB, Mayo PH, Slonim AD, editors. Critical care ultrasonography, 2e. New York, NY: McGraw-Hill Education; 2015.
9. McGahan JP. Kidney and renal transplant. In: McGahan JP, Schick MA, Mills LD, editors. Fundamentals of emergency ultrasound. Fundamentals of radiology. 1st ed. Maryland Heights: Elsevier; 2019. p. 210–57.
10. Standring S. Kidney and ureter. In: Standring S, editor. Gray's anatomy: the anatomical basis of clinical practice. 42nd ed. New York: Elsevier; 2021. p. 1259–75.
11. Takata T, Koda M, Sugihara T, Sugihara S, Okamoto T, Miyoshi K, et al. Left renal cortical thickness measured by ultrasound can predict early progression of chronic kidney disease. Nephron. 2016;132(1):25–32. https://doi.org/10.1159/000441957.
12. Standring S. Bladder, prostate, and urethra. In: Standring S, editor. Gray's anatomy: the anatomical basis of clinical practice. 42nd ed. New York: Elsevier Limited; 2021. p. 1276–91.
13. McAchran SE, Hartke DM, Nakamoto DA, Resnick MI. Sonography of the urinary bladder. Ultrasound Clin 2007;2(1):17–26. https://doi.org/10.1016/j.cult.2007.01.010.
14. Prentice DM, Sona C, Wessman BT, Ablordeppey EA, Isakow W, Arroyo C, et al. Discrepancies in measuring bladder volumes with bedside ultrasound and bladder scanning in the intensive care unit: a pilot study. J Intensive Care Soc. 2018;19(2):122–6. https://doi.org/10.1177/1751143717740805.
15. Schallom M, Prentice D, Sona C, Vyers K, Arroyo C, Wessman B, et al. Accuracy of measuring bladder volumes with ultrasound and bladder scanning. Am J Crit Care. 2020;29(6):458–67. https://doi.org/10.4037/ajcc2020741.
16. Noble VE, Nelson B, Sutingco AN. Renal and bladder. In: Noble VE, Nelson B, Sutingco AN, editors. Manual of emergency and critical care ultrasound. 1st ed. Cambridge: Cambridge University Press; 2007. p. 119–33.
17. Dillman JR, Kappil M, Weadock WJ, Rubin JM, Platt JF, DiPietro MA, et al. Sonographic twinkling artifact for renal calculus detection: correlation with CT. Radiology. 2011;259(3):911–6. https://doi.org/10.1148/radiol.11102128.
18. Brandon C, Mailhot T, Seif D, Swadron SP. Renal. In: Ma OJ, Mateer JR, Reardon RF, Byars DV, Knapp BJ, Laudenbach AP, editors. Ma and Mateer's emergency ultrasound. 4th ed. New York, NY: McGraw-Hill Education; 2021.
19. Wong C, Teitge B, Ross M, Young P, Robertson HL, Lang E. The accuracy and prognostic value of point-of-care ultrasound for nephrolithiasis in the emergency department: a systematic review and meta-analysis. Acad Emerg Med. 2018;25(6):684–98. https://doi.org/10.1111/acem.13388.

20. Barozzi L, Valentino M, Santoro A, Mancini E, Pavlica P. Renal ultrasonography in critically ill patients. Crit Care Med. 2007;35(5 Suppl):S198–205. https://doi.org/10.1097/01.CCM.0000260631.62219.B9.
21. Ninet S, Schnell D, Dewitte A, Zeni F, Meziani F, Darmon M. Doppler-based renal resistive index for prediction of renal dysfunction reversibility: a systematic review and meta-analysis. J Crit Care. 2015;30(3):629–35. https://doi.org/10.1016/j.jcrc.2015.02.008.
22. Beaubien-Souligny W, Rola P, Haycock K, Bouchard J, Lamarche Y, Spiegel R, et al. Quantifying systemic congestion with point-of-care ultrasound: development of the venous excess ultrasound grading system. Ultrasound J. 2020;12(1):16. https://doi.org/10.1186/s13089-020-00163-w.

Gastric, Biliary, and Hepatic Ultrasound in the ICU

44

Maha Salama and Amira Mohamed

Learning Objectives

1. Examine POCUS findings consistent with liver cirhossis
2. Review the key POCUS findings associated with acute cholycystitis
3. Understand the utility of point of care ultrasound in the identification of abdominal pathology
4. Learn the techniques required in the assessment of stomach, liver, and gallbladder as well as their associated pathologies using point of care ultrasound

Indications and Limitations

Gastric and biliary pathologies in the ICU are common problems and are ones that could be detrimental if missed. US diagnosis of GI dysfunction has been widely used for decades; however, it is only recently that it is being utilized by the intensivist. Free air, free fluid, and even biliary obstruction can be identified on an ultrasound exam but guidelines regarding the interpretation and diagnostic utility of these findings are lacking.

Patient positioning, surgical incisions, and other factors may be barriers to obtaining complete studies; however, any information obtained could be valuable, especially in an ICU. Just as with other parts of the POCUS (point of care ultrasound) exam, any images obtained should be interpreted together with the patient's overall clinical picture, and in some cases confirmed with additional imaging studies prior to making clinical decisions.

Anatomy and Technique

Stomach

The stomach is situated in the left upper quadrant of the abdomen anterior to the spleen. It is divided into three parts: the antrum, body, and the fundus. It can be visualized with the patient in multiple positions: supine, right lateral decubitus, sitting, and semi sitting, with the antrum being the easiest to visualize in most patients. In the critically ill patient, only the supine position is usually feasible and therefore we will focus on that position in this section.

M. Salama (✉)
Cardiothoracic ICU Lenox Hill Hospital NYC, Emergency Medicine Jacobi Medical Center/North Central Bronx, Bronx, NY, USA
e-mail: Msalama4@northwell.edu

A. Mohamed
Critical Care Medicine Fellowship Program, Albert Einstein College of Medicine, Bronx, NY, USA

Division of Critical Care Medicine, Montefiore Medical Center, Bronx, NY, USA
e-mail: ammohamed@montefiore.org

M. J. Lanspa, A. T. Levinson (eds.), *Echocardiography and Ultrasonography in the ICU*, Respiratory Medicine, https://doi.org/10.1007/978-3-031-80038-2_44

A low frequency probe is used and placed in the epigastric area in a longitudinal plane with the probe marker towards the patient's right side. You may be able to see the liver, pancreas, and antrum in this view (Fig. 44.1). Other landmarks that may be seen include the IVC (Inferior Vena Cava), the aorta, the superior mesenteric vein, and the superior mesenteric artery.

The gastric body and fundus are harder to examine due to their deep location and presence of air which may obstruct ultrasound waves. The low frequency probe can be placed in the subcostal margin or in the left mid-axillary line in a longitudinal plane to see the gastric body and fundus, respectively.

A high frequency probe can also be placed in the epigastric region to assess the five layers of the stomach wall which are best seen in the antrum, especially in thinner patients.

Liver

The liver is divided into the left lobe, the right lobe, and the caudate lobe. The left and right lobes are separated by the main lobar fissure which connects the gallbladder fossa and the IVC, while the caudate lobe is posteriorly located between the IVC and the fissure of the ligamentum venosum.

The best location to obtain ultrasound images of the liver is the right subcostal approach with the patient in a supine position. If the patient is awake, asking them to take a deep breath which will displace the liver downwards, enhancing the view.

Holding the low frequency probe in a longitudinal plane with the probe marker towards the patient's right side left of the midline and moving along the right subcostal margin laterally, the left lobe of the liver is seen at the same plane as the aorta followed by the caudate lobe, then the right lobe and the inferior vena cava in the same plane (Fig. 44.2). Moving further laterally, the gallbladder fossa is seen posterior to the right lobe, and the kidney inferiorly and laterally.

The liver is normally homogenous and is divided into eight segments, each with its own blood supply, lymphatics, and biliary drainage. The portal vein branch is centralized and surrounded by the hepatic veins in each segment. The most common measurement of the liver is in the midclavicular line and ranges between 12 and 16 cm.

Medially at the porta hepatis, the portal vein can be measured at about 10–15 mm and, using color doppler, the flow is seen with a velocity of 16–40 cm/s. The hepatic venous system will be covered elsewhere.

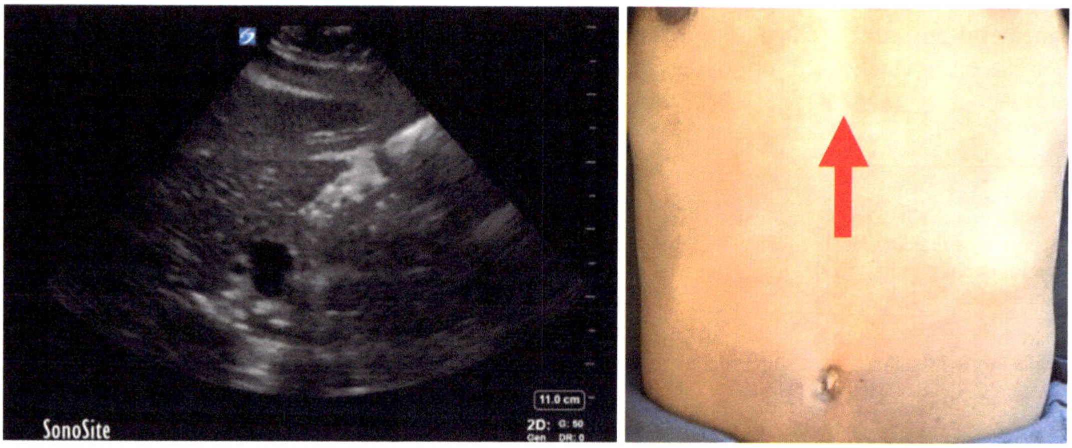

Fig. 44.1 The left lobe of the liver is seen with the antrum laterally. Stomach contents are seen in the antrum

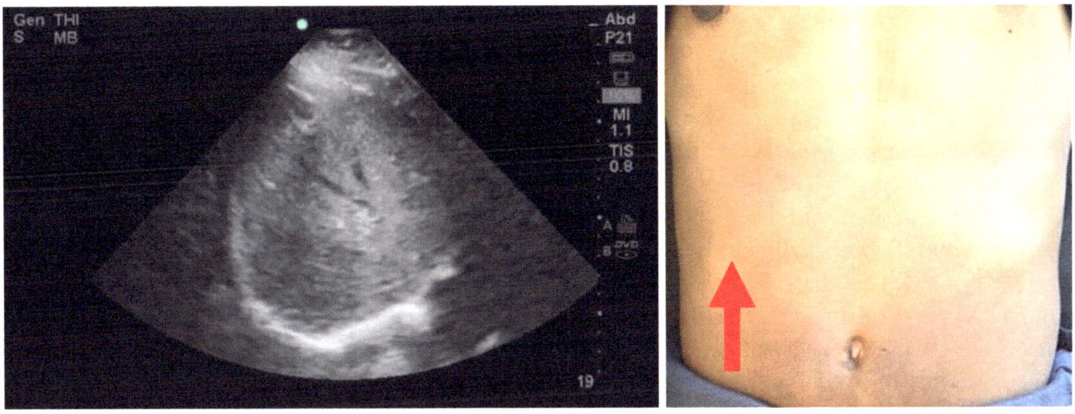

Fig. 44.2 A normal homogenous looking liver seen from the subcostal view

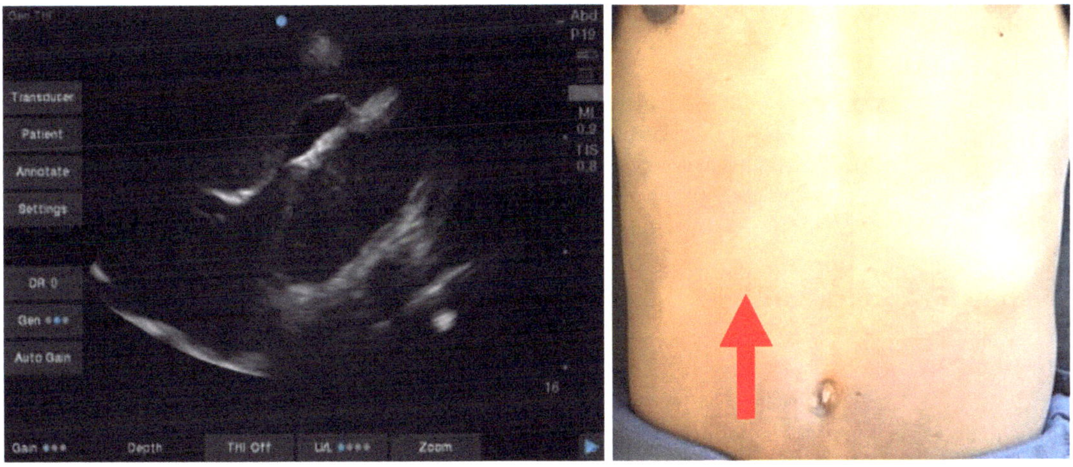

Fig. 44.3 A normal appearing gall bladder and common bile duct with no obvious stones

Biliary System

The gallbladder is situated in the gallbladder fossa of the posterior right hepatic lobe lateral to the second part of the duodenum and anterior to the kidney. It is divided into four parts: fundus, body, infundibulum, and neck. Using a low frequency probe, the biliary system can be visualized with the patient lying supine and the probe placed in the longitudinal plane in the right subcostal margin moving laterally until the gallbladder is seen.

Normally, the gallbladder will contain bile which appears anechoic and clear with no echoes. A normal gallbladder measured longitudinally is 8–12 cm, while the gallbladder wall thickness is normally 1–3 mm. It is recommended that the patient be fasting for around 6 h prior to imaging, otherwise the gallbladder wall may appear thickened due to contraction. However, this is often not feasible when assessing a patient in the ICU.

Landmarks that help with the identification of the gallbladder include the portal vein, common bile duct (CBD), and the hepatic artery or the portal triad which is also known as the "Mickey Mouse sign". Using color doppler to differentiate between the flow types, the hepatic artery and portal vein can be easily identified, while the CBD will not have any flow (Fig. 44.3). The main lobar fissure can be traced from the neck of the gallbladder to the portal triad which also makes it a useful landmark.

The common bile duct is divided into segments with the first or most proximal segment lying anterior to the portal vein, the second segment travels between the porta hepatis and the head of the pancreas, while the third segment is entirely intrapancreatic. The right and left hepatic ducts which converge into the CBD can also be visualized on US, but should be <2 mm in size. The measurement of the CBD should be done from the largest visualized portion in the longitudinal plane and its upper normal limit is 6–10 mm, being closer to 10 in older patients.

Pro Tip Call-Out
Gallbladder wall thickness of more than 4 mm is abnormal.

Pro Tip Call-Out
Add 1 mm for every decade; the patient is over 40 years old. Normal CBD is <4 mm for patients under 40. For a 50-year-old patient, a normal CBD is <5 mm!

Diagnostic Applications

Stomach

Clinical decision making, including intubation, could depend on the patient's stomach contents and therefore assessing gastric distention in the ICU is beneficial. This is best done by measuring the antrum size in the epigastric area. If the antrum is collapsed and the gastric walls are touching, then the stomach is most likely empty. In case of stomach fullness, the antrum would be distended and rounder and the stomach wall would be thinner.

The contents could be quantified by calculating the cross-sectional area of the antrum (CSA) using the formula of the area of an ellipse ($\prod \times r1 \times r2$) where r1 is the anterolateral radius and r2 is the craniocaudal radius.

If the stomach is distended, the decision to empty the stomach to decrease the risk of peri-intubation aspiration, for example by inserting an NG tube prior to intubation, could be made. Other situation where stomach distension may be of value is in patient with delayed gastric emptying, where feeding is discontinued or restarted depending on the findings on the US. In ileus and bowel obstruction, the antrum is severely distended with very thin walls and lack of peristalsis can also be noted.

The appearance of the gastric contents could also be of value, although reliability is limited. For example, in a patient with undifferentiated shock, a distended stomach on ultrasound could signal upper gastrointestinal bleeding as the cause. If blood is present in the stomach, the antrum would be distended, and the fluid would have a heterogenous appearance to the hypoechoic or anechoic appearance of simple fluid.

Air around the stomach has the appearance of A lines similar to the A line pattern visualized while performing lung ultrasound. An A line pattern around the stomach can be a sign of viscous perforation, in the right clinical scenario. If clinically indicated, further imaging with an upright CXR should be obtained.

Liver

In a diseased liver, the most noticeable change is usually the loss of homogeneity. In cirrhosis, the liver has a coarsened echotexture and nodular appearance with or without surrounding ascites. Elevated liver enzymes can signal acute hepatitis which can be further confirmed with an US. The most sensitive sign for hepatitis is hepatomegaly of over 16 cm and attenuated brightness sometimes described as a "starry sky". Hepatomegaly with increased echogenicity is seen in hepatic steatosis where liver enzymes are normal or mildly elevated.

A mass seen on the liver has a wide differential (Fig. 44.4). Clear, anechoic mases are more likely to be cysts while heteromorphic masses with or without air are more likely to be abscesses. Hypoechoic hepatic focal lesions in high-risk patients are suspicious for hepatocellular carcinoma or metastasis and may be associated with enlarged porta hepatic lymph nodes or para-aortic lymph nodes. Using color flow doppler, the vas-

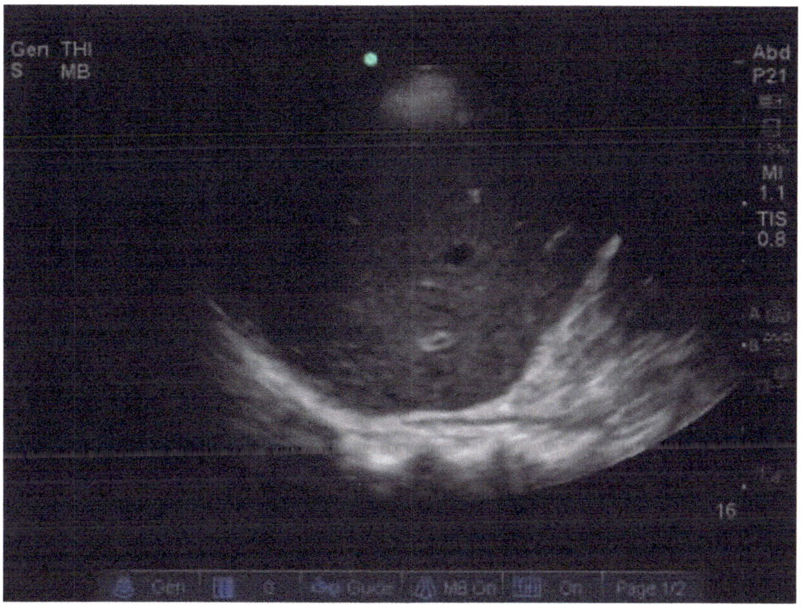

Fig. 44.4 A liver mass is seen. Color doppler can be used to assess its vascularity and help characterize it further

cularity of these masses can be analyzed and can show neovascularization.

The portal vein flow can be abnormal with low velocity combined with increased caliber being diagnostic in portal hypertension. Advanced disease leading to stagnation or even reversal of flow in the portal vein is a sign of grave prognosis.

Biliary System

Gall stones can be seen in the gallbladder as hyperechoic structures with hypoechoic shadowing. They may be asymptomatic or may cause biliary colic that resolves spontaneously. Repositioning the patient while looking at the stones to ensure they are mobile and moving freely is sometimes useful. Stones that migrate to the CBD can cause bile stasis and subsequent cholecystitis.

Even if the probe is not able to detect actual stones in the CBD due to poor visualization, CBD dilation of over 10 mm is sometimes enough for a diagnosis. A double channel or parallel channel sign often results when the CBD is distended and represents the hepatic artery. In this case, color doppler may be needed to differentiate between the two. In cases of severe obstruction, the biliary structure proximal to the CBD can also be visualized including intrahepatic ducts.

Other findings that may point towards gallstones include gallbladder sludge which is heterogenous fluid within the gallbladder. Gallbladder sludge is often a precursor to stones.

Cholecystitis or inflammation of the gallbladder can be calculous or, more commonly in the ICU, acalculous, without gallstones. Acalculous cholecystitis is associated with sepsis, blood transfusions, shock, major surgery, and trauma.

When the gallbladder is inflamed, it will appear distended (>12 mm) and its walls will appear thick (>3 mm) (Fig. 44.5). Gallbladder sludge or stones may be seen as well as fluid between the gallbladder and the liver or pericholecystic fluid. If the patient is awake, asking them to take a deep breath with the probe in place while pressing on the gall bladder using the US probe will illicit Murphy's sign and they will feel pain on inspiration.

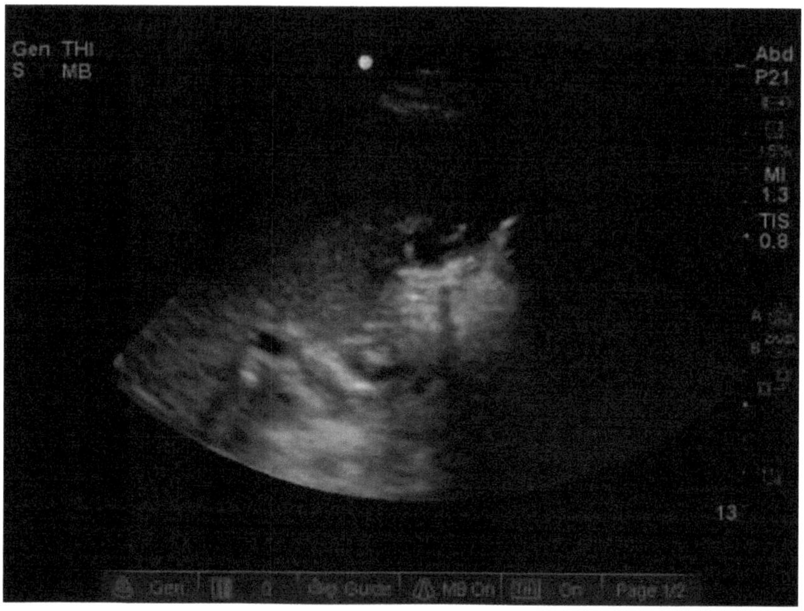

Fig. 44.5 A gall bladder with thickened walls. Measuring the wall diameter can help narrowing the diagnosis

Summary Points

- POCUS can have diagnostic utility for the intensivist in the evaluation of abdominal pathology
- POCUS can be used to identify abnormal stomach contents and perforated viscous
- Acute cholecystitis is demonstrated by sonographic Murphy's sign, dilated CBD, gallbladder wall thickening, and gallbladder sludge, +/− gallstones
- Loss of liver homogeneity is a sign of a hepatic pathology and warrants additional workup

Question(s)

A 38-year-old female presents to the Emergency Department with abdominal cramping, nausea, and decreased oral intake. Her vitals are HR 95, BP 118/56, RR 18, Temp 100.8. A POCUS is performed demonstrating acute cholecystitis. Which of the following ultrasound findings is not consistent with a diagnosis of acute cholecystitis?

A. Presence of gallstones
B. Heterogeneous fluid in the gallbladder
C. Gallbladder wall measurement of 5 mm
D. Common bile duct measurement of 4 mm

Answer: (D). Visualizing gallstones on ultrasound in a symptomatic patient is supportive of a diagnosis of acute cholecystitis. Hetergenous fluid in the gallbladder is consistent with gallbladder sludge, another finding in acute cholecystitis. Normal gallbladder wall size is less than 4 mm, therefore in a 48 year old female, a size of 5mm is abnormal and consistent with acute cholecystitis. Normal CBD measurement is less than 6mm, a CBD measuring 4mm would therefore not be consistent with a diagnosis of acute cholecystitis.

45 Ultrasound Guidance for Abdominal Procedures

Belal Noureddine and Kristin Dwyer

Learning Objectives

1. Describe how to perform paracentesis using ultrasound guidance
2. Examine the use of ultrasound to help place Blakemore and Minnesota Tubes

Paracentesis

Paracentesis is a bedside procedure in which ascitic fluid is obtained from the peritoneal space. The goal is either therapeutic, large volume removal of ascites to relieve symptoms of abdominal pain, early satiety, and shortness of breath caused by increased intraabdominal pressure, or diagnostic, small volume fluid removal aimed at assessing infection such as spontaneous bacterial peritonitis (SBP), malignancy, or cirrhosis. Paracentesis is not indicated for patients with concern for a surgical abdomen. Relative contraindications include evidence of increased risk for bleeding complications such as an international normalized ratio (INR) >2.0 or platelets <20,000 10^9/L. Additionally, caution should be taken with patients with distended bowel due to the risk of bowel injury as well as in patients with overlying cellulitis.

Ultrasound-guided paracentesis allows the operator to visualize the deepest and most favorable pocket of peritoneal fluid to avoid bowel and other intra-abdominal organs, offering a superior safety profile to the blind approach [1]. In addition, abdominal ultrasound can identify as little as 100 mL of intra-abdominal free fluid, allowing the operator to confirm the presence of ascites in the setting of abdominal pain and distention before inserting a needle unnecessarily (Fig. 45.1).

The use of ultrasound has been shown to increase the likelihood of success for paracentesis from 61% to 91% [1], and to significantly reduce the incidence of adverse events including infection, hematoma, and seroma from 4.7% to 1.4% [2, 3].

Supplementary Information The online version contains supplementary material available at https://doi.org/10.1007/978-3-031-80038-2_45.

B. Noureddine
Internal Medicine Group, Orlando Health, Orlando, FL, USA
e-mail: belaln@umich.edu

K. Dwyer (✉)
Emergency Medicine, Warren Alpert Medical School of Brown University, Providence, RI, USA

M. J. Lanspa, A. T. Levinson (eds.), *Echocardiography and Ultrasonography in the ICU*, Respiratory Medicine, https://doi.org/10.1007/978-3-031-80038-2_45

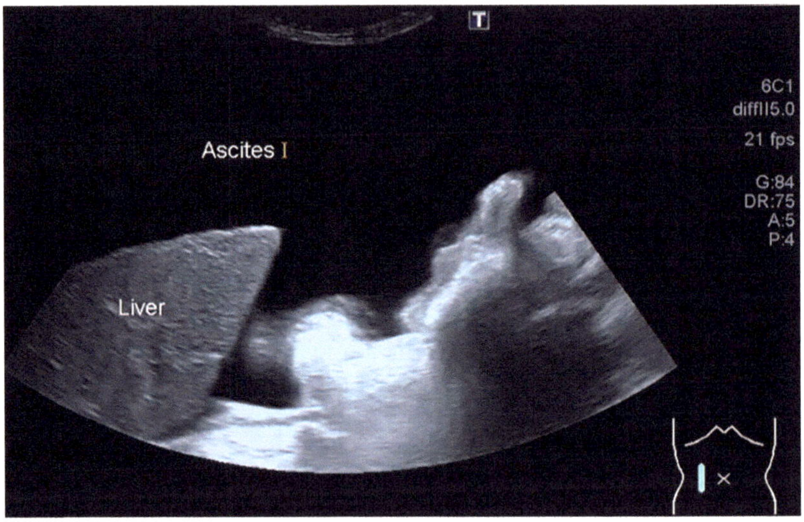

Fig. 45.1 Ultrasound image of ascites fluid

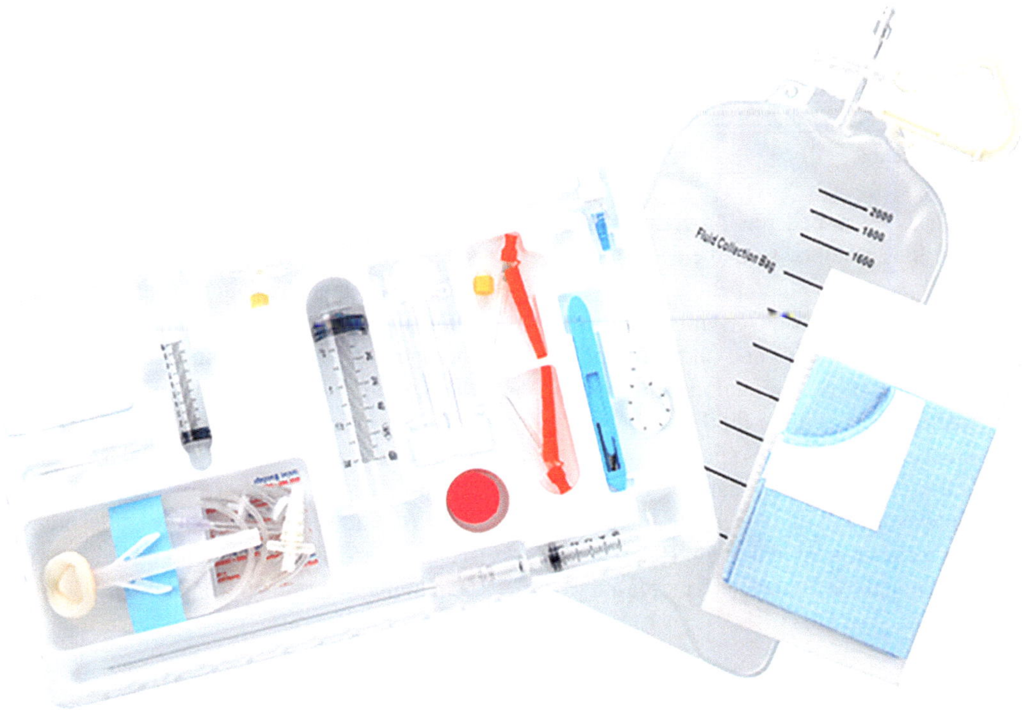

Fig. 45.2 Paracentesis kit

Technique

After obtaining informed consent, collect the materials/kit (Fig. 45.2) for the procedure. Not all below listed materials are required for a diagnostic paracentesis:

- Local anesthetic, needle, and syringe
- Antiseptic solution
- Fenestrated drape
- Paracentesis needle
- Scalpel
- 3-way stopcock

Table 45.1 Ascitic fluid analysis

Test	Causes of ascites Cirrhosis	Congestive Heart Failure (CHF)	Malignancy	SBP	Pancreatitis
Appearance	Clear straw or milky	Clear to pale yellow	Milky or bloody	Cloudy or turbid	Milky, cloudy or turbid
Total protein	<25 g/L	<25 g/L	≥25 g/L	≥25 g/L	≥25 g/L
Serum-ascites albumin gradient (SAAG)	≥1.1 g/dL	≥1.1 g/dL	<1.1 g/dL	<1.1 g/dL	<1.1 g/dL
LDH	↓	↓ or N	↑	↑ or N	↑ or N
Glucose	N	N	↓	↓	↓
Cell counts	≥250/μL or N			≥250/μL	
Bacterial culture	+ or −			+	

- 50 mL syringe
- Tubing set with rolling clamp
- Drainage bag
- Specimen vials
- Collection bottles

Before commencing, instruct the patient to empty their bladder. Place the patient in the supine or lateral decubitus position. The lower lateral quadrant is preferred and placing the patient on their side may aid in identifying the largest pocket.

To evaluate for ascites, the operator can use the curvilinear or phased array probes, which are both high penetration, low-frequency probes. Place the transducer in the transverse position with the orientation marker facing the operator's left. Slide the probe up and down the abdomen in a lawnmower-type motion to find a suitable pocket. Prep and drape the skin in the usual sterile fashion and administer local anesthetic to the skin, subcutaneous tissue, and down to the peritoneum. Ultrasound guidance decreases the likelihood of hitting an abdominal vessel or other abdominal contents such as the viscera [4, 5].

The operator can either insert their needle at the pre-marked location or they can use direct ultrasound visualization for real-time procedure guidance. Insert the needle or catheter perpendicular to the skin and consider using the z-track technique: once the skin is punctured, lift the skin caudally and then advance the needle. If a catheter is being inserted, the operator should make a small nick with an 11 blade in the skin and soft tissue to allow for catheter passage. Pull back on the syringe the needle/catheter as you advance until ascitic fluid begins to fill the syringe. Advance the catheter into the peritoneal cavity and withdraw the needle. If performing a diagnostic paracentesis, withdraw the catheter once an adequate specimen volume has been obtained. If performing a therapeutic tap, connect the tubing to remove larger volumes of ascites. For large volume paracentesis >5 liters, strong consideration should be given to administering albumin.

The specimen should be sent to the lab for analysis of cell count with differential, gram stain, and culture. Additional analysis to consider includes albumin, protein, glucose, lactate dehydrogenase (LDH), and cytology. SBP is diagnosed with an ascitic fluid absolute polymorphonuclear neutrophil (PMN) count >250 cells/mm^3 or a positive fluid culture. Traditional empiric treatment includes coverage for Escherichia. Coli and Klebsiella Pneumoniae with a third-generation cephalosporin, such as ceftriaxone. Prophylactic antibiotics should be considered for patients with ascitic fluid protein concentration <1 g/dL, variceal bleed, or prior SBP [6, 7] (Table 45.1).

Complications from paracentesis are uncommon but include persistent ascitic leak, abdominal wall hematoma, bladder or bowel perforation, vessel injury, hypotension, or infection [8].

Blakemore/Minnesota Tubes

A Blakemore tube is a tube that can be inserted through the oropharynx or nasopharynx, typically in the intubated patient, and advanced into the stomach to tamponade gastric or esophageal bleeding. This is generally reserved for use in unstable patients with uncontrolled bleeding, usually from gastric or esophageal varices, who are unable to get to the endoscopy suite. A Blakemore tube has three ports (gastric balloon, esophageal balloon, and gastric suction port) on one end and two balloons on the other end. A Minnesota tube is similar to a Blakemore tube; however, it has a larger gastric balloon and both gastric and esophageal aspiration ports [9]. Endoscopy by a gastroenterologist is the gold standard for treating acute variceal bleeding, but the Blakemore/Minnesota tube can be used as a rescue measure if endoscopy is unsuccessful or unavailable (Fig. 45.3).

To place a Blakemore tube, first secure the patient's airway and elevate the head of the bed if possible. Deflate and lubricate the tube after inflating to confirm that there are no balloon leaks. Mark the tube before insertion to identify how far to insert it (~50 centimeters (cm) above the esophageal balloon). The tube is advanced until the operator is confident that one balloon is in the stomach and the other balloon is in the esophagus.

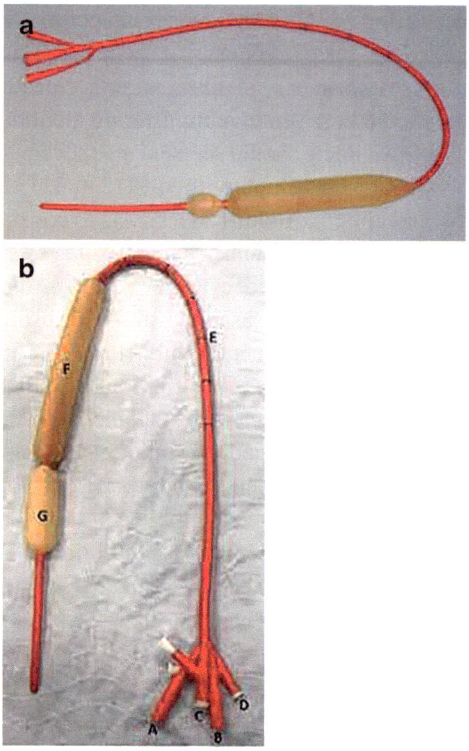

Fig. 45.3 (**a**) Blakemore tube (**b**) Minnesota tube

Next, fill the gastric balloon with approximately 50 milliliters (mL) of air through the port while auscultating over the stomach and lungs. Traditionally, a chest radiograph (X-ray) is obtained to confirm balloon placement in the stomach before inflating with an additional 200 mL of air. Ultrasound can be used instead to assess balloon placement and inflation. Next, apply traction to aid the inflated balloon in the tamponade of the bleeding vessel. Ensure that the tube does not move more than an inch with traction, as this may indicate more inflation is required. Using the gastric suction port, evaluate for ongoing bleeding below the gastric balloon. With continued gastric bleeding, consider additional balloon inflation. To evaluate esophageal bleeding, a nasogastric (NG) tube must be inserted to identify continued bleeding above the gastric balloon.

A Minnesota tube, functionally similar to a Blakemore tube with the exception an expanded 500 mL gastric balloon capacity and inclusion of both gastric and esophageal suction ports, may also be used to tamponade emergent bleeding. Additionally, the presence of the esophageal suction port obviates the need for separate NG tube insertion. The esophageal balloon can be inflated to a pressure of 20–40 millimeters of mercury (mmHg).

While the standard of care is to confirm gastric balloon placement with X-ray before inflation, this results in significant delays to therapeutic tamponade. In a hemodynamically unstable patient, bedside ultrasound may be able to more rapidly confirm placement and location of the balloon, as well as provide assistance with real-time position adjustments. At present, there is little evidence to support the use of ultrasound for balloon localization, as this is such an infrequently performed procedure [10, 11].

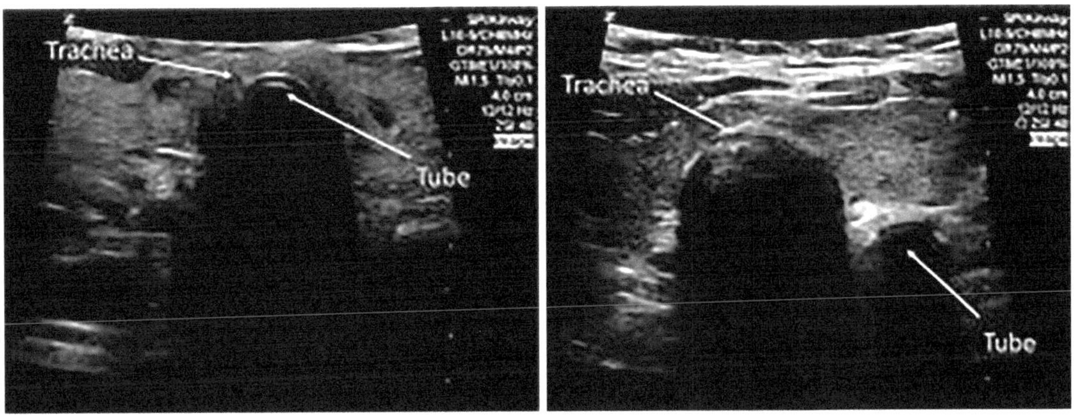

Fig. 45.4 Ultrasound images of the trachea and esophagus during tube placement

To locate the tube with ultrasound, use a high-penetration low-frequency probe, such as the curvilinear or phased array probe. Place the probe in the sagittal plane in the mid-epigastrium aiming to the patient's left to find the gastroesophageal junction (GEJ). Rotate counterclockwise, and this view will confirm the passing of the tube through the lower esophageal sphincter (LES) into the stomach [10]. In the hemorrhaging patient, the stomach is likely full of blood, allowing for better identification of the balloon as blood provides a good medium for ultrasound waves. Anteriorly in the supine patient, there may be interference from air which will obscure the operator's view. To find the best view, slide along the costal margin aiming towards the stomach. In the lateral view, the operator can confirm that the balloon is located below the diaphragm as it is being inflated [12].

Further, as the Blakemore or Minnesota tube is being advanced, the linear probe can be placed on the anterior neck in the transverse view with the marker to the patient's right. In this view, the trachea and esophagus can be visualized and passage of the tube through the esophagus can also be viewed [10] (Fig. 45.4).

Potential complications of this procedure include inflating the gastric balloon above the diaphragm, resulting in damage or rupture of the esophagus or trachea. In addition, prolonged placement (>24–36 hours) may result in pressure necrosis, and 50% of patients will experience rebleeding [13, 14].

Gastrostomy Tube

A Gastrostomy tube (G-tube) allows for enteral nutrition, as an alternative to parenteral nutrition, in patients with the inability to tolerate oral intake due to obstruction from head and neck tumors, neurologic decline, or esophageal damage due to stricture formation, obstructive malignancy, trauma, or surgery. A G-tube has three ports (medicine, feeding, balloon) on one end and one balloon with a bumper on the other end [15, 16] (Fig. 45.5).

G-tubes can be placed percutaneously via endoscopy, radiologically, or with ultrasound. G-tube placement may be performed transorally in the anterograde "pull-type" route or transabdominally in the retrograde "push-type" fashion. Of these percutaneous modalities, ultrasound is emerging as the favored technique in conjunction with radiologic placement via the "push-type" route, as ultrasound allows for real-time visualization of abdominal structures, thereby decreasing fluoroscopy time and minimizing radiation exposure to both the patient and the operator [18]. Endoscopic G-tube placement is limited by the requirement of deep sedation and is contraindicated in the setting of head and neck malignancy due to obstruction and the risk of gastric seeding.

Placing a G-tube in the retrograde abdominal fashion begins with the patient in the supine position. Using a curvilinear low-frequency ultrasound probe, hold the transducer in the transverse

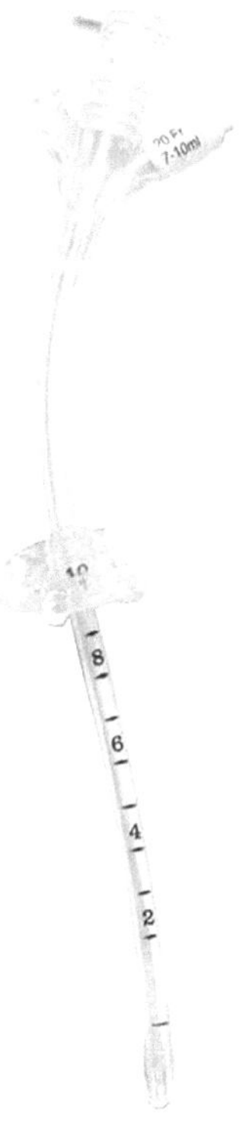

Fig. 45.5 A standard gastrostomy tube (from Cook et al. [17])

position with the orientation marker facing the operator's left. Fan the probe to identify key abdominal structures, including the margins of the liver and the gastric antrum, and mark them on the skin. An NG tube is inserted, and carbon dioxide is administered through it for insufflation of the stomach [18, 19].

Following gastric insufflation, fanning of the probe can locate a percutaneous access window, favored near the linea alba. A gastropexy device is then, under ultrasound guidance, placed to internally affix the stomach against the anterior abdominal wall. With the stomach in view, a large-bore needle is inserted in the center of the gastropexy site, visualized in real-time with ultrasound. Under continuous fluoroscopy, a guidewire is inserted, the needle entry tract is dilated, and then the G tube is inserted. After this, the G tube balloon is inflated, and contrast is inserted to confirm its placement.

Potential complications of this procedure include through-and-through puncture of the colon, and less frequently, the liver. Additionally, puncture of the liver increases the risk of abscess formation via the introduction of skin flora. The use of ultrasound both before the procedure to survey the liver margins and during the procedure to guide needle placement in real-time can help to mitigate these severe complications [20, 21].

Summary Points

- Ultrasound guidance for therapeutic and diagnostic paracentesis increases procedural safety by identifying the best ascites pocket to avoid injury to bowel and intra-abdominal organs.
- Placement of balloon tamponade devices for unstable patients with massive upper gastrointestinal bleeds is an uncommon procedure. Traditionally balloon placement is confirmed by X-ray, but more data are needed to determine whether a bedside ultrasound can more rapidly confirm balloon location accurately.
- Gastrostomy tubes are most commonly performed percutaneously with radiologic guidance. There is emerging evidence that this procedure can be augmented with ultrasound guidance.

Questions

1. A 31-year-old female with a past medical history of chronic Hepatitis C infection, intravenous drug abuse, and bipolar disorder presents after being found down for an unknown amount of time. Initial vitals are BP 96/43 mmHg, HR 63 bpm, RR 7 bpm, Temp 95.7 F, and 92% O_2 saturation on room air. On visual inspection, the patient appears in pain and is holding her abdomen, which on physical exam is noted to be grossly rigid and distended with localized epigastric erythema, and tender to palpation in all quadrants.

   Bedside ultrasound is performed and shows a shrunken liver and a large ascites pocket with an air fluid level. Complete blood count is notable for Hemoglobin 10.6 g/dL, Hematocrit 35%, White Blood Cells

27×10^9/L, and Platelets 12×10^9/L. The remaining lab work is in process. Urine HCG is positive.

As part of the infectious workup, the patient is planned for bedside paracentesis under point-of-care ultrasound (POCUS) guidance. While POCUS guidance increases the safety of paracentesis, which of the following is an absolute contraindication to paracentesis in this patient?

A. Pregnancy
B. Abdominal Cellulitis
C. Severe Thrombocytopenia
D. Concern for Peritonitis
E. Hypotension

Answer: (D). Pregnancy, abdominal cellulitis, thrombocytopenia, and hypotension are all relative contraindications that require careful consideration prior to performing a paracentesis. However, the presence or strong suspicion of a surgical abdomen is an absolute contraindication to performing a paracentesis.

2. A 56-year-old male presents to the emergency room overnight with 3 days of progressively worsening nausea and vomiting, which has been mostly yellow liquid. Past medical history is notable for chronic marijuana use, osteoarthritis managed with daily ibuprofen, and alcohol use disorder. While history is being obtained, the patient experiences an aggressive episode of vomiting which develops into persistent bouts of large volume hematemesis.

The patient reports feeling lightheaded and subsequently stops answering questions. Stat vitals are notable for BP 83/29 mmHg, HR 125 bpm, RR 14 bpm, and 89% peripheral O_2 saturation. Central access is rapidly obtained, four units of O-negative packed red blood cells are ordered stat, and a 2-L crystalloid bolus begins infusing. The patient is intubated for airway protection and the gastroenterologist on-call is paged for urgent endoscopic intervention but has to travel from offsite.

Despite fluid resuscitation and ongoing blood transfusion, repeat blood pressure is 75/21 mmHg and HR is 127 bpm. The decision is made to place a Minnesota tube to tamponade the bleeding until the gastroenterologist arrives. Which of the following is true about point-of-care ultrasound (POCUS) guidance for balloon tamponade placement in the unstable patient?

A. POCUS is established as superior to X-ray for confirming balloon placement in the stomach prior to inflation
B. POCUS may be able to save time as an alternative to X-ray for confirming balloon placement in the unstable patient
C. Balloon tamponade should be used for all hematemesis patients with a blood pressure of <90 mmHg, even if endoscopy is available
D. All of the above

Answer: (B). There is emerging evidence that POCUS may be able to expedite confirmation of gastric balloon placement and miniize radiation expsoure; however, at the time of writing, X-ray remains the gold standard. Additionally, when readily available, endoscopy is the superior modality for locating and treating upper gastrointestinal bleeds in both stable and unstable patients.

References

1. Nazeer SR, Dewbre H, Miller AH. Ultrasound-assisted paracentesis performed by emergency physicians vs the traditional technique: a prospective, randomized study. Am J Emerg Med. 2005;23(3):363–7. https://doi.org/10.1016/j.ajem.2004.11.001.
2. Patel PA, Ernst FR, Gunnarsson CL. Evaluation of hospital complications and costs associated with using ultrasound guidance during abdominal paracentesis procedures. J Med Econ. 2012;15(1):1–7. https://doi.org/10.3111/13696998.2011.628723.
3. Rodriguez Lima DR, Yepes AF, Birchenall Jiménez CI, Díaz MAM, Rojas DIP. Real-time ultrasound-guided thoracentesis in the intensive care unit: prevalence of mechanical complications. Ultrasound J. 2020;12:25. https://doi.org/10.1186/s13089-020-00172-9.
4. Hatch N, Wu TS, Barr L, Roque PJ. Advanced ultrasound procedures. Crit Care Clin. 2014;30(2):305–29, vi. Erratum in: Crit Care Clin. 2014 Oct;30(4):xi. https://doi.org/10.1016/j.ccc.2013.10.005.
5. Mayeaux EJ. Abdominal paracentesis [Internet]. 5MinuteConsult.com. [cited 2022 Jan 30]. Available from: https://5minuteconsult.com/

collectioncontent/30-156350/procedures/abdominal-paracentesis
6. Andreu M, Sola R, Sitges-Serra A, Alia C, Gallen M, Vila MC, et al. Risk factors for spontaneous bacterial peritonitis in cirrhotic patients with ascites. Gastroenterology. 1993;104(4):1133–8. https://doi.org/10.1016/0016-5085(93)90284-j.
7. Rasaratnam B, Kaye D, Jennings G, Dudley F, Chin-Dusting J. The effect of selective intestinal decontamination on the hyperdynamic circulatory state in cirrhosis. A randomized trial. Ann Intern Med. 2003;139(3):186–93. https://doi.org/10.7326/0003-4819-139-3-200308050-00008.
8. Aponte EM, Katta S, O'Rourke MC. Paracentesis. In: StatPearls [Internet]. Treasure Island (FL): StatPearls Publishing; 2021 Sep 8.
9. Powell M, Journey JD. Sengstaken-Blakemore tube. In: StatPearls [Internet]. Treasure Island (FL): StatPearls Publishing; 2021 Jul 27.
10. Farkas J. Pulmcrit Wee: ultrasound-guided Blakemore tube placement [Internet]. EMCrit Project. Metasin LLC; 2016 [cited 2022Jan31]. Available from: https://emcrit.org/pulmcrit/pulmcrit-wee-ultrasound-guided-blakemore-tube-placement/
11. Lock G, Reng M, Holstege A, Schölmerich J, Grüne S, Messman H. Inflation and positioning of the gastric balloon of a Sengstaken-Blakemore tube under ultrasonographic control [Internet]. Gastrointestinal Endoscopy; 1997 [cited 2022 Jan 31]. Available from: https://www.giejournal.org/article/S0016-5107(97)70194-9/fulltext
12. Weingart S, Guthrie JM. How to place a Blakemore tube in an ED patient with upper GI bleeding from esophageal varices [Internet]. ACEP Now; 2015 [cited 2022 Jan 31]. Available from: https://www.acepnow.com/article/place-blakemore-tube-ed-patient-upper-gi-bleeding-esophageal-varices/
13. Chong CF. Esophageal rupture due to Sengstaken-Blakemore tube misplacement. World J Gastroenterol. 2005;11(41):6563–5. https://doi.org/10.3748/wjg.v11.i41.6563.
14. Vlavianos P, Gimson AE, Westaby D, Williams R. Balloon tamponade in variceal bleeding: use and misuse. BMJ. 1989;298(6681):1158. https://doi.org/10.1136/bmj.298.6681.1158.
15. Ho SG, Marchinkow LO, Legiehn GM, Munk PL, Lee MJ. Radiological percutaneous gastrostomy. Clin Radiol. 2001;56(11):902–10. https://doi.org/10.1053/crad.2001.0782.
16. Wollman B, D'Agostino HB, Walus-Wigle JR, Easter DW, Beale A. Radiologic, endoscopic, and surgical gastrostomy: an institutional evaluation and meta-analysis of the literature. Radiology. 1995;197(3):699–704.
17. Cook F, Rodriguez J, McCaul L. Malnutrition, nutrition support and dietary intervention: the role of the dietitian supporting patients with head and neck cancer. Br Dent J. 2022;233:757–64. https://doi.org/10.1038/s41415-022-5107-8.
18. Shukla PA, Kolber MK, Tapnio R, Zybulewski A, Kumar A, Patel RI. Safety and feasibility of ultrasound-guided gastric access for percutaneous transabdominal gastrostomy tube placement. Gastroenterol Res. 2019;12(3):115–9. https://doi.org/10.14740/gr1136.
19. Wu TS, Leech SJ, Rosenberg M, Huggins C, Papa L. Ultrasound can accurately guide gastrostomy tube replacement and confirm proper tube placement at the bedside. J Emerg Med. 2009;36(3):280–4. https://doi.org/10.1016/j.jemermed.2007.11.064.
20. Lorentzen T, Nolsøe CP, Adamsen S. Percutaneous radiologic gastrostomy with a simplified gastropexy technique under ultrasonographic and fluoroscopic guidance: experience in 154 patients. Acta Radiol. 2007;48(1):13–9. https://doi.org/10.1080/02841850601045120.
21. Covarrubias DA, O'Connor OJ, McDermott S, Arellano RS. Radiologic percutaneous gastrostomy: review of potential complications and approach to managing the unexpected outcome. AJR Am J Roentgenol. 2013;200(4):921–31. https://doi.org/10.2214/AJR.11.7804.

Vascular Access

46

Hallie Brown and Viveta Lobo

Learning Objectives

1. Describe how the utilization of ultrasound guidance to guide vascular access has been shown to improve first attempt success rates and reduce procedure-related complications
2. Explore how to use ultrasound to place catheters in the subclavian vein and the radial artery

Internal Jugular (IJ)

Ultrasound-guided internal jugular access has become the standard of care when achieving central venous access. In this section, we will review the basics of this technique.

Using a linear probe, in transverse orientation and indicator to the patient's left, pre-scan the neck with ultrasound. The IJ is lateral and anterior to the carotid artery in most cases. Pick the side where puncture will be direct and superficial and chances of a mistaken arterial puncture are lower. Avoid applying too much pressure to inadvertently collapse the IJ, especially in hypovolemic patients. Placing these patients in the trendelenburg position can be especially helpful to engorge the IJ for better visualization. Try to position the IJ in the center of your screen and note its depth. Your catheter should be approximately at least 1.5 times the depth of the IJ in length.

Once the operator is gowned and gloved, apply sterile gel to the ultrasound probe, and with the assistance of another person the ultrasound probe is placed in the sterile sheath and secured with sterile rubber bands. Apply more sterile gel to the top of the covered probe and place in the sterile field. The patient's neck should be draped and cleaned. The ultrasound is held in your non-dominant hand and the anesthetic-filled syringe and needle in your dominant hand. Scan the neck perpendicular to the skin and center the IJ on the screen, finding it in the most directly accessible and superficial position. Approach the neck with your anesthetic needle at a 45° angle, deposit the anesthesia just under the skin superficially creating a "wheal" under the skin, and continue to advance and deposit anesthesia deeper while maintaining negative pressure on the syringe. Once all the anesthesia is deposited, continue by inserting your introducer needle and syringe, and approach the skin in the same manner at a 45° angle. Puncture the skin angling your needle tip to be directly underneath the ultrasound probe. Locate the needle tip on the screen and follow it as you advance your needle slowly observing as

Supplementary Information The online version contains supplementary material available at https://doi.org/10.1007/978-3-031-80038-2_46.

H. Brown · V. Lobo (✉)
Stanford University School of Medicine, Palo Alto, CA, USA
e-mail: vlobo@stanford.edu

M. J. Lanspa, A. T. Levinson (eds.), *Echocardiography and Ultrasonography in the ICU*, Respiratory Medicine, https://doi.org/10.1007/978-3-031-80038-2_46

it indents the IJ wall (Video 46.1). Once the IJ is punctured, identify your needle tip within the vessel (Video 46.2); nonpulsatile dark blood is drawn back into your syringe; drop the ultrasound probe on the field and continue with placing the guidewire. Prior to dilating the vessel and placing the catheter and removing the guidewire, scan the neck over the puncture site to confirm guidewire location and placement in the correct vessel (Video 46.3). Once the procedure is complete, you may use ultrasound again to confirm catheter placement (ECHO), rule out pneumothorax, arterial puncture, and/or local hematoma.

Femoral Vein

Femoral venous cannulation is a relatively superficial and easily accessed vein. Unlike upper neck anatomy that is complex, the femoral vascular structures are relatively isolated. However, femoral central venous catheters have higher risks of infection and thrombosis. We recommend that femoral sites only be used in a true emergent situation during active cardiopulmonary resuscitation (and then later exchanged for a line above the diaphragm) or when other sites are not accessible. Ultrasound guidance for placement of femoral lines increases the likelihood of successful cannulation and reduces the risk of complications [7].

The femoral vein and artery are accessible within the femoral triangle, which is defined by the inguinal ligament superiorly, the adductor longus muscle medially, and the sartorius muscle laterally. The femoral vein is imaged medially adjacent to the artery. Place the patient supine or in a slight reverse Trendelenburg position to distend the femoral vein and prevent air embolism. Comfortably abduct and externally rotate the leg. Perform a non-sterile prescan of the femoral vein 1 to 2 cm inferior to the inguinal ligament and determine whether the vein is suitable for cannulation. Use a short-axis view. Evaluate for its position relative to the femoral artery and ensure there is no thrombosis (the vein should be fully compressible, and no echogenicities seen within the vessel, Video 46.4). Known thrombosis is a contraindication to cannulation. Once the operator is gowned and gloved, apply sterile gel to the ultrasound probe, and with the assistance of another person the ultrasound probe is placed in the sterile sheath and secured with sterile rubber bands. Apply more sterile gel to the top of the covered probe and place in the sterile field. Disinfect the skin. Using your high frequency transducer, obtain a short axis image of the femoral vein. Slide the probe transversely as needed to place the imaged vein at the center of the ultrasound screen. Take note of the depth of the vein under the skin, you will enter the skin the same distance distal from the probe. At this level, inject your local anesthesia creating a "wheal" under the skin before injecting more anesthesia deeper. Then, follow with inserting your introducer needle into the skin pointed caudally at a 45° angle directed toward the midpoint of the probe. Tilt your probe towards your patient's feet to identify and visualize your needle tip at all times. Keep gentle negative pressure on the syringe plunger as you advance your needle. Slowly advance your needle, until you see the superficial wall of the vein indent as it enters the vessel accompanied by a flash of dark nonpulsatile blood into your syringe. As soon as you see the flash, stop advancing the needle and securely hold your needle hub in place. Continue to draw back on your syringe and draw blood to ensure placement. Once confirmed, drop the ultrasound probe on the field and continue with placing the guidewire. Prior to dilating the vessel and placing the catheter and removing the guidewire, scan the region over the puncture site to confirm guidewire location and placement in the correct vessel. Complete the procedure.

Subclavian

There are several factors that guide the practitioner in their selection and desired location of CVC placement, and while ultrasound-guided internal jugular CVC placement has become the current standard, there are several advantages to subclavian vein CVC placement. Subclavian CVCs have been associated with reduced infection rates when compared to IJ and femoral CVC placement, increased patient comfort, and increased ease of placement in the setting of trauma involving the neck and cervical spine or other atypical neck anatomy [8–10]. In this section, we will review the technical approach to ultrasound-guided subclavian CVC placement.

The subclavian vein originates at the lateral border of the first rib, as a continuation of the axillary vein. It runs laterally to medially passing over the first rib anterior to the subclavian artery, joining the internal jugular vein at the medial end of the clavicle. It is covered anteriorly by the clavicle and sits directly on top of the pleura [11]. Traditionally, subclavian central venous line placement has been performed via landmark identification. However, an ultrasound-guided approach to CVC placement in the subclavian is possible and has been associated with fewer complications including pneumothorax and arterial puncture [12].

The subclavian vein can be visualized from both infraclavicular and supraclavicular placement of the ultrasound probe; both techniques will be discussed below. To begin, the patient should be placed in the supine position with the arms down by the patient's side. A high frequency linear array probe should be selected. Usual sterile technique should be observed including sterile ultrasound gel and probe cover. Similar to the IJ and femoral approaches, the ultrasound probe should be manipulated with the operator's non-dominant hand and with the needle and syringe in the dominant hand.

From the infraclavicular approach, the infraclavicular fossa (triangular area of depression below the clavicle between the deltoid and pectoralis major muscles) should be identified by palpation and direct visualization, usually found along the lateral third of the clavicle. The probe should be placed in the infraclavicular fossa with the indicator pointed to the patient's right side. The subclavian vein can be visualized in both the short and long access from this position.

To obtain a long access view from the infraclavicular fossa, the probe should be oriented with the long access of the probe parallel to the course of the vessel. The operator may need to rotate/fan the medial end of the probe until the subclavian vein falls into view. The vein can be differentiated from the artery due to compressibility, lack of pulsations, and respiratory variation in the diameter of the vessel. As the subclavian artery is not visualized in the same plane as the subclavian vein in this view, the operator must confirm correct identification of the vein using the features listed above prior to puncturing the vessel. From this long access view, the tip of the needle should enter the skin laterally and in-plane with the subclavian vein at approximately a 45° angle. Keeping both the needle and the vessel in view in real time, the needle should be advanced medially and inferiorly towards the vessel. The needle tip should be directly visualized as it enters the subclavian vein. Once the needle has entered the vessel and blood is easily returned into the syringe, the ultrasound probe should be dropped onto the sterile field. The guidewire should then be inserted through the needle into the vessel and advanced without resistance. Once the guidewire has been advanced and the needle removed, confirmation of the guidewire in the subclavian vein can be obtained by placing the probe back on the patient in the long access orientation. The guidewire should then be visualized within the lumen of the subclavian vein.

From the infraclavicular fossa, a short access view of the subclavian vein as well as the artery and adjacent pleura can also be obtained. With the probe in the infraclavicular fossa with the long access of the probe perpendicular to the course of the vessel and the indicator again oriented towards the patient's right side, the medial of the probe can be rotated towards the clavicle until the subclavian vein and artery are in view. In the short access, the subclavian artery should be more inferior and lateral than the vein. As the subclavian vein is deeper and the needle tip is not visualized entirely prior to entry into the subclavian vein, there is an increased risk of complication including arterial puncture and pneumothorax from this approach [8].

From the supraclavicular approach, the probe is placed in the supraclavicular fossa with the long access of the probe parallel to the clavicle, probe indicator oriented to the patients' right.

Alternatively, the operator may start by placing the probe in a more superior position to first identify the internal jugular vein and then trace it distally to identify where it joins the subclavian vein. Once the subclavian vein has been identified, the operator should attempt to obtain a view with the subclavian vein directly in the middle of the screen. Once this view is obtained, the needle should enter the skin in the middle of the ultrasound probe (often indicated by a marking on the probe itself). The needle should be advanced until the needle tip is visualized puncturing the vein and blood is returned easily into the syringe. The guidewire can then be advanced into the vessel (Video 46.5). Once the guidewire has been advanced, its placement can be confirmed by visualizing the wire in the lumen of the vessel from the same short access view (Video 46.6).

The posterior location of the subclavian artery can lead to unrecognized arterial puncture, which can be difficult to control as it is a noncompressible site. Additionally, as the pleura is directly adjacent to the subclavian vein, there is an increased risk of pneumothorax when compared to IJ CVC placement. If the needle tip is not appropriately visualized upon entering the vessel, the pleura can easily be punctured, leading to pneumothorax [13]. While the risk of these complications is still present with an ultrasound-guided approach, they may be minimized. In their 2015 meta-analysis, Lalu et al. found that the overall complication rates were reduced when an ultrasound-guided approach to Subclavian CVC placement was performed in comparison to landmark-guided placement [13].

Radial Artery Cannulation

The radial artery is a small vessel commonly cannulated for placement of an arterial blood pressure monitor. Here the technical approach and additional considerations for ultrasound-guided cannulation of the radial artery are reviewed.

The radial artery is a bifurcation of the brachial artery, supplying blood to the anterior compartment of the forearm. The axillary artery bifurcates into the radial and ulnar arteries in the cubital fossa, from there the radial artery runs laterally along the forearm. Its course is superficial, and pulsation of the vessel is easily palpated just proximal to the wrist [14]. When cannulating the radial artery, usual sterile precautions should be observed.

A high frequency linear probe should first be selected by the operator. Prior to setting up the sterile field, the operator should use the ultrasound to identify and confirm an adequate target for cannulation. Additionally, prior to cannulation of the radial artery, the operator should ensure adequate collateral circulation to the hand via the ulnar artery, as placement of a catheter into this small vessel can compromise distal arterial flow. This can be done at the bedside using the Allen test.

Once the above has been completed, attention should be directed to appropriate positioning of the patient and setup for the procedure. The patient's arm should be supinated and secured, often a table or mayo stand can be used to stabilize the patient's arm. Using tape or adherent wrap to help secure the thumb is often helpful in maintaining a truly supinated forearm. After adequate positioning, usual sterile setup with adequate skin preparation and draping of the arm should be performed and a sterile cover should be placed over the ultrasound probe.

Using the nondominant hand, the high frequency linear array probe should be placed along the lateral and distal forearm with the probe indicator directed towards the patient's right side. From here, a short access view of the artery should be obtained. Once the artery is identified as a small, noncompressible, and pulsatile structure, the vessel should be traced both superiorly and inferiorly. Of note, the vessel is often identified quite superficially. Once identified, the practitioner should aim to maintain the radial artery image directly in the center of the screen. From here, the needle tip should enter the skin the middle of the probe and should enter the skin at approximately a 45° angle. Given the very superficial nature of the radial artery, once through the skin the angle at which the needle is advanced may need to be decreased.

The needle tip should be directly visualized as it punctures the artery. Bright red blood should be returned through the needle and should be pulsatile. Next, the guidewire should be advanced through the needle into the vessel. Correct placement of the wire within the artery can be confirmed with ultrasound. The radial artery catheter is then advanced over the wire and the wire is removed. Dilation of the radial is not generally needed.

Summary Points

Pro-Tips (Call-Out)

- A linear array transducer (frequency 7.5–10 MHz) should be used with a sterile cover and sterile gel.
- Position the machine in front and to the right of the operator where the ultrasound screen is within direct visibility.
- Predetermine the best choice for vascular access by pre scanning all options bilaterally.
- Ultrasound-guided vascular access should be performed using dynamic real-time approach (not using a static approach—where you only use ultrasound to localize the vein, then perform the procedure "blind").
- Once completed, check for any associated complications such as pneumothorax, hematoma, arterial puncture, or catheter malposition.

Pro Tips

- Scanning for appropriate targets on bilateral sides of the IJ, femoral, or subclavian vein to help map out anatomy and identify the best target prior to setting up the sterile field helps ensure best first attempt success.
- When using an ultrasound-guided approach to subclavian vein cannulation, the vein should be approached with a steeper angle than a blind/landmark-guided approach in which the subclavian vein is accessed more medially, as compared to this more lateral ultrasound-guided approach [15].
- During cardiopulmonary arrest, or even with low blood pressure and hypoxia, arterial blood may be dark and not pulsatile and may be mistaken for venous blood.
- If the carotid or femoral artery is errantly cannulated by either the tissue dilator or the CVC, leave the dilator or catheter in place and obtain vascular consultation for possible surgical removal.
- Insertion of local anesthetic, especially around small superficial vessels such as the radial artery, can obscure anatomy and is best done under ultrasound guidance to identify proximity to desired target vessel.

Evolving Evidence Call-Out

- A 2015 meta-analysis found that the overall complication rates were reduced when an ultrasound-guided approach to Subclavian CVC placement was performed in comparison to the landmark-guided placement.

Question

When placing an ultrasound-guided subclavian central venous catheter, the pleura is best visualized in which of the following views?

A. Supraclavicular short access
B. Supraclavicular long access
C. Infraclavicular short access
D. **Infraclavicular long access**

Answer: D. In the infraclavicular long access approach, the ultrasound probe is placed parallel to the clavicle in the infraclavicular region. This allows the operator to visualize the needle as it advances toward the vein in real time, and it provides a better view of deeper structures, including the pleura and lung apex. Visualizing the pleura is critical for avoiding pneumothorax, a key complication of subclavian line placement.

References

1. Troianos CA, Hartman GS, Glas KE, et al. Special articles: guidelines for performing ultrasound guided vascular cannulation: recommendations of the American Society of Echocardiography and the Society of Cardiovascular Anesthesiologists. Anesth Analg. 2012;114:46.
2. Lamperti M, Bodenham AR, Pittiruti M, et al. International evidence-based recommendations on ultrasound-guided vascular access. Intensive Care Med. 2012;38:1105.

3. Bouaziz H, Zetlaoui PJ, Pierre S, et al. Guidelines on the use of ultrasound guidance for vascular access. Anaesth Crit Care Pain Med. 2015;34:65.
4. Saul T, Doctor M, Kaban NL, et al. The ultrasound-only central venous catheter placement and confirmation procedure. J Ultrasound Med. 2015;34:1301.
5. Stone MB, Nagdev A, Murphy MC, Sisson CA. Ultrasound detection of guidewire position during central venous catheterization. Am J Emerg Med. 2010;28(1):82–4. https://doi.org/10.1016/j.ajem.2008.09.019.
6. Lichtenstein D, Mezière G, Biderman P, Gepner A. The comet-tail artifact: an ultrasound sign ruling out pneumothorax. Intensive Care Med. 1999;25:383.
7. Alten JA, Borasino S, Gurley WQ, et al. Ultrasound-guided femoral vein catheterization in neonates with cardiac disease. Pediatr Crit Care Med. 2012;13(6):654–9. https://doi.org/10.1097/PCC.0b013e318250af0c.
8. Shah A, Smith A, Panchatsharam S. Ultrasound-guided subclavian venous catheterisation - is this the way forward? A narrative review. Int J Clin Pract. 2013;67(8):726–32.
9. Pronovost P, Needham D, Berenholtz S, et al. An intervention to decrease catheter-related bloodstream infections in the ICU. N Engl J Med. 2006;355:2725–32.
10. Ruesch S, Walder B, Tramer MR. Complications of central venous catheters: internal jugular versus subclavian access – a systematic review. Crit Care Med. 2002;30:454–60.
11. Capobianco SM, Fahmy MW, Sicari V. Anatomy, thorax, subclavian veins. In: StatPearls. StatPearls Publishing; 2021 July 26.
12. Fragou M, Gravvanis A, Dimitriou V, et al. Real-time ultrasound-guided subclavian vein cannulation versus the landmark method in critical care patients: a prospective randomized study. Crit Care Med. 2011;39(7):1607–12.
13. Lalu MM, Fayad A, Ahmed O, et al. Ultrasound-guided subclavian vein catheterization: a systematic review and meta-analysis. Crit Care Med. 2015;43(7):1498–507.
14. Marchese RM, Geiger Z. Anatomy, shoulder and upper limb, forearm radial artery. In: StatPearls. StatPearls Publishing; 2021 July 25.
15. Bodenham AR. Ultrasound-guided subclavian vein catheterization: beyond just the jugular vein. Crit Care Med. 2011;39(7):1819–20.

47 Echocardiographic Guidance of Mechanical Circulatory Support (ECMO, IABP, REBOA)

Matthew J. Griffee, Mina Khorashadi, and Linda Nguyen

Learning Objectives

1. Review key steps for echo-guided placement of veno-venous and venoarterial extracorporeal membrane oxygenation (VV and VA ECMO), intra aortic balloon pump (IABP) support, and related devices.

Supplementary Information The online version contains supplementary material available at https://doi.org/10.1007/978-3-031-80038-2_47.

M. J. Griffee (✉)
Department of Anesthesiology and Perioperative Medicine, School of Medicine, University of Utah, Salt Lake City, UT, USA
e-mail: matthew.griffee@hsc.utah.edu

M. Khorashadi
Department of Anesthesia and Perioperative Care, University of California San Francisco, San Francisco, CA, USA

L. Nguyen
PeaceHealth St. Joseph Medical Center, Bellingham, WA, USA

Bellingham Anesthesia Associates, Bellingham, WA, USA

Tips for Identifying a Cannulation Wire on Ultrasound

A fundamental skill for ultrasound (US) guidance for intravascular devices is correct identification of a guidewire within a great vessel or in the right atrium (RA). In the aorta, the identification of a wire must be distinguished from reverberation artifacts from the layers of the aortic wall or from atheromas or calcium deposits in the wall of the aorta. Aortic wall reverberation artifacts start in the near-field, at the wall, and do not extend completely across the aorta. Imaging of a mural atheroma reveals a discrete echodense structure spanning only a short segment, arising from the aortic wall itself, with little to no far-field reverberation artifacts (see Video 47.1). By contrast, US reflecting on a wire within the aorta does not emanate from an abnormality of the aortic wall—instead, the wire is free floating within the lumen, is a bright, linear echodensity, with a prominent reverberation artifact ringing down nearly the entire vessel width (see Video 47.2). Ideally, identification of the J-point at the tip of a wire, with dynamic motion of the tip when the wire is manipulated, will confirm that a wire is present. Biplane of a guidewire within a target vessel will reveal that the structure is linear and is not restricted to atheromas/calcifications of the vessel wall.

M. J. Lanspa, A. T. Levinson (eds.), *Echocardiography and Ultrasonography in the ICU*, Respiratory Medicine, https://doi.org/10.1007/978-3-031-80038-2_47

Call-Out Pro-Tip

- Beware of interpreting calcified atheromas as wires; use biplane to identify the linear nature of a suspected wire running within a vessel; strive to identify a J-tip whenever possible, and note that the reverberation artifact should start at the depth of the wire, not the near-field vessel wall. Be sure to do a baseline exam to identify catheters or pacing wires already present prior to guidewire insertion.

Echo Guidance for VV ECMO Cannulation

Echocardiography is essential for guidance and troubleshooting of venovenous extracorporeal membrane oxygenation cannulation (VV ECMO) [1–4]. While there are multiple cannulation configurations possible for VV ECMO, this chapter focuses on echo for guidance of the dual-lumen, bicaval cannula via the right internal jugular vein. This cannula is designed to have the tip draining the inferior vena cava (IVC), beyond the hepatic vein, with return flow directed from the upper RA, across the tricuspid valve (Fig. 47.1, center). The position of the distal drainage orifices, and the position and direction of return flow, is essential to prevent recirculation.

The steps involved to guide cannulation are summarized in Table 47.1, and cannula position examples are illustrated in Fig. 47.1. Whether using TTE, TEE, or a combination, a focused baseline exam is important to identify the optimal windows [4]. The superior vena cava (SVC) to RA junction and posterior interatrial septum are best visualized by TEE. The junction of the hepatic vein, IVC, and inferior right atrium in some cases is well demonstrated in a transgastric TEE window, but some patients have a suitable subcostal window of this anatomy. The baseline exam should include evaluation of biventricular function. In cases of left ventricular failure, a multidisciplinary discussion should be held to decide whether to continue with VV ECMO or to change the strategy to VA ECMO [6]. Additional goals of the baseline exam are to evaluate any pericardial fluid, to interrogate the interatrial septum for an atrial septal defect or large patent foramen ovale, and to determine the baseline tricuspid regurgitation (TR). Evaluation of flow across the septum and TR may be difficult after cannulation and initiation of ECMO flow. Signs that cannulation may be difficult include a prominent Eustachian valve or Chiari network (which may block wire and cannula passage out of the RA), a prominent angle between the RA and IVC, bulging of the interatrial septum from left to right, and hyperdynamic cardiac function [7, 8]. Conversely, a straight and unobstructed path between the inferior RA and IVC is favorable anatomy for successful cannulation.

The next steps for echo guidance are confirmation of J-tipped guidewire passage from the SVC, across the RA, and into the IVC (see Video 47.3). When the J-tip is deflected from the IVC by a Eustachian valve, maneuvers to consider include increasing or decreasing airway pressure, rotation of the wire, using an angled wire, directional catheter, or coronary catheter, and using a stiff wire [9, 10]. Communication between the echocardiographer and surgeon is essential, because correct wire position leads to proper cannula position, and incorrect wire position can lead to injury of the heart or great vessels, with a risk of RV perforation and tamponade [11]. The tip of the wire should be several centimeters beyond the IVC-hepatic vein confluence, but the very long guidewire should not be advanced liberally because this leads to looping in the right atrium and in the right ventricle.

Call-Out Pro-Tip

- Even if the guidewire tip is within the IVC, a loop within the RA or RV will lead the cannula into the right heart, with a risk of perforation.

Signs of looping include resistance to wire advancement, PVCs, and the appearance of multiple reverberation artifacts in the RA, RV, or both. A crucial safety step, before proceeding with serial dilation and cannula placement, is to rule out loops.

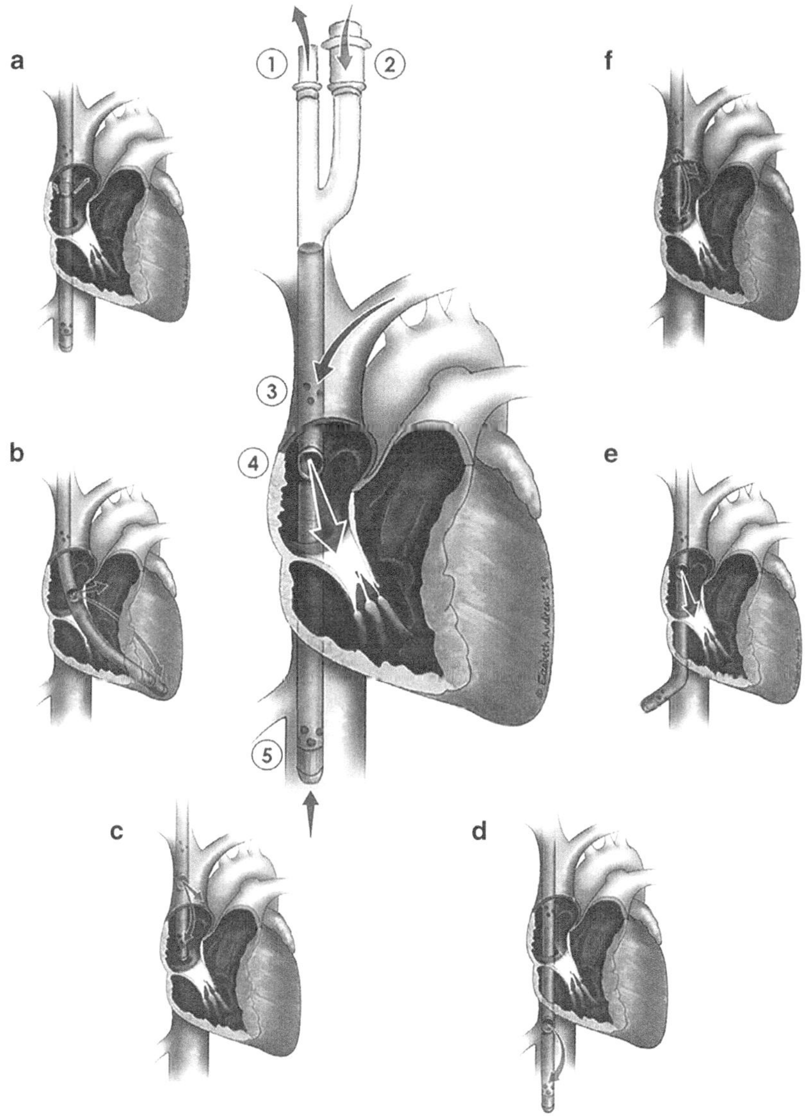

Fig. 47.1 Dual lumen venovenous cannula position examples. Central Figure, Correct cannula position. (1) drainage returning from IVC and SVC drain orifices, flow is going to ECMO; (2) return of oxygenated blood from ECMO; (3) SVC drainage orifices; (4) Return flow of oxygenated blood, originating from upper RA at level of upper fossa ovalis, towards tricuspid valve (anterior and leftward jet); (5) Distal tip with multiple orifices and distal drainage opening for drainage from IVC, distal tip beyond hepatic vein. Malposition Illustrations: (**a**) Return flow directed towards interatrial septum, leading to recirculation; (**b**) Cannula in RV, resulting in recirculation, arrhythmias, and risk of RV perforation; (**c**) Shallow cannula, outflow in SVC, resulting in recirculation, outflow difficult to image; (**d**) Deep cannula, outflow within IVC, leading to recirculation; (**e**) Tip of cannula in hepatic vein, resulting in collapse of vein around distal cannula, line chatter, and limited flow; (**f**) Cannula shallow, in this case, outflow at level of SVC/RA junction, visible on TEE. Source: MG hired Elizabeth Andreas to make this figure for our article cited in Griffee et al. [5]

Table 47.1 Steps and checklist items for echo-guided VV ECMO cannulation

Steps of US guidance	Checklist
1. Pre-cannulation evaluation	RIJ patent (vascular probe) Window evaluation – Midesophageal bicaval – Midesophageal modified bicaval (tricuspid) – Transgastric 2 chamber (RA, TV, RV) – Transgastric IVC long-axis, identify HV – 4 Chamber Baseline cardiac structure and function – RV function, LV function – Location and grading of TR – Presence of PFO, size and direction of shunt – Rule-out ASD – Size and hemodynamic consequences of pericardial effusion – Wires or lines in great vessels prior to cannulation Difficulty of cannulation – Hyperdynamic RV function – Large Eustachian valve or Chiari network – Angle between RA and IVC
2. Guidewire placement	Confirm passage of J tip of guidewire SVC->RA->IVC Rule out looping in RA or RV Confirm location of distal guidewire in IVC Rule out tip in hepatic vein Time out: Recheck RA and RV for loops Signs of looping: – PVCs – Multiple linear echodensities in RA or RV – Resistance to wire advancement Options for difficult passage from RA to IVC – Stiffer guidewire – Angled guidewire – Rotation of guidewire – Placement of long dilator/introducer to prevent looping in RA – Changing airway pressure
3. Serial dilation	Verify tip of wire remains in IVC beyond hepatic vein Verify no loops in RA or RV Rule out pericardial effusion
4. Cannula advancement	Follow cannula from SVC to RA to IVC – No looping, bending, or kinking – Tip in IVC beyond hepatic vein – Check for pericardial effusion
5. Cannula position with ECMO flows started; verify position stable after suturing of cannula.	Tip in IVC, 2–5 cm beyond HV Return flow originates from upper RA (upper fossa ovalis) Flow directed anteriorly, away from IAS Flow across/towards TV Evaluate biventricular function Rule out new pericardial effusion Rule out malposition

Table 47.2 Examples of malposition type and correction needed

Figure 47.1 example	Problem	Correction
A	Return flow posterior or lateral	Rotate cannula until return flow is directed towards tricuspid valve
B	Tip of cannula in RV	Pull back cannula, advance into IVC, may require starting over or placing guidewire from femoral vein [12]
C	Tip of cannula in RA (shallow)—no return flow visible	Advance until tip in IVC and flow across TV
D	Deep cannula, outflow in IVC	Pull back until return flow across TV
E	Tip of cannula in hepatic vein	Pull back and then advance tip into IVC; ignore if flows are adequate and ECMO working well (when hepatic vein drainage is an incidental finding, avoiding cannula adjustment may be safest option)
F	Tip of cannula in RA (shallow)—return flow visible, but high in RA	Advance until tip in IVC and flow across TV

Call-Out Pro-Tip

- After confirming distal wire location in IVC, recheck the RA and RV to rule out any loops. DO NOT PROCEED if there is any doubt about loops of wire. Watch for PVCs as a sign of wire loops entering RV. Do not count on the heavy, stiff cannula to "straighten out" loops and find its way into the IVC.

Any loops should be removed by pulling back the wire until it follows a single, straight course across the back of the right atrium, terminating in the IVC. Even if the J-tip is definitely within the IVC, an extra safety check should be carried out, involving looking at the right atrium in multiple planes and multiple views to rule out looping and confirm any loops have been corrected.

The final step is echo verification that the cannula follows the intended path (SVC to RA to IVC), again without looping or angling anteriorly (see Video 47.4). The tip of the cannula must be confirmed to be in the IVC, and not in a hepatic vein, or the RA or RV, prior to wire removal (see Videos 47.5 and 47.6). Wire removal prior to confirmation of cannula depth and course leads to time-consuming and dangerous repositioning efforts, if the cannula is misplaced [12]. After commencement of ECMO flow, the return jet (of oxygenated blood) should be evaluated. The outflow should originate from the upper RA, at the level of the upper fossa ovalis, and should be directed anteriorly, towards the TV (see Video 47.7). The jet is a high velocity pyramid which has a narrow origin and spreads slightly as it moves inferiorly to cross into the RV. Malposition examples and the maneuvers needed to correct the cannula position are illustrated in Fig. 47.1 and described in Table 47.2 [5]. A final exam of cannula tip, return flow jet, pericardial effusion, and biventricular function should be done after the cannula is sutured in place.

Echo Guidance for VA ECMO Cannulation

In patients with cardiogenic shock and in patients with concomitant respiratory failure and heart failure, V-A ECMO can be used when medical therapy fails [13–16]. Echocardiography plays a key role for V-A ECMO: to determine the appropriateness of therapy, to guide the cannulation process, and for cardiac evaluation during the ECMO run as well as during turndown assessments.

Cannulation

The common femoral artery or the axillary artery can be accessed either with an open surgical approach or with a percutaneous approach using the Seldinger technique [13–23]. Doppler ultrasound should be used before vascular access is established to assess the vessels for patency and significant atheroma in the artery [18, 24]. The venous cannula may be placed via the femoral or the internal jugular veins. Ultrasound should be used to avoid local complications. Once the vessel has been accessed, a guidewire is placed in the vein. The echocardiographer must confirm the presence of the wire in the RA and exclude its presence in the left atrium when an interatrial septal defect such as ASD or PFO is present. Visualization of the end of the guidewire (the J-tip) is particularly important in patients who possess right-sided intracardiac devices such as a pacemaker or defibrillator as these devices may easily be confused with the guidewire.

Call-Out Pro-Tip

- Strive to find the J-tip of a guide wire during US guidance of cannulation in the context of catheters or pacing wires already present in the right atrium; identify lines and pacing wires present prior to the guidewire and cannula advancement.

In the case of cannulation via the femoral vein, the guidewire often may be visualized in the IVC and entering the RA by TTE using a subcostal window. If TTE windows are inadequate, TEE should be considered. The mid-esophageal bicaval view typically provides excellent visualization of the guidewire in the RA (see Video 47.8). Following the placement of the guidewire, the proceduralist uses serial dilators to expand the vessel prior to placement of the cannula. It is possible for the guidewire to kink, move out of the RA, or traverse the tricuspid valve during this process. Therefore, the guidewire position should be reconfirmed just prior to placement of the venous cannula. The tip of the venous cannula should be placed just distal to the superior cavo-atrial junction without abutting the walls of the atrium, the interatrial septum, or the tricuspid valve to ensure optimal drainage [22–25] (see Video 47.9). The aortic cannula is placed via the femoral artery and the tip is located in the abdominal aorta [26]. After femoral arterial puncture, a guidewire is placed in the aorta. The guidewire can be visualized in the abdominal aorta using TTE and in the descending thoracic aorta when using TEE (see Video 47.2). The location of the wire should be confirmed after vessel dilation and just prior to cannula placement. The tip of the cannula is typically placed in the abdominal aorta or the distal descending thoracic aorta and is not always visualizable by echocardiography [26, 27]. Thus, confirming the presence of the guidewire just prior to cannulation is crucial.

Monitoring

Once V-A ECMO flow has been established, echocardiography should be used whenever a clinical need arises to monitor cardiac function, detect complications, and to assess myocardial recovery [24]. In the case of peripheral V-A ECMO, the high pressure return flow jet in the aorta may increase LV afterload, with increasing flow increasing the afterload proportionately [14, 15].

Call-Out Pro-Tip

- Higher ECMO flow results in higher LV afterload and can compromise both hemodynamics and cardiac recovery if the LV is dilated and under pressure in the context of myocardial injury. In particular, when there is little native LV contractility, the return flow can prevent aortic valve opening which can lead to LV distention and increase the risk of thrombus formation and significant cardiogenic pulmonary edema.

Blood stasis, which presents itself as spontaneous echo contrast in cardiac chambers, indicates a very high risk of thrombus formation. When signs of LV distention and thrombus formation become apparent on echo, measures such as increasing inotropic support or placement of mechanical devices such as a transaortic LV mechanical circulatory assist device or intra-aortic balloon pump should be considered to help unload the LV [25, 28]. When a patient becomes hemodynamically unstable while on ECMO, a bedside exam should be performed to rapidly diagnose and treat complications such as tamponade, LV thrombus, displaced venous cannula, shunting across the interatrial septum, or inadequate preload. Finally, early detection of myocardial recovery by echocardiography is crucial in order to minimize the time on ECMO. An area for future research is to determine whether outcomes are better with a daily (or otherwise regularly scheduled) surveillance echo, versus with echo evaluation performed only on as-needed basis.

Weaning

Some echocardiographic parameters have been shown to be useful in identifying patients who are likely to be successfully weaned from ECMO support [29], including LV ejection fraction (LVEF), LV outflow tract velocity time integral (LVOT VTI), and lateral mitral annular peak systolic velocity [16, 17]. Interestingly, Doppler measures of LV filling pressures have *not* been shown to predict weaning outcomes [17]. In terms of RV function, RV ejection fraction (RVEF), RV fractional area change (RV FAC), and an increase in magnitude of RV longitudinal strain correlate with successful weaning [23, 30]. Tricuspid annular plane systolic excursion (TAPSE) and the degree of tricuspid regurgitation are not as useful in predicting weaning outcomes [23, 30].

Weaning trials are essential to evaluate cardiac function before separation from ECMO. During a weaning trial, ECMO flows are reduced in a stepwise fashion and LV and RV function and volumes are assessed under the varying loading conditions [31, 32]. The weaning trial should be terminated if there is LV or RV dilation or sudden reduction in systolic function. Once it is established that the patient can maintain normal hemodynamic parameters without chamber dilation and on minimal flows (no more than 0.5 L/min), with inotropic requirements in a low range, it is reasonable to consider decannulation [19].

Echo Guidance for IABP and REBOA Placement

Echocardiography is a valuable tool for guidance of intra-aortic balloon pump (IABP) placement in the intraoperative and critical care setting. Aside from the advantages of the avoidance of radiation and portability of this imaging modality, the identification of contraindications during the preplacement exam, real-time visualization of the thoracic aorta and the ability to assess left ventricular systolic function after intervention is especially vital [33].

General considerations of the indications for IABP and risks are reviewed elsewhere [34]. The pre-procedure exam includes assessment of LV systolic function, ruling out moderate or severe aortic insufficiency (AI) and identifying severe aortic pathologies such as mobile atheromas or aortic dissection [35] We present a proposed TEE exam sequence for evaluating the aortic valve and aorta prior to wire and balloon placement in Fig. 47.2. Whether using TTE or TEE, emphasis

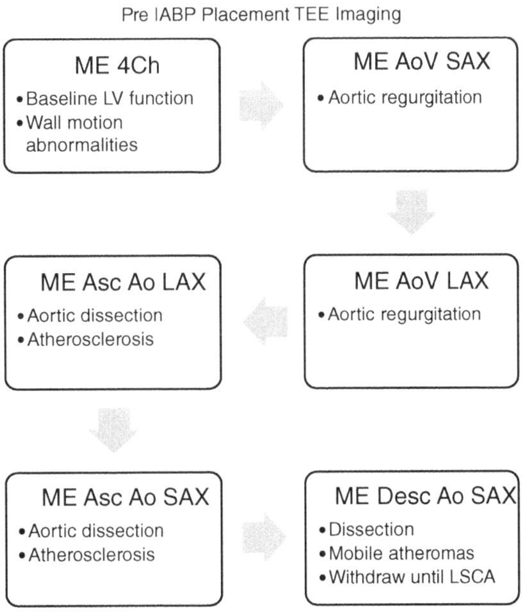

Fig. 47.2 Proposed imaging strategy starting from a mid-esophageal 4-chamber view to evaluate baseline LV systolic function. The following images are to assess presence of more than mild AI and mobile atheromas. Abbreviations: *4Ch* four-chamber, *AoV* aortic valve, *SAX* short axis, *LAX* long axis, *Ao* aorta, *LSCA* left subclavian artery. Source: Original work of Linda Nguyen

should be placed on ensuring that the balloon tip is 1–2 cm distal to the origin of the left subclavian artery (LSCA) to avoid critical limb or brain ischemia. TTE of the aorta (from suprasternal and subxiphoid windows) may be of limited value due to body habitus, supine positioning, and limited views of the descending aorta.

Femoral IABP Placement Guidance

Steps for placement are summarized in Table 47.3. For a TEE-guided femoral approach, obtain the descending aorta short axis (SAX) view to first identify the IABP pumping within the aorta (see Video 47.10). Then, change to a long axis view and slowly withdraw until the LSCA at the level of the aortic arch is seen (see Videos 47.11 and 47.12). Verify that the area of the transition from the transverse to the descending arch does not have the dynamic balloon within it [35] (see Video 47.13 (Note: this is a supplementary TTE view, showing the anatomy of the transverse to descending aorta and a balloon just past the transition)). Acoustic shadowing and reverberation artifacts will be seen as the balloon inflates during diastole and collapses during systole; the balloon cycling disappears as the probe is pulled up from the descending aorta to the transverse aorta (see Video 47.14).

An exam after IABP placement should ensure that there is effective LV counterpulsation by assessing LV systolic function and potential changes to wall motion. Examine the aorta to assess for dissection or hematoma. Exclude new aortic regurgitation. A physical exam should be performed to ensure that there is no upper extremity ischemia, mental status changes, excessive bleeding, arrhythmias, or hypotension.

In one CT case series, the distal IABP compromised at least one abdominal visceral branch of the aorta in 97% of patients, despite nearly all of the CXRs showing an appropriate proximal position [36]. In another series, abnormal renal artery doppler ultrasound was observed in 6 of 12 patients with IABP, with normalization of flow after balloon removal [37].

Axillary IABP Placement Guidance

In one retrospective case review, the most common minor adverse event in patients with percutaneous axillary IABP was device malposition,

Table 47.3 IABP placement checklist

Steps of US guidance	Checklist
1. Prior to IABP placement	Evaluate aorta for dissection or mobile atheroma – Midesophageal long axis view – Descending Aorta short axis – Descending Aorta long axis Evaluate for evidence of more than mild AI – Midesophageal long axis view – Aortic valve short axis view – Deep transgastric 5 chamber – Transgastric long axis view Evaluate baseline LV systolic function – Midesophageal 4 Ch, 2 Ch, LAX views – Transgastric LV short axis view
2. IABP placement	Balloon tip identified in descending aorta SAX Change to aorta SAX view or use Bi-plane Withdraw probe slowly until LSCA observed at level of aortic arch, note depth difference. Balloon tip should be 1–2 cm distal to origin of LSCA
3. Inflation of balloon	Observe for reverberation and acoustic shadowing artifacts due to balloon inflation
4. Evaluate for complications	Evaluate LV systolic function and wall motion Examine aorta for dissection or hematoma Examine for left arm, brain, renal, and mesenteric ischemia Ensure adequate diastolic augmentation

occurring in 22 of 50 patients [38]. Migration of the device can occur distally into the descending aorta or proximally to the level of arch vessels. Case reports of subclavian IABP malposition include one case with ultrasound identification of the balloon entering and obstructing the superior mesenteric artery [39]. Patients with IABP and concomitant VA-ECMO can propel the IABP catheter across the aortic arch and potentially into the LV cavity, due to retrograde aortic blood flow from the aortic ECMO cannula [38].

The distal balloon should terminate above the mesenteric and renal arteries. If the balloon covers the origin of aortic branches below the diaphragm, there should be consideration for removing helium, using a smaller balloon, and the position should be double checked, to ensure the tip is close to the left subclavian artery. Further research is needed to determine whether point-of-care abdominal ultrasound can be used to reliably evaluate the abdominal aorta branch patency in patients supported with IABPs. There is a definite need for such research, given the data suggesting that mesenteric ischemia may be common, and that the predicted distance from the subclavian artery to the mesenteric and renal arteries (based on patient height) does not correlate well with clinical observations [36, 37]. Key elements of the pre- and post-balloon placement exams are summarized in Fig. 47.3.

Ultrasound for REBOA

Resuscitative endovascular balloon occlusion of the aorta (REBOA) has typically been placed by fluoroscopy guidance for control of massive subdiaphragmatic hemorrhage [40]. One article described the use of abdominal sonography to verify the presence of the guidewire in the abdominal aorta and subsequently, the placement of the catheter tip above the diaphragm with target position of the balloon between the LSCA and the celiac trunk [40, 41]. Limitations to adequate imaging may include body habitus, transverse colon shadowing the window, and the presence of gas in the stomach. At this time, there is little literature on ultrasound guidance of the REBOA procedure and this is an area for further study.

Summary Points

- Beware of interpreting calcified atheromas as wires; use biplane to identify the linear nature of a suspected wire running within a vessel; strive to identify a J-tip whenever possible, and note that the reverberation artifact should start at the depth of the wire, not the near-field vessel wall. Be sure to do a baseline exam to identify catheters or pacing wires already present prior to guidewire insertion.
- During VV ECMO guidance, even if the guidewire tip is within the IVC, a loop within the RA or RV may lead the cannula into the right heart, with a risk of perforation. After confirming distal wire location in IVC, recheck the RA and RV to rule out any loops. Stop if there is any doubt about loops of wire. Watch for PVCs as a sign of wire loops entering the RV.

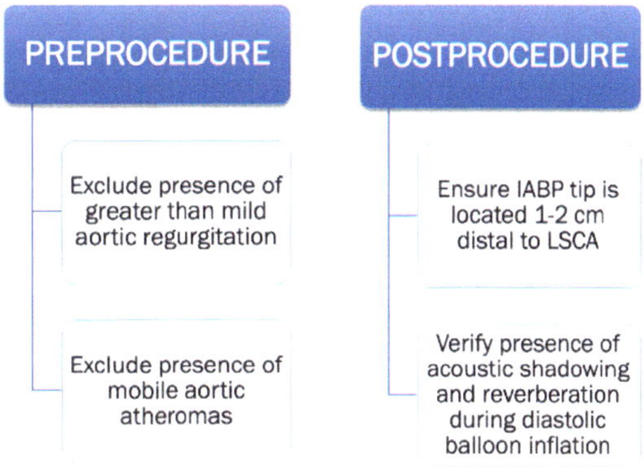

Fig. 47.3 Key points for IABP placement. Source: Original work of Linda Nguyen

- Higher VA ECMO flow results in higher LV afterload and can compromise both hemodynamics and cardiac recovery if the LV is dilated and under pressure in the context of myocardial injury. In particular, when there is little native LV contractility, the return ECMO flow can prevent aortic valve opening which can lead to LV distention and increase the risk of thrombus formation and cardiogenic pulmonary edema.
- During turndown trials of VA ECMO, robust LVEF, RVEF, and LVOT VTI correlate with good chances of successful weaning. Dilation of the ventricles and sustained hypotension during weaning should result in termination of the turndown trial.
- Intra-aortic balloon placement involves the risks of atheroma embolization and occlusion of branches of the aorta. The balloon should be just distal to the left subclavian artery.
- Clinical research is needed to define the role of echocardiography for management of patients supported with mechanical circulatory support. Key questions are about protocols for early identification of complications during ECMO, ultrasound-based diagnosis of ischemia in aortic branches during IABP support, and the role of echo in REBOA.

Questions

1. A 43-year-old woman with no significant past medical history presents with 2 months of increasing fatigue, shortness of breath, and orthopnea. She reports having a mild respiratory illness just prior to the onset of these symptoms. On exam, she is found to have heart rate 126, blood pressure 78/46, and oxygen saturation 83% on room air. An urgent echocardiogram shows LV ejection fraction <20% and a dilated RV with severely reduced systolic function. She is started on milrinone and vasopressin and given IV furosemide. Despite increasing doses of pressors and inotropes, she continues to be hypotensive and has increasing O2 requirement and reduced urine output. Which of the following is the best next step in therapy?
   A. Impella
   B. Durable surgically implanted LVAD
   C. V-A ECMO
   D. IABP
   E. V-V ECMO

   Suggested answer: C. This patient has concurrent hypoxic respiratory failure and severe cardiogenic shock and is failing medical therapy (diuresis and inotropic support). Key concept: V-A ECMO provides both circulatory support and oxygenation.

   Answer A is less favorable support because while an Impella will provide circulatory support for the LV, it does not support the RV or augment oxygenation. Answer B (Durable LVAD) is not indicated because this patient is in acute heart failure that may be reversible. An IABP will offload the LV but will not support the RV or help with oxygenation. While V-V is an appropriate treatment for this patient's respiratory failure, it is not sufficient in this case due to concurrent acute cardiogenic shock (with significant LV dysfunction).
2. A 58-year-old woman is placed on V-A ECMO in the setting of stress cardiomyopathy. Her hemodynamic parameters and cardiac function as assessed on serial echo exams have been improving over the last 5 days with decreasing pressor and inotrope requirements. Which of the following parameters is the best predictor of successful weaning from V-A ECMO?
   A. Minimal tricuspid regurgitation
   B. LVOT VTI > 20 cm
   C. Normal mitral inflow velocities
   D. TAPSE >18 mm
   E. Lateral mitral annulus peak velocity < 5 cm/s

   Correct answer: B. The degree of tricuspid regurgitation, TAPSE, and LV filling pressures (assessed by mitral inflow velocities and mitral annular tissue Doppler) have not been shown to correlate well with successful weaning from V-A ECMO. Lateral mitral annulus peak systolic velocity ≥6 cm/s is a predictor of successful weaning.

3. What is considered a contraindication for placing an intra-aortic balloon pump?
   A. Grade V aortic atheroma.
   B. Aortic regurgitation Doppler pressure half time 300 ms.
   C. Uncontrolled sepsis.
   D. Severe peripheral arterial disease.
   E. All of the above.

   Answer: E (all of the above). Contraindications for IABP placement include mobile atheromas (Grade V), more than mild AI (pressure half time of 300 ms suggests moderate AI), uncontrolled sepsis (the introduction of an intravascular device in a patient with potential bacteremia is contraindicated), and severe peripheral arterial disease.

References

1. Griffee MJ, Tonna JE, McKellar SH, Zimmerman JM. Echocardiographic guidance and troubleshooting for venovenous extracorporeal membrane oxygenation using the dual-lumen bicaval cannula. J Cardiothorac Vasc Anesth. 2018;32(1):370–8.
2. Dolch ME, Frey L, Buerkle MA, Weig T, Wassilowsky D, Irlbeck M. Transesophageal echocardiography-guided technique for extracorporeal membrane oxygenation dual-lumen catheter placement. ASAIO J. 2011;57(4):341–3.
3. Hemamalini P, Dutta P, Attawar S. Transesophageal echocardiography compared to fluoroscopy for Avalon bicaval dual-lumen cannula positioning for venovenous ECMO. Ann Card Anaesth. 2020;23(3):283–7.
4. Yastrebov K, Manganas C, Kapalli T, Peeceeyen S. Right ventricular loop indicating malposition of J-wire introducer for double lumen bicaval venovenous extracorporeal membrane oxygenation (VV ECMO) cannula. Heart Lung Circ. 2014;23(1):e4–7.
5. Griffee MJ, Zimmerman JM, McKellar SH, Tonna JE. Echocardiography-guided dual-lumen venovenous extracorporeal membrane oxygenation cannula placement in the ICU-A retrospective review. J Cardiothorac Vasc Anesth. 2020;34(3):698–705.
6. Kon ZN, Bittle GJ, Pasrija C, Pham SM, Mazzeffi MA, Herr DL, et al. Venovenous versus venoarterial extracorporeal membrane oxygenation for adult patients with acute respiratory distress syndrome requiring precannulation hemodynamic support: a review of the ELSO registry. Ann Thorac Surg. 2017;104(2):645–9.
7. Stechert MM, London MJ. Functional separation of the right atrium by an elongated eustachian valve. Anesth Analg. 2009;108(2):443–5.
8. Walpot J, Storm C, Bosmans J, Paelinck BP, Pasteuning WH, Wielenga J, et al. Right atrial inflow obstruction of the inferior vena cava due to atrial septal aneurysm and an elongated Eustachian valve. Eur J Echocardiogr. 2008;9(6):861–4.
9. Berdajs D. Bicaval dual-lumen cannula for venovenous extracorporeal membrane oxygenation: Avalon© cannula in childhood disease. Perfusion. 2015;30(3):182–6.
10. Trimlett RH, Cordingley JJ, Griffiths MJ, Price S, Hunter DN, Finney SJ. A modified technique for insertion of dual lumen bicaval cannulae for venovenous extracorporeal membrane oxygenation. Intensive Care Med. 2011;37(6):1036–7.
11. Hirose H, Yamane K, Marhefka G, Cavarocchi N. Right ventricular rupture and tamponade caused by malposition of the Avalon cannula for venovenous extracorporeal membrane oxygenation. J Cardiothorac Surg. 2012;7:36.
12. Tanaka D, Pitcher HT, Cavarocchi N, Hirose H. Migrated Avalon veno-venous extracorporeal membrane oxygenation cannula: how to adjust without interruption of flow. J Card Surg. 2015;30(11):865–8.
13. Le Gall A, Follin A, Cholley B, Mantz J, Aissaoui N, Pirracchio R. Veno-arterial-ECMO in the intensive care unit: from technical aspects to clinical practice. Anaesth Crit Care Pain Med. 2018;37(3):259–68.
14. Abrams D, Combes A, Brodie D. Extracorporeal membrane oxygenation in cardiopulmonary disease in adults. J Am Coll Cardiol. 2014;63(25):2769–78.
15. Combes A, Brodie D, Chen Y-S, Fan E, Henriques JPS, Hodgson C, et al. The ICM research agenda on extracorporeal life support. Intensive Care Med. 2017;43(9):1306–18.
16. The International ECMO Network (ECMONet) and The Extracorporeal Life Support Organization (ELSO), Abrams D, Garan AR, Abdelbary A, Bacchetta M, Bartlett RH, et al. Position paper for the organization of ECMO programs for cardiac failure in adults. Intensive Care Med. 2018;44(6):717–29.
17. Aissaoui N, Luyt C-E, Leprince P, Trouillet J-L, Léger P, Pavie A, et al. Predictors of successful extracorporeal membrane oxygenation (ECMO) weaning after assistance for refractory cardiogenic shock. Intensive Care Med. 2011;37(11):1738–45.
18. Danial P, Hajage D, Nguyen LS, Mastroianni C, Demondion P, Schmidt M, et al. Percutaneous versus surgical femoro-femoral veno-arterial ECMO: a propensity score matched study. Intensive Care Med. 2018;44(12):2153–61.
19. Aissaoui N, El-Banayosy A, Combes A. How to wean a patient from veno-arterial extracorporeal membrane oxygenation. Intensive Care Med. 2015;41(5):902–5.
20. Cavarocchi NC, Pitcher HT, Yang Q, Karbowski P, Miessau J, Hastings HM, et al. Weaning of extracorporeal membrane oxygenation using continuous hemodynamic transesophageal echocardiography. J Thorac Cardiovasc Surg. 2013;146(6):1474–9.
21. Pappalardo F, Pieri M, Arnaez Corada B, Ajello S, Melisurgo G, De Bonis M, et al. Timing and

strategy for weaning from venoarterial ECMO are complex issues. J Cardiothorac Vasc Anesth. 2015;29(4):906–11.
22. Platts DG, Sedgwick JF, Burstow DJ, Mullany DV, Fraser JF. The role of echocardiography in the management of patients supported by extracorporeal membrane oxygenation. J Am Soc Echocardiogr. 2012;25(2):131–41.
23. Donker DW, Meuwese CL, Braithwaite SA, Broomé M, van der Heijden JJ, Hermens JA, et al. Echocardiography in extracorporeal life support: a key player in procedural guidance, tailoring and monitoring. Perfusion. 2018;33(1_suppl):31–41.
24. Firstenberg MS, Orsinelli DA. ECMO and ECHO: the evolving role of quantitative echocardiography in the management of patients requiring extracorporeal membrane oxygenation. J Am Soc Echocardiogr. 2012;25(6):641–3.
25. Vieillard-Baron A, Millington SJ, Sanfilippo F, Chew M, Diaz-Gomez J, McLean A, et al. A decade of progress in critical care echocardiography: a narrative review. Intensive Care Med. 2019;45(6):770–88.
26. Levy B, Bastien O, Bendjelid K, Cariou A, Chouihed T, Combes A, et al. Experts' recommendations for the management of adult patients with cardiogenic shock. Ann Intensive Care. 2015;5(1):17.
27. Bonello L, Delmas C, Schurtz G, Leurent G, Bonnefoy E, Aissaoui N, et al. Mechanical circulatory support in patients with cardiogenic shock in intensive care units: a position paper of the "Unité de Soins Intensifs de Cardiologie" group of the French Society of Cardiology, endorsed by the "Groupe Athérome et Cardiologie Interventionnelle" of the French Society of Cardiology. Arch Cardiovasc Dis. 2018;111(10):601–12.
28. Levitov A, Frankel HL, Blaivas M, Kirkpatrick AW, Su E, Evans D, et al. Guidelines for the appropriate use of bedside general and cardiac ultrasonography in the evaluation of critically ill patients—part II: cardiac ultrasonography. Crit Care Med. 2016;44(6):1206–27.
29. Bailleul C, Aissaoui N. Role of echocardiography in the management of veno-arterial extra-corporeal membrane oxygenation patients. J Emerg Crit Care Med. 2019;3:25.
30. Huang K-C, Lin L-Y, Chen Y-S, Lai C-H, Hwang J-J, Lin L-C. Three-dimensional echocardiography–derived right ventricular ejection fraction correlates with success of decannulation and prognosis in patients stabilized by venoarterial extracorporeal life support. J Am Soc Echocardiogr. 2018;31(2):169–79.
31. Aissaoui N, Guerot E, Combes A, Delouche A, Chastre J, Leprince P, et al. Two-dimensional strain rate and doppler tissue myocardial velocities: analysis by echocardiography of hemodynamic and functional changes of the failed left ventricle during different degrees of extracorporeal life support. J Am Soc Echocardiogr. 2012;25(6):632–40.
32. Aissaoui N, Caudron J, Leprince P, Fagon J-Y, Lebreton G, Combes A, et al. Right–left ventricular interdependence: a promising predictor of successful extracorporeal membrane oxygenation (ECMO) weaning after assistance for refractory cardiogenic shock. Intensive Care Med. 2017;43(4):592–4.
33. Klopman MA, Chen EP, Sniecinski RM. Positioning an intraaortic balloon pump using intraoperative transesophageal echocardiogram guidance. Anesth Analg. 2011;113:40–3.
34. Parissis H, Graham V, Lampridis S, Lau M, Hooks G, Mhandu PC. IABP: history-evolution-pathophysiology-indications: what we need to know. J Cardiothorac Surg. 2016;11:122. https://doi.org/10.1186/s13019-016-0513-0.
35. Nicoara A, Skubas N, Ad N, Finley A, Hahn RT, Mahmood F, et al. Guidelines for the use of transesophageal echocardiography to assist with surgical decision-making in the operating room: a surgery-based approach. J Am Soc of Echocardiogr. 2020;33(6):692–734.
36. Rastan AJ, Tillmann E, Subramanian S, Lehmkuhl L, Funkat AK, Leontyev S, et al. Visceral arterial compromise during intra-aortic balloon counterpulsation therapy. Circulation. 2010;122(11 Suppl):S92–9.
37. Sukhodolya T, Damjanovic D, Beyersdorf F, Benk C, Heilmann C, Blanke P, et al. Standard intra-aortic counterpulsation balloon may cause temporary occlusion of mesenterial and renal arteries. ASAIO J. 2013;59(6):593–9.
38. Estep JD, Cordero-Reyes AM, Bhimaraj A, Trachtenberg B, Khalil N, Loebe M, et al. Percutaneous placement of an intra-aortic balloon pump in the left axillary/subclavian position provides safe, ambulatory long-term support as bridge to heart transplantation. JACC Heart Fail. 2013;1:382–8.
39. Tabit CE, Onsager DR, Kim GH, Jeevanandam V, Fedson SE. Positional obstruction of the superior mesenteric artery by an intra-aortic balloon pump placed through subclavian artery approach. Circ Heart Fail. 2014;7(5):864–7.
40. Ogura T, Lefor AK, Nakamura M, Fujizuka K, Shiroto K, Nakano M. Ultrasound-guided resuscitative endovascular balloon occlusion of the aorta in the resuscitation area. J Emerg Med. 2017;52(5):715–22.
41. Goldstein SA, Evangelista A, Abbara S, Arai A, Asch FM, Badano LP, et al. Multimodality imaging of diseases of the thoracic aorta in adults: from the American Society of Echocardiography and the European Association of Cardiovascular Imaging. J Am Soc Echocardiogr. 2015;28:119–82.

Deep Venous Thrombosis

48

Megan Trieu and Nida Qadir

Learning Objectives

1. Explore how the accurate and rapid identification of DVT can be accomplished at the bedside through the use of point-of-care ultrasound
2. Review the lower extremity venous anatomy, with an emphasis on the major venous branch-points which are the most common sites of thrombi
3. Understand the common causes of diagnostic error

Background

Venous thromboembolism (VTE), including pulmonary embolism (PE) and deep venous thrombosis (DVT), is a common complication of critical illness. Compared to other hospitalized patients, critically ill patients are at increased risk of DVT due to additional risk factors, including sepsis, prolonged immobilization, mechanical ventilation, vascular injury from indwelling central venous catheters, and other invasive interventions [1]. The incidence of DVT among medical-surgical intensive care unit (ICU) patients is estimated between 5% and 33%, depending on patient characteristics, use of thromboprophylaxis, and method of diagnosis [2–11]. Development of DVT has been associated with longer duration of mechanical ventilation, ICU stay, and hospital stay [12].

Although the gold standard for diagnosis of DVT is contrast venography, its invasiveness limits its utility. In practice, formal whole-leg duplex ultrasonography, which combines B-mode and doppler imaging, is the diagnostic modality of choice. However, point-of-care ultrasound (POCUS) has various notable benefits. POCUS enables physicians to make faster diagnosis and expedite treatment [13, 14]. While formal whole-leg duplex ultrasound exams are precluded by patient transport and the availability of professional ultrasonographers and radiologists to obtain and interpret the study, POCUS DVT exams can be performed readily and accurately. A meta-analysis of 16 studies demonstrated the accuracy of POCUS performed by trained non-radiologists in the diagnosis of lower extremity

Supplementary Information The online version contains supplementary material available at https://doi.org/10.1007/978-3-031-80038-2_48.

M. Trieu
Department of Medicine, Division of Pulmonary, Critical Care, and Sleep Medicine, University of California, San Diego, La Jolla, CA, USA
e-mail: metrieu@health.ucsd.edu

N. Qadir (✉)
Division of Pulmonary and Critical Care Medicine, David Geffen School of Medicine at UCLA, Los Angeles, CA, USA
e-mail: nqadir@mednet.ucla.edu

M. J. Lanspa, A. T. Levinson (eds.), *Echocardiography and Ultrasonography in the ICU*, Respiratory Medicine, https://doi.org/10.1007/978-3-031-80038-2_48

DVT with a pooled sensitivity of 96.1% and specificity of 96.8% [15].

Point-of-care compression DVT ultrasound has been validated across multiple settings, including the emergency department, inpatient wards, and critical care units [15–18], demonstrating that with dedicated training, POCUS can be adopted by clinicians from multiple specialties as an effective diagnostic tool for DVT [16–20]. In this chapter, we will first focus on the different approaches to lower extremity compression DVT ultrasound and review components of venous Doppler assessment. Finally, we will discuss the evaluation of upper extremity DVT.

Anatomy

In ultrasound evaluation of the lower extremity deep venous system, veins are assessed proximal to distal, opposite to the normal direction of venous blood flow. Therefore, it is useful to review the lower extremity vascular anatomy in this orientation. Merging of veins is thus often described as "branching" or "splitting," and the junctions, at which this occurs, are described as "branchpoints."

The lower extremity deep venous system includes the external iliac, common femoral, deep femoral, femoral, popliteal, anterior tibial, posterior tibial, and peroneal veins (Fig. 48.1). At the inguinal ligament, the external iliac vein becomes the common femoral vein. The common femoral vein runs medial to the common femoral artery, and several branchpoints follow. First, the greater saphenous vein adjoins the common femoral vein anteromedially. Just distal to this point, the adjacent common femoral artery splits into the deep and superficial femoral arteries. Next, the lateral perforator vein branches laterally and runs between the deep and superficial femoral arteries. Then, the common femoral vein splits into the deep femoral and femoral veins. The femoral vein, formerly known as the superficial femoral vein, is a deep vein that runs anteriorly in the distal thigh to the adductor canal, which it subsequently exits as the popliteal vein. The popliteal vein travels superficial to the popliteal artery in the popliteal fossa until the vein trifurcates into the anterior tibial, posterior tibial, and peroneal veins.

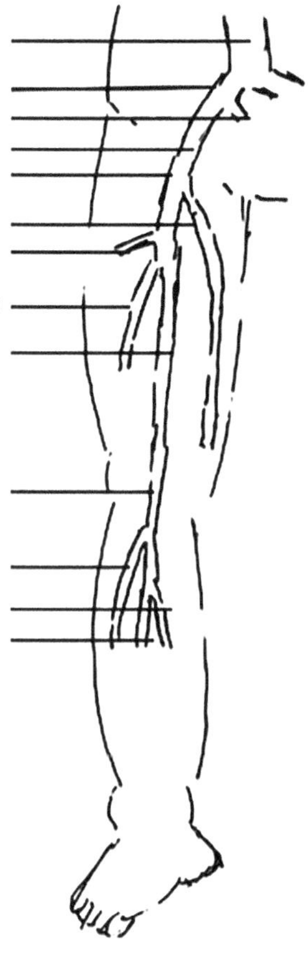

Fig. 48.1 Lower extremity deep venous system. The lower extremity deep venous system includes the external iliac, common femoral, deep femoral, femoral, popliteal, anterior tibial, posterior tibial, and peroneal veins

Pro-Tip Call-Out

- The major branch points of the lower extremity venous system are frequent sites of thrombi and must be visualized during DVT ultrasound assessment.

Image Acquisition

The linear array transducer is used to evaluate vasculature in most patients because its higher frequency (5–12 MHz) provides better resolution of superficial structures. However, in patients with obesity or edema, the lower frequency

(1–5 MHz) curvilinear transducer may be necessary to provide sufficient depth to evaluate deep veins.

To scan the lower extremity deep venous system, the patient may be positioned either standing, with leg straight, flexed, or supported, or more commonly, supine with the hip externally rotated and knee flexed (Fig. 48.2). The ultrasound machine should ideally be placed on the ipsilateral side to the provider and site of examination. With the screen marker on the left, the transducer marker should be oriented toward the patient's right. The transducer is placed in transverse orientation, centering the vasculature in the middle of the screen. Veins can be differentiated from arteries based on several characteristics. Veins are typically thin-walled and ovoid in cross-section. Valves may be visualized in veins, while calcified plaques can only be seen in arteries. Although veins are inherently nonpulsatile, pulsatility alone should not be used as a distinguishing characteristic, as pulsatility may be transduced from neighboring arteries. In situations where veins and arteries remain difficult to distinguish, color-flow Doppler may be utilized. With the transducer tilted towards the heart, venous blood flow traveling away from the transducer will appear blue.

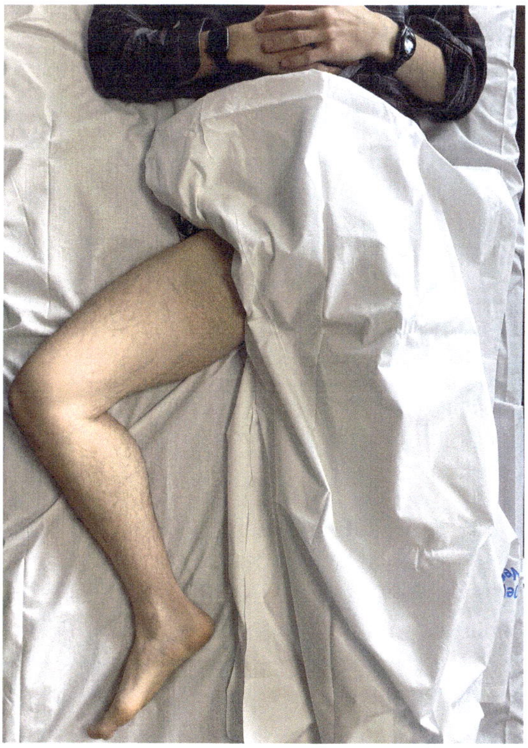

Fig. 48.2 Patient positioning. To scan the lower extremity venous system, the patient is most commonly positioned supine with the hip externally rotated and knee flexed

Starting above the inguinal ligament, the provider should observe for echogenic evidence of thrombus and compress the vein, applying enough downward pressure to cause slight arterial deformity or "winking" (Video 48.1.1). To avoid false-positive or false-negative scans, special attention should be paid to the manipulation of the transducer. First, the provider can brace their hand to avoid slipping. Second, both the angle of insonation and angle of compression should be perpendicular to the long-axis of the vein. If the transducer is titled away from the angle of compression, it is difficult to visualize venous collapse.

Pro-Tip

- In a normal vein, the anterior and posterior wall should meet when appropriately compressed. To ensure that sufficient pressure is being applied to the probe, look for "winking" of the neighboring artery.

While this process of observation and compression may be repeated every 1 centimeter (cm), sliding caudally along the lower extremity veins, it is most crucial to compress the vascular branchpoints, where DVTs most commonly occur due to turbulent blood flow and relative stasis (Fig. 48.3). Early studies demonstrated that most patients with symptomatic DVT were found to have extensive proximal vein thrombosis, rarely isolated to the superficial femoral vein alone [21, 22]. This data supports the use of a limited (two-zone or three-point) compression approach, focusing on the common femoral vein branchpoints and popliteal vein branchpoints.

To examine the femoral zone, start by visualizing the proximal common femoral vein near the inguinal crease (Video 48.1.1). Continuing distally, examine the greater saphenous vein branch-

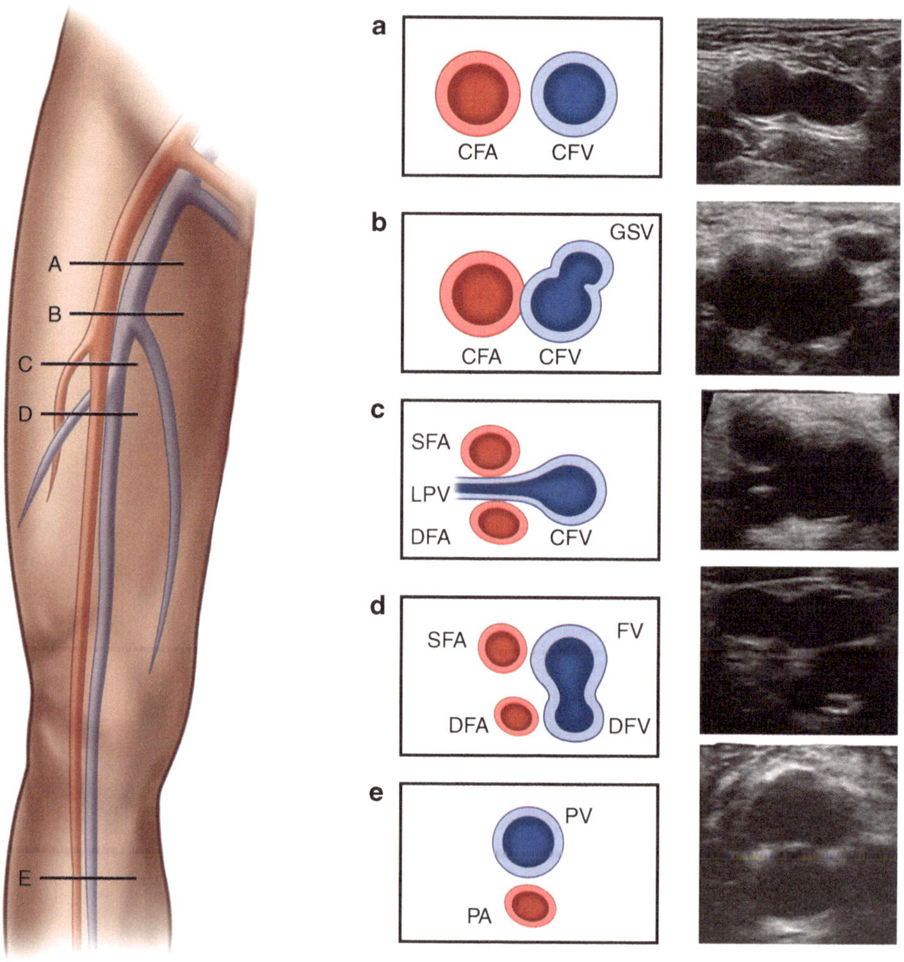

Fig. 48.3 Lower extremity vascular anatomy in cross-section. (**a**) Common femoral artery (CFA) and common femoral vein (CFV) visualized near the inguinal crease. (**b**) Greater saphenous vein (GSV) adjoins the CFV at the saphenofemoral junction. (**c**) CFA bifurcates into the superficial femoral artery (SFA) and deep femoral artery (DFA). The lateral perforator vein (LPV) branches from the CFV and traverses between the SFA and DFA. (**d**) CFV splits into the femoral vein (FV) and deep femoral vein (DFV). (**e**) Popliteal vein (PV) and popliteal artery (PA) visualized in the popliteal fossa

point (Video 48.1.2). Although the greater saphenous vein is a superficial vein, it is important to scan the proximal portion of the vein for thrombus given the high risk of extension into the common femoral vein. Following the common femoral vein further, visualize the lateral perforator vein branch laterally between the deep and superficial femoral arteries (Video 48.1.3). Finally, examine the common femoral vein as it splits into the deep femoral and femoral veins (Video 48.1.4).

In the popliteal zone, begin by identifying the popliteal vein in the popliteal fossa (Video 48.2.1). Using ample gel allows the provider to avoid applying excessive resting pressure, which could collapse the vein. If the popliteal vein remains difficult to visualize, squeezing the calf may help augment the venous return in the popliteal vein. After identifying the popliteal vein, examine the trifurcation into the anterior and posterior tibial and peroneal veins (Video 48.2.2). Beyond this junction, POCUS has lower diagnostic accuracy in detecting distal DVT. Given its low embolic potential and debated clinical relevance, examination of the distal deep veins of the calf is not included in the limited compression ultrasound approach [23, 24].

Extended Approach [Evolving Evidence Box]

- Recent studies suggest an incidence of isolated thrombi in the femoral vein between 5.5% and 22.3%, greater than previously described [25, 26]. Given the risk of missing a diagnosis of VTE, some clinicians recommend an extended compression ultrasound approach, scanning the femoral vein as it courses through the distal thigh into the adductor canal.

Image Interpretation

The ultrasound diagnosis of DVT requires either vein noncompressibility or visualization of echogenic thrombus. With the application of sufficient pressure to cause slight compression of the adjacent artery, normal veins should compress fully until anterior and posterior walls meet. Identification of a noncompressible vein is diagnostic of DVT even if an echogenic thrombus is not visible (Video 48.3.1). The chronicity of a thrombus affects its appearance on ultrasound. Acute DVT, which have not yet fully organized, may appear anechoic and may cause venous distension (Video 48.3.2). With time and increasing fibrin deposition, subacute and chronic DVT may generate more echogenicity. Chronic DVT are typically hyperechoic and often recanalize with development of collateral vessels (Video 48.3.3).

Pro-Tip

Acute thrombi are frequently anechoic and may manifest as venous noncompressibility alone.

Though POCUS DVT exams can be highly accurate, it is important to recognize the most common causes of false-positive and false-negative exams. Lymph nodes can often be mistaken for DVT given their similar hyperechoic appearance and noncompressibility. However, lymph nodes are generally ovoid, self-limiting structures that cannot be tracked proximally or distally (Video 48.4.1). They are typically more superficial and not paired with an adjacent artery. Popliteal cysts, or Baker's cysts, are noncompressible, anechoic structures found in the popliteal fossa. Compared to an acute thrombus, popliteal cysts often have posterior acoustic enhancement and a narrow passage of fluid connecting it to the joint space (Video 48.4.2). Smoke, or spontaneous echo contrast, is caused by rouleaux phenomenon, which can occur in the setting of a low-flow state (Video 48.4.3). Though not intrinsically pathogenic, smoke may suggest the presence of a more proximal DVT causing distal venous stasis. A variety of provider- and patient-dependent factors may lead to false-negative exams. Body habitus, edema, dressings, and contractures may make it difficult to examine the deep venous system. Additionally, improper technique, including inadequate depth, tangential compression, or probe migration, can result in both false-positive or false-negative exams.

Doppler Evaluation

The Doppler evaluation, which consists of color-flow Doppler imaging and spectral Doppler waveform analysis, is not a routine part of the POCUS DVT exam, but may be useful in select patients. In addition to differentiating veins and arteries, color-flow Doppler can be used to assess for patency of venous segments. Filling defects or complete absence of color-flow suggests partial or complete thrombosis of the vein. The spectral Doppler waveform from a normal, patent lower extremity should demonstrate phasicity due to respiratory variation (Fig. 48.4). Loss of respiratory phasicity suggests the presence of an occlusive thrombus cranial to the level of insonation. The augmentation maneuver can also be used to assess for patency of veins. Augmentation is performed by squeezing the leg distal to the level of

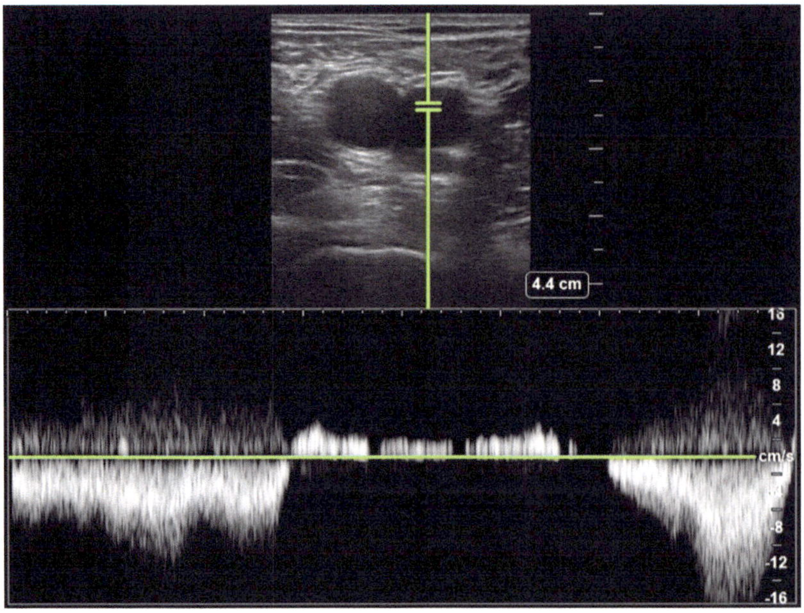

Fig. 48.4 Phasicity. The spectral Doppler waveform from a normal, patent lower extremity should demonstrate phasicity due to respiratory variation

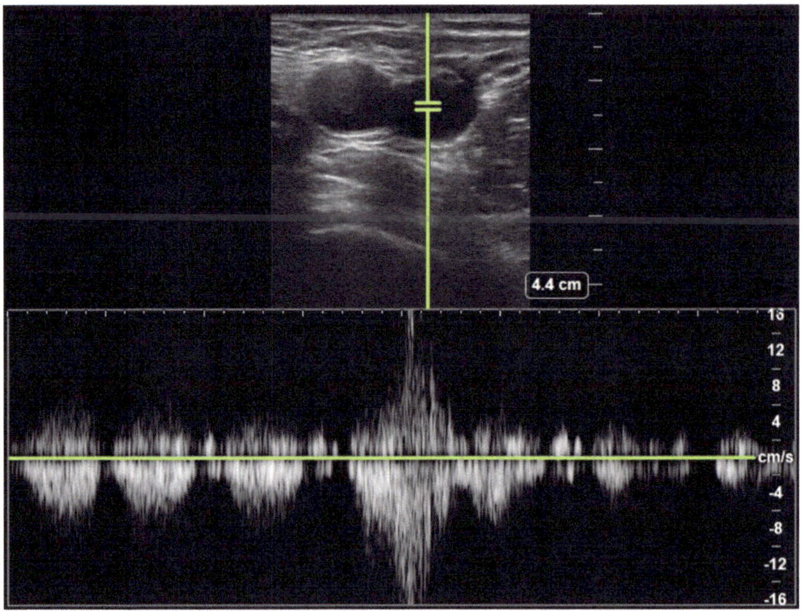

Fig. 48.5 Augmentation. Augmentation is performed by squeezing the leg distal to the level of insonation, resulting in increased anterograde venous flow on either color-flow or spectral Doppler. Absence or blunting of this response suggests presence of an occlusive thrombus between the level of augmentation and insonation

insonation (such as the distal thigh or calf), resulting in increased anterograde venous flow on either color-flow or spectral Doppler (Fig. 48.5 and Video 48.5). Absence or blunting of this response suggests presence of an occlusive thrombus between the level of augmentation and insonation.

Compared to compression B-mode ultrasonography, Doppler evaluation has not been shown to significantly add to the accuracy of the DVT POCUS exam [27]. For this reason, these techniques may be better utilized as diagnostic adjuncts in difficult or inconclusive cases.

Upper Extremity

DVT ultrasound evaluation of the upper extremity, typically only conducted pre-procedurally or in patients with high clinical suspicion for upper extremity DVT, shares many of the same principles to that of the lower extremity. The upper extremity deep venous system includes the brachiocephalic, internal jugular, subclavian, axillary, brachial, radial, and ulnar veins (Fig. 48.6). The distal paired veins, radial and ulnar, are less frequently involved with DVT.

The patient should be positioned with arm abducted and externally rotated. The proximal veins that are easily compressible, including jugular, axillary, and paired brachial veins, are amenable to evaluation by compression B-mode technique. Each vein should be accessed with compression at 1-cm intervals. Contrastingly, the subclavian and brachiocephalic veins are often inaccessible by compression due to the clavicle and, therefore, are better suited for Doppler evaluation. To visualize the subclavian vein, the transducer should be placed directly inferior to the clavicle with the transducer marker-oriented cephalad. The patient may also be asked to sniff to demonstrate venous collapsibility. To visualize the brachiocephalic vein, the transducer should be placed in transverse orientation above the supraclavicular space and tilted inferiorly.

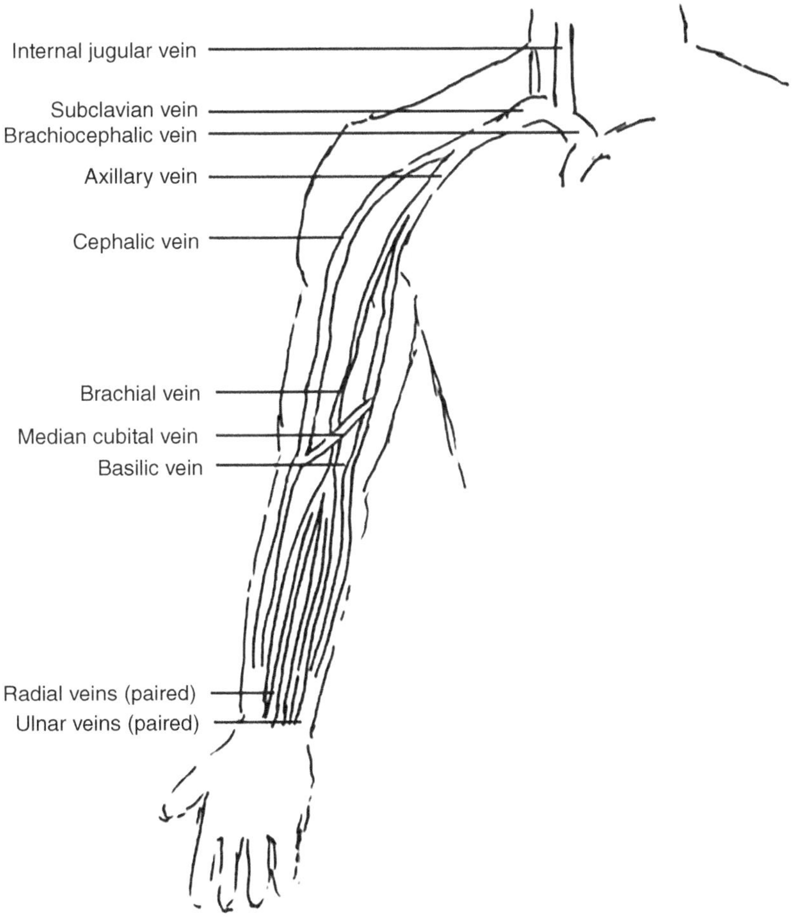

Fig. 48.6 Upper extremity deep venous system. The upper extremity deep venous system includes the brachiocephalic, internal jugular, subclavian, axillary, brachial, radial, and ulnar veins

Summary Points

- POCUS can be used to rapidly and accurately diagnosis DVTs in critically ill patients.
- DVT assessment requires knowledge of both vascular anatomy and an understanding of appropriate compression technique.
- DVTs most commonly occur at vascular branchpoints due to turbulent blood flow and relative stasis.
- The ultrasound diagnosis of DVT requires either vein noncompressibility or visualization of echogenic thrombus.
- While not routinely performed, doppler assessment and augmentation may be useful as diagnostic adjuncts in challenging cases.

Questions

1. In order to avoid false-positive scans, enough downward pressure should be applied with the transducer to cause:
   A. Mild patient discomfort
   B. **Slight arterial deformity or "winking"**
   C. Full arterial collapse
   D. Downward movement of the vein by at least 1 cm

   The anterior and posterior wall of the vein should meet when appropriately compressed. To ensure that sufficient pressure is being applied to the probe to result in normal venous compression, there should be a slight arterial deformity noted on compression.
2. What finding is seen in both acute and chronic DVT?
   A. Visualization of an echogenic clot
   B. Visualization of inflammation surrounding the vein
   C. **Noncompressibility of the vein**
   D. Pain with compression of the vein

   Both acute and chronic DVT have vein noncompressibility. The chronicity of a thrombus affects its appearance on ultrasound. Acute DVT, which have not yet fully organized, may appear anechoic and may cause venous distension.
3. What is the echogenicity of an acute DVT?
   A. **Anechoic**
   B. Hypoechoic
   C. Isoechoic
   D. Hyperechoic

   Acute DVT is anechoic. Subacute and chronic DVT are echogenic.
4. In the popliteal fossa, the popliteal vein is _______ to the popliteal artery.
   A. Lateral
   B. Medial
   C. **Superior**
   D. Inferior

   The popliteal vein travels superficial to the popliteal artery in the popliteal fossa until the vein trifurcates into the anterior tibial, posterior tibial, and peroneal veins.
5. Loss of respiratory phasicity suggests:
   A. Absence of an occlusive thrombus
   B. **Presence of an occlusive thrombus proximal to the level of insonation**
   C. Presence of an occlusive thrombus distal to the level of insonation
   D. Presence of a pulmonary embolism

   Loss of respiratory phasicity suggests the presence of an occlusive thrombus cranial to the level of insonation.

Acknowledgments Figure 48.3(d), Video 48.4.2, and Video 48.4.3 were provided by Dr. Brian Trieu, Department of Radiology, University of Texas Medical Branch.

References

1. Attia J, Ray JG, Cook DJ, Douketis J, Ginsberg JS, Geerts WH. Deep vein thrombosis and its prevention in critically ill adults. Arch Intern Med. 2001;161(10):1268–79. https://doi.org/10.1001/archinte.161.10.1268.
2. Moser KM, LeMoine JR, Nachtwey FJ, Spragg RG. Deep venous thrombosis and pulmonary embolism. Frequency in a respiratory intensive care unit. JAMA. 1981;246(13):1422–4.
3. Cade JF. High risk of the critically ill for venous thromboembolism. Crit Care Med. 1982;10(7):448–50. https://doi.org/10.1097/00003246-198207000-00006.
4. Hirsch DR, Ingenito EP, Goldhaber SZ. Prevalence of deep venous thrombosis among patients in medical intensive care. JAMA. 1995;274(4):335–7.
5. Marik PE, Andrews L, Maini B. The incidence of deep venous thrombosis in ICU patients. Chest. 1997;111(3):661–4. https://doi.org/10.1378/chest.111.3.661.
6. Kapoor M, Kupfer YY, Tessler S. Subcutaneous heparin prophylaxis significantly reduces the incidence of venous thromboembolic events in the critically ill. Crit Care Med. 1999;27(12):A69.

7. Fraisse F, Holzapfel L, Couland JM, Simonneau G, Bedock B, Feissel M, et al. Nadroparin in the prevention of deep vein thrombosis in acute decompensated COPD. The Association of Non-University Affiliated Intensive Care Specialist Physicians of France. Am J Respir Crit Care Med. 2000;161(4 Pt 1):1109–14. https://doi.org/10.1164/ajrccm.161.4.9807025.
8. Ibrahim EH, Iregui M, Prentice D, Sherman G, Kollef MH, Shannon W. Deep vein thrombosis during prolonged mechanical ventilation despite prophylaxis. Crit Care Med. 2002;30(4):771–4. https://doi.org/10.1097/00003246-200204000-00008.
9. Cook D, Crowther M, Meade M, Rabbat C, Griffith L, Schiff D, et al. Deep venous thrombosis in medical-surgical critically ill patients: prevalence, incidence, and risk factors. Crit Care Med. 2005;33(7):1565–71. https://doi.org/10.1097/01.ccm.0000171207.95319.b2.
10. PROTECT Investigators for the Canadian Critical Care Trials Group and the Australian and New Zealand Intensive Care Society Clinical Trials Group, Cook D, Meade M, Guyatt G, Walter S, Heels-Ansdell D, et al. Dalteparin versus unfractionated heparin in critically ill patients. N Engl J Med. 2011;364(14):1305–14. https://doi.org/10.1056/NEJMoa1014475.
11. Gibson CD, Colvin MO, Park MJ, Lai Q, Lin J, Negassa A, et al. Prevalence and predictors of deep vein thrombosis in critically ill medical patients who underwent diagnostic duplex ultrasonography. J Intensive Care Med. 2020;35(10):1062–6. https://doi.org/10.1177/0885066618813300.
12. Malato A, Dentali F, Siragusa S, Fabbiano F, Kagoma Y, Boddi M, et al. The impact of deep vein thrombosis in critically ill patients: a meta-analysis of major clinical outcomes. Blood Transfus. 2015;13(4):559–68. https://doi.org/10.2450/2015.0277-14.
13. Blaivas M, Lambert MJ, Harwood RA, Wood JP, Konicki J. Lower-extremity Doppler for deep venous thrombosis--can emergency physicians be accurate and fast? Acad Emerg Med. 2000;7(2):120–6. https://doi.org/10.1111/j.1553-2712.2000.tb00512.x.
14. Theodoro D, Blaivas M, Duggal S, Snyder G, Lucas M. Real-time B-mode ultrasound in the ED saves time in the diagnosis of deep vein thrombosis (DVT). Am J Emerg Med. 2004;22(3):197–200. https://doi.org/10.1016/j.ajem.2004.02.007.
15. Pomero F, Dentali F, Borretta V, Bonzini M, Melchio R, Douketis JD, Fenoglio LM. Accuracy of emergency physician-performed ultrasonography in the diagnosis of deep-vein thrombosis: a systematic review and meta-analysis. Thromb Haemost. 2013;109(1):137–45. https://doi.org/10.1160/TH12-07-0473.
16. Fischer EA, Kinnear B, Sall D, Kelleher M, Sanchez O, Mathews B, et al. Hospitalist-operated compression ultrasonography: a point-of-care ultrasound study (HOCUS-POCUS). J Gen Intern Med. 2019;34(10):2062–7. https://doi.org/10.1007/s11606-019-05120-5.
17. Mumoli N, Vitale J, Giorgi-Pierfranceschi M, Sabatini S, Tulino R, Cei M, et al. General practitioner-performed compression ultrasonography for diagnosis of deep vein thrombosis of the leg: a multicenter, prospective cohort study. Ann Fam Med. 2017;15(6):535–9. https://doi.org/10.1370/afm.2109.
18. Kory PD, Pellecchia CM, Shiloh AL, Mayo PH, DiBello C, Koenig S. Accuracy of ultrasonography performed by critical care physicians for the diagnosis of DVT. Chest. 2011;139(3):538–42. https://doi.org/10.1378/chest.10-1479.
19. Jang T, Docherty M, Aubin C, Polites G. Resident-performed compression ultrasonography for the detection of proximal deep vein thrombosis: fast and accurate. Acad Emerg Med. 2004;11(3):319–22. https://doi.org/10.1111/j.1553-2712.2004.tb02220.x.
20. Javaudin F, Seon J, Le Bastard Q, Cabiot A, Pes P, Arnaudet I, et al. Evaluation of short training session for venous limited compression ultrasonography: prospective multicenter study. Ultrasound J. 2020;12(1):5. https://doi.org/10.1186/s13089-020-0155-2.
21. Cogo A, Lensing AW, Prandoni P, Hirsh J. Distribution of thrombosis in patients with symptomatic deep vein thrombosis. Implications for simplifying the diagnostic process with compression ultrasound. Arch Intern Med. 1993;153(24):2777–80.
22. Pedraza García J, Valle Alonso J, Ceballos García P, Rico Rodríguez F, Aguayo López MÁ, Muñoz-Villanueva MDC. Comparison of the accuracy of emergency department-performed point-of-care-ultrasound (POCUS) in the diagnosis of lower-extremity deep vein thrombosis. J Emerg Med. 2018;54(5):656–64. https://doi.org/10.1016/j.jemermed.2017.12.020.
23. Garry J, Duke A, Labropoulos N. Systematic review of the complications following isolated calf deep vein thrombosis. Br J Surg. 2016;103(7):789–96. https://doi.org/10.1002/bjs.10152.
24. Righini M, Paris S, Le Gal G, Laroche JP, Perrier A, Bounameaux H. Clinical relevance of distal deep vein thrombosis. Review of literature data. Thromb Haemost. 2006;95(1):56–64.
25. Maki DD, Kumar N, Nguyen B, Langer JE, Miller WT Jr, Gefter WB. Distribution of thrombi in acute lower extremity deep venous thrombosis: implications for sonography and CT and MR venography. AJR Am J Roentgenol. 2000;175(5):1299–301. https://doi.org/10.2214/ajr.175.5.1751299.
26. Adhikari S, Zeger W, Thom C, Fields JM. Isolated deep venous thrombosis: implications for 2-point compression ultrasonography of the lower extremity. Ann Emerg Med. 2015;66(3):262–6. https://doi.org/10.1016/j.annemergmed.2014.10.032.
27. Poppiti R, Papanicolaou G, Perese S, Weaver FA. Limited B-mode venous imaging versus complete color-flow duplex venous scanning for detection of proximal deep venous thrombosis. J Vasc Surg. 1995;22(5):553–7. https://doi.org/10.1016/s0741-5214(95)70037-4.

Carotid Sonography in Critical Care

49

James Kornfield and Christopher Shaw

Learning Objectives

1. Describe how to obtain sonographic measurements of carotid blood flow
2. Explain the clinical significance of respiratory variation of peak carotid velocity

Introduction

Sonographic assessment of the carotid arteries has historically been utilized to evaluate cerebrovascular ischemia in the context of transient ischemic attack or stroke. More recently in the realm of critical care medicine, several carotid artery assessments have been described as potential tools for predicting fluid responsiveness, as well as assessing changes in cardiac output for patients in shock. These exams have significant logistical advantages when compared to transthoracic echocardiography (TTE), which explains in part the vigor with which they have been investigated. TTE acquisition in the critically ill can be challenging due to significant pulmonary disease, obesity, inability to take the left lateral decubitus position, use of prone position, and the presence of chest drains. Further, echocardiography requires significant training, whereas novice operators have demonstrated acceptable performance of carotid US after minimal instruction [1]. The relatively large caliber and superficial location of the carotid arteries, along with their anatomic consistency, make for a simple sonographic target. These vessels lie deep to the internal jugular vein in the anterior cervical triangle and can be easily visualized in both the axial and sagittal planes using a linear probe at ~5–10 MHz frequency.

We will spend the remainder of this chapter detailing the technique, physiologic underpinnings for, and literature describing the most promising of these exams: carotid blood flow, corrected carotid flow time, and respiratory variation of peak carotid velocity.

Carotid Blood Flow

Many therapeutic interventions in critical care aim to augment cardiac output (CO) as a means of optimizing perfusion. Thus, quantifying CO at the bedside to assess therapeutic efficacy has become a key task for the modern intensivist. The carotid arteries supply the majority of the cerebral circulation, which comprises approximately 20% of CO [2]. Given the proximity to the aorta, quantification of blood flow through the carotid artery may serve as an acceptable proxy for CO.

J. Kornfield (✉) · C. Shaw
OHSU Pulmonary, Allergy and Critical Care Medicine, Portland, OR, USA
e-mail: Kornfiel@ohsu.edu; Shawchr@ohsu.edu

M. J. Lanspa, A. T. Levinson (eds.), *Echocardiography and Ultrasonography in the ICU*, Respiratory Medicine, https://doi.org/10.1007/978-3-031-80038-2_49

Carotid blood flow (CBF) can be measured utilizing integration of the pulse wave doppler (PWD) function, similar to the left ventricular outflow tract velocity time integral (VTI). To determine CBF, both the diameter of the blood vessel and the VTI are required (Formula 49.1).

$$\mathrm{CBF} = \left[\mathrm{pi}\left({}^{D}/_{2}\right)^{2}\right] \times \mathrm{VTI} \times \mathrm{HR} \qquad (49.1)$$

Formula 49.1. Carotid blood flow is determined by the area of the vessel, calculated using the diameter (D), the distance the blood travels during a cardiac cycle (VTI), and the number of cardiac cycles per minute (HR).

The luminal diameter of the vessel, from intimal edge to intimal edge, should be measured in the axial dimension and confirmed in the sagittal plane. Different investigators have utilized a variety of locations for recording vessel diameter, including the level of the thyroid cartilage [2] or a predetermined distance inferior to the carotid bulb [1, 3, 4]. The PWD sample volume is placed into the middle of the lumen where the diameter measurement was obtained, and subsequently activated, which should produce a tracing similar to Fig. 49.1. It is essential that the angle of correction used is 60 degrees or less, as recommended by the American Institute for Ultrasound in Medicine, as larger angles increase the potential for error [5]. The VTI is recorded by tracing the contour of the resulting envelope (Fig. 49.1). Additionally, the carotid diameter may change over time, requiring repeat measurements with each assessment.

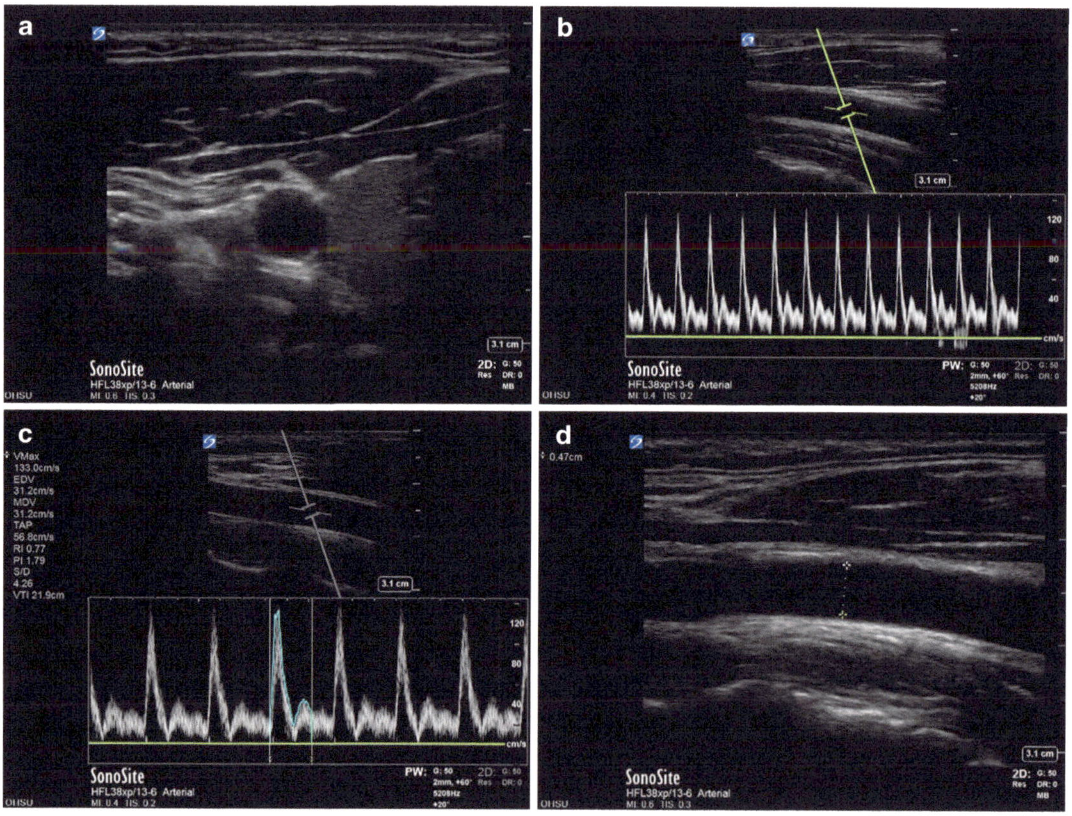

Fig. 49.1 The steps required for calculation of CBF. First the carotid artery is identified (**a**), then visualized in longitudinal plane placing the PWD gate in the center of the vessel with a correction angle <60° (**b**). PWD is activated and a velocity time integral is obtained. A single envelope is traced from initiation to dicrotic notch (**c**) and the ejection time, encompassed by the vertical bars, can be used to calculate FTc. Heart rate can be obtained from the same view and a diameter should be measured from intima to intima at the same location (**d**)

Edge of Evidence

Data corroborating CBF as a reliable surrogate for CO are promising. In 18 patients presenting for elective coronary artery bypass grafting, CBF demonstrated a moderate correlation with CO measured invasively by a pulse contour catheter in the femoral artery, although there was significant imprecision [6]. In a group of 36 mixed medical-surgical intensive care patients, estimated CO from CBF utilizing a standard multiplier based on physiologic assumptions found that carotid flow highly correlated with CO determined by either femoral artery pulse counter analysis or pulmonary artery catheter (PAC) [2]. Carotid flow moderately correlated to CO calculated using left ventricular outflow tract VTI in 20 healthy individuals [4]. Further, CBF moderately correlated with CO determined by thermodilution in 51 patients undergoing right heart catheterization [7]. Conversely, while both CBF and CO—as assessed by TTE—increased with the addition of norepinephrine in a small cohort of patients with suspected septic shock, there was no significant correlation between the two [8].

Significant challenges still exist for bringing CBF to the bedside. There are no published normal values for CBF, nor an agreed upon threshold for determining fluid responsiveness. It has been proposed that an increase of 20% in CBF after fluid administration or passive leg raise be used to indicate a positive response [9]. Perhaps the primary barrier may be the complex physiology regulating cerebral blood flow—the reason that patients with TBI are universally excluded from these studies. Lastly, there are no data confirming that the correlation between CBF and CO can add to the standard clinical assessment of the critically ill.

Evolving Evidence Call-Out
Significant challenges exist for bringing carotid blood flow to the bedside. There are no published normal values for carotid blood flow, nor an agreed upon threshold for determining fluid responsiveness.

Corrected Carotid Flow Time

While CBF may serve as a correlate for CO, the corrected carotid flow time (FTc) assesses ejection time as an indirect proxy of CO. Assuming that contractility remains relatively stable over a given period, a longer ejection time should produce a larger stroke volume [10].

The method for obtaining FTc is similar to CBF, utilizing PWD; however, the vessel diameter is not required. The PWD sample should be placed in the middle of the lumen, proximal to the carotid bulb to avoid excessive turbulent flow. Once the PWD tracing is obtained, the systolic time is recorded—from the initial upstroke of the doppler waveform to the dicrotic notch (Fig. 49.1). This value is used to calculate FTc as seen in Formula (49.2).

$$\text{FTc} = \text{systolic time} / \left(\text{HR}^{1/2}\right) \quad (49.2)$$

Formula 49.2. FTc is calculated using the systolic time, obtained from the PWD, and the heart rate (HR) at the time of evaluation. The formula displayed is Bazett's formula; Wodey's formula has been offered as an alternative [11].

Edge of Evidence

FTc has primarily been investigated as a predictor of fluid responsiveness. Initial observations found that FTc tended to be lower in hypovolemic healthy volunteers [12, 13], and higher in patients with volume excess [14]. FTc was also shown to increase significantly with fluid administration in patients determined to be volume depleted by clinical evaluation [15], and to decrease in patients with end-stage renal disease receiving dialysis in a dose dependent manner [15].

Although FTc seems to correlate with intravascular volume, data regarding its efficacy in predicting fluid responsiveness are mixed. Authors have offered different absolute or relative changes as thresholds for determining fluid responsiveness [9, 12, 16]. FTc did identify fluid responders in a heterogenous group of studies including patients undergoing elective neurosurgeries who received a fluid challenge [8], critically ill patients with invasive arterial lines [17], and in ICU patients with undifferentiated shock [16]. However, FTc failed to predict fluid responsiveness in patients with suspected sepsis [3], or suspected circulatory failure based on clinical and laboratory data [18]. Lastly, poor interrater reliability has been demonstrated in publications utilizing nonexpert sonographers [19].

Respiratory Variation in Carotid Peak Systolic Velocity

Physiologic respiratory variation in the pulse pressure has frequently been utilized to evaluate response to fluid administration. While other methods of pulse pressure variation can be challenging in novice hands or require invasive tools (arterial catheters, transesophageal probes), carotid doppler is both simple and noninvasive. Measurement of the change in carotid doppler peak velocity (ΔCDPV) can be performed at the bedside utilizing the same techniques described above. A PWD of the common carotid artery is obtained, setting the sweep speed to obtain an appropriate respiratory cycle (Fig. 49.2). The maximum and minimum peak velocities are recorded and the variability calculated using Formula (49.3), with values above 15% suggesting that fluid administration could increase stroke volume.

$$\Delta CDPV = 100 \times (\text{max peak velocity} - \text{min peak velocity}) / (\text{mean peak velocity}) \quad (49.3)$$

Formula 49.3. Variability in the carotid peak systolic velocities is measured using the difference between with minimum and maximum identified velocities, which is then divided by the mean peak velocity. Mean peak velocity is obtained by dividing the sum of the maximum and minimum velocities by 2.

There are several factors to account for when applying ΔCDPV in a clinical context. As stated previously, measures of carotid flow are subject

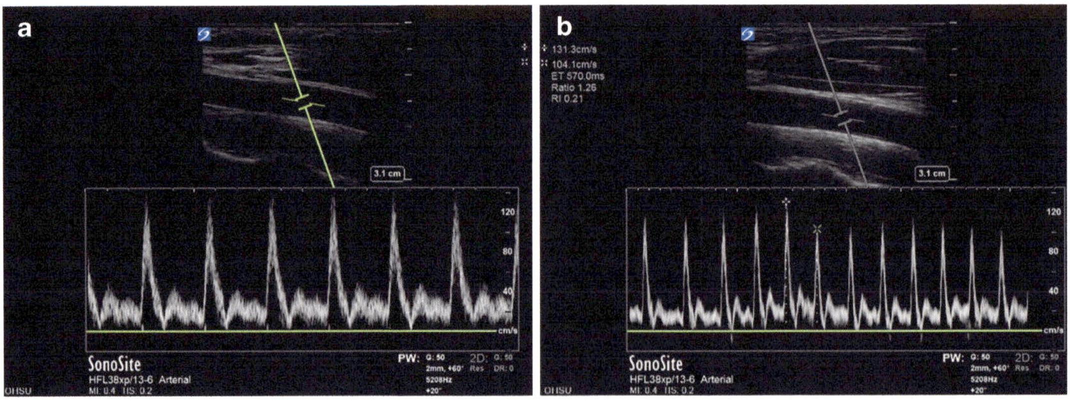

Fig. 49.2 Demonstration of carotid peak systolic velocity variation measurement. A PWD tracing of the carotid artery is obtained (**a**) but the sweep speed must be optimized to review sufficient waveforms to appreciate respiratory variation (**b**). The maximal and minimal peak velocities are then measurement and the values are plugged into Formula (49.3) to obtain a percent variation

to the unique factors that regulate cerebral blood flow. Additionally, as respiratory variation is affected by patients' effort, many studies were performed specifically on mechanically ventilated patients, limiting generalizability. Carotid flow will vary substantially with underlying cardiovascular pathology such as arrhythmia, valvular disease, and carotid stenosis, which complicate the bedside utility of ΔCDPV.

Edge of Evidence

ΔCDPV values have often been compared to measurements obtained using PAC (stroke volume index, cardiac output, or cardiac index). One study of 59 fluid challenges in 19 patients found a sensitivity and specificity of 86% for ΔCDPV when distinguishing patients who would be 'fluid responders,' defined as a >15% increase in stroke volume index (SVI) [20]. Similarly, small cohorts of mechanically ventilated patients with septic shock [21] and those undergoing coronary artery bypass grafting [22] demonstrated a correlation between ΔCDPV and an increase in cardiac index or SVI after fluid administration. As with CBF and FTc, there are no values that have been validated to predict an increase in CO after giving fluids—a range of >11–15% ΔCDPV has often been used to indicate a positive test.

Summary Points

- Carotid arteries are easily visualized in most critically ill patients
- Obtaining a carotid artery pulse wave doppler waveform allows for calculation of the carotid blood flow (CBF), carotid flow time (FTc), and respiratory variation of the carotid peak systolic velocity (ΔCDPV)
- CBF can be used as a surrogate for cardiac output
- ΔCDPV may be useful in predicting an increase in stroke volume if intravenous fluids are given
- Further studies are required to validate the use of CBF, FTc, and ΔCDPV in clinical decision making and to identify standard reference range values

Question

A 57-year-old female patient is transferred to the intensive care unit from the emergency room (ER) for septic shock. She has a past medical history of obesity, hypertension, and recurrent urinary tract infections and presented to the ER with fever of 102° F and several days of abdominal pain. Her workup is significant for a serum lactate 5.4 mmol/L, white blood cell count of 24.2 k with 88% neutrophils, an elevated creatinine 1.5 mg/dL with a BUN 44 mg/dL, a high-sensitivity troponin 32 ng/L, and NT-pro-BNP 521 pg/mL. EKG shows sinus tachycardia. She became progressively more somnolent in the ER and was intubated for airway protection. She received a total of 3 L of intravenous lactated ringers and one dose of vancomycin and piperacillin-tazobactam. On arrival to the intensive care unit, her blood pressure is 83/47 with a heart rate of 117. A bedside ultrasound is performed, but cardiac views are difficult to obtain. A carotid doppler is performed and shows a carotid blood flow of 350 mL/min. Which of the following would be an appropriate next step based on the carotid doppler findings:

A. Obtain formal TTE prior to next intervention
B. Start epinephrine given low carotid blood flow
C. Give a fluid bolus of 250–500 mL of lactated ringers and remeasure carotid blood flow
D. Give 1 L of lactated ringers and repeat blood pressure in 1–2 h
E. Place a pulmonary artery catheter to better assess cardiac output

Answer: C. The patient presents with septic shock, likely urinary in origin. She has received a fluid challenge, but remains hypotensive. It is unclear if she would benefit from further volume expansion or if she should be started on vasoactives. Determining response to fluid should be accomplished with dynamic assessments, which includes iterative measurements of CBF (C). Waiting for a sonographer-performed TTE (A) prior to treatment would be inappropriate given the patient's critical illness. Epinephrine may be a feasible next step (B), but norepinephrine is the consensus first-line vasopressor for septic shock and fluid responsiveness should be assessed first. Blood pressure is a blunt tool for assessment of fluid responsiveness and should not be used in isolation (D). PAC have not been shown to improve outcomes in mixed critical care populations and should be avoided in situations where cardiogenic shock or RV failure is not the primary differential (E).

References

1. Stolz L, Mosier J, Gross A, Douglas M, Blaivas M, Adhikari S. Can emergency physicians perform common carotid doppler flow measurements to assess volume responsiveness? West J Emerg Med. 2015;16(2):255–9.
2. Gassner M, Killu K, Bauman Z, Coba V, Rosso K, Blyden D. Feasibility of common carotid artery point of care ultrasound in cardiac output measurements compared to invasive methods. J Ultrasound. 2015;18(2):127–33.
3. Liteplo AS, Schleifer J, Marill KA, Huang CK, Gouker SK, Ratanski D, et al. Carotid ultrasound in assessing fluid responsiveness in patients with hypotension and suspected sepsis. Shock. 2021;56(3):419–24. https://doi.org/10.1097/SHK.0000000000001755.
4. Sidor M, Premachandra L, Hanna B, Nair N, Misra A. Carotid flow as a surrogate for cardiac output measurement in hemodynamically stable participants. J Intensive Care Med. 2020;35(7):650–5.
5. The AIUM practice parameter for the performance of an ultrasound examination of the extracranial cerebrovascular system. J Ultrasound Med. 2022;41(4):E21–7.
6. van Houte J, Mooi FJ, Montenij LJ, Meijs LPB, Suriani I, Conjaerts BCM, et al. Correlation of carotid doppler blood flow with invasive cardiac output measurements in cardiac surgery patients. J Cardiothorac Vasc Anesth. 2022;36(4):1081–91.
7. Ma IWY, Caplin JD, Azad A, Wilson C, Fifer MA, Bagchi A, et al. Correlation of carotid blood flow and corrected carotid flow time with invasive cardiac output measurements. Crit Ultrasound J. 2017;9(1):10.
8. Kim D-H, Shin S, Kim N, Choi T, Choi SH, Choi YS. Carotid ultrasound measurements for assessing fluid responsiveness in spontaneously breathing patients: corrected flow time and respirophasic variation in blood flow peak velocity. Br J Anaesth. 2018;121(3):541–9.
9. Marik PE, Levitov A, Young A, Andrews L. The use of bioreactance and carotid doppler to determine volume responsiveness and blood flow redistribution following passive leg raising in hemodynamically unstable patients. Chest. 2013;143(2):364–70.
10. Barjaktarevic I, Chiem A, Cannesson M. Time to correct the flow of corrected flow time. Crit Ultrasound J. 2017;9(1):18.
11. Hossein-Nejad H, Banaie M, Davarani SS, Mohammadinejad P. Assessment of corrected flow time in carotid artery via point-of-care ultrasonography: reference values and the influential factors. J Crit Care. 2017;40:46–51.
12. Shokoohi H, Berry GW, Shahkolahi M, King J, King J, Salimian M, et al. The diagnostic utility of sonographic carotid flow time in determining volume responsiveness. J Crit Care. 2017;38:231–5.
13. Mackenzie DC, Khan NA, Blehar D, Glazier S, Chang Y, Stowell CP, et al. Carotid flow time changes with volume status in acute blood loss. Ann Emerg Med. 2015;66(3):277–282.e1.
14. Hossein-Nejad H, Mohammadinejad P, Lessan-Pezeshki M, Davarani SS, Banaie M. Carotid artery corrected flow time measurement via bedside ultrasonography in monitoring volume status. J Crit Care. 2015;30(6):1199–203.
15. Blehar DJ, Glazier S, Gaspari RJ. Correlation of corrected flow time in the carotid artery with changes in intravascular volume status. J Crit Care. 2014;29(4):486–8.
16. Barjaktarevic I, Toppen WE, Hu S, Aquije Montoya E, Ong S, Buhr R, et al. Ultrasound assessment of the change in carotid corrected flow time in fluid responsiveness in undifferentiated shock. Crit Care Med. 2018;46(11):e1040–6.
17. Jalil B, Thompson P, Cavallazzi R, Marik P, Mann J, El-Kersh K, et al. Comparing changes in carotid flow time and stroke volume induced by passive leg raising. Am J Med Sci. 2018;355(2):168–73.
18. Abbasi A, Azab N, Nayeemuddin M, Schick A, Lopardo T, Phillips GS, et al. Change in carotid blood flow and carotid corrected flow time assessed by novice sonologists fails to determine fluid responsiveness in spontaneously breathing intensive care unit patients. Ultrasound Med Biol. 2020;46(10):2659–66.
19. Doctor M, Siadecki SD, Cooper D, Rose G, Drake AB, Ku M, et al. Reliability, laterality and the effect of respiration on the measured corrected flow time of the carotid arteries. J Emerg Med. 2017;53(1):91–7.
20. Ibarra-Estrada MÁ, López-Pulgarín JA, Mijangos-Méndez JC, Díaz-Gómez JL, Aguirre-Avalos G. Respiratory variation in carotid peak systolic velocity predicts volume responsiveness in mechanically ventilated patients with septic shock: a prospective cohort study. Crit Ultrasound J. 2015;7(1):12.
21. Lu N, Xi X, Jiang L, Yang D, Yin K. Exploring the best predictors of fluid responsiveness in patients with septic shock. Am J Emerg Med. 2017;35(9):1258–61.
22. Song Y, Kwak YL, Song JW, Kim YJ, Shim JK. Respirophasic carotid artery peak velocity variation as a predictor of fluid responsiveness in mechanically ventilated patients with coronary artery disease. Br J Anaesth. 2014;113(1):61–6.

Optic Nerve Assessment

50

Carla Venegas, Kimberly McPhearson, and Aarti Sarwal

Learning Objectives

1. Understand the sono-anatomy of Optic nerve sheath diameter (ONSD)
2. Describe the indications and limitations of this technique
3. Describe step by step the technique
4. Review the evidence on the efficacy of ONSD in the evaluation of neurocritical patients to identify intracranial hypertension

Background

Multiple traumatic and nontraumatic brain injuries can cause elevated intracranial pressure (ICP), a complication that requires early recognition and management due to its associated poor prognosis. The gold standard noninvasive diagnostic tool is CT scan of the head, but limitations in obtaining this study include availability at the treating center, immediate interpretation lecture by a radiologist, and increased risk of transportation due to hemodynamic instability. The most reliable diagnostic tool is invasive ICP monitoring with an external ventricular device (EVD) or fiber optic brain monitoring, but it requires a bedside neurosurgical team available [1], and it is not exempt of complications like infection, hemorrhage, or catheter malfunction, which range between 6% and 33% [2].

Optic nerve sheath diameter (ONSD), which can be visualized and measured utilizing ultrasonography, can reflect changes in cerebrospinal fluid (CSF) pressure [3]. The use of optic ultrasound in neurocritical care medicine varies between centers. Experience is growing since the onset of the COVID pandemic where bedside ultrasonographic evaluation has facilitated triaging of patients, evaluation with telemedicine technologies or in community centers as a triaging tool for referrals, and even in large tertiary care centers where access to external ventricular drains (EVD) is not readily available. For the neurointensivist, ultrasound can act as a tracking tool that provides a one-time measure and gives valuable information as a follow-up regarding response to therapeutic measurements [1].

Understanding Sono-Anatomy of ONSD

The optic nerve sheath (ONS) is contiguous with the dura mater, which communicates with the subarachnoid space and, therefore, will increase

C. Venegas (✉) · K. McPhearson
Department of Critical Care Medicine, Mayo Clinic, Jacksonville, FL, USA
e-mail: Venegas.Carla@mayo.edu; McPhearson.Kimberly@mayo.edu

A. Sarwal
Division of Neurocritical Care Chief, Virginia Commonwealth University, Richmon, VA, USA
e-mail: ASarwal@wakehealth.edu

M. J. Lanspa, A. T. Levinson (eds.), *Echocardiography and Ultrasonography in the ICU*, Respiratory Medicine, https://doi.org/10.1007/978-3-031-80038-2_50

in size with increased ICP. Because the eye is a fluid-filled structure, ultrasound waves can easily travel and identify the eyelid, anterior chamber, iris, lens, vitreous body, and retina. The optic nerve (ON), located posterior to the globe and perpendicular to the posterior wall, appears hypoechoic while the core is anechoic, and the sheath surrounding it appears hyperechoic (See Fig. 50.1 and Picture 50.1).

Ultrasonographic visualization of the ONS was initially described in 1994, using B-mode and standardizing the measurement of the most significant degree of distension of the sheath at 3 mm behind the optic globe [3]. The technique for ocular sonography is quickly learned. Reports describe a need for ten studies for an experienced ultrasound operator or 25 for a novice, and evaluation of both eyes takes about 4 min [4].

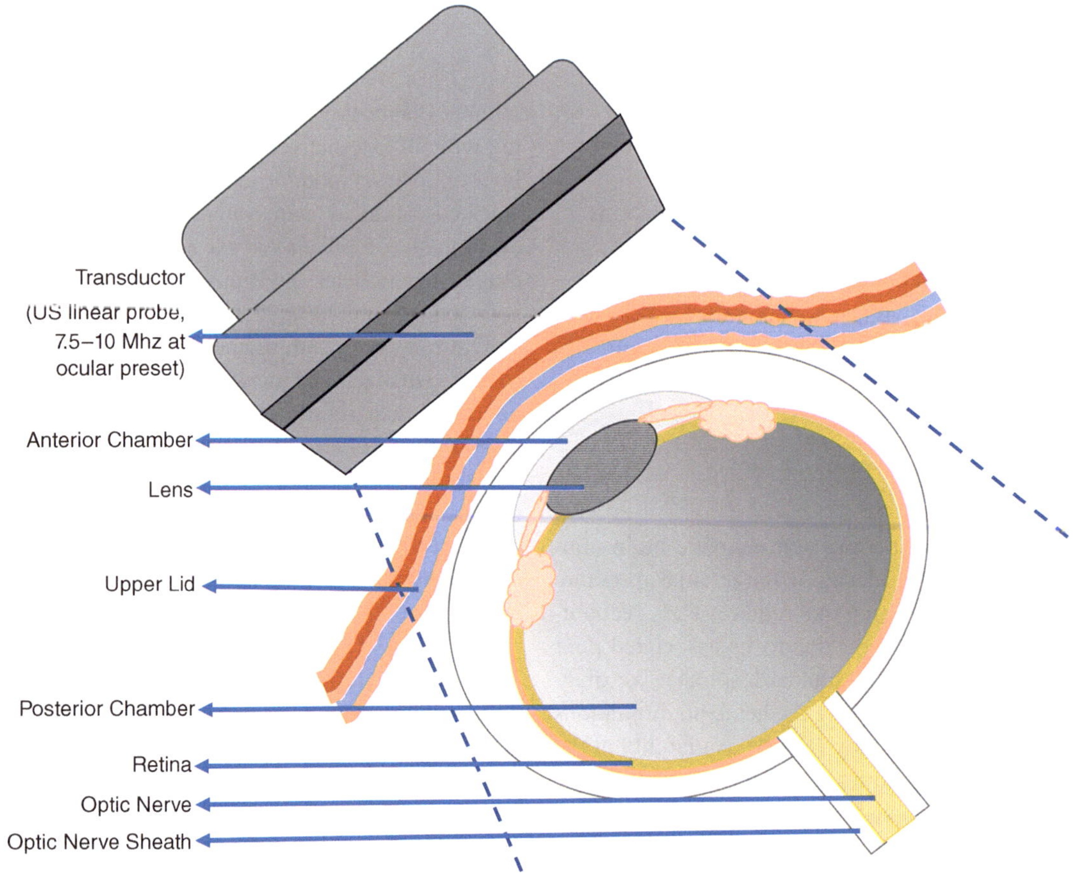

Fig. 50.1 Diagram of optic nerve sono-anatomy

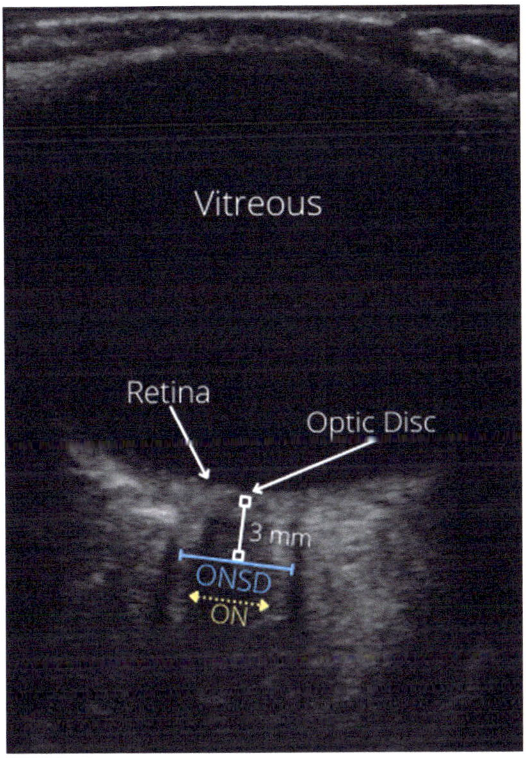

Picture 50.1 Ultrasound view of optic nerve sheath and its measurement. Ultrasonographic image of the eye and optic nerve. *ONSD* Optic nerve sheath diameter, *ON* Optic nerve. Measurement is taken 3 mm behind the globe of the eye to the edges of the optic nerve sheath (ONS)

Indications

Ultrasound is an excellent diagnostic tool for the eye given that it is a fluid-filled structure and thus straightforward to image. It has a place in traumatic and nontraumatic settings as long as globe rupture is not suspected, the one contraindication to ocular ultrasound. Ultrasound can be used to evaluate many ocular pathologies including acute change in vision, eye trauma or pain, or suspected foreign body [5].

The primary use in the critical care setting is for evaluation of the ONSD with suspected elevated ICP. Elevated ICP can cause the optic disc to bulge (papilledema) which can be seen on ultrasound. Papilledema is confirmed on ultrasound when the optic disc is elevated from the retina more than 0.6 mm [6]. Optic neuritis should be considered with unilateral increase accompanied by painful eye movement and monocular vision loss [7].

Limitations

In studies that compared invasive ICP monitoring with ONSD, there was dissimilarity in the optimal ONSD measurement indicative of elevated ICP [1]. There are likely multiple variables that contribute to this including the patient's baseline ONSD, acute versus acute-on-chronic disease processes (such as in acute-on-chronic liver failure), as well as the cause of the elevated ICP (ONSD is likely less reliable in subarachnoid patients). This study is operator-dependent, and given the minute measurements being taken, there can be some inter-rater reliability issues.

Technique Including Crescent Sign/ CRAO

- This study requires the use of a linear probe. It is recommended to use a 7.5–10 MHz frequency with the ocular preset, if available. If unavailable, opt for a superficial preset.
- Set imaging depth to approximately 4 cm with the gain initially at zero.
- The patient should be placed in a supine position with the head of the bed at 20–30 degrees (this is primarily for patient comfort and some evidence of no change in ONSD with changes in the elevation of the head, though this concept is still controversial).
- If the patient is conscious, have them fix their gaze forward.
- With a closed eye, place a protector tape and a thick layer of ultrasound gel.
- Hold the probe in a pencil grip, place it in a transverse manner on the temporal portion of the upper eyelid with minimal pressure exerted on the eye. (See Picture 50.2).
- Using minute caudad and cephalad movements, bring the globe of the eye into view.

Identify the ocular anatomy including eyelid, anterior chamber, iris, lens, vitreous body, and

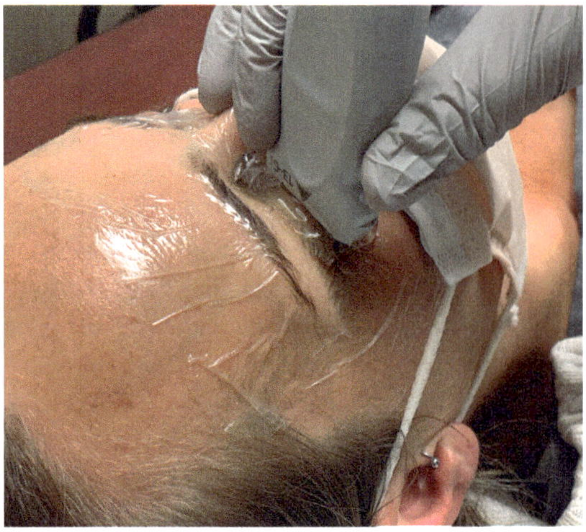

Picture 50.2 Ideal position for performing ocular ultrasound. Image showing how to perform ONSD measurement with proper placement of a Tegaderm dressing over the eye and a linear probe lightly placed with an abundance of ultrasound gel over the closed eye with fingers resting on the bridge of the nose for stability

retina (See Fig. 50.1 and Picture 50.1). Find the optic nerve (ON) which is posterior to the globe and perpendicular to the posterior wall. The ON is hypoechoic, the core is anechoic, and the sheath surrounding it appears hyperechoic. Center the ON in the field of view and then freeze the frame on the clearest image.

- Scroll through the frames to find the image with the cleanest margins for measurement.
- Using the calipers, measure 3 mm back from the globe. This area is the bulbous portion of the ON and is the most sensitive to ICP changes.
- Once a depth of 3 mm is identified, measure perpendicular to that across from each outer edge of the hyperechoic area which will be the diameter of the ONS. (See Fig. 50.1).
- Once the measurement has been obtained in the transverse view, reorient the probe in the sagittal view and obtain another measurement, this time using small movements nasally and temporally to again bring the ONS into view.

If unable to obtain a transverse view secondary to a prominent brow, then it is recommended to obtain a second transverse measurement. Once two measurements are obtained, take the mean to determine the ONSD. Then repeat the process on the opposite eye.

Identification of papilledema can lend value supporting the likelihood of elevated ICP. Unfortunately, there is a paucity of studies looking at papilledema as a sign of acute elevation of ICP, but there is more supportive data on the presence of papilledema as reflection of elevated ICP as a chronic process due to the fact that the development of papilledema takes time [8].

Papilledema can be seen on ocular ultrasound anterior to the ON, where the elevated optic disk can be visualized in the posterior globe as a convexity protruding into the vitreous. Sometimes when measuring the ONSD, an increase in the subarachnoid fluid surrounding the ON can be seen as an echolucent circle, which is termed the crescent sign. While there are limited data on the value of this finding in the critical care setting, there are ophthalmology publications correlating the crescent sign with papilledema and one study showed that the crescent sign had a lower sensitivity compared to ONSD but did have high specificity for papilledema [9].

Another useful tool is using doppler to find the central retinal artery (CRA) which lies in the center of the ON. This can help ensure ONSD measurements are taken in the correct plane. Identification of the CRA can be of benefit when a patient presents with monocular vision loss. The presence of a retrobulbar spot sign (RBSS), which is a hyperechoic spot in the center of the ON, can indicate a central retinal artery occlusion (CRAO), a well-known ophthalmologic emergency. The RBSS represents high specificity for CRAO, but its absence has low sensitivity. Sometimes optic nerve drusen can be mistaken for RBSS, but drusen usually lie at the head of the ON and is much larger than the RBSS, which lies within the ON [10].

Tricks to Obtain Proficiency

Even though this procedure can be learned with a short period of training and performed by any healthcare provider [11], the technique can be challenging. The evaluated structure has millimetric measurements, it could be moving, and miscalculation within the 0.1 of a millimeter can be significant, which calls for perfect proficiency [12]. There are some tricks which can facilitate the learning curve and decrease the inter-rater variance:

- If there is difficulty acquiring an image, the answer is often more gel. It is even more important to have a thick layer of gel in ocular ultrasound as the window is small and the pressure that can be applied is minimal.
- Placing a Tegaderm over the eye can also be of benefit as well as improve patient comfort, just ensure when placing the dressing that there is no air between the Tegaderm and the skin.
- Hand stabilization while performing ocular ultrasound is also vital and this can be accomplished by anchoring the hand on the patient's forehead, bridge of the nose, or midface. This helps avoid overt pressure on the eye that could distort the anatomy or cause eye injury.
- Another tip to help bring the ONSD into focus is to start with the gain at zero to find the globe of the eye, and then as the focus is brought onto the ONS, gradually increase the gain to help sharpen the ONS outline.
- Too much gain can be detrimental since it can cause artifacts when working in millimeters and it is generally not recommended to increase the gain above 60%.

Evolving Evidence

Literature supporting the use of ultrasound for the evaluation of ONSD includes a recent meta-analysis of 40 studies involving more than 5100 patients comparing the accuracy of physical examination, CT head findings, sonography of the ONSD, and transcranial Doppler pulsatility index (TCD-PI) for the diagnosis of elevated ICP in critically ill patients [12]. They found ONSD with a pooled area under the ROC curve of 0.94 (0.91–0.96, I2 = 60.9%), suggesting the optimal cut-off for ONSD of 5 mm and ONSD sonography as a diagnostic alternative, but further studies are needed.

Another meta-analysis including 71 studies found ONSD with a pooled sensitivity, specificity, the positive and negative likelihood ratio of 94%, 87%, 7.23, and 0.07, respectively, for diagnosing increased ICP in all patients, with increased sensitivity for patients with traumatic brain injury (97%), but less sensitivity (92%) when applied to nontraumatic patients, highlighting the importance of the pretest probability on the analysis of the findings [13]. Similar sensitivity was reported by a different meta-analysis (95%) but with higher specificity (92%) and a positive likelihood ratio of 12.5 (95% CI, 4.16–37.5). The high sensitivity and specificity of this study highlights the importance of population selection and group risk stratification [14].

A different study that focused on the reproducibility and accuracy of ONSD compared repeated measurements of the ONSD on 15 healthy volunteers measured by ultrasound (in B-mode using a 9–3 MHz linear array transducer) versus MRI (performed on a 3 T whole-body scanner using a 32-channel phased-array head coil and a rapid T2-weighted half-Fourier acquisition single-shot turbo spin-echo (HASTE) sequence optimized for quantification). They found that comparing ultrasound and MRI there is an acceptable reproducibility ($r > 0.75$, $p \leq 0.001$, mean differences <2%), measurement accuracy ($r = 0.72$, $p = 0.002$, mean difference <5%), and interobserver agreement ($r > 0.82$, $p < 0.001$, mean differences <5%) between the two techniques measuring the ONSD at 3 mm depth behind the papilla [15]. This high intra- and interobserver reliability was also described when comparing ONSD versus ONS measurement [16].

A prospective blinded observational study correlated the ONSD threshold of 5 mm measured by ocular US with a 10(−5) MHz linear probe, compared with ICP >20 cm H_2O measured directly by ventriculostomy. The association between ONSD and ICP was assessed with the Spearman rank correlation coefficient demonstrating a significant positive correlation (0.59 ($p < 0.0005$)) and ROC curve (0.93 (95% confidence interval [CI] = 0.84–0.99)) to distinguish abnormal ICP at this specific cut-off of

5 mm with a sensitivity of 88% (95% CI = 47–99%) and specificity of 93% (95% CI = 78–99%) [17].

In another study, the ONSD measurement was evaluated in 3 point-of-care ultrasound views (inferior, sagittal, and transverse planes) and compared with MRI measurements in 51 healthy patients. In this particular population, wide variability in the correlation (range of 0.1–0.8) between different ultrasound views was found, where the inferior and transverse views achieved the best image quality and highlighted the importance of pretest probability [18].

Ultrasonographic measurement of the ONSD to evaluate the ICP is rapid, accessible, reliable, accurate, noninvasive, easy to learn, and easy to perform. This technique can be used as a screening method before obtaining a brain image (CT or MRI) and a serial follow-up once management has been initiated [2]. Given ocular ultrasound is easy to perform at the bedside, it is a potential tool in the ER or ICU setting [19, 20].

Summary Points

- Understanding the value and limitations of ONSD evaluation is essential for patients with traumatic and nontraumatic brain injury who would benefit from a prompt referral, may or not need emergency treatment, and may or not require invasive therapeutic modalities.
- It is necessary to understand that in neurocritical care the value of ONSD is not in a single measurement or an absolute value in a point of time, but is valuable as a strong tool during daily clinical monitoring to detect raised intracranial pressure and to suspect clinical deterioration, particularly in neurocritical patients, sedated and mechanically ventilated or when invasive ICP monitoring is not available.
- An appropriate technique for ultrasound evaluation of ONSD can be quickly learned and used as an excellent bedside, noninvasive diagnostic tool in the early identification of intracranial hypertension during routine evaluation of neurocritical patients.

Questions

1. A 28-year-old male has a traumatic brain injury as a consequence of a motor vehicle accident. He is transferred to ICU due to altered mental status. During his ocular ultrasound evaluation, the optic nerve sheath diameter (ONSD) measurements in both eyes are as follow: 5.7 mm and 6.2 mm (left eye) and 5.8 mm and 6.2 mm (right eye) in both orientations. Does this patient have intracranial pressure (ICP) elevation?
   A. Yes
   B. No
   Answer: A.
2. Current available evidence about the diagnostic performance of ocular ultrasound in the evaluation of elevated intracranial pressure is true, except:
   A. Bilateral ultrasonographic findings of papilledema are common in patients with elevated intracranial pressure, but absent in normal patients, representing high sensitivity and low specificity.
   B. Ocular sonography should not be performed by emergency physicians due to the poor correlation of their measurement with optical coherence tomography.
   C. Papilledema outperformed optic nerve sheath diameter with high sensitivity lower specificity using a cutoff value of >5.8 mm.
   D. The ideal point for measuring the ONSD is the bulbous portion of the optic nerve 3 mm back from the globe.
   Answer: B.

References

1. Moretti R, Pizzi B. Ultrasonography of the optic nerve in neurocritically ill patients. Acta Anaesthesiol Scand. 2011;55(6):644–52. https://doi.org/10.1111/j.1399-6576.2011.02432.x.
2. Jeon JP, Lee SU, Kim SE, Kang SH, Yang JS, Choi HJ, et al. Correlation of optic nerve sheath diameter with directly measured intracranial pressure in Korean adults using bedside ultrasonography. PLoS One. 2017;12(9):e0183170.

3. Hansen HC, Helmke K. Validation of the optic nerve sheath response to changing cerebrospinal fluid pressure: ultrasound findings during intrathecal infusion tests. J Neurosurg. 1977;87(1):34–40. https://doi.org/10.3171/jns.1997.87.1.0034.
4. Tayal VS, Neulander M, Norton HJ, Foster T, Saunders T, Blaivas M. Emergency department sonographic measurement of optic nerve sheath diameter to detect findings of increased intracranial pressure in adult head injury patients. Ann Emerg Med. 2007;49(4):508–14. https://doi.org/10.1016/j.annemergmed.2006.06.040.
5. Blaivas M, Theodoro D, Sierzenski PR. A study of bedside ocular ultrasonography in the emergency department. Acad Emerg Med. 2002;9(8):791–9. https://doi.org/10.1111/j.1553-2712.2002.tb02166.x.
6. Teismann N, Lenaghan P, Nolan R, Stein J, Green A. Point-of-care ocular ultrasound to detect optic disc swelling. Acad Emerg Med. 2013;20(9):920–5. https://doi.org/10.1111/acem.12206.
7. Lochner P, Leone MA, Coppo L, Nardone R, Zedde ML, Cantello R, et al. B-mode transorbital ultrasononography for the diagnosis of acute optic neuritis. A systematic review. Clin Neurophysiol. 2016;127(1):803–9. https://doi.org/10.1016/j.clinph.2015.05.005.
8. Steffen H, Eifert B, Aschoff A, Kolling GH, Völcker HE. The diagnostic value of optic disc evaluation in acute elevated intracranial pressure. Ophthalmology. 1996;103(8):1229–32. https://doi.org/10.1016/s0161-6420(96)30518-6.
9. Mohson KI, Auday N. Role of orbital ultrasound in the assessment of clinically detected papilledema. J Med Ultrasound. 2019;27(3):135–40. https://doi.org/10.4103/JMU.JMU_70_18.
10. Smith AT, Wilbert CD, Ferre RM. Using the retrobulbar spot sign to assist in diagnosis and management of central retinal artery occlusions. J Ultrasound Med. 2020;39(1):197–202. https://doi.org/10.1002/jum.15073.
11. Zeiler FA, Ziesmann MT, Goeres P, Unger B, Park J, Karakitsos D, et al. A unique method for estimating the reliability learning curve of optic nerve sheath diameter ultrasound measurement. Crit Ultrasound J. 2016;8(1):9. https://doi.org/10.1186/s13089-016-0044-x.
12. Fernando SM, Tran A, Cheng W, Rochwerg B, Taljaard M, Kyeremanteng K, et al. Diagnosis of elevated intracranial pressure in critically ill adults: systematic review and meta-analysis. BMJ. 2019;366:l4225. https://doi.org/10.1136/bmj.l4225.
13. Koziarz A, Sne N, Kegel F, et al. Bedside optic nerve ultrasonography for diagnosing increased intracranial pressure: a systematic review and meta-analysis. Ann Intern Med. 2019;171:896–905.
14. Ohle R, McIsaac SM, Woo MY, Perry JJ. Sonography of the optic nerve sheath diameter for detection of raised intracranial pressure compared to computed tomography: a systematic review and meta-analysis. J Ultrasound Med. 2015;34(7):1285–94. https://doi.org/10.7863/ultra.34.7.1285.
15. Bäuerle J, Schuchardt F, Schroeder L, Egger K, Weigel M, Harloff A. Reproducibility and accuracy of optic nerve sheath diameter assessment using ultrasound compared to magnetic resonance imaging. BMC Neurol. 2013;13:187. https://doi.org/10.1186/1471-2377-13-187.
16. Lochner P, Coppo L, Cantello R, Nardone R, Naldi A, Leone MA, et al. Intra- and interobserver reliability of transorbital sonographic assessment of the optic nerve sheath diameter and optic nerve diameter in healthy adults. J Ultrasound. 2016 mar;19(1):41–5.
17. Kimberly HH, Shah S, Marill K, Noble V. Correlation of optic nerve sheath diameter with direct measurement of intracranial pressure. Acad Emerg Med. 2008;15(2):201–4. https://doi.org/10.1111/j.1553-2712.2007.00031.x.
18. Raval R, Shen J, Lau D, Ferguson N, Kelly T, Daniels J, et al. Comparison of three point-of-care ultrasound views and MRI measurements for optic nerve sheath diameter: a prospective validity study. Neurocrit Care. 2020;33(1):173–81. https://doi.org/10.1007/s12028-019-00881-7.
19. Oberfoell S, Murphy D, French A, Trent S, Richards D. Inter-rater reliability of sonographic optic nerve sheath diameter measurements by emergency medicine physicians. J Ultrasound Med. 2017;36(8):1579–84. https://doi.org/10.7863/ultra.16.05055.
20. Toscano M, Spadetta G, Pulitano P, Rocco M, Di Piero V, Mecarelli O, et al. Optic nerve sheath diameter ultrasound evaluation in intensive care unit: possible role and clinical aspects in neurological critical patients' daily monitoring. Biomed Res Int. 2017;2017:1621428. https://doi.org/10.1155/2017/1621428.

Transcranial Ultrasound

51

Nina Massad and Shivani Ghoshal

Learning Objectives

1. Identify indications for the use of transcranial Doppler
2. Understand TCD metrics and modes
3. Appreciate limitations in TCD
4. Understand anatomical landmarks and technique

Indications

Transcranial Doppler (TCD) is a non-invasive, cost-effective point-of-care tool to help evaluate and understand cerebral hemodynamics, using a 2 MHz frequency phased array ultrasound probe. This is especially useful in the neurocritical care patient, in which varying degrees of consciousness may cloud the intensivist's ability to follow the neurologic exam. TCD can be used to evaluate and trend information on intracranial blood flow in a variety of conditions.

TCD is especially useful in neurocritical care when evaluating for cerebral vasospasm, cerebral vasculopathy, and ischemic stroke. It also has broader utility when investigating the effects of systemic critical illness on the central nervous system. Examples of this include ICP monitoring in acute liver failure, dialysis disequilibrium, and cerebral circulatory arrest. This chapter will focus on the application and interpretation of TCD in adults with critical illness.

An important distinction should be established between non-imaging transcranial Doppler with color M-mode and transcranial color-coded duplex sonography (TCCS), the latter of which can be readily utilized at the bedside in the ICU. TCCS provides direct visualization of brain structures and the major cerebral vessels compared with non-imaging TCD. Once landmarks are identified using grey-scale (B-mode), color flow Doppler can be used to identify blood vessels of interest, as it is color-coded to demonstrate the direction of flow to and away from the transducer. From there, a pulsed wave Doppler can be implemented to investigate cerebral hemodynamics by using pulses to measure flow in a vessel of interest.

TCD Measurements

Notable metrics in transcranial Doppler include the TCD waveform, mean flow velocity, and pulsatility index, which are important to define. The **TCD waveform** (Fig. 51.1) typically shows a sharp systolic upstroke and stepwise deceleration with positive end-diastolic flow. The first peak on the waveform is the peak systolic velocity (PSV), typically a rapid upstroke and measured in cm/s. When there is low resistance in intracranial arte-

N. Massad · S. Ghoshal (✉)
Department of Neurology, Columbia University, New York, NY, USA
e-mail: sg3450@cumc.columbia.edu

M. J. Lanspa, A. T. Levinson (eds.), *Echocardiography and Ultrasonography in the ICU*, Respiratory Medicine, https://doi.org/10.1007/978-3-031-80038-2_51

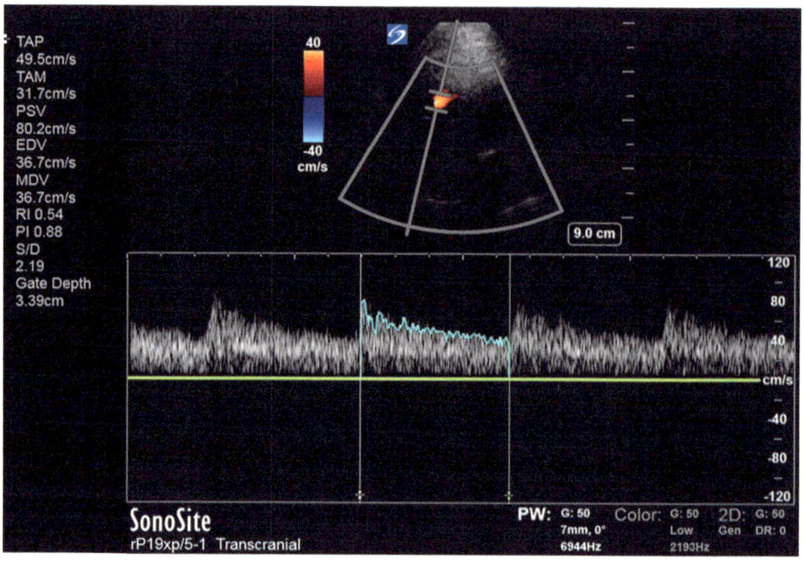

Fig. 51.1 TCD waveform of the MCA, with a sharp systolic upstroke and stepwise deceleration with positive end-diastolic flow

rial flow, the end-diastolic velocity falls under 30% of the PSV value. The **mean flow velocity (MFV)** can be derived from the following equation. Normal MFV varies based on the vessel; it is typically highest in the middle cerebral artery (MCA) and is normally <80 cm/s.

$$\text{Mean Flow Velocity} = \text{End Diastolic Velocity} + \frac{1}{3}\left(\text{Peak Systolic Velocity} - \text{End Diastolic Velocity}\right)$$

Per the Monro-Kellie doctrine, given that the skull is a rigid structure containing three components (brain parenchyma, blood, and cerebrospinal fluid), increasing ICP causes the narrowing of cerebral vessels. This results in the increase of systolic peak flows along with the blunting of diastolic flow. The **pulsatility index (PI)** can be used as a helpful tool for the estimation of ICP. PI reflects flow resistance; this is calculated with the following equation. The normal PI is ≤1.2 for intracranial circulation [1–7].

$$\text{Pulsatility Index} = \frac{\text{Peak Systolic Velocity} - \text{End Diastolic Velocity}}{\text{Mean Flow Velocity}}.$$

Cerebral Vasospasm

Cerebral vasospasm is a major complication of aneurysmal subarachnoid hemorrhage (SAH). Its risk is highest between 3 and 14 days after hemorrhage, though it may extend up to 21 days after the event. Arteriolar cerebral vasospasm in subarachnoid hemorrhage can lead to the development of delayed cerebral ischemia and poor neurologic outcomes. Daily serial TCDs are a standard of care non-invasive measure, in conjunction with the neurologic exam, to assess the risk of vasospasm.

TCDs in subarachnoid hemorrhage involve daily assessment of mean flow velocity, particularly in the MCA, but also extracranial internal carotid arteries, anterior cerebral arteries, and basilar and vertebral arteries. In vasospasm, the diameter of the tube decreases. Based on **Bernoulli's**

principle with respect to the conservation of mass, the velocity of the blood must increase as the same volume of blood must pass through a smaller caliber tube. In this way, the mean velocity of blood increases to 120–159 cm/s in mild vasospasm, 160–199 cm/s in moderate vasospasm, and over 200 cm/s in severe vasospasm.

In the setting of a hyperdynamic state, flow velocities will also be higher. This becomes relevant in the SAH patient, in which blood pressure is often targeted to therapeutic hypertension once the aneurysm is secured. Other physiologic factors can affect flow velocity, such as age, pCO_2, and hematocrit in addition to mean arterial pressure. To help distinguish hyperemia from cerebral vasospasm, a useful concept is the **Lindegaard ratio**.

$$\text{Lindegaard Ratio} = \frac{\text{MCA mean flow velocity}}{\text{Ipsilateral extracranial ICA mean flow velocity}}$$

A Lindegaard ratio >3 is suggestive of vasospasm, with 3–5 more consistent with mild to moderate vasospasm, and a ratio >6 typically indicating severe vasospasm. When concerned for vasospasm based on TCD and clinical examination, this can be further evaluated with a CT angiogram (CTA) of the head and neck with perfusion, but the gold standard remains a conventional angiogram.

Cerebral Vasospasm: Limitations

It is important to note that other entities can increase MFV. For example, intracranial atherosclerosis causes vessel narrowing and increased MFV. Because of this, the trend in flow velocities over time with serial TCDs tends to be more useful than absolute values. Assessing for cerebral vasospasm is also more difficult for the posterior circulation, specifically the vertebral and basilar arteries, and often waveforms cannot be obtained. Visualization of these arteries is done using the transforaminal window, where the skull is much thicker than the transtemporal window. Of course, like many aspects of point-of-care ultrasound, accurate measurement is operator-dependent and requires proper vessel identification.

Cerebral Autoregulation

Cerebral autoregulation is a homeostatic process where cerebral blood vessels can maintain constant cerebral blood flow across a range of systemic blood pressures. TCD can be used to assess cerebral autoregulation in conditions with concern for cerebral vasculopathy and, in situations of impairment, can be used to determine optimal target blood pressure to optimize autoregulation. **The mean flow index (Mx)** can be used to monitor dynamic autoregulation; this is calculated as the coefficient index between cerebral perfusion pressure and flow velocity. Negative Mx values or Mx values that approach zero indicate intact cerebral autoregulation, while positive values that approach 1.0 indicate impaired autoregulation.

TCD also has utility in assessing cerebral hemodynamics in patients with Moyamoya disease and is used in some centers to assess patients before and after surgical intervention. To evaluate these patients' cerebrovascular autoregulation and reserve, vasodilation is induced by acetazolamide or inhaled CO_2.

Assessment of Intracranial Pressure

TCD can be used as a non-invasive tool to identify patients at risk for developing increased **intracranial pressure (ICP)**. This can be applied to common disease states in neurology, such as traumatic brain injury or intracranial hemorrhage, but also cardiac arrest and hepatic encephalopathy. In the setting of intact autoregulation, when systemic blood flow is decreased, there is compensatory vasodilatation in the brain to maintain cerebral blood flow, and with this, decreased flow velocities while overall maintaining PI. Conversely, when there is impaired autoregulation, increased ICP is reflected by a high pulsatility index, indicating worsened cerebral perfusion pressure.

Although parenchymal or intraventricular monitors remain the gold standard for assessment of ICP, TCD, along with other non-invasive assessments of ICP, such as pupillometry and optic nerve sheath diameter, can be valuable in clinical decision-making. TCD trends can be valuable in decision-making, both to help tailor clinical interventions (such as hyperosmolar therapy and target cerebral perfusion pressure) and to help decide if an invasive monitor should be placed.

Assessment of Intracranial Pressure: Limitations

TCD can provide a general estimate for ICP but should not be interpreted as a surrogate for an invasive ICP monitor. Like with mean flow velocity, there is an age effect on flow PI, where increasing age results in significantly higher flow PI. Other factors that might affect blood vessel diameter, such as intracranial atherosclerosis, can affect the PI. Again, similar to flow velocities in cerebral vasospasm, the absolute values are less meaningful than serial monitoring and observing trends over time.

Increased mean arterial pressure and decreased pCO_2 can alter the PI and should be taken into consideration. Additionally, patients who are on assistive cardiac devices will not have an interpretable pulsatility index on TCD. This includes patients on V-A extracorporeal membrane oxygenation or patients on left ventricular assist devices.

Cerebral Circulatory Arrest

Transcranial Doppler can be used as a bedside ancillary test when suspecting brain death. While the determination of brain death is typically a clinical diagnosis, certain circumstances necessitate the use of ancillary studies to confirm the diagnosis. Continued and refractory increases in intracranial pressure can ultimately lead to **cerebral circulatory arrest (CCA),** or brain death. Pathophysiologically, cytotoxic swelling causes progressive cerebral edema, lack of adequate oxygenation of neuronal tissue leading to further edema, increased cerebrovascular flow resistance due to mass effect, and decrease in perfusion, herniation, and eventually complete cessation of blood flow to the brain.

Brain death on TCD is essentially a continuation of the findings that can be seen with high ICP. There is an initial increase in flow velocity during systole with a corresponding decrease, or blunting, of diastolic flow. In CCA, after severe blunting of diastolic flow, there is a reversal of diastolic flow near equal to the systolic forward flow, known as **reverberating flow**. Finally, there is progression to the absence of diastolic flow with small systolic spikes followed by complete absence of flow. Of note, in most medical jurisdictions, TCD cannot be used as an official ancillary test but can help as an adjunct to determine if an accepted confirmatory ancillary test should be performed.

Cerebral Circulatory Arrest: Limitations

Especially when concerned about brain death, it is important to understand the limitations of transcranial Doppler. Here, operator experience is critical, as having suboptimal windows could easily be misinterpreted as an absence of intracranial vascular flow and misdiagnosis of brain death. Additionally, up to 10% of patients may not have adequate transtemporal windows. For this reason, in places where TCD is an acceptable diagnostic tool to declare death, a second TCD must be repeated 30 min later to confirm cessation of blood flow.

Ischemic Stroke

Transcranial Doppler can be used in the setting of acute ischemic stroke to demonstrate an arterial occlusion. Advantages of this over other imaging modalities are that it is rapidly obtained at the bedside and is a non-invasive tool. The **thrombolysis in brain ischemia (TIBI) score** was developed to grade Doppler flow and determine clinical severity in patients with ischemic stroke following treatment with tPA. In some settings, TCD can be used in patients with large vessel occlusion to assess for recanalization in real-time during endovascular treatment.

TCDs can also be useful after the acute setting in investigating the etiology of ischemic stroke. Detection of micro-emboli in the intracranial cerebral arteries suggests an underlying embolic etiology of ischemic stroke and indicates an increased risk of recurrent stroke. **High-intensity transient signals** can indicate either gaseous or solid micro-emboli. These can be detected by insonating an artery, typically middle cerebral arteries, for an extended period of time in color M-mode if using non-imaging TCD, or in pulsed wave Doppler in TCCS. Micro-emboli will appear as very brief vertical signals and emit a very brief "chirp" sound.

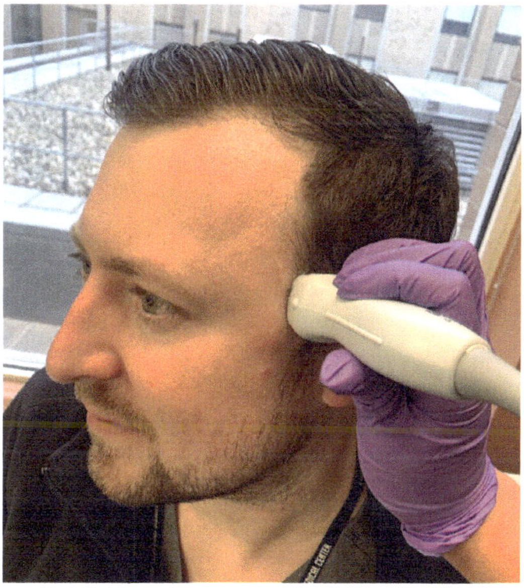

Fig. 51.2 The transtemporal window is obtained by placing a probe on the temporal bone at the level of the pterion, with the probe marker oriented anteriorly

Ischemic Stroke: Limitations

Limitations of this certainly depend on the amount of time the probe remains in place to insonate the vessel in question. Vessel insonation is typically done for 30 min, which is a limitation depending on time and resource availability. Artifact is also commonly seen and, at times, can be hard to distinguish from the true high-intensity transient signal.

Anatomical Landmarks and Technique

Transcranial Doppler allows the examiner to directly visualize the major cerebral vessels but requires familiarity and understanding of the anatomy of cerebral vasculature in order to perform. There are three transcranial windows used in comprehensive TCD: **transtemporal, transorbital**, and **transforaminal (or suboccipital)**. A **submandibular** approach can also be used to evaluate the terminal internal carotid artery; however, it is not always performed in point-of-care TCD.

The **transtemporal** window is obtained (Fig. 51.2) by insonating the temporal bone at the level of the pterion, where the skull is the thinnest. A starting depth of 12–16 cm should be employed until the hyperechoic, curvilinear contralateral temporal bone is visualized.

The examiner should place the probe on the temporal bone anterior to the ear and adjust the device until the cerebral peduncles of the midbrain are identified—these appear hypoechoic with a butterfly-shaped appearance (Fig. 51.3). Just anterior to the peduncles at a depth of 6–8 cm is the third ventricle with characteristically hyperechoic borders.

Using **a color Doppler** at this point will allow the examiner to visualize the circle of Willis (Fig. 51.4). The MCA should be readily identified as a linear, nearly vertical structure with blood flow toward the transducer in a red color Doppler signal. In the transtemporal window, a slight adjustment of the insonation angle can help capture the anterior and posterior cerebral arteries as well. The anterior cerebral artery flows away from the transducer (blue Doppler signal) at a depth of 6–7 cm, while the posterior cerebral arteries angulate posteriorly and away (with blue Doppler signal) at a 6–6.5 cm depth. After obtaining the desired information, this is then repeated contralaterally for the opposite hemisphere.

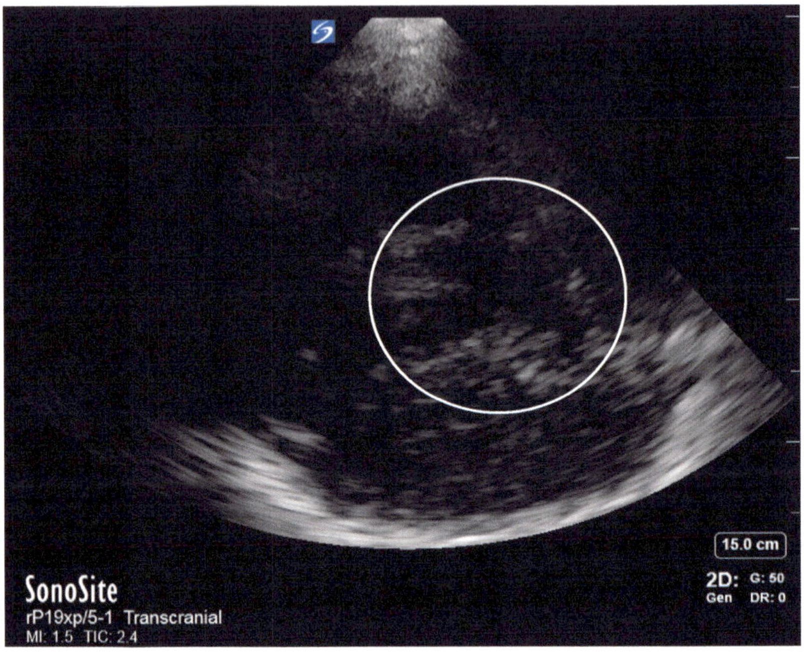

Fig. 51.3 The transtemporal window demonstrating the hypoechoic butterfly-shaped appearance of the midbrain

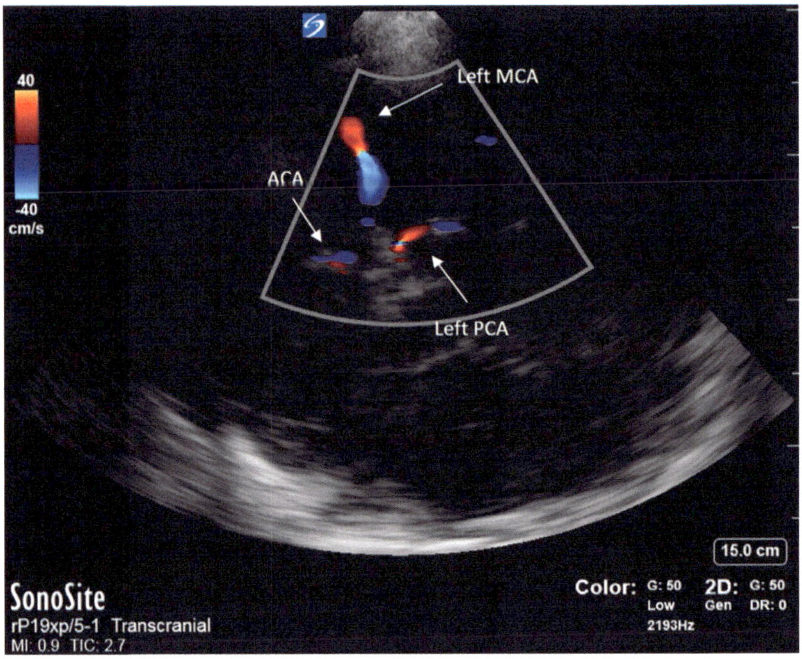

Fig. 51.4 The transtemporal window using the color Doppler

The **transforaminal** or suboccipital window is obtained by placing the transducer at the junction between the occiput and posterior midline of the neck and the occiput at a starting depth of 10–12 cm, with the probe directed toward the foramen magnum. On color Doppler, the vertebral arteries will be visible coursing away from the probe around 6.5–7 cm deep and joining as the basilar artery, which courses at a depth of 8–10 cm; this appears blue with a Y-shaped appearance. The **transorbital** window is used primarily to insonate the ophthalmic artery; this is visualized in the same window used to obtain optic nerve sheath diameter. Ophthalmic artery flow reversal can be seen in the setting of high-grade internal carotid artery occlusion or stenosis and therefore can provide insight into hemodynamics.

Visualization of the extracranial internal carotid, necessary for the Lindegaard ratio calculation, is done using the **submandibular window**. The ultrasound probe should be placed on the patient's neck with the marker directed cranially until the carotid artery is identified as pulsatile and noncompressible relative to the compressible internal jugular vein. Slide the probe up until the carotid bifurcation is identified and the internal carotid is in view; mean velocity can then be calculated using pulsed-wave Doppler.

When obtaining all windows, consideration must be made regarding the relative direction of the probe relative to the direction of blood flow in a particular vessel. Along with the probe's relative direction and position in a particular window and depth of insonation, one should be able to identify vessels in the major branches of the circle of Willis.

Summary Points

- Notable metrics in transcranial Doppler include the TCD waveform, mean flow velocity, and pulsatility index.
- TCD can be used as a non-invasive tool to identify patients at risk for developing increased **intracranial pressure (ICP)**. This can be applied to common disease states in neurology, such as traumatic brain injury or intracranial hemorrhage, but also cardiac arrest and hepatic encephalopathy.
- Transcranial Doppler allows the examiner to directly visualize the major cerebral vessels but requires familiarity and understanding of the anatomy of cerebral vasculature in order to perform.

Questions

1. What is the optimal transcranial window used to measure the mean velocity of the extracranial internal carotid artery?
   A. Transtemporal
   B. Suboccipital
   C. Submandibular
   D. Transorbital
   Answer: C
2. Which of the following physiologic factors does NOT result in increased TCD flow velocity?
   A. Increased $PaCO_2$
   B. Increase in cardiac output
   C. Low blood viscosity
   D. Decreased mean arterial pressure
   Answer: D

References

1. Klein SP, Depreitere B, Meyfroidt G. How I monitor cerebral autoregulation. Crit Care. 2019;23:160. https://doi.org/10.1186/s13054-019-2454-1.
2. Lau V, Arntfield R. Point of care transcranial Doppler by intensivists. Crit Ultrasound J. 2017;9:21. https://doi.org/10.1186/s13089-017-0077.
3. Lau VI, Jaidka A, Wiskar K, Packer N, Elaine Tang J, Koenig S, et al. Better with ultrasound - transcranial Doppler. Chest. 2019;157:142. https://doi.org/10.1016/j.chest.2019.08.2204.
4. Purkayastha S, Sorond F. Transcranial Doppler ultrasound: technique and application. Semin Neurol. 2012;32(4):411–20. https://doi.org/10.1055/s-0032-13318129.
5. Reynolds PS, Greenberg JP, Lien LM, Meads DC, Myers LG, Tegeler CH. Ophthalmic artery flow direction on color flow duplex imaging is highly specific for severe carotid stenosis. J Neuroimaging. 2002 Jan;12(1):5–8. https://doi.org/10.1111/j.1552-6569.2002.tb00082.x.
6. Roach ES, Golomb MR, Adams R, Biller J, Daniels S, Deveber G, et al. Management of stroke in infants and children: a scientific statement from a Special Writing Group of the American Heart Association Stroke Council and the Council on Cardiovascular Disease in the Young. Stroke. 2008;39:2644.
7. Robba C, Taccone FS. How I use transcranial Doppler. Crit Care. 2019;23:420. https://doi.org/10.1186/s13054-019-2700-6.

Part IV

Complex Clinical Scenarios

Diagnostic Approach to Patient in Shock

52

Jan Kasal and Chakra Venkata

Learning Objectives

1. Recognize the image patterns for different types of shock.
2. Understand basic and advanced techniques to characterize different types of shock.
3. Review different ultrasound protocols for assessing patients in shock.

Key Points

- The echocardiographic approach to undifferentiated shock starts with the recognition of image patterns of hypovolemia, LV failure, RV failure, tamponade, valvular pathology, and decreased vasomotor tone.
- The objectives are to rapidly identify the shock mechanism, narrow down the etiology of shock, choose treatments, monitor the effectiveness of therapies, and avoid potentially harmful interventions.
- The process of obtaining the correct diagnosis, identifying the best therapeutic options, and delivering the appropriate therapies in shock is often done simultaneously, at the bedside, by an ICU practitioner.
- There are many described protocolized ultrasound approaches. While the evidence for echocardiography in shock is evolving, the ICU community has embraced the widespread use of point-of-care ultrasound in shock.

J. Kasal (✉)
Washington University School of Medicine, St. Louis, MO, USA
e-mail: jankasal@wustl.edu

C. Venkata
Saint Louis University/Mercy Hospital St. Louis, St. Louis, MO, USA
e-mail: Chakradhar.Venkata@mercy.net

Introduction

Echocardiography is an essential tool in the initial assessment of patients with cardiopulmonary instability [1]. This principle applies especially to patients with undifferentiated hypotension (hypotension without known cause) but also holds for patients with a preexisting working diagnosis of the underlying mechanism responsible for hypotension.

The traditional categories of shock [2] **and the categories based on echocardiographic examination largely overlap, but they are not synonymous**. Under the conventional classification, shock can be hypovolemic, cardiogenic, obstructive, or distributive. Echocardiography allows rapid identification of patterns that are based primarily on visual findings. Hypovolemia, left ventricular (LV) failure, right ventricular (RV) failure, tamponade, and valvular pathology have unique characteristics, while the pattern of decreased vasomotor tone (distributive shock) is not specific. The echocardiographic approach may yield more granular information than the traditional classification. Echocardiography-

M. J. Lanspa, A. T. Levinson (eds.), *Echocardiography and Ultrasonography in the ICU*, Respiratory Medicine, https://doi.org/10.1007/978-3-031-80038-2_52

based diagnoses sometimes require dramatically different treatments within a single traditional shock category. For example, a patient with tamponade and a patient with acute pulmonary embolism would be classified as an obstructive shock in the traditional sense. Still, these patients would look vastly different on echocardiography and receive different therapies.

The degree of severity of findings in patients in shock varies. The practitioner must tailor the echocardiography approach to the urgency of the situation. Cardiac arrest from hemorrhage is an extreme form of hypovolemic shock. A brief echocardiographic exam would show the extreme signs of hypovolemia on the 2D exam without the need for further quantification and Doppler. On the other hand, a patient with sepsis who has received initial fluid resuscitation yet still needs vasopressors and still manifests hypoperfusion is on the opposite end of the spectrum of hypovolemia. The echocardiographic exam, in that case, would require advanced techniques, including quantitative Doppler, looking for preload responsiveness.

The examination should start with a working list of possible mechanisms and causes of shock. The knowledge of the clinical information about the patient should drive the drafting of the pretest differential diagnostic list. In addition, the different clinical settings will mean different pretest probabilities of individual types of shock. For example, in an emergency department setting, the most common cause of undifferentiated hypotension is sepsis, while tamponade is uncommon [3]. However, the same may not be accurate for other settings (e.g., medical ICU, surgery ICU, cardiothoracic ICU).

Principles of Echocardiographic Approach to Shock

At its core, there may be only a limited number of basic echocardiographic patterns encountered in hypotensive patients. These patterns are **(1) small and hyperdynamic LV (usually reflecting hypovolemia)**, **(2) LV failure**, **(3) RV failure**, **(4) tamponade**, **(5) valvular pathology**, and **(6) no specific echocardiographic finding (reflecting decreased vasomotor tone)**. We will discuss details of individual findings in the following sections.

The goals of echocardiography during shock will depend on the timing of the exam. The initial goal of echocardiography is to identify the mechanism responsible for circulatory failure and select the most appropriate treatments. Subsequently, during the later phase, the goal shifts toward using echocardiography to guide and titrate treatments (e.g., fluid, vasopressor, inotropic therapy). Repeated echocardiographic evaluation is critical if there is a lack of improvement despite appropriate treatments and unexpected hemodynamic worsening.

Examiners must address immediately life-threatening problems first. These (tamponade, tension pneumothorax, aortic dissection, and acute valvular regurgitation) need specific interventions and early referrals.

For conceptual ease, one can view the echocardiographic techniques as either basic or advanced. The degree of complexity ranges from focused cardiac ultrasound to more complex applications. Focused cardiac ultrasound is goal- and problem-oriented, limited in scope, simplified, qualitative, or semiquantitative [1]. With the increased availability of ultrasound education and increased availability of technology, many practitioners are becoming proficient in techniques beyond the focused exam. In reality, one must seamlessly move between the basic and advanced techniques depending on the clinical situation and either be skilled in the technique or refer further. For example, TEE may be necessary for the postpericardiotomy shock of unclear etiology and non-diagnostic TTE.

Once the examiner identifies the basic echocardiographic pattern, he/she should generate a **differential list of possible causes** of this pattern (Table 52.1) because the reasons (and treatments required) may differ (Table 52.2). An example would be RV failure caused by acute pulmonary embolism or ARDS, processes with the same echo appearance but drastically different treatment approaches.

Table 52.1 Differential list of common ICU causes of shock based on echo finding

Echocardiographic finding	Etiology
LV failure	Global dysfunction (dilated cardiomyopathy; myocarditis; sepsis) Regional dysfunction (myocardial ischemia; tako-tsubo cardiomyopathy)
RV failure	Acute cor pulmonale (pulmonary embolism; ARDS) Acute on chronic cor pulmonale RV infarction Biventricular failure
Hypovolemia	Bleeding; sepsis (early phase) LVOT obstruction
Tamponade	Pericardial circumferential effusion (bleeding, uremia, malignancy, autoimmune) Regional compression (hematoma s/p cardiothoracic surgery; hemothorax/pleural effusion; solid masses)
Valvular pathology	Mitral regurgitation: Endocarditis, myocardial ischemia, trauma, myxomatous disease Aortic regurgitation: Endocarditis, aortic dissection, myocardial ischemia Aortic stenosis
Decreased vasomotor tone	Sepsis; adrenal insufficiency; end-stage liver disease; vasodilators

Table 52.2 Echocardiographic findings and therapeutic considerations

Echo finding	Therapeutic considerations
LV failure	Inotrope Regional wall motion abnormalities: Revascularization Mechanical circulatory support
RV failure	Inotrope Vasopressor Adjust mechanical ventilation setting (PEEP, tidal volume) Anticoagulation/thrombolysis/embolectomy Pulmonary vasodilator ECMO
Hypovolemia	Crystalloid Colloid Blood product LVOT obstruction: Volume, alpha mimetic, avoid inotrope
Tamponade	Pericardiocentesis/pericardial window Resternotomy post pericardiotomy Evacuation of hemothorax, pleural effusion
Valvular pathology	Cardiothoracic surgery consultation Mechanical circulatory support (no IABP if AR)
Decreased vasomotor tone	Vasopressor Stress dose hydrocortisone Source control in sepsis Antidote in calcium channel overdose

Technical aspects of image acquisition must be kept in mind. Examinations should be focused but systematic, using several standard echocardiographic views. These views are parasternal long axis (PLAX), parasternal short axis (PSAX), apical four-chamber (A4C), and subcostal (SC). In an extreme emergency (e.g., arrest), one key view (e.g., SC) is sufficient. In the case of repeated serial examinations, one view may be adequate [1]. One should use the same machine, settings, and sector size to reduce between-exams variability. The degree of complexity ranges from basic findings (qualitative, semiquantitative) to advanced (quantitative).

An essential part of the examination is carefully **considering all available ultrasound modalities.** The evaluation usually starts with an echo-centered approach with further inputs from lung/vascular/abdominal ultrasound as needed. Some authors proposed approaches based primarily on non-cardiac modalities such as lung ultrasound [4].

TEE is necessary for the minority but significant group of patients with shock. The indications for TEE are either because TTE views are not available or because TTE is inherently limited in identifying the pathology. In patients with surgical wounds/dressings/devices, lung hyperinflation from PEEP/asthma/COPD, and obesity, TTE views may not be possible. In patients with aortic dissection, papillary muscle rupture, prosthetic valve endocarditis/clot, or tamponade after cardiothoracic surgery, even good TTE may not yield sufficient information. The most important aspect is recognizing the indication to move beyond the TTE; practitioners may perform TEE or refer patients for TEE.

Examination Techniques and Specific Findings

Identifying the basic echocardiographic pattern is just an initial step of evaluating the patient in shock in the hands of an experienced practitioner. After recognizing the basic pattern, the practitioner should perform a detailed examination utilizing advanced echocardiographic techniques. However, this may ultimately depend on time limitations, urgency, operator skills, available windows, clinical background, and the clinical questions asked. The specific techniques and findings are listed in Table 52.3. Major points and caveats will be discussed in the next section; further details can be found in other chapters.

LV Failure

Finding acute LV dysfunction should trigger a search for the cause. LV dysfunction can be **global or regional**. Usually (but not always), the regional wall motion abnormalities in ICU may be caused by coronary artery disease or Takotsubo cardiomyopathy, while global LV dysfunction is caused by sepsis or myocarditis.

This approach should not be confused with the classification based on morphofunctional phenotype under the MOGES classification. Within that framework, the cardiomyopathies are dilated, hypertrophic, restrictive, arrhythmogenic RV cardiomyopathy, and noncompaction of myocardium [5].

Myocardial ischemia may manifest with regional wall motion abnormalities or global LV dysfunction and other acute complications not appearing as acute LV systolic dysfunction. These complications (LV free wall rupture with pseudoaneurysm and hemopericardium, ventricular septal rupture, papillary muscle rupture, ischemic mitral regurgitation, RV infarction) may present with shock. The mechanisms of shock in these cases are different from acute LV systolic dysfunction.

Takotsubo cardiomyopathy (stress-induced cardiomyopathy) can mimic acute coronary artery syndrome in the setting of normal epicardial coronary arteries. The transient wall motion abnormalities may be typical (apical) or atypical (midventricular or basal) and extend beyond specific coronary artery distribution.

Additional findings to consider include **wall thickness** (for cardiomyopathy or hypertensive heart disease), **excessive trabeculations** (noncompaction), **aneurysm** (CAD, arrhythmogenic cardiomyopathy), **valvular abnormalities** (MR is present in ischemic cardiomyopathy), **pulmonary artery pressure**, and **RV function** (may be reduced in patients with ischemic cardiomyopathy).

Heart failure with reduced EF (HFrEF) is said to be present if LVEF is 40% or less. However, in shock management, one must realize there may be patients with low LVEF in whom the cause of shock is actually not the low EF with low cardiac output, while other patients with normal LVEF may be in cardiogenic shock. We discussed the role of the **loading conditions** when interpreting ventricular function under the general limitations section. **LVOT VTI** offers the advantage of good repeatability in ICU patients [6], assesses stroke volume under varying preload, inotrope, and heart rate, and is available even if there is no parasternal view in ICU patients [7].

Table 52.3 Basic and advanced examination techniques

Basic techniques	Advanced techniques
LV failure	
Visual estimation of LV EF (normal, reduced) (2D)	**Visual estimation of LV EF** (<30%, 30–40%, 40–50%, 50–70%, >70%) **Regional wall motion abnormalities** (2D) **Signs of chronicity** (thin LV walls; dilatation of LV (LVIDd >6 cm); LV hypertrophy) (2D or M-mode) **LVOT VTI** (estimate of stroke volume) (PW) **Diastolic evaluation** (mitral E, A, E/A; mitral annulus lateral and medial e'; E/e') (PW/tissue Doppler)
RV failure	
RV dilatation (in A4C) (ratio >0.6, severe if >1.0. **Interventricular septal flattening** (in PSAX) (all 2D) **Clot in transit** (2D)	**RV dilatation** in A4C (base diameter of RV (RVDD) >4.1 cm) (2D) **RV function**: TAPSE (M-mode), S' (tissue Doppler) **RV hypertrophy** (>5 mm) (2D) **Aneurysms** **LV systolic dysfunction** **Displaced septal position of tricuspid valve** **Regional wall motion: McConnell sign** (RV hypokinesis with apical sparing) (2D) **60/60 sign** (PASP <60 mmHg/RVOT AT <60 ms) (CW/PW)
Hypovolemia	
***Gross signs of hypovolemia*:** **Hyperdynamic small LV** **Kissing papillary muscles** **Small collapsible IVC** (all 2D)	***Preload responsiveness*:** **Distensibility of IVC** (>12–18%)* **Collapsibility of IVC** (≥48%) **Collapsibility of SVC** (>36%)* **Variability of aortic flow velocity** (>12–18%)* **Increase of LVOT VTI** (passive leg raise or fluid bolus) (>12.5%) **Mini-fluid challenge** **End-expiratory to end-inspiratory occlusion change of LVOT VTI** (>13%)* *requires passive mechanical ventilation
Tamponade	
Pericardial effusion (circumferential) **Cardiac chamber collapse** **Dilated IVC** **Pleural effusion, solid mass** (causing cardiac chamber compression) (all 2D)	***TTE*:** **Systolic collapse of RA** (2D) **Diastolic collapse of RV** (2D) **Variability of tricuspid valve and mitral valve inflow** (variability of inflow more than 30% (MV), 60% (TV)) (PW) ***TEE after pericardiotomy:*** **Pericardial effusion (localized)/hematoma with cardiac chamber compression**

(continued)

Table 52.3 (continued)

Basic techniques	Advanced techniques
Valvular pathology	
Severe mitral regurgitation	
Severe regurgitation (color Doppler, A4C) **Grossly abnormal MV appearance** (e.g., mass, vegetation, flail, or prolapsed leaflet) (2D) Secondary LV changes: Normal/hyperdynamic LV EF and LV size (acute MR) vs. dilated LA/LV (chronic MR) (2D)	**Severe valve lesions** (papillary muscle rupture, flail leaflet, severe retraction, large perforation; severe tenting, poor leaflet coaptation) (2D) **Large central jet** (>50% LA) **or eccentric wall impinging jet of variable size** (color Doppler) **Large** (>1 cm) **flow convergence MR throughout systole** (color Doppler) **Vena contracta width** ($\geq$7 mm) (color Doppler) **Holosystolic/dense triangular jet** (CW) **PV systolic flow reversal** (PW)* *TEE
Severe aortic regurgitation	
Severe regurgitation (color Doppler, PLAX) **Grossly abnormal AV appearance** (e.g., flail leaflet or coaptation defect) (2D) Secondary LV changes: Normal LV size (acute AR) vs. dilated LV (chronic AR) (2D)	**Severe valve lesions** (abnormal/flail, or wide coaptation defect) (2D) **Large jet width** (color Doppler); **AR jet width** (PLAX) (jet width/LVOT width >65%) (color Doppler); **AR jet area** (PSAX) (jet area/LVOT area >60%) (color Doppler) **Large flow convergence** (color Doppler) **Vena contracta width** (>6 mm) (color Doppler) **Dense jet** (CW) **Steep deceleration** (pressure half time <200 ms) (CW) **Prominent descending aorta holodiastolic flow reversal** (PW)
Severe aortic stenosis	
Grossly abnormal AV appearance (valve thickening, calcification, restricted mobility) (2D)	**AV jet peak velocity** (Vmax >4 m/s) (CW) **AV mean gradient** (>40 mmHg) (CW) **AV area** (<1.0 cm^2, indexed <0.6 cm^2/m^2) (PW/CW) **Velocity ratio (LVOT V_{max}/AV V_{max})** <0.25 (PW/CW)
LVOT obstruction	
Systolic anterior motion of mitral anterior leaflet (2D) Hyperdynamic LV EF (2D)	**Associated mitral regurgitation** (color Doppler) **Late-peaking velocity curve**: Concave upward in early systole ("dagger" shaped appearance) of LVOT outflow (CW)
Aortic dissection	
Ascending aortic flap (PLAX) (2D) **Pericardial effusion** (2D)	***TEE:*** **Ascending aortic flap** (2D) **Segmental wall motion abnormalities** (2D) **Aortic regurgitation** (color Doppler)
Decreased vasomotor tone	
No specific pathological findings Normal/hyperdynamic LV EF LVEDA not at extremes (LV end-diastolic area >5.5 cm^2, absence of kissing papillary muscles) IVC not at extremes (not very small and completely collapsible) (all 2D)	**Absence of preload responsiveness** suggests purely distributive shock without hypovolemia

It is crucial to consider the possibility of **diastolic dysfunction** with normal LV systolic function as the cause of low cardiac output. The discussion of hypertrophic cardiomyopathy, hypertensive cardiomyopathy, cardiac amyloidosis, eosinophilic myocarditis, and others is beyond the scope of the chapter. If associated with hypertrophic cardiomyopathy, hypovolemia may result in hemodynamic instability due to **LVOT or midventricular obstruction**.

RV Failure

The general considerations start with recognizing the phenotype of RV failure [8]. Questions that may help to differentiate include the following: Is RV failure acute or acute-on-chronic? Is it predominantly RV or biventricular failure? Are there clues of specific etiology (e.g., clot in transit)?

Finding a **dilated RV** should trigger consideration of either acute cor pulmonale, acute on chronic cor pulmonale, or RV infarct.

Acute cor pulmonale is caused by an acute increase of RV afterload [9, 10]. Its echocardiographic manifestations are septal dyskinesia, RV dilatation, and intraventricular septal flattening.

The causes of acute cor pulmonale include embolism or hypoxemic respiratory failure/ARDS. Embolism is usually synonymous with thromboembolic disease, but other forms of embolism (fat, air, amniotic fluid) can present in the same manner. McConnel's [11] and 60/60 [12] signs have been proposed to assist in diagnosing embolism. Another chapter will discuss their limitations. Of note, preserved apical contraction can also be seen in RV MI [8]. **Sepsis** is another common cause of RV dysfunction, being present in almost half of patients with sepsis [13].

Echocardiography is limited in definitively diagnosing pulmonary embolism. The clot in transit is an example of when the diagnosis can be made with confidence. Finding new RV dysfunction in a patient with a high probability is highly suggestive. On the other hand, a patient with shock and a normal RV echo appearance is not unstable because of massive PE, and the examiner should seek another explanation for shock.

Acute cor pulmonale secondary to hypoxemic respiratory failure is not uncommon, including in COVID-19 patients [14]. The treatments should be focused on reducing RV afterload by excellent management of hypoxemia, including pulmonary vasodilators, pruning, adjusting mechanical ventilator settings to avoid excessive intrathoracic pressures, fluid management, and ECMO, if applicable.

The identification of acute-on-chronic cor pulmonale may be challenging. It is helpful to review past echocardiograms, if available. RV-free wall thickness >5 mm is a marker of long-standing pulmonary hypertension. A severely increased PASP is not caused solely by an acute process because an unconditioned RV would not tolerate a PASP much higher than 60 mmHg [5].

Other findings may become relevant. LV enlargement suggests chronic LV failure; LV dysfunction may also be decreased in the presence of severe RV failure. Aneurysm suggests arrhythmogenic RV cardiomyopathy. The displaced septal position of the TV is suggestive of Ebstein's anomaly.

Hypovolemia

Hypovolemia may present as a **small hyperdynamic LV**. However, other conditions may manifest in the same manner. Differential diagnosis of hyperdynamic LV includes decreased LV preload (absolute fluid loss, e.g., bleeding, or relative fluid loss caused by fluid shifts and decreased vasomotor tone, e.g., sepsis) or decreased afterload (sepsis, adrenal insufficiency, end-stage liver disease, and vasodilators). Other causes of hyperdynamic LV include severe diastolic dysfunction, LVOT obstruction, acute cor pulmonale, tamponade, acute MR, or tension pneumothorax. In those conditions, there will be other prominent echo findings.

Preload responsiveness techniques may be of limited value in a patient in shock with gross signs of hypovolemia on 2D images. On the other hand, as an initial step, checking preload responsiveness is an excellent objective measure when uncertainty about preload deficit exists. The reader can find a detailed discussion about the advantages and limitations of individual preload responsiveness techniques [15–17] in Chap. 53: Assessment of Fluid Responsiveness.

A small and fully collapsible IVC is useful as a gross sign of hypovolemia. Beyond the extreme scenario, one cannot use it to predict the response to preload. Other limitations of interpreting IVC exist. IVC size will depend on spontaneous/active vs. mechanical ventilation/passive breathing, mechanical ventilation setting (tidal volume, PEEP), lung stiffness, right heart failure, tamponade, abdominal compartment, and open chest.

Tamponade

Cardiac tamponade is one of the immediately life-threatening findings in shock. **Echocardiographic findings may be limited** due to several factors. Echocardiographic signs of tamponade may be less susceptible to collapse in patients with pulmonary hypertension (RV will remain distended) [18] and more sensitive to collapse in LV dysfunction [19]. Respiratory variability of mitral inflow may be minimal under positive airway pressure in mechanically ventilated patients [20]. Pleural effusion, epicardial fat, LV pseudoaneurysm, and pericardial cysts can mimic pericardial effusion. Tamponade may occur from pleural effusion and even solid masses. Tamponade after cardiac surgery requires the practitioner to maintain a high level of suspicion and utilize TEE.

Valve Pathology

The goal of initial ICU echocardiography is to **recognize the valvular problem and refer for further imaging or perform advanced examination**. A detailed discussion of advanced techniques is beyond the scope of the chapter [21, 22].

In acute regurgitations, patients will present with **acute onset pulmonary edema** due to increased left atrial pressure (in mitral regurgitation) or increased LV end-diastolic pressure (in aortic regurgitation). The etiology of lung infiltrates is often initially not recognized and may be misdiagnosed as ARDS/pneumonia.

Assessing LV/LA volumes is useful. Enlarged chamber volumes suggest chronic regurgitations. Chronic severe MR almost always leads to dilated LV and LA. Likewise, chronic severe AR almost always leads to dilated LV.

Acute severe MR (due to flail MV or ruptured papillary muscle) and **acute severe AR** are more challenging to diagnose than chronic severe MR and AR, particularly with color Doppler (very eccentric regurgitation, short duration, tachycardia, low MR or AR velocity) [21]. Therefore, one should maintain a high index of suspicion with a low threshold to perform TEE.

In patients with **aortic stenosis**, usually, some other event, other than AS, is responsible for the shock. The AS and its consequences may complicate the management of the shock. EF is load-dependent, and the increase in LV afterload associated with AS may decrease the EF. Ventricular hypertrophy typically results in a small ventricular cavity with thick walls and diastolic dysfunction [22].

Decreased Vasomotor Tone

Sepsis is the most common cause of undifferentiated hypotension [3]. For our purpose, we use sepsis as an example of distributive shock, acknowledging that sepsis may present in various types of shock [23–25]. Remarkably, distributive shock does not have any unique echocardiographic correlate. The decreased vasomotor tone is a diagnosis of exclusion. The presence or absence of hyperdynamic LV function is not required for the diagnosis, as both patterns were described in sepsis patients [24].

Its diagnosis requires careful consideration because decreased vasomotor tone may be the primary etiology of shock despite the presence of other echocardiographic findings (e.g., LV systolic dysfunction, RV dysfunction) suggestive of different shock types.

Diagnosing preload deficit in distributive shock does not necessarily mean the preload deficit has to be completely corrected. The risk of excessive cumulative fluid balance is a genuine concern. An example of complex decision-making would be a sepsis patient with high cardiac output, who remains preload responsive, yet who has adequate tissue perfusion and exhibits pulmonary congestion based on diffuse interstitial syndrome on lung ultrasound.

Non-Echocardiography Ultrasound Modalities

Ultrasound in shock heavily relies on echocardiography. However, the non-echocardiography ultrasound modalities may yield critical information that significantly impacts decision-making in specific scenarios. The information may even present as a standalone finding sufficient for decision-making. For shock diagnosis and management, the ultrasound findings and the relevant shock patterns include:

Lung ultrasound: absent sliding, absent lung pulse, and absent vertical artifacts strongly suggest tension pneumothorax while the lung point is diagnostic of it; bilateral B-lines (diffuse interstitial syndrome) may be significant in LV failure. On the other hand, bilateral A-lines with sliding (normal lung pattern) will be present in multiple shock patterns.

Vascular ultrasound: aortic flap is diagnostic of aortic dissection; noncompressible veins (DVT) are highly suggestive of thromboembolism as the cause of acute cor pulmonale.

Abdominal ultrasound: a positive FAST (free intra-abdominal fluid) is a critical finding in a hypovolemic trauma patient.

Limitations and Caveats

The most significant risk of echocardiography in the management of critically ill patients with shock stems from making incorrect conclusions and making clinical decisions based on these conclusions. Diagnostic and management errors are either caused by inadequate echocardiographers' competence, including the interpretation and image acquisition skills, or by failure to recognize the limitations inherent to echocardiography itself. It is imperative for practitioners to be aware of these limitations.

The vividness of visual images may activate the availability heuristic (availability bias), leading to diagnostic errors [26, 27]. Such danger is real and may lead to fatal missteps during management: administering a thrombolytic for acute cor pulmonale that was caused by ARDS, inserting a chest tube based on a lack of lung sliding that turned out to be caused by a massive lung bulla without pneumothorax, or a fatal pericardiocentesis for pericardial effusion while missing the aortic dissection.

Systematic consideration of all possibilities is needed when multiple possible mechanisms compete for the same echocardiographic end result. For example, not considering the possibility of hypovolemia and not testing preload responsiveness in a patient with LV dysfunction may lead to the erroneous application of inotropes while missing the opportunity to simply correct preload deficit with fluids.

One should interpret the ventricular function with the clinical background knowledge, including the loading conditions. LV ejection fraction (EF) is a complex variable and results from contractility influenced by therapies (e.g., inotropes) and manipulations of the afterload and preload. Vasopressors will increase afterload and make LV EF appear worse; vasodilation from sepsis/vasodilators will decrease afterload and make LV EF appear normal even in case of reduced baseline LV EF. RV function may worsen from high RV afterload related to increased intrathoracic pressure (from high PEEP/tidal volume) and hypoxemic pulmonary vasoconstriction. Mechanical circulatory support (intra-aortic balloon pump, temporary or permanent ventricular assist devices) may be a factor driving the echocardiographic appearance of the ventricular function.

Failure to recognize chronic conditions will result in incorrect conclusions. Examiners should be aware of the implications and limitations of such conditions. They should stay systematic during the examination and implement advanced quantitative techniques when appropriate. The scenarios of chronic diseases and their implications include

1. Dilated and thin LV (clue of chronic cardiomyopathy): hypovolemia may never manifest with small hyperdynamic LV; the cause of hemodynamic collapse may be a distinct, separate process (e.g., sepsis) rather than the cardiomyopathy itself.
2. LV hypertrophy: patients may have inadequate preload; severe diastolic dysfunction may be present and complicate the management (a small stiff LV impairs the ability to increase stroke volume by fluid administration); a concomitant problem may be present (severe aortic stenosis, left ventricular outflow tract obstruction).
3. RV hypertrophy (a clue of long-standing pulmonary hypertension): the cause of RV dilatation is not just an acute process; a dilated IVC may not ensure adequate LV preload.
4. Dilated atria (a clue of chronically increased ventricular pressure): there may be underlying diastolic dysfunction, restrictive cardiomyopathy, or a significant valvular regurgitation present.

Not obtaining a follow-up study may result in missing subsequent changes in dynamic pathological processes. A patient may initially present with hypovolemia during the initial sepsis phase and later develop cardiogenic shock from new LV dysfunction that has not been recognized because of not obtaining a repeat study.

Misusing echocardiographic techniques without knowing their specific limitations will result in wrong conclusions. A patient with significant variability of pulse pressure on the ICU monitor due to RV dysfunction caused by acute cor pulmonale due to acute asthmatic exacerbation and very high intrathoracic pressure should not be evaluated for preload responsiveness (e.g., breath-to-breath variability in LVOT VTI, distensibility index of IVC) because these techniques are not applicable in RV dysfunction.

The basic examination is excellent in producing several specific findings (hypovolemia, LV failure, RV failure, gross valvular disease, overt cardiac masses, and pericardial effusion). **However, even a high-quality basic examination may not yield sufficient information for appropriate management**. For example, findings of LV failure will point the examiner in the correct direction. Still, advanced examination showing regional wall motion abnormality will be much more specific for the etiology (coronary artery disease) and will steer the management toward revascularization.

Echocardiography may not discern a single etiology of shock when several simultaneous processes are present. A patient with concurrent reduced vasomotor tone from sepsis and poor cardiac output from stress cardiomyopathy is an example of such a challenging situation.

Even when echocardiographic examination identifies a singular shock mechanism, it may not yield any information pointing toward the specific etiology. A patient with reduced vasomotor tone will look identical on echo to a patient with adrenal insufficiency, a patient with end-stage liver disease-related vasodilated state, or a patient who received vasodilators.

The patient's anatomy may limit the number of available views. The examiner may need to rely on limited information obtained from a single view in such situations. Subcostal short-axis view may sometimes provide the same information as the parasternal short axis. It is helpful for practitioners to be familiar with this and other alternative echocardiographic views [28]. Noncardiac ultrasound modalities complement TTE and sometimes provide the critical information necessary for management. A trauma patient with an initially unclear cause of shock and inadequate echo windows, who turns out to have free fluid on repeat abdominal FAST examination, is an example of the indispensable role of leveraging all available ultrasound modalities.

Echocardiography is not an ICU hemodynamic monitor. Other devices (PA catheter, PICCO) are more appropriate. Comparing small interval changes of quantitative data is less useful (e.g., small changes of PASP or E/e') than comparing qualitative, categorical changes (e.g., PASP <40 mm Hg vs. PASP >60 mm Hg; E/e' <8 vs. E/e' >14) [29].

Evolving Evidence

Ultrasound Protocols

Many excellent protocols using the ultrasound approach to shock have been published over the last two decades. This literature is challenging to interpret due to no direct comparison between the individual methods and no rigorous data on patient outcomes. However, it is helpful to be familiar with the published protocols because these are useful to organize and focus the examiner's approach. Indeed, the use of a systematic approach to shock is recommended in guidelines [1], utilizing specific views in a recent consensus statement [30].

The protocols generally tend to share the common trait of leveraging multiple ultrasound modalities. The focus of published protocols ranges from those heavily based on echocardiography (FATE) [7] to those spanning across all ultrasound modalities (RUSH) [31] to those primarily focused on lung ultrasound (FALLS) [4]. The protocols tend to use basic echocardiographic findings as opposed to advanced techniques. One of the recent novel protocols (EASy) [32] suggests using only the subcostal view combined with anterior lung views while still capturing all basic shock scenarios (Fig. 52.1).

Evidence Supporting Use of Echocardiography in Shock

Echocardiography is a powerful tool that enables practitioners to accurately evaluate the structures, e.g., LV function [33–35]. In addition, there is good evidence that the practitioners can narrow down the differential diagnosis [3, 36–39] and often change their management [40–42].

These positive intermediary outcomes commonly used in the ultrasound literature are somewhat tempered by the relative lack of and conflicting data about echocardiography and ultrasound's impact on hard outcomes such as mortality and morbidity. Most of the evidence supporting the use of echocardiography in shock currently comes from retrospective studies, including large patient cohorts. Echocardiography was associated with decreased mortality in critically ill patients ($N = 220$) [43], in sepsis patients from the MIMIC III database ($N = 6361$) [44] and ($N = 3191$) [45]. In addition, echocardiography was associated with decreased mortality in five of six leading diagnoses (including sepsis) in the Nationwide Inpatient Sample ($N = 256{,}148$) [46]. Against that evidence, an association was found between echocardiography, increased care delays, and increased mortality in ED ($N = 5441$) [47].

There are very few prospective, randomized controlled trials. A small feasibility study found no difference in mortality in ICU patients ($N = 30$) [48] and a larger study found no difference in ED patients ($N = 270$) [3]. There are many potential reasons why it is difficult to establish evidence for echocardiography on patient centered outcomes through randomized trials [49].

Although the impact of echocardiography has not been shown yet in a randomized trial, the ICU community will undoubtedly continue to use it widely. The reasons include its capacity to expedite the diagnosis of shock mechanisms, identify high-risk patients, select appropriate therapy, monitor the effectiveness of treatment, and avoid potentially harmful interventions.

Summary Points

Evaluation of shock of undifferentiated etiology using ultrasound should consist of the following:

(a) Have a working list of possible causes of shock in mind prior to starting the echo examination.
(b) Exclude sequentially:
  - Immediately life-threatening conditions:
    - Tamponade
    - Severe valve pathology (severe valve regurgitation, LVOT obstruction)
    - Tension pneumothorax
  - Hypovolemia
  - LV failure
  - RV failure
  - Decreased vasomotor tone

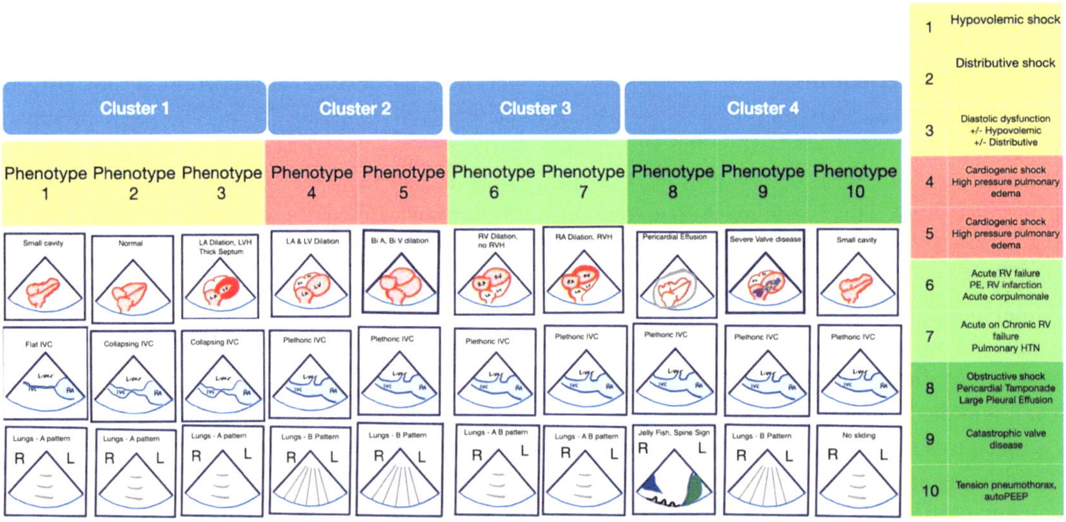

Fig. 52.1 EASy phenotypes. EASy phenotypes are based on the subcostal four-chamber view (top row), subcostal IVC view (middle row), and lung evaluation in the upper lung fields (bottom row). Phenotypes 1 to 3 are grouped within cluster 1, phenotypes 4 and 5 are part of cluster 2, phenotypes 6 and 7 are part of cluster 3, and phenotypes 8–10 are part of cluster 4. In general, cardiac assessment assesses myocardial performance, IVC evaluation provides the estimate of fluid responsiveness, and lung examination defines fluid tolerance (A-profile) and intolerance (B-profile). Phenotype 1 describes the patient with hypovolemic shock with small diastolic ventricular chamber size, collapsed IVC with significant variability in its diameter throughout the respiratory cycle, and A-profile on lung examination. Phenotype 2 is consistent with distributive shock in adequately fluid-resuscitated patients with good cardiac filling, normal IVC size, and A-profile on lung examination. Phenotype 3 describes a patient with hypertrophic LV, commonly dilated left atrium, small and collapsible IVC, and A-profile on lung examination. Phenotypes 4 and 5 describe patients with isolated LV (phenotype 4) and biventricular (phenotype 5) dysfunction, usually plethoric IVC and B-profile on lung examination. Phenotype 6 most commonly describes patients with ARDS complicated by RV dysfunction. These patients demonstrate enlarged RV, plethoric IVC, and B-profile on lung examination more commonly reflecting nonhydrostatic edema. Phenotype 7 includes patients with underlying pulmonary hypertension and RV hypertrophy who develop acute or chronic RV failure. These patients have enlarged and hypertrophic RV, plethoric IVC, and variable lung profile (B-profile shown here). Phenotype 8 shows pericardial tamponade, phenotype 9 shows severe valvular regurgitation, and phenotype 10 shows tension pneumothorax with loss of lung sliding and a small LV cavity. Bi A, Bi atrial; Bi V, Bi ventricular; HTN, hypertension; LA, left atrium; LVH, left ventricular hypertrophy; RA, right atrium; RVH, right ventricular hypertrophy. (Courtesy of N. Bughrara, MD, Albany, NY)

(c) Start with pattern recognition and basic techniques; add advanced techniques as applicable depending on indications, time limitations, and examiner's skills.
(d) Implement non-cardiac ultrasound (lung, venous, FAST) when appropriate.
(e) Repeat examination at any point to evaluate the effect of therapies, if changes in patient condition, or as routine follow-up.

Call-Out: Pro-Tip

- The initial goal of echocardiography is to identify the mechanism responsible for circulatory failure and select the most appropriate treatments. Subsequently, during the later phase, the goal shifts toward using echocardiography to guide and titrate treatments.

Questions

1. Which of the following features on ultrasound suggest hypovolemia as the likely cause of shock?
   A. Hyperdynamic LV
   B. Small and collapsed IVC
   C. Absence of B-lines in anterior lung zones
   D. Decreased LVOT VTI
   Answer: B

Rationale: All the above ultrasound features can be present in a patient with hypovolemia. However, only the small and completely collapsed IVC can suggest hypovolemia as the likely cause of shock. Hyperdynamic LV can be present in many other conditions, including decreased vasomotor tone (sepsis), obstructive shock (tension pneumothorax), LVOT obstruction, severe diastolic dysfunction, etc. The presence of B-lines in the lung ultrasound suggests hydrostatic pulmonary edema and points towards cardiogenic shock in the context of decreased LV systolic function. However, the absence of B lines will not suggest hypovolemic shock. The FALLS protocol incorporates lung ultrasound in diagnosing and managing undifferentiated shock. Once obstructive and cardiogenic shock types are ruled out using a schematic approach of the FALLS protocol, the presence of an A-profile in lung ultrasound narrows down the shock etiology to either hypovolemic or distributive shock. These will be differentiated by the presence of clinical improvement with the administration of fluid boluses (likely hypovolemic shock) versus lack of improvement or development of B-lines (distributive/septic shock). LVOT VTI is a surrogate for stroke volume, and a decreased LVOT VTI is seen in decreased LV or RV function and tamponade, besides hypovolemia.

2. Which of the following clinical scenarios would NOT require TEE guidance in circulatory shock management?
   A. Undifferentiated shock in a post-cardiotomy patient in the immediate post-operative period
   B. Undifferentiated shock in a trauma patient with extensive subcutaneous emphysema
   C. Assessment of respiratory variation of SVC diameter
   D. Assessment of respiratory variation of IVC diameter

   Answer: D

   Rationale: An essential part of ultrasound examination in diagnosing and managing shock is to consider all the available ultrasound modalities. TEE is of significant value in a select patient population when adequate TTE views are unavailable (e.g., in patients with chest dressings, extensive subcutaneous emphysema, lung hyperinflation, etc.) or in specific scenarios (e.g., localized tamponade in post-cardiac surgery). Respiratory variation of SVC diameter is a high specificity indicator to predict fluid responsiveness in mechanically ventilated patients with circulatory failure. This assessment requires the use of TEE. In contrast, respiratory variation of IVC diameter can be assessed with a TTE probe in the subcostal view (e.g., EASy protocol).

3. Which of the following features noted on echocardiography suggests acute PE as the likely cause of acute RV failure?
   A. Clot in transit in the RV
   B. McConnel's sign
   C. Mid-systolic notching of RVOT Doppler profile
   D. RV: LV end-diastolic area ratio >1

   Answer: A

   Rationale: Echocardiography is limited in definitively diagnosing acute PE as the cause of acute RV dysfunction. Seeing a clot in transit in the right heart chamber is the most definitive way to diagnose acute PE as the likely cause of acute RV dysfunction. McConnel's sign can be seen in other conditions of acute cor pulmonale (e.g., ARDS) and is not specific for acute PE. The presence of early or mid-systolic notching of the RVOT Doppler profile can be seen in acute PE. However, it can also be seen in other conditions with increased pulmonary vascular resistance and RV dysfunction (e.g., PAH). The presence of dilated RV on echocardiography should trigger consideration of acute cor pulmonale or acute on chronic cor pulmonale or RV infarction.

References

1. Via G, Hussain A, Wells M, et al. International evidence-based recommendations for focused cardiac ultrasound. J Am Soc Echocardiogr. 2014;27:683.e1–683.e33.
2. Weil MH, Shubin H. Proposed reclassification of shock states with special reference to distributive defects. Adv Exp Med Biol. 1971;23:13–23.

3. Atkinson PR, Milne J, Diegelmann L, et al. Does point-of-care ultrasonography improve clinical outcomes in emergency department patients with undifferentiated hypotension? An international randomized controlled trial from the SHoC-ED investigators. Ann Emerg Med. 2018;72:478–89.
4. Lichtenstein D. Fluid administration limited by lung sonography: the place of lung ultrasound in assessment of acute circulatory failure (the FALLS-protocol). Expert Rev Respir Med. 2012;6:155–62.
5. Oh JK, Kane GC, Seward JB, Tajik AJ. The echo manual. 4th ed. Wolters Kluwer; 2019.
6. Bergenzaun L, Gudmundsson P, Ohlin H, et al. Assessing left ventricular systolic function in shock: evaluation of echocardiographic parameters in intensive care. Crit Care. 2011;15:R200.
7. Jensen MB, Sloth E, Larsen KM, Schmidt MB. Transthoracic echocardiography for cardiopulmonary monitoring in intensive care. Eur J Anaesthesiol. 2004;21:700–7.
8. Vieillard-Baron A, Naeije R, Haddad F, et al. Diagnostic workup, etiologies and management of acute right ventricle failure: a state-of-the-art paper. Intensive Care Med. 2018;44:774–90.
9. Jardin F, Dubourg O, Bourdarias JP. Echocardiographic pattern of acute cor pulmonale. Chest. 1997;111:209–17.
10. Vieillard-Baron A, Prin S, Chergui K, et al. Echo-Doppler demonstration of acute cor pulmonale at the bedside in the medical intensive care unit. Am J Respir Crit Care Med. 2002;166:1310–9.
11. McConnell MV, Solomon SD, Rayan ME, et al. Regional right ventricular dysfunction detected by echocardiography in acute pulmonary embolism. Am J Cardiol. 1996;78:469–73.
12. Kurzyna M, Torbicki A, Pruszczyk P, et al. Disturbed right ventricular ejection pattern as a new Doppler echocardiographic sign of acute pulmonary embolism. Am J Cardiol. 2002;90:507–11.
13. Lanspa MJ, Cirulis MM, Wiley BM, et al. Right ventricular dysfunction in early sepsis and septic shock. Chest. 2021;159:1055–63.
14. Venkata C, Aruchamy S, Kasal J. Acute right ventricular dysfunction in a critically ill patient with COVID-19. CASE (Phila). 2020;4:474–6.
15. Vignon P, Repesse X, Begot E, et al. Comparison of echocardiographic indices used to predict fluid responsiveness in ventilated patients. Am J Respir Crit Care Med. 2017;195:1022–32.
16. Vieillard-Baron A, Evrard B, Repessé X, et al. Limited value of end-expiratory inferior vena cava diameter to predict fluid responsiveness impact of intra-abdominal pressure. Intensive Care Med. 2018;44:197–203.
17. Monnet X, Teboul JL. Assessment of fluid responsiveness: recent advances. Curr Opin Crit Care. 2018;24:190–5.
18. Leimgruber PP, Klopfenstein HS, Wann LS, et al. The hemodynamic derangement associated with right ventricular diastolic collapse in cardiac tamponade: an experimental echocardiographic study. Circulation. 1983;68:612–20.
19. Hoit BD, Gabel M, Fowler NO. Cardiac tamponade in left ventricular dysfunction. Circulation. 1990;82:1370–6.
20. Faehnrich JA, Noone RB Jr, White WD, et al. Effects of positive-pressure ventilation, pericardial effusion, and cardiac tamponade on respiratory variation in transmitral flow velocities. J Cardiothorac Vasc Anesth. 2003;17:45–50.
21. Zoghbi WA, Adams D, Bonow RO, et al. Recommendations for noninvasive evaluation of native valvular regurgitation: a report from the American Society of Echocardiography developed in collaboration with the Society for Cardiovascular Magnetic Resonance. J Am Soc Echocardiogr. 2017;30:303–71.
22. Baumgartner H, Hung J, Bermejo J, et al. Recommendations on the echocardiographic assessment of aortic valve stenosis: a focused update from the European Association of Cardiovascular Imaging and the American Society of Echocardiography. J Am Soc Echocardiogr. 2017;30:372–92.
23. Pulido JN, Afessa B, Masaki M, et al. Clinical spectrum, frequency, and significance of myocardial dysfunction in severe sepsis and septic shock. Mayo Clin Proc. 2012;87:620–8.
24. Geri G, Vignon P, Aubry A, et al. Cardiovascular clusters in septic shock combining clinical and echocardiographic parameters: a post hoc analysis. Intensive Care Med. 2019;45:657–67.
25. Lafon T, Appert A, Hadj M, et al. Comparative early hemodynamic profiles in patients presenting to the emergency department with septic and nonseptic acute circulatory failure using focused echocardiography. Shock. 2020;53:695–700.
26. Brown SM, Kasal J. Bedside ultrasound in the intensive care unit: where is the evidence? Semin Respir Crit Care Med. 2015;36:878–89.
27. Redelmeier DA. Improving patient care. The cognitive psychology of missed diagnoses. Ann Intern Med. 2005;142:115–20.
28. Mitchell C, Rahko PS, Blauwet LA, et al. Guidelines for performing a comprehensive transthoracic echocardiographic examination in adults: recommendations from the American Society of Echocardiography. J Am Soc Echocardiogr. 2019;32:1–64.
29. Porter TR, Shillcutt SK, Adams MS, et al. Guidelines for the use of echocardiography as a monitor for therapeutic intervention in adults: a report from the american society of echocardiography. J Am Soc Echocardiogr. 2015;28:40–56.
30. Atkinson P, Bowra J, Milne J, et al. International Federation for Emergency Medicine Consensus statement: sonography in hypotension and cardiac arrest (SHoC): an international consensus on the use of point of care ultrasound for undifferentiated hypotension and during cardiac arrest. CJEM. 2017;19:459–70.
31. Perera P, Mailhot T, Riley D, Mandavia D. The RUSH exam: rapid ultrasound in SHock in the evalu-

ation of the critically Ill. Emerg Med Clin North Am. 2010;28:29–56, vii.
32. Bughrara N, Diaz-Gomez JL, Pustavoitau A. Perioperative management of patients with sepsis and septic shock, part II: ultrasound support for resuscitation. Anesthesiol Clin. 2020;38:123–34.
33. Jones AE, Craddock PA, Tayal VS, Kline JA. Diagnostic accuracy of left ventricular function for identifying sepsis among emergency department patients with nontraumatic symptomatic undifferentiated hypotension. Shock. 2005;24:513–7.
34. Lucas BP, Candotti C, Margeta B, et al. Diagnostic accuracy of hospitalist-performed hand-carried ultrasound echocardiography after a brief training program. J Hosp Med. 2009;4:340–9.
35. Kimura BJ, Yogo N, O'Connell CW, et al. Cardiopulmonary limited ultrasound examination for "quick-look" bedside application. Am J Cardiol. 2011;108:586–90.
36. Jones AE, Tayal VS, Sullivan DM, Kline JA. Randomized, controlled trial of immediate versus delayed goal-directed ultrasound to identify the cause of nontraumatic hypotension in emergency department patients. Crit Care Med. 2004;32:1703–8.
37. Shokoohi H, Boniface KS, Pourmand A, et al. Bedside ultrasound reduces diagnostic uncertainty and guides resuscitation in patients with undifferentiated hypotension. Crit Care Med. 2015;43:2562–9.
38. Shokoohi H, Boniface KS, Zaragoza M, et al. Point-of-care ultrasound leads to diagnostic shifts in patients with undifferentiated hypotension. Am J Emerg Med. 2017;35:1984.e3–7.
39. Ahn JH, Jeon J, Toh HC, et al. SEARCH 8Es: a novel point of care ultrasound protocol for patients with chest pain, dyspnea or symptomatic hypotension in the emergency department. PLoS One. 2017;12:e0174581.
40. Breitkreutz R, Price S, Steiger HV, et al. Focused echocardiographic evaluation in life support and peri-resuscitation of emergency patients: a prospective trial. Resuscitation. 2010;81:1527–33.
41. Mayron R, Gaudio FE, Plummer D, et al. Echocardiography performed by emergency physicians: impact on diagnosis and therapy. Ann Emerg Med. 1988;17:150–4.
42. Haydar SA, Moore ET, Higgins GL 3rd, et al. Effect of bedside ultrasonography on the certainty of physician clinical decisionmaking for septic patients in the emergency department. Ann Emerg Med. 2012;60:346–58.e4.
43. Kanji HD, McCallum J, Sirounis D, et al. Limited echocardiography-guided therapy in subacute shock is associated with change in management and improved outcomes. J Crit Care. 2014;29:700–5.
44. Feng M, McSparron JI, Kien DT, et al. Transthoracic echocardiography and mortality in sepsis: analysis of the MIMIC-III database. Intensive Care Med. 2018;44:884–92.
45. Lan P, Wang TT, Li HY, et al. Utilization of echocardiography during septic shock was associated with a decreased 28-day mortality: a propensity score-matched analysis of the MIMIC-III database. Ann Transl Med. 2019;7:662.
46. Papolos A, Narula J, Bavishi C, et al. U.S. hospital use of echocardiography: insights from the nationwide inpatient sample. J Am Coll Cardiol. 2016;67:502–11.
47. Mosier JM, Stolz U, Milligan R, et al. Impact of point-of-care ultrasound in the emergency department on care processes and outcomes in critically ill non-traumatic patients. Crit Care Explor. 2019;1:e0019.
48. Lanspa MJ, Burk RE, Wilson EL, et al. Echocardiogram-guided resuscitation versus early goal-directed therapy in the treatment of septic shock: a randomized, controlled, feasibility trial. J Intensive Care. 2018;6:50.
49. Vignon P. Critical care echocardiography: diagnostic or prognostic? Ann Transl Med. 2020;8:909.

53 Assessment of Fluid Responsiveness

Xavier Monnet

Learning Objectives

1. Describe the tests and indices that have been developed to assess fluid responsiveness.
2. Review the tests and indices that can be performed with echocardiography to assess fluid responsiveness.
3. Examine the evidence supporting the use of various echocardiographic techniques to evaluate fluid responsiveness.
4. List the respective advantages and limitations of the various echocardiographic techniques.

Introduction

Volume expansion is the first step when treating a majority of patients with shock. Its purpose is to increase cardiac preload, with the aim of increasing cardiac output, and ultimately, arterial oxygen delivery [1]. However, the inconsistent response to this treatment and the risks associated with excessive fluid administration have led to the development of methods that can predict the hemodynamic effectiveness of a fluid bolus before infusing it [2]. Over the past 20 years, several tests and indices have been developed to achieve this prediction in a "dynamic" way, that is, by testing the responsiveness of the cardiovascular system to a transient change in cardiac preload [3].

In this chapter, we will review the tests and indices that can be performed with echocardiography. We will detail the physiological principles underlying them, describe their practical performance, and list their respective advantages and limitations.

What Is the Concept of Detection of Preload Responsiveness?

Fluid therapy for the purpose of expanding the vascular content poses two fundamental problems [2]. On the one hand, its effectiveness is inconsistent. Because of the curvilinear relationship between stroke volume and cardiac preload, the response of cardiac output to a fluid bolus is not always present. Indeed, if the right and left ventricles work on the flat part of the Frank-Starling curve (Fig. 53.1), i.e., if they are both preload unresponsive, the increase in cardiac preload induced by the fluid bolus does not lead to the increase in cardiac output that was expected from it. In critically ill patients, volume expansion induces a significant increase in cardiac output in only half of the cases [2].

X. Monnet (✉)
AP-HP, Service de médecine intensive-réanimation, Hôpital de Bicêtre, DMU 4 CORREVE, Inserm UMR S_999, FHU SEPSIS, CARMAS, Université Paris-Saclay, Le Kremlin-Bicêtre, France
e-mail: xavier.monnet@aphp.fr

M. J. Lanspa, A. T. Levinson (eds.), *Echocardiography and Ultrasonography in the ICU*, Respiratory Medicine, https://doi.org/10.1007/978-3-031-80038-2_53

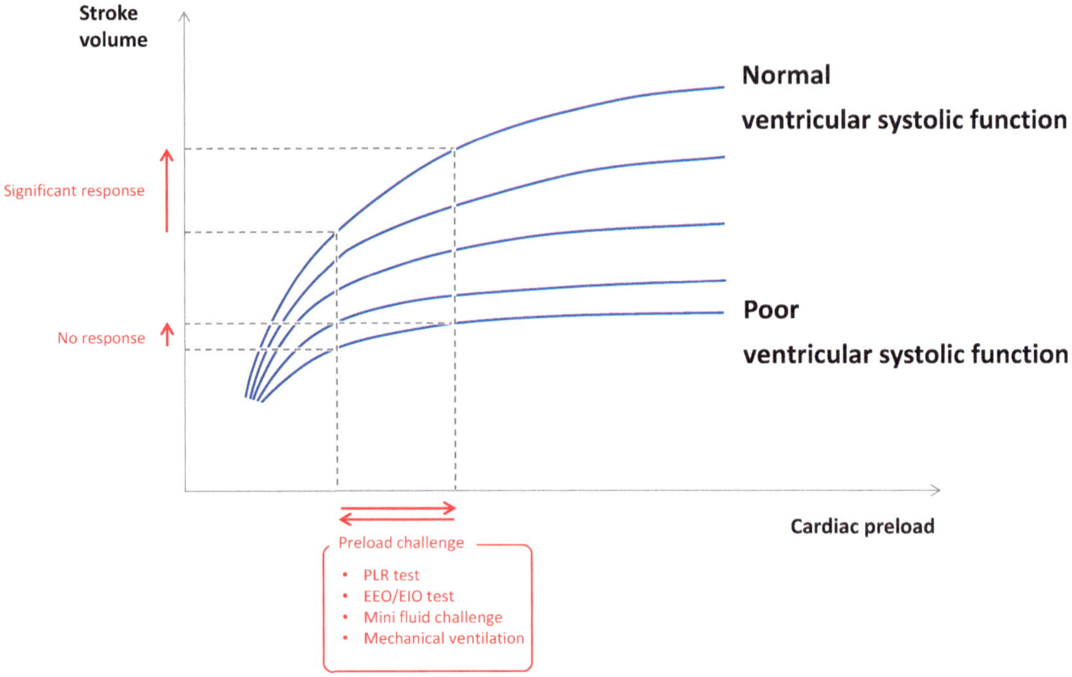

Fig. 53.1 Frank-Starling relationship and principles of the dynamic prediction of fluid responsiveness
The slope of the Frank-Starling curve reflects the degree of preload responsiveness. It is indicated by the response of stroke volume to changes in cardiac preload, either spontaneous during mechanical ventilation or induced by passive leg raising (PLR), end-expiratory occlusion (EEO), end-inspiratory occlusion (EIO), or a mini-fluid challenge

On the other hand, the toxicity of fluids in critically ill patients and in the perioperative context is now clearly demonstrated. An increased fluid balance is a factor that independently increases mortality in critically ill patients, especially in cases of septic shock [4] and acute respiratory distress syndrome (ARDS) [5]. In the perioperative setting, it is associated with an increased rate of complications after surgery [6].

Thus, fluids are drugs, the response to which is inconsistent, the side effects numerous, and the overdose dangerous [2]. This is the theoretical basis that justifies predicting the response to volume expansion before deciding to perform it, in order to avoid fluid infusion in patients that will not benefit from it.

Static or Dynamic Indices?

For many years, to decide whether or not to administer a fluid bolus, clinicians have relied on "static" indices, that is, variables that estimate an absolute value of cardiac preload. Central venous pressure has been widely used for this purpose. However, none of these variables reliably predict fluid responsiveness. This is mainly explained by the fact that the slope of the Frank-Starling curve is variable depending on the contractility of the ventricles. A given value of cardiac preload can correspond to a variable degree of preload responsiveness (Fig. 53.1): preload is not preload responsiveness.

This is the case for all the echocardiographic variables that estimate the right (diameter of the inferior vena cava) or left (ratio of E over e' waves of the mitral Doppler, end-diastolic area, or volume of the left ventricle) cardiac preload. For example, the diameter of the inferior vena cava, which is an estimate of the central venous pressure, is not different between patients who will respond and others who will not respond to volume expansion by a significant increase in cardiac output. Even extreme values have a poor predictive value, which is even worse in the case of intra-abdominal hypertension [7].

Conversely, dynamic estimation of preload responsiveness consists of observing the effect on stroke volume, cardiac output, or their surrogates of changes in cardiac preload induced spontaneously by artificial ventilation or intentionally by specific tests [8, 9] (Fig. 53.1).

Passive Leg Raising Test

What Is the Principle of the Test?

Transferring a patient from a semi-recumbent position at 30–45° to a position in which the trunk is horizontal and the lower limbs elevated at 30–45° induces the transfer of venous blood from the lower limbs and the vast splanchnic territory to the heart chambers. The passive leg raising (PLR) test mimics the effects of volume expansion. It increases the average systemic pressure, the upstream pressure of systemic venous return [10]. The volume of blood transferred to the intrathoracic blood volume is equivalent to a volume expansion of approximately 300 mL [11], even if this volume is very variable from one patient to another.

Compared to a fluid challenge, the great advantage of the PLR test is of course that it is completely reversible. Another major advantage is that it remains reliable in conditions where the respiratory variability of stroke volume or its surrogate (see below) cannot be used, such as cardiac arrhythmias, spontaneous ventilation, or ARDS [12].

Numerous clinical studies [13] and some meta-analyses [14, 15] have demonstrated that the PLR test is reliable in detecting preload dependence. The diagnostic threshold for increased stroke volume or cardiac output is 10%.

How to Perform the Test in Practice?

A few practical rules must be followed when carrying out the PLR test [16] (Table 53.1, Fig. 53.2). The initial position of the patient should not be horizontal but semi recumbent at 30–45°. Thus, the large blood volume of the splanchnic territory is mobilized, which enhances the PLR-induced increase in cardiac preload [11]. Then, the maneuver should not be performed by manually raising the lower limbs of the patient so as not to create pain that would interfere with the hemodynamic effect of the test. The automatic system of electric beds should be preferred. Also, it must be ensured after the test that the cardiac output returns to its initial value in order to verify that the patient is hemodynamically stable and that the changes observed are indeed due to the PLR test alone [16].

With echocardiography, the effects of the PLR test are estimated on changes in velocity time integral (VTI) in the left ventricular outflow tract (LVOT) (Table 53.1, Fig. 53.2). Since the heart

Table 53.1 Passive leg-raising test

What does it consist of?	• Place the patient in the semi-recumbent position at 30–45°. • Measure VTI at baseline. • Move the patient to the PLR position. • Measure VTI after 30–60 s.
What is the diagnostic threshold?	↗ VTI ≥10%
What are the limitations?	• Contra-indicated in case of intracranial hypertension. • False negatives in case of intra-abdominal hypertension (likely).

PLR passive leg raising test; *VTI* velocity time integral

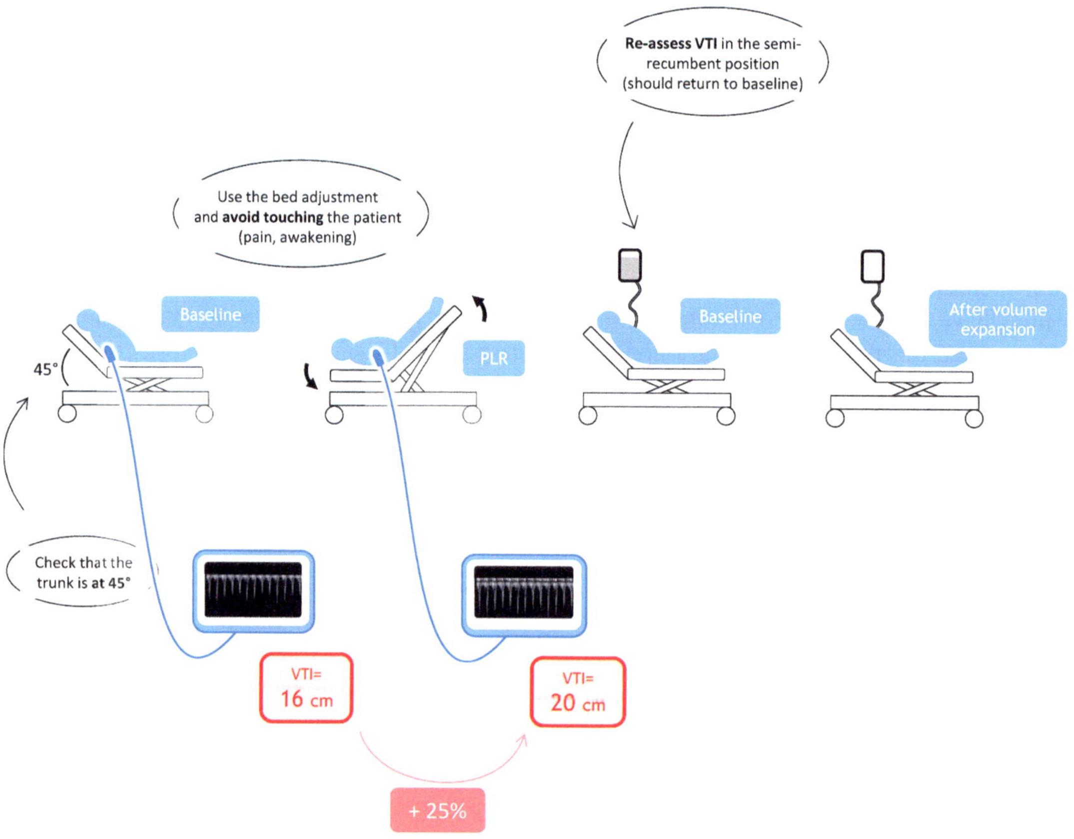

Fig. 53.2 The passive leg-raising test

The increase in the velocity time integral (VTI) in the left ventricular outflow tract during passive leg raising (PLR) indicates preload responsiveness. Preload responsiveness is likely if the PLR-induced increase in VTI is ≥10%

rate changes little, and since the diameter of the LVOT remains constant, changes in LVOT VTI are proportional to those in cardiac output. Nevertheless, the diagnostic threshold is close to the smallest significant change [17]. In order to ensure the reproducibility of the LVOT VTI measurement, it is preferable to keep the probe in contact with the patient and the ultrasound beam in the LVOT during the postural maneuver [17]. Thus, the test is easier to perform if a second operator changes the position of the bed.

Some studies have suggested that velocity changes measured in the femoral or carotid artery with vascular Doppler have the same diagnostic value [18]. However, other studies have found opposite results [19, 20]. More generally, doubts exist regarding the ability of carotid blood flow to track changes in cardiac output [21, 22]. One should thus be cautious before considering this technique as reliable.

What Are the Limitations of the Test?

The PLR test is contraindicated in cases of intracranial hypertension. It is obviously not feasible during surgery. The presence of venous compression stockings is probably responsible for false negatives because they reduce the mobilized blood volume [8] (Table 53.1). Finally, a study showed that intra-abdominal hypertension is also probably responsible for false negatives because it decreases splanchnic blood volume, which plays an important role in the hemodynamic effects of the test [23]. The results of this single study need to be confirmed [24], but, in the meantime, it is reasonable to advise caution in interpreting the PLR test in cases of intra-abdominal hypertension (Table 53.1).

Respiratory Occlusion Tests

What Is the Principle of the Tests?

Under positive pressure ventilation, each insufflation increases the intrathoracic pressure. After transmission to the thin right atrium, this decreases the pressure gradient of systemic venous return and decreases cardiac preload. Thus, the interruption of ventilation at the end of expiration stops the cyclic impediment to systemic venous return and temporarily increases cardiac preload. If stroke volume and cardiac output increase subsequently, both ventricles must be in a preload-responsive state [25].

Conversely, during respiratory occlusion at the end of insufflation, the prolonged increase in intrathoracic pressure lowers cardiac preload and decreases stroke volume and cardiac output in the event of preload responsiveness [25]. The occlusions must be sufficiently prolonged, longer than 12 s, to allow changes in stroke volume induced on the right side to be transmitted to the left side after the lung transit time [25].

It has been demonstrated that an increase in cardiac output measured continuously, for example, with pulse wave contour analysis, of more than 5% during an end-expiratory occlusion test allows the detection of preload responsiveness with very good diagnostic reliability [26–28]. With echocardiography, the hemodynamic effect might be assessed through changes in LVOT VTI, which are proportional to changes in cardiac output. Nevertheless, this diagnostic threshold is too low compared to the smallest significant change in LVOT VTI measurable by echocardiography [17]. This is why our group has suggested adding a 15-s end-expiratory occlusion and a 15-s end-inspiratory occlusion and summing the changes in LVOT VTI (in absolute value) observed during each occlusion. The amplitude of the change is larger, and the diagnostic threshold, which is 13%, is compatible with the reproducibility of echocardiography [29].

How to Perform the Tests in Practice?

After an initial LVOT VTI measurement, an end-expiratory occlusion is performed for 15 s (Table 53.2; Fig. 53.3). The change in LVOT VTI is measured at the end of the occlusion. After resuming normal ventilation for a few seconds, a 15-s end-of-inspiratory occlusion is performed using the same procedures. The absolute value of the observed changes is added. As with the PLR test, changes in LVOT VTI are proportional to changes in cardiac output [25]. The diagnostic threshold is 13% [29].

What Are the Limitations of the Test?

In patients who have too strong spontaneous breathing activity, end-inspiratory or end-expiratory occlusions may be interrupted before the required 15 s, and the test is not feasible (Table 53.2).

Table 53.2 Respiratory occlusion tests

What does it consist of?	• Measure VTI at baseline. • Perform EEO for 15 s and measure VTI at the end (keep the probe on the patient). • Let ventilation resume. • Perform EIO for 15 s and measure VTI at the end (keep the probe on the patient).
What is the diagnostic threshold?	Some of the change in VTI (↗ during EEO and ↘ during EIO) ≥13%.
What are the limitations?	Cannot be performed if the patient interrupts the 15-s EEO or EIO.

EEO end-expiratory occlusion; *EIO* end-inspiratory occlusion; *VTI* velocity time integral

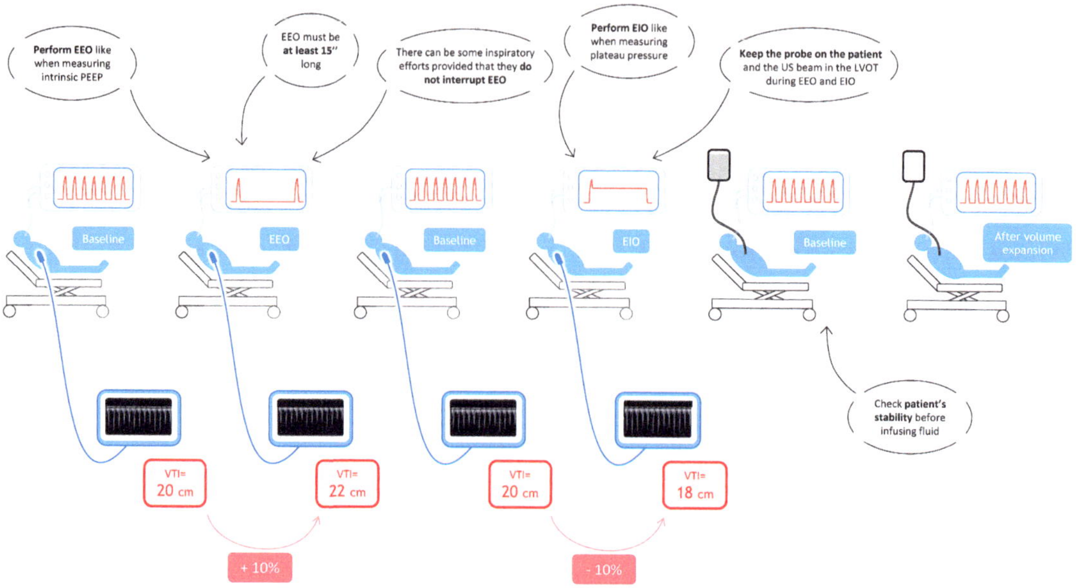

Fig. 53.3 The end-expiratory and end-inspiratory occlusion tests
Under mechanical ventilation, preload responsiveness is associated with a significant increase in the velocity time integral (VTI) in the left ventricular outflow tract (LVOT) during a 15-s end-expiratory occlusion (EEO) and with a significant decrease in VTI during a 15-s end-inspiratory occlusion (EIO). Preload responsiveness is likely if the sum of both changes (in absolute value) is ≥13%

One study reported that the end-tidal occlusion test was reliable at 8 mL/kg Vt but not at 6 mL/kg Vt [30]. However, several other studies that clearly demonstrated the validity of the test had included ventilated patients with a Vt of less than 8 mL/kg, or even less than 7 mL/kg [25, 31]. This was even recently confirmed by a meta-analysis that only included studies performed under conditions of low Vt [32]. In addition, the EEO test has been shown to be reliable regardless of the level of respiratory driving pressure [33]. Thus, low Vt ventilation is likely not a limitation of the respiratory occlusion tests.

Two studies also suggested that the end-expiratory occlusion test was unreliable in a prone position [34, 35]. In one of the studies, reliability was only acceptable in patients whose central venous pressure increased during end-expiratory occlusion [34]. However, there is no obvious reason why the test should be less reliable in a prone than in a supine position, and this point also needs confirmation.

Respiratory Variation of Stroke Volume

What Is the Principle of the Index?

As we have seen, during positive pressure ventilation, each inflation increases the right atrial pressure and decreases cardiac preload. If the right ventricle operates on the ascending portion of the Frank-Starling curve, its stroke volume decreases. In addition to this phenomenon, there is an inspiratory increase in right ventricular afterload. After 2–4 heartbeats, which corresponds to the pulmonary transit time, the preload of the left ventricle in turn decreases. If the left ventricle is also preload responsive, stroke volume decreases. Because of lung transit time, this decrease occurs during expiration. Added to this phenomenon, the inspiratory drop in left ventricular afterload tends to increase the left ventricular stroke volume on inspiration, independently of preload responsiveness. In turn, stroke volume increases on inspiration and decreases on expiration, and the phenomenon is amplified if both ventricles are preload responsive [36].

How to Measure the Index in Practice?

If the arterial pressure waveform can be collected through an arterial catheter, the pulse pressure variation (PPV) reflects the stroke volume variability and indicates preload responsiveness. PPV is the index of preload responsiveness that has received the strongest evidence in terms of diagnostic reliability [36].

In the absence of a blood pressure curve, the variability of the stroke volume can be estimated by echocardiography through the maximal velocity of the systolic Doppler signal in the LVOT [37] (Table 53.3, Fig. 53.4). It has been shown that if this variability is greater than 12–15%, it is very likely that cardiac output will increase in response to volume expansion [37, 38].

It should be noted that this measurement can be complicated because it is necessary to ensure that the ultrasound beam remains in the axis of the LVOT in spite of the respiratory movements (Table 53.3, Fig. 53.4). Without this, the peak velocity in the LVOT might only be related to the cyclic deviation of the ultrasound beam from the left ventricular ejection flow.

What Are the Limitations of the Index?

Beyond the fact that it is rather difficult to measure with echocardiography, the respiratory variability of stroke volume has many limitations due to some very strict conditions of use [36] (Table 53.3). Cardiac arrhythmias are responsible for false positives, since in these cases the variability is not related to preload responsiveness but to rhythm irregularity. The presence of spontaneous ventilation may also create false positives, due to the irregularity of alveolar pressure changes, even though PPV and the variability of the peak velocity in the LVOT have been demonstrated to remain valid [38].

A low tidal volume (Vt), less than 8 mL/kg, on the contrary, creates false negatives because the variation in intrathoracic pressure is too small to create significant variations in preload [36]. Similarly, if lung compliance is low, as in ARDS, the transmission of intrathoracic pressure changes to the heart chambers is weaker [39] (Table 53.3).

In turn, the respiratory stroke volume, assessed by the variability of the peak velocity in the LVOT with echocardiography, can only be used in a minimal proportion of patients, particularly in the intensive care unit.

Table 53.3 Respiratory variation of the peak velocity in the left ventricular outflow tract

What does it consist of?	• Check the validity conditions. • Measure the highest and lowest Vpeak in the LVOT over one respiratory cycle and calculate the respiratory variation: (highest value -lowest value) / mean of both values. • Repeat the measurement over 3 respiratory cycles and average the results.
What is the diagnostic threshold?	Respiratory variation of Vpeak ≥15%.
What are the limitations?	• False positives in case of cardiac arrhythmias and spontaneous breathing. • False negatives in case of low tidal volume (≤8 mL/kg) and low respiratory system compliance (≤30 mL/mmHg).

LVOT left ventricular outflow tract; *Vpeak* peak velocity

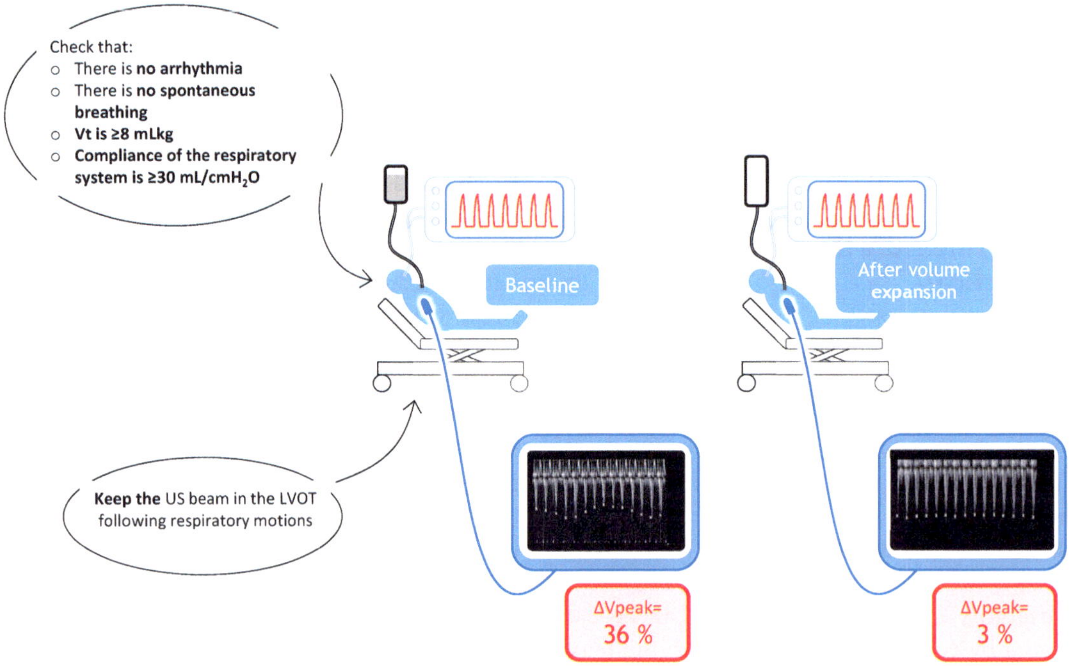

Fig. 53.4 Respiratory variation in the peak velocity in the left ventricular outflow tract
Under mechanical ventilation, the respiratory variation of the peak velocity (ΔVpeak) in the left ventricular outflow tract (LVOT) is high at baseline, indicating preload responsiveness. Fluid infusion leads to an increase in stroke volume, as reflected by the velocity time integral in the left ventricular outflow tract, and a reduction in ΔVpeak. Preload responsiveness is likely ΔVpeak before fluid infusion is ≥12%

Tidal Volume Challenge

What Is the Principle of the Test?

As stated above, the respiratory variability of the stroke volume and PPV is not valid if Vt is smaller than 8 mL/kg. The Vt challenge makes it possible to circumvent this limitation. It consists of increasing the Vt from 6 to 8 mL/kg for 1 min and measuring the changes induced by PPV. If PPV increases significantly, it implies that both ventricles are preload responsive [30]. The advantage of the test is that, provided that PPV is measured through an arterial line, it does not require any device for measuring cardiac output.

The Vt challenge has been validated by far fewer studies than the PPV or the PLR test; for example, even if its reliability has been confirmed in a recent meta-analysis [32]. Moreover, the diagnostic thresholds differ slightly between the few available studies [30].

How to Carry Out the Test in Practice? What Are the Limitations of the Test?

The simplest and most validated method of performing the Vt challenge is to observe changes in PPV [32], which requires an arterial curve, obtained invasively or through the volume clamp method. In the absence of an arterial line, could ultrasound represent a valid alternative? The diagnostic value of Vt challenge-induced changes in the respiratory variation of the peak velocity in the LVOT has not been tested. In contrast, the changes in respiratory variability of inferior vena cava diameter during Vt challenge have been demonstrated to be poorly reliable for detecting preload responsiveness [40]. This is probably explained by the low diagnostic value of the distensibility of the inferior vena cava itself, as we will see below.

Mini-Fluid Challenge

What Is the Principle of the Test?

Intuitively, the easiest way to detect preload responsiveness is to infuse a fluid bolus and observe the induced change in cardiac output [41]. However, the classic fluid challenge, with the infusion of 300–500 mL of fluid, is not a "challenge" but the treatment itself. If cardiac output does not increase in response, the fluid administered in excess cannot be withdrawn. It exerts its deleterious effects without inducing any benefit.

This is why the idea was born of administering a lower volume of fluid so that the deleterious effects are less in the absence of preload responsiveness [42]. It has been shown that if stroke volume or cardiac output increases by more than 5% in response to the infusion of 100–150 mL of solute crystalloid or colloid, cardiac output is likely to increase significantly in response to the administration of a full bolus [28]. After relatively small studies, two recent meta-analyses confirmed the reliability of the mini-fluid challenge [28, 32]. They have been confirmed by a multicenter study involving more than 100 patients in the operating theater [43].

How to Carry Out the Test in Practice?

The mini-fluid challenge requires direct estimation of cardiac output or stroke volume; that is, it cannot be done by just measuring arterial pressure changes [44, 45]. Echocardiography is one of the means that can be used. As the diameter of the LVOT remains constant during the infusion of a fluid bolus, and since heart rate does not change to a significant extent [46], changes in LVOT VTI induced by a mini fluid challenge are proportional to changes in cardiac output (Table 53.4, Fig. 53.5). Nevertheless, the diagnostic threshold of the mini fluid challenge (5% [28]) is smaller than the smallest significant change in LVOT VTI detectable by echocardiography [17]. Thus, care must be taken to perform a very careful measurement of the LVOT VTI. The accuracy of transthoracic echocardiography is greater when changes are measured when keeping the hand on the thorax with the ultrasound beam in the LVOT [17] (Table 53.4, Fig. 53.5). Thus, the results of the mini fluid challenge will be more reliable if the injection is performed quickly, for example, by means of two boluses of 50 mL of fluid infused with a syringe, keeping the hand on the patient without interrupting the measurement of the LVOT VTI.

What Are the Limitations of the Test?

The majority of studies that have investigated the reliability of the mini-fluid challenge pose a methodological problem [47]. Indeed, these studies used as an evaluation criterion not the response to the volume administered after the mini-fluid challenge but the response to the total volume infused, including that already administered during the test itself. Thus, the challenge mini-fluid primarily predicts

Table 53.4 Mini fluid challenge

What does it consist of?	• Measure VTI at baseline. • Infuse 100–150 mL fluid rapidly (typically with 50 mL syringes) while keeping the probe on the patient. • Measure VTI at the end of the infusion.
What is the diagnostic threshold?	↗ VTI ≥5%
What are the limitations?	• Small threshold compared to the least significant change in VTI. Rely only on "good" VTI measurements in echogenic patients. • May induce fluid overload if repeated.

VTI velocity time integral

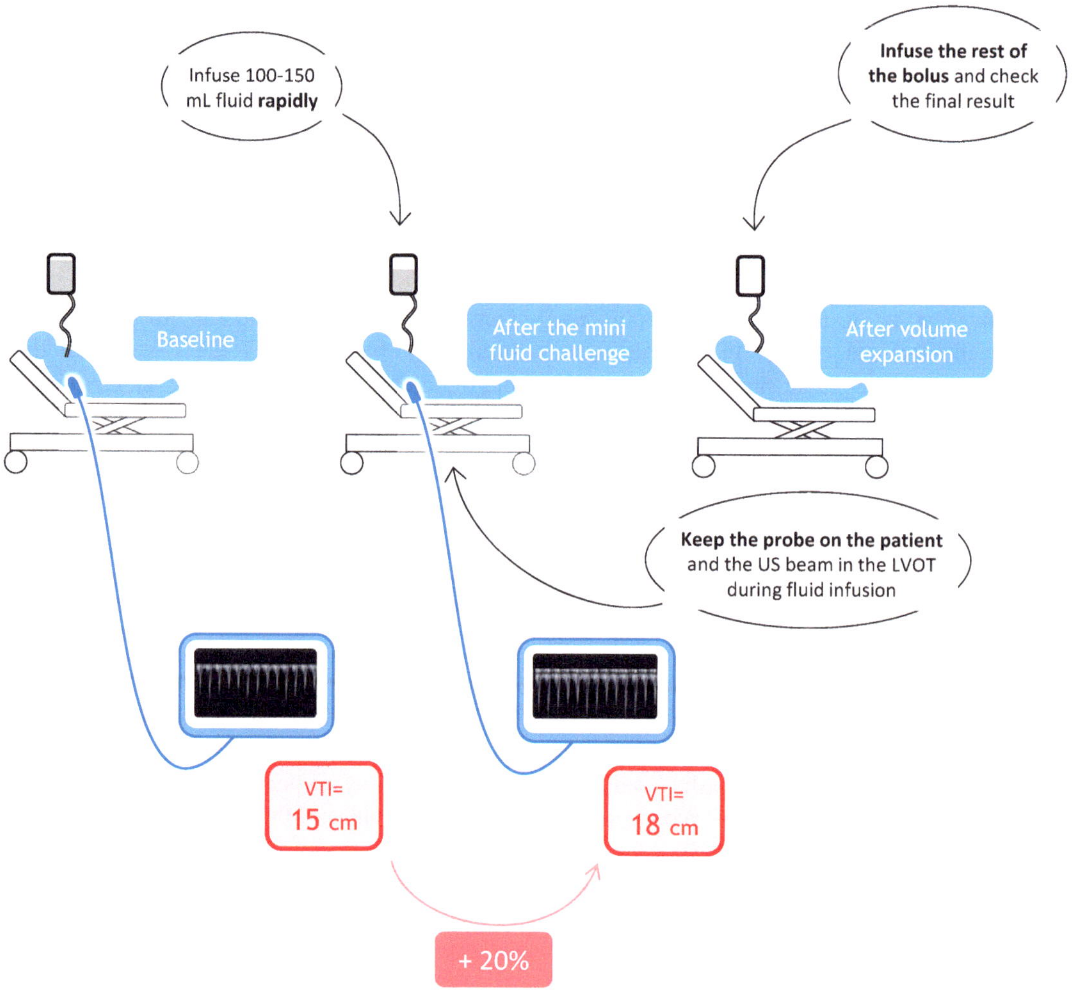

Fig. 53.5 Mini-fluid challenge
The effects of the infusion of a bolus of 100–150 mL bolus of fluid on the velocity time integral (VTI) measured in the left ventricular outflow tract (LVOT) is predictive of the subsequent effect of the rest of a 500 mL-fluid bolus on cardiac output. The diagnostic threshold is a 5% increase in VTI

the effects of the challenge mini-fluid itself. This could have led to an overestimation of the reliability of the test [48]. Further studies should clarify whether this is an important limitation.

Beyond this possible methodological limitation, the major drawback of the mini-fluid challenge is that it still involves the infusion of fluid, which cannot be evacuated if it proves to be ineffective. If repeated, it inherently induces fluid overload, although the risk is less than with a classic fluid challenge.

Variation in the Diameter of the Vena Cava

What Is the Principle of the Index?

Under mechanical ventilation, in the event of preload responsiveness, the central venous pressure, i.e., the intramural pressure of the vena cava, varies significantly during breathing [49], inducing a variation in its diameter. However, other phenomena are also involved. In the case of hypovolemia, the compliance of the vessels is higher, favoring the variation of their diameter during ventilation. Also, for the inferior vena cava, respiratory variations in intra-abdominal pressure, linked to thoraco-abdominal transmission of changes in intrathoracic pressure, influence respiratory changes in diameter.

How to Measure the Index in Practice?

Variations in the diameter of the inferior vena cava are measured on a subcostal section in transthoracic ultrasound. The vessel can be identified by two-dimensional ultrasound in the retro-hepatic pathway, upstream of its drainage into the right atrium. Motion mode allows an accurate measurement of inferior vena cava diameter over time and facilitates the calculation of its respiratory variability. The measurement must be taken in the last centimeters of the vein before it enters the right atrium. The diagnostic value retained is a variation greater than 15% (Table 53.5).

Respiratory variations of the superior vena cava are only measurable by transesophageal echocardiography. The section is obtained from the section of the basal vessels by centering the image on the superior vena cava in transverse section and then by turning the multiplane probe up to approximately 90° in order to obtain a longitudinal section of this vein. The threshold values used for diagnosis are more variable, ranging from 12% to 36% [50].

What Are the Limitations?

The respiratory variability of the diameter of the vena cava shares the limitations of PPV and its surrogates, apart from cardiac arrhythmia. In the case of spontaneous ventilation, low tidal volume, and/or low pulmonary compliance, the diagnostic value is less. Also, this index is not valid in the case of intra-abdominal hypertension [51] (Table 53.5).

The fact that, as we have seen, the variability of the diameter of the vena cava depends on many factors that are not related to the degree of preload responsiveness probably explains why this index is the least reliable of all the methods predicting the response to the volume expansion (Table 53.5). This has been demonstrated by numerous small studies, included in meta-analyses [52–55]. This was also demonstrated in a study that included a large number of patients, which showed that the diagnostic value of the variability in the diameter of the vena cava, in particular the inferior vena cava, is low for detecting preload responsiveness [51]. Only the extreme values, observed in very few patients, were informative [51].

What Is the Practical Use of Preload Responsiveness Tests and Indices?

No Magic Value!

It should be kept in mind that no diagnostic test or index has perfect reliability. The diagnostic thresholds found by the studies, even if they were

Table 53.5 Respiratory changes in venae cavae diameter

What does it consist of?	• Measure the diameter of the vena cava at expiration and at inspiration (inferior vena cava: transthoracic echography, superior vena cava: transoesophageal echography). • Calculate the respiratory variation: (largest diameter—smallest diameter) / mean of both diameters.
What is the diagnostic threshold?	Superior vena cava: variability ≥15% Inferior vena cava: variability ≥15–36%
What are the limitations?	• Less reliable than other indices and tests. • False positives in case of spontaneous breathing. • False negatives in case of low tidal volume (≤8 mL/kg) and low respiratory system compliance (≤30 mL/mmHg). • Unreliable in case of intra-abdominal hypertension.

numerous and solid, should not be considered as "magic" values. In addition, for the purpose of studies, the preload responsiveness state is described in a binary way (response, no response). However, the Frank-Starling relation shows that the preload responsiveness state is a continuous variable (Fig. 53.1). Some patients are non-responders, others are very responsive, and others are poor responders. Thus, the higher the value of the index, the further the test result is from the diagnostic threshold described, and the greater the probability of the presence or absence of preload responsiveness.

Test the Preload Responsiveness: Not Always!

The clinical context in which volume expansion is intended is important to consider. In cases where profound hypovolemia is certain, such as during severe extracellular dehydration, hemorrhage, or in the initial phase of septic shock before any fluid infusion, the patient is definitely in a preload responsiveness state. In these cases, it is useless to search for it, and performing tests and measuring indices can only delay processing unnecessarily.

Also, the positivity of a test or index of preload responsiveness should not systematically lead to the infusion of fluid. First of all, it should be remembered that preload responsiveness is physiological. A positive test or index should lead to volume expansion only if it seems necessary to increase cardiac output, i.e., if there are arguments that it is too low (oliguria, elevation of blood lactate, or of the veno-arterial gradient in partial pressure of carbon dioxide, lengthening of the capillary refill time, etc.) Then, the decision to perform a volume expansion must also take into account the risks to which it exposes the patient. Even in the case of preload responsiveness, the severity of ARDS or the obvious elevation of the pulmonary hydrostatic pressure may lead to preferring to restore the hemodynamic state rather than by fluid treatment [2].

Test Preload Responsiveness, Not Just to Decide to Infuse Fluid!

The most important interest of the tests and indices that we have described is to avoid infusing fluid into patients who will not benefit from it. However, they can also be used to guide the decision to withdraw fluid.

During the de-escalation phase of shock, fluid withdrawal is another means of reducing the cumulative fluid balance. However, the fear is always that the depletion of fluid exceeds its goal and deteriorates the hemodynamic condition. However, cardiac output only decreases in response to fluid withdrawal if it is dependent on preload. This is another advantage of estimating preload responsiveness. It has been shown that when the PLR test is negative, fluid withdrawal is unlikely to lead to a drop in cardiac output and blood pressure [56].

Conclusion

To guide the fluid therapy decision process, many tests and indices are now available to test preload responsiveness. Their use should reasonably lead to the administration of the fluid only in patients who will benefit from it in terms of cardiac output and to lower the total fluid balance. Most of these tests and indices can be measured or performed with echocardiography, even if for some an adaptation is necessary because of the reproducibility of ultrasound, which is less than that of other techniques for measuring cardiac output.

References

1. Monnet X, Teboul JL. My patient has received fluid. How to assess its efficacy and side effects? Ann Intensive Care. 2018;8:54.
2. Malbrain M, Van Regenmortel N, Saugel B, De Tavernier B, Van Gaal PJ, Joannes-Boyau O, et al. Principles of fluid management and stewardship in septic shock: it is time to consider the four D's and the four phases of fluid therapy. Ann Intensive Care. 2018;8:66.

3. Monnet X, Marik PE, Teboul JL. Prediction of fluid responsiveness: an update. Ann Intensive Care. 2016;6:111.
4. Tigabu BM, Davari M, Kebriaeezadeh A, Mojtahedzadeh M. Fluid volume, fluid balance and patient outcome in severe sepsis and septic shock: a systematic review. J Crit Care. 2018;48:153–9.
5. Jozwiak M, Silva S, Persichini R, Anguel N, Osman D, Richard C, et al. Extravascular lung water is an independent prognostic factor in patients with acute respiratory distress syndrome. Crit Care Med. 2013;41:472–80.
6. Messina A, Robba C, Calabro L, Zambelli D, Iannuzzi F, Molinari E, et al. Perioperative liberal versus restrictive fluid strategies and postoperative outcomes: a systematic review and metanalysis on randomised-controlled trials in major abdominal elective surgery. Crit Care. 2021;25:205.
7. Vieillard-Baron A, Evrard B, Repesse X, Maizel J, Jacob C, Goudelin M, et al. Limited value of end-expiratory inferior vena cava diameter to predict fluid responsiveness impact of intra-abdominal pressure. Intensive Care Med. 2018;44:197–203.
8. Monnet X, Teboul JL. Prediction of fluid responsiveness in spontaneously breathing patients. Ann Transl Med. 2020;8:790.
9. Jozwiak M, Monnet X, Teboul JL. Prediction of fluid responsiveness in ventilated patients. Ann Transl Med. 2018;6:352.
10. Guerin L, Teboul JL, Persichini R, Dres M, Richard C, Monnet X. Effects of passive leg raising and volume expansion on mean systemic pressure and venous return in shock in humans. Crit Care. 2015;19:411.
11. Jabot J, Teboul JL, Richard C, Monnet X. Passive leg raising for predicting fluid responsiveness: importance of the postural change. Intensive Care Med. 2009;35:85–90.
12. Mesquida J, Gruartmoner G, Ferrer R. Passive leg raising for assessment of volume responsiveness: a review. Curr Opin Crit Care. 2017;23:237–43.
13. Pickett JD, Bridges E, Kritek PA, Whitney JD. Passive leg-raising and prediction of fluid responsiveness: systematic review. Crit Care Nurse. 2017;37:32–47.
14. Monnet X, Marik P, Teboul JL. Passive leg raising for predicting fluid responsiveness: a systematic review and meta-analysis. Intensive Care Med. 2016;42:1935–47.
15. Cherpanath TG, Hirsch A, Geerts BF, Lagrand WK, Leeflang MM, Schultz MJ, et al. Predicting fluid responsiveness by passive leg raising: a systematic review and meta-analysis of 23 clinical trials. Crit Care Med. 2016;44:981–91.
16. Monnet X, Teboul JL. Passive leg raising: five rules, not a drop of fluid! Crit Care. 2015;19:18.
17. Jozwiak M, Mercado P, Teboul JL, Benmalek A, Gimenez J, Depret F, et al. What is the lowest change in cardiac output that transthoracic echocardiography can detect? Crit Care. 2019;23:116.
18. Barjaktarevic I, Toppen WE, Hu S, Aquije ME, Ong S, Buhr R, et al. Ultrasound assessment of the change in carotid corrected flow time in fluid responsiveness in undifferentiated shock. Crit Care Med. 2018;46:e1040–e6.
19. Girotto V, Teboul JL, Beurton A, Galarza L, Guedj T, Richard C, et al. Carotid and femoral Doppler do not allow the assessment of passive leg raising effects. Ann Intensive Care. 2018;8:67.
20. Chowhan G, Kundu R, Maitra S, Arora MK, Batra RK, Subramaniam R, et al. Efficacy of left ventricular outflow tract and carotid artery velocity time integral as predictors of fluid responsiveness in patients with sepsis and septic shock. Indian J Crit Care Med. 2021;25:310–6.
21. van Houte J, Mooi FJ, Montenij LJ, Meijs LPB, Suriani I, Conjaerts BCM, et al. Correlation of carotid Doppler blood flow with invasive cardiac output measurements in cardiac surgery patients. J Cardiothorac Vasc Anesth. 2021;36:1081.
22. Roehrig C, Govier M, Robinson J, Aneman A. Carotid Doppler flowmetry correlates poorly with thermodilution cardiac output following cardiac surgery. Acta Anaesthesiol Scand. 2017;61:31–8.
23. Beurton A, Teboul JL, Girotto V, Galarza L, Anguel N, Richard C, et al. Intra-abdominal hypertension is responsible for false negatives to the passive leg raising test. Crit Care Med. 2019;47:e639–e47.
24. Minini A, Abraham P, Malbrain M. Predicting fluid responsiveness with the passive leg raising test: don't be fooled by intra-abdominal hypertension! Ann Transl Med. 2020;8:799.
25. Gavelli F, Teboul JL, Monnet X. The end-expiratory occlusion test: please, let me hold your breath! Crit Care. 2019;23:274.
26. Gavelli F, Shi R, Teboul JL, Azzolina D, Monnet X. The end-expiratory occlusion test for detecting preload responsiveness: a systematic review and meta-analysis. Ann Intensive Care. 2020;10:65.
27. Si X, Song X, Lin Q, Nie Y, Zhang G, Xu H, et al. Does end-expiratory occlusion test predict fluid responsiveness in mechanically ventilated patients? A Systematic Review and Meta-Analysis. Shock. 2020;54:751–60.
28. Messina A, Dell'Anna A, Baggiani M, Torrini F, Maresca GM, Bennett V, et al. Functional hemodynamic tests: a systematic review and a metanalysis on the reliability of the end-expiratory occlusion test and of the mini-fluid challenge in predicting fluid responsiveness. Crit Care. 2019;23:264.
29. Jozwiak M, Depret F, Teboul JL, Alphonsine JE, Lai C, Richard C, et al. Predicting fluid responsiveness in critically ill patients by using combined end-expiratory and end-inspiratory occlusions with echocardiography. Crit Care Med. 2017;45:e1131–e8.
30. Myatra SN, Prabu NR, Divatia JV, Monnet X, Kulkarni AP, Teboul JL. The changes in pulse pressure variation or stroke volume variation after a "tidal volume challenge" reliably predict fluid responsiveness during low tidal volume ventilation. Crit Care Med. 2017;45:415–21.

31. Biais M, Larghi M, Henriot J, de Courson H, Sesay M, Nouette-Gaulain K. End-expiratory occlusion test predicts fluid responsiveness in patients with protective ventilation in the operating room. Anesth Analg. 2017;125:1889–95.
32. Alvarado Sanchez JI, Caicedo Ruiz JD, Diaztagle Fernandez JJ, Amaya Zuniga WF, Ospina-Tascon GA, Cruz Martinez LE. Predictors of fluid responsiveness in critically ill patients mechanically ventilated at low tidal volumes: systematic review and meta-analysis. Ann Intensive Care. 2021;11:28.
33. Silva S, Jozwiak M, Teboul JL, Persichini R, Richard C, Monnet X. End-expiratory occlusion test predicts preload responsiveness independently of positive end-expiratory pressure during acute respiratory distress syndrome. Crit Care Med. 2013;41:1692–701.
34. Yonis H, Bitker L, Aublanc M, Perinel RS, Riad Z, Lissonde F, et al. Change in cardiac output during Trendelenburg maneuver is a reliable predictor of fluid responsiveness in patients with acute respiratory distress syndrome in the prone position under protective ventilation. Crit Care. 2017;21:295.
35. Messina A, Montagnini C, Cammarota G, Giuliani F, Muratore L, Baggiani M, et al. Assessment of fluid responsiveness in prone neurosurgical patients undergoing protective ventilation: role of dynamic indices, tidal volume challenge, and end-expiratory occlusion test. Anesth Analg. 2020;130:752–61.
36. Teboul JL, Monnet X, Chemla D, Michard F. Arterial pulse pressure variation with mechanical ventilation. Am J Respir Crit Care Med. 2019;199:22–31.
37. Feissel M, Michard F, Mangin I, Ruyer O, Faller JP, Teboul JL. Respiratory changes in aortic blood velocity as an indicator of fluid responsiveness in ventilated patients with septic shock. Chest. 2001;119:867–73.
38. Lanspa MJ, Grissom CK, Hirshberg EL, Jones JP, Brown SM. Applying dynamic parameters to predict hemodynamic response to volume expansion in spontaneously breathing patients with septic shock. Shock. 2013;39:155–60.
39. Monnet X, Bleibtreu A, Ferré A, Dres M, Gharbi R, Richard C, et al. Passive leg raising and end-expiratory occlusion tests perform better than pulse pressure variation in patients with low respiratory system compliance. Crit Care Med. 2012;40:152–7.
40. Taccheri T, Gavelli F, Teboul JL, Shi R, Monnet X. Do changes in pulse pressure variation and inferior vena cava distensibility during passive leg raising and tidal volume challenge detect preload responsiveness in case of low tidal volume ventilation? Crit Care. 2021;25:110.
41. Vincent JL, Cecconi M, De Backer D. The fluid challenge. Crit Care. 2020;24:703.
42. Muller L, Toumi M, Bousquet PJ, Riu-Poulenc B, Louart G, Candela D, et al. An increase in aortic blood flow after an infusion of 100 ml colloid over 1 minute can predict fluid responsiveness: the mini-fluid challenge study. Anesthesiology. 2011;115:541–7.
43. Messina A, Lionetti G, Foti L, Bellotti E, Marcomini N, Cammarota G, et al. Mini fluid chAllenge aNd End-expiratory occlusion test to assess flUid responsiVEness in the opeRating room (MANEUVER study): A multicentre cohort study. Eur J Anaesthesiol. 2021;38:422–31.
44. Monnet X, Letierce A, Hamzaoui O, Chemla D, Anguel N, Osman D, et al. Arterial pressure allows monitoring the changes in cardiac output induced by volume expansion but not by norepinephrine*. Crit Care Med. 2011;39:1394–9.
45. Pierrakos C, Velissaris D, Scolletta S, Heenen S, De Backer D, Vincent JL. Can changes in arterial pressure be used to detect changes in cardiac index during fluid challenge in patients with septic shock? Intensive Care Med. 2012;38:422–8.
46. Ait-Hamou Z, Teboul JL, Anguel N, Monnet X. How to detect a positive response to a fluid bolus when cardiac output is not measured? Ann Intensive Care. 2019;9:138.
47. Vistisen ST, Scheeren TWL. Challenge of the mini-fluid challenge: filling twice without creating a self-fulfilling prophecy design. Anesthesiology. 2018;128:1043–4.
48. Enevoldsen J, Scheeren TWL, Berg JM, Vistisen ST. Existing fluid responsiveness studies using the mini-fluid challenge may be misleading: methodological considerations and simulations. Acta Anaesthesiol Scand. 2021;66(1):17–24.
49. Magder S, Georgiadis G, Cheong T. Respiratory variations in right atrial pressure predict the response to fluid challenge. J Crit Care. 1992;1992:76–85.
50. Shi R, Monnet X, Teboul JL. Parameters of fluid responsiveness. Curr Opin Crit Care. 2020;26:319–26.
51. Vignon P, Repesse X, Begot E, Leger J, Jacob C, Bouferrache K, et al. Comparison of echocardiographic indices used to predict fluid responsiveness in ventilated patients. Am J Respir Crit Care Med. 2017;195:1022–32.
52. Zhang H, Zhang Q, Chen X, Wang X, Liu D. Chinese Critical Ultrasound Study G. Respiratory variations of inferior vena cava fail to predict fluid responsiveness in mechanically ventilated patients with isolated left ventricular dysfunction. Ann Intensive Care. 2019;9:113.
53. Long E, Oakley E, Duke T, Babl FE. Paediatric Research in Emergency Departments International C. Does respiratory variation in inferior vena cava diameter predict fluid responsiveness: a systematic review and meta-analysis. Shock. 2017;47:550–9.
54. Das SK, Choupoo NS, Pradhan D, Saikia P, Monnet X. Diagnostic accuracy of inferior vena caval respiratory variation in detecting fluid unresponsiveness: A systematic review and meta-analysis. Eur J Anaesthesiol. 2018;35:831–9.
55. Huang H, Shen Q, Liu Y, Xu H, Fang Y. Value of variation index of inferior vena cava diameter in predicting fluid responsiveness in patients with circulatory shock receiving mechanical ventilation: a systematic review and meta-analysis. Crit Care. 2018;22:204.
56. Monnet X, Cipriani F, Camous L, Sentenac P, Dres M, Krastinova E, et al. The passive leg raising test to guide fluid removal in critically ill patients. Ann Intensive Care. 2016;6:46.

54 Assessment of Venous Congestion with Ultrasound

Korbin Haycock

Learning Objectives

1. Review how point of care ultrasound (POCUS) can be used to assess for venous congestion in various ways.
2. Understand how to use Doppler techniques such as the venous excess with ultrasound score (VExUS) and femoral vein pulsatility to assess for venous congestion.
3. Compare the utility and applications of Doppler techniques to assess venous congestion with IVC collapsibility.

Introduction

Venous congestion is gaining increasing recognition as an important component of hemodynamics. Central venous pressure (CVP) has largely been regarded as a surrogate of ventricular preloading conditions in the past, rather than being seen in the context of a final downstream detriment to the systemic circulation of blood [1, 2]. In addition to being the primary impedance to venous return to the heart, elevations in venous pressure also serve as a terminal outflow interference for perfusing blood flow through the organs, as well as to decrease the lymphatic clearance of interstitial fluid. Furthermore, increased congestive forces combined with diminished lymphatic drainage of the organs promote elevated interstitial pressures that reduce the transcapillary flux of nutrients to the tissues [1, 3–5]. Increases in venous congestion and interstitial pressure are particularly detrimental to perfusion in encapsulated organs such as the kidneys or the brain [6–9].

While assessment of venous congestion with ultrasound is a new and evolving area, the harmful effects of excess venous pressures on multiple organ systems have been well documented. A positive fluid balance has been associated with adverse outcomes in multiple studies [10–17]. Portal vein pulsatility in the context of venous hypertension has been linked with encephalopathy and ICU delirium. In addition, portal hypertension in venous congested states leads to malnutrition, inflammation, bacterial translocation, and promotion of sepsis syndromes [18–22]. The kidneys, as encapsulated organs, are particularly vulnerable to congestion [6, 7]. Poor renal and other outcomes have been demonstrated in the environment of renal venous congestion in both acutely ill and chronic cardiorenal syndromes [10, 15, 17, 23–29].

K. Haycock (✉)
Emergency Medicine and Pediatrics, Loma Linda University School of Medicine, Loma Linda, CA, USA

Department of Emergency Medicine, Riverside University Health System Medical Center, Moreno Valley, CA, USA

Department of Emergency Medicine, Loma Linda University Medical Center, Loma Linda, CA, USA

Department of Emergency Medicine, Desert Regional Medical Center, Palm Springs, CA, USA

M. J. Lanspa, A. T. Levinson (eds.), *Echocardiography and Ultrasonography in the ICU*, Respiratory Medicine, https://doi.org/10.1007/978-3-031-80038-2_54

An important point is that once venous congestion has been appreciated, the clinician should consider the cause of the congestion and what approach is best to manage the condition. Venous congestion can be the result of volume overload, right ventricular dysfunction, or a combination of both. Furthermore, right ventricular dysfunction may be the result of volume overloading, valve dysfunction, infarction, acute or chronic pre-capillary pulmonary hypertension, or left ventricular failure.

Point of care ultrasound (POCUS) can be used to assess for venous congestion in various ways. The most basic and popular method historically was to assess the inferior vena cava (IVC) for size and amount of IVC collapse with spontaneous respiration or the release of ventilator-delivered breaths. However, an IVC that appears to suggest elevated CVP does not necessarily mean there is venous congestion, nor can it quantify the degree of congestion. More recently, Doppler techniques such as the venous excess with ultrasound score (VExUS) and femoral vein pulsatility have been used, which, while more technically challenging, provide more information about actual venous congestion than 2D POCUS of the IVC alone.

IVC

The IVC can be viewed in multiple windows. The most common approach is the subcostal echocardiographic view, with the probe rotated counterclockwise until the indicator is directed toward the patient's head, giving a long-axis view. With a 90-degree rotation, the IVC can be seen in the short axis from the subcostal view as well. An alternative to the subcostal window is a transhepatic approach from the lateral upper abdomen. Here, with the indicator to the head, the IVC can be seen on a long axis (with the right side of the IVC in the near field and the left side in the far field), and with the indicator pointed to the ceiling, the indicator side of the sector indicates the anterior IVC and the non-indicator side is the posterior IVC.

Ultrasonographic evaluation of the IVC is affected by multiple factors. Because the IVC is measured as it transits through the liver and on the abdominal side of the diaphragmatic border between the abdomen and the thorax, the size and collapsibility are essentially determined between differences in compressive intraabdominal pressures (which tend to collapse the IVC), and pressures inside the IVC (which tend to distend the IVC) which rise with increasing CVP. While intrabdominal pressures are relatively static, CVP is more dynamic and affected by the sum of interactions of those factors promoting venous return, right heart function, and intrathoracic pressures [30, 31].

The primary driving forces for venous return to the heart are the sum of the pressures exerted by the elastic recoil of the small veins and venules and the elastic recoil of the arterial system that fills the venous side when blood transits the capillary beds. Because the capacitance of the venous circulation is much higher than the arterial side of the circulation, most of the blood volume resides in the venous compartment, and the upstream filling pressure of the heart—the mean systemic filling pressure (Pmsf)—is closer to venous rather than arterial pressures as well. A higher Pmsf will promote IVC distension [31, 32].

Right heart function will lower the CVP when the heart can effectively translate the forces promoting venous return into forward flow. This is because the flow that the upstream Pmfs generates that fills the right ventricle is efficiently ejected forward, and thus the residual downstream pressure at the right atrium is lowered. However, when the right ventricle starts to fail to deal with venous return, the result is a buildup of backpressure which is the CVP [31]. This will increase the pressure gradient between the pressures inside the IVC and the intra-abdominal pressures, thus promoting IVC distension.

Finally, the most dynamic influence of CVP is intrathoracic pressures. With spontaneous inspiration, intrathoracic pressure drops. This will increase the pressure gradient between the combined intra-abdominal pressure, the Pmfs, and the intrathoracic pressure, thus lowering the CVP and encouraging venous return as long as the right ventricle can accommodate the increase in flow [30, 33]. The effect of this is a tendency for the IVC to dynamically decrease in size with inspiration. Conversely, with exhalation, the intrathoracic pressure becomes more positive, and venous return will decrease as the pressure difference between the upstream pressure and downstream pressure decreases. This will tend to increase the size of the IVC with exhalation. When the patient is mechanically ventilated, however, the intrathoracic pressure rises with a breath delivery, and the gap between downstream and upstream pressure narrows, decreasing venous return and increasing IVC distension. The opposite is true when a breath delivery is released [30, 33]. The caveat to these situations in mechanical ventilation is that this assumes the patient is not initiating spontaneous breaths, which would have a modifying effect on ventilator-induced dynamics.

Because the IVC's appearance and collapsibility are so multifactorial, unless the clinician has a thorough grasp on all real-time factors affecting the IVC during a POCUS evaluation, extreme caution must be taken regarding the interpretation of the IVC's appearance in isolation. Other pitfalls in the evaluation of the IVC include an off-true long-axis insonation, where the IVC is seen to seem smaller in size than it actually is, and differential collapse along the length of the IVC in the short axis [34]. Thus, a biplane (both short and long axis) evaluation of the IVC is highly recommended. Although distension of the IVC usually indicates either some right ventricular dysfunction and/or volume overload, it does not necessarily imply clinically relevant venous congestion. Rather, an IVC that appears full should caution the clinician that a state of volume intolerance exists, and administration of IVF should be given only with careful consideration.

VExUS

The VExUS exam consists of pulsed wave (PW) Doppler evaluation of a hepatic vein, the portal vein, and an intrarenal vein when the IVC is plethoric. Each vein is given an assigned value as normal, a mild abnormality, or a severe abnormality depending on the Doppler pattern. Depending on the number and severity of total Doppler patterns, the VExUS is scored as Grade 0 (IVC <2 cm), Grade 1 (IVC >2 cm and only normal or mild abnormalities), Grade 2 (IVC >2 cm and one severe abnormality), or Grade 3 (IVC >2 cm and 2 or more severe abnormalities) [35] (Fig. 54.1). Grade 3 VExUS scores have been associated with increased rates of kidney injury in both cardiac surgical and general intensive care populations [35, 36]. In patients with cardiorenal syndrome, an improvement in VExUS scores was associated with the resolution of acute kidney injury [37]. Further research into the clinical utility of VExUS in both the inpatient and outpatient settings is ongoing.

Hepatic vein Doppler is the first component of the VExUS exam. The PW Doppler pattern of the hepatic vein mirrors the jugular venous waveform and consists of the A wave, S wave, V wave, and D wave (corresponding to the A wave, X descent, V wave, and Y descent of the jugular waveform). These waveforms represent flow from the hepatic vein towards or away from the IVC and the right atrium, with above the baseline PW Doppler signals representing retrograde flow up the hepatic vein and below the baseline

Fig. 54.1 VExUS grading system depending on the number of Doppler findings of normal, mild, or severe abnormalities

VExUS Grade	Doppler Patterns from HVD, PVD, and IRVD
0	IVC < 2 cm
1	IVC > 2 cm, Normal or Mild abnormalities only
2	IVC > 2 cm, One severe abnormality
3	IVC > 2 cm, At least two severe abnormalities

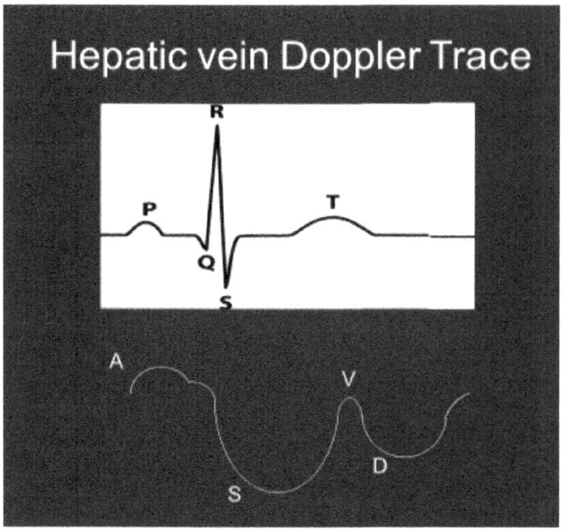

Fig. 54.2 Hepatic vein Doppler trace showing the relationship of the A, S, V, and D waves to the ECG tracing

Doppler signifying flow toward the right atrium (Fig. 54.2).

The A wave is generated by atrial contraction. Because there is no effective valve between the right atrium and the IVC, some of the pressure generated by atrial contraction will result in retrograde flow into the hepatic vein, even though most of the blood flow generated by the contraction is usually directed into the right ventricle at end-diastole. The S wave is determined primarily by three events during right ventricular systole. First atrial relaxation, early in systole, generates a negative pressure gradient that promotes forward flow from the IVC and hepatic vein. Second, the ejection of blood from the ventricles makes room for further blood entry into the atria, which is otherwise limited within the confines of the pericardial sac. Finally, the apical motion of the tricuspid annulus during right ventricular contraction promotes further atrial filling. As the right atria fills to its limit of compliance, the forward flow slows and may reverse as the v wave. With the onset of diastole, the tricuspid valve opens, and the atrium becomes a conduit for blood entry from the IVC to the right ventricle. The normal PW Doppler waveform should have a small A wave, an insignificant V wave (or a V inflection that does not cross the baseline at all), and an S wave with greater peak velocity and velocity time integral than the D wave.

As venous congestion increases, several changes to the hepatic vein waveform occur. The A and V waves will become more prominent, and the S wave will initially become less prominent than the D wave and eventually reverse to an above-the-baseline trace, often fusing with the A and V waves. In the VExUS classification, an S wave greater than a D wave is "normal," an S wave less than a D wave is a "mild abnormality," and an S wave reversal is a "severe abnormality" (Fig. 54.3).

The hepatic vein can be evaluated in the subcostal view with the indicator pointing to the patient's head (as in the evaluation of the IVC in the long axis) or from a transhepatic view. Hepatic veins are identified either by their entry into the IVC or by their non-echogenic walls. It is highly recommended that an ECG trace be utilized when interrogating the hepatic vein so that the timing of the cardiac cycle can be used to correctly identify the Doppler waveforms.

The portal vein drains most of the abdominal organs, and through it, this venous drainage runs into the liver, where blood is delivered to the hepatic sinusoids, which are lined by specialized fenestrated endothelial cells that freely filter plasma into the space of Disse, where much of the hepatic function can then take place by the hepatocytes. The hepatic sinusoids drain into hepatic veins, which progressively merge into the three main hepatic veins that then drain into the IVC. Portal blood flow is characterized by nonpulsatile, undulating forward flow at about 20 cm/sec. Venous pulsations that are transmitted up the hepatic veins are normally dampened by the compliant hepatic sinusoids and thus do not affect the portal flow. However, when hepatic venous congestion from elevated CVP is severe enough to distend the sinusoids to their limit of compliance, the venous pulsations are transmitted to the portal vein, and the normal undulating forward flow becomes pulsatile. Initially minor pulsatility in the portal vein is encountered due to higher amplitude A waves reflecting back to the liver, but the pulsatility increases as A waves become more prominent and the S wave reverses, further interrupting the continuous portal flow.

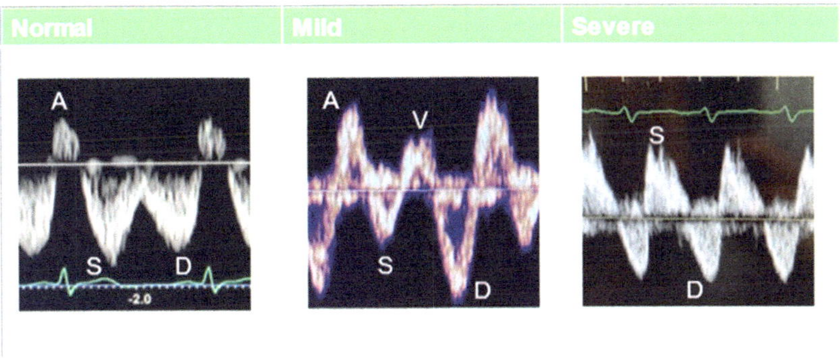

Fig. 54.3 Hepatic vein Doppler with normal, mild, and severe abnormalities within the VExUS classification

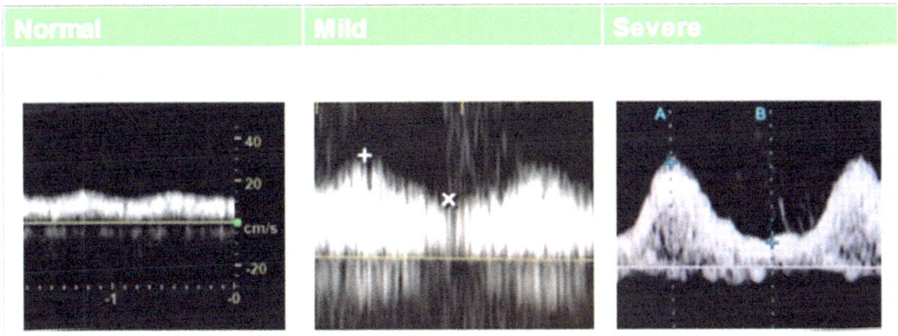

Fig. 54.4 Portal vein Doppler with normal, mild, and severe abnormalities within the VExUS classification

The degree of portal vein pulsatility is determined by taking the peak velocity, subtracting the lowest velocity, and dividing by the peak velocity. This gives a "pulsatility index" or "PI." A PI of less than 0.3 is "normal," a PI of 0.3–0.49 is a "mild abnormality," and a PI greater than 0.5 is a "severe abnormality" in the VExUS system (Fig. 54.4).

Using an upper abdominal window near the anterior axillary line, the right branch of the main portal vein can usually be seen with excellent Doppler angles. Alternatively, the portal vein can often also be seen in the anterior right side of the abdomen, under the costal margin (very similar to where the gallbladder is usually imaged). The portal vein is identified by its echogenic borders, due to its envelopment in Glisson's capsule. Branches of the proper hepatic artery and the bile ducts run along with the portal vein in the portal triad, and occasionally arterial "crosstalk" may be encountered as the artery may fall within or near the PW gate.

The final component of the VExUS exam is intrarenal venous Doppler (IVRD). The venous flow pattern in the renal parenchymal veins has characteristics of both the hepatic and portal veins. Typical venous flow is continuous and undulating, very similar to normal portal flow. With the onset of congestion, the flow begins to become pulsatile but still maintains a continuous forward direction. As congestion worsens, the flow becomes interrupted, having a forward systolic and diastolic component, which can be appreciated by comparison with the above baseline intrarenal arterial flow that accompanies the below baseline venous trace. The systolic component of venous flow is generated by the same factors that are responsible for the hepatic vein S wave, and the diastolic flow represents the hepatic D wave. Progressive congestion will diminish the size of the intrarenal S wave until it disappears completely from below the baseline trace, leaving only the D wave's forward diastolic flow.

VExUS categorizes continuous and uninterrupted pulsatile flow as "normal," interrupted flow with both an S and D wave as a "mild abnormality," and diastolic-only flow as a "severe abnormality." For the purposes of VExUS, the arterial trace is not considered but usually shows wider gaps between the peak systolic flow veloc-

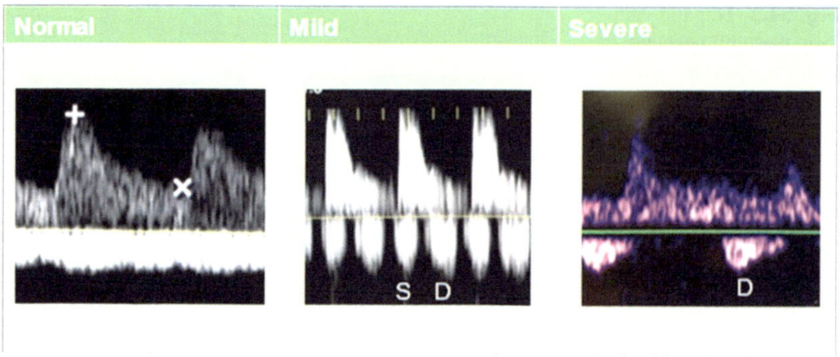

Fig. 54.5 Intrarenal vein and artery Doppler with normal, mild, and severe abnormalities within the VExUS classification

ity and the end-diastolic velocity as congestion worsens (Fig. 54.5).

To image the intrarenal vein, it is important to place the PW Doppler gate over either an interlobar or arcuate vein. Placing the gate too near the hilum will show a venous trace very similar to the hepatic vein trace and will not yield much additional information regarding renal congestion. Interlobar veins can be interrogated by first placing a color Doppler box over the renal parenchyma, finding the vascular bundle traveling between the medullary pyramids, and then placing the PW gate over the vessels. If there is difficulty finding the vessels with color Doppler, the sonographer can decrease the color Doppler scale or, additionally, turn up the color Doppler gain.

Femoral Vein Doppler

Normal femoral venous flow is respirophasic and continuous. Interruption of venous flow with respiration suggests IVC collapse and could represent hypovolemia or vasodilation in an unstable patient, whereas a lack of respirophasic variation in flow can represent venous thrombosis downstream from the site of femoral Doppler evaluation. With mild right ventricular dysfunction, the femoral venous pattern becomes cardiophasic, pulsatile, and even mildly bidirectional. Significant bidirectional cardiophasic patterns (peak retrograde velocity > 10 cm/sec or > 50% forward velocity) likely represent significant right ventricular dysfunction [38].

Summary Points

- Venous congestion is an important, underappreciated clinical entity.
- The IVC, VExUS score, and femoral vein pulsatility are useful tools to assess for the presence of venous congestion.
- VExUS utilizes the hepatic, portal, and intrarenal veins to quantify the degree of venous congestion.

Questions

1. VExUS uses PW Doppler to determine the severity of venous congestion using which vessels?
   A. Hepatic vein, Splenic vein, Portal vein
   B. Hepatic vein, Portal vein, Femoral vein
   C. Hepatic vein, Portal vein, Intrarenal vein
   D. Hepatic vein, Portal vein, Intrarenal vein, and Renal arterial resistive index
   Correct Answer: C
2. A patient that has a plethoric IVC, S wave reversal wave on hepatic vein Doppler, portal pulsatility index 0.4, and D wave only on IRVD has a VExUS grade?
   A. Zero

B. One
C. Two
D. Three

Correct Answer: D

A plethoric IVC will be found in VExUS grades one, two, and three. S wave reversal of the hepatic vein is a severe abnormality. Portal pulsatility more than 0.3 but less than 0.5 is a mild abnormailty. An intrarenal D wave only is a severe abnormality. Therefore the patinet has two severe abnormalities and VExUS grade 3 is two or more severe Doppler findings.

References

1. Berlin DA, Bakker J. Starling curves and central venous pressure. Crit Care. 2015;19:55.
2. Shah P, Louis MA. Physiology, central venous pressure. StatPearls. Treasure Island; (FL)2022.
3. Woodcock T. Plasma volume, tissue oedema, and the steady-state Starling principle. BJA Edu. 2016;17(2):74–8.
4. Vellinga NA, Ince C, Boerma EC. Elevated central venous pressure is associated with impairment of microcirculatory blood flow in sepsis: a hypothesis generating post hoc analysis. BMC Anesthesiol. 2013;13:17.
5. Su L, Pan P, Li D, Zhang Q, Zhou X, Long Y, et al. Central Venous Pressure (CVP) reduction associated with higher Cardiac Output (CO) favors good prognosis of circulatory shock: a single-center, retrospective cohort study. Front Med (Lausanne). 2019;6:216.
6. Cruces P, Salas C, Lillo P, Salomon T, Lillo F, Hurtado DE. The renal compartment: a hydraulic view. Intensive Care Med Exp. 2014;2(1):26.
7. Winton FR. The influence of venous pressure on the isolated mammalian kidney. J Physiol. 1931;72(1):49–61.
8. Dabrowski W, Kotlinska E, Rzecki Z, Czajkowski M, Stadnik A, Olszewski K. Raised jugular venous pressure intensifies release of brain injury biomarkers in patients undergoing cardiac surgery. J Cardiothorac Vasc Anesth. 2012;26(6):999–1006.
9. Lahiri S, Schlick KH, Padrick MM, Rinsky B, Gonzalez N, Jones H, et al. Cerebral pulsatility index is elevated in patients with elevated right atrial pressure. J Neuroimaging. 2018;28(1):95–8.
10. Bouchard J, Mehta RL. Fluid accumulation and acute kidney injury: consequence or cause. Curr Opin Crit Care. 2009;15(6):509–13.
11. Boyd JH, Forbes J, Nakada TA, Walley KR, Russell JA. Fluid resuscitation in septic shock: a positive fluid balance and elevated central venous pressure are associated with increased mortality. Crit Care Med. 2011;39(2):259–65.
12. Kasotakis G, Sideris A, Yang Y, de Moya M, Alam H, King DR, et al. Aggressive early crystalloid resuscitation adversely affects outcomes in adult blunt trauma patients: an analysis of the Glue Grant database. J Trauma Acute Care Surg. 2013;74(5):1215–21. discussion 21-2.
13. Silva JM Jr, de Oliveira AM, Nogueira FA, Vianna PM, Pereira Filho MC, Dias LF, et al. The effect of excess fluid balance on the mortality rate of surgical patients: a multicenter prospective study. Crit Care. 2013;17(6):R288.
14. Mitchell KH, Carlbom D, Caldwell E, Leary PJ, Himmelfarb J, Hough CL. Volume overload: prevalence, risk factors, and functional outcome in survivors of septic shock. Ann Am Thorac Soc. 2015;12(12):1837–44.
15. Zhang L, Chen Z, Diao Y, Yang Y, Fu P. Associations of fluid overload with mortality and kidney recovery in patients with acute kidney injury: a systematic review and meta-analysis. J Crit Care. 2015;30(4):860:e7–13.
16. Danziger J, Chen K, Cavender S, Lee J, Feng M, Mark RG, et al. Admission peripheral edema, central venous pressure, and survival in critically ill patients. Ann Am Thorac Soc. 2016;13(5):705–11.
17. Woodward CW, Lambert J, Ortiz-Soriano V, Li Y, Ruiz-Conejo M, Bissell BD, et al. Fluid overload associates with major adverse kidney events in critically ill patients with acute kidney injury requiring continuous renal replacement therapy. Crit Care Med. 2019;47(9):e753–e60.
18. Valentova M, von Haehling S, Bauditz J, Doehner W, Ebner N, Bekfani T, et al. Intestinal congestion and right ventricular dysfunction: a link with appetite loss, inflammation, and cachexia in chronic heart failure. Eur Heart J. 2016;37(21):1684–91.
19. Sandek A, Swidsinski A, Schroedl W, Watson A, Valentova M, Herrmann R, et al. Intestinal blood flow in patients with chronic heart failure: a link with bacterial growth, gastrointestinal symptoms, and cachexia. J Am Coll Cardiol. 2014;64(11):1092–102.
20. Byrne L, Obonyo NG, Diab SD, Dunster KR, Passmore MR, Boon AC, et al. Unintended consequences: fluid resuscitation worsens shock in an ovine model of endotoxemia. Am J Respir Crit Care Med. 2018;198(8):1043–54.
21. Niebauer J, Volk HD, Kemp M, Dominguez M, Schumann RR, Rauchhaus M, et al. Endotoxin and immune activation in chronic heart failure: a prospective cohort study. Lancet. 1999;353(9167):1838–42.
22. Sundaram V, Fang JC. Gastrointestinal and liver issues in heart failure. Circulation. 2016;133(17):1696–703.
23. Iida N, Seo Y, Sai S, Machino-Ohtsuka T, Yamamoto M, Ishizu T, et al. Clinical implications of intrarenal hemodynamic evaluation by Doppler ultrasonography in heart failure. JACC Heart Fail. 2016;4(8):674–82.
24. Ahmad T, Jackson K, Rao VS, Tang WHW, Brisco-Bacik MA, Chen HH, et al. Worsening renal function

in patients with acute heart failure undergoing aggressive diuresis is not associated with tubular injury. Circulation. 2018;137(19):2016–28.
25. Hanberg JS, Sury K, Wilson FP, Brisco MA, Ahmad T, Ter Maaten JM, et al. Reduced cardiac index is not the dominant driver of renal dysfunction in heart failure. J Am Coll Cardiol. 2016;67(19):2199–208.
26. Gambardella I, Gaudino M, Ronco C, Lau C, Ivascu N, Girardi LN. Congestive kidney failure in cardiac surgery: the relationship between central venous pressure and acute kidney injury. Interact Cardiovasc Thorac Surg. 2016;23(5):800–5.
27. Maxwell MH, Breed ES, Schwartz IL. Renal venous pressure in chronic congestive heart failure. J Clin Invest. 1950;29(3):342–8.
28. Nijst P, Martens P, Dupont M, Tang WHW, Mullens W. Intrarenal flow alterations during transition from euvolemia to intravascular volume expansion in heart failure patients. JACC Heart Fail. 2017;5(9):672–81.
29. Nijst P, Verbrugge FH, Martens P, Dupont M, Tang WHW, Mullens W. Renal response to intravascular volume expansion in euvolemic heart failure patients with reduced ejection fraction: mechanistic insights and clinical implications. Int J Cardiol. 2017;243:318–25.
30. Bodson L, Vieillard-Baron A. Respiratory variation in inferior vena cava diameter: surrogate of central venous pressure or parameter of fluid responsiveness? Let the physiology reply. Crit Care. 2012;16(6):181.
31. Funk DJ, Jacobsohn E, Kumar A. The role of venous return in critical illness and shock-part I: physiology. Crit Care Med. 2013;41(1):255–62.
32. Guyton AC, Lindsey AW, Abernathy B, Richardson T. Venous return at various right atrial pressures and the normal venous return curve. Am J Phys. 1957;189(3):609–15.
33. Grinnan DC, Truwit JD. Clinical review: respiratory mechanics in spontaneous and assisted ventilation. Crit Care. 2005;9(5):472–84.
34. Wallace DJ, Allison M, Stone MB. Inferior vena cava percentage collapse during respiration is affected by the sampling location: an ultrasound study in healthy volunteers. Acad Emerg Med. 2010;17(1):96–9.
35. Beaubien-Souligny W, Rola P, Haycock K, Bouchard J, Lamarche Y, Spiegel R, et al. Quantifying systemic congestion with Point-Of-Care ultrasound: development of the venous excess ultrasound grading system. Ultrasound J. 2020;12(1):16.
36. Spiegel R, Teeter W, Sullivan S, Tupchong K, Mohammed N, Sutherland M, et al. The use of venous Doppler to predict adverse kidney events in a general ICU cohort. Crit Care. 2020;24(1):615.
37. Bhardwaj V, Vikneswaran G, Rola P, Raju S, Bhat RS, Jayakumar A, et al. Combination of inferior vena cava diameter, hepatic venous flow, and portal vein pulsatility index: Venous Excess Ultrasound Score (VEXUS Score) in predicting acute kidney injury in patients with cardiorenal syndrome: a prospective cohort study. Indian J Crit Care Med. 2020;24(9):783–9.
38. Denault AY, Aldred MP, Hammoud A, Zeng YH, Beaubien-Souligny W, Couture EJ, et al. Doppler interrogation of the femoral vein in the critically ill patient: the fastest potential acoustic window to diagnose right ventricular dysfunction? Crit Care Explor. 2020;2(10):e0209.

Pulmonary Embolism and Acute Cor Pulmonale

55

Achikam Oren-Grinberg and Akiva Leibowitz

Learning Objectives

1. Review the echocardiographic and ultrasound findings that are used to evaluate patients suspected of having a VTE.
2. Understand the information that is required to suggest the presence of PE.
3. Examine the limitations of ultrasound when used to evaluate for the presence of PE.

Introduction

Venous thromboembolism (VTE)—the third most frequent diagnosis among cardiovascular disorders—is a spectrum of disease ranging from deep vein thrombosis (DVT) to pulmonary embolism (PE) [1]. It is estimated that the incidence of PE is approximately 100–400 cases per 100,000 people per year [2, 3], leading to anticipated 60,000–100,000 deaths annually in the USA. VTE is a major cause of hospitalization, morbidity, and mortality. For example, one-third to one-half of patients who have had DVT will develop long-term complications [4].

Pathophysiology

The primary cause of death in PE is acute right-sided heart failure due to increased pulmonary vascular resistance (PVR) [5]. Acute and profound increase in right ventricular afterload leads to acute RV failure, RV dilatation, and shock, which can eventually lead to death.

Under normal conditions, PVR is low due to high compliance of the pulmonary vessels. When more than 30% of the pulmonary arterial vasculature is occluded by thromboemboli the pulmonary artery pressure starts to increase [5].

In addition to anatomical obstruction of blood flow by an embolus, vasoactive mediators released mainly by activated platelets lead to vasoconstriction, which in return further increases PVR. Thromboxane A2 and serotonin are likely the two most important pulmonary vasoconstrictors in this context [6]. This significant hemodynamic effect can be reversed by vasodilators [7, 8].

This sudden and significant increase in PVR can have a devastating effect on the right heart.

The right ventricular free wall is a thin structure and therefore cannot withstand sudden pressure overload. Therefore, when exposed to high-pressure conditions it dilated, which in turns leads to increased wall tension and myocardial

Supplementary Information The online version contains supplementary material available at https://doi.org/10.1007/978-3-031-80038-2_55.

A. Oren-Grinberg (✉) · A. Leibowitz
Department of Anesthesia, Critical Care and Pain Medicine, Harvard Medical School, Beth Israel Deaconess Medical Center, Boston, MA, USA
e-mail: agrinbe1@bidmc.harvard.edu; aleibow1@bidmc.harvard.edu

M. J. Lanspa, A. T. Levinson (eds.), *Echocardiography and Ultrasonography in the ICU*, Respiratory Medicine, https://doi.org/10.1007/978-3-031-80038-2_55

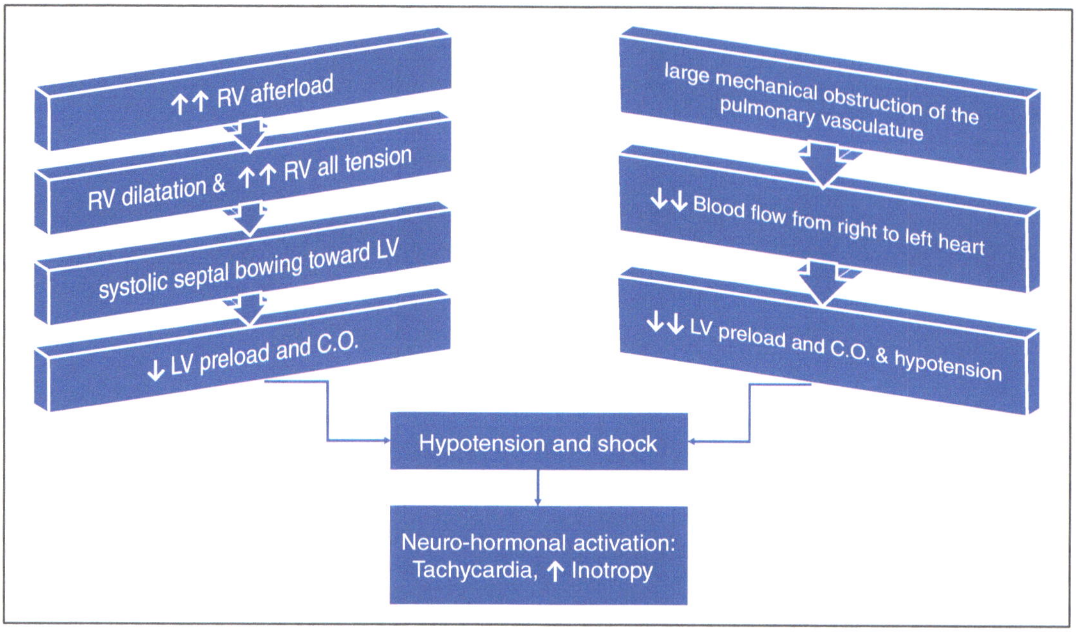

Fig. 55.1 Summary of PE pathophysiology. A large mechanical obstruction of the pulmonary vasculature prevents blood movement from the right ventricle to the left heart. This leads to decreased LV preload, cardiac output, and hypotension. In addition, the sudden and significant increase in RV afterload leads to RV dilatation (which, in turn likely lead to tricuspid insufficiency) and increased RV wall tension. RV pressure overload also leads to septal bowing to the left ventricle, further decreasing LV preload and cardiac output. Finally, it also activates the neurohormonal axis as a compensatory mechanism (e.g., catecholamine release) leading to tachycardia and increased inotropy. These processes cause an increase in RV oxygen demand and ischemia, which eventually leads to decreased RV contractility, decreased RV cardiac output, hemodynamic collapse, and death

stretch. Both processes affect the contractile properties of the right ventricular myocardium. While increased catecholamine levels may temporarily help compensate by increasing heart rate and contractility, the right ventricle eventually fails.

Since RV infarction is uncommon in the setting of acute PE, the presence of elevated levels of myocardial biomarkers (e.g., troponin) suggests RV ischemia because of an imbalance between oxygen supply and demand [9, 10], which further exacerbates RV systolic function and contributes to hemodynamic instability.

Hemodynamic instability in acute and severe PE occurs from significant reduction in cardiac output (C.O.) due to two, parallel processes. First, the mechanical obstruction of the pulmonary vasculature reduces passage of blood from the right to the left heart, reducing left ventricular preload, and C.O. Second, the same process leads to prolonged contraction time, which extends into early diastole of the left ventricle. This leads to interventricular septum shift toward the left ventricle [11], further reducing left ventricular preload and cardiac output [12] (Fig. 55.1).

Role of Echocardiography in the Diagnosis of Pulmonary Embolism

Diagnostic strategy: Computed tomographic angiography (CTA) is the gold standard imaging modality for the diagnosis of pulmonary embolism. It allows for adequate visualization of the pulmonary arteries down to the segmental level and potentially beyond [13, 14]. However, the diagnostic strategy for suspected PE might differ based on availability of CT scan and hemodynamic status of the patient being examined. For example, a patient may not have access to CTA due to lack of a CT scanner in the treating facility, contraindications such as renal insufficiency, allergy to intravenous contrast, or profound hemodynamic instability preventing transport of the patient to a remote CT scanner. It is ***only*** in the setting of shock with hemodynamic instability severe enough to prevent safe transport of the patient to the CT scan and HIGH suspicion of acute PE that echocardiography can be recommended to suggest the presence of acute PE [15, 16].

It is important to realize that there is very little published data on the efficacy of echocardiography for the initial management of acute PE despite its widespread use in this setting. This may explain the recommendation by several societies not to use echocardiography to establish the diagnosis of acute PE [17]. However, strategies that exclude bedside echocardiography from the diagnostic algorithm fail to provide guidance or useful information for patients with life-threatening shock and high probability of PE who cannot be safely transported to radiology. Echocardiography, which looks at direct and indirect signs of PE, is an accepted alternative strategy in such cases [15, 16].

Since up to 50% of patients with PE have also DVT, [18–20] adding lower body compression ultrasonography to the workup of PE may be valuable in this setting, While not as prevalent, it is important to also investigate for upper extremity DVT, which accounts for 10% of all DVT cases [21]. This is especially true with the increasing use of peripherally inserted central catheters (PICC), which appear to increase the prevalence of upper extremity DVT [22].

Echocardiographic Findings in Acute PE Leading to Hemodynamic Instability

Direct thrombus visualization: In patients with acute and severe shock and high suspicion for PE, visualization of a mobile thrombus likely confirms the diagnosis of acute PE (Clip 55.1). TTE visualization of thrombi (usually in the right atrium or ventricle but not in the pulmonary arteries) occurs in about 5% of patients with acute PE [23]. Occasionally, a thrombus can be seen in the pulmonary artery either partially or completely obstructing the artery (Clips 55.2 and 55.3).

Indirect signs: Since visualization of mobile thrombi is rare, the suggestion of the presence of acute PE most often relies on indirect echocardiographic signs.

I. *RV strain*: RV strain refers to right ventricular dysfunction, usually in the absence of an underlying cardiomyopathy. Echocardiographic findings of RV strain include RV dilatation and free wall hypokinesis (Clip 55.4). Since acute and severe PE leads to RV failure (acute dilatation and hypokinesis), PE as a cause of shock can be ruled out patients with normal RV size and function.

II. *Septal dyskinesia*: Dyskinesia refers to the paradoxical (outward) motion of a segmental wall during systole. In the context of septal motion, in the presence of RV pressure or volume overload, septal dyskinesis refers to the abnormal motion of the septum toward the LV. In pure RV pressure overload, the interventricular septum is pushed toward the LV in systole leading to a D-shape of the left ventricle in a cross-sectional view (Clip 55.5, Fig. 55.2). In pure RV volume overload, the interventricular septum is pushed toward the LV in diastole, leading to left ventricular D-shaped in diastole (Clip 55.6, Fig. 55.3). As stated above, acute PE leading to shock and hemodynamic instability is expected to have pressure (and often also volume) overload (Clip 55.7). Therefore, when evaluating a patient in shock with echocardiography, it is expected to see sign of pressure and volume overload. The best views to look for RV pressure and volume overload is the parasternal and subcostal short-axis view (TTE) and mid-esophageal short-axis view (TEE).

McConnell's sign: McConnell's sign is a unique regional wall motion abnormality of the RV free wall. It includes severe RV free wall hypokinesis or akinesis, with normal, and often hyperdynamic motion of the RV apex (Clip 55.8). This pattern is often referred to "RV free wall

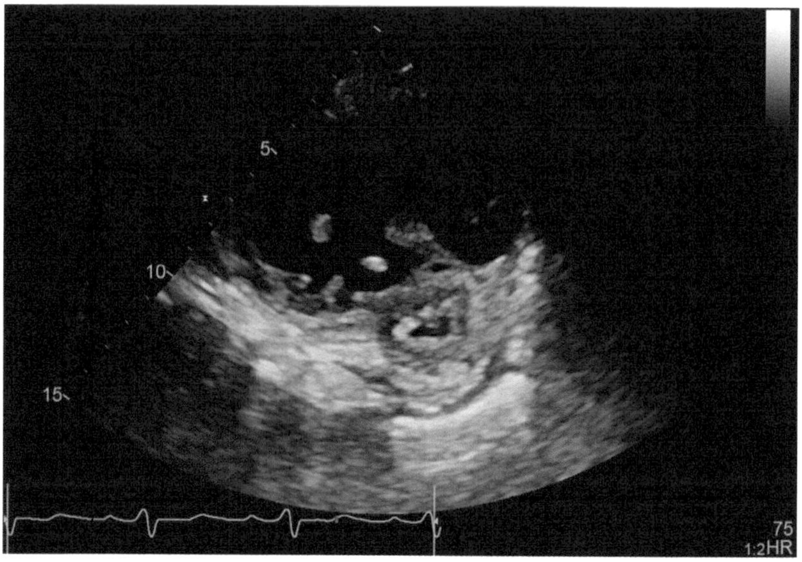

Fig. 55.2 An image of the PSAX view of the mid-papillary section stopped in systole (red bar on the ECG tracing), demonstrating D-shaped left ventricle due to RV pressure overload

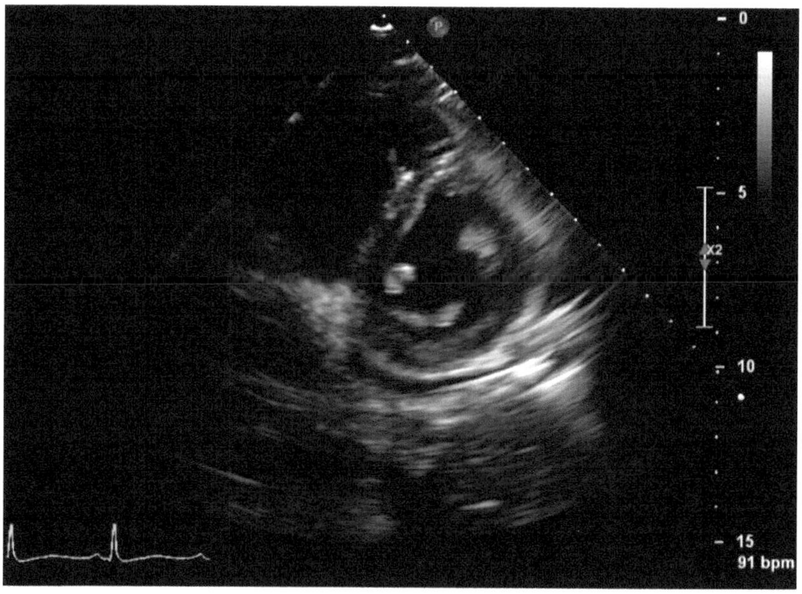

Fig. 55.3 An image of the PSAX view of the mid-papillary section stopped in diastole, demonstrating D-shaped left ventricle due to RV volume overload

hypokinesis with apical sparing." That is, the RV apex is spared from hypokinesis/akinesis and contracts normally or hyperdynamic [24]. Following the original publication, the McConnell's sign was regarded for years as a highly specific echocardiographic finding in acute pulmonary embolism. However, it is now well accepted that the McConnell's sign has poor positive predictive value for diagnosis of acute PE, [25, 26] and can be seen in other instances of acute cor pulmonale (e.g., RV infarction and acute respiratory distress syndrome). Therefore, the McConnell's sign should not be used in isolation for the diagnosis of acute PE.

Doppler Signs of PE:

(a) *Pulmonary artery pressure*: In patients without pre-existing cardiopulmonary disease, pulmonary artery pressure (PAP) starts to rise once about 25–30% of the pulmonary vasculature is occluded [5]. The RV can compensate until greater than 50–75% of the pulmonary vasculature is obstructed by emboli, with ability to mildly increase PAP. As the process continues, the RV dilates when afterload reaches a critical level. Eventually the RV fails due to the combination of increased afterload and RV ischemia, which in turn occurs due to reduced coronary perfusion in the setting of low cardiac output, hypotension, and increased RV pressure. Once the RV fails, it has limited ability to increase pressure in the pulmonary artery. Therefore, contrary to common belief, PA pressure can only mildly increase in patients without pre-existing cardiac disease who have acute and severe PE.

(b) *Echocardiographic estimation of PA systolic pressure*: Assuming no pulmonic valve stenosis, right ventricular systolic pressure and pulmonary artery systolic pressure (sPAP) are equal (equalization of systolic pressures when the pulmonic valve is open). Echocardiography can be used to estimate sPAP using the continuous wave Doppler modality using the simplified Bernoulli equation, which relates flow across a valve to the pressure difference between two chambers. The simplified Bernoulli equation is $P = 4\ V^2$ where P is pressure gradient and V is the maximum velocity across the valve.

In the presence of tricuspid regurgitation, the pressure gradient between the right ventricle and atrium can be estimated using the Simplified Bernoulli equation. The tricuspid valve is interrogated with continuous wave Doppler in the A4CH or RV inflow-outflow views, and the pressure gradient between the two chambers is estimated: $P = 4\ V^2$, where P is the pressure difference between the RV and RA and V is the peak velocity of flow across the tricuspid valve.

It is important to understand that this pressure difference between the RV and RA is "against" a fixed pressure, which is the pressure in the right atrium. Using this concept, the pulmonary artery systolic pressure (sPAP) can be estimated with echocardiography:

$$RVSP = 4\left(TR_{velocity}\right)^2 + P_{RA}$$

where the RVSP is the RV systolic pressure, $TR_{velocity}$ is the maximal velocity of the TR jet (in meters per second) and the P_{RA} is an estimate (or measured, when the CVP is available) of the right atrial pressure (Clip 55.9, Fig. 55.4). In the absence of pulmonary stenosis, the RVSP equals PA systolic pressure. This approach provides a simple and usually accurate estimation of the presence and severity of PA hypertension [27].

(c) *60/60 Sign*: Pulse wave Doppler of the RVOT creates a typical spectral display (Fig. 55.5). The acute development of high pulmonary artery pressure can affect this pattern and typically will shorten RVOT acceleration time (the time from the beginning to peak RVOT flow, Fig. 55.6). In acute PE, RVOT acceleration time is much shorter than in other causes of pulmonary hypertension [28]. Typically, in acute and massive PE, RVOT acceleration time is less than 60 milliseconds (Fig. 55.7).

Coexistence of these two Doppler signs—RVOT acceleration time and TR peak jet gradient—has been described as the "60/60 sign"; RVOT acceleration time of less than 60 milliseconds in the presence of TR pressure gradient of less than 60 mmHg (Fig. 55.8). While the "60/60 sign" is not very sensitive, it is very specific (94%) for the diagnosis of acute PE [29].

(d) Early systolic "notch": Acute development of high pulmonary artery pressure (acute cor pulmonale in massive and submassive PE) can also affect the shape of the RVOT spectral display. "Early" systolic "notching" pattern (spike and dome, or "M" morphology) is a frequently observed (92%) in patients with massive and submassive PE [30] (Fig. 55.9).

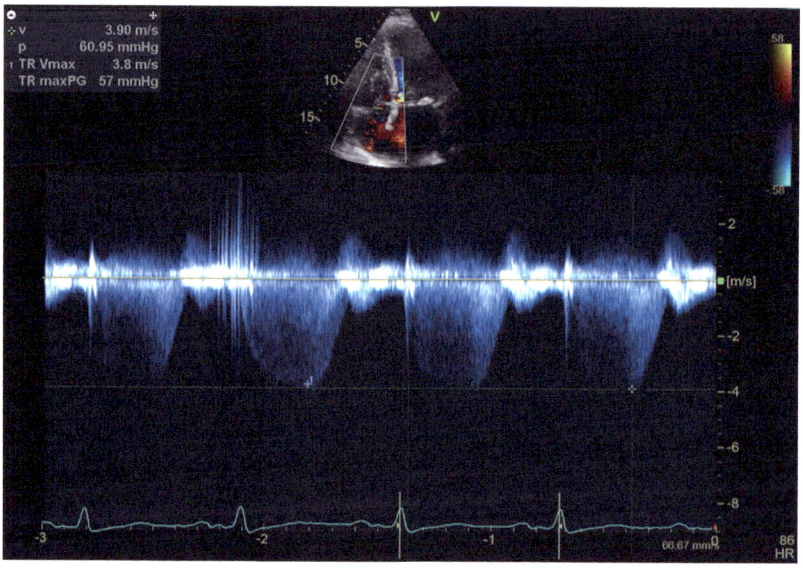

Fig. 55.4 An image of the apical 4-chamber view with continuous wave Doppler interrogation of the tricuspid valve. In the presence of tricuspid regurgitation, a characteristic spectral display is recorded. Using the simplified Bernoulli's equation ($p = 4\ V^2$, p = pressure gradient, V = peak velocity), the peak flow across the valve is converted to pressure gradient from the RV to the LV. In this case, the pressure gradient was calculated by the computer to be 61 mmHg ($p = 4 \bullet 3.9^2 = 61$)

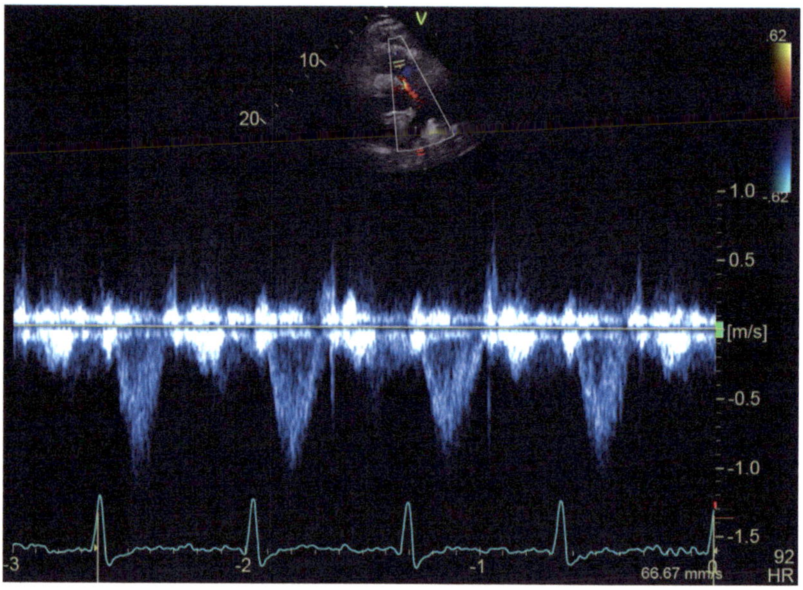

Fig. 55.5 An image of the RV inflow-outflow focusing in the RVOT and main PA. The pulse wave Doppler is used to interrogate the RVOT, creating a characteristic spectral display similar to the pulse wave interrogation of the LVOT

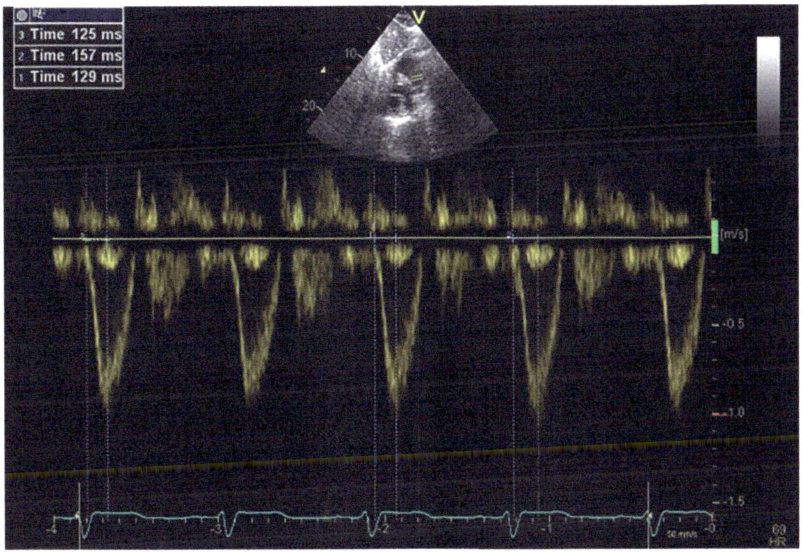

Fig. 55.6 An image of the RV inflow-outflow focusing in the RVOT and main PA with pulse wave interrogation of the RVOT. The RVOT acceleration time (the time from the beginning to peak RVOT flow) is measured and found to be between 125 ms and 157 ms

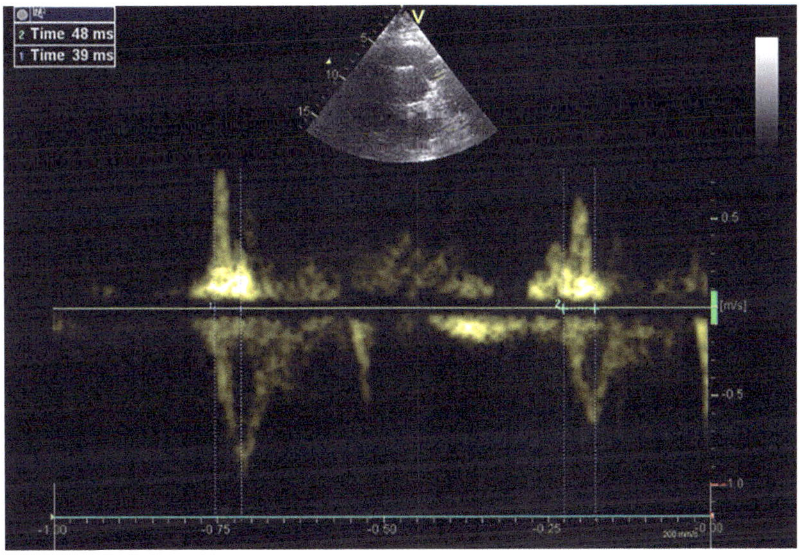

Fig. 55.7 An image of the RV inflow-outflow focusing in the RVOT and main PA with pulse wave interrogation of the RVOT. The RVOT acceleration time is measured and was found to be between 39 ms and 48 ms

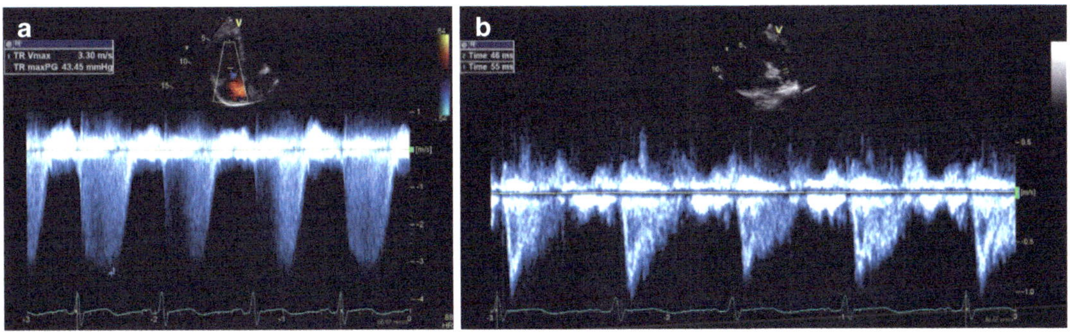

Fig. 55.8 The "60/60 sign". (**a**) Apical 4-chamber view continuous wave Doppler interrogation of the tricuspid valve. The pressure gradient is 43 mmHg (smaller than 60 mmHg). (**b**) RV inflow-outflow view with pulse wave interrogation of the RVOT. RVOT acceleration time is 46 ms and 55 ms, both of which are lower than 60 ms. The 60/60 sign very specific for the diagnosis of acute PE

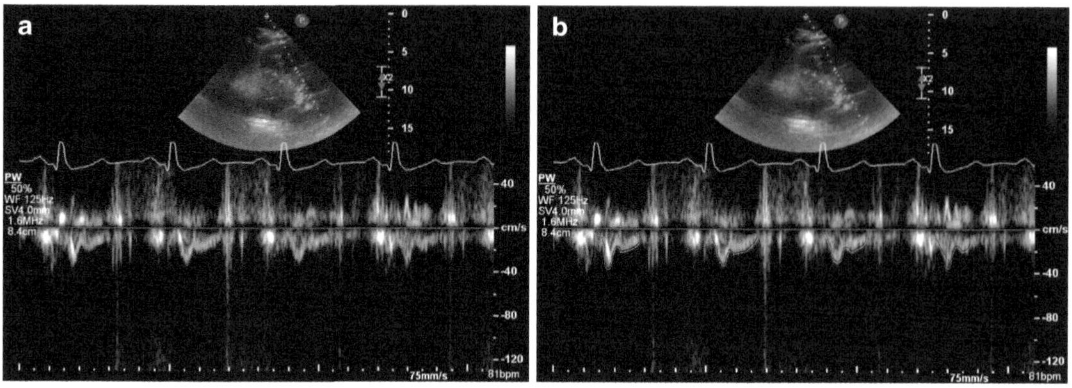

Fig. 55.9 (**a**) Early "systolic notch" of the RVOT spectral display due to acute cor pulmonale, likely from pulmonary embolism (92% specificity). (**b**) Same image with red tracing of the spectral display, demonstrating the "M pattern" of the spectral display

Medical Management of Pulmonary Embolism

The medical management of pulmonary embolism is driven by risk stratification. Patients with low-risk PE are usually treated with anticoagulation. Within the low-risk category, patients with a single sub-segmental PE who have no DVT, active cancer, or symptoms may not require anticoagulation [31]. On the other extreme, high-risk patients with massive PE, defined by hemodynamic instability with sustained systolic blood pressure (SBP) <90 mmHg or a decrease in SBP by ≥40 mmHg from baseline, require immediate intervention which may include thrombolytics and/or thrombectomy and may also require mechanical hemodynamic support.

Patients with intermediate risk (sometimes refer to "submassive PE") defined by hemodynamic stability with SBP ≥90 mmHg and features of right heart dysfunction would benefit from risk stratification using clinical scores such as the Pulmonary Embolism Severity Index (PESI), [32] using 11 clinical criteria, or its simplified version sPESI, [33] biomarkers, and imaging modalities that detect RV strain. Generally, the presence of RV strain (which can be seen on various imaging modalities or with elevated biomarkers) indicates a high-risk, submassive PE and associated with worse prognosis, which may require more aggressive treatment [34].

While the details of the management of patients with PE are beyond the scope of this chapter, it is important to mention that systemic thrombolysis is considered standard aggressive therapy for high-risk patients with PE, but controversial for intermediate risk patients. In this patient population, usually a conservative therapy with anticoagulation is most commonly used.

Pulmonary Infarct

Occlusion of the distal pulmonary arteries may lead to ischemia, hemorrhage, and ultimately necrosis of the lung parenchyma (pulmonary infarction). While it is thought that the dual blood supply to the lungs (pulmonary and the bronchial circulation) is protective against pulmonary ischemia, pulmonary infarction can be found in 10 to 50% of all patients with PE [35].

"Pulmonary infarction" implies necrosis of lung tissue, yet the definition of pulmonary infarction in the literature is mixed. Three different types of definitions are generally used: a histological phenomenon, a radiological finding, and a clinical syndrome. The histological definition is primarily based on autopsy findings with the classical finding of area of 'coagulative necrosis' of lung parenchyma within a hemorrhage region, which is usually next to the pleura. Both radiological finding and the clinical syndrome reflect tissue necrosis.

Pathophysiology: The pulmonary artery system, which is a low-pressure high flow circulation, supplies the lungs with deoxygenated blood, while the bronchial arteries supply the lungs with oxygenated blood at systemic pressure (6 times that of the pulmonary arteries). The bronchial circulation supplies oxygenated blood to the bronchial walls, the visceral pleura, and the lung parenchyma. While this dual blood supply has been thought to be protective against ischemic injuries of the lungs, obstruction of a pulmonary artery by acute PE can cause pulmonary infarction. Sometimes, though, the process is reversible when the intra-alveolar blood is resorbed in 2–4 days, avoiding necrosis or residual damage. In cases where the obstructing thrombus is not absorbed, erythrocytes extravasate into the lung parenchyma and break down into hemosiderin within 1–2 days. Usually at that point, necrosis of the lung parenchyma starts and leads to lung infarction. Eventually, the infarcted area is replaced by a fibrotic scar over a period of weeks (histologically) to months (radiologically) [36, 37].

Thromboembolism in distal pulmonary branches is more likely to cause pulmonary infarction when compared with extensive or central obstructions [36]. This is because when a main pulmonary artery is obstructed, the collateral flow from the bronchial circulation enters the pulmonary circulation distal to the obstructed area [38]. The high-pressure blood flow from the bronchial arteries is distributed throughout the entire arterial bed of that lung, allowing to absorb this abrupt influx of bronchial blood distal to the obstructed central pulmonary artery. In contrast, in distal PE, the pressure of the bronchial arterial inflow distal to the obstructed area may be much greater than the ability of the small, distal arterial segment can accommodate.

In addition to the increased bronchial arteries blood flow, local transient capillary ischemia (from the transient collateral circulation circulatory failure) leads to increased vascular permeability, [39] due to ischemia-induced inflammatory response which, in turn, leads to endothelial barrier dysfunction [40, 41]. The end result of the two processes is increased vascular permeability causes extravasation of red blood cells into the alveoli [36]. While the resulting intra-alveolar hemorrhage resembles an infarct, the lung architecture can be restored once the blood is resorbed. If, however, the intra-alveolar hemorrhage cannot be resorbed, lung tissue infraction is likely to occur [37, 38].

Summary Points

- CTA is the gold standard diagnostic modality for acute pulmonary embolism.
- Echocardiography should be discouraged from routine use for the diagnosis of acute PE.
- Echocardiography has a role **only** in patients with acute shock and high pre-test probability for massive PE, who do not have access to CTA.
- Indirect echocardiographic signs of acute PE include RV strain (RV dilatation, severe RV free wall hypokinesis, or akinesis) and septal flattening, indicating RV pressure and volume overload. These echocardiographic findings are consistent with acute cor pulmonale.
- McConnell's sign—severe hypokinesis of the RV free wall with apical sparing is a non-specific sign for elevated pulmonary pressure (acute cor pulmonale). It is also seen in ARDS and RV infarction.
- The "60–60 sign"—RVOT acceleration time shorter than 60 milliseconds AND TR pressure gradient of smaller than 60 mmHg—is specific but not sensitive sign for acute PE.
- The decision on how to manage patients with high probability for acute and massive PE and echocardiographic evidence of PE (e.g., thrombolytic therapy) should be made only after multidisciplinary discussion with experts in managing patients with pulmonary embolism.

Pro-Tip Callout

In acute PE, RVOT acceleration time is much shorter than in other causes of pulmonary hypertension [28]. Typically, in acute and massive PE, RVOT acceleration time is less than 60 milliseconds.

Evolving evidence: There is very little published data on the efficacy of echocardiography for the initial management of acute PE despite its widespread use in this setting. This may explain the recommendation by several societies not to use echocardiography to establish the diagnosis of acute PE.

Questions

1. The etiology of acute hypotension and desaturation in this patient is (Only ONE answer is correct):
   A. Acute PE
   B. ARDS
   C. Severe hypovolemia
   D. Cannot tell

   Answer: D. This clip of the apical 4-chamber view demonstrates massively dilated and severely hypokinetic right ventricle. The combination of these two findings is often refers to RV strain. The clip also demonstrates McConnell's sign, which consists of moderate-to-severe RV free wall hypokinesis and normal and frequently hyperkinesis RV apex.

   While this pattern is seen in acute and massive PE, it is not a specific sign for PE and seen also in ARDS and other causes of acute cor pulmonale.

   In this case, the patient had ARDS from aspiration pneumonitis.

2. An 84-year-old male suffered unwitnessed fall 2 stairs at home and was found down by family. He was brought by ambulance to the hospital and trauma protocol was activated. His injuries included subarachnoid hemorrhage overlying the left cerebral hemisphere, small bilateral subdural hematomas, bilateral small hemorrhagic contusions in the frontal lobes, as well as a minimally displaced left temporal bone fracture. In addition, he was found to have left 4–6 rib fractures.

   He was stable hemodynamically and on hospital day # 2 he had an echocardiogram done. Based on these images, PE can be excluded:
   A. True
   B. False

   Answer: B: False echocardiography cannot be used to rule out pulmonary embolism. In hemodynamically unstable patients with high pre-test probability and inability to mobilize patients to get a CTA done echocardiography may demonstrate indirect signs of acute cor pulmonale and Doppler signs that may highly suggest PE as the cause of shock. However, it can never rule out the presence of PE. When this patient was sent for chest CTA, large thrombus was seen in the right main pulmonary artery.

3. A 41-year-old female underwent uneventful esophagectomy due to esophageal cancer. Her post-op care was uneventful. On day six post-surgery she underwent evaluation with physical therapy just before getting discharged from the hospital.

   She developed sudden and acute episode of shortness of breath and tachypnea. ABG on non-rebreather face mask with FiO_2 1.0 was 7.45/41/58/29/+3. Within an hour she was in the ICU intubated and in refractory shock. Her systolic blood pressure was in the mid-50 s despite maximum dose of phenylephrine, norepinephrine, and vasopressin.

   Based on the clip recorded during the echocardiogram exam in the ICU, it should be recommended to:
   A. Start systemic anticoagulation therapy with heparin drip
   B. Initiate thrombolysis
   C. Initiate systemic heparin therapy and thrombolysis
   D. None of the above—echocardiography should not be used to diagnose PE

   Answer: C. While echocardiography should not be used to make the diagnosis of PE in most cases, it can greatly help in cases where the patient has no access to CTA, which is the gold standard modality for the diagnosis of PE.

   In this case, the patient cannot be mobilized to the radiology suite to undergo chest CTA due to the severe refractory shock which, if untreated, would likely lead to the patient's demise.

   The TTE clip of the RV inflow-outflow showing the main PA and its bifurcation demonstrates a mass, which is likely a clot in transit, in the right pulmonary artery.

The patient has risk factors for the development of DVT and PE; cancer and recent surgery. The pre-test probably is high given the story of development of acute respiratory distress, severe hypoxemia, and rapid deterioration of her condition and development of refractory shock despite maximum support.

In this setting, finding of a mobile mass in the heart is highly suggestive of PE as the cause of shock. Management decision should be made quickly in a multidisciplinary discussion, including the surgeon and aggressive therapy with thrombolysis and systemic heparin should be recommended, since the patient is in such severe shock that she would unlikely be able to survive this insult without attempting to treat the likely massive pulmonary embolism.

References

1. Huisman MV, Klok FA. Current challenges in diagnostic imaging of venous thromboembolism. Blood. 2015;126(21):2376–82.
2. Bonderman D, et al. Risk factors for chronic thromboembolic pulmonary hypertension. Eur Respir J. 2009;33(2):325–31.
3. Deitelzweig SB, et al. Prevalence of clinical venous thromboembolism in the USA: current trends and future projections. Am J Hematol. 2011;86(2):217–20.
4. Beckman MG, et al. Venous thromboembolism: a public health concern. Am J Prev Med. 2010;38(4 Suppl):S495–501.
5. McIntyre KM, Sasahara AA. The hemodynamic response to pulmonary embolism in patients without prior cardiopulmonary disease. Am J Cardiol. 1971;28(3):288–94.
6. Smulders YM. Pathophysiology and treatment of haemodynamic instability in acute pulmonary embolism: the pivotal role of pulmonary vasoconstriction. Cardiovasc Res. 2000;48(1):23–33.
7. Delcroix M, et al. Effects of vasodilators on gas exchange in acute canine embolic pulmonary hypertension. Anesthesiology. 1990;72(1):77–84.
8. Huet Y, et al. Cardiopulmonary effects of ketanserin infusion in human pulmonary embolism. Am Rev Respir Dis. 1987;135(1):114–7.
9. Lankeit M, et al. Predictive value of the high-sensitivity troponin T assay and the simplified Pulmonary Embolism Severity Index in hemodynamically stable patients with acute pulmonary embolism: a prospective validation study. Circulation. 2011;124(24):2716–24.
10. Mehta NJ, Jani K, Khan IA. Clinical usefulness and prognostic value of elevated cardiac troponin I levels in acute pulmonary embolism. Am Heart J. 2003;145(5):821–5.
11. Marcus JT, et al. Interventricular mechanical asynchrony in pulmonary arterial hypertension: left-to-right delay in peak shortening is related to right ventricular overload and left ventricular underfilling. J Am Coll Cardiol. 2008;51(7):750–7.
12. Mauritz GJ, et al. Prolonged right ventricular post-systolic isovolumic period in pulmonary arterial hypertension is not a reflection of diastolic dysfunction. Heart. 2011;97(6):473–8.
13. Ghaye B, et al. Peripheral pulmonary arteries: how far in the lung does multi-detector row spiral CT allow analysis? Radiology. 2001;219(3):629–36.
14. Patel S, Kazerooni EA, Cascade PN. Pulmonary embolism: optimization of small pulmonary artery visualization at multi-detector row CT. Radiology. 2003;227(2):455–60.
15. Konstantinides SV, et al. 2014 ESC Guidelines on the diagnosis and management of acute pulmonary embolism: the Task Force for the Diagnosis and Management of Acute Pulmonary Embolism of the European Society of Cardiology (ESC)Endorsed by the European Respiratory Society (ERS). Eur Heart J. 2014;35(43).3033–80.
16. Konstantinides SV, et al. 2019 ESC Guidelines for the diagnosis and management of acute pulmonary embolism developed in collaboration with the European Respiratory Society (ERS): the Task Force for the diagnosis and management of acute pulmonary embolism of the European Society of Cardiology (ESC). Eur Heart J. 2019;41(4):543–603.
17. Patel MR, et al. ACCF/SCAI/AATS/AHA/ASE/ASNC/HFSA/HRS/SCCM/SCCT/SCMR/STS 2012 appropriate use criteria for diagnostic catheterization: a report of the American College of Cardiology Foundation Appropriate Use Criteria Task Force, Society for Cardiovascular Angiography and Interventions, American Association for Thoracic Surgery, American Heart Association, American Society of Echocardiography, American Society of Nuclear Cardiology, Heart Failure Society of America, Heart Rhythm Society, Society of Critical Care Medicine, Society of Cardiovascular Computed Tomography, Society for Cardiovascular Magnetic Resonance, Society of Thoracic Surgeons. J Thorac Cardiovasc Surg. 2012;144(1):39–71.
18. Righini M, et al. Diagnosis of pulmonary embolism by multidetector CT alone or combined with venous ultrasonography of the leg: a randomised non-inferiority trial. Lancet. 2008;371(9621):1343–52.
19. Kearon C, Ginsberg JS, Hirsh J. The role of venous ultrasonography in the diagnosis of suspected deep venous thrombosis and pulmonary embolism. Ann Intern Med. 1998;129(12):1044–9.
20. Perrier A, Bounameaux H. Ultrasonography of leg veins in patients suspected of having pulmonary

embolism. Ann Intern Med. 1998;128(3):243. author reply 244-5
21. Engelberger RP, Kucher N. Management of deep vein thrombosis of the upper extremity. Circulation. 2012;126(6):768–73.
22. Muñoz FJ, et al. Clinical outcome of patients with upper-extremity deep vein thrombosis: results from the RIETE registry. Chest. 2008;133(1):143–8.
23. Cohen R, et al. Echocardiographic findings in pulmonary embolism: an important guide for the management of the patient. World J Cardiovasc Dis. 2012;02(03):4.
24. McConnell MV, et al. Regional right ventricular dysfunction detected by echocardiography in acute pulmonary embolism. Am J Cardiol. 1996;78(4):469–73.
25. Casazza F, et al. Regional right ventricular dysfunction in acute pulmonary embolism and right ventricular infarction. Eur J Echocardiogr. 2005;6(1):11–4.
26. Vaid U, et al. Poor positive predictive value of McConnell's sign on transthoracic echocardiography for the diagnosis of acute pulmonary embolism. Hosp Pract (1995). 2013;41(3):23–7.
27. Armstrong WF, Ryan T. Specialized echocardiographic techniques and methods. In: Fingenbaum's echocardiography. 7th ed. Lippincott Williams & Wilkins; 2010.
28. Kitabatake A, et al. Noninvasive evaluation of pulmonary hypertension by a pulsed Doppler technique. Circulation. 1983;68(2):302–9.
29. Kurzyna M, et al. Disturbed right ventricular ejection pattern as a new Doppler echocardiographic sign of acute pulmonary embolism. Am J Cardiol. 2002;90(5):507–11.
30. Afonso L, et al. A Doppler echocardiographic pulmonary flow marker of massive or submassive acute pulmonary embolus. J Am Soc Echocardiogr. 2019;32(7):799–806.
31. Kearon C, et al. Antithrombotic therapy for VTE disease: CHEST guideline and expert panel report. Chest. 2016;149(2):315–52.
32. Aujesky D, et al. Derivation and validation of a prognostic model for pulmonary embolism. Am J Respir Crit Care Med. 2005;172(8):1041–6.
33. Jiménez D, et al. Simplification of the pulmonary embolism severity index for prognostication in patients with acute symptomatic pulmonary embolism. Arch Intern Med. 2010;170(15):1383–9.
34. Stein PD, et al. Outcome in stable patients with acute pulmonary embolism who had right ventricular enlargement and/or elevated levels of troponin I. Am J Cardiol. 2010;106(4):558–63.
35. Cha S-I, et al. Clinical relevance of pulmonary infarction in patients with pulmonary embolism. Thromb Res. 2012;130(3):e1–5.
36. Dalen JE, et al. Pulmonary embolism, pulmonary hemorrhage and pulmonary infarction. N Engl J Med. 1977;296(25):1431–5.
37. Hampton AO, Castleman BL. Correlation of postmortem chest teleroentgenograms with autopsy findings with special reference to pulmonary embolism and infarction. AJR; 1940.
38. Virchow R. Gesammelte abhandlungen zur wissenschaftlichen medizin. Meidinger; 1856.
39. Wagenvoort C. Pathology of pulmonary thromboembolism. Chest. 1995;107(1):10S–7S.
40. Matot I, et al. Fluorescence imaging of lipid peroxidation in isolated rat lungs during non-hypoxic lung ischemia. Free Radic Biol Med. 2003;34(6):785–90.
41. Chatterjee S, et al. Shear stress-related mechanosignaling with lung ischemia: lessons from basic research can inform lung transplantation. Am J Phys Lung Cell Mol Phys. 2014;307(9):L668–80.

The Critically Ill Patient with Pulmonary Hypertension

56

Karim El-Kersh and Bilal Athar Jalil

Learning Objectives

1. Understand pathophysiology of right ventricular failure.
2. Know the limitations of commonly used dynamic parameters for predicting fluid responsiveness in PH patients.
3. Recognize atypical cardiac tamponade in setting of PH.
4. Identify common ultrasound parameters that are used to assess PH decompensation and response to treatment.

Common Pathologic Presentations

It is important to understand the differences between systemic and pulmonary circulations when managing critically ill PH patients. These differences include the vascular circuits and the perfusing pump (left ventricle vs. right ventricle). A normal pulmonary circulation is a low-pressure circuit that can accommodate a significant increase in cardiac output through pulmonary vascular recruitment with a minimal increase in pulmonary artery pressure via a decrease in pulmonary vascular resistance [1]. In PH patients with pulmonary vascular remodeling, there is a decrease in pulmonary arterial compliance and an increase in pulmonary vascular resistance leading to impairment of this pulmonary circuit physiologic response. It is important to note the differences between the right ventricle (RV) and the left ventricle (LV) as they have different embryological origins, structures, and physiology. The right ventricle is thin, heavy trabeculated, crescentic in shape in cross-section, with predominantly longitudinal myocyte orientation leading to peristaltic-like contractility from RV inlet to outlet and a bellows-like movement of the free wall toward the septum [2]. This unique RV structure results in functional differences from the LV in response to sudden increases in preload or afterload. In contrast to the LV, the normal compliant RV poorly tolerates sudden increases in afterload and can better handle an increase in preload [1]. In setting of PH with reduced RV compliance and impaired ventricular function, there is a further compromise in the ability to tolerate a sudden increase in afterload and/or preload. It is essential to consider the interaction of

Supplementary Information The online version contains supplementary material available at https://doi.org/10.1007/978-3-031-80038-2_56.

K. El-Kersh
Division of Pulmonary, Critical Care, and Sleep Medicine, Department of Medicine, University of Arizona of College of Medicine, Phoenix, AZ, USA
e-mail: Karimelkersh@arizona.edu

B. A. Jalil (✉)
Divisions of Cardiovascular Critical Care and Advanced Heart Failure, Heart and Vascular Institute, West Virginia University, Morgantown, WV, USA
e-mail: bilal.jalil@hsc.wvu.edu

M. J. Lanspa, A. T. Levinson (eds.), *Echocardiography and Ultrasonography in the ICU*, Respiratory Medicine, https://doi.org/10.1007/978-3-031-80038-2_56

the cardiopulmonary unit's two components, i.e., the RV and pulmonary arterial vessels, and be cognizant of the concept of "coupling" to distinguish between an adaptive and maladaptive RV. The adaptive RV increases its contractility (homeometric phase) to adapt to the increase in afterload and to preserve ventriculoarterial coupling (RV end-systolic elastance (Ees) adapts to the increased pulmonary vascular afterload, the arterial elastance (Ea), with an efficient energy transfer) [3]. In a maladaptive RV, there is a loss of this coupling and RV dilation (heterometric phase) to maintain stroke volume via the Frank-Starling mechanism. An illustration of the pathophysiology of RV failure is depicted in Fig. 56.1.

A broad categorization of clinical presentations includes patients without a known diagnosis of PH (new patients), specifically, group I pulmonary arterial hypertension (PAH), and patients with a known PH diagnosis who present with decompensated PH, or with a concurrent etiology that triggers clinical decompensation such as sepsis, arrhythmias, bleeding, pulmonary embolism, hyperthyroidism, pregnancy, sudden treatment interruption, an accidental bolus of parenteral vasodilators among others. Due to improved diagnosis and treatment of PAH patients, ICU admissions with undiagnosed group I PAH have decreased considerably [1]. If the patient has a known underlying PAH, it is useful to review the most recent medical records that may include functional class, brain natriuretic peptide or N-terminal pro-brain natriuretic peptide level, 6-min walk distance, cardiac echocardiography, and right heart catheterization hemodynamic data among other data that may be available. This allows the recognition of the patient's most recent risk status, which can be low, intermediate, or high risk [4]. If the patient is receiving pulmonary artery vasodilator therapy, it is important to inquire about any treatment interruption, and to review medications and their doses, specifically doses of parenteral therapies.

A study that included PAH patients admitted to the ICU for RV decompensation found a triggering factor in 41% of the cases [2]. Common insults in critically ill PH patients relate to their fluid status. More commonly, the PH patients can present with volume overload due to various reasons, including disease progression, non-adherence to diuretics and/or pulmonary artery vasodilators, or indiscretion of dietary sodium and fluid intake. Also, PH patients may suffer an insult that causes hypovolemia, such as bleeding or excessive fluid loss due to vomiting and/or diarrhea, causing a decrease in preload. Sepsis

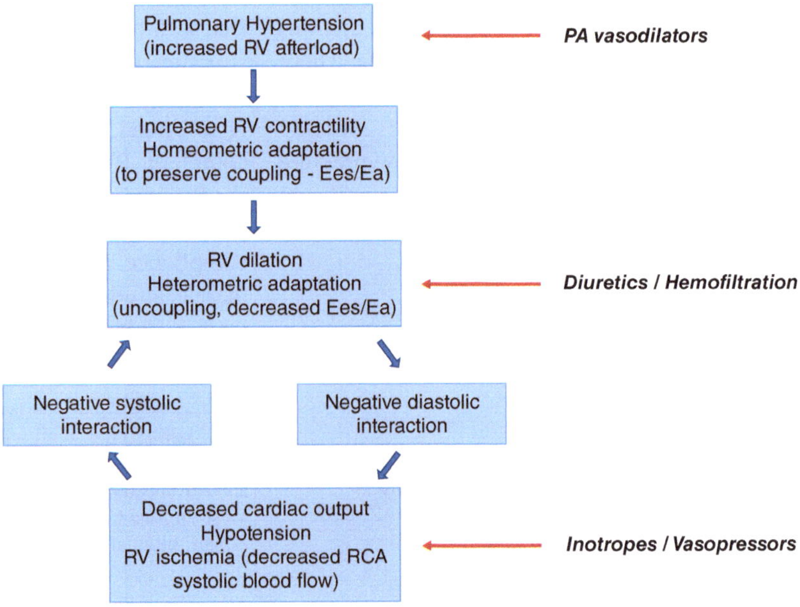

Fig. 56.1 Pathophysiology of RV failure (*PA* pulmonary artery, *Ees* end-systolic elastance, *Ea* arterial elastance, *RCA* right coronary artery)

in patients with pre-existing PH is not well tolerated as the decrease in the systemic vascular resistance can result in a decrease in preload, worsening of RV ischemia, and worsening of the already compromised RV function [5]. It is difficult to predict fluid responsiveness using conventional measurements, as discussed in the next section of this chapter. Atrial tachyarrhythmias can be detrimental in PH patients as the augmented atrial contractility is an essential compensatory mechanism in setting of decreased RV compliance. The loss of this atrial contractility can precipitate RV failure in patients with advanced PH [6].

PH patients do not tolerate mechanical ventilation well. An increase in intrathoracic pressure with positive pressure mechanical ventilation may result in an abrupt increase in RV afterload, which, when coupled with systemic hypotension related to induction agents, is not tolerated and can result in hemodynamic compromise shortly after intubation [7]. If intubation is not avoidable, then hypotension during the procedure must be prevented, and the proactive use of catecholamines can be considered to prevent it [6]. Etomidate may be considered for induction due to its minimal effect on cardiac contractility and vascular tone [6]. Correction of hypoxia and acidosis while avoiding high positive end-expiratory pressure and utilization of low tidal volumes can be challenging but helps to minimize the expected increase in RV afterload in mechanically ventilated patients [1].

Besides treating the triggering factors for RV decompensation in PH patients, volume optimization is an essential part of management. In case of hypervolemia, this can be achieved by diuresis or hemofiltration when applicable. Reducing RV afterload by utilizing pulmonary artery vasodilators for approved indications, optimizing cardiac output by inotropic support, and optimizing the systemic blood pressure by vasopressors as needed are key factors for supporting the decompensated PH patient (Fig. 56.1). If there is an insufficient response, and in the presence of realistic chances for recovery or lung transplantation, extracorporeal lung support can be considered in highly selected cases [8].

Difficulties of Hemodynamic Assessment

Fluid responsiveness and venous congestion are important to evaluate in critically ill patients. Indices to assess fluid responsiveness are grouped into static and dynamic parameters, where dynamic parameters are generally more reliable and accurate measures of fluid status in critically ill patients. Dynamic indices rely on heart-lung interactions that generate respirophasic variations in parameters. The goal is to identify patients on the ascending portion of the Frank-Starling curve who would be deemed to have "preload reserve." [9].

Echocardiography is a commonly used non-invasive tool to assess hemodynamic parameters in the ICU, specifically in predicting fluid responsiveness. The classic index of right ventricular preload is right atrial pressure and measured as central venous pressure (CVP). Echocardiography can be used to non-invasively estimate CVP using a combination of size and collapsibility or distensibility of the inferior vena cava (IVC). Collapsibility or distensibility of the IVC has also been used to predict fluid responsiveness in critically ill patients, but due to venous backflow and right ventricular stiffness [10], patients with right ventricular failure are expected to have persistent distention of the IVC, which would preclude collapsibility or distensibility as an index of predicting fluid responsiveness. Hepatic vein Doppler and IVC size have been studied to assess venous congestion but are also deemed invalid due to venous backflow and altered RV dynamics [11].

The non-echocardiographic dynamic measures of fluid responsiveness that rely on respirophasic interactions such as pulse pressure variation (PPV) and stroke volume variation (SVV) have been well-studied in critically ill patients. In patients without PH, the SVV and PPV denote variations in RV preload. However, in patients with PH, the variation in pulse pressure and stroke volume represents variations in RV afterload instead of RV preload [12, 13].

Pulmonary hypertension makes evaluating fluid status very difficult, and multiple indices used to assess preload and to predict fluid responsiveness have several limitations in PH patients. Thus, it is important to be mindful of the presence of PH while assessing preload and predicting fluid responsiveness.

Echocardiographic Protection from Tamponade

The development of pericardial effusion portends a poor prognosis in patients with pulmonary arterial hypertension [14]. The presence of a pericardial effusion is associated with the severity of right ventricular dysfunction. Effusion size usually correlates with the mean right atrial pressure elevation, which likely contributes to impairment in reabsorption of pericardial fluid through venous and lymphatic channels [4]. Alternatively, in patients with PAH associated with connective tissue disease, the underlying inflammatory condition can independently affect the pericardium resulting in the development of pericardial effusion (Fig. 56.2, Video 56.1). Cardiac tamponade is a clinical syndrome in which the intrapericardial pressure exceeds the intracardiac pressure leading to compromise of cardiac filling [15]. In pulmonary hypertension, the significant elevation in right atrial and ventricular pressures can "protect" from the rising intrapericardial pressure and maintain the right ventricular output even with the intrapericardial pressure elevation [15]. In this setting, the classic echocardiographic signs of cardiac tamponade can be concealed (Fig. 56.3, 56.4, and 56.5; Videos 56.2 and 56.3) [15, 16]. Previous studies have revealed poor accuracy of classic echocardiographic signs of tamponade such as right atrial collapse, right ventricular diastolic collapse, trans-mitral Doppler flow velocity variation, and inferior vena cava plethora in setting of pulmonary hypertension [17].

For example, in pulmonary hypertension, right atrial and/or right ventricular collapse may be absent in setting of a pericardial tamponade that is already compromising the left side, causing left atrial and/or ventricular collapse when the intrapericardial pressure exceeds the left ventricular diastolic pressure [16]. Also, a significant decrease in right ventricular compliance with limitation in changing its volume in response to respiratory cycle can mask pulsus paradoxus clinically, and transvalvular Doppler flow velocity variation on echocardiography [15].

Pericardial drainage should be done with extreme caution in patients with pulmonary hypertension. Rapid drainage of a large volume of pericardial fluid in pulmonary hypertension patients is hypothesized to possibly result in a transmural pressure increase and rapid increase in systemic venous return causing the right ventricle to dilate acutely and the cardiac output to decrease, which may explain the hemodynamic

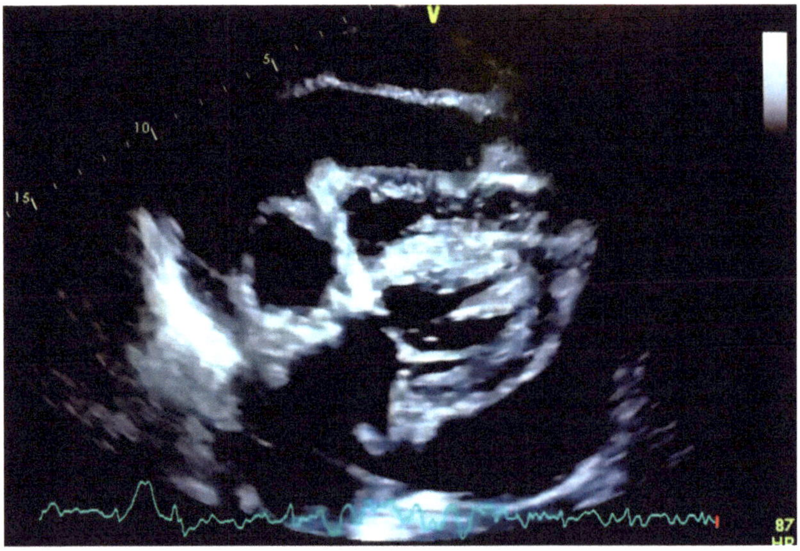

Fig. 56.2 and Video 56.1 Large circumferential pericardial effusion causing cardiac tamponade in PAH patient with associated connective tissue disease. The pericardial effusion was due to the associated connective tissue disease. The patient was treated with pericardiocentesis and immunotherapy with no recurrence of pericardial effusion

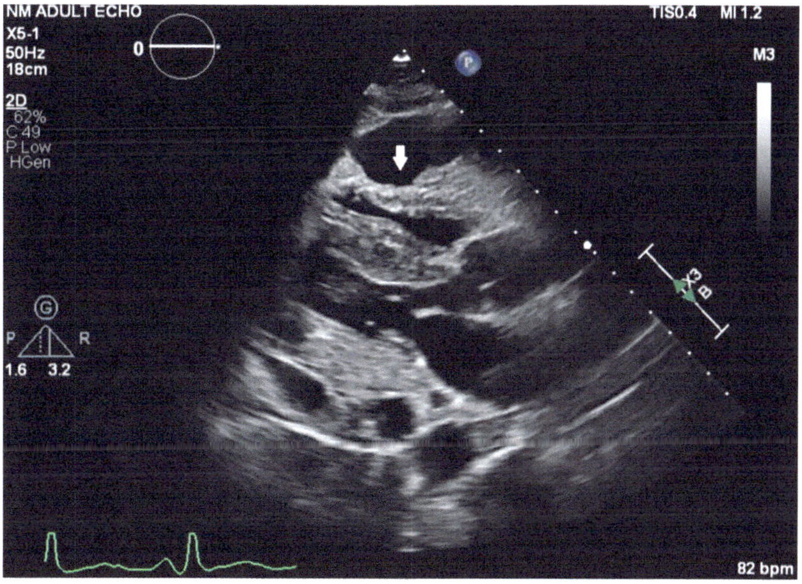

Fig. 56.3 and Video 56.2 Left PLAX view in non-PH patient showing pericardial effusion with diastolic RV free wall collapse, annotated by the arrow

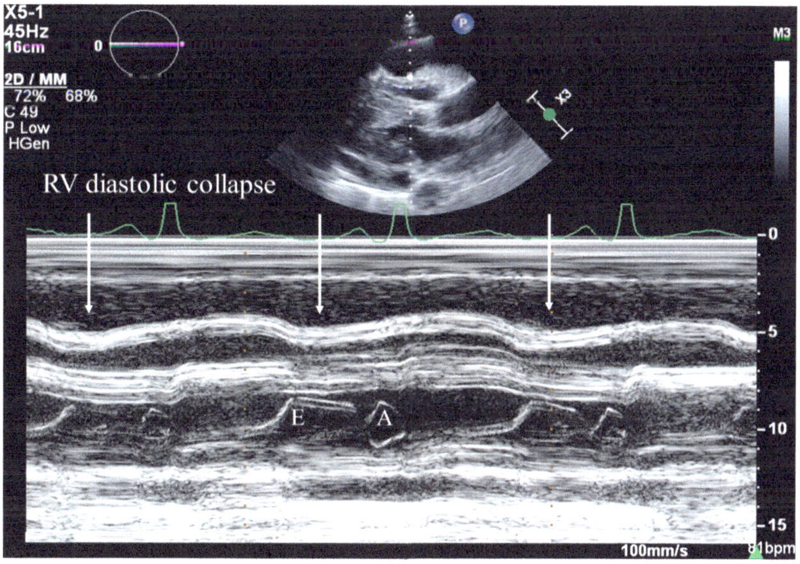

Fig. 56.4 M-mode of left PLAX in non-PH patient showing pericardial effusion and diastolic (note EKG timing and mitral valve opening) RV free wall collapse (arrows) consistent with tamponade physiology (E and A points of anterior mitral valve leaflet are shown)

compromise observed in some pulmonary hypertension patients post pericardiocentesis. A careful adaptive approach that utilizes simultaneous monitoring of pericardial pressure, intracavitary pressure, and cardiac output has been previously described to mitigate this possible risk [18].

Finally, cardiac tamponade remains a clinical diagnosis. A careful consideration of the clinical picture in constellation with multiple echocardiographic and hemodynamic parameters can help establish the diagnosis in this unique situation.

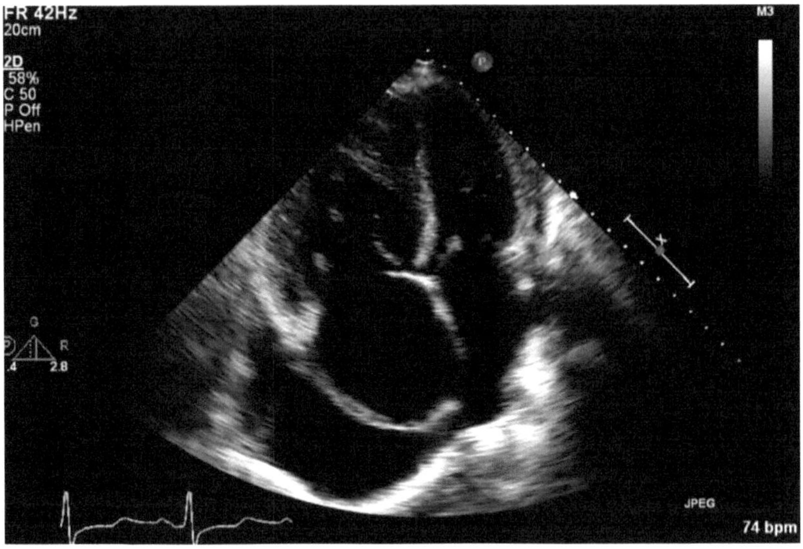

Fig. 56.5 and Video 56.3 Apical 4-chamber view in PAH patient shows right atrial dilation, severe right ventricular enlargement, pericardial effusion, and absence of right atrial collapse

Ultrasound Evaluation in Acute Decompensation, Vasodilator Titration

Bedside echocardiography is a valuable tool in monitoring and managing PH patients with acute decompensation. It allows assessment of right-sided pressures, right atrial and right ventricular size, right ventricular function, and pericardial effusion. These parameters help in the initial assessment and follow-up of decompensated PH patients during treatment. Due to the unique RV geometry, it is important to examine all the available right ventricular windows and views. Apical 4-chamber, RV-focused apical 4-chamber, left parasternal long-axis (PLAX) and parasternal short-axis (PSAX), left parasternal RV inflow, and subcostal views allow for comprehensive RV evaluation [19].

Right ventricular systolic pressure (RVSP) can be estimated using the maximum tricuspid regurgitation (TR) velocity via the modified Bernoulli equation (Fig. 56.6), adding this value to the estimated right atrial (RA) pressure where RVSP = 4(V)2 + RA pressure (V is the peak TR velocity in m/sec, and RA pressure is estimated from IVC diameter and associated respiratory variations). In the absence of obstruction at the level of the pulmonary valve or RVOT, the systolic pulmonary artery pressure is equal to RVSP [19]. The pulmonary artery diastolic pressure (PADP) can be estimated from the maximum pulmonary regurgitant velocity at end-diastole using the modified Bernoulli equation as well (Fig. 56.7) where PADP = 4 x (end-diastolic pulmonary regurgitant velocity)^2 + RA pressure [19].

Optimizing the RV-focused apical four-chamber view is critical to obtain accurate RV dimensions, as minor rotations can cut the RV in different planes leading to an underestimation of RV size. Normally, in the apical 4-chamber view, the RV size is not more than two-thirds the size of the left ventricle, and an end-diastolic basal diameter >4.1 cm in the RV-focused view suggests RV dilatation (Fig. 56.8) [19, 20]. It is important to pay close attention to the shape of the RV during an examination. In advanced PAH, the RV becomes spherical, and the interventricular septum protrudes toward the left ventricle resulting in a D-shaped LV seen in a PSAX view (Fig. 56.9, Video 56.4) [19]. This sign can be noted in both systole and diastole in pressure overload and in diastole in volume overload [19].

RV function can be evaluated either globally by calculating the fractional area change (end-diastolic area—end-systolic area) / end-diastolic area x 100) (Fig. 56.10), the RV index of myocardial performance (RIMP/Tei Index), or regionally through measuring tricuspid annular plane systolic excursion (TAPSE) by M-mode, RV sys-

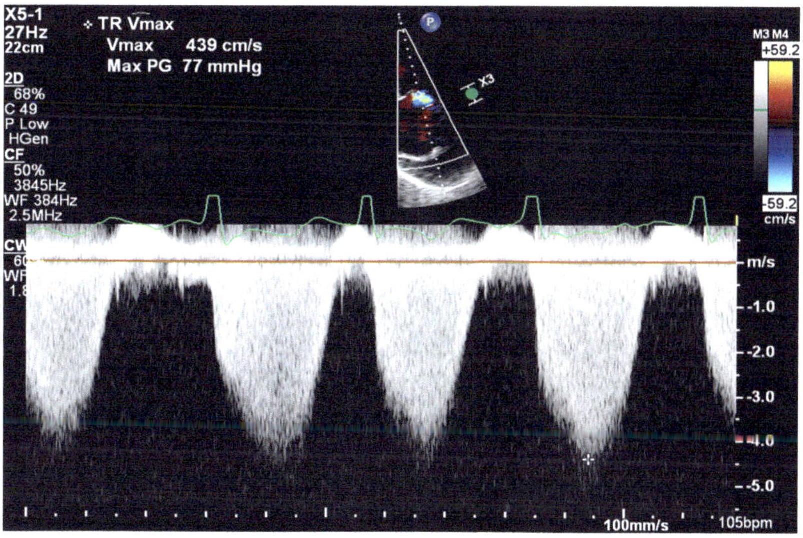

Fig. 56.6 Continuous wave Doppler of TR with TR velocity of 4.39 m/sec giving a pressure gradient of 77 mmHg, with added RA pressure of 15 mmHg, the RVSP (PASP) is 92 mmHg

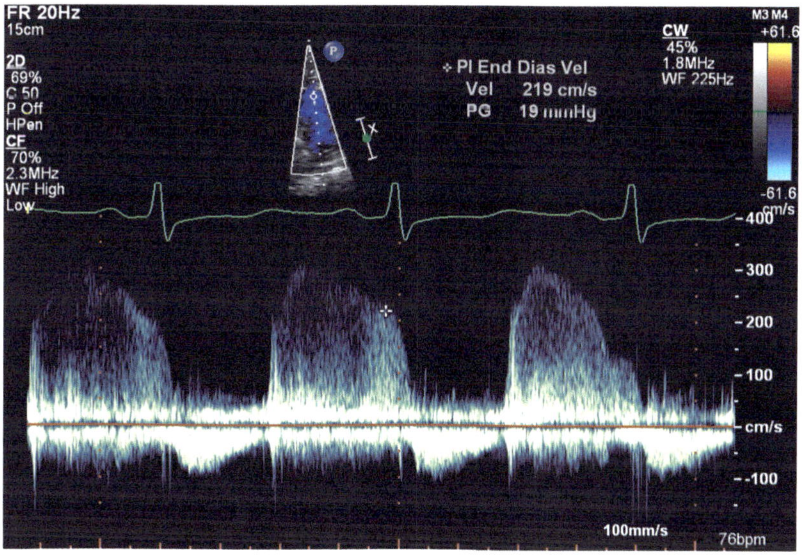

Fig. 56.7 End-diastolic PR velocity of 2.19 m/sec giving a pressure gradient of 19 mmHg, with added RA pressure of 15 mmHg, the PADP is 34 mmHg

tolic S' velocity by tissue Doppler (Figs. 56.11 and 56.12) [19]. A TAPSE value less than 1.8 cm has an estimated 87% accuracy in predicting a stroke volume index <29 ml/m2 and is associated with an increased rate of right-sided heart failure hospitalization and decreased survival in PAH patients. An S′ less than 10 cm/sec has an 89% sensitivity and 87% specificity in predicting a cardiac index <2.0 l/min/m2 [21].

Recent studies proposed TAPSE/PASP ratio for assessing RV-arterial coupling in PH and as a prognostic marker that was significantly associated with outcome, hemodynamics, and functional class in PAH patients. A TASPE/PASP ratio threshold of 0.31 mm/mmHg was 87.5% sensitive and 75.9% specific in discriminating RV-arterial uncoupling. The utilization of this ratio is yet to be validated in acute PAH decompensation [22, 23].

While in PH decompensation, we can see an increase in right-sided pressures, increase in RA and RV sizes, and decrease in RV function and improvement of these parameters with volume offloading, inotropic support, and titration of pulmonary artery vasodilators, it is important to note that in some patients with progressive and

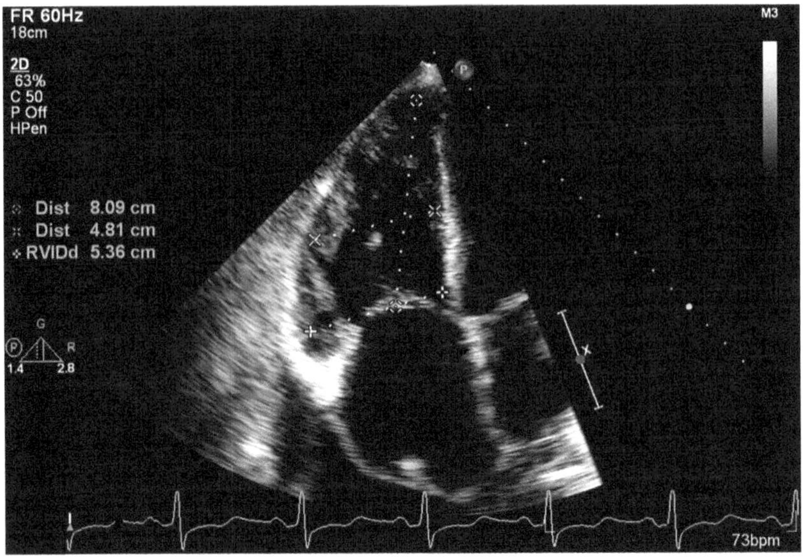

Fig. 56.8 RV-focused view showing RV dilation with a basal diameter of 5.36 cm

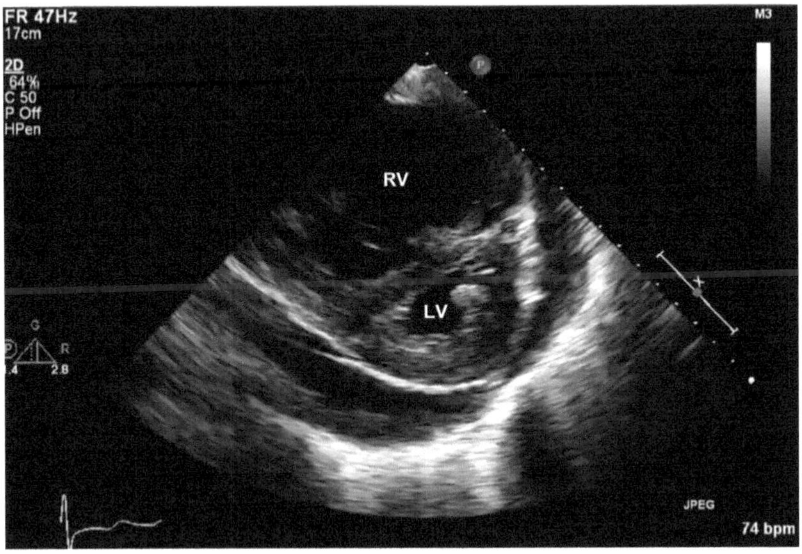

Fig. 56.9 and Video 56.4 PSAX view at the level of papillary muscles shows dilated RV, pericardial effusion, and flattening of the interventricular septum with LV D-shape sign

severe RV failure, the pulmonary artery pressure (and RVSP) may not be significantly elevated because of a decrease in cardiac output and inability of the failing RV to generate sufficient pressure. Thus, it is important to note all these parameters during evaluation and treatment and not focus solely on RVSP (PASP) for monitoring.

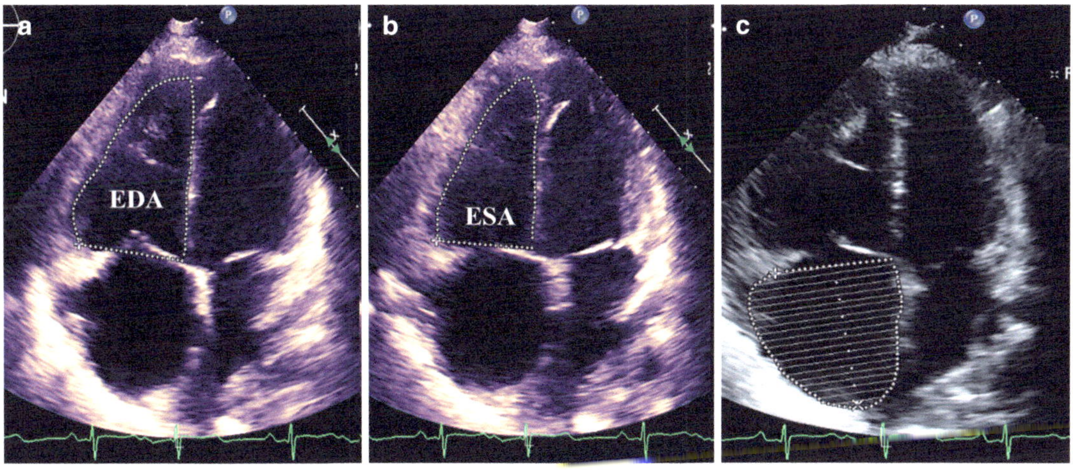

Fig. 56.10 Apical 4-chamber views showing: (**a**) End-diastolic area (EDA), (**b**) End-systolic area (ESA) with a calculated FAC of 15%. (**c**) RA dilation with an RA area of 25.4 cm2

Fig. 56.11 M-mode showing significant reduction in TAPSE (0.8 cm) in patient with severe PAH

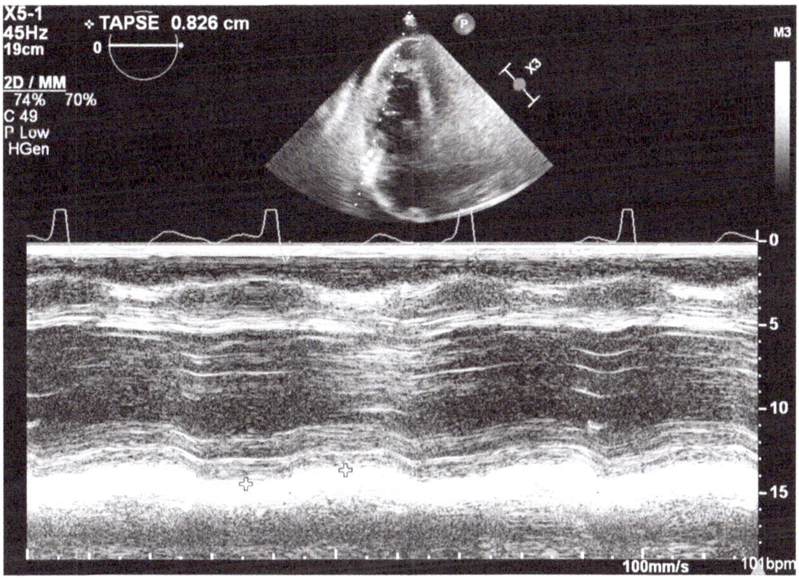

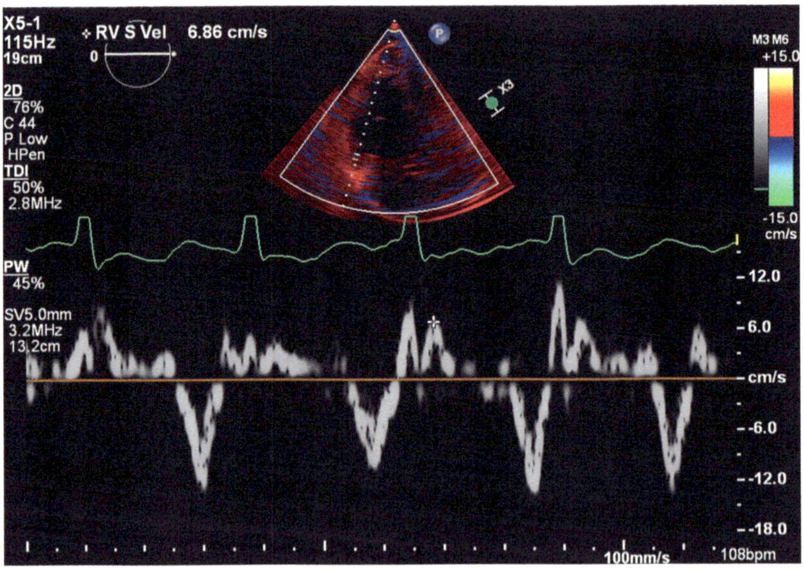

Fig. 56.12 Tissue Doppler imaging of the lateral tricuspid annulus showing significant reduction in S' (6.9 cm/sec) in a patient with severe PAH

Summary Points

- Identify and treat triggers of RV failure in decompensated PH patient.
- Management of decompensated PH patients includes volume optimization, reducing RV afterload, inotropic, and vasopressor support as needed.
- Commonly used parameters for predicting fluid responsiveness have limitations in PH patients.
- Due to elevated right-sided pressures and reduced RV compliance, classic echocardiographic tamponade signs can be concealed in setting of PH.
- When evaluating acute decompensation and response to treatment by echocardiography, it is important to be comprehensive and to consider different parameters of morphology, size, function, and pressure rather than focusing on one parameter.

Evolving Evidence

"Robust data from large prospective clinical trials focusing on critical care management of PH patients are not available. Thus, most of the recommendations for management of critically ill PH patients are based on expert consensus and experience."

Pro-Tip

"Optimizing the RV-focused apical four-chamber view is critical to obtain accurate RV dimensions, as minor rotations can cut the RV in different planes leading to an underestimation of RV size."

Board-Style Questions

Question 1:

A 34-year-old female with a known history of group I PAH associated with scleroderma on triple combination pulmonary artery vasodilator therapy that includes intravenous epoprostenol at 30 ng/kg/min, oral macitentan at 10 mg daily, and oral tadalafil at 40 mg daily was just emergently intubated in the ER for acute hypoxic respiratory failure. Etomidate and rocuronium were used for the intubation. Upon physical examination, the patient was still paralyzed on controlled mechanical ventilation with FIO2 of 60% and PEEP of 16 cm H_2O with a saturation of 98%. She had regular rhythm, an accentuated pulmonary component of S2, grade III systolic murmur best heard at the left lower sternal border, bilateral lower extremities +2 pitting edema. The arterial line showed BP of 80/40 mmHg with pulse pressure variation (PPV) of 20%. Bedside echocardiography examination showed basal RV diameter of 5 cm, TAPSE of 1.2 cm, RVSP of

50 mmHg, trace pericardial effusion, plethoric IVC with a diameter of 2.2 cm without respiratory variations.

1. What should you do next?
   A. Intravenous lactated Ringer's solution 500 cc bolus and subsequent fluid infusion due to the noted high PPV.
   B. Emergent pericardiocentesis.
   C. Decrease PEEP as tolerated.
   D. Decrease the epoprostenol dose to 10 ng/kg/min due to hypotension.

   Answer for question 1: C

   Although high pulse pressure variation has been used to predict fluid responsiveness in mechanically ventilated patients without cardiac arrhythmia or spontaneous breaths, RV dysfunction could result in false-positive values for PPV. In such cases, the PPV can be high despite fluid unresponsiveness. The failing RV is very sensitive to an increase in afterload; thus, the RV stroke volume decreases during insufflation resulting in a decrease in LV preload and a decrease in LV stroke volume. Decreasing PEEP as tolerated will help reduce some of the RV afterload induced by positive mechanical ventilation, especially in the setting of significant RV dilation and dysfunction (answer A). The patient has underlying group I PAH complicated by fluid overload based on physical and echocardiographic examination. The noted high PPV is related to underlying RV dysfunction, so intravenous fluid is not indicated (answer A). The trace pericardial effusion is unlikely to be causing tamponade in this PAH patient, and pericardiocentesis is not recommended (answer B). A sudden decrease in epoprostenol dose in patients with PAH can be detrimental and should be avoided (answer D).

Question 2:

A 50-year-old female with a known history of group I idiopathic PAH presented with increased shortness of breath, hypotension, and tachycardia. Examination revealed distant heart sounds, jugular venous distension, and bilateral lower extremities pitting edema. Bedside echocardiography examination showed a large circumferential pericardial effusion with a dilated IVC at 2.5 cm without respiratory variations. There was no evidence of right atrial or right ventricular collapse, no significant respiratory variations in trans-mitral Doppler flow velocity.

2. Which of the following statements is correct?
   A. The absence of right atrial collapse rules out cardiac tamponade.
   B. The absence of right ventricular collapse rules out cardiac tamponade.
   C. The absence of significant respiratory variations in trans-mitral Doppler flow velocity rules out cardiac tamponade.
   D. None of the above criteria in isolation can rule out cardiac tamponade in this patient.

   Answer for question 2: D

   The typical echocardiographic signs of cardiac tamponade can be concealed in PH patients. Due to the significant increase in right-sided pressures, right atrial and/or right ventricular collapse may be absent (answers A and B). Also, the significant decrease in RV compliance can result in limitations in changing its volume in response to the respiratory cycle, which can conceal significant transvalvular Doppler flow velocity variation (answer C). The diagnosis of cardiac tamponade remains a clinical diagnosis. It cannot be ruled out in PH patients based merely on the absence of right atrial, right ventricular collapse, or absence of significant respiratory variations in trans-mitral Doppler flow velocity (answer D).

References

1. Ventetuolo CE, Klinger JR. Management of acute right ventricular failure in the intensive care unit. Ann Am Thorac Soc. 2014;11(5):811–22.
2. Friedberg MK, Redington AN. Right versus left ventricular failure: differences, similarities, and interactions. Circulation. 2014;129(9):1033–44.
3. Vonk Noordegraaf A, et al. Pathophysiology of the right ventricle and of the pulmonary circulation in pulmonary hypertension: an update. Eur Respir J. 2019;53(1):1801900.

4. Hinderliter AL, et al. Frequency and prognostic significance of pericardial effusion in primary pulmonary hypertension. PPH Study Group. Primary pulmonary hypertension. Am J Cardiol. 1999;84(4):481–4. A10
5. Lanspa MJ, et al. Right ventricular dysfunction in early sepsis and septic shock. Chest. 2021;159(3):1055–63.
6. Hoeper MM, Granton J. Intensive care unit management of patients with severe pulmonary hypertension and right heart failure. Am J Respir Crit Care Med. 2011;184(10):1114–24.
7. Hohn L, et al. Circulatory failure after anesthesia induction in a patient with severe primary pulmonary hypertension. Anesthesiology. 1999;91(6):1943–5.
8. Hoeper MM, et al. Intensive care, right ventricular support and lung transplantation in patients with pulmonary hypertension. Eur Respir J. 2019;53(1):1801906.
9. Jalil BA, Cavallazzi R. Predicting fluid responsiveness: a review of literature and a guide for the clinician. Am J Emerg Med. 2018;36(11):2093–102.
10. Marcus JT, et al. Vena cava backflow and right ventricular stiffness in pulmonary arterial hypertension. Eur Respir J. 2019;54(4):1900625.
11. Fadel BM, et al. Spectral Doppler of the hepatic veins in pulmonary hypertension. Echocardiography. 2015;32(1):170–3.
12. Teboul JL, et al. Arterial pulse pressure variation with mechanical ventilation. Am J Respir Crit Care Med. 2019;199(1):22–31.
13. Magder S. Further cautions for the use of ventilatory-induced changes in arterial pressures to predict volume responsiveness. Crit Care. 2010;14(5):197.
14. Benza RL, et al. Predicting survival in patients with pulmonary arterial hypertension: the REVEAL risk score calculator 2.0 and comparison with ESC/ERS-based risk assessment strategies. Chest. 2019;156(2):323–37.
15. Dudzinski DM, Mak GS, Hung JW. Pericardial diseases. Curr Probl Cardiol. 2012;37(3):75–118.
16. Gollapudi RR, Yeager M, Johnson AD. Left ventricular cardiac tamponade in the setting of cor pulmonale and circumferential pericardial effusion. Case report and review of the literature. Cardiol Rev. 2005;13(4):214–7.
17. Plotnick GD, et al. Pulmonary hypertension decreases the predictive accuracy of echocardiographic clues for cardiac tamponade. Chest. 1995;107(4):919–24.
18. Ruopp NF, Schoenberg NC, Farber HW. Swan-Ganz and pericardial pressure-guided pericardiocentesis in pulmonary arterial hypertension-associated cardiac tamponade. Ann Am Thorac Soc. 2019;16(9):1189–91.
19. Rudski LG, et al. Guidelines for the echocardiographic assessment of the right heart in adults: a report from the American Society of Echocardiography endorsed by the European Association of Echocardiography, a registered branch of the European Society of Cardiology, and the Canadian Society of Echocardiography. J Am Soc Echocardiogr. 2010;23(7):685–713; quiz 786–8.
20. Lang RM, et al. Recommendations for cardiac chamber quantification by echocardiography in adults: an update from the American Society of Echocardiography and the European Association of Cardiovascular Imaging. Eur Heart J Cardiovasc Imaging. 2015;16(3):233–70.
21. Roberts JD, Forfia PR. Diagnosis and assessment of pulmonary vascular disease by Doppler echocardiography. Pulm Circ. 2011;1(2):160–81.
22. Tello K, et al. Validation of the tricuspid annular plane systolic excursion/systolic pulmonary artery pressure ratio for the assessment of right ventricular-arterial coupling in severe pulmonary hypertension. Circ Cardiovasc Imaging. 2019;12(9):e009047.
23. Tello K, et al. Relevance of the TAPSE/PASP ratio in pulmonary arterial hypertension. Int J Cardiol. 2018;266:229–35.

57 ARDS and Respiratory Failure

Imrana Qawi and Kathleen M. Waybill

Learning Objectives
1. Application of point of care ultrasound in ARDS.
2. Stages of ARDS. Lung ultrasound may help in following progression of ARDS.
3. LUNG US Scoring system: Evolving data.
4. POCUS in open lung strategy and prone position ventilation.

Lung ultrasonography has demonstrated diagnostic utility in respiratory failure. However, there is marked variability in the clinical utilization of ultrasound to help guide diagnosis and treatment, ranging from extensive sonographic examinations of patients with respiratory symptoms to use only for procedural guidance. Studies over the last decade support the use in select groups of patients to improve the diagnosis and management of ARDS patients (Fig. 57.1) [1, 2].

I. Qawi (✉) · K. M. Waybill
Division of Pulmonary, Critical Care and Sleep Division, Tufts Medical Center, Boston, MA, USA
e-mail: Imrana.Qawi2@tuftsmedicine.org

M. J. Lanspa, A. T. Levinson (eds.), *Echocardiography and Ultrasonography in the ICU*, Respiratory Medicine, https://doi.org/10.1007/978-3-031-80038-2_57

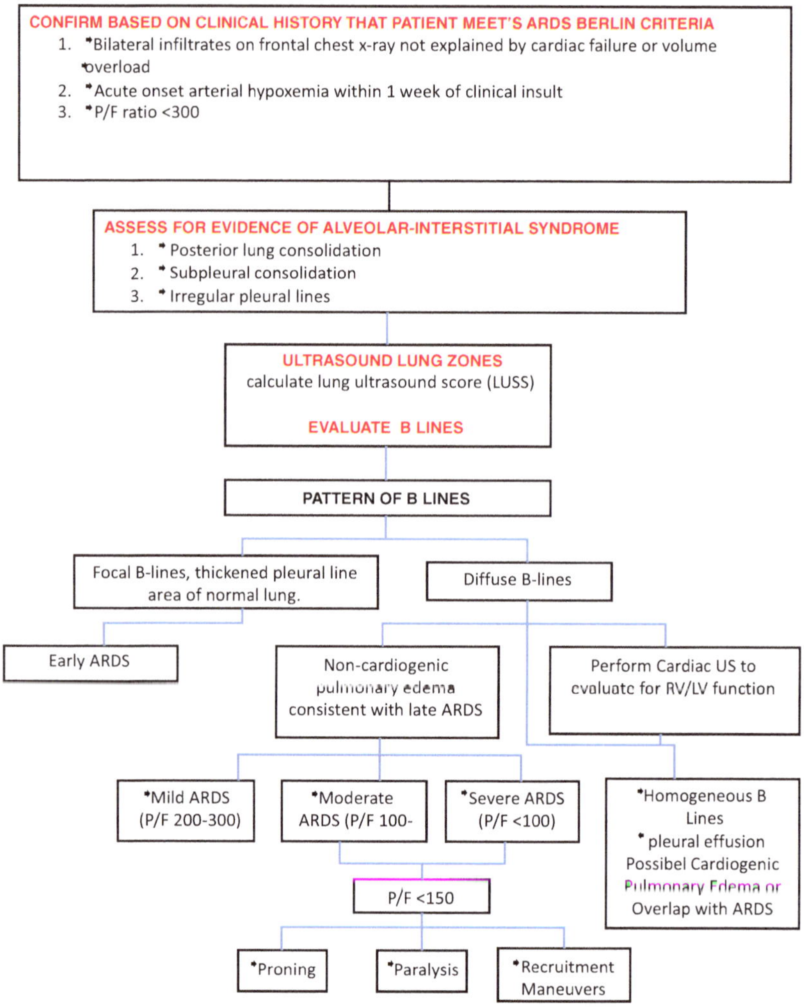

Fig. 57.1 Proposed algorithm to apply lung ultrasound in ARDS

Stages of ARDS

ARDS typically shows bilateral multilobar ground-glass opacities and/or consolidative opacities with a peripheral dominance, usually in a posterior distribution. In the early stages, focal B lines are the main pattern (Image 57.1). In the progressive stage that follows, thickened pleural lines, multiple, or fused B-lines, and subpleural non-homogeneous consolidations are the main features (Images 57.2 and 57.3). In advanced ARDS, multiple continuous hypoechoic consolidations combined with the hepatization sign, diffuse B-lines, and extensive air bronchograms are prominent features (Image 57.4). LUS has some limitations, and CT may be required for diagnosis. For example, in patients who have underlying chronic lung conditions like pulmonary fibrosis or other interstitial lung diseases, CT is the definitive modality to better elucidate acute and chronic processes.

Image 57.1 Early ARDS on Lung US: Focal B Lines, heterogenous area of normal lungs and area of consolidation. In comparison, cardiogenic pulmonary edema has usually homogenous thin, pleural lines with B lines and pleural effusions

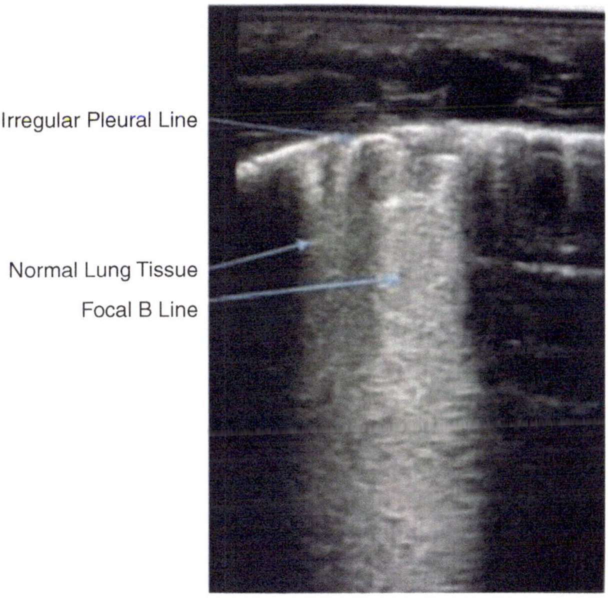

Image 57.2 Alveolar interstitial syndrome Alveolar Interstitial Syndrome is the main feature in Moderate to Severe ARDS. Note Subpleural consolidations, the irregular pleural line, and confluent B lines

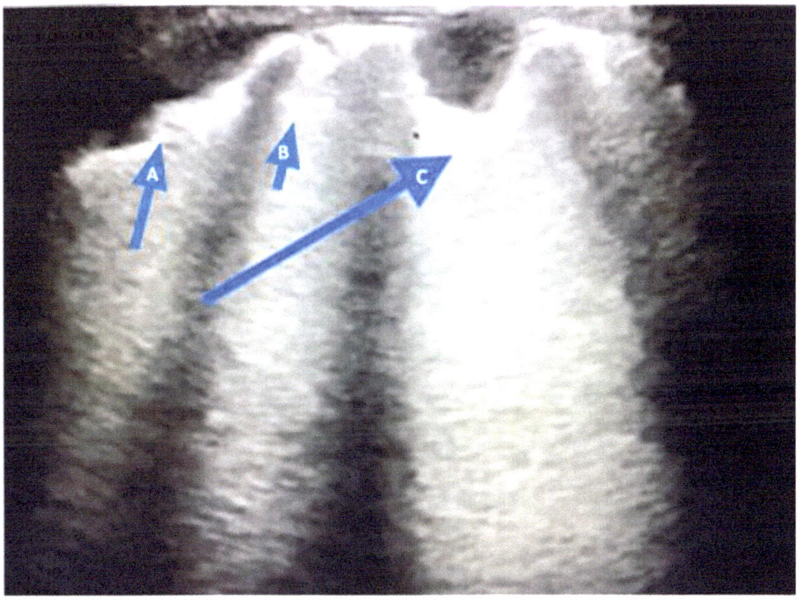

Lung Findings in advanced ARDS: A. Irregular Pleural lines; B. Confluent homogenous B Lines; C. Subpleural consolidation and thickened pleura

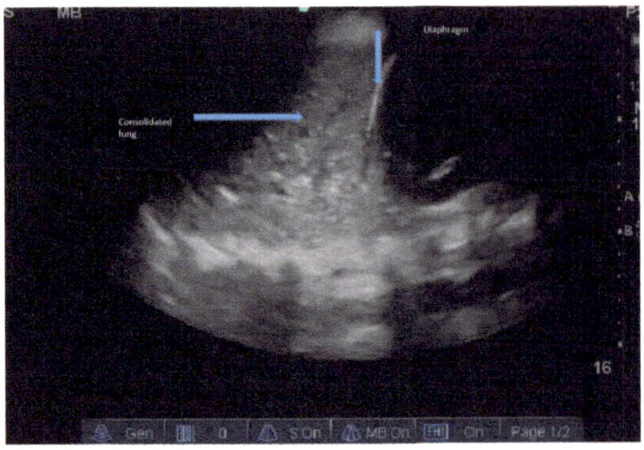

Image 57.3 Subpleural consolidations
Small Subpleural consolidations separated from aerated Lung with irregular Margins, like a shredded tissue paper hence called "Shred sign." First described by Lichtenstein in 2009. The shred sign helps differentiate consolidation from passive atelectasis
BLUE ARROW DOWN: LIVER, BLUE ARROW UP: DIAPHRAGM, GREEN ARROW: SHRED SIGN (PNEUMONIA)
(Image from op)

Image 57.4 Lung consolidation in late-stage ARDS
Consolidated Lung in late stage of ARDS. The air bronchogram is located inside the consolidation and consists of branching and various shaped hyperechoic areas
Air bronchograms can be either resorptive atelectasis or dynamic (air movement within bronchogram) in pneumonic consolidation . Dynamic air bronchograms are much more rare in resportive atelectasis than in alveolar processes such as ARDS or infectious causes

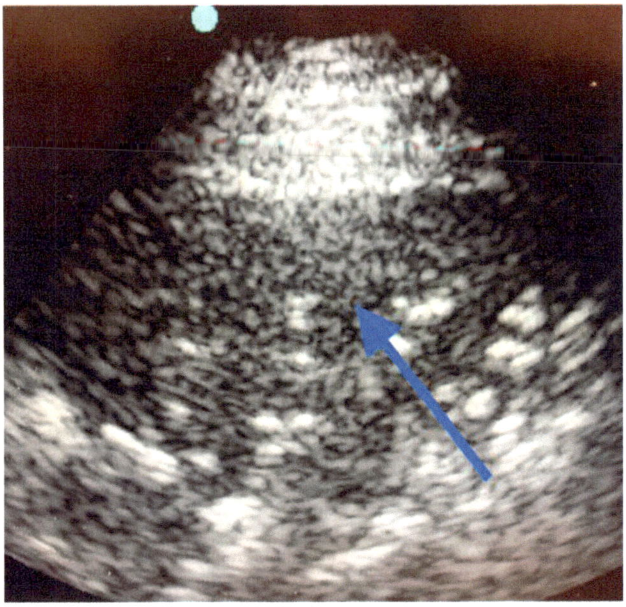

Example of posterior lung consolidation

Lung Ultrasound Scoring Systems (LUS)

Recent studies have proposed lung ultrasound scoring systems (LUSS) which may help to assess early changes in ARDS and predict severity and progression. It is based on examination of 12 thorax regions to assess lung aeration changes specifically prior to intubation, and after various therapeutic interventions in mechanically ventilated patients. It can help with the monitoring of regional lung aeration changes resulting from prone positioning, volume overload, positive end-expiratory pressure, and drainage of large pleural effusions. In ventilated critically ill patients with ARDS or multilobar pneumonia, a rapid decrease in the LUS score indicates successful intervention and improved lung aeration, whereas an increase in the LUS indicates worsening respiratory failure. Such scoring systems (Fig. 57.2) are operator dependent and require the competence to recognize normal aeration, interstitial syndrome, alveolar edema, and lung necessary to calculate the LUS score.

Lung Consolidation Score
0= A lines, no B lines
1 = Multiple B lines (regularly/irregularly placed no consolidation
2 = comet tails on the pleural surface
3 = one location of consolidation ≥1 cm
SCORE 0-36

Fig. 57.2 Lung consolidation score

Ventilation Support and Open Lung Strategy

Optimal mechanical ventilation support remains the cornerstone of treatment in moderate to severe ARDS. Lung ultrasound can be used to evaluate the impending respiratory failure requiring intubation and subsequent ventilator interventions in early stages of ARDS. A recent study showed that a LUSS ≥ 25 on admission had 90% specificity for predicting subsequent need for intubation, in COVID-19 ARDS patients. Per ARDS Net lung protective ventilation strategies with low tidal volume ventilation have shown mortality benefits. However, very high high PEEP associated with the management of severe ARDS has the potential for worsening V/Q (ventilation/perfusion) mismatch by worsening pulmonary compliance and causing or worsening right heart strain. With patients exhibiting high driving pressures ($\Delta P = V_T/C_{RS}$), evaluating right ventricular function may help optimize the balance between open lung strategies and and preventing or worsening RV dysfunction. With P/F ratio 150 mmHg, or less prone positioning and recruitment maneuvers (RM) should be considered. Prone position ventilation can improve ventilator-related lung injury in dependent regions and unload the right ventricle, while aiding in correcting hypoxemia in patients with severe ARDS (Image 57.5). In the Proning Severe ARDS Patients (PROSEVA) trial, patients who were randomized to prone-positioning for 16 h showed reduced 28-day mortality compared to leaving patients in the supine position. Lung ultrasound allows for an easily available bedside assessment to monitor improvement in aeration in lateral and posterior regions of the thorax while proned [3, 4].

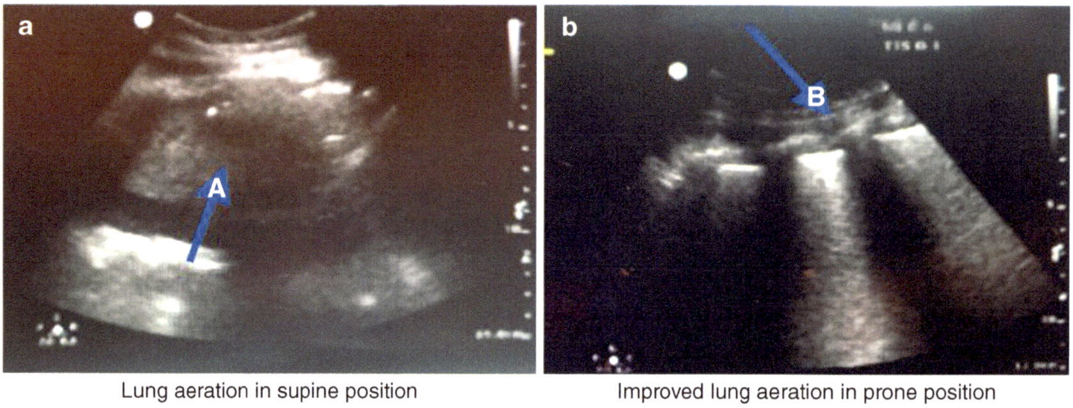

Image 57.5 Lung aeration in supine vs. prone position

Lung Ultrasound in Extubation

For patients recovering from respiratory failure, earlier liberation from invasive mechanical ventilation reduces the incidence of ventilator-associated complications. POCUS can help predict extubation success through cardiac, lung, and diaphragmatic dysfunction parameters. Systolic ejection fraction <35%, diaphragmatic weakness, and diastolic dysfunction increase the risk of extubation failure .

Right Ventricular Dysfunction in ARDS

Of all hospitalized patients with moderate-to-severe ARDS, 20–30% will have right ventricular (RV) dysfunction (Image 57.6). Apical 4-chamber view or parasternal short-axis view can give an "eyeball estimate" of moderate-severe dysfunction. A 4-chamber view interpreted by an experienced operator can compare the right ventricular end diastolic area (RVEDA) with the left ventricular end diastolic area (LVEDA). Right ventricular dilation is defined as moderate when RVEDA/LVEDA ratio is between 0.6 and 1 and is severe when the ratio is more than 1.0. Similarly, left ventricular function can be assessed on parasternal short axis or 4-chamber view [5, 6]. Assessing RV and LV dysfunction is discussed in other chapters.

Summary Points

- In early ARDS, LUS typically shows bilateral multilobar ground-glass opacities and/or consolidative opacities with a peripheral dominance.
- In ARDS, progression thickened pleural lines, multiple, or fused B-lines, and subpleural non-homogeneous consolidations are the main features.
- In advanced ARDS, multiple continuous hypoechoic consolidations combined with the hepatization sign, diffuse B-lines, and extensive air bronchograms are prominent features.
- Lung ultrasound scoring systems (LUSS) may may help to assess early changes in ARDS and predict severity and progression.
- Evaluating right ventricular function can optimize the balance between open lung strategies for patients on mechanical ventilation and preventing or worsening RV dysfunction.

Evolving Evidence

Lung ultrasound in early ARDS patients has recently shown to help predict respiratory.

Pro-Tips

TIP 1: US sonographic B-lines are produced by diseases that affect the interstitium and alveoli hence can be seen in pulmonary edema or focal or generalized inflammation. History and clinical presentation are important to

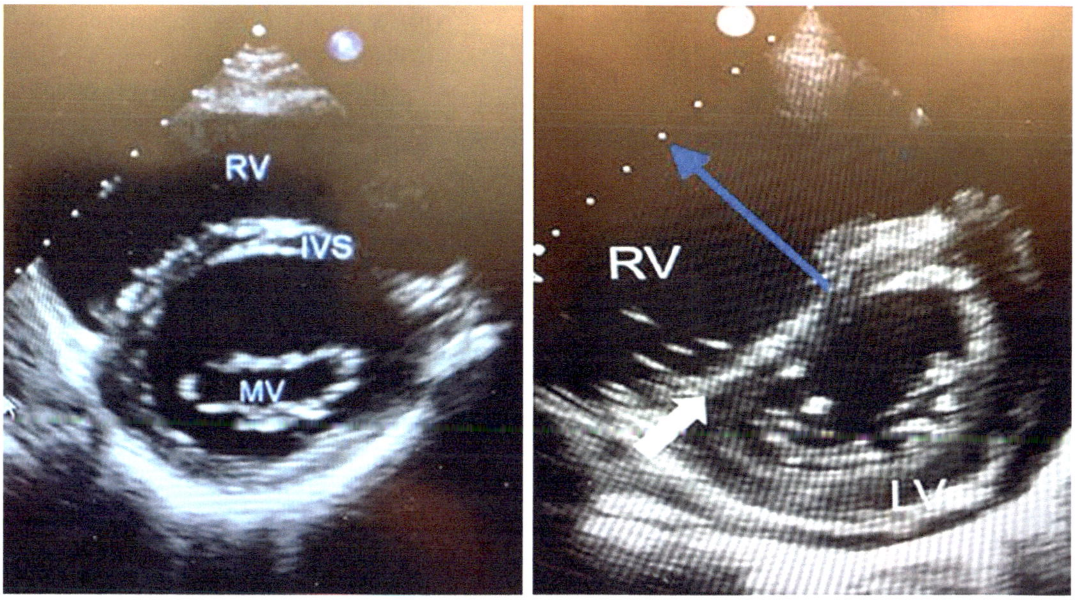

Image 57.6 Normal vs. dilated right ventricle
PARASTERNAL SHORT AXIS (PSAX): LEFT IMAGE NORMAL PSAX AT THE LEVEL OF MITRAL VALVE, RIGHT IMAGE: DILATED RIGHT VENTRICLE, FLATTENED SEPTUM

clinch the diagnosis. Lung ultrasound helps in rapid bedside assessment and is a more superior diagnostic tool than a chest radiograph.

TIP 2: ARDS /Pneumonia: On lung ultrasound look for dependent consolidations, possible adjacent B-lines, or a parapneumonic effusion.

TIP 3: Pulmonary fibrosis or other Interstitial lung disease produces very similar appearances to ARDS. Always look at clinical context and history of your patient when interpreting your lung findings.

TIP 4: In patient who have high driving pressure (DP) on ventilator, application of recruitment maneuvers can be assessed with cardiac ultrasound to evaluate RV function.

Questions

1. A 35-year-old present to emergency room with 2 days of high fever, cough productive of yellow green phlegm and dyspnea on exertion. Chest X-ray shows bilateral ground glass opacities. Vital Temp 39.2, HR 120 s sinus, BP 90/60 mmHg, RR 30 /min, O2 sats 86% on RA. The ER Physician performs lung ultrasound.

   Laboratory data: WBC 24 K, H/H 11.2/36.9, PLT 139, BUN 35, CR 1.0, Lactate 4.1.

   CXR:

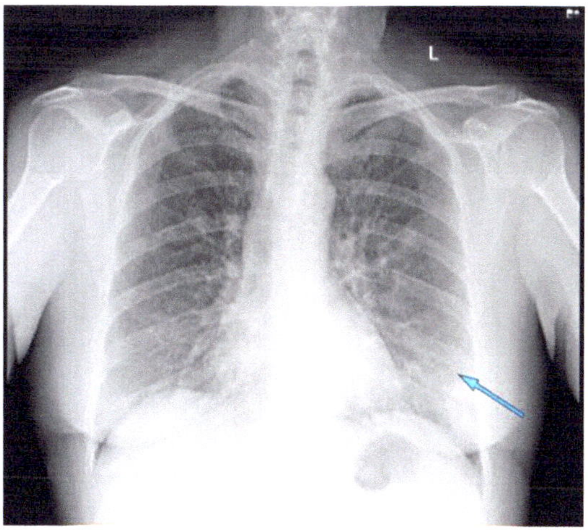

LUNG ULTRASOUND: LEFT LUNG ZONE

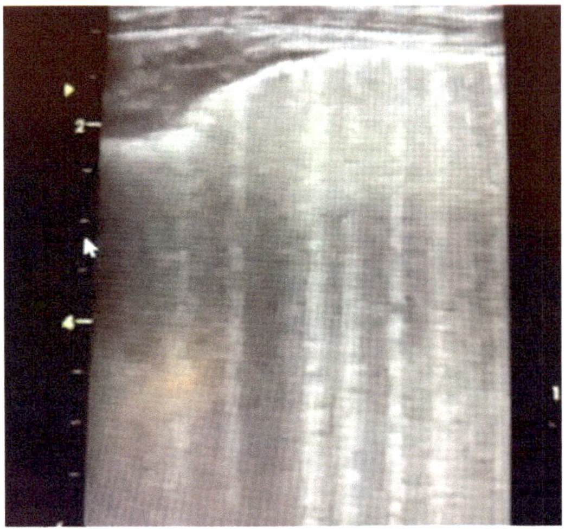

LEFT LUNG ZONE 12

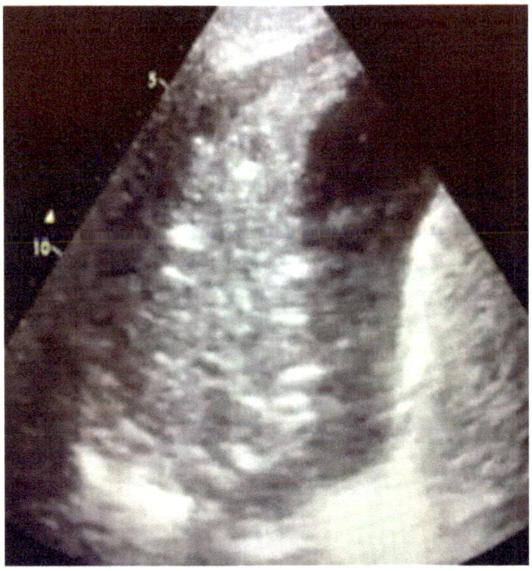

What is the diagnosis for respiratory distress in this patient

A. Left lobar pneumonia with early ARDS
B. Cardiogenic Pulmonary edema
C. Pulmonary embolism
D. Asthma exacerbation

2. 39-year-old female, smoker since age 20 1 PPD, h/o asthma, obesity presents to emergency room with acute onset of shortness of breath × 12 h. She denies any sick contact. Endorses 4/10 mid-chest pain with no specific radiation. She was on business trip to California and returned 2 days back to Boston. On clinical exam she is anxious, HR 120–122 Sinus, BP 100/70 mmHg, RR 24–26 O2 sats 88% RA. Her chest is clear to auscultate. Left extremity has 1 + pedal edema.

LABS: WBC 11.2, HB 9.9, PLT 196, K 3.9, BUN 20, CR 0.9, Lactate 2.9

CXR:

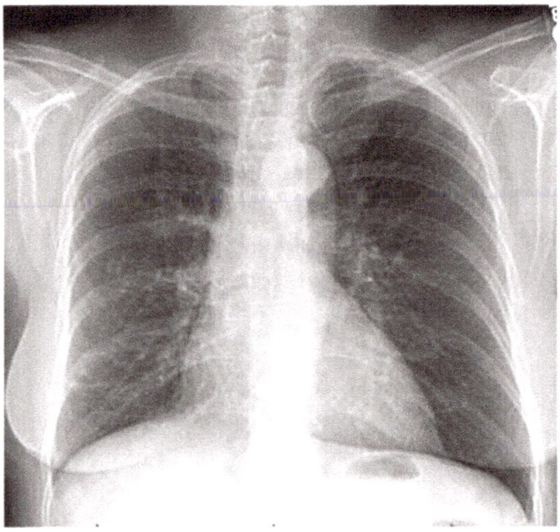

LUNG US: BOTH LUNG SHOW A LINES

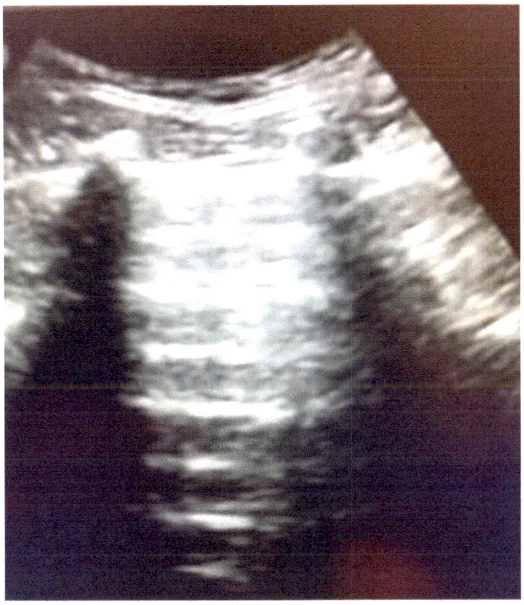

2a) WHAT IS PROBABLE DIAGNOSIS FOR THIS PATIENT'S RESPIRATORY DISTRESS

A. CARDIOGENIC PULMONARY EDEMA
B. MULTILOBAR PNEUMONIA
C. PANIC ATTACK
D. PULMONARY EMBOLISM

2b) WHAT IS THE NEXT DIAGNOSTIC MODALITY?

A. CHEST CT NON-CONTRAST
B. CHEST CT WITH PE PROTOCOL
C. ECHOCARDIOGRAPHY
D. ANTIBIOTICS AND FLUIDS

3. 56-year-old man with h/o uncontrolled HTN, CAD with HFpEF, paroxysmal atrial fibrillation presents with progressive dyspnea over a week. He endorses nonproductive cough for 2–3 days. No sick contact. No recent travels. He is a smoker with 50 pack years of smoking. IN The emergency room he is in mild distress an using accessory neck muscles. Heart rate 120–125 irregular, BP 120/66 mmHg, JVD ~ 5–6 cm. On chest auscultation, he has scant expiratory wheeze bilateral and diminished breath sounds at the bases.

LABS: WBC 11.1, HB 10.9, PLT 198, BUN 25, CR 1.9 (baseline 1.5), K 5.0, Cl 110, HCO3 27, INR 1.6.

CXR

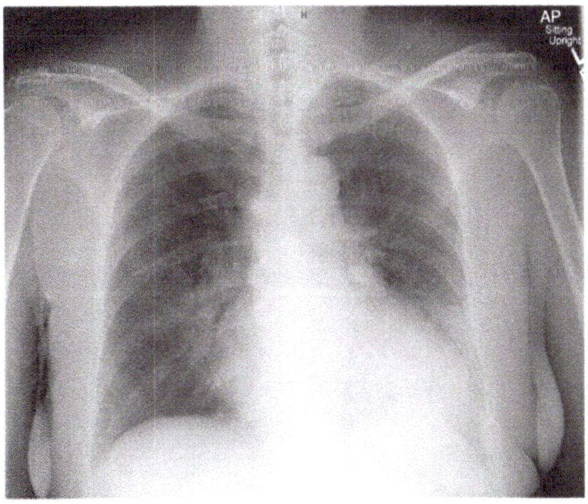

LUNG ULTRASOUND IS PERFORMED

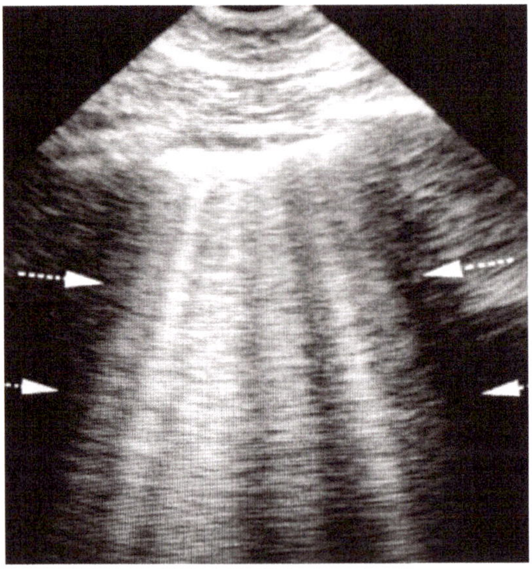

3a) WHAT ARE THE ARROWS POINTING AT

A. A LINES
B. B LINES
C. Z LINES
D. PLEURAL LINES

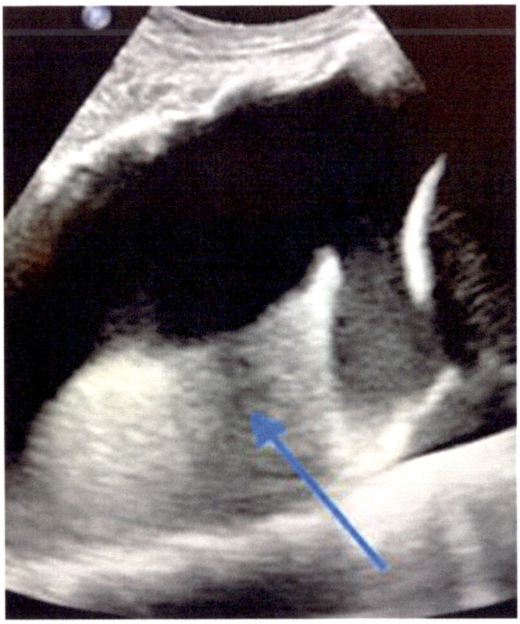

3b) WHAT IS THE ARROW POINTING AT

A. DIAPHRAGM
B. PLEURAL EFFUSION
C. ATELECTATIC LUNG
D. ASCITES

3c) WHAT IS NEXT STEP IN MANAGEMENT OF RESPIRATORY DISTRESS

A. Antibiotics and fluids
B. Diuretics and rate control
C. Chest tube drainage
D. Lytic therapy

Question 4:

You are assessing a patient in respiratory distress. The anterior lung zones show bilateral B lines with area of normal zones in left hemithorax.

4a) Are B lines

A. An artifact
B. Are formed due increase of density due to loss of aeration
C. Is due to Pulmonary edema or inflammation
D. A, B
E. A, B and C

4b) Differential Diagnosis in unilateral B lines include all except

A. Aspiration Pneumonia
B. Alveolar hemorrhage
C. Pulmonary Contusion
D. Pulmonary Fibrosis

Correct answers

1)a

2a) d 2b) b

3a) b 3b) c 3c)b

4a) e 4b) c

References

1. Utility of Point-of-Care Lung Ultrasound for Initial Assessment of Acute Respiratory Distress Syndrome Patients in the Emergency Department. J Emerg Trauma Shock. 2019;12(4):248–53.
2. Lung ultrasound: predictor of acute respiratory distress syndrome in intensive care unit patients. Saudi J Anaesth. 2018;12(3):457–461.
3. Boumans MMA, Aerts W, Pisani L, Bos LDJ, Smit MR, Tuinman PR. Diagnostic accuracy of lung ultrasound in diagnosis of ARDS and identification of focal or non-focal ARDS subphenotypes: a systematic review and meta-analysis. Crit Care. 2024;28(1):224.
4. Ultrasonography for the assessment of lung recruitment maneuvers. Crit Ultrasound J. 2016;8(1):8.
5. Applicability of lung ultrasound in COVID-19 diagnosis and evaluation of the disease progression: a systematic review. Pulmonology. 2021;27(6):529–62.
6. Zochios V, Yusuff H, Schmidt M; Protecting the Right Ventricle Network (PRORVnet). Acute right ventricular injury phenotyping in ARDS. Intensive Care Med. 2023;49(1):99–102.

US, Diuresis, and Weaning from Mechanical Ventilation

58

Kathryn Hendrickson and Ellie Hirshberg

Learning Objectives

1. Review how ultrasound and echocardiography are helpful in guiding clinicians in managing patients with shock
2. Explain how lung ultrasound looking for B lines and pleural effusions can suggest pulmonary edema
3. Describe how E/e' measurement, passive leg raise, and end-expiratory occlusion pressure can predict the fluid status of critically ill patients and guide management

Diuresis, a Necessary Consequence of Volume Resuscitation

The first-line treatment for acute circulatory failure is to increase cardiac output and oxygen delivery through volume expansion with volume resuscitation. Rivers et al. described the benefit of early fluid resuscitation in patients with sepsis and septic shock [1]. The patients who received early goal-directed therapy with large volume fluid resuscitation in the first 6 h of presentation to the hospital had a lower in-hospital mortality than patients who did not. More recently; however, multiple studies concluded increased mortality in patients with sepsis and excessive volume administration [2, 3]. Excessive volume administration can also produce poor outcomes in patients with acute respiratory distress syndrome (ARDS), abdominal compartment syndrome, and renal failure [4–6]. Volume overload is associated with worse outcomes in patients requiring mechanical ventilation or with cardiac dysfunction and is a leading cause of failure to wean from mechanical ventilation [7]. Ideal volume resuscitation and intravascular effective arterial blood volume are essential to optimize outcomes in critically ill patients. In this chapter, we will discuss tools and methods to evaluate a patient's intravascular volume status to guide diuresis and weaning from mechanical ventilation.

Static Measures

Static measures of fluid balance reflect a single point in time and are used to estimate volume status in critically ill patients. Historically, static measures such as vital signs, physical exam, central venous pressure (CVP) measurement, and pulmonary capillary wedge pressure modalities are not consistently accurate in diagnosing intravascular volume status [8]. Ultrasound static measures, including left ventricular end diastolic volume (LVEDV), E/e', and B lines (on lung ultrasound), are easy to perform and while not

K. Hendrickson
Pulmonary and Critical Care, The Oregon Clinic, Portland, OR, USA

E. Hirshberg (✉)
Intermountain, Salt Lake City, UT, USA
e-mail: Ellie.hirshberg@imail.com

M. J. Lanspa, A. T. Levinson (eds.), *Echocardiography and Ultrasonography in the ICU*, Respiratory Medicine, https://doi.org/10.1007/978-3-031-80038-2_58

accurate in assessing volume status per se, can be helpful in guiding diuresis.

Vital Signs

Vital signs have been used to attempt to understand cardiac output in the past. Unfortunately this does not correlate reliably with cardiac output in patients with critical illness [9].

Physical Exam

Physical exam is a pillar of the clinical work up for any patients, including critically ill patients. Grissom et al. showed in 2009 that capillary refill, knee mottling, and cool extremities are not useful predictors of low cardiac output [8].

CVP

Central venous pressure (CVP) is a commonly used parameter for determining cardiac output; however, its practical, clinical use has not borne out in the literature. Multiple meta-analyses/systematic reviews have shown no correlation with CVP and fluid responsiveness in critically ill patients. A static CVP should not be used to guide volume resuscitation in critically ill patients [10, 11].

B Lines and Pleural Effusions on US

Ultrasound is a useful tool to assist clinicians in the evaluation of critically ill patients in respiratory failure. Ultrasound is accurate in diagnosing the cause of respiratory failure by assisting clinicians to rapidly begin appropriate therapy. The presence of lung sliding and B lines has a 95% specificity and 97% sensitivity for the presence of pulmonary edema [12]. Lichtenstein et al. established US can be more accurate in the diagnosis of pulmonary edema and pleural effusions than lung auscultation and chest radiography [13]. B lines are comet-tail lines that span vertically from the pleura to the bottom of the US screen. They slide with lung sliding if present and three or more B lines in the space between ribs indicates the presence of pulmonary edema [13]. Lung ultrasound is non-invasive, has reproducible patterns, and can be completed and interpreted rapidly, in real time at the bedside.

E/e′

Left ventricular systolic and diastolic dysfunction is associated with ventilator weaning failure in critically ill patients. E/e' is a cardiac ultrasound parameter that helps in the assessment of diastolic dysfunction and can be thought of as a non-invasive pulmonary wedge pressure. Mitral inflow velocity (E) is usually measured in the apical 4 chamber view using pulse wave (PW) Doppler. The sample volume is placed between the mitral tips during diastole. Mitral inflow velocity can then be measured at end-expiration. E' is measured using annular pulsed wave Doppler tissue imaging in the apical 4 chamber view with averaging of the e' velocity from the septum and lateral mitral annulus [14]. Elevated E/e' correlates with risk of weaning failure in ventilated patients [15, 16]. An E/e' of 7 or less indicates the patient has a higher likelihood of successfully weaning from the ventilator [17, 18].

Dynamic Measures

Dynamic measures of fluid responsiveness are much more accurate in determination of fluid status and need for diuresis in critically ill patients. Recall that dynamic measures produce a change in cardiac preload and then measure a change in cardiac output or a surrogate measure of cardiac output. Although IVC diameter with respiratory variation can be tricky in critically ill patients, its use with appropriate context or in addition to passive leg raise (PLR), and end-expiratory occlusion pressure can predict fluid responsiveness in patients with respiratory failure and guide clinicians with diuresis and weaning off mechanical ventilation.

Change in IVC Diameter

IVC change in diameter with respiratory variation is a commonly used and easily obtained parameter to evaluate which patients will respond to volume resuscitation using bed-side echocardiography. It can also be used to help predict hemodynamic stability during diuresis or dialysis. The change in IVC diameter with respiration reflects a change in intrathoracic pressure and right atrial preload. Therefore, patient conditions will alter the thoracic pressure changes. In mechanically ventilated patients, change in IVC diameter with respiration is most reliable when patients are receiving neuromuscular blockade and Assist control ventilation with a tidal volume large enough to engage intraventricular dependence and perturbation of cardiac preload. In spontaneously breathing patients on the ventilator, change in IVC diameter has limited positive predictive value in predicting volume responsiveness in the ICU setting because the change in thoracic pressure is not consistent. However, Lanspa et al. demonstrated that volume responsiveness may be more accurately predicted in patients whose IVC variation with respiration is ≥42% [19]. Positive pressure mechanical ventilation increases the intrathoracic pressure in the chest resulting in a mean airway pressure greater than non-intubated patients. Because of this increase in intrathoracic pressure the IVC can appear dilated on ultrasound regardless of volume status. Therefore, a dilated IVC without respiratory variation in mechanically ventilated patients does not have adequate positive predictive value of volume overload. However, if there is respiratory variation of IVC diameter with tidal breathing of a patient on positive pressure ventilation, the patient is more likely to be volume responsive and therefore they are unlikely to tolerate diuresis [20].

Passive Leg Raise

Passive leg raise (PLR) is used as a reversible "preload challenge" of about 300 ml of blood to test volume responsiveness in critically ill patients, both ventilated and non-ventilated. If a patient is determined not to be volume responsive, they are likely to tolerate diuresis. The effects of PLR must be measured continuously with measure of cardiac output. This can be done non-invasively using echocardiography with the change in velocity-time integral in the left ventricular outflow tract, change in peak aortic pressure, change in IVC diameter, change in pulse pressure, or change in cardiac index (CI) during PLR [21]. Change in CVP with PLR is not a measure of cardiac output, and is not a reliable indicator of preload responsiveness [22]. Critically ill patients who are determined to be volume responsive with PLR do not tolerate dialysis, and PLR is able to predict preload and hemodynamic tolerance to fluid removal during dialysis [23].

End-Expiratory Occlusion Pressure

In mechanically ventilated patients, end-expiratory occlusion pressure can be used to measure changes in cardiac output. Echocardiography is used to measure the cardiac index (CI) and velocity time integral (VTI) before and after end-expiratory occlusion. Change in CI ≥4% or a change in VTI ≥5% is a reliable marker of fluid responsiveness in critically ill, mechanically ventilated patients [24, 25].

Conclusion

Two Cases Are Illustrative of the Utility of Using Ultrasound to Guide Fluid Management in Patients in Shock

Case 1: A 55-year-old woman was admitted to the ICU for septic shock and respiratory failure due to Streptococcus pneumoniae pneumonia. She required intubation and mechanical ventilation, antibiotics, and 5 L of crystalloid volume resuscitation as well as peripheral pressors for a short time. Her shock quickly resolved, and the physician team wanted to work toward extubation. Lung US was performed which showed lung sliding and > 3 B lines present. Critical care ECHO was performed with a left ventricular ejection fraction (LVEF) of 60%. IVC diameter was 2.5 cm with

25% change in diameter with inspiration. E/e' was measured as 26.7. PLR was performed with no change in IVC or left ventricular velocity-time integral. The patient was given diuresis and was net fluid negative 2 liters in the next 24 h. She performed well on her spontaneous breathing trial and was successfully extubated the following day.

Case 2: A 76-year-old man with history of HFrEF, baseline ejection fraction of 30%, and mild dementia presented to the hospital with hypotension and confusion. He was found to have a urinalysis positive for infection. The emergency department gave him 1 liter of crystalloid, antibiotics, started on 2 L nasal cannula oxygen, and he was admitted to the ICU with ongoing hypotension requiring pressors. Critical care ECHO revealed LVEF of 25% and an IVC diameter of 2.0 cm with 50% collapse with inspiration. E/e' was measured as 7.1 with noticeable change in IVC and pulse pressure with PLR. An expiratory hold was performed with VTI change of 5%. Lung US revealed no evidence of pleural effusions and 2 B lines seen with good lung sliding. The patient was given an additional 1.5 liters of crystalloid and pressors were weaned off quickly. He was transferred out of the ICU the next day.

A positive fluid balance in critically ill patients leads to prolonged ventilation and increased mortality [26]. Because of this, determining the volume status of critically ill patients to guide diuresis is important. Ultrasound and echocardiography are helpful in guiding clinicians in these complex decisions. Lung ultrasound looking for B lines and pleural effusions suggests pulmonary edema. E/e' measurement, passive leg raise, and end-expiratory occlusion pressure are all accurate ways to predict the fluid status of critically ill patients. Using these techniques can help clinicians wean for mechanical ventilation faster, and reduce overall mortality.

Summary Points

- Determining the volume status of critically ill patients to guide diuresis is important.
- Ultrasound and echocardiography are helpful in guiding clinicians in these complex decisions.
- Lung ultrasound looking for B lines and pleural effusions suggests pulmonary edema.
- E/e' measurement, passive leg raise, and end-expiratory occlusion pressure are all accurate ways to predict the fluid status of critically ill patients.
- Using ultrasound techniques to assess volume status can help clinicians wean patients from mechanical ventilation, guide ongoing resuscitation, and reduce overall mortality.

References

1. Rivers E, et al. Early goal-directed therapy in the treatment of severe sepsis and septic shock. N Engl J Med. 2001;345(19):1368–77.
2. Vincent JL, et al. Sepsis in European intensive care units: results of the SOAP study. Crit Care Med. 2006;34(2):344–53.
3. Boyd JH, et al. Fluid resuscitation in septic shock: a positive fluid balance and elevated central venous pressure are associated with increased mortality. Crit Care Med. 2011;39(2):259–65.
4. National Heart L, et al. Comparison of two fluid-management strategies in acute lung injury. N Engl J Med. 2006;354(24):2564–75.
5. Kirkpatrick AW, et al. Intra-abdominal hypertension and the abdominal compartment syndrome: updated consensus definitions and clinical practice guidelines from the World Society of the Abdominal Compartment Syndrome. Intensive Care Med. 2013;39(7):1190–206.
6. Bouchard J, et al. Fluid accumulation, survival and recovery of kidney function in critically ill patients with acute kidney injury. Kidney Int. 2009;76(4):422–7.
7. Boles JM, et al. Weaning from mechanical ventilation. Eur Respir J. 2007;29(5):1033–56.
8. Grissom CK, et al. Association of physical examination with pulmonary artery catheter parameters in acute lung injury. Crit Care Med. 2009;37(10):2720–6.
9. Wo CC, et al. Unreliability of blood pressure and heart rate to evaluate cardiac output in emergency resuscitation and critical illness. Crit Care Med. 1993;21(2):218–23.
10. Marik PE, Baram M, Vahid B. Does central venous pressure predict fluid responsiveness? A systematic review of the literature and the tale of seven mares. Chest. 2008;134(1):172–8.
11. Marik PE, Cavallazzi R. Does the central venous pressure predict fluid responsiveness? An updated meta-analysis and a plea for some common sense. Crit Care Med. 2013;41(7):1774–81.
12. Lichtenstein DA, Meziere GA. Relevance of lung ultrasound in the diagnosis of acute respiratory failure: the BLUE protocol. Chest. 2008;134(1):117–25.
13. Lichtenstein D, et al. Comparative diagnostic performances of auscultation, chest radiography, and lung

ultrasonography in acute respiratory distress syndrome. Anesthesiology. 2004;100(1):9–15.
14. Papanikolaou J, et al. New insights into weaning from mechanical ventilation: left ventricular diastolic dysfunction is a key player. Intensive Care Med. 2011;37(12):1976–85.
15. de Meirelles Almeida CA, et al. Diastolic dysfunction as a predictor of weaning failure: a systematic review and meta-analysis. J Crit Care. 2016;34:135–41.
16. Sanfilippo F, et al. Association of weaning failure from mechanical ventilation with transthoracic echocardiography parameters: a systematic review and meta-analysis. Br J Anaesth. 2021;126(1):319–30.
17. Caille V, et al. Echocardiography: a help in the weaning process. Crit Care. 2010;14(3):R120.
18. Haji K, et al. The impact of heart, lung and diaphragmatic ultrasound on prediction of failed extubation from mechanical ventilation in critically ill patients: a prospective observational pilot study. Crit Ultrasound J. 2018;10(1):13.
19. Airapetian N, et al. Does inferior vena cava respiratory variability predict fluid responsiveness in spontaneously breathing patients? Crit Care. 2015;19:400.
20. Vignon P, et al. Comparison of echocardiographic indices used to predict fluid responsiveness in ventilated patients. Am J Respir Crit Care Med. 2017;195(8):1022–32.
21. Monnet X, Marik PE, Teboul JL. Prediction of fluid responsiveness: an update. Ann Intensive Care. 2016;6(1):111.
22. Hamzaoui O, et al. Increase in central venous pressure during passive leg raising cannot detect preload unresponsiveness. Crit Care Med. 2020;48(8):e684–9.
23. Monnet X, et al. The passive leg raising test to guide fluid removal in critically ill patients. Ann Intensive Care. 2016;6(1):46.
24. Jozwiak M, et al. Predicting fluid responsiveness in critically ill patients by using combined end-expiratory and end-inspiratory occlusions with echocardiography. Crit Care Med. 2017;45(11):e1131–8.
25. Monnet X, et al. Passive leg-raising and end-expiratory occlusion tests perform better than pulse pressure variation in patients with low respiratory system compliance. Crit Care Med. 2012;40(1):152–7.
26. Micek ST, et al. Fluid balance and cardiac function in septic shock as predictors of hospital mortality. Crit Care. 2013;17(5):R246.

59 Ultrasound Diagnosis of Acute Respiratory Failure and the BLUE-Protocol

Daniel A. Lichtenstein

Learning Objectives

1. Describe the key components of the BLUE-protocol
2. Review the five profiles of the fast-track BLUE-protocol
3. Examine misconceptions about the BLUE-protocol

The lung is the most vital organ. Respiratory failure is therefore one of the heaviest concerns in acute medicine, but also an extreme suffering [1]. Physicians face a situation where a diagnosis must be done urgently. This exercise is difficult, and generates deleterious issues [2]. The BLUE-protocol is proposed as a possible help.

The BLUE-protocol is one particular application of lung ultrasound, a part of holistic whole body critical ultrasound (HWBCU), a recent use of ultrasound summarizing a life's research. Ultrasound created a too discrete revolution in medicine [3]. The images were impossible to understand, then real time came, but new imaging methods also came, such as CT [4]. Therefore, ultrasound remained a rather minor technique in medicine, usually confided to the radiologist. The use of HWBCU, held by the first-line doctor, changed the very definition of ultrasound [5]. The consideration of the lung made the big part of HWBCU. Critical ultrasound was a nice cake, the lung was the cherry. The community had just to accept two concepts simultaneously (to see ultrasound used by non-radiologists, and mostly to see the lung insonated) [6].

The BLUE-protocol is a synthesis of lung ultrasound in the critically ill (LUCI), enabling users to develop it through at least 15 medical disciplines [7].

D. A. Lichtenstein (✉)
Medical intensivist, Ambroise-Paré hospital, Paris-West university, France

Definition and Principles

The BLUE-protocol is a fast protocol devoted to patients with acute respiratory failure. This is a structured way to standardize lung ultrasound data. E.g., when LUCI says "interstitial syndrome," the BLUE-protocol specifies its origin, e.g., acute hemodynamic pulmonary edema (AHPE). Three sectors are considered. LUCI (logical, this is the suffering organ). The venous system (because when pulmonary embolism is suspected, veins are analyzed). The heart (the BLUE-protocol simplifies echocardiography to the point that the heart is not included; it can and must be studied, but this is done outside the BLUE-protocol).

A principle of the BLUE-protocol is to consider gravity (practically, by distinguishing anterior from posterior analysis) and to associate one (sometimes two) sign, the whole generating profiles. This approach gives an overall 90.5% accu-

M. J. Lanspa, A. T. Levinson (eds.), *Echocardiography and Ultrasonography in the ICU*, Respiratory Medicine, https://doi.org/10.1007/978-3-031-80038-2_59

racy for the main diagnoses. The BLUE-protocol is just a protocol, which only suggests (from strongly to very strongly) a pathway, highly improved when basic clinical data are considered (history, fever, physical examination, and simple tests—ECG, D-dimers…).

Eight profiles are described. They are simply but strictly defined. Any patient can be classified in one of these profiles, and only one (there is a hierarchy, C-profile is over B-prime-profile, B-prime-profile over B-profile, B-profile over A-profile). Their labels are codes, enabling to share many information in a minimal timing.

All profiles imply first a work at the ground level (where gravity works), a patient in the supine (or semirecumbent) position, an anterior analysis, focused on the four anterior BLUE-points. In addition, the term A-profile implies predominant A-lines, plus, of critical importance although not in the short label A-profile, the conservation of lung sliding. The suffix "prime" is inserted when lung sliding is abolished, see below. No consolidation, even trace, should be seen. One B-line per point (even two) is accepted.

The BLUE-protocol is a completely qualitative tool. No measurement is done. The BLUE-protocol is not a score.

One trace consolidation has the same value than a huge one or multiple ones.

Last, the BLUE-protocol does not prevent from traditional management (CT if judged necessary). Just, blood gases may be asked less often (see Conclusions).

Patients, Tools Used, User Guide of the BLUE-Protocol

Patients Were all (adult) 301 patients seen in the ER, admitted to the ICU for respiratory failure, and benefiting from a diagnosis in the final report of medical intensivists of a university-affiliated teaching hospital. For obvious methodological reasons, patients with no diagnosis (5%) or double diagnoses (5%), or rare diagnoses (3%) were excluded. The 260 remaining patients had 6 diseases: pneumonia, AHPE, asthma, eCOPD, pulmonary embolism, and pneumothorax.

Tools In the current era of laptops or even cellphones, we advise simple cart-based equipment, much easier for multiple ergonomic reasons in case of hospital use. Artificial intelligence is not required if simple machines are used. Sophisticated machines add filters which make the analysis more difficult (and therefore require "helps" such as AI). With a single, well-designed probe, we can scan the lungs and the veins (BLUE-protocol), and we perform simple emergency cardiac sonography (see below).

The abdomen, all procedures (venous, pleural, peritoneal) pertain to this probe. The machine we use is a 1992 technology which is compact, easy-to-clean, easy-to-buy, fast to switch-on: 7 s (currently the fastest of the world).

User Guide How is the BLUE-protocol integrated in the usual management? After the clinical step (history, physical examination), we make a BLUE-protocol each time there is the slightest doubt on the diagnosis (that is, almost always), and ask for very basic tests (EKG, D-dimers if needed…). Waiting for their results, we can perform the simple emergency cardiac sonography (or ask for a conventional echocardiography, read below).

How to Learn the BLUE-Protocol

The BLUE-protocol may appear complex for some, it just superposes several layers of things to know, each being of immediate understanding. Only the number is high, this is why these points must be learned sequentially, quietly.

We advise to begin by the simplest, and the most profitable clinically: AHPE. Once the principle is understood, other applications come more easily.

Just note that the current knowledge for diagnosing the cause of a dyspnea requires long studies for understanding the lung anatomy, physiology, pathology, physical examination, radiology, biology… The BLUE-protocol aims at lightening some fields which are both the less important and the most difficult.

Technique

The probe is applied anteriorly (with three corrections enabling to acquire the bat sign, that is, symmetrical ribs, horizontal pleural line, and thin pleural line). If no anomaly is detected (A-profile), it is then applied on strategic zones of the venous system, then if no DVT is found, at the (accessible) posterior lung. The BLUE-protocol is performed without changing the position of the patient (semirecumbent if dyspneic, supine position if already intubated).

We find safer to remind (rapidly) the BLUE-points. One lung has at the anterior chest wall the projection of two hands (of the patient's size), from the clavicula. The probe is applied (roughly) at the center of each of these four areas, defining upper BLUE-point and lower BLUE-point. The PLAPS-point (PosteroLateral Alveolar and/or Pleural Syndrome) is a semiposterior point obtained from the transversal continuation of the lower BLUE-point, as posterior as possible in patients who can be ventilated.

Profiles of the BLUE-Protocol

The Five Profiles of the Fast-Track BLUE-Protocol

The anterior wall is the main area, enabling to define five of eight profiles. This analysis is sufficient in 46% of cases, defining the fast-track BLUE-protocol.

The A-profile, described above, implies further analysis and is not part of the fast-track BLUE-protocol. It defines only a normal lung *surface,* and is seen in diseases. It generates three sub-profiles, see below.

The B-Profile Lung sliding conserved, associated with lung rockets at the four anterior BLUE-points. No consolidation (even millimetric) should be seen. It indicates AHPE with 97% sensitivity and 95% specificity (see below). The 95% specificity can be easily improved using clinical and simple biological data plus, at this step, a simple look at the heart. Standard timing: 30 s (Fig. 59.1).

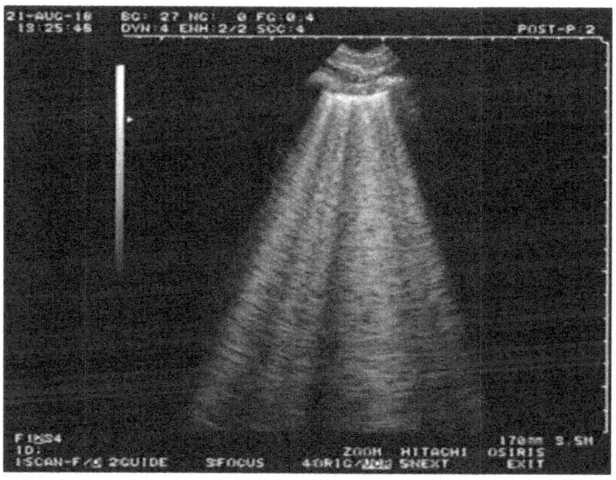

Fig. 59.1 B-profile (partial and static view)
Lung rockets in a patient with hemodynamic pulmonary edema. One can count seven or eight B-lines in the rib short-axis view (which generates a standardized, constant length of pleural line of 25+/−3 mm in adults, here 28 mm). These are glass-rockets, indicating ground-glass areas on CT (septal rockets mean three B-lines, indicating thickened interlobular septa)
Note six of the seven criteria of the B-line (in our recommended order): comet-tail artifact; arising from the pleural line (not visible in this frozen view: moving with lung-sliding); usually well-defined laser-ray like; usually long (ten-cm are required, making vascular probes less suitable for this criterium); usually erasing A-lines; usually hyperechoic
Colleagues can take any article and compare the image quality and clarity. Hitachi-405 (1992–2010) with microconvex probe. This machine was 32-cm width, making the current revolution possible long before the era of laptops

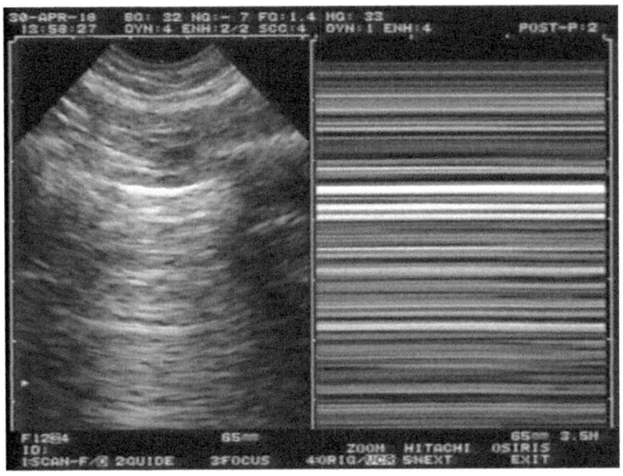

Fig. 59.2 A-prime profile (first step for the diagnosis of pneumothorax)
A typical A-prime profile, fully sensitive for pneumothorax, not specific (very suggestive, but only the lung-point is 100% specific). Note basic points: (1) Non-vascular probe, but a perfect contact with the intercostal space, a range enabling to visualize superficial as well as deep regions, a total control (this probe can be inserted posteriorly, at the apex…). This probe is suitable for basic heart, abdomen, veins, and procedures (e.g., venous canulation). (2) Both images are side-by-side. (3) Not only they are side-by-side, but exactly side-by-side. This simple requirement, possible since 1992, and even before, enables to locate exactly the pleural line on the right image. This critical detail makes much easier diagnosis even in dyspneic patients. (4) Left, real time (static image). This A-line is a constant and mandatory sign. Right, M-mode: abolished lung-sliding: stratosphere sign (not barcode sign, a term able to generate deadly confusions in view of the new barcodes). (5) This image, at the anterior wall, has a name in the BLUE-protocol: the A-prime-profile

The B-prime-profile is a B-profile with impaired (up to abolished) lung sliding. It is a usual marker of pneumonia. Standard timing: a few seconds.

The C-profile simply indicates anterior consolidation(s), *regardless number and size* (this includes therefore Cm-lines). It indicates almost always pneumonia (including in recent pandemia). Standard timing: from a few seconds up to 1 min.

The A/B-profile is basically a half A-profile and a half B-profile. It indicates almost always pneumonia. The mini-A/B-profile (one pattern at upper BLUE-point, the other at lower BLUE-point), the micro-A/B-profile (in the same length of pleural line, one area full of B-lines, one devoid of B-line) are variants. Standard timing: a few seconds.

The A-prime-profile is an A-profile with exclusive (not predominant) A-lines plus full abolition of lung sliding. This is the first step for diagnosing pneumothorax (the second step is active search for a lung point). Standard timing: a few seconds (Fig. 59.2).

Profiles of the BLUE-Protocol

The Three Last Profiles (Comprehensive BLUE-Protocol)

The A-profile is seen in asthma, COPD, pulmonary embolism, and some posterior pneumonias. Standard timing: 30 s.

A-DVT-Profile Defines pulmonary embolism. The detection of lung rockets, especially bilateral, glass-rockets, is exceptional in pulmonary embolism occurring on healthy lungs. Facing an A-profile, the user should urgently rule in pulmonary embolism. Here, the veins are scanned (posterior scanning of the lung will not add discriminative elements). The sequence A-profile plus positive DVT, defining the A-DVT-profile, is 99% specific (this specificity raises the question of the opportunity of an immediate therapy in unstable patients).

The sequential venous analysis of the BLUE-protocol is still under submission. Meanwhile, users can read [8] or choose any existing protocol, the specificity will be unchanged, only the sensitivity is impacted.

The venous step is the longest part of the BLUE-protocol, yet the approach is sequential: following an order, it can be achieved in a few seconds in the best cases, up to a bit less than 2 min if none of the five sites (per side) is positive. The principle is, again, qualitative: as soon as one area of DVT is detected, the BLUE-protocol is over. BLUE-protocol takes high consideration to calf veins, using a simple protocol. Jugular, subclavian veins are under focus. A negative venous scan decreases the probability of embolism, without ruling it out (when clinical data indicate a possibility of embolism, physicians are of course invited to go beyond). Echocardiography can be done at will, just note that dilated right ventricle is seen at various degrees in all cases of respiratory failure not originating from the left heart [9].

A-V-PLAPS-Profile Suggests posterior pneumonia. When no DVT is detected, the posterior lung (PLAPS-point) is under analysis. A consolidation and/or an effusion defines a PLAPS (*regardless volume, regardless if unilateral*). The sequence is labeled A-V-PLAPS-profile (meaning, first detection of an A-profile, then negative search for DVT, then a PLAPS found). Standard timing: between 2 and 3 min.

Nude Profile Usually indicates asthma and COPD (two diagnoses put together, given their similitude in pathophysiology). It associates A-profile, no DVT, no PLAPS. Standard timing: the longest, roughly 3 min. If a trace PLAPS has been detected (i.e., no longer a nude profile), the diagnosis is pneumonia (decompensating COPD), very schematically. In the case of a nude profile, the simple stethacoustic detection of wheeze decreases again the likeliness of embolism.

The BLUE-protocol has variable geometry In case of A profile, the sequence is the anterior wall (half a minute), then, if needed, the venous system (2 min at worst), then, if needed, one PLAPS-point (less than 30″), then if negative, the contralateral PLAPS-point.

Decision Tree of the BLUE-Protocol (Fig. 59.3, Table 59.1)

The decision tree published in 2008 shows the six usual diagnoses of 97% of patients. Minor adaptations came: at the far left, instead of "pulmonary edema," we specified "hemodynamic." At the far right, the sequence lung sliding abolished then exclusive A-lines has a name: the A-prime-profile.

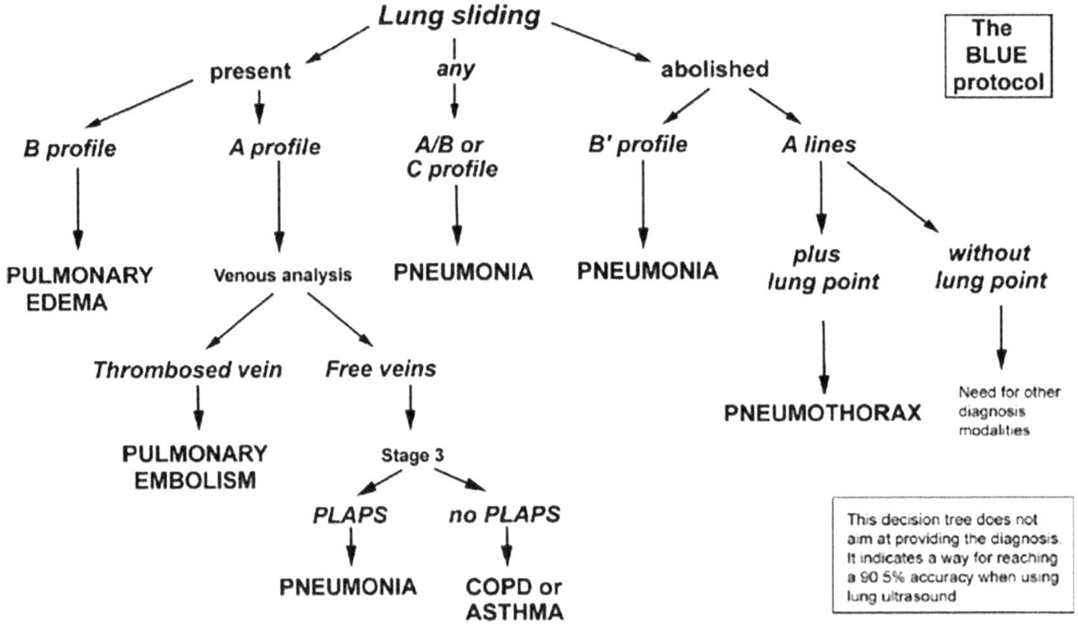

Fig. 59.3 Decision tree of the BLUE-protocol
The main changes from the original Figure from Chest 2008;136:117–125. With permission of Elsevier

Table 59.1 Accuracy of the profiles of the BLUE-protocol

Mechanism of dyspnea	Profiles of BLUE-protocol	Sensitivity	Specificity	Positive predictive value	Negative predictive value
Acute hemodynamic pulmonary edema	*B-profile*	97%	95%	87%	99%
Pneumonia (assimilated to ARDS, see text)	*The four profiles*[a]	89%	94%	88%	95%
	B′-profile	11%	100%	100%	70%
	A/B profile	14.5%	100%	100%	71.5%
	C-profile	21.5%	99%	90%	73%
	A-V-PLAPS profile	42%	96%	83%	78%
Exacerbated COPD or severe acute asthma	*Nude profile (A-profile with no DVT*[b] *and no PLAPS)*	89%	97%	93%	95%
Pulmonary embolism	*A-profile with DVT*	81%	99%	94%	98%
Pneumothorax	*A'-profile (with lung point)*	88%	100%	100%	99%

[a]The sensitivity is calculated by totalling the sensitivity of each profile
[b]*DVT* deep venous thrombosis

BLUE-Protocol and ARDS

There is not one word to add regarding ARDS. ARDS is a pneumonia in most cases (a severe, extensive, deadly pneumonia, but a pneumonia). ARDS is assimilated to pneumonia in the BLUE-protocol. The four profiles of pneumonia (B′-profile, A/B-profile, C-profile, A-[V]-PLAPS-profile) are found again in infectious ARDS in most cases [10]. Secondary ARDS cannot yet be dealt with (work in progress).

Terms familiar in literature (irregular pleural line, spared areas, abolished lung sliding) are replaced, in the nomenclature of the BLUE-protocol, by more informative labels, respectively, C-profile, A/B-profile, and B-prime profile.

Regarding the extension/monitoring of ARDS, we use the Pink-protocol, a BLUE-protocol with two modifications. First, it is comprehensive: the six BLUE-points & PLAPS-points are at least studied. Second, Pink-protocol introduces quantitative assessment (on submission).

The B-Profile, a Focus on AHPE and the Distinction with Other Disorders (Mainly ARDS)

The B-profile is connected with AHPE with a 97% sensitivity and 95% specificity. AHPE is a didactic model of interstitial syndrome.

Because AHPE is first an interstitial syndrome, it will generate lung rockets. An A-profile, even with PLAPS, cannot be seen.

Because AHPE is a transudative disorder, lung sliding is preserved (a data that neither radiographs nor even CT can show). The B-prime-profile is therefore not consistent with AHPE.

Because the whole (or at least large symmetrical parts) of the interstitial sector is filled with fluid, this makes a bilateral, symmetrical, homogeneous pattern. The A/B-profile is therefore not consistent with AHPE.

Because the interstitial sector is first saturated, before the alveolar sector, there is no reason to see in a semirecumbent/lying patient any anterior alveolar syndrome. The slightest anterior consolidation (even 1 cm-line) generates the C-profile, regardless of surrounding B-lines. The C-profile rules out AHPE. We do not remind what is a B-line, nor its hierarchized seven criteria enabling to avoid any confusion with others comet-tail artifacts (Fig. 59.1).

The B-profile rules out pneumothorax (using lung sliding and/or the B-lines). It rules out COPD and asthma.

BLUE-Protocol and Weaning-Induced Pulmonary Edema (WIPO)

We were asked to deal with WIPO (a probably underestimated cause of weaning failure). We saw it in half cases where spontaneous breathing trials failed [11]. Here, patients have usually sequelae with multiple B-lines here and there. We have defined the delta-B-lines for circumventing this issue. It indicates the number of B-lines which appear from a given number of B-lines, at strictly determined points (the four BLUE-points). The value of six (that is, the theoretical value of 1,5 line per BLUE-point) gave a 88% sensitivity and a 91% specificity for WIPO.

Note that this threshold of two, and even one B-line differ from the traditional value of three B-lines for being able to speak of interstitial syndrome. First, because the intensivist is present for detecting WIPOs at very early stages. Second, because WIPO usually occurs on already damaged lungs. Note however that the delta-B lines was >6 in most cases with WIPO.

Pearls

Some teams make comprehensive analysis for ruling in, or out, pneumothorax. They can do this, provided time is not an issue. In case of hurry, using principle 2 of LUCI, one point speaks for the whole lung: the most dominant in the sky/earth axis (approximately the lower BLUE-point in supine patients, the upper BLUE-point in semirecumbent patients). At this point, lung sliding rules out pneumothorax [12]. Abolished lung sliding is a 100% sensitive sign of clinical pneumothorax.

Regarding pneumothorax again, it is surprising to read concerns in literature about "search for solutions" for improving the diagnosis. In the CEURF world, there is no problem since three decades. Possibly, machines used by the new generation of doctors are not adapted, generating confusions responsible for this situation.

Subpleural consolidations are not sought for in pulmonary embolism. First, this term is not useful (all consolidations seen with ultrasound are subpleural). Second, their sensitivity is low (6% of cases seen anteriorly [13]). Third, their specificity is low (they are found, posteriorly, in pneumonia, AHPE, contusion, and other conditions, even pneumothorax [14, 15].

Some colleagues say that it is no longer useful to auscultate, etc. We hope these are only corridor talks. As to usual tests (BNP, TTE or expert TEE, helical CT…), they can be done at will of course.

Some Other Misconceptions

We were asked to comment the misconceptions in LUCI. This is not possible in the assigned volume, so we made a random selection of 10% of the comments found in [16].

Comment #13. "Pleural effusions are anechoic." Only anechoic effusions are anechoic—and severe cases are echoic (this is why we defined the quad sign, a universal sign which works for both)

Comment # 15. "the spine sign": we never used it (we describe a universal sign).

Comment #24. "The terms 'B1-profile' and 'B2-profile'" often seen in literature. These terms suppose that in these studies, lung-sliding was carefully studied and all these patients had conserved lung-sliding? Likely lung-sliding was not measured in these articles, with the risk to confuse B-profile and B-prime-profile (and give the wrong therapy). Better is to replace the terms "B1-profile," "B2-profile" by septal-rockets and glass-rockets, terms which have the advantage of being independent from lung-sliding—and easier for the memory (Fig. 59.1).

Comment #43. "LUS." LUS means, burned forever on the marble, Lung Ultrasound Score. We write lung ultrasound, or, more specific, LUCI.

Some Among Many Frequently Asked Questions on the BLUE-Protocol

Does the BLUE-protocol work in trauma?

Of course it does, especially for pneumothorax.

The pericardial tamponade was forgotten?

Pericardial tamponade, easy to assess, is not in the decision tree, just because it does not, to our knowledge, generate acute respiratory failure. This being said, this rare but easy diagnosis can be sought for before or after the BLUE-protocol.

Can we do the BLUE-protocol with traditional laptop machines and traditional probes?

Yes. It will be harder, longer, less precise, more costly, more operator dependent, less clean but yes, one must always try.

The heart is not included in the decision tree. Why?

We will make extremely short. Echocardiographic data are welcome. Echocardiography can be performed at will before the BLUE-protocol, or after, but is not included in the BLUE-protocol. The non-inclusion of the "peri-heart" (pericardium) was already explained. Regarding the very heart, studying the suffering organ (the lung) provides direct data. The left heart cannot show "pulmonary edema," it shows the cardiac function, a fine but indirect sign of pulmonary edema. In practice, we get clinical data, of prime importance, perform the BLUE-protocol, make at will simple emergency cardiac sonography (a simple protocol of CEURF centered to right ventricle volume), manage the patient, and ask for an expert echocardiography, if indicated, in a relieved patient.

For Knowing More

Like everything, the BLUE-protocol can hold in a short book chapter, or in a more comprehensive, 400-page volume [8]. Doctors have currently the choice between many textbooks; they can also enjoy subtleties such as unusual approaches (apical analysis), signs (peculiarities of pneumothorax in dyspneic patients), applications (the hemodynamic power of the B-line, or the Pink-protocol, LUCI in ARDS) among others.

Concluding Remarks and Future Perspectives

The BLUE-protocol was conceived in the years 1990. Each brick of LUCI had to be submitted several times before we could submit the BLUE-protocol. Time was irreversibly lost (with consequences on the currently used equipment). Time was lost at times where even CT was not available The positive point was a 18-year experience when it was published. This is for the past. Regarding the future, we expect two major outcomes, apart from the prompt relief of the dyspnea. First, a decrease in irradiating or painful tests (see below). Second, the medicolegal issues may one day be inverted in light of LUCI. One example among hundred is the radiography done for excluding pneumothorax (after for instance manipulation of chest tube), given the proven weakness of bedside radiographies. We hope that this update will enable those physicians who discover the potentials of the BLUE-protocol, to fully enjoy it [17–20].

The last word will regard the future of blood gases, precisely given the accuracy of the BLUE-protocol [21]. We reserve this painful test to the really difficult cases, we hope it will be exceptionally required in the future for respiratory diagnoses (*circulatory* applications are something different). If this succeeds, it will be the best contribution of our research.

With the BLUE-protocol, critical ultrasound shows, again, its pertinence regarding an application which was not supposed to be feasible [22].

Summary Points

- The lung is the most vital organ. A simple equipment is the best for analyzing both artifacts and structural disorders, enabling to build one of the eight profiles of the BLUE-protocol for better knowing the origin of an acute respiratory failure.
- Analyzing the anterior wall is sufficient in half cases for building a profile of pneumonia (B-prime, C, A/B), of hemodynamic pulmonary edema (B-profile), of pneumothorax (A-prime-profile).
- A normal anterior lung surface associated with a DVT generates the A-DVT-profile, almost specific to pulmonary embolism.
- The BLUE-protocol is only a protocol, it is of course contextualized using simple elements from history and clinical examination.
- The BLUE-protocol is purely qualitative. Based on variable geometry, it is concluded after a minimum of a few seconds, a maximum of 3 min.
- Those discovering the BLUE-protocol should first study only the B-profile, which is probably the most useful and the simplest. It helps to understand the spirit of the BLUE-protocol.
- For studying ARDS, an extension of the BLUE-protocol is done, the Pink-protocol. This is a comprehensive BLUE-protocol (all sites are studied), with quantitative measurements.
- Echocardiography is not included in the BLUE-protocol. It matters to understand this choice, and to understand that echocardiography can be performed at will, before or after.

References

1. Irwin RS, Rippe JM. Intensive care medicine. 6th ed. Philadelphia: Lippincott Williams & Wilkins; 2008. p. 491–6.
2. Ray P, Birolleau S, Lefort Y, Becquemin MH, Beigelman C, Isnard R, Teixeira A, Arthaud M, Riou B, Boddaert J. Acute respiratory failure in the elderly: etiology, emergency diagnosis and prognosis. Crit Care. 2006;10(3):R82.
3. Dénier A. Les ultrasons, leur application au diagnostic. Presse Méd. 1946;22:307–8.

4. Hounsfield GN. Computerized transverse axial scanning. Brit J Radiol. 1973;46:1016–22.
5. Lichtenstein D, Axler O. Intensive use of general ultrasound in the intensive care unit, a prospective study of 150 consecutive patients. Intensive Care Med. 1993;19:353–5.
6. Weinberger SE, Drazen JM. Diagnostic procedures in respiratory diseases. In: Harrison's principles of internal medicine. 15th ed. New York: McGraw-Hill; 2001. p. 1454.
7. Lichtenstein D, Malbrain ML. Lung Ultrasound in the Critically Ill (LUCI): a translational discipline. Anaesthesiol Intensive Ther. 2017;49(5):430–6. https://doi.org/10.5603/AIT.a2017.0063. ISSN 0209-1712.
8. Lichtenstein D. Lung ultrasound in the critically ill. The BLUE-protocol. Heidelberg: Springer; 2016.
9. Jardin F, Dubourg O. L'exploration échocardiographique en médecine d'urgence. Paris and New York: Masson; 1986. p. 1–154.
10. Pesenti A, Musch G, Lichtenstein D, Mojoli F, Amato M, Cinnella G, Gattinoni L, Quintel M. Imaging in acute respiratory distress syndrome. Intensive Care Med. 2016;42:686–98. https://doi.org/10.1007/s00134-016-4328-1.
11. Ferré A, Guillot M, Lichtenstein D, Mezière G, Richard C, Teboul JL, Monnet X. Lung ultrasound allows the diagnosis of weaning-induced pulmonary edema. Intensive Care Med. 2019;45(5):601–8. https://doi.org/10.1007/s00134-019-05573-6.
12. Lichtenstein D, Holzapfel L, Frija J. Projection cutanée des pneumothorax et impact sur leur diagnostic échographique. Réan Urg. 2000; 9(Suppl 2):138s.
13. Mathis G, Blank W, Reißig A, Lechleitner P, Reuß J, Schuler A, Beckh S. Thoracic ultrasound for diagnosing pulmonary embolism. Chest. 2001;128:1531–8.
14. Reissig A, Kroegel C. Relevance of subpleural consolidations in chest ultrasound. Chest. 2009;136:1706. https://doi.org/10.1378/chest.08-2541.
15. Lichtenstein D, Mezière G. Response. Chest. 2009;136:1706–7. https://doi.org/10.1378/chest.09-2550.
16. Lichtenstein D. Current Misconceptionsl in lung ultrasound. A short guide for experts (Commentary). Chest. 2019;156(1):21–5. https://doi.org/10.1016/j.chest.2019.02.332. Epub 2019 Mar 11. PMID: 30872018.
17. Bekgoz B, Kilicaslan I, Bildik F, Keles A, Demircan A, Hakoglu O, Coskun G, Demir HA. BLUE-protocol ultrasonography in emergency department patients presenting with acute dyspnea. Am J Emerg Med. 2019;S0735-6757(19):30112–3.
18. Islam M, Levitus M, Eisen L, Shiloh AL, Fein D. Lung ultrasound for the diagnosis and management of acute respiratory failure. Lung. 2020;198(1):1–11.
19. Patel CJ, Bhatt HB, Parikh SN, Jhaveri BN, Puranik JH. BLUE-protocol as a diagnostic tool in patients of acute respiratory distress presenting to emergency department. J Emerg Trauma Shock. 2018;11(2):125–9.
20. Seyedhosseini J, Bashizadeh-Fakhar G, Farzaneh S, Momeni M, Karimialavijeh E. The impact of the BLUE-protocol ultrasonography on the time taken to treat acute respiratory distress in the ED. Am J Emerg Med. 2017;35:1815–8.
21. Lichtenstein D, Mezière G. Relevance of lung ultrasound in the diagnosis of acute respiratory failure. The BLUE-protocol. Chest. 2008;134:117–25.
22. van der Werf TS, Zijlstra JG. Ultrasound of the lung: just imagine. Intensive Care Med. 2004;30:183–4.

Acute Coronary Syndrome

60

Christopher W. Hoeger and Eli V. Gelfand

Learning Objectives

1. Examine how bedside echocardiography is an essential tool in triaging the critically ill patient with chest pain.
2. Describe echocardiographic findings suggestive of mechanical complications from acute MI.

Pathophysiology/Diagnosis

Myocardial infarction is a process of irreversible myocardial injury due to ischemia, usually due to thrombotic occlusion of an epicardial coronary artery. This often, but not always, occurs at the site of an atherosclerotic plaque. The coronary thrombus may be occlusive, as is typically the case in ST-elevation myocardial infarction, or non-occlusive, in non-ST-elevation myocardial infarction. Myocardial injury results in cell death and release of cardiac enzymes into the blood. These enzymes, including cardiac troponin, can be measured and are essential in diagnosing a myocardial infarction. Myocardial infarction is diagnosed in a patient with an elevation of cardiac troponin above the 99th percentile of the upper reference limit with an acute rise or fall. This is accompanied by one or more of the following: symptoms of myocardial ischemia, dynamic ischemic electrocardiogram (ECG) changes, or development of pathological Q waves, imaging evidence of new loss of viable myocardium, or new regional wall motion abnormality in a pattern consistent with an ischemic etiology.

Supplementary Information The online version contains supplementary material available at https://doi.org/10.1007/978-3-031-80038-2_60.

C. W. Hoeger · E. V. Gelfand (✉)
Cardiovascular Division, Beth Israel Deaconess Medical Center, Harvard Medical School, Boston, MA, USA
e-mail: cwhoeger@bidmc.harvard.edu; egelfand@bidmc.harvard.edu

Coronary Anatomy

Knowledge of typical coronary anatomy is important in understanding typical patterns of wall motion abnormality consistent with myocardial ischemia. The coronary arteries supply blood to the myocardial segments along their course, and occlusion of any of these arteries results in a typical pattern of abnormal wall motion correlating to the ischemic segments.

The left coronary artery divides into the left anterior descending (LAD) and left circumflex (LCx) arteries. The LAD travels down the anterior intraventricular grove to the apex of the left ventricle (LV), while the LCx travels laterally through the atrioventricular groove. The LAD gives off diagonal and septal branches that supply the anterior 2/3 of the intraventricular septum.

M. J. Lanspa, A. T. Levinson (eds.), *Echocardiography and Ultrasonography in the ICU*, Respiratory Medicine, https://doi.org/10.1007/978-3-031-80038-2_60

The distal LAD most often supplies the apex of the left ventricle (LV). The LCx gives off obtuse marginal (OM) branches that supply the lateral territories of the heart. The right coronary artery (RCA) travels medially through the atrioventricular groove and supplies the right ventricle (RV). In the majority (80%) of patients, the RCA supplies blood to the posterior of the heart via the posterior descending artery (PDA). This is termed a "right dominant" coronary circulation. In a minority of patients, the PDA is supplied by the LCx, in which case the coronary circulation is termed "left dominant," or in equal parts by the RCA and LCx ("co-dominant" circulation).

17-Segment Model of the LV

In an attempt to standardize assessment of regional wall motion and allow correlation with vascular territories and comparison between different imaging modalities, a model of the LV has been developed that divides the myocardium into 17 segments [1]. These segments correlate with standard echocardiographic views of the left ventricle from the apical and parasternal windows. The LV is divided into six longitudinal walls, correlating with the walls seen in the 4-chamber, 2-chamber, and long-axis (3-chamber) windows. Moving clockwise, the walls are termed: anterior, anterolateral, inferolateral (posterior), inferior, inferoseptal, and anteroseptal. These walls are then segmented lengthwise into 3 sections, termed basal, mid, and apical. The LV tapers towards the apex, thus the apex is split into 4 segments: anterior, lateral, posterior, and septal. The tip of the apex is a single segment.

An assessment for segmental wall motion abnormality by echocardiography should ideally include visualization of all 17 segments of the LV. This can be accomplished via acquisition of apical 4-chamber (anterolateral, inferoseptal walls, apex), 2-chamber (anterior, inferior walls, apex), and 3-chamber (inferolateral, anteroseptal walls, apex) images. Care must be taken to avoid foreshortening of the LV in the apical windows. The parasternal long axis allows for visualization of the basal and mid segments of the inferolateral and anteroseptal walls. The parasternal short axis allows circumferential imaging of the myocardium at the basal, mid, and apical sections of the LV. From the parasternal short view, if the ultrasound probe is angled towards the apex, off-axis images may result in visualization of the basal portions of the anterior LV with apical portions of the posterior walls. The critically ill patient may have suboptimal windows for a variety of reasons, including pulmonary disease, suboptimal patient positioning, surgical dressings, and lines or tubes obscuring the field of view. In these cases, assessment of wall motion via subcostal windows may be helpful. A 4-chamber view via the subcostal approach highlights the inferoseptal and anterolateral walls. Through counterclockwise rotation of the transducer in the subcostal position, short-axis views can be obtained, which will show the inferior and inferolateral walls closest to the ultrasound transducer, in contrast to parasternal windows, where the anterior and anterolateral walls are closest.

Image depth and width should be minimized to maximize frame rate and thus temporal resolution for assessment of wall motion.

Wall Motion Assessment

A normal myocardial wall segment demonstrates both inward motion and wall thickening in systole. A segment is termed "hypokinetic" if the degree of inward motion and/or wall thickening are reduced. If these are absent, the segment is "akinetic." A wall that moves paradoxically, or outward, in systole is considered "dyskinetic." This is usually associated with myocardial scar and thinning of the wall segment. Finally, if a dyskinetic segment has an abnormal contour in diastole, it is termed "aneurysmal."

Patterns of Wall Motion Abnormality by Coronary Lesion

Wall motion abnormalities in patients with ACS correlate with the vascular territory of the affected vessel (Fig. 60.1, Video 60.1). There is variability

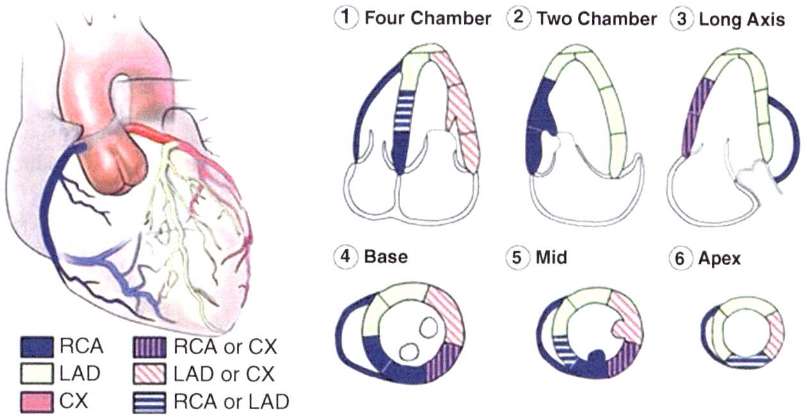

Fig. 60.1 17-segment model of the left ventricle with associated vascular territories. (Reference for figure: [2])

based on variations in patient anatomy as well as the location of obstruction within a coronary artery. Lesions in a branch or a distal segment of a coronary artery will generally cause abnormal wall motion in a smaller and more distal area of myocardium.

Lesions in the LAD will often cause abnormal motion of the anterior septum via septal perforator arteries, basal to apical anterior wall, and apex. If the LAD is a large vessel that wraps around the apex, the distal inferior wall can also be affected. The LAD may give off large diagonal branches to the anterolateral wall, in which case anterolateral wall motion abnormalities can be seen.

Lesions in the LCx will most often cause wall motion abnormalities in the anterolateral and inferolateral LV walls, with the extent being dependent on the size of the vessel and the dominance of the coronary circulation. Even a complete LCx coronary occlusion may sometimes present with subtle ECG changes, and thus echocardiography is a helpful diagnostic tool in these cases.

Lesions in the RCA will generally affect the inferoseptal, inferior, and inferolateral walls, with the latter being dependent on the size of the RCA and the coronary circulation being right dominant. RV involvement can be seen with proximal RCA disease.

Bedside Echocardiography in ACS

Diagnostic assessment of the critically ill patient with chest pain

Apart from myocardial ischemia, commonly encountered causes of chest pain in a critically ill patient include pulmonary embolism, aortic dissection, myocarditis or pericarditis, musculoskeletal discomfort (including costal pain following cardiopulmonary resuscitation), and gastrointestinal disorders including esophagitis and biliary colic (Table 60.1). As a first step in evaluating any patient with suspected ACS, a 12-lead ECG and measurement of blood level of cardiac troponin should be performed (Table 60.2). An ECG meeting diagnostic criteria for ST-elevation MI should prompt immediate consideration for coronary angiography and possible percutaneous coronary intervention [3]. Bedside echocardiography can be helpful to assess for ventricular function and to rule out mechanical complications of MI but should not delay treatment.

If the ECG is non-diagnostic and initial cardiac troponin is negative, an alternative diagnosis should be considered. If suspicion remains high for ACS despite a negative initial workup, measurement of cardiac troponin should be repeated, as blood levels may be normal in the earliest phases of an MI. In the critically ill patient with suspected ACS but a non-diagnostic ECG, an elevated cardiac tro-

Table 60.1 Differential diagnosis of chest pain in the critically ill patient

Differential diagnosis for chest pain in the critically ill patient
Acute coronary syndrome
Aortic dissection
Arteritis
Cocaine use
Costochondritis
Gastroesophageal disorders
Hypertensive crisis
Pulmonary embolism
Pericarditis/Myopericarditis
Pleuritis
Stress (Takatsubo) cardiomyopathy

ponin should prompt suspicion for non-ST-elevation MI and further evaluation with bedside echocardiography for LV wall motion assessment, ideally via parasternal and apical windows to allow for complete LV assessment. A focal wall motion abnormality in this setting should prompt treatment for non-ST-elevation MI. A globally hypokinetic LV should prompt evaluation and treatment for non-ischemic causes of heart failure. If the LV assessment is normal, alternative diagnoses should be considered. Formal echocardiography can be of utility in this case to rule out a subtle wall motion abnormality and for comprehensive assessment of cardiac morphology and function.

If a diagnosis of ACS is made, further assessment should be made with bedside echocardiography to assess for complications of MI, especially in an unstable patient. A pericardial effusion may be seen in cases of pericarditis or a free wall rupture. If an effusion is seen, M-mode echocardiography (if available) and IVC assessment can be used to assess for evidence of cardiac tamponade. RV function can be assessed from the apical 4-chamber view. A hypokinetic RV can be seen in cases of RV MI, which is sometimes seen with proximal RCA disease. Color doppler should be placed over the intraventricular septum in this view to assess for a ventricular septal defect.

Table 60.2 Acute coronary syndrome algorithm with ultrasound

Concern for ACS
ECG meets STEMI criteria
Cardiology consult
Bedside echocardiogram to assess for mechanical complications of MI, time permitting
ECG non-diagnostic and troponin negative
Consider alternative diagnosis
Repeat troponin if high suspicion for ACS
ECG non-diagnostic and troponin positive
Perform bedside echocardiogram
LV function and wall motion normal
Consider alternative diagnosis
LV function is globally reduced
Consider non-ischemic etiology of heart failure
Focal wall motion abnormality present
Treat for ACS
If ACS diagnosed, assess for complications of MI
Pericardial effusion present
Small pericardial effusion—Post-MI pericarditis or myopericarditis
Large pericardial effusion—Consider free wall rupture
M-mode assessment for tamponade
Cardiac surgery consult
LV aneurysm or large area of akinesis
Assess for LV thrombus
Formal echocardiogram with endocardial definition agent more sensitive for detection of thrombus
Color flow across IVS
VSR—Cardiac surgery consult
Significant MR
Assess for ischemic leaflet restriction and papillary muscle rupture
Cardiac surgery consult if papillary muscle rupture seen
Formal echocardiogram to quantify MR
RV hypokinesis
Consider RV MI and other causes of RV failure, such as pulmonary embolism or pulmonary hypertension

ECG electrocardiogram, *STEMI* ST-elevation myocardial infarction, *MI* myocardial infarction, *ACS* acute coronary syndrome, *LV* left ventricular, *IVS* intraventricular septum, *VSR* ventricular septal rupture, *MR* mitral regurgitation, *RV* right ventricular

Takotsubo (Stress) Cardiomyopathy

It is important to consider a diagnosis of takotsubo (stress) cardiomyopathy in a patient with suspected ACS [4]. Stress cardiomyopathy is often triggered by intense physical or emotional stress and presents most commonly with acute-onset chest pain, though dyspnea and syncope can also be seen. In more severe cases, patients can present with heart failure or cardiogenic shock. Patients may have an elevated cardiac troponin and ST-segment elevations, depressions, or T wave inversions on ECG in a similar fashion to ACS. On echocardiography, focal wall motion abnormalities are seen and the LVEF is usually reduced. There are a number of patterns of wall motion abnormality seen. The most common phenotype is the apical form, which is seen as ballooning of the LV apex with abnormal wall motion of the mid, distal, and apical segments of the LV. This pattern can be consistent with either a non coronary distribution or LAD-territory ischemia, depending on the specific segments involved. The base of the LV may be hyperdynamic, and a dynamic LV outflow tract (LVOT) obstruction can result. This can be detected via segmental pulse wave doppler across the LVOT from the apical 5-chamber view. Less commonly, stress cardiomyopathy can present with wall motion abnormalities limited to the mid ventricle, base, focal segments, or global hypokinesis. Often, distinguishing a stress cardiomyopathy from ACS can be difficult on the basis of point of care echocardiography, cardiac biomarkers, and ECG alone, and further evaluation with coronary angiography should be considered.

Mechanical Complications of MI

Development of hemodynamic instability in an ICU patient with a recent diagnosis of acute coronary syndrome, especially when accompanied by recurrent discomfort and/or ECG changes, should prompt an expeditious search for a mechanical complication [5], (Table 60.3).

Mitral Regurgitation

Mitral regurgitation most often complicates an acute inferior wall MI and occurs as a result of one of two etiologies. Systolic tethering of the posterior leaflet to a hypo- or a-kinetic inferolateral wall causes eccentric mitral regurgitation, which can be significant, but is rarely acutely severe. Treatment is focused on revascularization and subsequent post-MI medical therapy. Conversely, an inferoposterior MI may lead to a partial or complete rupture of the posteromedial papillary muscle, with resultant flail posterior leaflet and severe mitral regurgitation. In the latter case bedside echocardiography will typically

Table 60.3 Mechanical complications of myocardial infarction

Complication	Echo findings
Pseudoaneurysm	Focal area of wall thinning and akinesis with an acute takeoff from normal myocardium and a thin neck with neck: pseudoaneursm ratio <0.5
Aneurysm	Focal area of wall thinning/scarring and dyskinesis with neck: aneurysm ratio >0.5
Pericarditis	Pericardial effusion, possible pericardial thickening
Free wall rupture	Circumferential pericardial effusion
Ventricular septal defect	Color or continuous wave Doppler flow across intraventricular septum in systole, interruption of intraventricular septum not always seen
Ischemic mitral leaflet restriction	Restricted movement of posterior mitral valve leaflet with failure of mitral valve coaptation, posteriorly directed regurgitant jet
Papillary muscle rupture	Mitral leaflet flail with prolapse of papillary muscle fragment into left atrium in systole
Right ventricular infarct	Hypokinetic right ventricle, usually with inferior wall motion abnormality
Left ventricular thrombus	Echodense structure in ventricle distinct from myocardium

reveal a highly eccentric jet of severe mitral regurgitation, with a flail posterior leaflet and a mobile mass attached to the flail chorda tendinae (Fig. 60.2, Videos 60.2 and 60.3). This scenario necessitates an urgent surgical evaluation for mitral valve repair or replacement. Transesophageal echocardiography may be needed to confirm the complication and clarify the mechanism of mitral regurgitation.

Ventricular Septal Rupture

Infarction of a portion of the intraventricular septum can cause myocardial necrosis and ventricular septal rupture (VSR) (Fig. 60.3, Videos 60.4 and 60.5). With RCA-territory MI, the VSR will appear basal, located close to the atrioventricular valves and often serpiginous in appearance. Doppler flow across the interventricular septum confirms the diagnosis. With LAD-territory infarction, the VSR may be located in the mid- or distal portion of the interventricular septum and may be missed if the apical views are foreshortened. A helpful clue to the presence of an apical VSR may be brisk systolic flow in the *right ventricular* apex, unmasking apical left-to-right shunting.

Free Wall Rupture

Ischemia and necrosis of the free wall of the LV may result in a free wall rupture. This is most commonly seen in anterior and lateral MI (LAD or LCx territories). Free wall rupture results in

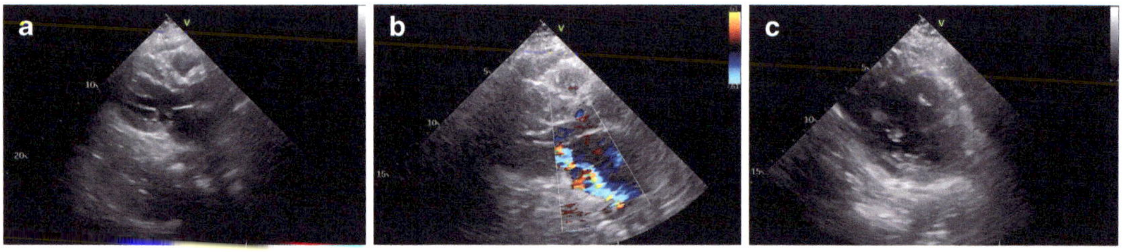

Fig. 60.2 Transthoracic echocardiogram images demonstrating rupture of the posteromedial papillary muscle with flail and severe mitral regurgitation in a patient with an inferior myocardial infarction. (**a**) Parasternal long axis images. (**b**) Parasternal long axis images with color doppler over the mitral valve showing a posteriorly-directed jet of mitral regurgitation. (**c**) Parasternal short axis images

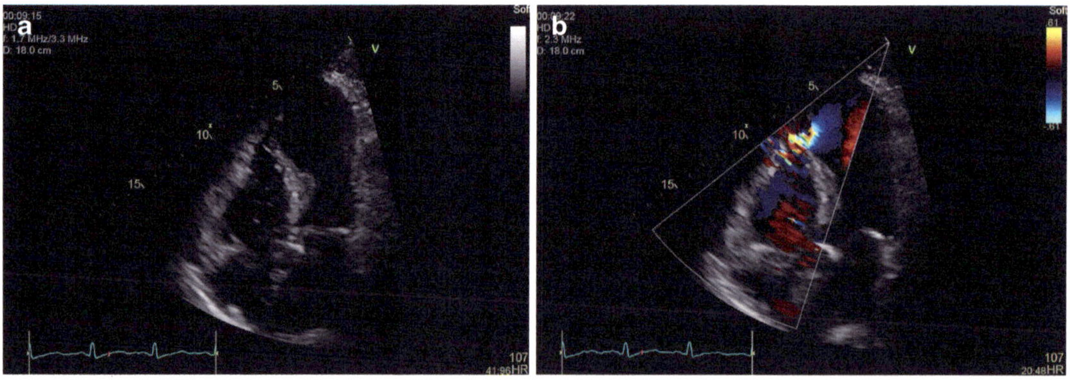

Fig. 60.3 Ventricular septal rupture in a patient with an anterior ST-elevation myocardial infarction due to occlusion of the left anterior descending artery. (**a**) Transthoracic echocardiogram images from the apical 4-chamber view demonstrating akinesis of the distal anterolateral wall, apex, and distal inferoseptum. (**b**) Apical 4-chamber images with color doppler across the intraventricular septum demonstrating color flow across the distal inferoseptum between the left and right ventricles

blood flow into the pericardial space, which will be seen on bedside ultrasound as a pericardial effusion. Since the pericardial accumulation will consist entirely of arterial blood which will coagulate rapidly, it may appear echogenic and may occasionally be misdiagnosed as pericardial or epicardial fat pad. Because development of cardiac tamponade in these cases is typically rapid, hemodynamic instability and death typically ensue, unless a rapid surgical intervention is undertaken.

Aneurysm and Pseudoaneurysm

Occasionally, a small free wall rupture will be contained by adherent pericardial tissue and thrombus and result in a pseudoaneurysm. Unlike a *true ventricular aneurysm*—a late complication of acute MI—a *pseudoaneurysm* carries a high risk of rupture and often requires urgent surgical treatment (Fig. 60.4, Video 60.6). A pseudoaneurysm is characterized by a ratio of the width of the interface between the LV and the pseudoaneurysm, termed the "neck" of less than 0.5. Color doppler flow may be seen across the neck and thrombus may be seen in the cavity. The transition between normal myocardium and the thin-walled pseudoaneurysm cavity is abrupt. An aneurysm, on the other hand, is most often seen at the LV apex, or less commonly near the basal inferolateral wall, and has a neck to cavity ratio of greater than 0.5, with a gradual tapering of the healthy myocardium to aneurysm wall.

Pericardial Effusion

A pericardial effusion can develop after MI as a consequence of the inflammatory response to myocardial injury. These effusions may be associated with a syndrome of pericarditis, but are frequently clinically silent. Rarely, cardiac tamponade may develop; however, a finding of a large pericardial effusion in the setting of ACS should prompt consideration of alternative explanation, such as a free wall rupture or an aortic dissection.

Left Ventricular Thrombus

Areas of akinetic myocardium may be associated with the formation of thrombus in the hours to days after an MI. This is most commonly seen with infarction of the apex and may be associated with aneurysm formation. An LV thrombus is seen on bedside echocardiography as an echogenic mass that is distinct from the myocardium. The finding of a thrombus should result in con-

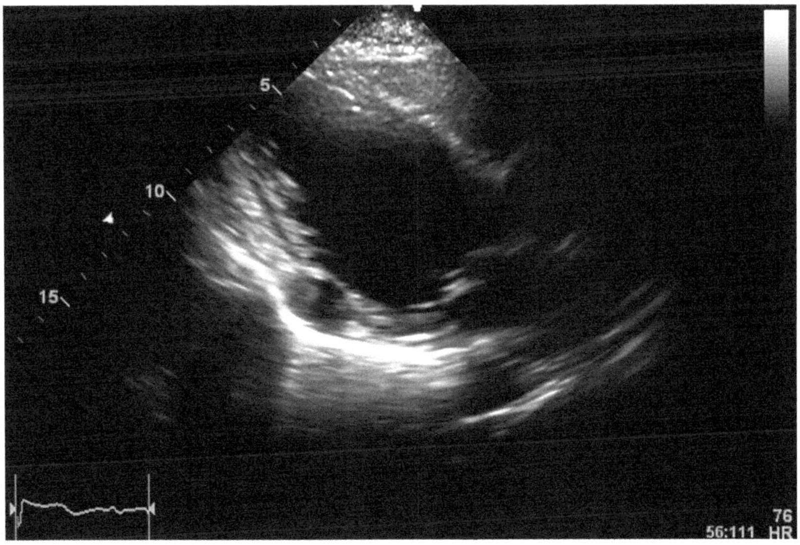

Fig. 60.4 Transthoracic echocardiogram images from the parasternal long-axis view in a patient with coronary artery disease demonstrating a pseudoaneurysm of the basal-mid inferolateral wall as well as akinesis of the basal-mid inferolateral wall and basal anteroseptum

sideration of systemic anticoagulation due to the risk of systemic embolization of the thrombus. Formal echocardiography with administration of an endocardial definition agent may be necessary to adequately assess for thrombus if not seen on bedside echocardiography in a patient with ACS and akinetic myocardium.

Right Ventricular Infarction

Inferoposterior MI, often due to occlusion of the RCA, may result in infarction of the RV, which will manifest as RV hypokinesis on echocardiography. The RV may or may not be dilated depending on the acuity of MI, volume status, and presence of pre-existing pulmonary disease.

Incorporation of Formal Echocardiography

Formal echocardiography complements the bedside echocardiographic evaluation and should be performed in all patients with confirmed or suspected ACS. While the goal of point-of-care cardiac ultrasound in ACS primarily assists with initial triage and rapid assessment for ACS complications, formal echocardiography utilizes high temporal and spatial resolution, in concert with techniques such as speckle tracing, tissue Doppler, and ultrasound contrast to provide comprehensive myocardial and valvular assessment and risk stratification of patients following myocardial infarction.

Summary Points

- The diagnosis of myocardial infarction requires an elevated troponin level with an acute rise or fall as well as other evidence of cardiac ischemia, which can include a new regional wall motion abnormality on echocardiography.
- The left ventricle is by convention divided into 17 segments that should be imaged ideally via the parasternal long and short axes as well as the apical 4-, 2-, and 3-chamber views for complete wall motion abnormality assessment.
- The three major coronary arteries supply distinct territories of myocardium. Abnormal patterns of wall motion due to ischemia should follow these patterns.
- Wall motion is abnormal if the degree of inward motion and/or wall thickening is reduced as compared to normal myocardium.
- Patients with suspected acute coronary syndrome in the intensive care unit should undergo bedside echocardiography to assess for wall motion, global biventricular function, and for mechanical complications of myocardial infarction.

Questions

1. Which of the following echocardiographic findings would be typical of an acute ST-elevation myocardial infarction due to occlusion of the left anterior descending artery?
   A. Hypokinesis of the basal and mid inferoseptum and inferior walls with a hypokinetic right ventricle.
   B. Akinesis of the anteroseptum, anterolateral wall, and apex.
   C. Severe mitral regurgitation with posterior leaflet flail and a mobile echodensity seen in the left atrium in systole.
   D. A small circumferential pericardial effusion without tamponade physiology and aortic regurgitation with a dilated aortic root and normal left ventricular systolic function.

   Answer: B. Acute occlusion of the LAD classically presents as an anterior ST-elevation MI, with wall motion abnormalities in the anterior wall, septum, and apex. A. describes typical changes seen with an inferior MI with RV involvement, typically due to occlusion of the RCA. C. represents findings typical of a papillary muscle rupture, which can be a complication of MI but is typically due to inferior/posterior MI. D. findings are classic for an ascending aortic dissection with involvement of the aortic root. An aortic dissection can cause coronary ischemia, but this more commonly results in RCA occlusion as opposed to the LAD or LCx. Additionally, a LAD occlusion would be likely to result in ischemia, infarction, and resulting wall motion abnormality.

2. What is the most accurate term to describe the following findings on a bedside echocardiogram of a patient admitted to the ICU 1 week after first experiencing unrelenting chest pain at rest: "An aneurysmal appearing lateral wall of the left ventricle with an abrupt transition from normal myocardium to aneurysmal wall, a ratio between cavity neck to cavity diameter of 0.3, and color doppler flow across the cavity neck. No pericardial effusion."?
   A. Uncontained free wall rupture.
   B. Left ventricular aneurysm.
   C. Left ventricular pseudoaneurysm.
   D. Ventricular septal rupture.

   Answer: C. The findings are classic for a pseudoaneurysm, which has the following characteristics: An abrupt transition from normal myocardium to a thin wall, a ratio of pseudoaneurysm neck width to pseudoaneurysm diameter of <0.5, acute angle between normal myocardium and pseudoaneurysm wall, and partial filling of the pseudoaneurysm with thrombus. Color flow may be seen across the pseudoaneurysm neck. A. While a pseudoaneurysm is technically a form of contained free wall rupture, an uncontained free wall rupture is associated with a circumferential pericardial effusion. B. A true ventricular aneurysm, in contrast to a pseudoaneurysm, has a gradual transition from normal myocardium to thinned and scarred myocardium with a wide neck. This is most often seen at the apex of the left ventricle, and less commonly, at the basal inferolateral wall. D. A ventricular septal defect results in a communication between the left and right ventricles, which is most commonly seen as doppler flow across the intraventricular septum in systole.

3. Which of the following techniques would be LEAST useful to identify a subtle LV wall motion abnormality?
   A. Increase probe beam depth and width.
   B. Administer intravenous endocardial definition agent.
   C. Acquire subcostal long- and short-axis views in a patient with poor parasternal or apical windows.
   D. Disable color doppler prior to image acquisition.

   Answer: A. Increasing probe beam depth and width will decrease frame rate, which can make subtle changes in wall motion harder to detect. Instead, the depth and width should be minimized to acquire images of the structure of interest. B. Use of endocardial definition agents with formal echocardiography allows for improved visualization of wall motion. C. Subcostal long- and short-axis views provide good visualization of the left ventricle and can be a good alternative in a patient with other poor windows. D. Disabling color doppler will increase image framerate and which may help to visualize wall motion abnormalities.

References

1. Cerqueira MD, Weissman NJ, Dilsizian V, et al. Standardized myocardial segmentation and nomenclature for tomographic imaging of the heart. American Heart Association Writing Group on Myocardial Segmentation and Registration for Cardiac Imaging. Circulation. 2002;105:538–42.
2. Lang RM, Bierig M, Devereux RB, Flachskampf FA, Foster E, Pellikka PA, et al. Recommendations for chamber quantification: a report from the American Society of Echocardiography's Guidelines and Standards Committee and the Chamber Quantification Writing Group, developed in conjunction with the European Association of Echocardiography, a branch of the European Society of Cardiology. J Am Soc Echocardiogr. 2005;18:1440–63.
3. Amsterdam EA, et al. 2014 AHA/ACC guideline for the management of patients with non–ST-elevation acute coronary syndromes: a report of the American College of Cardiology/American Heart Association Task Force on Practice Guidelines. J Am Coll Cardiol. 2014;64(24):e139–228.
4. Lancellotti P, et al. The use of echocardiography in acute cardiovascular care: recommendations of the European Association of Cardiovascular Imaging and the Acute Cardiovascular Care Association. Eur Heart J Cardiovasc Imaging. 2015;16(2):119–46.
5. Gueret P, Khalife K, Jobic Y, et al. Echocardiographic assessment of the incidence of mechanical complications during the early phase of myocardial infarction in the reperfusion era: a French multicentre prospective registry. Arch Cardiovasc Dis. 2008;101:41–7.

61 Extracorporeal Life Support

Mark Caridi-Scheible

Learning Objectives

1. Describe how mechanical circulatory support devices rely on proper positioning and flow settings
2. Characterize how TTE can be used to evaluate and adjust the positioning of specific devices
3. Delineate how TTE and vascular ultrasound can diagnose common complications of assist devices, including chugging, suck-down, clot, drainage restrictions, poor decompression, distal limb malperfusion, and congestive hepatopathy

The use of mechanical circulatory support (MCS) for severe pulmonary, cardiac, or cardiopulmonary failure has been steadily increasing over the last 15 years. These modalities include venovenous extracorporeal membrane oxygenation (VV-ECMO), venoarterial ECMO (VA-ECMO), and an array of temporary or implanted ventricular assist devices. Indeed, it can be speculated that as technology improves, the use of these modalities will be as commonplace as continuous renal replacement therapy (CRRT) has become in the ICU. One of the limiting factors, however, of expanded use is the considerable amount of expertise required to manage these devices. This is in part due to the complexity of the physical implantation and maintenance of the devices, as well as the complexity of matching the device settings to the changing physiological needs of the patient. Ultrasound and echocardiography are essential tools that allow real-time assessment of the device function and its dynamic impact on the patient's cardiac and circulatory physiology. The potential downstream effects of more accurate monitoring of these parameters are shortened times on the device, lower resource utilization, fewer complications, and improved patient outcomes. Most of the views required for complete assessment of these devices are within the evolving scope of ultrasound by critical care providers, and the American Society of Echocardiography maintains additional comprehensive guidelines for echocardiography for MCS [1].

There exists a wide variety of designs, manufacturers, and configurations for circulatory assist devices, but they can be grouped into 2 main categories: isolated respiratory support (VV-ECMO) and cardiac or cardiopulmonary support (ventricular assist devices (VAD) and VA-ECMO). Combinations of these devices may also be used, but the ultrasound assessment of each remains the same. Each set of devices has a specific set of physiological goals which are important to understand before being able to interpret and apply

Supplementary Information The online version contains supplementary material available at https://doi.org/10.1007/978-3-031-80038-2_61.

M. Caridi-Scheible (✉)
Emory University Hospital, Atlanta, GA, USA
e-mail: mark.caridi-scheible@emory.edu

M. J. Lanspa, A. T. Levinson (eds.), *Echocardiography and Ultrasonography in the ICU*, Respiratory Medicine, https://doi.org/10.1007/978-3-031-80038-2_61

ultrasound results. To achieve these goals, they have specific mechanical properties that must be maintained, such as precise positioning and patent flow. Lastly, there are potential complications with each that must be monitored for.

In general, transthoracic echocardiography (TTE) is indicated; however, where limitations in provider skill, difficult windows, or the need for more accurate confirmation arise, transesophageal echocardiography (TEE) can be useful and provide better images (Videos 61.1, 61.2, 61.3, 61.4, 61.5, 61.6, 61.7, 61.8, 61.9, 61.10, 61.11, 61.12, 61.13, 61.14, 61.15, and 16.16) [2, 3]. Regardless of the modality used, it should be kept in mind that often it is dynamic changes that are of interest, so it is often quite helpful to have a good baseline exam to compare to. Whether by the bedside provider or echocardiography service, a full baseline echocardiogram should be obtained. Additional baseline images that a consult team or standard echocardiography is unlikely to acquire, such as vascular or abdominal imaging to assess placement, should be captured by the bedside provider.

Respiratory Support

VV-ECMO removes deoxygenated blood from the central venous space, externally oxygenates it, and removes carbon dioxide, then reintroduces the oxygenated blood downstream of the drainage closer to the heart. The net effect on the venous volume is therefore zero and there is no change in preload to the heart. The exception to this is V-PA or RA-PA configurations, such as with a Protek Duo® cannula, which bypass the RV but are functionally equivalent to other VV configurations in the absence of RV failure. Otherwise, there should be no hemodynamic changes as a consequence of changes in the flow of blood through the circuit. However, there is an interplay between the flow of blood through the circuit and the delivery rate of oxygen to the body. At any given speed, the flow is determined by adequate drainage of blood and then low impedance to its return. Arterial saturation is a function of flow, proportion of flow to overall cardiac output, and a low rate of recirculation (reinfused blood being pulled back into pump).

While there are many interventions to improve oxygenation in the setting of VV-ECMO that are beyond the scope of this book, there are several specific assessments by ultrasound that can help with common problems. Because they are so easily done, these assessments should be a routine part of bedside troubleshooting. Ultrasound for initial placement of percutaneous ECMO cannulas is discussed elsewhere in Chap. 46: Cannulation for intravascular devices, but common configurations are summarized in Table 61.1.

Probably, the most common complication in VV-ECMO (or any MCS modality that relies on a percutaneous drainage cannula) includes restrictions in drainage flow. This can manifest as continuously high negative pressures which can be caused by any continuous obstruction such as kinks, clots in the line, low volume, or extraluminal obstruction by DVT, vessel walls, or extravascular compression (tumor, ascites, etc.). It can also manifest as "chugging" or "chatter" wherein the caval wall suctions onto the catheter obstructing flow completely. This then releases the caval walls temporarily until suction builds again. This causes a rhythmic, visible swaying in the tubing leaving the patient and causes an oscillation in venous pressures and flows. Often, these manifestations are reflexively attributed to volume depletion. While volume usually will transiently reduce the symptoms, it may not completely solve them and often runs counter to therapeutic goals of reducing pulmonary edema and other consequences of volume overload.

A complete volume assessment using TTE, as described elsewhere in this book, can help to narrow the differential. If standard measures of hypovolemia are present, volume challenge is reasonable. If not present, then a mechanical problem with the cannula is more likely. TTE and abdominal ultrasound may visualize the cannulas along their path to look for extra-cannular clot or caval compression. Distal drainage cannulas such as in a fem-fem configuration may not be in a large enough caliber vessel portion, or the entire IVC may be too small for one or both cannulas. Fixing this may require replacing the cannula

Table 61.1 Common cannula configurations

Configuration (Cannula name)	Venous insertion site	Optimal position	Ultrasound views
Femoral-femoral	Drain: femoral	Tip distal to reinfusion cannula ports (ideally by approximately 10 cm)	Abdominal IVC (curvilinear probe)
	Reinfusion: contralateral femoral	Tip at or just past the IVC-RA junction	Subcostal IVC and 4-chamber views (TTE)
Femoral-IJ (or SC)	Drain: femoral	Tip below IVC-RA junction, preferably just distal to the hepatic vein and at least 10 cm from the tip of the reinfusion cannula	Subcostal IVC view (TTE)
	Reinfusion: internal jugular (IJ) or subclavian (SC)	Tip in proximal SVC just above SVC-RA junction	Subcostal bicaval, modified apical 5 chamber (TTE)
Dual lumen (Avalon or Crescent)	IJ or SC	Tip in the IVC. Widened part of cannula (beginning of dual lumen) should not enter IVC. Color doppler reinfusion jet in RA directed at Tricuspid Valve (TV).	Subcostal IVC, 4-chamber and bicaval views (TTE). Subcostal 4-chamber or parasternal short axis RVIO level views using color doppler.
Dual lumen RA-PA (Protek Duo)	IJ or SC	See cardiac support for more complete discussion	Parasternal long axis RVOT view, subcostal short axis RVOT view

with a deeper or smaller cannula. Extra-caval compression may require paralysis, abdominal drainage, laparotomy, or replacement of the cannula past the obstruction. Clots may require thrombectomy, cannula replacement, or more aggressive anticoagulation.

Recirculation is another common problem and is entirely related to the position of the cannula(s). In two-cannula configurations, recirculation occurs when the reinfusion cannula is too close to the drainage such that oxygenated blood is redirected back to the pump rather than the system circulation reducing effective oxygen delivery. This becomes more exaggerated as the pump speed is increased and greater suction towards the drainage is experienced. Even when the cannulas are an acceptable distance apart on x-ray, if the drainage cannula is too far towards or into the right atrium (RA), then mixed blood can be drawn towards the drainage. Similarly, if the reinfusion cannula is too far into the right atrium, the force of the outflow jet may direct the oxygenated blood directly towards the IVC and the drainage cannula. Echocardiographic guidance can be used to assess and pull back the problematic cannula using the views and landmarks in Table 61.1.

In single cannula configurations, the distance between the drainage and reinfusion cannulas is fixed, but the cannula is designed to be placed such that oxygenated blood is directed preferentially towards the RV and away from the SVC and IVC and any recirculation zones (Image 61.1). However, if the cannula is too deep or too shallow, such that the reinfusion port is in the cava, then turbulent mixing will occur within the cava and backflow of oxygenated blood into the drainage will occur. A cannula that is rotated such that the jet is directed to the atrial wall will also create turbulent mixing that can backflow. This may also result in higher reinfusion pressures and has the potential for shear and erosion through the atrial wall. Rotation should be corrected immediately. Subcostal IVC view is the highest yield view for aligning these cannulas; however, the cannula should be seen transiting the RA and the reinfusion jet should be seen pointed towards the tricuspid in multiple views, including the apical and subcostal 4-chamber views.

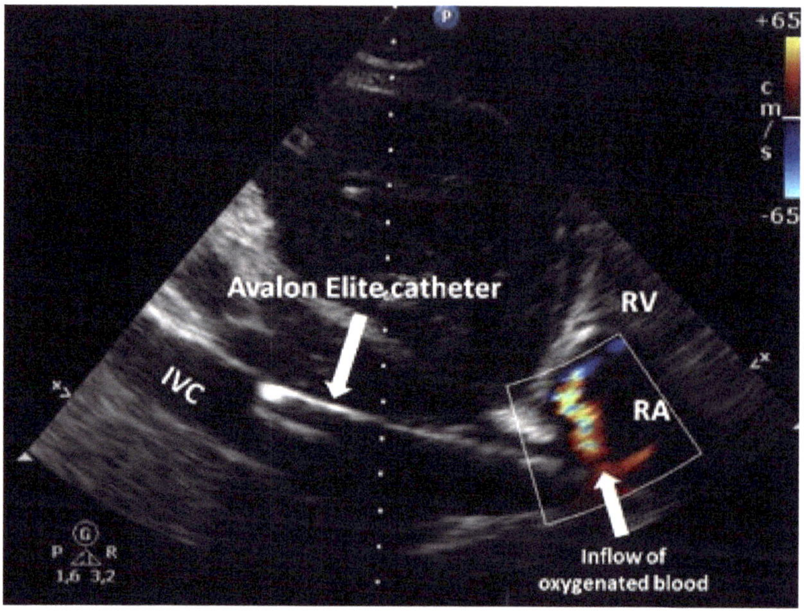

Image 61.1 Correct Avalon placement in subcostal IVC view with reinfusion jet directed towards the RV. (Source: Ref. [12])

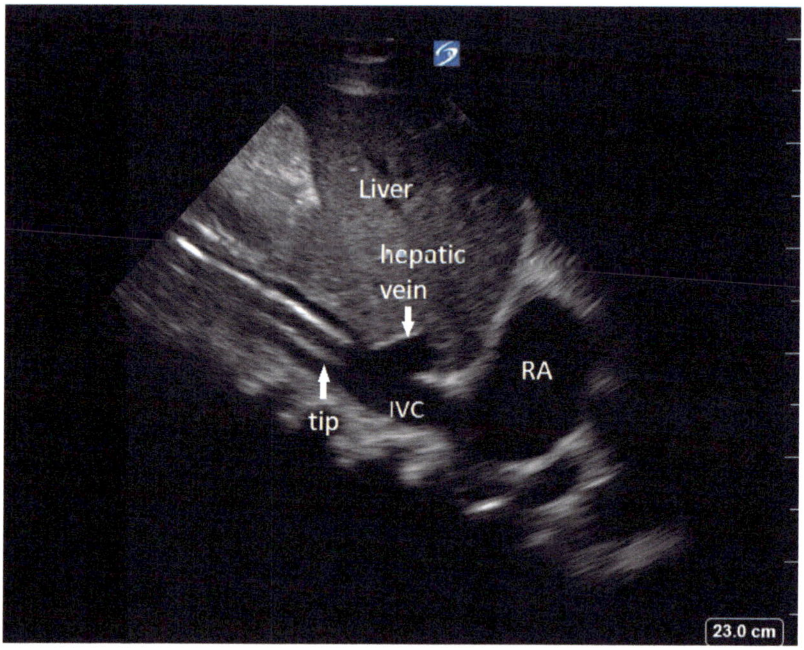

Image 61.2 Correct placement of VV-ECMO drainage cannula in the Subcostal IVC view with the tip of the cannula just distal to the hepatic vein

Congestive hepatopathy, as indicated by rising transaminases without other cause, is sometimes seen with ECMO support and is caused either by a drainage cannula obstructing or inserted into the outflow of hepatic vein, clot near the hepatic vein, or a reinfusion cannula either obstructing, inserted into, or with outflow jet oriented towards the hepatic vein. In all cases, this should be visible on subcostal IVC and abdominal ultrasound of the liver. Pulling back the offending cannula is the first step, but other revisions may be required if flows are insufficient with pulling back. Image 61.2 demonstrates optimal placement of venous drainage cannula to avoid recirculation and hepatic vein obstruction.

The final utility of echocardiography in VV-ECMO is the assessment of the need for transition to VA-ECMO in the case of shock. If the patient is hyperdynamic such as in septic shock, VA-ECMO will not improve either hemodynamics or oxygenation, which in fact could be made worse. In shock associated with profound hypoxia, even if heart function is compromised, the resolution to normoxia usually will normalize heart function as well. Although VA-ECMO will initially also restore normoxia, if the heart rapidly recovers and the lungs are failing, then the patient could develop severe north–south syndrome that in itself can cause cardiac ischemia However, if cardiogenic shock by echocardiographic assessment persists after VV-ECMO initiation, then in fact a transition to VA-ECMO may be indicated [4].

Cardiac Support

Mechanical assist devices for cardiac failure involve bypassing to some degree the right ventricle, the left ventricle, or both. Devices that shunt blood directly from the venous to the arterial system by necessity must have an oxygenator (VA-ECMO). Devices that reinfuse blood before or that drain blood after functional lungs do not require an oxygenator and are often not extracorporeal (e.g., Impella, durable or temporary left ventricular assist device (LVAD), or right ventricular assist device (RVAD)). The physiologic goal of this bypass is not to completely divert cardiac output, but to offload the failed ventricle(s) to allow rest and recovery or to minimize further deterioration until more durable solution (implanted VAD or transplant) can be found or until recovery occurs. In fact, diverting all flow from the heart is detrimental as even in the setting of systemic anticoagulation, blood that is static in the heart and pulmonary circulation will eventually clot. This can catastrophically limit later therapeutic options. With the exception of peripheral VA-ECMO, initial placement of all these devices requires fluoroscopy or surgery; however, most are subject to migration and amenable to adjustment at the bedside. Echocardiography is critical for confirming correct positioning of the device, titration of device speed to therapeutic goals, monitoring of complications, and assessing recovery in preparation for removal [4].

There are three modes of cardiac support: LVAD, RVAD, and biventricular assist device(s) (BIVAD). The mode can be achieved either through an externalized pump or through an inserted or implanted device designed for a specific ventricle (Table 61.2). Extracorporeal devices may utilize special cannulas (Protek Duo, Tandem Heart) or standard cannulas inserted peripherally or centrally (via sternotomy) or both. Biventricular support is achieved through either VA-ECMO or using both an LVAD and an RVAD device.

Implanted devices generally are positioned well intraoperatively with TEE confirmation and do not migrate, but appropriate position of and laminar flow into the inflow conduit to the pump can be confirmed using TTE apical views (ideal) or parasternal long axis or subcostal 4-chamber views. Flow should be laminar through the long axis of the ventricle using color doppler. The jet of the outflow conduit into the ascending aorta can generally be visualized in the parasternal long axis view using color doppler.

Femoral drain cannulas used in extracorporeal devices function similarly to those for VV-ECMO and can be assessed with the same views. Ideal positioning, however, is for the cannula tip to be into the RA or even the SVC for optimal drainage. Since there is no venous reinfusion cannula, recirculation is not an issue. The exception to this is V-A-V configuration wherein part of the oxygenated blood is returned arterially and part venous. This is uncommon but does have the same risk of recirculation and requires a drainage cannula in the standard VV position described earlier. Most often, a patient will start on VA and have the venous return added later as the heart recovers if the lungs are not functional. In this case, TTE can be used to pull back the femoral drain to the optimal position. Femoral or other peripheral arterial cannulas are generally short and lie in distal parts of the arteries or else in grafts attached to the arteries. They are not assessable by TTE, but as described later vascular

Table 61.2 Extracorporeal circulatory support

Mode	Configuration/ Device	Pump	Drainage	Reinfusion
RVAD	2 cannula RA-PA	External	Femoral vein or central (RA)	Central PA
	Protek Duo (RA-PA)	External	Single cannula, drain port in RA/RV	Single cannula, reinfusion port in PA
	Impella RP	Internal, inserted via femoral vein	RV	PA
LVAD	2 standard cannulas (LA-Ao)	External	Central drain in pulm vein, LA or LV	Central to ascending aorta or peripheral to femoral artery
	Tandem Heart	External	Venous insertion, transseptal puncture for LA drainage	Peripheral artery (usually femoral)
	Impella	Internal, inserted via femoral or axillary artery	LV	Aorta
	Heartmate 2, 3 Heartware	Internal, implanted	LV apex	Aorta
VA-ECMO (BIVAD)	2 cannula (V-A)	External	Femoral vein or central (RA)	Central to ascending aorta or peripheral to femoral artery

ultrasound is useful to monitor for complications. Other drainage and reinfusion sites using standard cannulas are surgically placed centrally and may have varying orientations and insertion sites. These require a discussion with the surgical team before interpreting appropriate positioning on TTE or TEE.

The specialty cannulas (ProtekDuo and TandemHeart) do require precise positioning to function correctly. The ProtekDuo is a dual-lumen cannula inserted generally into the right IJ and directed through the right ventricle and into the main PA. The drainage ports need to be located well before the pulmonic valve and the tip with several reinfusion fenestrations needs to be situated past the pulmonic valve. Otherwise, blood will just recirculate in the RV and not be moved into the pulmonary circulation as intended. If the tip, however, is too distal and enters the right or the left PA, then that lung may experience excessive blood flow and be prone to hemorrhage. The recommended positioning is for the tip of the cannula to be 2 cm past the pulmonic valve. The two views most amenable to confirming this positioning are the parasternal long-axis RVOT view and the parasternal short axis RVIO view. If a clear view into the main PA cannot be achieved but the cannula is noted to at least be past the valve, then confirming that there is no turbulent flow on color doppler in the RV itself or near the valve (not to be confused with pulmonary insufficiency (PI)) also indicates that the reinfusion port is well past the valve (Image 61.3). If there is significant PI, then there is a good likelihood that the pump will not be able to offload the RV and VA-ECMO should be considered to bypass the cardiopulmonary circulation entirely. The cannula tip and outflow jet should also be visible in the upper esophageal views with TEE (Image 61.4).

The TandemHeart is a drainage cannula that crosses the intra-atrial septum and drains blood from the left atrium. This blood is then reinfused arterially generally via a femoral cannula. There is usually no oxygenator attached, so the blood must all be oxygenated. If the cannula is malpositioned such that part or all of the multi-fenestrated end of the cannula is pulled back into the right atrium, a significant shunt of unoxygenated blood can occur. Excessive pump speeds can suction the LA down, creating chatter similar to VV-ECMO. This suctioning also encourages migration of the cannula or else can encourage shunting through the ASD created by the cannula

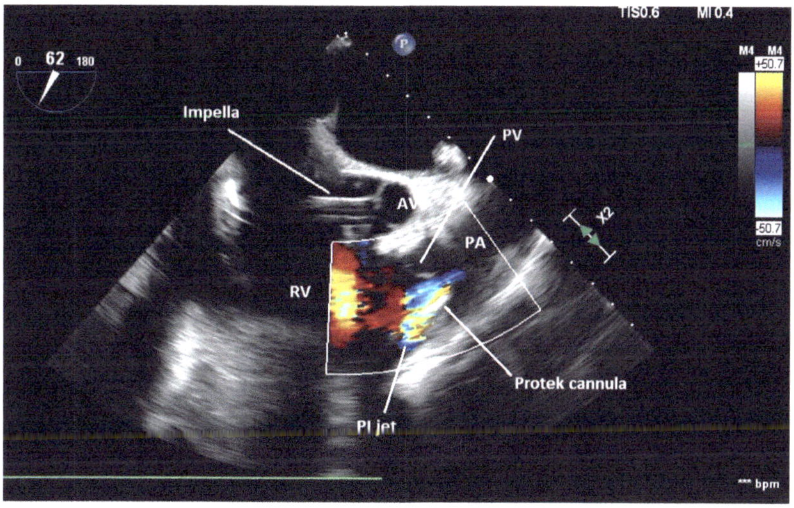

Image 61.3 Protek Duo cannula crossing the pulmonic valve into the PA in the Mid-esophageal RVIO view on TEE. A small PI jet is seen and is distinguished from outflow of the cannula by its presence only in diastole. A left-sided impella is also seen crossing the aortic valve

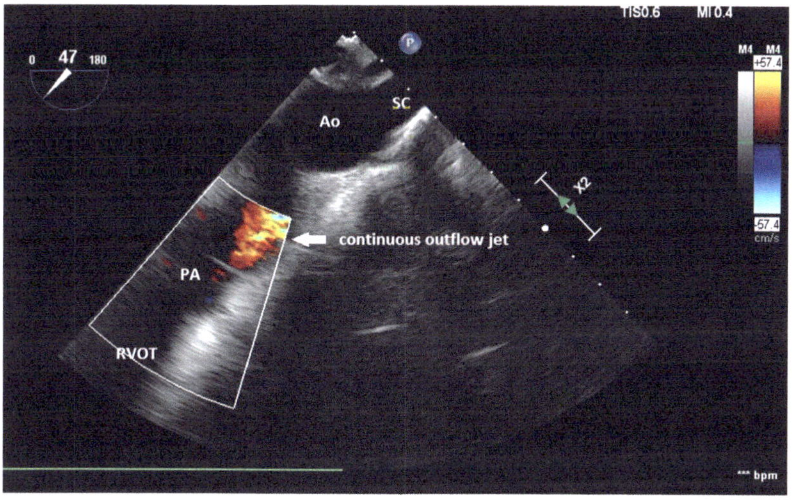

Image 61.4 Upper esophageal TEE view of the main PA with continuous outflow jet of the Protek Duo cannula

or a PFO. Chatter or hypoxia should prompt examination with TTE. The cannula is most likely to be seen in the apical 4-chamber view, but may also be visualized in the subcostal 4-chamber or parasternal short-axis RVIO view (Image 61.5). Even if the cannula itself is poorly visualized, color doppler can look for inflow or shunt jets that are inappropriate. It can also assess whether the left atrium is collapsed which should prompt a reduction in pump speed. A bubble study may also be useful to identify shunts, but extreme caution should be taken with bubble studies as some pumps will shut down if bubbles are detected in the circuit. This may be temporarily overridden but the risk/benefit of the study should be carefully considered. There should overall be a low threshold for using TEE instead as views of the device as it crosses through the septum are generally quite clear in the mid-esophageal bicaval views. All the fenestrations should be visualized past the septum.

Impella devices are miniature pumps that are placed endovascularly. One end of the pump lies in the ventricle that is dysfunctional and the other end is located after the outflow valve. If the device is located entirely in the ventricle, then the pump simply recirculates the blood in the ventricle and it will remain distended. A right-sided device that is too deep may direct excessive flow towards a single lung. A left-sided device that is

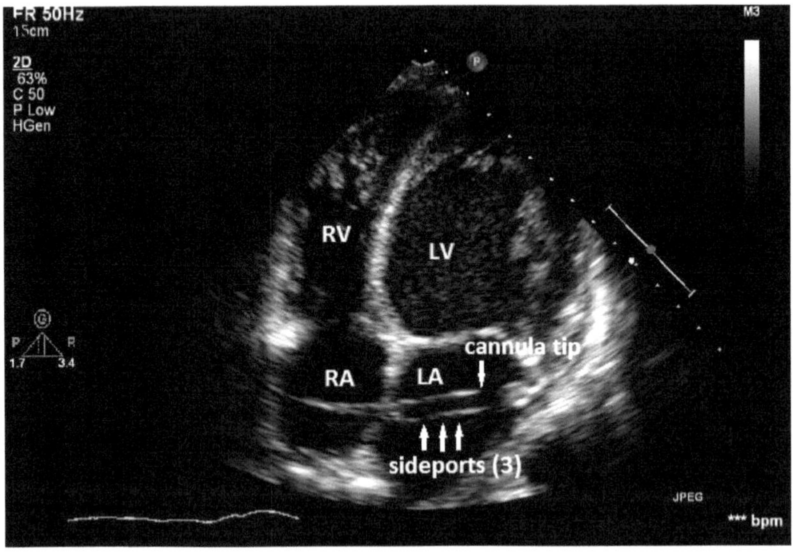

Image 61.5 TandemHeart crossing the interatrial septum in this Apical 4-Chamber view. All three sideports can be visualized appropriately in the left atrium. The LV remains dilated with a significant amount of spontaneous echo contrast concerning for stasis

too deep will suction against or otherwise mechanically irritate the endocardium and induce arrhythmias. The Impella RP is a right ventricular device and should be positioned such that the outflow port is 2 to 4 cm past the pulmonic valve [5]. The tip should not be confused with the protective pigtail on the end of the device. This pigtail will generally sit either just into the left or just into right PA when correctly positioned (Image 61.6). As with the ProtekDuo cannula, you should not see turbulent flow around the valve in the RVOT. Also as with the ProtekDuo, if severe pulmonary insufficiency (PI) is noted, then the ventricle is unlikely to be offloaded and VA-ECMO should be considered.

The left-sided Impellas must be even more precisely placed. The inflow port to the pump generally should be located in the LVOT with the device pigtail (if present) within the ventricle (Image 61.7). The recommended distance from the tip of the device to the aortic valve annulus is 4.0–4.5 cm [5]. This is generally assessed in the parasternal long-axis view. This distance does not include the pigtail extension which is not present on all models. There is also a fixed angle to the device that sits between the inflow and outflow ports. This angle should be in the aortic root or at the valve itself. Color doppler should be able to identify the outflow jet within the aorta and not in the LVOT. It is possible for the pigtail to become entangled in the chordae, so it is important to examine the sub-mitral apparatus and also evaluate for worsening mitral regurgitation (MR) [6]. The pigtail can also become wedged against the ventricular wall inducing arrhythmias. As with right-sided devices, if there is significant aortic insufficiency, then even a correctly placed device may simply recirculate the blood. Severe aortic insufficiency in the setting of any mechanical circulatory support can be difficult to manage [7].

As discussed before, there are three physiologic goals that must be achieved. First is maintaining adequate systemic perfusion, second is decompressing the bypassed ventricle(s), and third is preventing stasis through the heart that may lead to clot formation. Generally as speed of the device is increased to achieve systemic perfusion, there are consequent effects on the heart that may run counter to the other goals [8]. Although adjustments can be made clinically with experience, TTE remains the best modality to balance these effects or determine if a different modality is required.

The RVAD is the simplest case to consider. As flows are increased on the device, the RV should be seen to be decreasing in volume in the apical 4-chamber or subcostal 4-chamber views. These views are ideal as you can see consequent effects on the LV. If the LV dilates and LV function

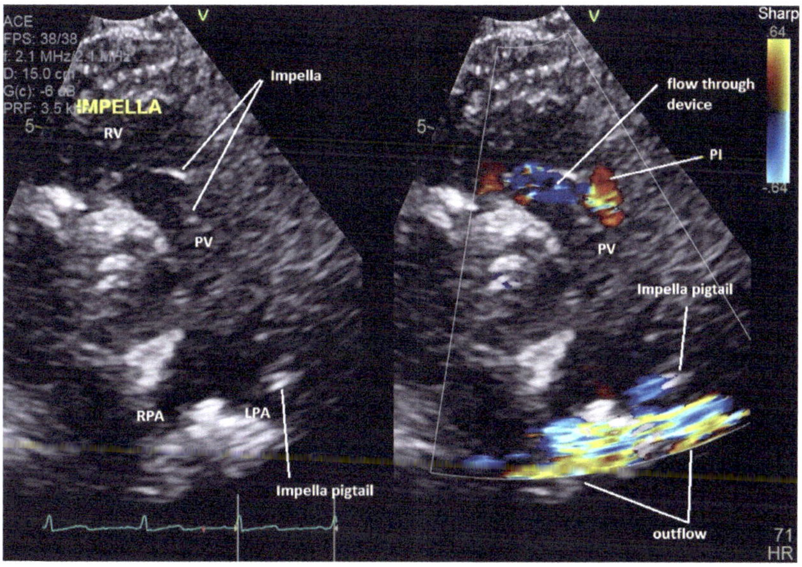

Image 61.6 RV Impella crossing the pulmonic valve in this Parasternal Short-Axis RVIO level view. Color doppler delineates the flow through the device as well as the distal outflow deep in the PA. The device's pigtail is appropriately sitting in the left PA. A small amount of PI is visible and acceptable

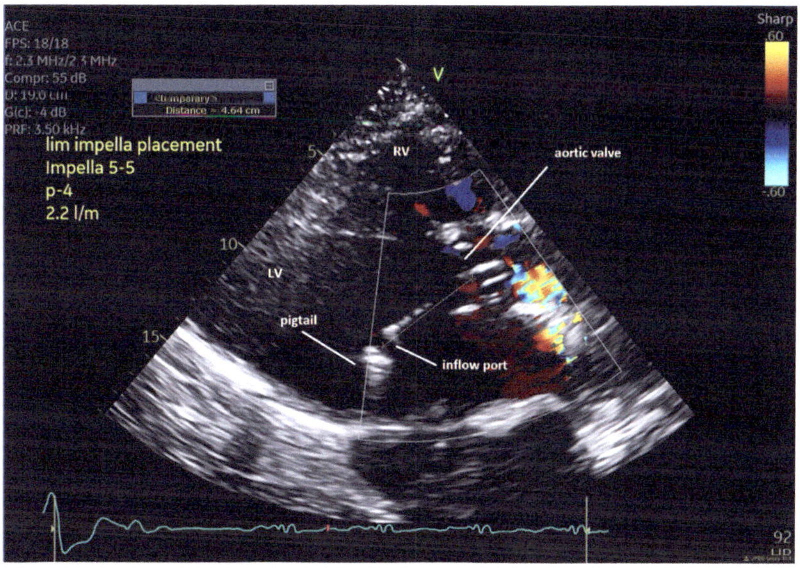

Image 61.7 Appropriate placement of left-sided Impella device in this Parasternal Long-Axis view. The angle of the device is just at the valve annulus and the distance from the annulus to the tip is appropriate. Turbulent flow can be seen in the root but not in the LVOT

reduces, then the LV is also failed and additional inotropy or a biventricular support mode should be considered. There should be minimal PI, and ideally, the pulmonic valve should be opening indicative of some flow through the right ventricle to prevent stasis. If the right ventricle, right atrium, or cava is collapsed, then volume may need to be given or else the speed needs to be reduced.

Many of the same considerations apply with left-sided devices. The speed should be increased sufficiently to decompress the ventricle. Ideally, this is to be less than the normal LVEDD cutoff of 5.5 cm measured in the parasternal short axis, but in a chronically dilated heart this is not likely achievable and 15% reduction in size is instead recommended under current LVAD management guidelines [9]. Additionally, tissue-doppler imaging (TDI) can be used to estimate LA pressures, although some devices measure this directly. Color doppler should be used to evaluate for excessive AI that may be contributing to dilation.

If max flows cannot be reached due to systemic hypertension, then afterload reducers should be employed. If the ventricle is unable to be decompressed with the device at max flows, then another approach or device should be considered in addition to aggressive volume removal.

Also critical on the left side is careful evaluation for stasis or clot in the LA, LV, or LVOT. Clot formation in any of these may preclude transplant or placement of durable LVAD. It also carries significantly increased risk of stroke. Suspicion of clot should be confirmed with echo contrast, but care should be taken with this as many devices will interpret contrast as air in the circuit and may shut down. Contrast use should be coordinated with the perfusionist. Spontaneous echo contrast (SAE), particularly in the LV apex, should merit monitoring. The aortic valve should be opening at least every few beats to eject static blood from the LVOT. SAE or lack of valve opening may be able to be addressed with additional inotropy, afterload reduction, and sometimes reducing pump speed.

Left-sided devices are also more likely to have deleterious effects on right-sided function. If the device over-suctions blood from the left ventricle, it may drop LV diastolic pressures to significantly below RV diastolic pressures and cause the septum to bow into the LV. This narrowing will induce a Venturi effect and cause even lower pressures leading to an eventually collapse of the LV and complete loss of flows (Image 61.8). This is commonly referred to as a "suck-down" event. Prior to LV collapse, the RV will also become volume overloaded as it loses contractility with the septal shift [8]. Changes to pump speed under echocardiographic guidance can be extremely advantageous to prevent the likelihood of suck-down events [10]. As flows are increased under the apical 4-chamber or the parasternal short axis views, the LV should become less dilated but the septum should remain flat. At the point that the septum starts to bow towards the LV, the speed should be reduced slightly and the two ventricles can be said to be in balance [9]. If the RV remains dilated and the septum bowed even when the speed is turned down, then septal shift likely occurred because of primary RV failure. In this case, additional inotropy, pulmonary afterload reduction, and biventricular support may be indicated. Suck-down can also occur with sudden volume loss such as with bleeding. Without TTE or TEE, it is extremely difficult to distinguish the various causes of suck-down in which the wrong therapy (e.g., speed reduction versus volume versus inotropy) can be catastrophic to the RV.

Biventricular support using VA-ECMO combines the same goals as either RVAD or LVAD sup-

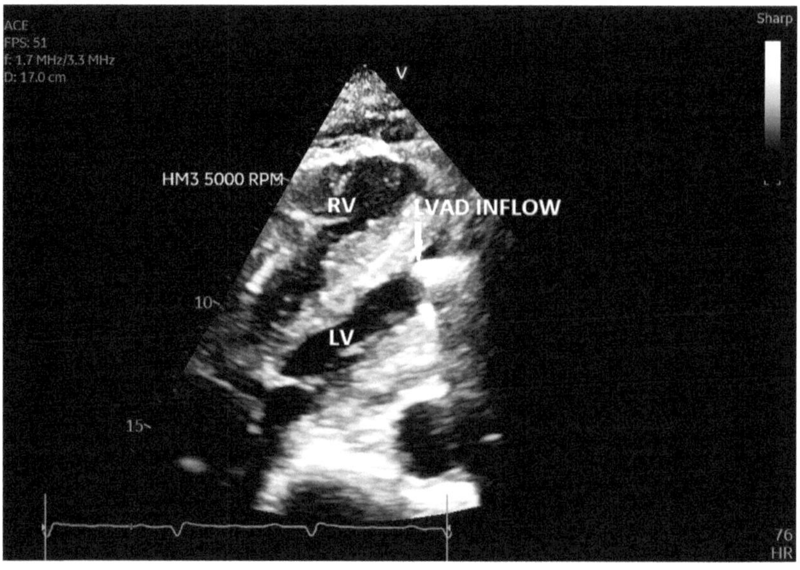

Image 61.8 Subcostal 4-Chamber view demonstrating extreme narrowing of the LV cavity and impingement on the LVAD cannula. The RV is dilated and the septum shifted towards the left

port. The ventricles should be appropriately decompressed but with enough flow to prevent stasis. Examinations for stasis and clot should be periodic. As flows are increased, the ECMO flow raises afterload on the heart which may be unable to eject, leaving it static and dilated. Again, ensuring some aortic valve opening and reaching diameter goals is critical. Inotropy can be added to help eject; however, if the function is too poor it may not be possible to both sufficiently decompress the heart and meet minimum systemic perfusion pressures. In this case, a second device must be added to directly vent the LV [11]. This often is an Impella device, but there are a variety of other common approaches.

Biventricular support using both an isolated RVAD and an isolated LVAD device has the same interdependency issues for the single device alone, but with some added flexibility. If the RV fails, causing suck-down on the LV, it is possible to increase the RV support speed. Particularly as one side of the heart or the other or both recover, the interplay between what is essentially four pumps can be quite dynamic. Assessing biventricular size and function in real-time can help with the frequent changes in LVAD or RVAD speed that may be required in response to highly dynamic loading conditions and hemodynamic changes. Again, this can be done clinically in experienced hands, but directly visualizing with TTE or TEE is simpler and much more reliable.

It is difficult to gauge the recovery of the heart while it is being fully supported as the loading conditions are held in an optimized state. The heart must be dynamically challenged with additional volume and workload to gauge recovery. The measurement of its success is often hemodynamics; however, these alone may fail to capture the ongoing strain on the heart. Turning down support under echocardiographic observation can pick up on signs such as worsening dilation and reduced function that may precede hemodynamic failure. It can also assess whether the other modifiable factors such as volume overload are contributing to the ongoing failure.

Vascular Ultrasound

With the exception of implanted VADs or centrally places cannulas, all mechanical assist devices involve the peripheral vasculature. For any venous indwelling device, DVT is a common complication as femoral or subclavian cannulas can obstruct distal venous flow causing stasis and thrombus, even in the setting of anticoagulation. Arterial cannulas that are not placed within chimney grafts or arterial devices that are indwelling such as an Impella run a risk of impeding flow to distal extremities causing ischemia that is potentially catastrophic. If arterial extracorporeal support is being used, there should be smaller distal perfusion cannula that reinfuses blood behind the main reinfusion cannula towards the distal extremity, but these are prone to misplacement and failure. Poor pulses, extremity discoloration, or swelling can be assessed with bedside vascular ultrasound to assess flow compromise or clot distal to the cannula. Any vascular compromise is an emergency and should prompt reconfiguration of the cannulas to allow for removal from the affected extremity. Vascular ultrasound at the insertion site can also be used to evaluate for hematoma, pseudoaneurysm, or active extravasation that may necessitate revision or open repair. Kinking of the cannula in the insertion tract may also be identified.

Summary Points

- Mechanical assist devices rely on proper positioning and flow settings
- Baseline exams are important
- Positioning is particular to specific devices, but all amenable to TTE evaluation
- TTE helps to assure physiologic goals of decompression of a failed ventricle
- TTE helps to assure adequate residual flow through the heart to prevent stasis and clot
- TTE and vascular ultrasound can diagnose common complications including chugging, suck-down, clot, drainage restrictions, poor decompression, distal limb malperfusion, and congestive hepatopathy
- TTE can aid in assessing recovery and weaning support

References

1. Stainback RF, Estep JD, Agler DA, Birks EJ, Bremer M, Hung J, et al. Echocardiography in the Management of Patients with Left Ventricular Assist Devices: recommendations from the American Society of Echocardiography. J Am Soc Echocardiogr. 2015;28(8):853–909.
2. Charron C, Repesse X, Bodson L, Au SM, Vieillard-Baron A. Ten good reasons why everybody can and should perform cardiac ultrasound in the ICU. Anaesthesiol Intensive Ther. 2014;46(5):319–22.
3. Schmidt S, Dieks JK, Quintel M, Moerer O. Critical care echocardiography as a routine procedure for the detection and early treatment of cardiac pathologies. Diagnostics (Basel). 2020;10(9).
4. Kon ZN, Bittle GJ, Pasrija C, Pham SM, Mazzeffi MA, Herr DL, et al. Venovenous versus venoarterial extracorporeal membrane oxygenation for adult patients with acute respiratory distress syndrome requiring precannulation hemodynamic support: a review of the ELSO registry. Ann Thorac Surg. 2017;104(2):645–9.
5. Impella® ventricular support systems for use during cardiogenic shock and high-risk PCI: Abiomed operating manual.: Abiomed; 2018.
6. Burzotta F, Trani C, Doshi SN, Townend J, van Geuns RJ, Hunziker P, et al. Impella ventricular support in clinical practice: collaborative viewpoint from a European expert user group. Int J Cardiol. 2015;201:684–91.
7. Fang JC, Wever-Pinzon O. Dealing with unintended consequences: continuous-flow LVADs and aortic insufficiency. JACC Cardiovasc Imaging. 2016;9(6):652–4.
8. Tchoukina I, Smallfield MC, Shah KB. Device management and flow optimization on left ventricular assist device support. Crit Care Clin. 2018;34(3):453–63.
9. William J, Mak V, Leet A, Kaye DM, Nanayakkara S. Optimal mechanical unloading in left ventricular assist device recipients relates to progressive up-titration in pump speed. J Am Soc Echocardiogr. 2020;33(5):583–93.
10. Bouchez S, Van Belleghem Y, De Somer F, De Pauw M, Stroobandt R, Wouters P. Haemodynamic management of patients with left ventricular assist devices using echocardiography: the essentials. Eur Heart J Cardiovasc Imaging. 2019;20(4):373–82.
11. Ricarte Bratti JP, Cavayas YA, Noly PE, Serri K, Lamarche Y. Modalities of left ventricle decompression during VA-ECMO therapy. Membranes (Basel). 2021;11(3).
12. Kalbhenn J, Maier S, Heinrich S, et al. Bedside repositioning of a dislocated Avalon-cannula in a running veno-venous ECMO. J Artif Organs. 2017;20:285–8. https://doi.org/10.1007/s10047-017-0961-x.

Ultrasound in Cardiac Arrest

62

Danie Leahy and Stephanie Cha

Learning Objectives

1. Describe how focused ultrasound protocols during PEA cardiac arrest may identify reversible etiologies for arrest.
2. Review the potential benefits of ultrasonography during cardiac arrest.
3. Examine how the use of ultrasound in cardiac arrest must center around minimization of no-flow-intervals.

Introduction

According to the American Heart Association (AHA), approximately 290,000 patients experience in-hospital cardiac arrest in the United States each year. Of these, approximately 80% present with a nonshockable rhythm such as asystole or pulseless electrical activity (PEA) [1]. Survival is poor at 18%, although outcomes are improving, and the majority of survivors do retain good neurologic function [2, 3]. High-quality chest compressions and early defibrillation when applicable are the cornerstones of management during cardiac arrest. However, point-of-care ultrasonography (POCUS) is emerging as a powerful tool that can aid bedside diagnosis as it may be helpful in identifying and treating reversible causes for arrest and guiding high-quality chest compressions or arrhythmia management. Furthermore, POCUS may enhance monitoring of high-risk pre-arrest care and optimize hemodynamic performance in postarrest care. The American Heart Association (AHA), European Resuscitation Council (ERC), and Society of Critical Care Medicine (SCCM) now support the use of POCUS integration into Advanced Cardiopulmonary Life Support (ACLS) for the identification of reversible etiologies of arrest and detection of cardiac standstill, with the caveat that integration of POCUS into ACLS requires "considerable training" [4–6]. In addition, POCUS may have utility in predicting outcomes in cardiac arrest, specifically in the case of cardiac standstill or appearance of postarrest hepatic gas patterns.

True vs. Pseudo-PEA

There are many challenges in the management of cardiac arrest. Clinicians are often unreliable in detecting mechanical pulse by palpation, and POCUS examination of the carotid or femoral arter-

Supplementary Information The online version contains supplementary material available at https://doi.org/10.1007/978-3-031-80038-2_62.

D. Leahy · S. Cha (✉)
Department of Anesthesiology and Critical Care Medicine, Johns Hopkins University School of Medicine, Baltimore, MD, USA
e-mail: Danielle.Leahy@spectrumhcp.com; scha4@jhmi.edu

M. J. Lanspa, A. T. Levinson (eds.), *Echocardiography and Ultrasonography in the ICU*, Respiratory Medicine, https://doi.org/10.1007/978-3-031-80038-2_62

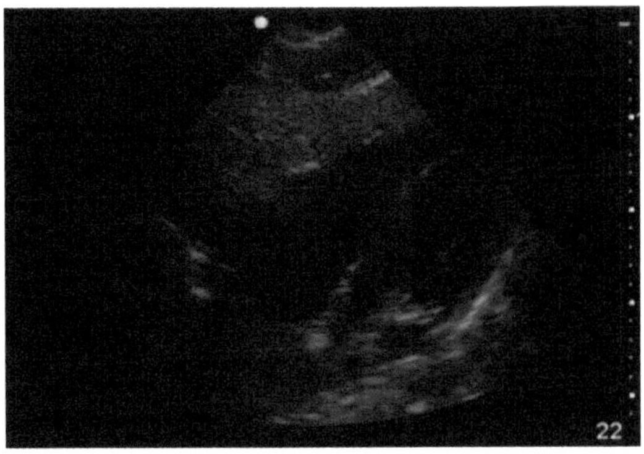

Fig. 62.1 A subcostal 4-chamber clip demonstrates "True"-PEA. Here, there is neither mechanical pulse detection nor spontaneous cardiac motion

ies may facilitate prompt cardiopulmonary resuscitation (CPR) [7–9]. Furthermore, PEA itself may be subdivided into two states- "true"-PEA, which is defined as the absence of pulse in addition to the absence of myocardial motion on echocardiography (see Fig. 62.1, Video 62.1), and "pseudo"-PEA, which is defined by absence of pulse with findings of spontaneous cardiac motion or cardiac activity on ultrasound. While "true"-PEA carries nearly 0% likelihood of return of spontaneous circulation, survival of "pseudo"-PEA is more favorable [6]. In a 2010 study of 204 patients arriving to the ED in cardiac arrest, "pseudo"-PEA represented the majority of PEA cases (58%) with a demonstrated survival to hospital admission of 55% compared to 8% in cases with "true"-PEA [10]. "Pseudo"-PEA may result from cardiac tamponade, myocardial ischemia, pulmonary embolism, tension pneumothorax, or severe hypovolemia [11]. Early identification of these causes is imperative for definitive treatment, such as in the case of pericardial tamponade requiring emergent pericardiocentesis or myocardial ischemia requiring emergent revascularization and common and underappreciated causes for arrest [12–14].

Practical Implementation

Utilization of POCUS during cardiac arrest must be performed in a trained and protocolized manner, taking care to minimize interruptions or interference to ongoing high-quality chest compressions. The subcostal 4-chamber view is recommended during ACLS because it can be obtained without interfering with sternal compressions, and it is the view most successfully performed with diagnostic quality, especially by novices [15]. Furthermore, US imaging during ACLS must be minimized to a standard of 10 s, also referred to as the "No-Flow Interval" (NFI), the maximum tolerated time to chest compression disruption, per Pediatric Advanced Life Support (PALS) guidelines, based on the rationale that brief interruptions to CPR are associated with improved success rate of defibrillation, improved coronary blood flow and post-arrest neurologic function in animal models of cardiac arrest, as well as improved survival to hospital discharge [1, 16, 17].

Common US Findings

Pericardial Tamponade

POCUS is more sensitive for the detection of pericardial tamponade than physical exam and electrocardiography alone and is identified in 5–22% PEA arrests (and perhaps more in special populations) [10]. The underlying mechanism leading to hemodynamic collapse is intrapericardial pressure buildup, leading to impaired ventricular filling and reduced cardiac output.

While the diagnosis of tamponade itself is made clinically, ultrasound findings of pericardial tamponade include visualization of pericardial fluid with evidence of right atrial systolic collapse, right ventricular diastolic collapse, a plethoric inferior vena cava, or doppler evidence of respirophasic transmitral (>30%) and transtricuspid (>60%) flow variation (see Fig. 62.2, Video 62.2). It is the rate of accumulation, rather than the absolute size of the effusion, that may predict tamponade physiology. In acute tamponade, as little as 50–100 cc of fluid may be enough to cause cardiovascular collapse, whereas in subacute tamponade, often greater than 1500 cc may accumulate before hemodynamic compromise is appreciated [18].

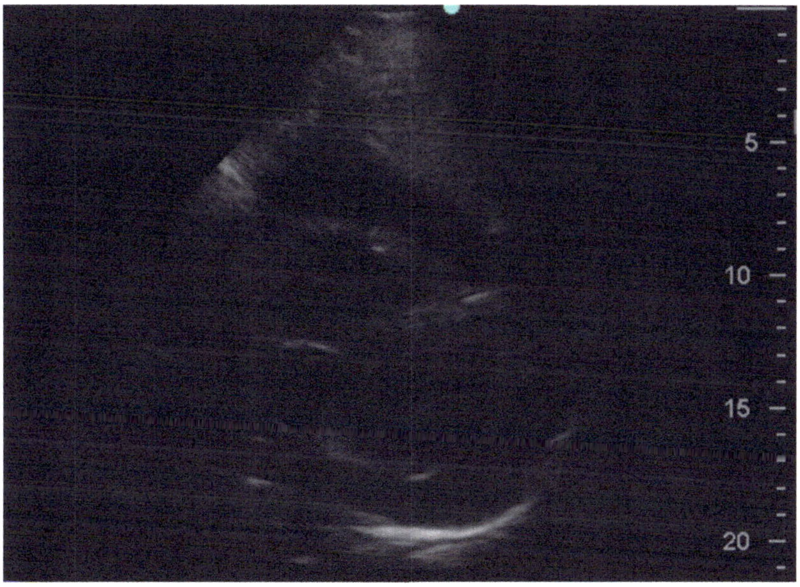

Fig. 62.2 A subcostal 4-chamber view demonstrates a large pericardial effusion causing cardiac tamponade

Tamponade is ultimately alleviated only by pericardiocentesis, although surgical exploration (i.e., sternotomy or pericardial window) may be necessary if the effusion is complex, loculated, or positioned posteriorly (i.e., post-cardiac surgery). In addition, pericardiocentesis guided by ultrasound is both effective (>90% success rate) and may be safer than the blind approach [11].

Myocardial Ischemia

Myocardial ischemia is often diagnosed by troponin leak, electrocardiographic ST-segment changes, and the presence of regional wall motion abnormalities (RWMAs). In cardiac arrest, myocardial ischemia may present as either PEA/asystole or ventricular fibrillation/tachycarda. Early detection is important to minimize time to coronary revascularization.

Ultrasound findings of myocardial ischemia include visualization of new RWMAs, although these are more likely to be observed after sustained return of spontaneous circulation (ROSC). POCUS examination may also be useful in recognizing complications of acute myocardial ischemia, including acute reduction of LV systolic function (see Fig. 62.3, Video 62.3), ischemic mitral insufficiency, mitral papillary muscule rupture, ventricular septal defect, RV infarction, or ventricular septal aneurysm/rupture.

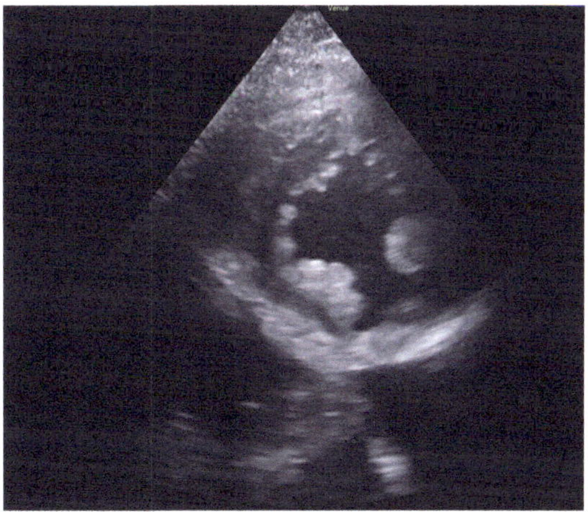

Fig. 62.3 A parasternal short-axis view demonstrates acute regional wall motion abnormalities primarily of anterior and septal walls in addition to global reduction in LV systolic function

Tension Pneumothorax

Tension pneumothorax should be considered in trauma or surgical patients with a suspicion for pleural injury, as well as in patients undergoing prolonged CPR with increased risk for iatrogenic injury. As the intrapleural pressure increases, the mediastinum shifts away from the affected lung, leading to decreased venous return and ultimately obstructive cardiovascular collapse. Prompt needle decompression or chest tube placement is

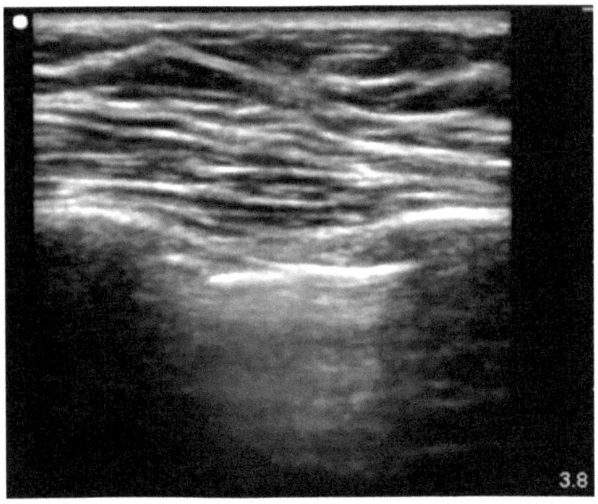

Fig. 62.4 A pleural view demonstrates presence of a "lung point," which is pathognomic for a pneumothorax

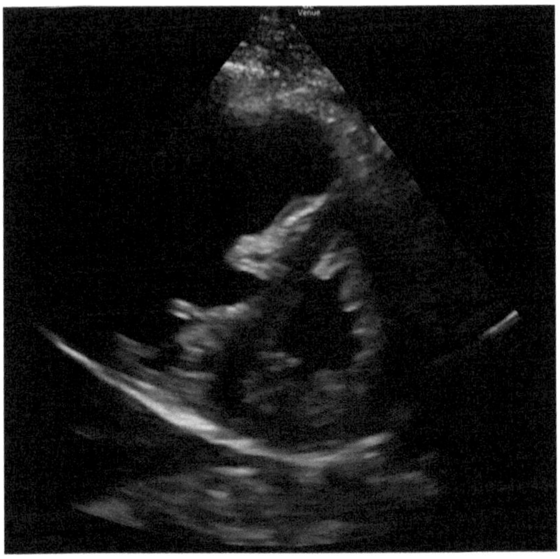

Fig. 62.5 A parasternal short-axis view demonstrates profound RV dilatation and interventricular septal deviation toward the LV. These findings, in addition to clinical suspicion for pulmonary embolism or additional ultrasound evidence for DVT, may suggest pulmonary embolism as a cause for cardiac arrest

necessary to relieve the increase in intrathoracic pressure. POCUS is useful in identifying pneumothorax and can be utilized during chest compressions by probe placement away from the sternum.

Ultrasound diagnosis of tension pneumothorax carries greater specificity than chest x-ray alone (100%) and can be identified by the presence of a "lung point" or absence of lung sliding, B-lines, and lung pulse (see Fig. 62.4, Video 62.4) [19]. While the absence of lung sliding alone does not diagnose pneumothorax, the presence of A-lines with absent lung sliding during cardiac arrest demonstrates a high sensitivity and specificity for pneumothorax [20].

Pulmonary Embolism

Pulmonary embolism is identified in 5% of PEA arrests each year in the US and continues to carry high mortality, in part due to delayed treatment. Definitive treatment includes systemic or local thrombolytic therapy and surgical or local thrombectomy to relieve right ventricular strain and improve the rate of ROSC. However, thrombolysis may also precipitate life-threatening bleeding (20% severe hemorrhage, 3–5% intracranial hemorrhage), and so direct ultrasound visualization of thrombus or identification of acute right ventricular dysfunction may inform this risk-benefit calculation [21].

While direct visualization of thrombus in the pulmonary arteries is uncommon, indirect findings such as deep venous thrombosis, acute dilatation of the right ventricle (RV) (see Fig. 62.5, Video 62.5), elevated pulmonary artery or right ventricular pressures, or interventricular septal deviation may suggest massive PE in the setting of cardiac arrest. POCUS may be misleading due to the following caveats—[1] Late visualization of right ventricular dilatation may be due to progressive effect of ongoing hypoperfusion and ultimately cardiac chamber pressure equalization, and [2] RV dilatation/dysfunction may be seen with other etiologies of right ventricular failure (i.e., chronic pulmonary hypertension). In the latter case, confirmation of right ventricular hypertrophy (right ventricular wall thickness >7 mm) may discern acute vs. chronic processes.

Severe Hypovolemia

Hypovolemia should be considered following exclusion of the above diagnoses, especially in the trauma or surgical patient. The findings of

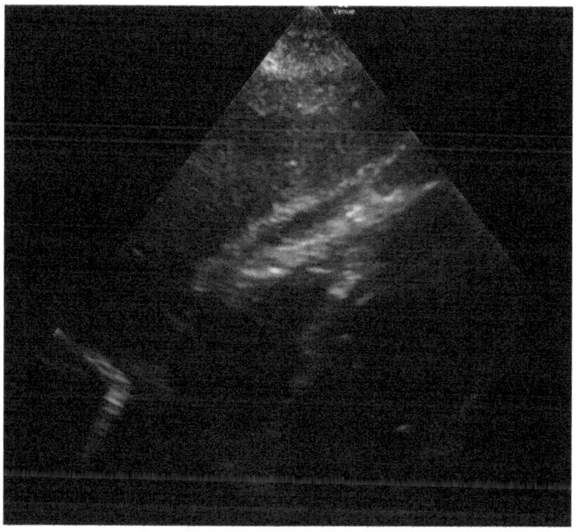

Fig. 62.6 A subcostal 4-chamber view demonstrates hyperdynamic ventricles, with small, or underfilled appearance of the RV, consistent with hypovolemia. In addition, there is a trace pericardial effusion without evidence of chamber collapse or clinical impact

small, hyperdynamic ventricles and the presence of indices suggesting volume responsiveness (i.e., superior vena cava or left ventricular outflow tract VTI variation, positive passive leg raise maneuver) may implicate hypovolemia as the cause of cardiac arrest (see Fig. 62.6, Video 62.6) [22]. In a trauma patient with undifferentiated hypotension, a "focused assessment with sonography in trauma" (FAST) exam can also be performed to assess for signs of intraabdominal or intrathoracic sources of bleeding. The response to fluid administration may also be observed by subsequent imaging of the heart throughout the resuscitation process.

Establishing a Protocol

In 2007, the Focused Echocardiographic Evaluation in Resuscitation (FEER) protocol was developed to guide POCUS during cardiac arrest [23]. Since that time, many other protocols have been established, including the Cardiac Arrest Ultrasound Exam (CAUSE), Cardiac Arrest Sonographic Assessment (CASA), and most recently Echocardiographic Assessment using Subcostal-only view in Advanced Life Support (EASy-ALS), all of which include whole-body imaging of cardiac structures, lung fields, abdomen, and/or vasculature. [24–26] While no single protocol has demonstrated superiority over any other, common features of all protocols include initial examination with subcostal 4-chamber view, rapid assessment of reversible etiologies of arrest, and strict adherence to ACLS guidelines so as not to prolong ultrasound examination, thereby disrupting CPR (see Fig. 62.7).

The FEER protocol guides the timeline and choreography of ultrasound examination during the no-flow-interval (NFI), or pulse/rhythm check portion of ACLS. It consists of four repeatable phases: [1] preparation of ultrasound, [2] ultrasound image acquisition, [3] resumption of CPR, and [4] interpretation of ultrasound results. The preparation phase occurs during the CPR cycle and includes readying and testing the ultrasound machine, placing gel on the ultrasound probe, and positioning the sonographer for subcostal examination as the CPR cycle is still ongoing, but coming to a close. Once chest compression ceases, a subcostal 4-chamber image of the heart should be acquired as rapidly as possible while a code timekeeper counts down the allotted 10 s for the NFI. CPR is then resumed with a verbal command by the code team leader. After resumption of CPR, the acquired images are interpreted and integrated into clinical management with the goal of identifying an etiology for arrest. The exam may be repeated throughout ACLS for every NFI, with the option to attempt different cardiac views if the subxiphoid view is difficult to obtain [23].

Transesophageal Echocardiography

Transthoracic echocardiography is a noninvasive technique with low risk of harm; however, there are some potential disadvantages that may render surface imaging unhelpful. Patient-related factors such as body habitus, gastric insufflation, lung disease, and defibrillation pad placement may make image acquisition challenging. In addition, by requiring probe placement in close proximity to sternal compressions, there is

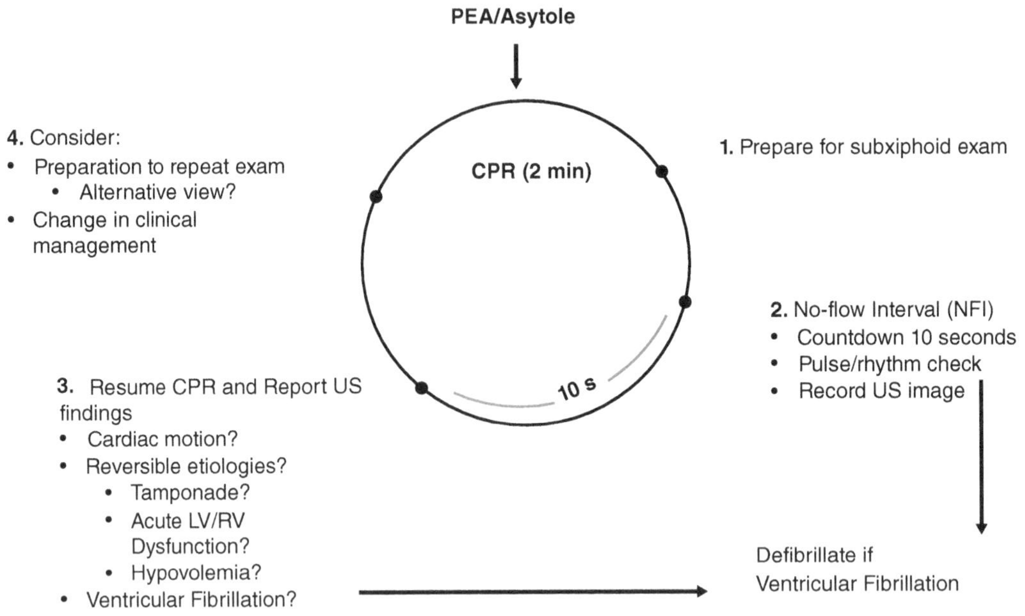

Fig. 62.7 Recommended implementation of POCUS in ACLS

potential for compromise to ongoing CPR. Therefore, there has been recent interest in the use of transesophageal echocardiography (TEE) as an alternative means to visualize cardiac structures during CPR.

Fair et al. demonstrated a reduction in mean pulse check duration (9 s with TEE vs 19 s with TTE) [27]. Furthermore, quality of CPR as gauged by blood flow through the left ventricular outflow tract (LVOT) and visualization of LV compression may be easier to assess with TEE [28]. Disadvantages of TEE include traumatic oropharyngeal or esophageal injury during TEE probe placement, cost, and the need for providers to undergo additional training. In addition, imaging of noncardiac structures, such as the lung, abdomen, or lower extremity vasculature, may not be possible.

Limitations

The risk of direct physical injury from transthoracic ultrasound is extremely low, yet there are two main potential harms from POCUS during cardiac arrest. First, image misinterpretation may result in incorrect or harmful management. For instance, if a small pericardial effusion is noted and interpreted as the cause for cardiac arrest, the decision to perform pericardiocentesis could lead to potentially greater complications such as myocardial perforation or effusion expansion resulting in tamponade. Second, and perhaps most important, is the potential for POCUS examination to delay NFIs. The proportion of time spent performing chest compressions during ACLS, known as the chest compression fraction (CCF), is independently associated with improved survival. A CCF of greater than 80% is considered optimal in both in-hospital and out-of-hospital cardiac arrest care [29]. In a prospective cohort study of patients in cardiac arrest, the use of POCUS demonstrated significantly increased mean duration of pulse checks compared to those without the use of POCUS (21 s vs 13 s, respectively) [30]. However, a more recent study demonstrated that proper use of an organized POCUS algorithm during cardiac arrest significantly decreased the duration of pulse checks [25]. Structured training of providers in the use POCUS during ACLS is therefore paramount to safe implementation.

Conclusion

POCUS remains a valuable tool in cardiac arrest to rapidly identify reversible etiologies for arrest and subsequently lead to prompt definitive treatment. POCUS may additionally be helpful with prognostication in the case of cardiac standstill or "True"-PEA, guidance of the quality ongoing chest compressions, and early recognition of fine ventricular fibrillation. While early investigations of the application of POCUS protocols in cardiac arrest suggested a harm of prolonged no-flow intervals, subsequent studies and provider training demonstrated no adverse compromise to the high-quality CPR.

However, linking POCUS application directly to improved clinical outcomes, especially survival, remains elusive. This likely stems from varied POCUS protocols applied to heterogeneous patient populations in the absence of a uniform clinical response to identified findings. In addition, POCUS providers comprise a diverse range of training backgrounds and levels, which emphasizes the need for best practice guidelines regarding training methods for ultrasound in ACLS. Over time, limited TEE examinations may supplant TTE protocols, although this requires additional expertise and training requirements.

Summary Points

- Focused ultrasound protocols during PEA cardiac arrest may identify reversible etiologies for arrest, including pericardial tamponade, myocardial ischemia, tension pneumothorax, pulmonary embolism, and severe hypovolemia.
- "Pseudo"-PEA occurs more frequently than "True"-PEA and carries a greater survival to hospital discharge
- Benefits of ultrasonography during cardiac arrest include guidance of CPR quality, prognostication, and identification of fine ventricular fibrillation.
- While many ultrasound protocols exist, execution of any one protocol must center around minimization of no-flow-intervals to <10 s, the current standard.

3 Board Questions

1. A 64-year-old female is admitted to the surgical ICU following an open ruptured AAA repair. She becomes acutely hypotensive and goes into cardiac arrest. ACLS is initiated and the code team leader requests an ultrasound at the bedside. Which of the following statements is true regarding ultrasound use during cardiac arrest?
   A. Chest compressions should be stopped as soon as the ultrasound is available
   B. Ultrasound exam of the lungs, abdomen, or lower extremities should not occur while chest compressions are ongoing
   C. Ultrasound images of the heart should occur primarily during pulse checks and not exceed the recommended 10-s no-flow-interval as to comply with ACLS guidelines
   D. The subxyphoid view is the only recommended cardiac view to obtain during cardiac arrest

   Answer: **C**. Ultrasound examination during CPR should not interfere with ACLS guidelines. This means that CPR should not be stopped solely for the purpose of obtaining an ultrasound view of the heart. Rather, cardiac imaging should occur during pulse checks, but should not exceed the recommended no-flow-interval of 10-s as to maintain an adequate chest compression fraction of >80%. The subxyphoid view is often the first view obtained and may be attempted while chest compressions are occurring if it does not interfere with the quality of compressions. Subsequent views may be obtained including apical 4-chamber and parasternal long or short-axis. Other areas such as lung, abdomen, and lower extremity vessels may be examined, while chest compressions are occurring as long as these exams do not interfere with CPR.
2. Which of the following ultrasound findings is not associated with cardiac tamponade?
   A. Right atrial systolic collapse
   B. Flattened inferior vena cava
   C. Right ventricular diastolic collapse
   D. Visualization of pericardial fluid

Answer: **B**. Typical ultrasound findings of hemodynamically significant cardiac tamponade include right atrial systolic collapse, right ventricular diastolic collapse, visualization of pericardial fluid, and a plethoric IVC. A flattened IVC would not be consistent with the high right heart filling pressures that are seen in cardiac tamponade.

3. Which of the following is not one of the potentially reversible etiologies of cardiac arrest that can be identified with POCUS?
   A. Severe hypovolemia
   B. Pulmonary emolism
   C. Tension pneumothorax
   D. Hyperkalemia

   Answer: **D**. While hyperkalemia is a potentially reversible cause of cardiac arrest, it is not one that is identifiable by ultrasound. Hyperkalemia may be identified by serum potassium levels. Severe hypovolemia may be identified on ultrasound by small, hyperdynamic ventricles. Pulmonary embolism may be identified by direct visualization of thrombus, acute dilation of right ventricle, or septal flattening. Tension pneumothorax may be identified by absence of lung slide with presence of A-lines or by the presence of lung point.

References

1. Andersen LW, Holmberg MJ, Berg KM, Donnino MW, Granfeldt A. In-hospital cardiac arrest: a review. JAMA. 2019;321(12):1200–10. https://doi.org/10.1001/jama.2019.1696.
2. Parish DC, Dinesh Chandra KM, Dane FC. Success changes the problem: why ventricular fibrillation is declining, why pulseless electrical activity is emerging, and what to do about it. Resuscitation. 2003;58(1):31–5. https://doi.org/10.1016/s0300-9572(03)00104-7.
3. Morrison LJ, Neumar RW, Zimmerman JL, Link MS, Newby LK, McMullan PW Jr, et al. Strategies for improving survival after in-hospital cardiac arrest in the United States: 2013 consensus recommendations: a consensus statement from the American Heart Association. Circulation. 2013;127(14):1538–63. https://doi.org/10.1161/CIR.0b013e31828b2770.
4. Berg KM, Soar J, Andersen LW, Böttiger BW, Cacciola S, Callaway CW, et al. Adult advanced life support: 2020 international consensus on cardiopulmonary resuscitation and emergency cardiovascular care science with treatment recommendations. Circulation. 2020;142(16_suppl_1):S92–S139. https://doi.org/10.1161/CIR.0000000000000893.
5. Soar J, Nolan JP, Böttiger BW, Perkins GD, Lott C, Carli P, et al. European resuscitation council guidelines for resuscitation 2015: section 3. Adult advanced life support. Resuscitation. 2015;95:100–47. https://doi.org/10.1016/j.resuscitation.2015.07.016.
6. Levitov A, Frankel HL, Blaivas M, Kirkpatrick AW, Su E, Evans D, et al. Guidelines for the appropriate use of bedside general and cardiac ultrasonography in the evaluation of critically ill patients-part II: cardiac ultrasonography. Crit Care Med. 2016;44(6):1206–27. https://doi.org/10.1097/ccm.0000000000001847.
7. Ochoa FJ, Ramalle-Gómara E, Carpintero JM, García A, Saralegui I. Competence of health professionals to check the carotid pulse. Resuscitation. 1998;37(3):173–5. https://doi.org/10.1016/s0300-9572(98)00055-0.
8. Eberle B, Dick WF, Schneider T, Wisser G, Doetsch S, Tzanova I. Checking the carotid pulse check: diagnostic accuracy of first responders in patients with and without a pulse. Resuscitation. 1996;33(2):107–16. https://doi.org/10.1016/s0300-9572(96)01016-7.
9. Badra K, Coutin A, Simard R, Pinto R, Lee JS, Chenkin J. The POCUS pulse check: a randomized controlled crossover study comparing pulse detection by palpation versus by point-of-care ultrasound. Resuscitation. 2019;139:17–23. https://doi.org/10.1016/j.resuscitation.2019.03.009.
10. Breitkreutz R, Price S, Steiger HV, Seeger FH, Ilper H, Ackermann H, et al. Focused echocardiographic evaluation in life support and peri-resuscitation of emergency patients: a prospective trial. Resuscitation. 2010;81(11):1527–33. https://doi.org/10.1016/j.resuscitation.2010.07.013.
11. White J. The value of focused echocardiography during cardiac arrest. J Diagn Med Sonogr. 2019;35(6):484–90. https://doi.org/10.1177/8756479319870171.
12. Atkinson PR, Beckett N, French J, Banerjee A, Fraser J, Lewis D. Does point-of-care ultrasound use impact resuscitation length, rates of intervention, and clinical outcomes during cardiac arrest? A study from the sonography in hypotension and cardiac arrest in the emergency department (SHoC-ED) investigators. Cureus. 2019;11(4):e4456. https://doi.org/10.7759/cureus.4456.
13. Lalande E, Burwash-Brennan T, Burns K, Atkinson P, Lambert M, Jarman B, et al. Is point-of-care ultrasound a reliable predictor of outcome during atraumatic, non-shockable cardiac arrest? A systematic review and meta-analysis from the SHoC investiga-

tors. Resuscitation. 2019;139:159–66. https://doi.org/10.1016/j.resuscitation.2019.03.027.
14. Tayal VS, Kline JA. Emergency echocardiography to detect pericardial effusion in patients in PEA and near-PEA states. Resuscitation. 2003;59(3):315–8. https://doi.org/10.1016/s0300-9572(03)00245-4.
15. Price S, Ilper H, Uddin S, Steiger HV, Seeger FH, Schellhaas S, et al. Peri-resuscitation echocardiography: training the novice practitioner. Resuscitation. 2010;81(11):1534–9. https://doi.org/10.1016/j.resuscitation.2010.07.001.
16. Soar J, Deakin CD, Nolan JP, Abbas G, Alfonzo A, Handley AJ, et al. European Resuscitation Council guidelines for resuscitation 2005. Section 7. Cardiac arrest in special circumstances. Resuscitation. 2005;67(Suppl 1):S135–70. https://doi.org/10.1016/j.resuscitation.2005.10.004.
17. Bobrow BJ, Clark LL, Ewy GA, Chikani V, Sanders AB, Berg RA, et al. Minimally interrupted cardiac resuscitation by emergency medical services for out-of-hospital cardiac arrest. JAMA. 2008;299(10):1158–65. https://doi.org/10.1001/jama.299.10.1158.
18. Ward RP, Lang RM. Chapter 56—Pericardial tamponade. In: Lang RM, Goldstein SA, Kronzon I, Khandheria BK, editors. Dynamic echocardiography. Philadelphia: W.B. Saunders; 2011. p. 250–3.
19. Lichtenstein DA. BLUE-protocol and FALLS-protocol: two applications of lung ultrasound in the critically ill. Chest. 2015;147(6):1659–70. https://doi.org/10.1378/chest.14-1313.
20. Husain LF, Hagopian L, Wayman D, Baker WE, Carmody KA. Sonographic diagnosis of pneumothorax. J Emerg Trauma Shock. 2012;5(1):76–81. https://doi.org/10.4103/0974-2700.93116.
21. Kürkciyan I, Meron G, Sterz F, Janata K, Domanovits H, Holzer M, et al. Pulmonary embolism as a cause of cardiac arrest: presentation and outcome. Arch Intern Med. 2000;160(10):1529–35. https://doi.org/10.1001/archinte.160.10.1529.
22. Ávila-Reyes D, Acevedo-Cardona AO, Gómez-González JF, Echeverry-Piedrahita DR, Aguirre-Flórez M, Giraldo-Diaconeasa A. Point-of-care ultrasound in cardiorespiratory arrest (POCUS-CA): narrative review article. Ultrasound J. 2021;13(1):46. https://doi.org/10.1186/s13089-021-00248-0.
23. Breitkreutz R, Walcher F, Seeger FH. Focused echocardiographic evaluation in resuscitation management: concept of an advanced life support-conformed algorithm. Crit Care Med. 2007;35(5 Suppl):S150–61. https://doi.org/10.1097/01.Ccm.0000260626.23848.Fc.
24. Hernandez C, Shuler K, Hannan H, Sonyika C, Likourezos A, Marshall J. C.A.U.S.E.: Cardiac arrest ultra-sound exam—a better approach to managing patients in primary non-arrhythmogenic cardiac arrest. Resuscitation. 2008;76(2):198–206. https://doi.org/10.1016/j.resuscitation.2007.06.033.
25. Clattenburg EJ, Wroe PC, Gardner K, Schultz C, Gelber J, Singh A, et al. Implementation of the Cardiac Arrest Sonographic Assessment (CASA) protocol for patients with cardiac arrest is associated with shorter CPR pulse checks. Resuscitation. 2018;131:69–73. https://doi.org/10.1016/j.resuscitation.2018.07.030.
26. Bughrara N, Herrick SL, Leimer E, Sirigaddi K, Roberts K, Pustavoitau A. Focused cardiac ultrasound and the periresuscitative period: a case series of resident-performed echocardiographic assessment using subcostal-only view in advanced life support. A A Pract. 2020;14(10):e01278. https://doi.org/10.1213/xaa.0000000000001278.
27. Fair J 3rd, Mallin MP, Adler A, Ockerse P, Steenblik J, Tonna J, et al. Transesophageal echocardiography during cardiopulmonary resuscitation is associated with shorter compression pauses compared with transthoracic echocardiography. Ann Emerg Med. 2019;73(6):610–6. https://doi.org/10.1016/j.annemergmed.2019.01.018.
28. Teran F, Prats MI, Nelson BP, Kessler R, Blaivas M, Peberdy MA, et al. Focused transesophageal echocardiography during cardiac arrest resuscitation: JACC review topic of the week. J Am Coll Cardiol. 2020;76(6):745–54. https://doi.org/10.1016/j.jacc.2020.05.074.
29. Meaney PA, Bobrow BJ, Mancini ME, Christenson J, Caen AR, Bhanji F, et al. Cardiopulmonary resuscitation quality: improving cardiac resuscitation outcomes both inside and outside the hospital. Circulation. 2013;128(4):417–35. https://doi.org/10.1161/CIR.0b013e31829d8654.
30. Huis In't Veld MA, Allison MG, Bostick DS, Fisher KR, Goloubeva OG, Witting MD, et al. Ultrasound use during cardiopulmonary resuscitation is associated with delays in chest compressions. Resuscitation. 2017;119:95–8. https://doi.org/10.1016/j.resuscitation.2017.07.021.

Part V

Ultrasound Education

63 Principles of Pedagogy

Christopher K. Schott and Mark M. Ramzy

Learning Objectives

1. Discuss three domains of learning related to Point of care Ultrasound (POCUS): cognitive, psychomotor, and affective.
2. Explore how the theory of Andragogy pertains to POCUS.
3. Examine how feedback provided to ultrasound learners can be specific, measurable, achievable, relevant, and timely (SMART).

Pedagogy and Andragogy

Point of Care Ultrasound (POCUS) is a relatively unique skill in medicine that requires simultaneous integration of multiple learning domains. In the 1950s, Benjamin Bloom led a group of educational psychologists to develop categories and models of learning and educational skills, known as Bloom's taxonomy [1, 2]. They identified three key domains. The **cognitive domain** refers to acquisition of new knowledge [1, 3]. For POCUS, this refers to the ability to understand how the devices work (i.e., a basic understanding of ultrasound physics), how to use the device to optimize images (i.e., "knobology"), identification of anatomic structures, and recognition of pathology or abnormal findings. The **psychomotor domain** refers to acquisition of new skills [4, 5]. This refers to the hand-eye coordination and probe manipulation skills for an individual to be able to locate views of relevant structures via standardized sonographic windows with fine motor adjustments to optimize the image. The **affective domain** refers to the intrinsic motivation to incorporate POCUS into clinical care [6]. This is the recognition that POCUS could be utilized in a clinical scenario, overcoming the initial practice inertia to begin implementation of a novel skill. In this chapter, we will address how educators can leverage many principles of adult learning to help learners across various training levels and medical specialties achieve competency in these complex skills.

POCUS and Adult Learning

Adults are driven to learn in unique ways that are readily applicable to POCUS. Malcolm Knowles' Andragogy demonstrates that adult learners (1) tend to be self-directed and intrinsically

C. K. Schott (✉)
Critical Care Medicine and Emergency Medicine, VA Pittsburgh Healthcare Sciences and University of Pittsburgh, Pittsburgh, PA, USA
e-mail: schottck@upmc.edu

M. M. Ramzy
Multidisciplinary Critical Care Training Program, University of Pittsburgh Medical Center, Pittsburgh, PA, USA
e-mail: ramzymm2@upmc.edu

M. J. Lanspa, A. T. Levinson (eds.), *Echocardiography and Ultrasonography in the ICU*, Respiratory Medicine, https://doi.org/10.1007/978-3-031-80038-2_63

motivated, (2) learn based on prior experiences, (3) are motivated to learn about things directly related to their needs or roles, (4) need to understand why they should learn the material, (5) tend to be more problem-, rather than topic-, focused, and (6) tend to learn through practice or by doing [7–9]. Curriculum Development for POCUS will be discussed in subsequent chapters. However, across the different forms of teaching POCUS, there is much commonality in how to optimize the learners' ability to achieve competency across each educational domain.

Cognitive

Regardless of exam type (cardiac, lung, vascular, etc.), it is essential for those learning POCUS to be able to demonstrate a basic understanding of ultrasound physics, knobology, the identification of normal anatomy, and recognition of abnormal or pathologic findings. This cognitive, or knowledge, domain can be provided in a variety of means. Group lectures, such as those provided at conferences or immersive workshops, are common ways to reach a large number of learners. However, they tend to be presenter-centric rather than learner-centric. In this model, there is a tendency towards passive learning among the participants as they listen to information provided by the presenter, often via PowerPoint slides. While this is easier on the presenter to develop and reach a larger audience of learners, it does not address the principles needed for adult learners to actively understand, retain, and apply novel information. A learner-centric approach is the ideal; however, this tends to be much more labor-intensive for the educators. Fortunately, there are ways to address this balance. One such approach is to provide the didactic content via a flipped-classroom model.

The **flipped-classroom** approach is one in which core materials are provided to students prior to the educational session [10–13]. The learners are able to view the content, as often as needed, asynchronously and when convenient for their needs. The availability can also provide "just in time" resources as the learners begin to apply content. Pre-course materials may include prerecorded video lectures or reading for the learner. This is particularly applicable to POCUS, where the inherent visual nature of the medium may easily be translated to digital content. While developing the content may initially be time-consuming for the instructor, the upfront investment provides many downstream benefits. Although occasional updates are needed, the material may be provided to large groups of learners without the need to schedule instructors to periodically provide the content in real-time. Care should be given to develop content that has appropriate scaffolding to previously known content (**scaffolding, zone of proximal development**) with the right amount of material to challenge the learner but not overwhelm them (**cognitive load theory, desirable difficulty, and goldilocks effect**) [14–23].

Once learners have been able to review the content, this provides the opportunity to optimize the direct interactions between the instructor and learners. This may include practice cases, simulation, or other means of allowing the learner to "play" with the novel content in active ways to better understand and retain the material (**experiential learning**) [24]. In terms of POCUS, this may include having learners view prerecorded lectures with subsequent time spent between the instructor and learners to more efficiently focus on the psychomotor skills of image acquisition with direct formative feedback.

Psychomotor

The psychomotor domain, referring to the hands-on skills to manipulate the probe to obtain optimal ultrasound views, is perhaps one of the most challenging aspects of POCUS. POCUS hinges on this domain: without the ability to obtain images, the ability to interpret and utilize this information is rendered useless. Work has demonstrated that trainees can learn the cognitive elements of POCUS, but require deliberate practice with formative feedback to be able to grow towards competency [25]. This may be achieved through workshops with hands-on scanning sessions, immersive rotations (i.e., a POCUS elective rotation), or longitudinal experiences over prolonged periods of training. Work has demonstrated that participants are able to retain image acquisition skills at least 6–9 months following short courses for in-practice physicians [26]. However, longitudinal experiences appear to demonstrate even greater growth towards achieving competency, as these incorporate the adult learning principles of **spaced repetition, perceptual motor grounding, feedback effects**, and **generation effects** [25, 27–32]. The role of archiving studies for Quality Assurance (QA) and indirect formative feedback, as related to aiding learners in the development of their image acquisition skills, is discussed later. Additionally, the combinations of methods to address the psychomotor domain address **dual code and multimedia effect** principles of adult learning to further enhance correlation to the cognitive elements via **scaffolding** and **contiguity** to improve achievement of POCUS competency [33–36].

Affective

One of the most challenging barriers to implement novel skills is practice inertia [37, 38]. Moreover, the amount of time needed to practice and build confidence in their skills, balanced against competing demands, may preclude providers from achieving competency in the complex skills of POCUS [39–41]. A recently published retrospective review of mid- to late-career nonacademic Emergency Medicine demonstrated that, despite a period of focused education in POCUS, many physicians did not complete the training for hospital credentialing in these skills for clinical use [42]. The affective domain refers to education specifically to address the learner's feelings, value, and motivation to use the material. Although adult learners are noted to typically have more intrinsic motivation, there are additional ways to enhance the likelihood that providers will not only participate in POCUS training, but begin to utilize it in clinical practice.

Adult learners are most successful when they are able to take an idea, manipulate it, and see how it applies in multiple situations (**experiential learning**) [24]. It is also beneficial to build on existing knowledge (**scaffolding**) while being challenged (**cognitive flexibility & desirable difficulties**) to generate their own conclusions (**generation effect**) [14, 16, 19–21, 41]. Additionally, stories, explanations, and multiple examples help adults learn novel concepts as well as seeing how it is relevant to their needs. In terms of POCUS, this can be done in several ways. One such way is a presentation of cases that utilized POCUS. This can be done as (1) interactive cases during initial learning, (2) case-based conferences, (3) sharing of cases through social media or other digital platforms, or (4) simulation [44–48]. Simulation can range from low to high-fidelity, with several commercially available ultrasound simulators that allow a learner to practice image acquisition and interpretation, inclusive of example pathologies. Multiple publications have demonstrated the impact of using simulation for POCUS education [49–55]. A key component among these is the need for an interactive element to challenge the learner with questions to help them think through the application of POCUS to clinical scenarios.

Another possibility, which may initially serve as more of an extrinsic motivation, is the requirement to develop and submit a portfolio of studies. This can provide deliberate practice with formative feedback, QA, and tracking of progress with tangible demonstration of competence to aid credential and privileging processes. Throughout practice, learners are not only able to develop competency and efficiency in their skills, but will begin to see how POCUS can be applied to their clinical practice. This is augmented with proper formative feedback to improve the learners' skills while cultivating their intrinsic motivation (**feedback effect**) [25, 31, 32].

Feedback

Defined as a supportive discussion clarifying a learner's awareness and continued improvement of their skills, feedback plays a vital role in many areas of POCUS [56]. Formative feedback can enhance a learner's motivation towards skill mastery and challenge them to set specific objectives for improvement [57]. Similar to George Doran's method of setting objectives, formative feedback as it relates to POCUS should be specific, measurable, achievable, relevant, and timely (SMART) [58].

S—Specific

Specific formative feedback in POCUS should describe a very clear, recognizable behavior that is either positive or requires improvement. It should be directly tailored to the learner and a desired objective. Examples range from acquiring a particular number of organ-specific exams to directionally manipulating the probe to optimize a certain view during a POCUS cardiac exam. Instead of "*Apical-four chamber view needs improvement*", the feedback should be "*Rotate probe counter-clockwise to better visualize the right ventricle in this apical four-chamber view*".

M—Measurable

Measurable feedback should attempt to quantify the desired change in behavior to determine whether or not the learner has achieved the objective. Continuing along with the examples aforementioned, measurable feedback would be to obtain five complete POCUS cardiac exams with as many views optimized as possible. Instead of "*Additional practice is needed for competency when performing POCUS cardiac exams*", the feedback should be "*Obtain five complete POCUS cardiac exams with clear visualization of the right ventricle in the apical-four chamber view*".

A—Achievable

The achievable portion of feedback should be possible within the learner's time and resource constraints. In addition to being unrealistic, setting unachievable goals may actually de-motivate the learner. Each piece of formative achievable feedback should be specific to the singular behavior or skill improvement desired. A step-by-step approach should be utilized with frequent check-ins and reevaluations to ensure the learner is on track to achieving the desired goal.

R—Relevant

Feedback needs to be relevant to the objectives and goals desired by the learner. This feature of formative feedback directly ties to the third feature of Malcolm Knowles' Andragogy of adult learning discussed earlier. Adult learners regularly exposed to POCUS cardiac exams in their practice are more motivated to improve their image acquisition as it directly relates to their needs.

T—Timely

In order to be effective and relevant, feedback needs to be done in a time-sensitive manner. While there is no consensus on a particular time frame for feedback, immediate corrective action following a behavior was shown to be more effective in preventing future occurrences of the erroneous action [59]. Therefore, a learner performing a scan is more likely to remember the behavioral actions that need to be changed or continued when the SMART feedback discussion is held sooner rather than later.

Hand-on workshops utilizing the flipped classroom model and personalized bedside scanning sessions both provide excellent avenues for delivering SMART feedback. Although discussed in greater depth later, feedback via QA can serve as another, arguably primary, route for measuring specific and achievable objectives in a timely manner.

Summary Points

- POCUS requires education across three domains of learning: Cognitive (knowledge regarding ultrasound physics, anatomy and pathology), psychomotor (hands-on skills of image acquisition), and affective (how ultrasound relates to the learner's feelings, value, and motivation to use the material).
- The theory of Andragogy pertains to POCUS in that adult learners tend to be self-directed, learn from prior experiences, learn things directly related to their needs, and need to understand why the material should be learned.
- Feedback provided to ultrasound learners should be an objective-driven tailored discussion that is specific, measurable, achievable, relevant, and timely (SMART). This can be done during workshops, bedside scanning sessions or via QA.

References

1. Taxonomy of educational objectives. A committee of college and university examiners. Bloom BS. The classification of educational goals. Handbook 1: cognitive domain. New York: Longman; 1956. p. 120–200.
2. Anderson LW, Krathwohl DR, Airasian PW, Cruikshank KA, Mayer RE. A taxonomy for learning, teaching and assessing: a revision of Bloom's taxonomy of educational objectives. (Anderson LW, Krathwohl DR, Airasian PW, Cruikshank KA, Mayer RE, eds.). Longman: Pearson; 2001.
3. Orgill BD, Nolin J. Learning taxonomies in medical simulation. In: StatPearls. Treasure Island, FL: StatPearls Publishing; 2021.
4. Adams NE. Bloom's taxonomy of cognitive learning objectives. J Med Libr Assoc. 2015;103(3):152–3. https://doi.org/10.3163/1536-5050.103.3.010.
5. Weeks KW, Coben D, O'Neill D, et al. Developing and integrating nursing competence through authentic technology-enhanced clinical simulation education: pedagogies for reconceptualising the theory-practice gap. Nurse Educ Pract. 2019;37:29–38. https://doi.org/10.1016/j.nepr.2019.04.010.
6. Krathwohl DR, Bloom BS, Masia BB. Taxonomy of educational objectives: the classification of educational goals. Handbook II: affective domain. New York, NY: David McKay; 1964.
7. Knowles EFHMS, Swanson RA. The adult learner: the definitive classic in adult education and human resource development. 7th ed. Oxford: Elsevier; 2011.
8. McBride M, Almodovar MC, Florez AR, Imprescia A, Su L, Allan CK. Applying educational theory to interdisciplinary education in pediatric cardiac critical care. World J Pediatr Congenit Heart Surg. 2019;10(6):742–9. https://doi.org/10.1177/2150135119881370.
9. Bryan RL, Kreuter MW, Brownson RC. Integrating adult learning principles into training for public health practice. Health Promot Pract. 2009;10(4):557–63. https://doi.org/10.1177/1524839907308117.
10. Young TP, Bailey CJ, Guptill M, Thorp AW, Thomas TL. The flipped classroom: a modality for mixed asynchronous and synchronous learning in a residency program. West J Emerg Med. 2014;15(7):938–44.
11. Horn M. The transformational potential of flipped classrooms: different strokes for different folks. Educ Next. 2013;13(3):78–9.
12. King A, Boysen-Osborn M, Cooney R, et al. Curated collection for educators: five key papers about the flipped classroom methodology. Cureus. 2017;9(10):e1801. https://doi.org/10.7759/cureus.1801.
13. Menashe S, Otjen J, Thapa MM. Techniques for creating video content for radiology education. Radiographics. 2014;34(7):1819–23.
14. Tawfik AA, Kolodner JL. Systematizing scaffolding for problem-based learning: a view from case-based reasoning. Interdiscip J Probl-Based Learn. 2016;10(1). Available at: https://doi.org/10.7771/1541-5015.1608.
15. Vygotsky L. Mind and society: the development of higher mental processes. Cambridge: Cambridge University Press; 1978.
16. Sanders D, Welk DS. Strategies to scaffold student learning: applying Vygotsky's Zone of Proximal Development. Nurse Educ. 2005;30(5):203–7. https://doi.org/10.1097/00006223-200509000-00007.
17. Young JQ, Van Merrienboer J, Durning S, Ten Cate O. Cognitive load theory: implications for medical education: AMEE Guide No. 86. Med Teach. 2014;36(5):371–84. https://doi.org/10.3109/0142159X.2014.889290.
18. van Merriënboer JJ, Sweller J. Cognitive load theory in health professional education: design principles and strategies. Med Educ. 2010;44(1):85–93. https://doi.org/10.1111/j.1365-2923.2009.03498.x.
19. Bereiter C, Scardamalia M. Cognitive coping strategies and the problem of "inertknowledge". In: Chipman SF, Segal JW, Glaser R, editors. Thinking and learningskills: Vol. 2. Current research and open questions. Hillsdale, NJ: Erlbaum; 1985. p. 65–80.
20. Bjork RA. Retrieval practice and maintenance of knowledge. In: Gruneberg MM, Morris PE, Sykes RN, editors. Practical aspects of memory: current

research and issues, vol. 1. New York: Wiley; 1988. p. 396–401.
21. Bjork RA. Assessing our own competence: heuristics and illusions. In: Gopher D, Koriat A, editors. Attention and performance XVII: cognitive regulation of performance: interaction of theory and application. Cambridge, MA: MIT press; 1999. p. 435–59.
22. Metcalfe J, Kornell N. A region of proximal learning model of study time allocation. J Mem Lang. 2005;52(4):463–77. https://doi.org/10.1016/j.jml.2004.12.001.
23. Schreiner M, Rehder B, Laham D, et al. Learning from text: matching readers and texts by latent semantic analysis. Discourse Process. 2003;25:309–36.
24. Kolb DA. Experiential learning: experience as the source of learning and development. Englewood Cliffs, NJ: Prentice-Hall; 1984.
25. Schott CK, Kode KR, Mader MJ. Teaching vs learning: impact of deliberate practice and formative feedback on developing point of care ultrasound skills. J Clin Ultrasound. 2020;48(8):437–42. https://doi.org/10.1002/jcu.22878.
26. Schott CK, LoPresti CM, Boyd JS, et al. Retention of point-of-care ultrasound skills among practicing physicians: findings of the VA national POCUS training program. Am J Med. 2020;134(3):391–399.e8. https://doi.org/10.1016/j.amjmed.2020.08.008.
27. Tabibian B, Upadhyay U, De A, Zarezade A, Schölkopf B, Gomez-Rodriguez M. Enhancing human learning via spaced repetition optimization. Proc Natl Acad Sci USA. 2019;116(10):3988–93. https://doi.org/10.1073/pnas.1815156116.
28. Glenberg AM, Kaschak MP. Grounding language in action. Psychon Bull Rev. 2002;9(3):558–65. https://doi.org/10.3758/bf03196313.
29. Abrahamse E, Braem S, Notebaert W, Verguts T. Grounding cognitive control in associative learning. Psychol Bull. 2016;142(7):693–728. https://doi.org/10.1037/bul0000047.
30. McCurdy MP, Viechtbauer W, Sklenar AM, Frankenstein AN, Leshikar ED. Theories of the generation effect and the impact of generation constraint: A meta-analytic review. Psychon Bull Rev. 2020;27(6):1139–65. https://doi.org/10.3758/s13423-020-01762-3.
31. Wulf G, Shea C, Lewthwaite R. Motor skill learning and performance: a review of influential factors. Med Educ. 2010;44(1):75–84. https://doi.org/10.1111/j.1365-2923.2009.03421.x.
32. Jimenez-Diaz J, Chaves-Castro K, Morera-Castro M. Effect of self-controlled and regulated feedback on motor skill performance and learning: A meta-analytic study. J Mot Behav. 2021;53(3):385–98. https://doi.org/10.1080/00222895.2020.1782825.
33. Chang HY, Wu HF, Chang YC, Tseng YS, Wang YC. The effects of a virtual simulation-based, mobile technology application on nursing students' learning achievement and cognitive load: randomized controlled trial. Int J Nurs Stud. 2021;120:103948. https://doi.org/10.1016/j.ijnurstu.2021.103948.
34. Choe RC, Scuric Z, Eshkol E, et al. Student satisfaction and learning outcomes in asynchronous online lecture videos. CBE Life Sci Educ. 2019;18(4):ar55. https://doi.org/10.1187/cbe.18-08-0171.
35. Moreno R, Valdez A. Cognitive load and learning effects of having students organize pictures and words in multimedia environments: the role of student interactivity and feedback. Educ Technol Res Dev. 2005;53(3):35–45.
36. Healey MK, Long NM, Kahana MJ. Contiguity in episodic memory. Psychon Bull Rev. 2019;26(3):699–720. https://doi.org/10.3758/s13423-018-1537-3.
37. Phillips LS, Branch WT, Cook CB, et al. Clinical inertia. Ann Intern Med. 2001;135(9):825–34. https://doi.org/10.7326/0003-4819-135-9-200111060-00012.
38. Cabana MD, Rand CS, Powe NR, et al. Why don't physicians follow clinical practice guidelines? A framework for improvement. JAMA. 1999;282(15):1458–65. https://doi.org/10.1001/jama.282.15.1458.
39. Ablordeppey EA, Keating SM, Brown KM, Theodoro DL, Griffey RT, James AS. Implementation of ultrasound after central venous catheter insertion: A qualitative study in early adopters [published online ahead of print, 2021 Nov 11]. J Vasc Access. 2021:11297298211053447. https://doi.org/10.1177/11297298211053447.
40. Koratala A, Bhattacharya D, Kazory A. Point of care renal ultrasonography for the busy nephrologist: A pictorial review. World J Nephrol. 2019;8(3):44–58. https://doi.org/10.5527/wjn.v8.i3.44.
41. Jarwan W, Alshamrani AA, Alghamdi A, et al. Point-of-care ultrasound training: an assessment of interns' needs and barriers to training. Cureus. 2020;12(10):e11209. https://doi.org/10.7759/cureus.11209. Published 2020 Oct 28.
42. Smalley CM, Simon EL, Muir MR, Delgado F, Fertel BS. Letter point-of-care ultrasound training and credentialing for mid—late career emergency physicians: is it worth it? POCUS J. 2021;06(02):56–7.
43. Greenstein YY, Littauer R, Narasimhan M, Mayo PH, Koenig SJ. Effectiveness of a critical care ultrasonography course. Chest. 2017;151(1):34–40. https://doi.org/10.1016/j.chest.2016.08.1465.
44. Dinh VA, Giri PC, Rathinavel I, et al. Impact of a 2-day critical care ultrasound course during fellowship training: a pilot study. Crit Care Res Pract. 2015;2015:1–8. https://doi.org/10.1155/2015/675041.
45. Patrawalla P, Narasimhan M, Eisen L, Shiloh AL, Koenig S, Mayo P. A regional, cost-effective, collaborative model for critical care fellows' ultrasonography education. J Intensive Care Med. 2019;35:1447. https://doi.org/10.1177/0885066619828951.
46. Rajamani A, Shetty K, Parmar J, et al. Longitudinal competence programs for basic point-of-care ultrasound in critical care: a systematic review. Chest. 2020;158(3):1079–89. https://doi.org/10.1016/j.chest.2020.03.071.
47. Kanji HD, Mccallum JL, Bhagirath KM, Neitzel AS. Curriculum development and evaluation of

a hemodynamic critical care ultrasound: a systematic review of the literature. Crit Care Med. 2016;44(8):e742–50. https://doi.org/10.1097/CCM.0000000000001661.
48. Lewiss RE, Hoffmann B, Beaulieu Y, Phelan MB. Point-of-care ultrasound education: the increasing role of simulation and multimedia resources. J Ultrasound Med. 2014;33(1):27–32. https://doi.org/10.7863/ultra.33.1.27.
49. Knudson MM, Sisley AC. Training residents using simulation technology: experience with ultrasound for trauma. J Trauma. 2000;48(4):659–65. https://doi.org/10.1097/00005373-200004000-00013.
50. Damewood S, Jeanmonod D, Cadigan B. Comparison of a multimedia simulator to a human model for teaching FAST exam image interpretation and image acquisition. Acad Emerg Med. 2011;18(4):413–9. https://doi.org/10.1111/j.1553-2712.2011.01037.x.
51. Barsuk JH, McGaghie WC, Cohen ER, O'Leary KJ, Wayne DB. Simulation-based mastery learning reduces complications during central venous catheter insertion in a medical intensive care unit. Crit Care Med. 2009;37(10):2697–701.
52. Barsuk JH, Cohen ER, Vozenilck JA, O'Connor LM, McGaghie WC, Wayne DB. Simulation-based education with mastery learning improves paracentesis skills. J Grad Med Educ. 2012;4(1):23–7. https://doi.org/10.4300/JGME-D-11-00161.1.
53. Mendiratta-Lala M, Williams T, de Quadros N, Bonnett J, Mendiratta V. The use of a simulation center to improve resident proficiency in performing ultrasound-guided procedures. Acad Radiol. 2010;17(4):535–40. https://doi.org/10.1016/j.acra.2009.11.010.
54. Sekiguchi H, Bhagra A, Gajic O, Kashani KB. A general critical care ultrasonography workshop: results of a novel web-based learning program combined with simulation-based hands-on training. J Crit Care. 2013;28(2):217.e7. https://doi.org/10.1016/j.jcrc.2012.04.014.
55. Lefroy J, Watling C, Teunissen PW, Brand P. Guidelines: the do's, don'ts and don't knows of feedback for clinical education. Perspect Med Educ. 2015;4(6):284–99. https://doi.org/10.1007/s40037-015-0231-7. PMID: 26621488; PMCID: PMC4673072.
56. Roze des Ordons AL, Gaudet J, Grant V, Harrison A, Millar K, Lord J. Clinical feedback and coaching – BE-SMART. Clin Teach. 2020;17(3):255–60. https://doi.org/10.1111/tct.13084. Epub 2019 Aug 26
57. Doran GT. There's a S.M.A.R.T. way to write management's goals and objectives. Manag Rev. 1981;70(11):35–6.
58. Hattie J, Timperley H. The power of feedback. Rev Educ Res. 2007;77:81–112. https://doi.org/10.3102/003465430298487.

Curriculum Design

64

Drew Brotherston, Robert Jackson, and Alberto Goffi

Learning Objectives

1. Discuss how curriculum must be framed around a universal approach to ultrasound.
2. Explore content that includes both clinical applications and background physics, machine care, patient interaction, and administration.
3. Describe the importance of course structures with initial introductions, longitudinal mixed direct and remote supervision, and evaluation of competence.
4. Review the educational utility of archiving and reporting system.
5. Determine how the delivery of education can leverage the expertise of non-critical care professionals.

D. Brotherston
Department of Medicine, University of Toronto, Toronto, ON, Canada

Department of Medicine, St. Michael's Hospital, Unity Health Toronto, Toronto, ON, Canada
e-mail: Drew.Brotherston@unityhealth.to

R. Jackson
Interdepartmental Division of Critical Care Medicine, University of Toronto, Toronto, ON, Canada

A. Goffi (✉)
Department of Medicine, University of Toronto, Toronto, ON, Canada

Department of Medicine, St. Michael's Hospital, Unity Health Toronto, Toronto, ON, Canada

Interdepartmental Division of Critical Care Medicine, University of Toronto, Toronto, ON, Canada

Department of Critical Care Medicine, St. Michael's Hospital, Unity Health Toronto, Toronto, ON, Canada
e-mail: Alberto.Goffi@unityhealth.to

M. J. Lanspa, A. T. Levinson (eds.), *Echocardiography and Ultrasonography in the ICU*, Respiratory Medicine, https://doi.org/10.1007/978-3-031-80038-2_64

Introduction

The performance of ultrasound assessment at the point-of-care in Critical Care has been widely adopted. Since the ACCP/SRLF (American College of Chest Physicians/ La Société de Réanimation de Langue Française) original position statement in 2009, there have been several important guidelines and recommendations published [1–4]. These provide guidance regarding scope of critical care ultrasound (CCUS), but do not specifically address curriculum structure or design.

Additionally, the provision of ultrasound training remains significantly heterogenous with very few examples of operationalized programs making this perhaps one of the greatest barriers to the implementation of CCUS into critical care practice.

There are emerging nationally recognized certifications for critical care echocardiography (CCE) [5, 6]; however, ultrasound teaching is almost exclusively determined by individual programs.

The development of a local ultrasound curriculum contains many considerations, with a tailored approach based on local resources, target learners, local scope of practice/goals/circumstances, burden of diseases, equipment, and instructors available, being essential to the success of the program [1, 7, 8].

The aim of this chapter will be to provide a basic framework of the minimum components and delivery of CCUS curriculum as well as elements that can be added in institutions with robust resources.

Educational Model

Before even considering the scan application content of a CCUS curriculum, it is imperative to provide a universal model for how to approach ultrasound use. The I-AIM model, standing for indication, acquisition, interpretation, and management, is the only published educational model that addresses this need and provides both a cognitive aid and checklist function [9]. We suggest this model be the foundation upon which all US applications be taught to ensure trainees approach each scan systematically.

It begins by asking is ultrasound indicated or likely to be of use, is it within the scope of the sonographer's skill to perform, and are there alternatives? From an educator standpoint, this serves to build discussions of the utility and limitations of each application into course content.

The acquisition portion of the model is further broken down into four domains with a separate mnemonic, the 4 Ps: patient, probe, picture, and protocol. The patient component refers to appropriate positioning, lighting, and draping, analogous to efforts to optimize physical examination. The probe refers to selecting the appropriate transducer for the job considering the frequency, footprint, and how the probe is held/manipulated. Picture covers knobology relating to image optimization/measurements; alterations of depth, gain, focal zone, frequency range, tissue harmonics, color/power, or spectral Doppler. Lastly, there is the consideration of possible protocols involving multiple body locations or organ systems that, taken together, provide a more complete picture for clinical decision making.

Interpretation refers to the real-time assessment of the image for normal anatomy, pathology, as well as artifacts, and overall quality.

Finally, the management component of the model includes the ability to synthesize the interpreted ultrasound images into the patient's overall history, physical examination, and clinical trajectory to arrive at a management decision. An example of this complete process is shown in Fig. 64.1 for the indication of undifferentiated shock.

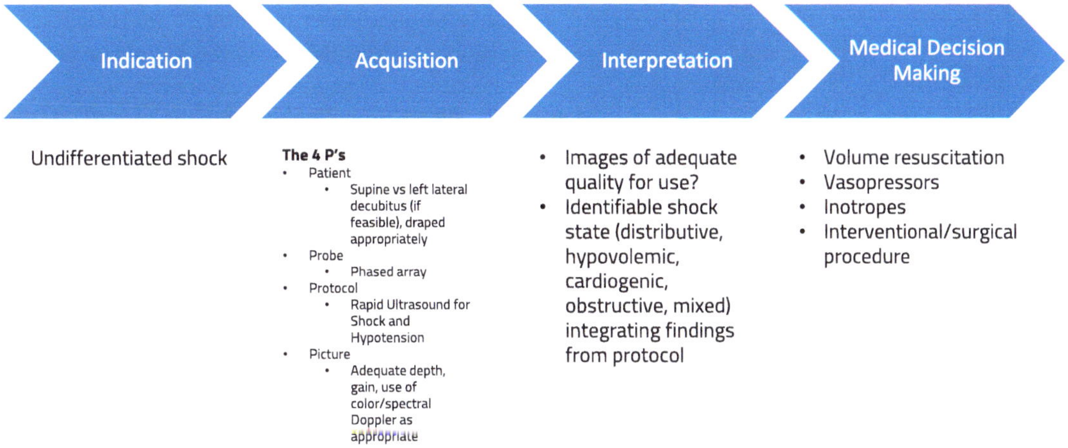

Fig. 64.1 I-AIM Framework for US assessment of undifferentiated shock

Ultrasound Applications

The ultrasound applications considered essential to CCUS have been outlined by numerous critical care groups to provide a baseline framework for the goals of CCUS curriculum; however, there is no universal agreement on what is considered essential [3, 4, 10–12].

A universally agreed upon baseline requirement of curriculum must include basic physics, knobology, and image artefacts as these are germane to all applications of US. Similarly, all major guidelines/consensus statements divide CCUS into two broad categories: CCE and general critical care ultrasonography (GCCUS). Overall, GCCUS encompasses lung, abdominal, vascular, and procedural ultrasound, while CCE refers to cardiac scanning and may include transesophageal in addition to transthoracic applications.

There is a further subdivision of CCE into basic and advanced applications. Conceptually, the division is to a certain extent arbitrary; however, there are generally agreed upon principles for this distinction.

For example, the International Federation of Emergency Medicine (IFEM) defines basic applications as being simple, easily learned, able to be performed quickly, and address questions that are common to the practice population [13]; this would include the evaluation for pleural effusion or abdominal-free fluid in GCCUS, or qualitative LV systolic function, or presence of pericardial effusion in CCE. There is generally good agreement across multiple societies regarding what is considered essential basic CCUS; these are summarized in Table 64.1.

Advanced applications as they pertain to CCUS are generally in the realm of CCE and include those applications that require established proficiency in ultrasound, are more difficult or more time-intensive to perform, and answer questions that are either less common or of higher complexity and more closely approximate formal echocardiography. Enhanced applications would include stroke volume estimation by left ventricular outflow tract velocity time integral or diastolic function assessment; noncardiac applications may include solid organ doppler for assessment of venous congestion or brain ultrasonography including transcranial Doppler.

The ceiling of advanced applications, and specifically echocardiography, is determined by the expertise of educators and the clinical needs of the institution; in this regard, all aspects of echocardiography can be considered for potential inclusion. Practically, however, given the intent of CCUS is to support patient management in a focused and time-sensitive fashion, while advanced quantitative techniques such as Simpson's biplane ejection fraction can be taught, these will be of less use clinically versus applications relevant to hemodynamics such as

Table 64.1 Recommended basic CCUS applications

System	Application
Echocardiography syndromes	Severe hypovolemia LV failure RV failure Tamponade Acute cor pulmonale Severe valvular abnormalities
Echocardiography	Qualitative LV size LV systolic function LV contraction pattern Valvular disease via 2D and color doppler Right ventricle size RV systolic function Pericardial effusion presence, RV/RA diastolic collapse Quantitative Inferior vena cava size and collapsibility[a]
Thoracic ultrasound syndromes	Consolidation Pleural effusion Interstitial syndrome Pneumothorax
Thoracic procedures	Pleural drainage
Abdominal[b]	Free fluid Bladder volume Hydronephrosis
Abdominal procedures	Ascitic drainage
Vascular ultrasound	Lower extremity compression ultrasound for DVT
Vascular access	Femoral vein Jugular vein Radial artery Femoral artery

[a] IVC measure quantitative
[b] All qualitative

stroke volume determination or left atrial pressure estimation. Based on the aggregate recommendations from major pulmonary, emergency, and critical care societies and our experience, we have assembled a list of recommended advanced applications; Table 64.2.

With respect to transesophageal echocardiography (TEE) in a center with adequate access to technology and skilled educators and in the population of patients who have a secure airway, it could be considered a basic CCE application. Its use to guide intra-arrest resuscitation for chest compression adequacy/placement, and for rapid evaluation for LV/RV function, pericardial effusion, or valvular catastrophe is not technically more difficult than transthoracic imaging in the intubated and sedated patient and may in fact be easier in many cases. Similarly, the use of transesophageal ultrasound for lung-ultrasonography (TELUS) can provide valuable information for the diagnosis of occult consolidation and effusion too medial to be detected by transthoracic lung ultrasound and should be considered an essential TEE application and skill set. The indications and key views of resuscitative or focused TEE are summarized in Table 64.3.

It is our recommendation that all programs strive to achieve the delivery of curriculum covering at minimum the basic applications outlined in Table 64.1 and striving to achieve those in Table 64.2 where they can be adequately supported with available training resources.

Table 64.2 Suggested advanced applications

System	Application
Echocardiography	Hemodynamics Stroke volume determination via LVOT VTI[a] LVOT VTI and AV VTI respiratory variability Systolic anterior motion of the mitral valve by 2D and M-mode Mid-cavity/LVOT continuous wave Doppler for peak gradient for dynamic obstruction grading Quantitative assessment of LV function Presence of regional wall motion abnormality Quantitative assessment of RV function TAPSE Fractional area change RV s' Pulmonary hypertension RVOT Doppler morphology for elevated PA pressures (e.g., early systolic notching) Pulmonary acceleration time for mPAP estimation TR Vmax for right ventricular systolic pressure estimate Tamponade Mitral/tricuspid inflow variability Right to left shunt IV bubble contrast Valvular assessment Aortic Aortic valve VTI/LVOT VTI for dimensionless index Aortic valve peak velocity Aortic valve mean gradient Pressure half time with aortic regurgitation Abdominal aorta diastolic flow reversal in AR Mitral Vena contracta Pulmonic Color Doppler for qualitative identification of severe regurgitation Tricuspid TR Doppler morphology/signal density for qualitative assessment for severe TR Diastology Mitral inflow E/A E/e' TR Vmax Left atrial volume Mitral inflow deceleration time ECMO [14][b] Pre-ECMO assessment During cannulation Patient monitoring during ECMO Weaning from ECMO Post-ECMO
Respiratory muscle function ultrasound	Diaphragm function (excursion/thickening) *Extra-diaphragmatic respiratory muscles*
Abdominal	Hepatic vein Doppler (qualitative, waveform assessment) Portal vein Doppler (qualitative, waveform assessment, and quantitively pulsatility index) Renal vein doppler (qualitative, waveform assessment)
Transcranial	Midline shift, 2D assessment Middle cerebral artery Doppler morphology and for intracranial pressure estimation

[a]Velocity time integral
[b]Extracorporeal membrane oxygenation

Table 64.3 Resuscitative transesophageal echocardiography

Resuscitative TEE	Competencies
Specific indications	All basic transthoracic CCE indications in the setting of absence or limited transthoracic windows in critically ill patient (due to trauma, devices, or patient factors) Intra-arrest compression optimization Support for extracorporeal membrane oxygenation cannulation
Basic views	Midesophageal four chamber Midesophageal long axis Bicaval view Transgastric short axis Descending aorta short axis and long axis Right and left lung
Applications	LV function RV function Severe valvular abnormality Pericardial effusion SVC variability Evaluate for LVOT compression during CPR Visualization of ECMO[a] cannula placement TELUS for assessment of basal lung consolidation

[a]Extracorporeal membrane oxygenation

Methodology

The goals of CCUS education are now established in major critical care society guidelines. However, the methods of delivering ultrasound curriculum in the critical care context have yet to be similarly defined. Models of education have been established in other disciplines such as emergency medicine and provide a framework for CCUS.

The specifics of curriculum content and delivery will be contingent on presence of trained faculty and number, patient population, commonness of certain disease entities (e.g., valvular heart disease versus ischemic disease, young versus elderly, medical versus surgical), machines factors (e.g., ultrasound machine numbers/capabilities, cart vs. handheld devices [15, 16]), and archiving (e.g., picture archiving and communication system, standalone database, cloud sharing [17]).

A needs assessment should be carried out to understand these individual institutional aspects before undertaking program design. This will involve the establishment of desired outcomes and identifications of barriers to implementation, creating a timeline for delivery and selecting the appropriate format for curriculum delivery. In this section, we will aim to describe practical aspects of these steps and potential solutions to common challenges.

Common to all curricula should be a process of initial induction, portfolio completion and formative assessment, competence assessment, followed by quality assurance/maintenance of competence which is the foundation of the ESCIM, ACCP, SCCM, FUSIC, ICARUS recommendations [2–4, 18, 19]. Overall, there is little evidence to guide specific methods for these phases; therefore, we provide a summary of our own experience and expert consensus from society guidelines and initiatives.

To effectively develop CCUS as part of clinical practice, it must be performed consistently. For the same reason, CCUS training must be longitudinal as well. While there is little evidence to make specific recommendations for program structure, trainees should generate studies for personal portfolio weekly with at most 1 month between studies.

While intensive rotations may be part of this training and serve as an opportunity to focus on acquiring and refining skills, this cannot be the only mechanism for teaching given the risk of skill decay, inability to generate an adequate portfolio, and challenges of clinical integration as on such rotations trainees are typically not directly managing patients.

Additionally, there is the consideration of the skill domains inherent to ultrasonography which include visual-cognitive, motor, and hand-eye coordination [20]. Motor and hand-eye coordination may be thought of as the act of scan performance, whereas visual-cognitive skills relate to interpretation/assessment of quality. Motor and hand-eye coordination skills invariably require hands-on practice in either simulated, normal models, or patients and all curricula must include regular opportunities to exercise these skills. Visual-cognitive skills can be taught separately using either facilitator-led image review or online modules [21] offering some flexibility for course designers when it comes to image interpretation, synthesis, and management skills teaching.

Personnel

Delivery of CCUS curriculum necessitates an ultrasound director who oversees the administration of the program and is responsible for infrastructure, training faculty/residents/fellows, curriculum development and evaluation, and QA. This individual must have externally recognized expertise in the form of fellowship training or certification in echocardiography or recognition by national or internal critical care societies as having expertise in CCUS [12].

In addition to the director, there must be additional faculty with sufficient training to support trainee oversight and curriculum development, generally at least 1–2 other individuals [22].

The establishment of an ultrasound fellow, a senior critical care trainee or recent graduate pursuing advanced training, may support and facilitate daily operations such as direct trainee supervision or remote quality assurance and ultrasound teaching. In this setting, it may be possible to offer an intensive rotation where trainees are entirely devoted to CCUS to supplement longitudinal curriculum.

Still more options exist where a multidisciplinary approach with contributions from other subspecialties and sonographers to provide teaching, mentoring, and/or support for curriculum development and assessment can be considered. For example, establishing an ultrasound education group including cardiology, anesthesia, radiology, echocardiographers, and sonographers can distribute teaching responsibilities and draw on the high-level expertise of these individuals in their respective fields [21, 23, 24].

Induction/Didactic Training

In broad terms, curricula should begin with an initial induction where learners are provided with foundational knowledge and skills [25–27]. This might take the form of a "bootcamp", an intensive potentially multiday course covering introduction to framework for performing scans, setting 'ground-rules' or expectations for scan conduct, goals for the program, and outline of the next steps.

There is a didactic component including an overview of fundamentals of operation and scan performance including ultrasound physics, knobology/machine operation, as well as image generation/optimization, and finally standards for image capture and documentation. A list of suggested topics is included in Table 64.4.

It is important at this stage to cover very practical aspects of training such as machine handling and infection protocols. For example, providing clear instruction on cleaning practices to prevent infection spread and also to avoid damage to machines.

Additionally, emphasis should be given on the importance of patient-centered approach to ultrasonography ensuring patients and/or families/decision makers are told the reason for the study (diagnostic vs educational), considerations of consent, and privacy. Privacy considerations specific to CCUS in the education setting are particularly relevant in the sharing of deidentified images for review. Deidentification of images is achieved when usual patient identifiers (name, date of birth, record number) as well as the institution where the study took place and the date (though not necessarily the time) are removed or masked from recorded images.

Induction should also include basic protocols and key pathology for the applications to be included. There must be sufficient time for 'hands-on' scanning where trainees are provided with access to either standardized patients, faculty/trainee volunteers, or high-fidelity models to practice motor skills.

Without regular use, skills and knowledge decay over time, therefore it is important to consider a

Table 64.4 Fundamental ultrasound competencies

Content Category	Competencies
Physics and knobology	• Components of ultrasound machine • Transducer types and characteristics • Probe frequency ranges effects on penetration and image quality • Ultrasound controls • Common artifacts and their etiology
Image generation	• Transducer manipulation • Ultrasound modes 2D, color/power Doppler, spectral Doppler • Types of resolution and methods for improvement
Indications and alternatives	• Clinical syndromes with CCUS indication • Limitations of US and role for other imaging modalities • Choice of TTE versus TEE
Administration and documentation	• Image recording during studies • Archiving of studies (using local systems) • Documentation of findings • Medicolegal aspects of findings and documentation
Patient-centered approach	• Obtaining patient consent • Communication with patients and family regarding findings • Anonymization of scans stored outside of archiving system (e.g., removal of patient identifiers including name, medical record numbers, and study date)
Machine handling/care	• General machine care to prevent damage (securing transducers, cords, shutting down machines after use, charging on surge protected electricity source) • Infection prevention and control, i.e., machine cleaning, policies on use on patients with precautions

longitudinal approach to didactic training. This can be accomplished through a schedule of teaching sessions throughout the academic year which can be in person or delivered virtually via webinar [21]. There are many free open-access medical education (FOAMED) platforms that are expertly reviewed and may serve as yet another method for delivery of ultrasound didactic content in the absence of traditional didactic lectures delivered locally.

Gaining Experience

All CCUS must include hands-on scan time on real patients within the critical care environment. Initially, we recommend there should be some form of direct supervision at the bedside. Owing to the substantial time required, it is pragmatic to augment supervised scanning with instruction by noncritical care professionals such as Echocardiographers and Sonographers or other subspecialty physicians.

As comfort in basic applications is established, trainees may perform studies on patients with indirect supervision in the form of review of images after the fact or with an expert repeating the study to verify findings.

The performance of CCUS as a dedicated rotation provides advantages to devote significant time to honing skills and increase experience and exposure rapidly over a short time. At the University of Western Ontario in Canada, there is an operationalized CCUS training model whereby critical care trainees perform CCUS studies on critical care patients as a consult service supervised by ultrasound leadership and CCUS fellows as part of an intensive month-long rotation. In this model, it is possible for trainees to be supervised directly or with near immediate feedback as their assessments are reviewed in similar manner to a case presentation as an inpatient consultation [28].

Regardless of the model of practical experience, it must be clear to trainees to not act on findings until they have been deemed sufficiently competent to do so by either the Ultrasound director or other program leads.

Formative Assessment/Portfolio Completion

An ultrasound portfolio refers to a compilation of scans acquired by the learner. A portfolio should not merely be a collection of images, but should also include a report including the context for the scan, interpretation, and actions based on the scan [29].

The creation of a personal portfolio of ultrasound cases is important not only for the purposes of quantifying the volume and types of scans performed, but also to allow for over-reading by educators/assessors as a method of competence assessment and for the learner to undergo self-reflection on scan performance, interpretation, and subsequent management after the fact [4].

There is no universal standard for how many scans should be captured in an individual portfolio; however, there is general guidance and data to support numbers compatible with minimum competence that can serve as a baseline. A minimum of 40–50 CCE studies for basic applications and 100 for advanced, 20 lung and pleural examinations, 10 assessments for abdominal free fluid, and 10 lower extremity DVT exams are a reasonable baseline for CCE and GCCUS as these are recommended by several major societies and international expert groups [5, 8, 24, 30–32].

Expert opinion in this area suggests that trainees should perform at least 80% of portfolio studies on critically ill patients [24]. This ensures acquisition of skills in a setting consistent with eventual practice and pathology and the unique challenges of scan performance in critically ill patients which are frequently technically difficult.

In tandem with the generation of portfolio, formative feedback should be provided by either the program lead or a mentor with expertise in CCUS. Feedback must include specific emphasis on acquisition and interpretation and determination of whether individual studies 'pass' or 'fail' [33, 34].

In a well-resourced program, the formative assessment and portfolio process is facilitated by an electronic archiving system whereby scans are captured and uploaded from the point-of-care device to a central database and are linked to an individual user profile (generally the user would input their credentials prior to beginning the scan) and a standardized report is written to accompany the images either immediately or shortly after the fact. Ideally, the report would be linked and editable alongside the captures. The images and report are then subsequently over-read, and feedback provided by an expert reviewer who may be local or remote, done in real-time or asynchronously. In such a system, trainees can seamlessly practice the use of POCUS and incorporate it into patient care while having their progress logged in a permanent record.

The main barriers to implementation of such a system are financial and information technology-related as there must be communication between the point of care device and the archiving system and ideally linkage between the archiving system and the patient chart. Such systems are available through several companies and require licensing fees and ongoing IT support.

In more resource-limited programs, it is possible to recreate some aspects of the systems presented above. For example, there are online tools for uploading and sharing anonymized scans that do not require a local technical solution at all. Similarly, scans may be loaded into local shared network drives with a basic report in a document file. Presently, there are emerging enterprises with remote teleguidance and image review possible by experts with no affiliation with the institution but who are still able to provide quality assurance and feedback [35].

Competency Assessment

There is currently no universally agreed upon standard for competency assessment in CCUS. There are, however, several agreed upon principles mainly that trainees should complete a certain number of scans and that these be over-read by an expert reviewer for both image quality and accuracy in interpretation and synthesis and potentially accompanied by formalized assessment of knowledge and scanning technique in an objective structured clinical examination (OSCE).

In highly resourced programs, assessment may be carried out by local educators and should include OSCEs on standardized patients and written exams [32, 36, 37].

Though there are not yet universally agreed upon test methods, there are emerging expert consensus-based tools for what constitutes the cut-off for a technically complete study [38–41] as well as general core skills in ultrasound use which may serve as the basis for locally developed clinical assessments [42].

A more resource-limited setting may rely on external certification or exams, to be challenged after completion of training. There are several emerging professional organizations that offer pathways to certifications in point-of-care ultrasound which could serve as the competence assessment for a program with limited faculty or limited experience in assessment [5, 6].

Quality Assurance/Maintaining Competence

Presently, there is not a universally agreed upon approach to quality assurance (QA) and maintenance of competence. There are, however, essential components for both with some guidance from professional societies and experience from established programs [3, 4, 10, 12, 43, 44].

Quality assurance (QA) refers to the process of scans performed by either trainees or experienced providers being over-read by experts at the institution to ensure appropriateness, technical adequacy, correct interpretation, and actions taken in response to the scan. This serves to maintain a degree of safety for patients, practitioner competence, as well as adherence to guidelines and local best practices.

Current professional recommendations are that all QA systems include digital archiving with patient demographic data, images, and interpretation documented, image review by a designated expert or ultrasound director, and documentation of the study within the patient chart [12].

From a curriculum standpoint, QA serves as a formative feedback tool to the ultrasound user on their image quality and interpretation. The methods for QA are varied but several central tenants apply.

First is that trainee scans are reviewed by an expert for both scan quality and interpretation accuracy and feedback provided. Oversight can be either in-person through direct observation or asynchronously through written feedback after the fact [34].

From a quality standpoint, the assessor should address both aspects of safety and technical adequacy. There are numerous potential scales against which a scan could be assessed [40–42, 45–50], but the general intention should be to stratify a study/practitioner into one of four categories. The first and most straightforward is a complete and well-performed study with no action required. The second is where general standards are maintained but there are technical aspects of the study or interpretation that need to be refined and feedback should be provided to the practitioner to address them for the future. Third is where standards are not met and there is a potential for patient risk which should prompt specific intervention to address skills/safety. Lastly and most significantly is where standards are not met with serious errors in acquisition or interpretation and patient harm results or would certainly result from acting on the interpretation necessitating removal of ultrasound privileges. While additional gradations could be added or subtracted, it is our opinion that QA must include some version of this assessment of studies and include mechanisms for intervening when patient safety is a concern.

Maintenance of competence is the final component of curriculum; however, it can also be the most nebulous. There are currently no universal standards for establishing competence in CCUS to begin with, let alone for maintenance of competence. In institutions with established ultrasound programs, maintenance of competence often becomes a matter of local consensus in adherence to minimum standards for scans with periodic review of scans done by independent practitioners or by a local expert who can then share feedback with practitioners [13, 31]. There are formal certifications and tracks for achieving these as either a learner or attending in the United States and Canada [6, 51, 52].

We recommend that programs/institutions should establish some mechanism for ensuring ongoing competence whether this is meeting a threshold of continuing medical education in ultrasound performance, periodic peer-review of ultrasound practice, simulation training, or a combination of these methods.

Adaptations to Learner Types

The bulk of this chapter has focused on the delivery of curriculum to subspecialty trainees in critical care; however, the need for CCUS curriculum for more junior leaners to attending level physicians is also of import. In the former case, the critical care environment provides an excellent opportunity for trainees to encounter pathology and to work through the challenges of integrating findings into patient management as well as the obvious procedural ultrasound where critical care may be the only opportunity to learn these skills practically. A comparison of these various tracks is outlined in Fig. 64.2.

Modifications to reduce the scope and scale of CCUS to high-yield applications and can reasonably be accomplished within a short rotation should be considered [53]. This largely excludes cardiac assessments, but diagnostic lung, abdomen for free fluid, and vascular access are reasonable objectives with reduced target numbers. Direct oversight by attending physicians or critical care trainees or verification of findings with supervisor performance is recommended. Assessment may be integrated into other rotation assessments (rotation exams or clinical rotation evaluations). Observed bedside assessment in a formalized fashion may be overly resource-intensive and can be forgone for this population.

In the case of teaching to attending physicians, this requires a unique approach, but it is of critical importance that there are training mechanisms for attending physicians not only to bolster the supply of local instructors for a program but also to embed a culture of ultrasound use into clinical practice. Even a well-established program with significant expertise among ultrasound educators can be undermined if there is not consistent familiarity with CCUS use among attending physicians.

In our view, attending level training should closely mirror that of subspecialty trainees in terms of content and criteria for assessment, however, with several important caveats. There must be considerably more flexibility in attending level education. For example, rather than a rigid timeline, physicians should be allowed the ability to receive training until competent. The

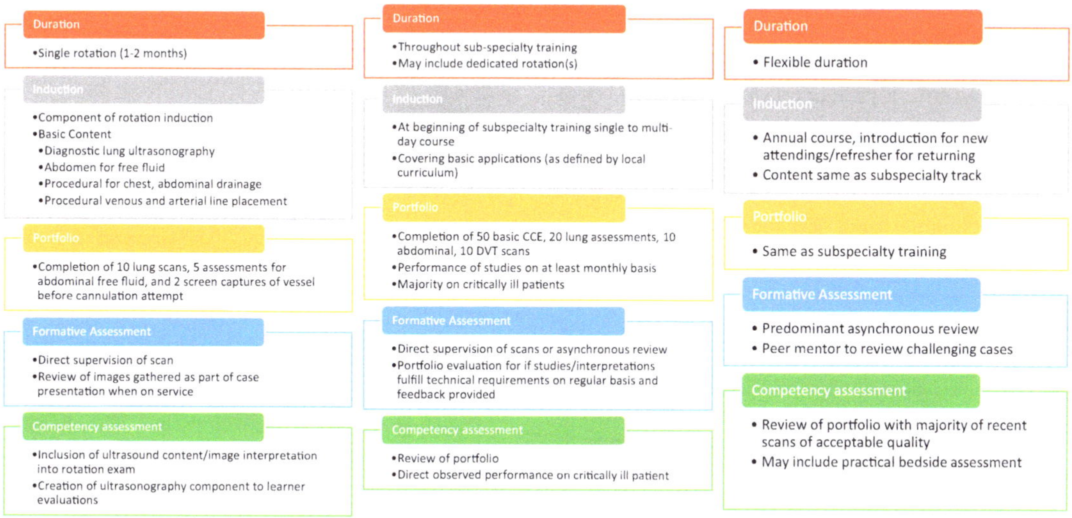

Fig. 64.2 Critical care ultrasound curriculum by learner type

question of competence assessment of whether to perform formalized evaluations versus assessment of study quality asynchronously depends on the resources of the institution and consensus within the department; at minimum, a review of recent portfolio scans should be the basic method for competence assessment and the ability to perform studies without overview by a local expert once deemed to be competent. Combined portfolio review and written testing has been implemented on a large scale mixed academic/community program for attending physicians [45]. The use of a direct OSCE style of assessment may be considered; however, we feel it is less critical at the attending level.

Summary Points

- POCUS curriculum should be taught within a universal framework such as the indication, acquisition, interpretation, and management (I-AIM) model, to build a systematic approach to all CCUS.
- CCUS includes both clinical applications such as focused echocardiography and general ultrasonography including lung, abdominal, vascular, and procedural guidance and physics, machine operation and care, patient consent and privacy, and administration.
- Curriculum design must ultimately follow a longitudinal structure with initial induction, followed by a system of gaining experience and competence assessment.
- A needs assessment should be completed prior to program implementation to identify program administration, technology requirements, educational resources, and trainer availability/ capacity barriers which can render a program unsustainable if not accounted for early.

References

1. Mayo PH, Beaulieu Y, Doelken P, Feller-Kopman D, Harrod C, Kaplan A, et al. American College of Chest Physicians/La Societe de Reanimation de Langue Francaise statement on competence in critical care ultrasonography. Chest. 2009;135(4):1050–60. https://doi.org/10.1378/chest.08-2305.
2. Wong A, Galarza L, Forni L, De Backer D, Slama M, Cholley B, et al. Recommendations for core critical care ultrasound competencies as a part of specialist training in multidisciplinary intensive care: a framework proposed by the European Society of Intensive Care Medicine (ESICM). Crit Care. 2020;24(1):1–6.
3. International consensus statement on training standards for advanced critical care echocardiography. Intensive Care Med. 2014;40(5):654–66. https://doi.org/10.1007/s00134-014-3228-5.
4. International expert statement on training standards for critical care ultrasonography. Intensive Care Med. 2011;37(7):1077–83. https://doi.org/10.1007/s00134-011-2246-9.
5. Critical Care Ultrasonography. https://www.chestnet.org/Learning/certificate-of-completion/Critical-Care-Ultrasonography (2022). Accessed 4 Sept 2022.
6. Panebianco NL, Mayo PH, Arntfield RT, Brown SM, Diaz-Gomez J, Hernandez A, et al. Assessing competence in critical care echocardiography: development and initial results of an examination and certification processes. Crit Care Med. 2021;49(8):1285–92. https://doi.org/10.1097/ccm.0000000000004940.
7. Burleson SL, Pigott DC, Gullett JP, Greene C, Gibson CB, Irvine S, et al. Point-of-care ultrasound in resource-limited settings: the PURLS fellowship. Ultrasound J. 2020;12(1):14. https://doi.org/10.1186/s13089-020-00159-6.
8. Price S, Via G, Sloth E, Guarracino F, Breitkreutz R, Catena E, et al. Echocardiography practice, training and accreditation in the intensive care: document for the World Interactive Network Focused on Critical Ultrasound (WINFOCUS). Cardiovasc Ultrasound. 2008;6(1):49. https://doi.org/10.1186/1476-7120-6-49.
9. Bahner DP, Hughes D, Royall NA. I-AIM: a novel model for teaching and performing focused sonography. J Ultrasound Med. 2012;31(2):295–300. https://doi.org/10.7863/jum.2012.31.2.295.
10. Mayo PH, Beaulieu Y, Doelken P, Feller-Kopman D, Harrod C, Kaplan A, et al. American College of Chest Physicians/La Société de Réanimation de Langue Française statement on competence in critical care ultrasonography. Chest. 2009;135(4):1050–60.
11. Wong A, Galarza L, Forni L, De Backer D, Slama M, Cholley B, et al. Recommendations for core critical care ultrasound competencies as a part of specialist training in multidisciplinary intensive care: a framework proposed by the European Society of Intensive Care Medicine (ESICM). Crit Care. 2020;24(1):393. https://doi.org/10.1186/s13054-020-03099-8.
12. Pustavoitau A, Blaivas M, Brown SM, Gutierrez C, Kirkpatrick AW, Kohl BA, et al. Recommendations for achieving and maintaining competence and credentialing in critical care ultrasound with focused cardiac ultrasound and advanced critical care echocardiography. Crit Care Med. 2016.
13. Atkinson P, Bowra J, Lambert M, Lamprecht H, Noble V, Jarman B. International Federation for Emergency

Medicine point of care ultrasound curriculum. Can J Emerg Med. 2015;17(2):161–70.
14. Doufle G, Roscoe A, Billia F, Fan E. Echocardiography for adult patients supported with extracorporeal membrane oxygenation. Crit Care. 2015;19(1):1–10.
15. Manasia AR, Nagaraj HM, Kodali RB, Croft LB, Oropello JM, Kohli-Seth R, et al. Feasibility and potential clinical utility of goal-directed transthoracic echocardiography performed by noncardiologist intensivists using a small hand-carried device (SonoHeart) in critically ill patients. J Cardiothorac Vasc Anesth. 2005;19(2):155–9.
16. Vignon P, Dugard A, Abraham J, Belcour D, Gondran G, Pepino F, et al. Focused training for goal-oriented hand-held echocardiography performed by noncardiologist residents in the intensive care unit. Intensive Care Med. 2007;33(10):1795–9.
17. Smith B. SonoClipShare. https://www.sonoclipshare.com/ (2016). Accessed 21 Aug 2022.
18. Miller A, Peck M, Clark T, Conway H, Olusanya S, Fletcher N, et al. FUSIC HD. Comprehensive haemodynamic assessment with ultrasound. J Inten Care Soc. 2021;23:17511437211010032.
19. Malbrain ML, De Tavernier B, Haverals S, Slama M, Vieillard-Baron A, Wong A, et al. Executive summary on the use of ultrasound in the critically ill: consensus report from the 3rd Course on Acute Care Ultrasound (CACU). Anaesthesiology intensive therapy. 2017;49(5):393.
20. Akhigbe T. Cognitivism and ultrasound skills in emergency medicine training: from theory to practice. Int J Med Rev. 2018;5(2):47–9. https://doi.org/10.29252/ijmr-050201.
21. Jackson R, Brotherston D, Jain A, Douflé G, Piquette D, Goffi A. Teaching ultrasound at the point of care in times of social distancing. ATS Scholar. 2021;2(3):341–52. https://doi.org/10.34197/ats-scholar.2021-0023PS.
22. Gaudreau-Simard M, Wiskar K, Kilabuk E, Walsh MH, Sattin M, Wong J, et al. An overview of internal medicine point-of-care ultrasound rotations in Canada. Ultrasound J. 2022;14(1):1–6.
23. Senthilnathan M, Kundra P, Mishra S, Velayudhan S, Pillai A. Competence of intensivists in focused transthoracic echocardiography in intensive care unit: a prospective observational study. Indian. J Crit Care Med. 2018;22(5):340.
24. Rajamani A, Galarza L, Sanfilippo F, Wong A, Goffi A, Tuinman P, et al. Criteria, processes, and determination of competence in basic critical care echocardiography training: a Delphi Process Consensus Statement by the Learning Ultrasound in Critical Care (LUCC) initiative. Chest. 2022;161(2):492–503. https://doi.org/10.1016/j.chest.2021.08.077.
25. Kanji HD, McCallum JL, Bhagirath KM, Neitzel AS. Curriculum development and evaluation of a hemodynamic critical care ultrasound: a systematic review of the literature. Crit Care Med. 2016;44(8):e742–e50. https://doi.org/10.1097/ccm.0000000000001661.
26. Townsend NT, Kendall J, Barnett C, Robinson T. An effective curriculum for focused assessment diagnostic echocardiography: establishing the learning curve in surgical residents. J Surg Educ. 2016;73(2):190–6.
27. Vignon P, Mücke F, Bellec F, Marin B, Croce J, Brouqui T, et al. Basic critical care echocardiography: validation of a curriculum dedicated to noncardiologist residents. Crit Care Med. 2011;39(4):636–42.
28. Cheng J, Arntfield R. Training strategies for point of care ultrasound in the ICU. Curr Opin Anesthesiol. 2021;34(5):654–8. https://doi.org/10.1097/aco.0000000000001042.
29. Mateer J, Plummer D, Heller M, Olson D, Jehle D, Overton D, et al. Model curriculum for physician training in emergency ultrasonography. Ann Emerg Med. 1994;23(1):95–102.
30. American College of Emergency Physicians Ultrasound guidelines: emergency, point-of-care and clinical ultrasound guidelines in medicine. Ann Emerg Med. 2017;69(5):e27–54.
31. Arntfield R, Millington S, Ainsworth C, Arora R, Boyd J, Finlayson G, et al. Canadian recommendations for critical care ultrasound training and competency. Can Respir J. 2014;21(6):341–5. https://doi.org/10.1155/2014/216591. 16339 [pii].
32. Chisholm CB, Dodge WR, Balise RR, Williams SR, Gharahbaghian L, Beraud A-S. Focused cardiac ultrasound training: how much is enough? J Emerg Med. 2013;44(4):818–22. https://doi.org/10.1016/j.jemermed.2012.07.092.
33. Reid G, Bedford J, Attwood B. Bridging the logistical gap between ultrasound enthusiasm and accreditation. J Intens Care Soc. 2018;19(1):15–8.
34. Arntfield RT. The utility of remote supervision with feedback as a method to deliver high-volume critical care ultrasound training. J Crit Care. 2015;30(2):441, e1–e6.
35. Butterfly TeleGuidance™ Beta: Remote ultrasound made simple. https://www.butterflynetwork.com/teleguidance (2022). Accessed 7 July 2022.
36. Beraud A-S, Rizk NW, Pearl RG, Liang DH, Patterson AJ. Focused transthoracic echocardiography during critical care medicine training: curriculum implementation and evaluation of proficiency. Crit Care Med. 2013;41(8):e179–e81.
37. Budhram G, Elia T, Rathlev N. Implementation of a successful incentive-based ultrasound credentialing program for emergency physicians. Western J Emerg Med. 2013;14(6):602.
38. Soni NJ, Nathanson R, Andreae M, Khosla R, Vadamalai K, Kode K, et al. Development of a multisystem point of care ultrasound skills assessment checklist. Ultrasound J. 2022;14(1):17. https://doi.org/10.1186/s13089-022-00268-4.
39. Desy J, Noble VE, Liteplo AS, Olszynski P, Buchanan B, Dversdal R, et al. Minimal criteria for lung ultraso-

nography in internal medicine. Can J Gen Intern Med. 2021;16(2):6–13.
40. Millington SJ, Arntfield RT, Hewak M, Hamstra SJ, Beaulieu Y, Hibbert B, et al. The rapid assessment of competency in echocardiography scale. J Ultrasound Med. 2016;35(7):1457–63. https://doi.org/10.7863/ultra.15.07083.
41. Millington SJ, Arntfield RT, Guo RJ, Koenig S, Kory P, Noble V, et al. The Assessment of Competency in Thoracic Sonography (ACTS) scale: validation of a tool for point-of-care ultrasound. Crit Ultrasound J. 2017;9(1):25. https://doi.org/10.1186/s13089-017-0081-0.
42. Ma IWY, Desy J, Woo MY, Kirkpatrick AW, Noble VE. Consensus-based expert development of critical items for direct observation of point-of-care ultrasound skills. J Grad Med Educ. 2020;12(2):176–84. https://doi.org/10.4300/jgme-d-19-00531.1.
43. Robba C, Wong A, Poole D, Al Tayar A, Arntfield RT, Chew MS, et al. Basic ultrasound head-to-toe skills for intensivists in the general and neuro intensive care unit population: consensus and expert recommendations of the European Society of Intensive Care Medicine. Intensive Care Med. 2021;47(12):1347–67.
44. Ultrasound guidelines: emergency, point-of-care and clinical ultrasound Guidelines in medicine. Ann Emerg Med. 2017;69(5):e27–54. https://doi.org/10.1016/j.annemergmed.2016.08.457.
45. Russell FM, Kennedy SK, Rood LK, Nti B, Herbert A, Rutz MA, et al. Design and implementation of a basic and global point of care ultrasound (POCUS) certification curriculum for emergency medicine faculty. Ultrasound J. 2022;14(1):10. https://doi.org/10.1186/s13089-022-00260-y.
46. Bell C, Wagner N, Hall A, Newbigging J, Rang L, McKaigney C. The ultrasound competency assessment tool for four-view cardiac POCUS. Ultrasound J. 2021;13(1):42. https://doi.org/10.1186/s13089-021-00237-3.
47. Adamson R, Morris AE, Sun Woan J, Ma IW, Schnobrich D, Soni NJ. Development of a focused cardiac ultrasound image acquisition assessment tool. ATS Scholar. 2020;1(3):260–77.
48. Nielsen DG, Gotzsche O, Eika B. Objective structured assessment of technical competence in transthoracic echocardiography: a validity study in a standardised setting. BMC Med Educ. 2013;13(1):1–10.
49. Patrawalla P, Eisen LA, Shiloh A, Shah BJ, Savenkov O, Wise W, et al. Development and validation of an assessment tool for competency in critical care ultrasound. J Grad Med Educ. 2015;7(4):567–73.
50. Tolsgaard MG, Todsen T, Sorensen JL, Ringsted C, Lorentzen T, Ottesen B, et al. International multispecialty consensus on how to evaluate ultrasound competence: a Delphi consensus survey. PLoS One. 2013;8(2):e57687.
51. Díaz-Gómez JL, Frankel HL, Hernandez A. National certification in critical care echocardiography: its time has come. Crit Care Med. 2017;45(11):1801–4.
52. Mayo PH, Koenig S. Advanced critical care echocardiography certification: an update. Chest. 2020;158(1):48–9.
53. Nelson BP, Hojsak J, Dei Rossi E, Karani R, Narula J. Seeing is believing: evaluating a point-of-care ultrasound curriculum for 1st-year medical students. Teach Learn Med. 2017;29(1):85–92. https://doi.org/10.1080/10401334.2016.1172012.

Near-Peer Education in Point-of-Care Ultrasound

65

Deepak Pradhan and Jordan Talan

Learning Objectives

1. Describe near-peer education strategies.
2. Examine the evidence for utilizing near-peer education.
3. Determine best practices for near-peer education.

Theory Behind Near-Peer Education

Near-peer education (NPE) is an effective and resource-efficient strategy that can be utilized to teach complex skills such as point-of-care ultrasound (POCUS). NPE refers to a senior student or trainee who has recently mastered a particular skill teaching it to someone more junior in status [1]. The senior near-peer teacher (NPT) and the junior near-peer learner (NPL) are separated by an "educational distance", and their interaction results in mutual benefit [2, 3]. There is cognitive congruence between the NPT and NPL as the former has recently learned the topical material and is therefore better able to relate the micro-steps necessary for a junior learner to progress towards successful adoption [4]. The NPT shares with the NPL similar cognitive schema and can more easily see the learner's zone of proximal development and help them scaffold new information onto their existing capabilities [5]. Social congruence also facilitates learning outcomes, as the junior learner fosters less anxiety and stress learning from someone less separated in educational distance and is more apt to ask questions without fear over evaluation and grading. Additionally, the NPT also gains educational benefits. They are motivated to conduct a successful teaching session, which leads to a second "bite of the apple" to relearn and reprocess previously learned material, improve on their teaching skills, and advance their professional identity as a content expert and educator [6]. Of note, while originally conceived as teaching from senior teacher to junior learner, this teaching strategy can also be utilized in situations with "reverse educational distance", where a junior teacher teaches a more senior audience [7]. While examples of successful near-peer educational initiatives abound in the literature, there are also excellent practical guides available to use for crafting a trainee-as-teacher curriculum [8, 9].

D. Pradhan (✉) · J. Talan
New York University Grossman School of Medicine, New York, NY, USA
e-mail: deepak.pradhan@nyulangone.org; jordan.talan@nyulangone.org

M. J. Lanspa, A. T. Levinson (eds.), *Echocardiography and Ultrasonography in the ICU*, Respiratory Medicine, https://doi.org/10.1007/978-3-031-80038-2_65

NPE in POCUS: Learners and Content

The vast majority of the literature on NPE in POCUS is focused within the undergraduate medical education (UME) setting. Approximately 25% of United States medical schools lack a specific ultrasound curriculum, and NPE is a response to growing interest among medical students and a perceived need for exposure to POCUS prior to entering residency [10, 11]. However, research in near-peer POCUS education in UME is not limited to the United States, and several international publications have emerged from Germany [12–16], Switzerland [11, 17, 18], Italy [19], and Spain [20]. Topics of instruction are primarily anatomical (including the identification of abdominal and pelvic structures) and echocardiographic, but have also included musculoskeletal ultrasound, lung ultrasound, and the use of various protocols including FAST [14, 21] and RUSH [22]. Although often no particular educational design methodology is specified, NPE is widely versatile and compatible with multiple design models including Kern's 6-Step approach to curriculum development and Peyton's 4-step teaching approach [14, 23]. In addition, NPE has shown promise in educational ultrasound studies involving various learner populations including the graduate medical education (GME) setting among radiology and physiatry residents [24, 25] as well as with physician assistant students [22], and even eighth-grade middle school students [21]. Despite this literature, NPE remains relatively unexplored in certain learning settings such as continuing medical education (CME), and many ultrasound examinations and protocols remain uncharacterized in this approach. It is also important to note that available research on NPE in POCUS is limited by heterogeneity of study populations, varying study methodologies, and a lack of validation in the assessment of learning outcomes. NPE therefore remains an emerging modality in POCUS education.

NPE in POCUS: Effectiveness, Enjoyability, and Efficiency

NPE as an instructional strategy offers many benefits when applied to POCUS. When evaluating the benefit of any instructional program, it is often helpful to consider three aspects:

- Effectiveness (Do the learners successfully learn?)
- Satisfaction (Do learners enjoy the program?)
- Efficiency (Does the program utilize an appropriate amount of resources?)

Regarding effectiveness, multiple studies have shown NPE to improve subjective learning outcomes including self-reported confidence and competence in POCUS skills [22, 24, 26–28]. In terms of more objective outcomes, NPE has led to improvement in tests of POCUS knowledge on multiple choice tests and image recognition assessments [23, 29–31]. Several studies have also evaluated practical performance in POCUS after an NPE teaching intervention through checklist scores or Objective Structured Clinical Examinations (OSCE). The overwhelming majority of evidence supports improved practical POCUS performance using NPE in comparison to no curriculum or pre-intervention scores [20, 23, 32–34]. Some studies also suggest that NPE is superior or non-inferior to traditional faculty teaching [29, 35], whereas other studies contest this finding [16, 36]. Data on skill retention using NPE are limited [31, 32].

Regarding satisfaction, the existing data are more mixed. Several studies comment on a general "acceptance" or positive ratings of the learner experience with NPE [14, 19, 27]. Other studies report that near-peer teaching was rated as "well-delivered" or that the peer instructors were perceived as "competent" [26, 37]. On the other hand, in some studies, students reported either perceiving faculty teachers as more competent than peer teachers [29] or a preference for faculty teaching [23]. Despite these data, evidence regarding satisfaction with NPE in POCUS is severely limited by heterogeneity of study setting, methodology, and the degree of NPT training. In the absence of generalizable data, an educational designer considering NPE of POCUS would benefit from analyzing the perceptions of NPE among stakeholders in their own educational setting.

Regarding efficiency, establishing an NPE program requires significant resource investment including time for curricular (re)design and the continuous recruitment and training of NPTs [13]. Conversely, however, NPE can also help to conserve faculty resources, reducing overall faculty teaching time while increasing capacity for exposure to the curriculum [10, 38]. NPE also has several other advantages in terms of efficiency. For example, while NPTs educate the learner population, they simultaneously improve their own teaching skills and mastery of the content [27, 38]. As an additional efficiency outcome, one study from an emergency department in Arizona reported increased billing of ultrasound examinations after a near-peer teaching intervention and revenue from POCUS billing increased significantly [39].

NPE in POCUS: Examples of Success

NPE is currently utilized in several POCUS curricula globally, and there is much to learn from the design and implementation of these programs. For example, peer-teaching is highly valued in the German-speaking medical education community, where in one study 26 out of 28 surveyed medical faculties offered undergraduate ultrasound courses and 24 out of the 26 found peer-teaching to be important in conveying ultrasound skills [15]. At Saarland University in Germany, an undergraduate elective course called "*sonoBYstudents*" has been successfully implemented for over 5 years. In this NPE concept, abdominal and emergency POCUS as well as echocardiography is taught to a total of 90 students per semester, and over the history of the program, over 30 student tutors have been trained. After each semester, 10–12 new tutors are recruited from the student population and receive a special skill and didactic session before offering their own teaching. The elective is split into small groups of 5 students with each NPT for 90-min sessions weekly over 8 weeks [13]. With some small adjustment to group size and use of an online didactic component, the program has safely and successfully continued through the COVID-19 pandemic, allowing education leaders to avoid restarting from scratch in the recruitment and training of student tutors.

Touro University College of Osteopathic Medicine in California began staged development of their undergraduate ultrasound curriculum in the 2011–2012 academic year with only one ultrasound machine and a supervising radiologist. As the program expanded to a longitudinal curriculum over all 4 years of medical school, there became a need for peer educators. NPTs were recruited either as third or fourth-year students participating in a 2- or 4-week radiology elective or as second year students with a particular ultrasound interest who were responsible for working with trainers asynchronously to develop sufficient expertise to teach. All NPTs were approved by the course supervisor, a board-certified radiology professor. It was found most efficient to train NPTs in group sessions and estimated that it required approximately 2 h of training before they were ready to teach any particular session. By 2018, the program had 4–10 NPTs at any given time and was able to offer a 1:8 student-to-educator ratio in the ultrasound curriculum without hiring any additional faculty [40].

The University of North Carolina School of Medicine developed the first ultrasound scholarly concentration track offered to medical students in the United States. The program was initiated and sustained by students and relies heavily on the benefits of NPE. Rising second-year students complete a 3-credit asynchronous and completely virtual *Ultrasound Fundamentals* course and are provided with a handheld ultrasound probe to complete scanning assignments. During the third and fourth year of medical school, students maintain a longitudinal scan portfolio, present at and attend monthly ultrasound case conferences, and practice near-peer teaching. The completion of the program requires a final scholarly ultrasound project. As of July 2021, there were 12 students enrolled from the class of 2023 and 10 from the class of 2024 [10].

Aside from these specific examples in the UME setting, NPE for POCUS has been extensively used in other settings as well. For example, in the GME setting, a 2021 survey of scholarly tracks in emergency medicine residency found that of 57 programs with POCUS tracks, approximately 84% require participants to present at least one POCUS lecture and 79% require residents to instruct hands-on POCUS workshops [41]. NPE is also a prominent strategy at the CME level. For example, in a study of practicing anesthesiologists in Ontario, roughly 67% of anesthesiologists practicing in academic hospitals and 46% practicing in community hospitals reported receiving peer-to-peer ultrasound training. For both groups, NPE was the most preferred method of improving ultrasound skills [42].

NPE in POCUS: Practical Guidance for Successful Implementation

Despite the theoretical underpinnings and literature of successful application to POCUS, NPE like any teaching strategy can result in suboptimal outcomes if poorly implemented. Here is some practical guidance to help foster success and avoid potential pitfalls emanating from review of the literature as well as our personal experience utilizing NPE in POCUS for many years.

First, ask "*Why are you using NPE?*" Acceptable answers include absence of sufficient faculty educators, in hopes of improving the performance and teaching skills of trainee teachers, or to motivate both NPTs and NPLs. If you have the available resources, consider using some local experts as well, as the combination can serve as a valuable expert support for both the learners and teachers, and foster a more collaborative educational environment ("best of both worlds").

Second, buy-in from both teachers and learners is of paramount importance to successful implementation. NPTs need to be motivated to engage passionately in the teaching effort, while NPLs need to embrace being taught by NPTs. Both groups need to understand the potential benefits of the NPE approach, as well as the time commitments. Make the case for the importance of NPE to training program leadership as well, for both protected time for teachers and for funding as needed. We often highlight that such innovative teaching methods are favorably viewed by trainees and can be a recruitment tool for future applicants. Also, do not be afraid to utilize NPTs from different disciplines, as they can enrich the learning environment through unique experiences and perspectives.

Third, preparation of NPTs, i.e., "train the trainers", is crucial to success. You must ensure that the NPT is competent in the relevant US knowledge, image acquisition, and image interpretation skills demanded by the course. We meet with new NPTs ahead of training sessions to discuss US concepts as well as specific US learning tasks/objectives for the course. Also, we will often pre-scan with them prior to the teaching session to improve their performance and foster their confidence. In addition to preparation as a content expert, they must also be prepared for being a teacher. This includes guidance on navigating logistical issues, answering questions, and resolving conflicts. One of our strategies is to observe novice NPTs during their teaching sessions and provide them with formative feedback post-session with the goal of improving their subsequent teaching skills. This up-front effort entailed to train NPTs is a valuable investment, particularly if you are to reuse NPTs longitudinally over time, as a strong foundation for a sustained NPE POCUS program.

Fourth, support the NPTs during the teaching session. Spend a few minutes at the beginning of the session creating a "safe environment" where everyone is valued, questions are encouraged, and mistakes are welcome. During the session, the NPT should not feel isolated. Consider pairing novice NPTs with a more seasoned NPT or a local expert initially. Questions that the NPT is unable to answer should be "parked" for later discussion potentially by a local expert. This way, the NPT is not stressed and at the same time the learners know their questions will be ultimately answered (thus mitigating some of the knowledge gap between NPTs and expert faculty).

Fifth, teaching is great but learning is better. Assess your POCUS program periodically to understand if it is resulting in intended learning outcomes [43]. This includes NPL assessment through OSCEs, MCTs, confidence-based surveys, performance logs, and/or portfolio review. Obtain feedback from NPTs and NPLs to better understand what is working and what needs improvement. You will not get it right the first time, but you can make it progressively better if you listen to programmatic feedback and outcomes.

Overall, NPE in POCUS has great potential downstream benefits–the ability for reproducibility across institutions, scalability to larger learner groups, and the sustainability of a longitudinal educational model.

Summary Points

- Near-peer education is an effective teaching strategy to facilitate transfer of complex skills between NPTs and NPLs, with theoretical and practical benefits to both groups.
- Near-peer education in POCUS has been used internationally, at the UME and GME levels, to teach a variety of POCUS examinations.
- Literature on NPE in POCUS has generally demonstrated effectiveness, learner satisfaction, and efficiency using this method, with caveats that we have highlighted.
- Successful implementation of NPE with POCUS requires buy-in from relevant stakeholders, preparation of NPTs in content and teaching skills, support of NPTs during teaching sessions, and attention to learner and programmatic assessment for iterative change.

References

1. Whitman NA. Peer teaching: to teach is to learn twice, ASHE-ERIC Higher Education. Washington DC: ERIC Clearinghouse on Higher Education; 1988.
2. Ten Cate O, Durning S. Dimensions and psychology of peer teaching in medical education. Med Teach. 2007;29(6):546–52. https://doi.org/10.1080/01421590701583816.
3. Ten Cate O, Durning S. Peer teaching in medical education: twelve reasons to move from theory to practice. Med Teach. 2007;29:591–9. https://doi.org/10.1080/01421590701606799.
4. Lockspeiser TM, O'Sullivan P, Teherani A, Muller J. Understanding the experience of being taught by peers: the value of social and cognitive congruence. Adv Health Sci Educ Theory Pract. 2008;13(3):361–72. https://doi.org/10.1007/s10459-006-9049-8.
5. Vygotskiy LS, Cole M. Mind in society: the development of higher psychological processes. Cambridge: Harvard Univ. Press; 1978.
6. Hall S, Harrison CH, Stephens J, Andrade MG, Seaby EG, Parton W, et al. The benefits of being a near-peer teacher. Clin Teach. 2018;15(5):403–7. https://doi.org/10.1111/tct.12784.
7. Ruano Cea E, Constantin E, Thomas A. Reverse educational distance: exploring a novel concept to enhance resident-as-teacher curricula. Med Teach. 2019;41(7):773–9. https://doi.org/10.1080/0142159X.2019.1578875. Epub 2019 Apr 16. PMID: 30990734.
8. Ramani S, Mann K, Taylor D, Thampy H. Residents as teachers: near peer learning in clinical work settings: AMEE Guide No. 106. Med Teach. 2016;38(7):642–55. https://doi.org/10.3109/0142159x.2016.1147540.
9. Messman A, Kryzaniak SM, Alden S, Pasirstein MJ, Chan TM. Recommendations for the development and implementation of a residents as teachers curriculum. Cureus. 2018;10(7):e3053. https://doi.org/10.7759/cureus.3053. PMID: 30276032; PMCID: PMC6160295.
10. Bacon DR, Cowles K, Thapa D, White A, Allen AJ, Doughton J, Beck Dallaghan G, Jordan SG. Creating an ultrasound scholarly concentration program for medical students. Adv Med Educ Pract. 2021;12:1103–10. https://doi.org/10.2147/AMEP.S330771. PMID: 34594147; PMCID: PMC8478088.
11. Hari R, Kälin K, Harris M, Walter R, Serra A. Comparing blended learning with faculty-led ultrasound training: protocol for a randomised controlled trial (the SIGNATURE trial). Praxis (Bern 1994).

2020;109(8):636–40. https://doi.org/10.1024/1661-8157/a003497. PMID: 32517596.
12. Celebi N, Zwirner K, Lischner U, Bauder M, Ditthard K, Schürger S, Riessen R, Engel C, Balletshofer B, Weyrich P. Student tutors are able to teach basic sonographic anatomy effectively – a prospective randomized controlled trial. Ultraschall Med. 2012;33(2):141–5. https://doi.org/10.1055/s--0029-1245837. Epub 2010 Nov 23. PMID: 21104601.
13. Nourkami-Tutdibi N, Hofer M, Zemlin M, Abdul-Khaliq H, Tutdibi E. TEACHING MUST GO ON: flexibility and advantages of peer assisted learning during the COVID-19 pandemic for undergraduate medical ultrasound education—perspective from the "sonoBYstudents" ultrasound group. GMS. J Med Educ. 2021;38(1):Doc5. https://doi.org/10.3205/zma001401. PMID: 33659610; PMCID: PMC7899109.
14. Celebi N, Griewatz J, Malek NP, Krieg S, Kuehnl T, Muller R, Pauluschke-Fröhlich J, Debove I, Riessen R, Zipfel S, Fröhlich E. Development and implementation of a comprehensive ultrasound curriculum for undergraduate medical students – a feasibility study. BMC Med Educ. 2019;19(1):170. https://doi.org/10.1186/s12909-019-1611-1. PMID: 31138197; PMCID: PMC6537195.
15. Wolf R, Geuthel N, Gnatzy F, Rotzoll D. Undergraduate ultrasound education at German-speaking medical faculties: a survey. GMS. J Med Educ. 2019;36(4):Doc34. https://doi.org/10.3205/zma001242. PMID: 31544134; PMCID: PMC6737263.
16. Kühl M, Wagner R, Bauder M, Fenik Y, Riessen R, Lammerding-Köppel M, Gawaz M, Fateh-Moghadam S, Weyrich P, Celebi N. Student tutors for hands-on training in focused emergency echocardiography – a randomized controlled trial. BMC Med Educ. 2012;12:101. https://doi.org/10.1186/1472-6920-12-101. PMID: 23107588; PMCID: PMC3532362.
17. Kaymak D, Räschle N, Serra A, Hari R. Einführung eines "Peer Tutoring" -basierten, Ultraschallkurses—ein Update zum "Blended-Learning" – Basiskurs Sonografie [Introduction of an ultrasound course based on peer-tutoring – an update on the blended learning basic course sonography]. Praxis (Bern 1994). 2020;109(8):577–82. https://doi.org/10.1024/1661-8157/a003494. German. PMID: 32517604.
18. Räschle N, Hari R. "Blended learning" – Basiskurs Sonografie [Blended learning basic course sonography – a SGUM accredited ultrasound course based on peer-tutoring]. Praxis (Bern 1994). 2018;107(23):1255–9. https://doi.org/10.1024/1661-8157/a003116. German. PMID: 30424697.
19. Serrao G, Tassoni M, Magenta-Biasina AM, Mantero AG, Previtera A, Turci MC, Biganzoli EM, Bertolini EAM. Virtual dissection by ultrasound: probe handling in the first year of medical education. Ultrasound Int Open. 2017;3(4):E156–62. https://doi.org/10.1055/s--0043-121983. Epub 2017 Dec 7. PMID: 29226274; PMCID: PMC5721288.
20. García de Casasola Sánchez G, González Peinado D, Sánchez Gollarte A, Muñoz Aceituno E, Peña Vázquez I, Torres Macho J. Teaching of clinical ultrasonography to undergraduates: students as mentors. Rev Clin Esp (Barc). 2015;215(4):211–6. https://doi.org/10.1016/j.rce.2014.11.023. Epub 2015 Jan 10. PMID: 25583252. English, Spanish.
21. Kwon AS, Lahham S, Fox JC. Can an 8th grade student learn point of care ultrasound? World J Emerg Med. 2019;10(2):109–13. https://doi.org/10.5847/wjem.j.1920-8642.2019.02.007. PMID: 30687447; PMCID: PMC6340824.
22. Garvick S, Smith I, Carter J, El Tannir Z, Gentile A, Jones G, Rogers L, Gillette C. Impact of peer-assisted learning on ultrasound. J Physician Assist Educ. 2021;32(4):253–6. https://doi.org/10.1097/JPA.0000000000000392. PMID: 34817430.
23. Gradl-Dietsch G, Menon AK, Gürsel A, Götzenich A, Hatam N, Aljalloud A, Schrading S, Hölzl F, Knobe M. Basic echocardiography for undergraduate students: a comparison of different peer-teaching approaches. Eur J Trauma Emerg Surg. 2018;44(1):143–52. https://doi.org/10.1007/s00068-017-0819-1. Epub 2017 Jul 17. PMID: 28717985.
24. Berko NS, Le JN, Thornhill BA, Wang D, Negassa A, Amis ES Jr, Koenigsberg M. Design and validation of a peer-teacher-based musculoskeletal ultrasound curriculum. Acad Radiol. 2019;26(5):701–6. https://doi.org/10.1016/j.acra.2018.09.001. Epub 2018 Sep 19. PMID: 30243892.
25. Luz J, Siddiqui I, Jain NB, Kohler MJ, Donovan J, Gerrard P, Borg-Stein J. Resident-perceived benefit of a diagnostic and interventional musculoskeletal ultrasound curriculum: a multifaceted approach using independent study, peer teaching, and interdisciplinary collaboration. Am J Phys Med Rehabil. 2015;94(12):1095–103. https://doi.org/10.1097/PHM.0000000000000337. PMID: 26098924; PMCID: PMC4710470.
26. Dickerson J, Paul K, Vila P, Whiticar R. The role for peer-assisted ultrasound teaching in medical school. Clin Teach. 2017;14(3):170–4. https://doi.org/10.1111/tct.12541. Epub 2016 Jun 27. PMID: 27350650.
27. Naeger DM, Conrad M, Nguyen J, Kohi MP, Webb EM. Students teaching students: evaluation of a "near-peer" teaching experience. Acad Radiol. 2013;20(9):1177–82. https://doi.org/10.1016/j.acra.2013.04.004. Epub 2013 Jun 28. PMID: 23810649.
28. Goodcoff A, Keane D, Bialczak A, Ziner E, Hanna JB. Point-of-care ultrasonography integration in undergraduate medical education: a student-driven approach. J Am Osteopath Assoc. 2019;119(3):e11–6. https://doi.org/10.7556/jaoa.2019.033. PMID: 30801119.

29. Knobe M, Münker R, Sellei RM, Holschen M, Mooij SC, Schmidt-Rohlfing B, Niethard FU, Pape HC. Peer teaching: a randomised controlled trial using student-teachers to teach musculoskeletal ultrasound. Med Educ. 2010;44(2):148–55. https://doi.org/10.1111/j.1365-2923.2009.03557.x. Epub 2009 Dec 21. PMID: 20040056.
30. Cremerius C, Gradl-Dietsch G, Beeres FJP, Link B, Hitpaß L, Nebelung S, Horst K, Weber CD, Neuerburg C, Eschbach D, Bliemel C, Knobe M. Team-based learning for teaching musculoskeletal ultrasound skills: a prospective randomised trial. Eur J Trauma Emerg Surg. 2021;47(4):1189–99. https://doi.org/10.1007/s00068-019-01298-9. Epub 2020 Jan 10. PMID: 31925451.
31. Jeppesen KM, Bahner DP. Teaching bedside sonography using peer mentoring: a prospective randomized trial. J Ultrasound Med. 2012;31(3):455–9. https://doi.org/10.7863/jum.2012.31.3.455. PMID: 22368136.
32. Nourkami-Tutdibi N, Tutdibi E, Schmidt S, Zemlin M, Abdul-Khaliq H, Hofer M. Long-term knowledge retention after peer-assisted abdominal ultrasound teaching: is PAL a successful model for achieving knowledge retention? Ultraschall Med. 2020;41(1):36–43. https://doi.org/10.1055/a--1034-7749. English. Epub 2019 Nov 19. PMID: 31745964.
33. Garcia-Casasola G, Sánchez FJ, Luordo D, Zapata DF, Frías MC, Garrido VV, Martínez JV, de la Sotilla AF, Rojo JM, Macho JT. Basic abdominal point-of-care ultrasound training in the undergraduate: students as mentors. J Ultrasound Med. 2016;35(11):2483–9. https://doi.org/10.7863/ultra.15.11068. Epub 2016 Oct 13. PMID: 27738292.
34. Arias Felipe A, Doménech García J, Sánchez Los Arcos I, Luordo D, García Sánchez FJ, Villanueva Martínez J, Forero de la Sotilla A, Villena Garrido V, Torres Macho J, García de Casasola Sánchez G. Teaching the basics of echocardiography in the undergraduate: Students as mentors. Rev Clin Esp (Barc). 2017;217(5):245–51. https://doi.org/10.1016/j.rce.2017.02.006. English. Spanish. Epub 2017 Mar 15. PMID: 28318521.
35. Ben-Sasson A, Lior Y, Krispel J, Rucham M, Liel-Cohen N, Fuchs L, Kobal SL. Peer-teaching cardiac ultrasound among medical students: a real option. PLoS One. 2019;14(3):e0212794. https://doi.org/10.1371/journal.pone.0212794. PMID: 30917143; PMCID: PMC6436682.
36. Knobe M, Sellei RM, Maus U, Mooij SC, Gradl G, Sopka S, Niethard FU, Pape HC. Kurrikulare Ultraschallausbildung am Bewegungsapparat: Einfluss der anatomischen Vorbildung auf die Weitergabe von Basis-Skills an der Schulter [Undergraduate curricular training in musculoskeletal ultrasound: the impact of preexisting anatomic knowledge]. Z Orthop Unfall. 2010;148(6):685–90. https://doi.org/10.1055/s-0030-1250378. German. Epub 2010 Oct 12. PMID: 20941690.
37. Ahn JS, French AJ, Thiessen ME, Kendall JL. Training peer instructors for a combined ultrasound/physical exam curriculum. Teach Learn Med. 2014;26(3):292–5. https://doi.org/10.1080/10401334.2014.910464. PMID: 25010242.
38. Jeker L, Birrenbach T, Walter R, Hari R. Peer-Teaching in der Ultraschall-Ausbildung—Eine Übersichtsarbeit [Peer teaching in ultrasound education – a narrative review]. Praxis (Bern 1994). 2020;109(8):631–5. https://doi.org/10.1024/1661-8157/a003498. German. PMID: 32517595.
39. Adhikari S, Fiorello A. Emergency ultrasound fellowship training: a novel team-based approach. J Ultrasound Med. 2014;33(10):1821–6. https://doi.org/10.7863/ultra.33.10.1821. PMID: 25253829.
40. Hendriksz T, Markman Z, Pera A. An Education in Osteopathic Ultrasonography (AEIOU) program: one Institution's approach to advancing an ultrasonography curriculum. J Am Osteopath Assoc. 2018;118(11):746–52. https://doi.org/10.7556/jaoa.2018.160. PMID: 30398572.
41. Alerhand S, Situ-Lacasse E, Ramdin C, Gottlieb M. National survey of point-of-care ultrasound scholarly tracks in emergency medicine residency programs. West J Emerg Med. 2021;22(5):1095–101. https://doi.org/10.5811/westjem.2021.5.52118. PMID: 34546885; PMCID: PMC8463042.
42. Matava C, Hayes J. A survey of ultrasound use by academic and community anesthesiologists in Ontario. Can J Anaesth. 2011;58(10):929–35. https://doi.org/10.1007/s12630-011-9555-x. Epub 2011 Jul 12. PMID: 21748662.
43. Van Der Vleuten CPM, Schuwirth LWT, Driessen EW, Govaerts MJB, Heeneman S. Twelve tips for programmatic assessment. Med Teach. 2015;37(7):641–6. https://doi.org/10.3109/0142159X.2014.973388. Epub 2014 Nov 20. PMID: 25410481.

Utilization of Echocardiographic Labs

66

James N. Kirkpatrick and Vidhushei Yogeswaran

Learning Objectives

1. Describe the different learning components of the echocardiographic laboratory.
2. Examine educational limitations for learning the echocardiographic laboratory for critical care trainees.

Introduction

The echocardiographic laboratory is an important source of learning for critical care practitioners planning to further their ultrasonographic skills. The echocardiographic laboratory has four main components: the physical laboratory location, equipment, sonographers, and cardiologists. Many laboratories host a range of physician and sonographer trainees. Echocardiographic examinations are performed by either a fully trained cardiac sonographer under the supervision of a physician, or a physician who has obtained training in independently performing echocardiograms [1], depending on the country or region. The Intersocietal Accreditation Commission (IAC) serves as the national accrediting organization for echocardiographic laboratories in the United States [2].

A critical care clinician working towards advancing pivotal skills in critical care echocardiography (CCE) must identify individual trainee goals. While some trainees will be focused on identifying and interpreting basic cardiac views to make rapid diagnoses in urgent or emergent settings, others will require a wider skillset. The American Society of Echocardiography (ASE) suggests a framework for different levels and durations of training, from Ultrasound Assisted Physician Examination (weeks) to CCE (months) [3]. In addition to critical care and emergency medicine ultrasound training program trainers, echocardiographic laboratory staff can work with CCE trainees towards their echocardiography goals.

Sonographers as Teachers

In countries where sonographers perform echocardiographic examinations, the cardiac sonographer's primary role in the laboratory is to obtain high quality cardiac echocardiographic images, using their understanding of the ultrasound principles, equipment, and cardiovascular pathophysiology. Sonographers learn their craft in specialized training programs that include an internship and are credentialed within 2-years of

The original version of the chapter has been revised. A correction to this chapter can be found at https://doi.org/10.1007/978-3-031-80038-2_74

J. N. Kirkpatrick (✉) · V. Yogeswaran
Division of Cardiology, University of Washington School of Medicine, Seattle, WA, USA
e-mail: kirkpatj@cardiology.washington.edu; vyoges@uw.edu

M. J. Lanspa, A. T. Levinson (eds.), *Echocardiography and Ultrasonography in the ICU*, Respiratory Medicine, https://doi.org/10.1007/978-3-031-80038-2_66

the start of employment. Sonographers maintain credentials through continuing education. Additionally, sonographers must adopt the specific protocols and procedures of individual laboratories [4]. The IAC requires that individual laboratories assess sonographer's exam completeness and image quality at quality assurance meetings [2].

Image acquisition in echocardiography is one of the most challenging steps for new trainees, and sonographers can play a key role in teaching scanning skills. The challenge in obtaining adequate cardiac images is multifactorial, involving hand-eye coordination and machine control setting, at a minimum. Observing sonographers is an important step in working towards competency in ultrasonography, but there is no substitute for performing proctored examinations. As scanning experts, many experienced sonographers can provide direction in probe positioning, machine setting optimization, identification of artifacts, and recognition of quality images. This is especially important in CCE, where goal-directed ultrasound examinations can be a useful initial test but are often technically challenging due to lung interference, mechanical ventilation, positioning, and situational urgency [5].

It should be noted that sonographers often use different ultrasound imaging systems than those that may be available in the critical care setting. Small portable or laptop-sized machines are generally simpler in terms of available settings and ability to optimize images. They usually lack the same quality of 2D image and color Doppler and may lack spectral Doppler entirely. Sonographers may not be familiar with these machines and therefore may not be an optimal resource for training in CCE instrumentation. Cardiac sonographers increasingly employ imaging techniques that are beyond the scope of CCE training (as well as machine capabilities), such as advanced Doppler quantification, speckle-tracking strain, and 3D echocardiography. Conversely, they may be unfamiliar with important extra-cardiac aspects of critical care ultrasound imaging, such as lung ultrasound examinations. Even though critical care trainees should recognize differences of their training and machines vis-à-vis those of sonographers, and despite the fact that suboptimal images are common in light of the exigencies of the critical care setting, trainees must be able to recognize high quality images as a standard to approximate.

Cardiologists as Teachers

In addition to sonographers, different levels of physicians in the echocardiographic laboratory can work with critical care trainees on a variety of different skills. Some physicians may teach scanning skills, but most will play the role of teachers of interpretation.

Depending on local requirements, patient population, and laboratory volume, there may be different categories of physician interpreters. As stipulated by the American College of Cardiology Core Cardiology Training Symposium (COCATS) requirements for cardiology fellows, there are three levels of physician training required to perform and interpret transthoracic echocardiograms. Level I requires 75 exams and 150 interpretations performed over 3- cumulative months of training. Level II requires 150 examinations and 300 interpretations performed over 6-cumulative months of training. Level III requires 300 examinations and 750 interpretations performed over 9-cumulative months. Level III training often requires additional subspecialty training in echocardiography after general cardiology fellowship [6]. Physicians need at least Level II COCATS training to independently interpret and bill for echocardiograms [2].

Learning to interpret cardiac ultrasound images in the echocardiography laboratory can take different forms. Trainees may discuss interesting image findings on their own and/or with an expert, review entire studies, or even generate preliminary reports. The images may be ones they have acquired or those acquired by sonographers. As with sonographers, the scope of echocardiographers' practice does not perfectly match critical care trainee needs. Cardiologists who formally interpret echocardiograms use different techniques for a wide variety of indications, some of which do not relate to critical care. In addition to attending cardiologists in academic centers, cardiology fellows can provide additional guidance and understanding of the anatomy, image acquisition, and interpretation of cardiovascular ultrasound for a wide variety of trainees. Additionally, it can be helpful to participate in conferences and other educational sessions.

It may be helpful to exchange training experiences with general cardiology and advanced imaging fellows. With the evolution of the contemporary cardiac intensive care unit (CICU), it has become increasingly important for cardiovascular practitioners to advance their critical care skills [7]. Exchanges can be helpful to furthering both trainees' career development [3]. In particular, most cardiology fellows will not have learned, much less mastered, lung or leg vein scanning and would benefit from learning these techniques.

It is also important to recognize the limitations of individual laboratory resources. Not all echocardiography laboratories will have the available personnel or equipment or space to accommodate trainees.

Working with the Echo Lab

There are many ways that critical care trainees can receive training from the echo lab. Traditional weeks- or month(s)- long formal rotations provide trainees the opportunity to experience the practice of echocardiography and "dwell" in valuable educational experiences. However, spending unstructured time is often inefficient and may not be advisable for trainees with limited time to spend. The echocardiographic laboratory is often a busy area with multiple types of studies being performed concurrently. Transthoracic echocardiograms (TTE), exercise and bicycle stress echocardiograms, dobutamine stress echocardiograms, and transesophageal echocardiograms (TEE) are all performed in large laboratories, often in multiple areas of the hospital, and most echocardiography laboratories perform at least TTEs and exercise stress echocardiography. Critical care trainees need not gain skills in performing all of these procedures, but should recognize that staff in the laboratory often have responsibilities that go beyond their training needs.

In particular, most sonographers' primary duty is the efficient performance of TTE, and busy cardiologists may have a large number of studies to interpret, in addition to other clinical and nonclinical duties. They may not be paid by hospitals to teach trainees, though some academic centers have dedicated sonographer trainers, and academic centers may provide attending physicians reimbursement for teaching responsibilities. It may be particularly difficult for sonographers to prioritize critical care training, especially in settings where they are also training sonographer interns.

Furthermore, critical care trainees come to the echo lab from a variety of backgrounds (pulmonary medicine, general intensivist medicine, emergency medicine, anesthesiology, etc.) and have a wide variety of prior experiences and levels of training in cardiac ultrasound. Different training programs may have different emphases and may allot different amounts of curriculum time for cardiac ultrasound training. There has been a proliferation of point of care ultrasound (POCUS) training in medical schools and residency programs, but its penetration is far from universal. Tailored training is challenging, and it behooves both trainer and trainee to assess the educational needs and background experience of the trainee. In some cases, a "pretest" of scanning ability and interpretive skills may help guide the training regimen.

Finally, there may be limitations to the training that specific echocardiographic laboratories can provide. Echocardiogram machines are used primarily for clinical care or cardiology and sonographer trainees and may not be available for use by critical care echocardiography trainees, at least during business hours. Likewise, interpretation stations may be occupied by sonographers or cardiology fellows performing preliminary reports or by cardiologists providing final interpretations. During a pandemic, social distancing rules and restrictions may further complicate the ability of an echocardiography laboratory to accommodate critical care echocardiography trainees.

Education in Echocardiography

Echocardiographic education has evolved in the last few decades to involve live media, including those on websites, formal courses, and simulation, the last of which may play a particularly important role in the setting of a pandemic. In addition to hands-on skills taught by sonographers, simulation programs can help trainees work on hand-eye coordination and improve knowledge of cardiac anatomy [8].

Other important tools include review of digital image repositories and the building of portfolios of scanned images. The standardization of digital storage and review has allowed for the facilitation of medical education as images can now routinely be reviewed and leveraged for educational purposes. Echocardiographic laboratories can develop repositories of annotated images. Reviewing a range of selected images can provide trainees with a breadth of knowledge on both normal and pathological conditions, while helping them recognize when they have obtained high quality images.

Additionally, through storing their own images and interpretations in portfolios, critical care trainees can elicit feedback from sonographers and echocardiographers. These portfolios can also assist with building interactive cases for education. In the critical care setting, these images can be used with interactive clinical cases to focus on cardiac ultrasonography skills [9].

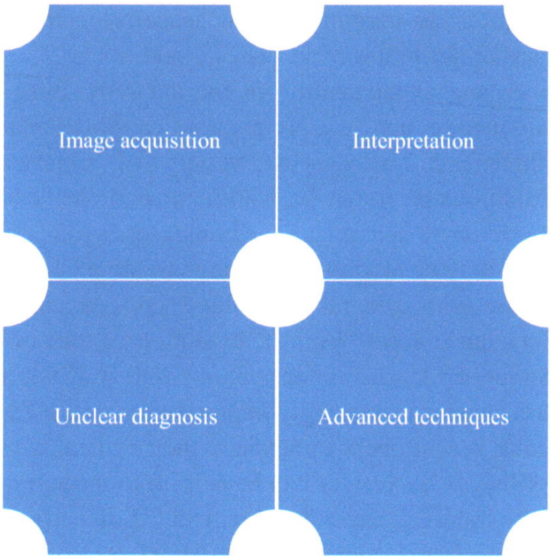

Fig. 66.1 Coordination of cardiac imaging between critical care and echocardiography laboratories

Coordination with the Echocardiographic Laboratory in Clinical Care

One of the core components of the functionality of the echocardiography laboratory is the appropriate selection of patients for different imaging modalities. Although this book focuses on education and skill training, it is important to continue the process of improving patient selection for echocardiography and maximize resource utilization. Appropriate Use Criteria [10] have been developed by cardiovascular societies for a number of clinical scenarios and help guide decisions to employ different cardiac imaging tests, and the Society of Critical Care Medicine (SCCM) has published guidelines on the appropriate use of bedside and cardiac ultrasonography in critically ill patients [9]. The criteria are a useful framework to guide trainees on the appropriate use of POCUS in the critical care unit.

There are several scenarios in which critical care practitioners and the echocardiographic laboratory must work together to further care in the critical care environment (Fig. 66.1). Although critical care practitioners often master basic cardiac ultrasonography, the reality of the critical care setting can make adequate image acquisition challenging. More experienced image-acquirers using more advanced machines may be necessary. Advanced echocardiographic techniques are quickly becoming a standard part of comprehensive echocardiography, including 3-dimensional (3D) imaging, speckle tracking strain, advanced Doppler, and the use of ultrasound enhancement agents (microbubble contrast). In particular, in patients with challenging images, the use of ultrasound enhancing agents may be necessary to detect regional wall motion abnormalities and accurately assess LVEF. 3D may assist in the accurate measurement of systolic function, and advanced Doppler can help delineate degrees of valvular abnormalities. In some situations, a limited critical care exam may not uncover pathology where there is ongoing suspicion for a cardiac etiology, such as in cases of intracardiac shunting or highly eccentric mitral regurgitation. In such situations, it is beneficial to have input from the echocardiographic laboratory.

CCE practitioners may acquire images with abnormal findings that require interpretive assistance. These findings may represent rare and unsuspected findings that the practitioner has not encountered, or they may be unusual artifacts. In some cases, saved images may contain important findings not recognized by critical care practitioners, and echocardiographers can assist in proposing next steps to evaluate these findings. There is therefore a strong argument for echocardiographers to have access to view critical care echocardiogram images for real-time clinical care, in addition to its potential to facility quality assurance. Ideally, there is capacity for real-time remote review while the scan is being performed, in addition to review of archived images. Importantly, the role of the echocardiographer is not to critique clinically acquired images or their interpretation, but to provide respectful, consultative assistance for the good of the patient. While such consultative work may be uncompensated, it is likely to be rewarded in the form of more efficient use of echocardiographic services.

Summary Points

- Critical care echocardiography trainees and practitioners should recognize the multiple components to most echocardiographic laboratories.
- Sonographers (in some regions) can be excellent teachers of image acquisition skills, and cardiologists who interpret echocardiograms can play a role as teachers of interpretation.
- In certain academic settings, general and advanced imaging cardiology fellows and sonographer trainers can also play a role in teaching scanning and interpretation.
- The practice and training of sonographers, cardiologists, and cardiovascular trainees includes elements that lie outside the necessary skills and knowledge of most critical care echocardiography trainees and lack other elements that are essential to critical care echocardiography.
- Critical care echocardiography trainees should recognize the specific time, staff, machine, reading station, and space limitations of echocardiographic laboratories.
- Digital archiving allows review of echocardiography laboratory image repositories as well as storage of trainees' images for subsequent expert adjudication.
- Scenarios in which ongoing collaboration with the echocardiography laboratory can facilitate patient care include assistance with image acquisition, interpretation, assistance with diagnoses, and deployment of advanced techniques.

References

1. Nicastro I, Barletta V, Conte L, Fabiani I, Morgantini A, Lastrucci G, et al. Professional education, training and role of the cardiac sonographer in different countries. J Cardiovasc Echogr. 2013;23(1):18–23.
2. Picard MH, Adams D, Bierig SM, Dent JM, Douglas PS, Gillam LD, et al. American Society of Echocardiography recommendations for quality echocardiography laboratory operations. J Am Soc Echocardiogr. 2011;24(1):1–10.
3. Kirkpatrick JN, Grimm R, Johri AM, Kimura BJ, Kort S, Labovitz AJ, et al. Recommendations for echocardiography laboratories participating in cardiac Point of Care Cardiac Ultrasound (POCUS) and critical care echocardiography training: report from the American Society of Echocardiography. J Am Soc Echocardiogr. 2020;33(4):409–22.e4.
4. Ehler D, Carney DK, Dempsey AL, Rigling R, Kraft C, Witt SA, et al. Guidelines for cardiac sonographer education: recommendations of the American Society of Echocardiography Sonographer Training and Education Committee. J Am Soc Echocardiogr. 2001;14(1):77–84.
5. Walley PE, Walley KR, Goodgame B, Punjabi V, Sirounis D. A practical approach to goal-directed echocardiography in the critical care setting. Crit Care. 2014;18(6):681.
6. Wiegers SE, Ryan T, Arrighi JA, Brown SM, Canaday B, Damp JB, et al. 2019 ACC/AHA/ASE advanced training statement on echocardiography (Revision of the 2003 ACC/AHA clinical competence statement on echocardiography): a report of the ACC Competency Management Committee. J Am Soc Echocardiogr. 2019;32(8):919–43.

7. Morrow DA, Fang JC, Fintel DJ, Granger CB, Katz JN, Kushner FG, et al. Evolution of critical care cardiology: transformation of the cardiovascular intensive care unit and the emerging need for new medical staffing and training models. Circulation. 2012;126(11):1408–28.
8. Dreyfus J, Donal E, Pezel T. Moving into a new era for echocardiography education with simulation and workshop-based training. JACC: Case Reports. 2020;2(3):505–7.
9. Levitov A, Frankel HL, Blaivas M, Kirkpatrick AW, Su E, Evans D, et al. Guidelines for the appropriate use of bedside general and cardiac ultrasonography in the evaluation of critically ill patients-part II: cardiac ultrasonography. Crit Care Med. 2016;44(6):1206–27.
10. Douglas PS, Khandheria B, Stainback RF, Weissman NJ, Brindis RG, Patel MR, et al. ACCF/ASE/ACEP/ASNC/SCAI/SCCT/SCMR 2007 appropriateness criteria for transthoracic and transesophageal echocardiography: a report of the American College of Cardiology Foundation Quality Strategic Directions Committee Appropriateness Criteria Working Group, American Society of Echocardiography, American College of Emergency Physicians, American Society of Nuclear Cardiology, Society for Cardiovascular Angiography and Interventions, Society of Cardiovascular Computed Tomography, and the Society for Cardiovascular Magnetic Resonance endorsed by the American College of Chest Physicians and the Society of Critical Care Medicine. J Am Coll Cardiol. 2007;50(2):187–204.

67 Utilization of Human Models, Patients, and Simulators

Valeria Santibanez and Paru Patrawalla

Learning Objectives

1. Describe the effective use of human models, real patients, and simulators for ultrasound training and assessment.
2. Examine effective strategies for the use of standardized patients and simulators for ultrasound learning and assessment.

Teaching Modalities and Definitions

Human Models

Human models include healthy volunteers and employed actors, such as standardized patients. Most often, human models do not have previously known pathology and are utilized to develop skills in image acquisition during introductory ultrasonography courses and for testing as part of competency-based assessments.

V. Santibanez (✉)
Division of Pulmonary, Critical Medicine and Allergy, Thomas Jefferson University, Philadelphia, PA, USA
e-mail: valeria.santibanez@jefferson.edu

P. Patrawalla
Division of Pulmonary and Critical Care Medicine, Icahn School of Medicine at Mount Sinai (Mount Sinai West/Morningside/Beth Israel), New York, NY, USA
e-mail: paru.patrawalla@mountsinai.org

Healthy volunteers can be recruited from local communities, medical schools, or other training programs. Curriculums utilizing medical student volunteers have shown favorable results both by helping students gain empathy for the role of a patient, and a greater understanding of anatomy, probe positioning, and technique [1]. Hiring costs of employed actors vary according to geography, hours, and number of subjects requested.

Human models should receive an introductory counseling session explaining their role followed by informed consent [2]. Ideally, all should have easily detectable structures, particularly for introductory training courses [2]. Scanning the human model prior to training can help identify the best ultrasound window, probe positioning, and any incidental findings.

Protocols for further investigation should be established if previously unknown abnormalities are identified in human models (i.e., contacting primary care physicians) [2]. If volunteers are students or trainees, special attention should be paid to preserve their privacy.

Participant's comfort and dignity should always be maintained. Gowns and bed sheets should be available to cover areas not being scanned and rooms should be at comfortable temperatures [2].

M. J. Lanspa, A. T. Levinson (eds.), *Echocardiography and Ultrasonography in the ICU*, Respiratory Medicine, https://doi.org/10.1007/978-3-031-80038-2_67

Real Patients

Real patients include humans with known pathology from many different healthcare settings; however, this chapter focuses primarily on the inpatient ward and intensive care unit (ICU).

Informed consent is recommended if patients will be scanned solely for educational purposes. The room layout should be optimized such that the trainer and learner are positioned with an unobstructed view of the ultrasound screen, with adequate and comfortable access to the machine controls [2]. Patient positioning is essential to optimize image quality, but it can be limited by surrounding devices (i.e., endotracheal tube, ventilator, drains). As with human models, the patient's dignity and privacy should be protected.

Simulators

Simulator refers to a physical object or technology that helps recreate an environment in which one or multiple tasks are carried out [3]. Simulation in medical education is defined as any educational activity that utilizes simulators to replicate clinical scenarios [4]. Simulation has been shown to improve operator confidence, skill, and patient outcomes for several ultrasound-guided procedures [5–9].

Simulators can be classified into low- and high-fidelity models and include [10, 11]:

- **Standardized patient**: an individual trained to portray a patient (see *Human Models*).
- **Partial task trainers (Phantom models)**: low-fidelity, life-like models of body parts, often used to improve procedural skills (e.g., blue phantom for pleural procedures) [5, 12]. They can be home-made [13, 14] or obtained commercially and are composed of synthetic skin, and structures mimicking the chest wall, pleural cavity, effusions, and blood (Fig. 67.1).
- **Hybrid simulators**: life-like body parts attached to standardized patients (e.g., wearable sleeves for venipuncture [15]).
- **Advanced task trainer:** body part model linked to a computer (e.g., Bronchoscopy simulator).

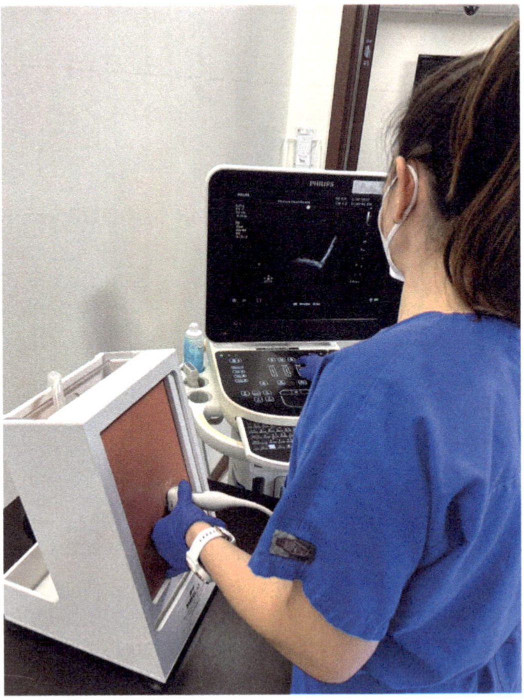

Fig. 67.1 Example of a partial task-trainer for pleural procedures. Demonstrator is holding ultrasound probe with her left hand as she scans the partial task-trainer during thoracentesis training. (Courtesy of Center of Advanced Medical Simulation, Mount Sinai West Hospital, New York)

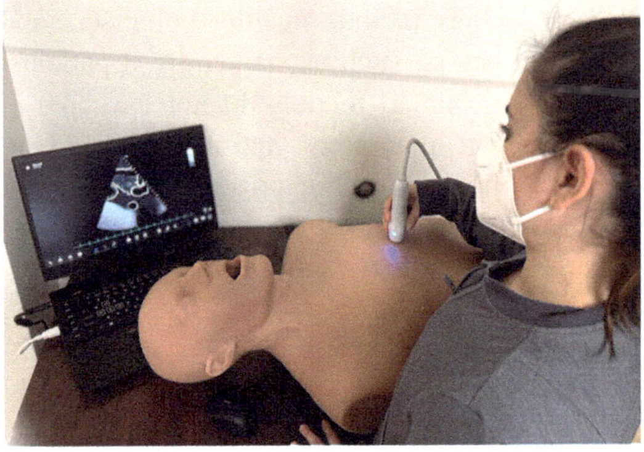

Fig. 67.2 Example of a High-fidelity ultrasound simulator. Demonstrator is using a high-fidelity mannequin to practice chest ultrasonography. (Courtesy of Center of Advanced Medical Simulation, Mount Sinai West Hospital, New York)

- **High-fidelity simulator**: a realistic computer-controlled patient simulation mannequin that can integrate ultrasound images. Cost may range from \$3000 (US) to more than \$50,000 [13] (Fig. 67.2).

- **Virtual reality simulators**: three-dimensional view interactive models.

Partial task trainers and high-fidelity simulators are the most described modalities for ultrasonography training.

Advantages and Disadvantages

Table 67.1 reviews advantages and disadvantages of each of these modalities.

Human Models

Advantages

- Healthy volunteers can provide real-time feedback (e.g., pressure applied, probe and body positioning) to improve image acquisition.
- Structures are easily identifiable, increasing novice learner confidence.
- Peer volunteers may see value in contributing to the education of trainees as well as increased empathy and understanding for the role of a patient.

Disadvantages

- Limited exposure to pathology and the challenges that will be encountered when scanning real patients.
- Bias can be introduced when recruiting only thin male models, minimizing exposure to diverse ultrasonographic anatomy such as obesity, female anatomy, and transgender population.
- Selection, recruitment, and model-training sessions can be challenging and not always possible due to time constraints or faculty availability [16].
- Potential for unknown abnormalities discovered in volunteers.
- Student or trainee volunteers may feel pressure to participate resulting in anxiety or increased vulnerability when being scanned.
- Elevated costs with paid actors and funding dependent on the institution's financial resources, grants, and sponsors [17].
- Access to companies that provide human models is limited by geography and local regulations.

Table 67.1 Advantages and disadvantages of utilizing human models, real patients, and simulators

	Advantages	Disadvantages
Human models	Real-time feedback Easily identifiable structures Increase novice learners' confidence Provide sense of value Increases patient perspective and empathy	Cost Requires training Time consuming Third party availability Anxiety provoking Selection, gender bias Lack of pathology
Real patients	Exposure to real-life scenarios Troubleshooting of body/devices positioning Prevents delay in care Correlation with ongoing clinical picture	Inability to ensure variety of disease exposure Anxiety provoking Longer study times Learner frustration with limited image acquisition Lack of cooperation if sedated
Simulators	Stress-free environment Unlimited hands-on training Minimizes patient's risks Practice of rare procedures Continuation of training	Cost of technology Access to simulation center and trained personnel Duty hour restrictions Faculty availability

Real Patients

Advantages

- Scanning real patients during training courses exposes learners to real-life conditions including environmental constraints to scanning, patient positioning, and suboptimal image acquisition [18].
- Provides an opportunity to learn methods to correct or adjust patient/device positioning prior to real encounters and may positively impact the learner's experience [19].
- Decreases delay in care, avoidance of transport of critically ill patients, and the opportunity to perform serial exams and rapid correlation with the clinical picture.
- Ability to acquire and interpret a variety of sonographic pathologies.

Disadvantages

- When performed in real-time, lack of knowledge of actual findings may lead to longer study times. Topics discussed will be biased towards conditions present in those patients [20].
- Time involved in appropriate positioning and troubleshooting can be discouraging and may decrease learner motivation. Some physicians experience frustration when scanning real patients given inability to obtain good images [19].
- Image acquisition may be limited secondary to mechanically ventilated overdistended lungs, surgical wounds, dressings, or devices attached to patients.
- Lack of cooperation in sedated patients can contribute to inadequate studies and learning.

Simulators

Advantages

- Provide opportunity for unlimited hands-on training enabling learning and mastery of procedural skills.
- Provides a stress-free environment for the learner without placing patients at risk for adverse events [21].
- Real life scenarios can be practiced before encountering them in practice. Rarely used, often emergent, procedures can be practiced with real-time feedback which enhances the learning process [10, 20, 22].
- Simulation-based ultrasonography can identify trainees who may benefit from additional instruction [23].
- Simulation-based training can accelerate initial learning, reducing the time to competence [24].
- Simulators are reusable, improving cost effectiveness.
- The importance of social distancing during the COVID-19 pandemic posed a barrier to in-person training with human models. Simulation-based experiences are safer for training during a pandemic [25].

Disadvantages

- Cost is the primary disadvantage. Some simulators cost over $100,000 and may be impractical to be used in large courses [5]. There are also costs related to simulator maintenance [26].
- A structured curriculum with a simulation facility, personnel, and expertise is required. This may be particularly difficult to achieve for smaller training programs [21].
- Other barriers include duty hour restrictions, scheduling conflicts, mannequin availability, and faculty availability.

Practical Implementations of Teaching Modalities

Human models are the most common teaching modality used for ultrasonography training in undergraduate medical education (UME) [27]. Students (33%) were the most frequent subjects scanned, followed by healthy volunteers (19%) and real patients (19%). Phantoms or simulators (27%) were also used, a third of which were "institution-made".

The American College of Graduate Medical Education (ACGME), the European Respiratory Society (ERS), and the American Board of

Internal Medicine (ABIM) strongly suggest including simulation in procedural training for pulmonary and critical care medicine [28, 29, 30].

Introductory Courses

Although there have been many published studies describing successful introductory courses, no standardized curriculum exists. The preferred modality often involves scanning human models with real-time feedback from trained faculty [17, 31, 32]. Not many curricula include scanning real patients as part of their introductory course [33, 34]. Only a minority of studies (<12%) used patients or subjects with known pathologies [35].

Small group session with a learner to faculty to human model ratio of 3:1:1 is preferable [17, 32]. Learners should rotate through various groups to scan different models [31, 32]. The characteristics or gender of the models used is not well described in literature.

Longitudinal Curriculums and Competency Acquisition

Little evidence exists supporting a specific modality to achieve ultrasound competency in critical care [35, 36]. Most curricula favor scanning patients with a clinical indication (45.2%). However, normal subjects and mannequins are still utilized for competency assessments [35] and the development of validated assessment tools [37].

Current guidelines emphasize the importance of scanning critically ill patients to obtain proficiency and the inability for other platforms to substitute for real patients [30, 36, 38–41].

Other Strategies to Consider

Strategies to maximize implementation include:

- When funding or lack of expert faculty are limited: developing a cost-sharing cooperative model with local teaching programs may be beneficial, mostly for fellowship programs without formal training [17].
- Designing educational models where trainees are recruited as volunteer models further adding to the educational experience [1].
- Building homemade phantoms or partial-task trainers in the absence of funding [14].
- Asking ultrasonography machine manufacturers to lend machines for training courses free of charge [17].
- Standardize teaching by holding faculty briefing sessions prior to the course [31, 32].
- Providing junior attendings and senior fellows faculty development to increase the number of voluntary faculty available to supervise sessions.

Barriers and Limitations

No specific guidelines or optimal curriculum exist for the implementation of these teaching modalities [42] and the lack of proficient faculty limits its implementation [43, 44].

Selection and Gender Bias

There is a lack of descriptive characteristics including gender, race, and body mass index of human models utilized in most training courses. Therefore, a definite assessment of an accurate representation of the patient population used for training cannot be made.

Selection and gender bias can be introduced by courses that recruit only slim male models for hands-on practice [2]. Female breasts and obesity can be significant challenges to performing thoracic and cardiac ultrasonography in real patients without prior training. Some ultrasonography teaching textbooks describe only normal male findings when utilizing ultrasonography in the ICU, further biasing representation of other genders [45]. Utilizing female and transgender human models to learn positioning and challenges directly related to their anatomy should be included as a best practice [46].

Final Thoughts

We suggest designing a longitudinal competency-based curriculum for ultrasound training that includes scanning live human models, real patients, or both, depending on local resources, funding, and expertise.

We recommend the implementation of a simulation-based mastery learning approach using partial task trainers for ultrasound-guided procedures.

If utilizing human models, we highly encourage including models of differing genders and body habitus to represent the diversity that will be seen with real patients.

Further research is needed to assess the effectiveness of the latest technologies available, to evaluate for selection or gender bias in the recruitment process of human models, and to validate assessment tools. There is a pressing need for explicit guidelines addressing the specific roles for each of these teaching modalities in a competency-based model for ultrasonography training.

Summary

- Ultrasound training can be performed by scanning human models, real patients, and simulators.
- Human models are the preferred modality for developing image acquisition skills in novice learners.
- Real patients offer the benefit of exposing and preparing learners for real life scenarios.
- Simulation-based training eliminates adverse patient events and may be preferred during the current COVID-19 pandemic.
- Medicine and critical care societies recommend a combination of these modalities for pulmonary and critical care training and competence-based assessment.
- There is a need for clear guidelines detailing the necessary training components and use of various teaching modalities.

Call-Outs Pro-Tips

- Incorporate and promote scanning of real patients in both introductory and competency-based training courses.
- Recruit human models of different gender identities and body types to better understand the specific skills required when scanning in real scenarios.
- Further research is needed to assess the effectiveness of the latest technologies available.
- Explicit guidelines addressing the specific roles for each of these teaching modalities are needed.

References

1. Blickendorf JM, Adkins EJ, Boulger C, Bahner DP. Trained simulated ultrasound patients: medical students as models, learners, and teachers. J Ultrasound Med. 2014;33:35–8.
2. Griksaitis MJ, Scott MP, Finn GM. Twelve tips for teaching with ultrasound in the undergraduate curriculum. Med Teach. 2014;36:19–24.
3. Cooper JB, Taqueti VR. A brief history of the development of mannequin simulators for clinical education and training. Postgrad Med J. 2008;84:563–70.
4. Al-Elq AH. Simulation-based medical teaching and learning. J Family Community Med. 2010;17:35–40.
5. McSparron JI, Michaud GC, Gordan PL, et al. Simulation for skills-based education in pulmonary and critical care medicine. Ann Am Thorac Soc. 2015;12:579–86.
6. Barsuk JH, Cohen ER, Potts S, Demo H, Gupta S, Feinglass J, McGaghie WC, Wayne DB. Dissemination of a simulation-based mastery learning intervention reduces central line-associated bloodstream infections. BMJ Qual Saf. 2014;23;749–56.
7. Barsuk JH, Cohen ER, Williams MV, Scher J, Jones SF, Feinglass J, McGaghie WC, O'Hara K, Wayne DB. Simulation-based mastery learning for thoracentesis skills improves patient outcomes: a randomized trial. Acad Med. 2018;93:729–35.
8. Huang GC, McSparron JI, Balk EM, Richards JB, Smith CC, Whelan JS, Newman LR, Smetana GW. Procedural instruction in invasive bedside procedures: a systematic review and meta-analysis of effective teaching approaches. BMJ Qual Saf. 2016;25:281–94.
9. Edrich T, Seethala RR, Olenchock BA, Mizuguchi AK, Rivero JM, Beutler SS, Fox JA, Liu X, Frendl G. Providing initial transthoracic echocardiography training for anesthesiologists: simulator training is not inferior to live training. J Cardiothorac Vasc Anesth. 2014;28:49–53.
10. Bangar M, Venegas-Borsellino C, Eisen LA. Simulation and education in the ICU. In: Oropello JM, Pastores SM, Kvetan V. eds. Critical care. McGraw-Hill Education; 2016.
11. Delisle M, Hannenberg AA. Alternatives to high-fidelity simulation. Anesthesiol Clin. 2020;38:761–73.

12. Singas E, Quintero LD, Dhar S, Tsegaye A, Finuf K, Pekmezaris R, Weitzen MS, Mayo PH (2021) Training pulmonary critical care medicine fellows in thoracentesis using a head-mounted video camera. ATS Scholar ATS–scholar.2021–0052IN.
13. Lewiss RE, Hoffmann B, Beaulieu Y, Phelan MB. Point-of-care ultrasound education. J Ultrasound Med. 2014;33:27–32.
14. Ramonell RP, Schimmel M, Greer M, Coleman CG, Bender WS, Daniels LM. Longitudinal trends using a point-of-care gelatin-based model for ultrasound-guided central venous catheter insertion. Med Educ Online. 2021;26:1924350.
15. Devenny A, Lord D, Matthews J, Tuhacek J, Vitlip J, Zhang M, Bucha AC, Wang L, Buckley JM, Cowperthwait A. Avstick: an intravenous catheter insertion simulator for use with standardized patients. Nurs Educ Perspect. 2018;39:102–4.
16. Bokken L, Rethans J-J, Jöbsis Q, Duvivier R, Scherpbier A, van der Vleuten C. Instructiveness of real patients and simulated patients in undergraduate medical education: a randomized experiment. Acad Med. 2010;85:148–54.
17. Patrawalla P, Narasimhan M, Eisen L, Shiloh AL, Koenig S, Mayo P. A regional, cost-effective, collaborative model for critical care fellows' ultrasonography education. J Intensive Care Med. 2020;35:1447–52.
18. Beaulieu Y, Marik PE. Bedside ultrasonography in the ICU. Chest. 2005;128:881–95.
19. Rajamani A, Miu M, Huang S, et al. Impact of critical care point-of-care ultrasound short-courses on trainee competence. Crit Care Med. 2019;47:e782–4.
20. Barrows HS, Others. An overview of the uses of standardized patients for teaching and evaluating clinical skills. Acad Med. 1993;68:443–51.
21. Aslam W, Lee HJ, Lamb CR. Standardizing education in interventional pulmonology in the midst of technological change. J Thorac Dis. 2020;12:3331–40.
22. Grenvik A, Schaefer JJ 3rd. Medical simulation training coming of age. Crit Care Med. 2004;32:2549–50.
23. Madsen ME, Nørgaard LN, Tabor A, Konge L, Ringsted C, Tolsgaard MG. The predictive value of ultrasound learning curves across simulated and clinical settings. J Ultrasound Med. 2017;36:201–8.
24. Vignon P, Pegot B, Dalmay F, Jean-Michel V, Bocher S, L'her E, Cros J, Prat G, EchoSimu Group. Acceleration of the learning curve for mastering basic critical care echocardiography using computerized simulation. Intensive Care Med. 2018;44:1097–105.
25. Jackson R, Brotherston D, Jain A, Douflé G, Piquette D, Goffi A. Teaching ultrasound at the point of care in times of social distancing. ATS Sch. 2021;2:341–52.
26. Asche CV, Kim M, Brown A, Golden A, Laack TA, Rosario J, Strother C, Totten VY, Okuda Y. Communicating value in simulation: cost-benefit analysis and return on investment. Acad Emerg Med. 2018;25:230–7.
27. Davis JJ, Wessner CE, Potts J, Au AK, Pohl CA, Fields JM. Ultrasonography in undergraduate medical education: a systematic review. J Ultrasound Med. 2018;37:2667–79.
28. Accreditation Council for Graduate Medical Education. (2020) ACGME program requirements for graduate medical education in pulmonary and critical care medicine. In: Accreditation Council for Graduate Medical Education. https://www.acgme.org/Portals/0/PFAssets/ProgramRequirements/156_PCCM_2021.pdf?ver=2021-06-23-150200-760. Accessed 25 Dec 2021.
29. Policies and Procedures for Certification November 2021. In: American Board of Internal Medicine. https://www.abim.org/Media/splbmcpe/policies-and-procedures.pdf. Accessed 5 Dec 2021.
30. Laursen CB, Clive A, Hallifax R, et al. European Respiratory Society statement on thoracic ultrasound. Eur Respir J. 2021;57:2001519. https://doi.org/10.1183/13993003.01519-2020.
31. Sarkar PK, Boivin M, Mayo PH. Effectiveness of an advanced critical care echocardiography course. J Intensive Care Med. 2020;35:1332–7.
32. Greenstein YY, Littauer R, Narasimhan M, Mayo PH, Koenig SJ. Effectiveness of a critical care ultrasonography course. Chest. 2017;151:34–40.
33. Kuza CM, Hanifi MT, Koç M, Stopfkuchen-Evans M. Providing transthoracic echocardiography training for intensive care unit trainees: an educational improvement initiative. J Surg Educ. 2018;75:1342–50.
34. Kanji HD, McCallum JL, Bhagirath KM, Neitzel AS. Curriculum development and evaluation of a hemodynamic critical care ultrasound: a systematic review of the literature. Crit Care Med. 2016;44:e742–50.
35. Rajamani A, Shetty K, Parmar J, Huang S, Ng J, Gunawan S, Gunawan G, SPARTAN Collaborative (Small Projects, Audits and Research Projects – Australia/New Zealand). Longitudinal competence programs for basic point-of-care ultrasound in critical care: a systematic review. Chest. 2020;158:1079–89.
36. Kumar A, Kugler J, Jensen T. Evaluation of trainee competency with point-of-care ultrasonography (POCUS): a conceptual framework and review of existing assessments. J Gen Intern Med. 2019;34:1025–31.
37. Patrawalla P, Eisen LA, Shiloh A, Shah BJ, Savenkov O, Wise W, Evans L, Mayo P, Szyld D. Development and validation of an assessment tool for competency in critical care ultrasound. J Grad Med Educ. 2015;7:567–73.
38. Icu ERT on E in, Expert Round Table on Echocardiography in ICU. International consensus statement on training standards for advanced critical care echocardiography. Intensive Care Med. 2014;40:654–66.
39. Expert Round Table on Ultrasound in ICU. International expert statement on training standards for critical care ultrasonography. Intensive Care Med. 2011;37:1077–83.

40. Arntfield R, Millington S, Ainsworth C, et al. Canadian recommendations for critical care ultrasound training and competency. Can Respir J. 2014;21:341–5.
41. Kirkpatrick JN, Grimm R, Johri AM, et al. Recommendations for echocardiography laboratories participating in cardiac point of care cardiac ultrasound (POCUS) and critical care echocardiography training: report from the American Society of Echocardiography. J Am Soc Echocardiogr. 2020;33:409–422.e4.
42. Rajamani A, Smith L, Gunawan S, Gunawan G, Parmar J, Arvind H, Huang S, SPARTAN Collaborative (Small Projects, Audits and Research Projects-Australia/New Zealand). Methodologic quality of guidelines for training or competence processes for basic point-of-care echocardiography in critical care: a systematic review of the literature. Chest. 2021;160:616–23.
43. Brady AK, Spitzer CR, Kelm D, Brosnahan SB, Latifi M, Burkart KM. Pulmonary critical care fellows' use of and self-reported barriers to learning bedside ultrasound during training: results of a national survey. Chest. 2021;160:231–7.
44. Hulett CS, Pathak V, Katz JN, Montgomery SP, Chang LH. Development and preliminary assessment of a critical care ultrasound course in an adult pulmonary and critical care fellowship program. Ann Am Thorac Soc. 2014;11:784–8.
45. Pakzad N, Kourouni I, Mathew JP, Narayanswami G. Non-cardiac point of care ultrasound in the CCU. In: Herzog E, Argulian E, editors. Echocardiography in the CCU. Cham: Springer International Publishing; 2018. p. 165–214.
46. Collett T, Kirvell D, Nakorn A, McLachlan JC. The role of living models in the teaching of surface anatomy: some experiences from a UK Medical School. Med Teach. 2009;31:e90–6.

68 Features of Successful Teaching Programs

Renee Dversdal and Paul Musgrave

Learning Objectives

1. Describe the features common to successful ultrasound teaching programs.
2. Detail effective strategies for the assessment of ultrasound skill and competency.

When considering features of successful point-of-care ultrasound (POCUS) and critical care echocardiography programs, a key task is to define *what* is success? However, an oft overlooked step is to identify *who* is defining success? There are many stakeholders in any clinical or educational program, and their priorities will likely vary. Fellows may prioritize fun hands-on experiences, although they are unlikely to master required skills in the image interpretation and clinical integration realms without additional didactic work and repetition. An intensive care unit medical director may prioritize clinical excellence; however, this can be challenging to assess and quantify. A program director may consider fellows passing the Critical Care Echocardiography boards as a measure that is objective and might also influence recruitment. However, the *when* now becomes important. When starting an ultrasound program, setting a goal of a certain percentage of fellows passing their echo boards might be too aggressive and increase the likelihood of the program being deemed a failure. Finally, division chiefs or department chairs may consider scholarly output such as peer-reviewed publication of educational methods and advance a measure of a successful training program. These activities can be excellent for later job recruitment and promotion, but are not appealing to all, and certainly are not required to become a competent clinician. Once the who, what, and when have been determined, the program is ready to address the *how*. This is quite variable, as there is no standardized curriculum for how to train learners in critical care ultrasound and echocardiography.

The first, and arguably most important, feature is the number of trained faculty available to educate, whether in formal educational sessions or during clinical care. When working with ultrasound-trained faculty, trainees are more likely to see ultrasound utilized to answer clinical questions. Image acquisition pearls will be learned, along with image interpretation and clinical integration, all "on the fly". Outside of clinical duties, all learners need dedicated time to practice performing ultrasound exams with trained faculty.

R. Dversdal
Department of Medicine, Division of Hospital Medicine, Oregon Health & Science University, Portland, OR, USA
e-mail: dversdar@ohsu.edu

P. Musgrave (✉)
Legacy Inpatient Medical Service, Legacy Health, Portland, OR, USA
e-mail: phmusgra@lhs.org

M. J. Lanspa, A. T. Levinson (eds.), *Echocardiography and Ultrasonography in the ICU*, Respiratory Medicine, https://doi.org/10.1007/978-3-031-80038-2_68

This is much more realistic and feasible if the burden does not fall upon one person to do all of the training. While it is optimal to have several trained faculty, even a single highly motivated faculty member (often described as the "POCUS champion") may be sufficient if there is also collaboration with other departments such as cardiology or radiology. Another approach that has been implemented by some programs is to have more experienced fellows involved with teaching beginning fellows, residents, and other trainees. The adage that "the best way to learn a topic is to teach it" applies here, and this has the added benefit of increasing instructors. If lack of trained fellows or faculty is a true limitation to program development, the "POCUS champion" may instead devote initial time and effort time to training faculty, as an investment in the program's future.

Next, almost all programs have some initial "bolus" training, implying stacked or more intensive ultrasound education in a dedicated period of time. Many programs have a core ultrasound rotation that all learners participate in at least once. The breakdown of the components of this rotation varies, but most have their trainees work directly with an expert for guided practice to hone image acquisition and interpretation skills. Programs which define success in part by fellows passing critical care echo boards design their ultrasound image acquisition opportunities to ensure fellows obtain the requisite number of guided and independently acquired images to qualify for the exam. Time for independent image acquisition is also a core part of many ultrasound rotations, as it is impossible to have constant supervision, and troubleshooting independently adds to skills as well. Independent practice is a critical component to develop this skill and forces learners to problem solve in order to reposition the patient, obtain adequate image windows, and identify anatomic landmarks. A learner portfolio to track the number of exams and assess image acquisition skill over time is common. In addition to learners interpreting their own images, interpreting images obtained by peers can be valuable to further strengthen learner pattern recognition. Either during this rotation, or in a separate rotation, many programs have their fellows spend time with cardiology reading comprehensive echocardiograms and shadowing echocardiographers and ultrasonographers to further refine skills.

Some programs are limited by time constraints and other challenges which may not afford dedicated time for a POCUS rotation. In these and other cases, programs have used more brief interventions such as intensive 1 or 2 day sessions to teach learners the necessary POCUS techniques. This can be done at the beginning of fellowship before clinical duties have begun and can be a great opportunity for learners to have guided practice with faculty to learn image acquisition techniques.

There are several studies that suggest that knowledge decay sets in quickly after intensive "boot-camp" style training sessions [1–3]. However, a significant challenge for many POCUS programs is determining how and when to create and support a longitudinal curriculum. Common barriers include identifying sufficient learner time, faculty time, and educational resources whether synchronous or asynchronous. Longitudinal curricula should take into account that to truly work towards competency, learners need to build on their image acquisition, image interpretation, and clinical integration skills. Strategies of successful programs vary, however all include some component of spaced learning to enhance retention of knowledge and skills.

Many programs allow for fellows to participate in an elective at some point after the core rotation. This allows trainees to hone skills as well as explore new techniques depending on their areas of interest. Collaboration across departments and divisions will be key to gaining access to the experts your learners may desire to learn with. For instance, a fellow who is interested in nerve blocks to reduce opioid use and delirium in the elderly may benefit from working with the regional anesthesia team. If your site has an interventional pulmonology service, ultrasound-guided pigtail catheter placement or pleural biopsies may be of interest. A learner passionate about advancing transesophageal echocardiogram (TEE) use in cardiac arrest situations could spend some time in perioperative cardiac surgeries. Nephrologists lead the way in the venous excess ultrasound examination (VExUS) at some sites, and the university or emergency medicine point-of-care ultrasound group may have an educational sonographer who could ensure they are truly solid in their technical skills. The possibilities are nearly endless.

If the desire goes beyond the capabilities of an elective, research projects on POCUS topics can further enrich the skills of the fellows beyond the core topics. Some programs have ongoing POCUS-related research projects that fellows assist with. Opportunities like this allow them to become content experts, gaining a deeper understanding of the material, and to become an expert on a focused topic. Working outside of your program as outlined above can contribute to your program's success while also expanding your network.

Not all programs will have the ability to offer POCUS electives or research projects, but rest assured, there are many other methods of ensuring longitudinal learning. Synchronous, or live, examples include regular image review conference, journal clubs, quality assurance sessions, dedicated POCUS didactics each month, clinical case discussions, dedicated image acquisition shifts, and more. In one program, senior fellows are the ones to give POCUS lectures and then receive feedback on their teaching skills. Asynchronous, or independent and self-timed, examples include interactive online modules where learners can work through the necessary steps for image acquisition, interpretation, and integration via example cases. Even if not built into an app or website, a diverse repository of pathological images and video clips can be compiled for rotators to review. These can be integrated with clinical information to have a series of case files that can be studied at any time. Finally, even if your program is starting from scratch, there is a plethora of Free Online, Open Access, Medical education (FOAMEd) content that can be utilized to enhance your curriculum.

Whether synchronous or asynchronous training is desired, if available, simulation centers may have a wealth of resources. Educational ultrasound machines, rooms with stretchers, standardized patients for proctored image acquisition, echocardiography and ultrasound simulators, ultrasound pathology phantoms, and procedure simulators can all be found in a well-equipped simulation center. One program integrates POCUS into an Advanced Cardiac Life Support (ACLS) and cardiac arrest training session occurring in their simulation center. Other programs utilize echocardiogram simulators in order to hone the basic skills of image acquisition and landmark identification. Some simulation centers, cardiology, or anesthesia groups will have TEE simulators, which are costly, but can provide invaluable practice experience. Reaching out to others in education to see which resources can be shared is always a good idea.

A strategy to support education outside of formal curricular elements involves tools for immediate, "just-in-time training" or "just-prior" reference. These tools are also known as Reusable Learning Objects (RLO) and vary from laminated cards attached to an ultrasound unit to easily accessible files downloaded to the user's phone to quick videos in an app. As an example, RLOs for POCUS exams may contain "Checklists" with the necessary views and information for image acquisition and interpretation. These can be created for specifics that a program desires and vary from focusing on the basics to advanced ultrasound examinations. Table 68.1 outlines various educational methods utilized by successful training programs.

While the following chapter will discuss assessment of competency in detail, one cannot omit this in a discussion of successful teaching programs. Until the development of the Critical care echocardiography board examination (CCEeXAM) in 2019, there was no validated and standardized method to assess critical care ultrasound and echocardiography knowledge in North America. Not every program desires their learners to prepare to this level, though, so additional evaluation methods are needed. There remain few validated tools to assess image acquisition, image interpretation, or clinical integration competency. There are, however, several strategies that many successful programs do have in common.

69 Training for the Critical Care Echocardiography Board Certification

Andrew T. Levinson

Learning Objectives

1. Review the definitions of certification and accreditation.
2. Describe key components of certification.
3. Assess the rationale for critical care echocardiography certification.
4. Discuss the National Board of echocardiography (NBE) examination of special competence in critical care echocardiography (CCEeXAM®).

Introduction

Critical care ultrasound, and specifically Critical Care Echocardiography (CCE), offers a powerful diagnostic tool to assist providers caring for critically ill patients. The primary objective of critical care ultrasound education, training, and certification is to ensure safety and clinical competency. Over the last decade, issues of certification have evolved and become more specified.

The levels of competency in point-of-care ultrasound and the extent of its utilization are highly variable—both broadly in terms of geography and between providers within the same institution. Given this diversity, the need for continued development of standardized training pathways for accreditation and certification in order to improve provider knowledge and patient care is crucial [1].

An essential role of critical care ultrasonography institutional accreditation and external certification is to ensure that the clinician utilizing the technology has the required skills, knowledge base, and technical expertise and is able to recognize the potential pitfalls and limitations of point-of-care ultrasound. To be successful, intensivists must be trained to understand their scope of practice and need to recognize when comprehensive formal ultrasound and echocardiographic studies are indicated [2].

Certification and Accreditation

Certification and accreditation are a means of assessing if a provider is well-trained and competent. The primary goal of training programs and curricula is to develop clinical competency. Certification is a statement that an individual completed a specified training curriculum and has a specified knowledge of a subject. Accreditation, in contrast, includes quantitative and qualitative demonstrations of competency [3].

A. T. Levinson (✉)
Division of Pulmonary, Critical Care, and Sleep Medicine, The Warren Alpert Medical School, Brown University, Providence, RI, USA
e-mail: andrew_levinson@brown.edu

M. J. Lanspa, A. T. Levinson (eds.), *Echocardiography and Ultrasonography in the ICU*, Respiratory Medicine, https://doi.org/10.1007/978-3-031-80038-2_69

General Certification in Critical Care Ultrasound

As critical care ultrasound education for intensivists became widespread, varying levels of competency and certification were delineated [4]. Specifically with regard to critical care echocardiography, a tiered system of demonstrated competency and accreditation was proposed [5]. International guidelines propose that all intensivists receive training in basic-level echocardiography and general critical care ultrasound. International guidelines further proposed that advanced-level education and training in critical care echocardiography should be optional in the training of all critical care physicians [6].

The specific components of tiered levels of competency have been identified in detail by international experts in critical care ultrasound. A joint consensus statement from the American College of Physicians /La Societe de Reanimation de Langue Francaise in 2009 recommended that critical care ultrasound and echocardiography competence be delineated into basic and advanced levels. Skills required to identify important clinical findings and answer basic clinical questions comprise the basic level of competence. The authors recommended that all intensivists be trained in general critical care ultrasound and basic critical care echocardiography. The consensus statement also proposed that general critical care ultrasound and basic critical care transthoracic echocardiography competency training be required components in the training of all intensivists [7]. Intensivists who desire further competence are encouraged to pursue additional training in advanced critical echocardiography, including TEE, emphasizing comprehensive evaluation of cardiac anatomy and function.

Certification in Critical Care Echocardiography

A comprehensive three-tiered system of critical care echocardiography accreditation and certification was first proposed in 2008 by the World Interactive Network Focused on Critical Ultrasound (WINFOCUS). The authors delineated four proposed levels of competency for the use of echocardiography by intensivists (Fig. 69.1). The levels of competency range from acquiring standard transthoracic views in a hemodynamically unstable patient (emergency echo) up to performing specialized comprehensive echocardiography exams (Level 3) [5].

Assessment required for certification "is necessary for proof of expertise in every domain that requires integration of cognitive and motor skills." Both European and American Critical Care Echocardiographers advocated for the development of a formal certification process specific for the practice of CCE [8].

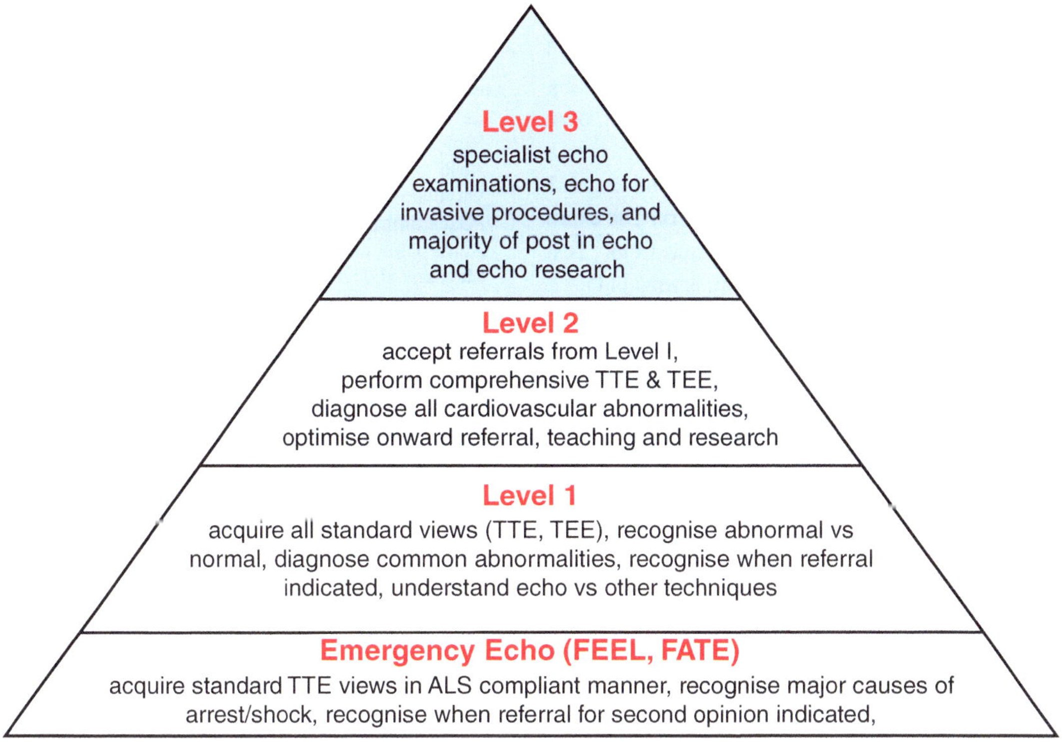

Fig. 69.1 Proposed levels of echocardiography in ICU [5]. (From first edition chapter 2, Fig. 2.1)

ASE Echocardiography

The National Board of echocardiography (NBE) since 2019 has administered the examination of special competence in critical care echocardiography (CCEeXAM®). The CCEXAM is a collaborative effort initially spear-headed by the Society of Critical Care Medicine (SCCM), American Society of Echocardiography (ASE), Society of Cardiovascular Anesthesiologists, American College of Chest Physicians, American Thoracic Society, American College of Emergency Physicians, Canadian Critical Care Society, and the World Interactive Network Focused on Critical Ultrasound [8]. The certification process requires both exam passage ("testamur status") and completion of performed echocardiograms reviewed by a mentor [9].

The NBE examination questions were developed and are maintained by a committee representing the sponsoring societies and diverse disciplines that perform critical care echocardiography as par their clinical care [10].

Rationale

The designers of the CCEeXAM state that "the primary aim of the NBE board examination is to provide physicians an objective means to demonstrate expertise and advanced knowledge in CCE." [10]

Eligibility

Candidates for the CCEeXAM must have a current medical license in good standing, have completed a critical care fellowship or currently be in practice using CCE, and document meeting certain requirements, including supervision, training, or practice-based experience with documented logs of performed and interpreted images [11]. Certification in advanced critical care echocardiography (ACCE) includes meeting both examination passage and attainment of a mentored image set [9].

The computer-based exam is administered 1 day annually at regional testing centers. The exam consists of 200 multiple choice questions. Test takers have 4.5 h to answer the questions [11].

Exam Content in the CCEeXAM®

There are four main content areas covered in the exam. The exam designers note that "although echocardiography is the focus, the examination also covers essential ultrasonography-related topics unique to critical care such as thoracic, abdominal, and vascular ultrasonography." [10]

First, test takers must have knowledge of functional anatomy seen on echocardiography, including the left ventricle, right ventricle, atria, valves, pericardium, and great vessels, as well as the ability to correctly identify congenital and anatomic abnormalities and pathology. Second, test takers must have a solid foundation in the use of both qualitative and quantitative methods for characterizing different types of shock, volume assessment, and acute cardiovascular presentations such as MI, pulmonary embolism, and aortic dissection. Third, candidates must demonstrate a thorough understanding of ultrasound physics, artifacts, and image acquisition. Finally, the integration of extra-cardiac imaging, including lung and pleura, vascular, and abdominal ultrasound, is required [12] (Table 69.1).

The NBE states that it "does not endorse or recommend any third-party review course or material. Any text in cardiovascular techniques and evaluation, cardiac patient care and management may be used. Current standards and guidelines endorsed by professional societies are also appropriate." There are several board review courses and materials for exam preparation sponsored by various professional societies.

Table 69.1 Exam content critical care echocardiography exam

Anatomy:
Left ventricle
Right ventricle
Atria
Valvular disease
Pericardium
Aorta/pulmonary artery/IVC/SVC
Mechanical devices
Intracardiac masses
Congenital defects
Diagnosis and management:
Shock
Volume assessment
Acute cardiovascular presentations
Trauma
Respiratory failure
Cardiac arrest
Image acquisition
Physics
Artifacts
Probe position and manipulation
Integrated ultrasound imaging:
Lung and pleura
Vascular/DVT
Abdominal

Adapted from: https://www.echoboards.org/wp-content/uploads/2022/11/CCEeXAM-Handbook-2022-22-1.pdf [12]

Initial Examination Results

The first year that the exam was offered, 43% of the candidates had clinical training in anesthesiology, 33% in pulmonary critical care, and 9% in emergency medicine. Over 70% of candidates had less than 6 years of CCE experience. Six hundred and twenty four candidates took the exam the first year, and the initial passage rate was 81% ($n = 436$) [10].

Key Points

- An essential role of critical care ultrasonography institutional accreditation and external certification is to ensure that the clinician utilizing the technology has the required skills, knowledge base, and technical expertise.

- Certification is a statement that an individual completed a specified training curriculum and has a specified knowledge of a subject. Accreditation includes quantitative and qualitative demonstrations of competency.
- National Board of Echocardiography CCE certification has two parts: (1) and (2).
- The CCEeXAM® has four main content areas.

References

1. Huang SJ, McLean AS. Do we need a critical care ultrasound certification program? Implications from an Australian medical-legal perspective. Crit Care. 2010;14:313.
2. Lau G, Swanevelder J. Echocardiography in intensive care—where we are heading? Anaesthesia. 2011;66:649–52.
3. Bennett S. Training guidelines for ultrasound: worldwide trends. Best Pract Res Clin Anaesthesiol. 2009;23:363–73.
4. Vieillard Baron A, Slama M, Cholley B, Janvier G, Vignon P. Echocardiography in the intensive care unit: from evolution to revolution? Intensive Care Med. 2008;34:243–9.
5. Price S, Via G, Sloth E, et al. Echocardiography practice, training and accreditation in the intensive care: document for the World Interactive Network Focused on Critical Ultrasound (WINFOCUS). Cardiovasc Ultrasound. 2008;6:49.
6. Expert Round Table on Ultrasound in ICU. International expert statement on training standards for critical care ultrasonography. Intensive Care Med. 2011;37:1077–83.
7. Mayo PH, Beaulieu Y, Doelken P, et al. American College of Chest Physicians/La Societe de Reanimation de Langue Francaise statement on competence in critical care ultrasonography. Chest. 2009;135:1050–60.
8. Diaz-Gomez JL, Frankel HL, Hernandez A. National certification in critical care echocardiography: its time has come. Crit Care Med. 2017;45:1801–4.
9. Mayo PH, Koenig S. Advanced critical care echocardiography certification: an update. Chest. 2020;158:48–9.
10. Panebianco NL, Mayo PH, Arntfield RT, et al. Assessing competence in critical care echocardiography: development and initial results of an examination and certification processes. Crit Care Med. 2021;49:1285–92.
11. Certification. 2024. Accessed 17 Feb 2024.
12. CCEeXAM Content. NAtional Board of Echocardiography, 2024. Accessed 16 Feb 2024.

Competence and Quality Assurance: How an Institution Can Assess Ongoing Competence of an Individual Practitioner

70

Stanley Abraham, Drew Brotherston, and Paul H. Mayo

Learning Objectives

1. Review strategies for the determination of competence and ongoing quality assurance (QA) with the use of critical care ultrasonography (CCUS).
2. Describe key components of an effective QA program.

Competence and Credentialing

In defining competence in CCUS, it is necessary to define those elements of ultrasonography that the intensivist would need to master. The ACCP/SRLF Statement on Competence in CCUS was written specifically to provide guidance in establishing a minimum standard for competence [1]. An international consensus statement on training in CCUS used the 2011 Statement as its foundation document [2]. An additional international statement on training in advanced critical care echocardiography (ACCE) served to define competence in this component of CCUS [3]. An international working group recently updated the 2011 Statement without much change in the requirements for competence [4]. These four documents provide a summary of what constitutes competence in CCUS and a guide to the goals of training and maintenance of competence of the individual practitioner.

The question is how to determine whether an intensivist is competent in CCUS. As there is no national level certification available for CCUS (except for ACCE), determination of competence is often through a local hospital credentialing committee. The privileges to perform CCUS are granted based on local rules that are variable and depend on input from different subspecialty services such as cardiology, radiology, or critical care. According to the American Medical Association's policy H-230.960 on ultrasound privileging [5], an administrative entity either grants privileges broadly (i.e., a specialty-based set of privileges encompassing a set of applications), or for individual applications (e.g., cardiac ultrasound for pericardial effusion, vascular ultrasound for deep vein thrombosis, etc.). Prior to being granted privileges, noncredentialed physicians should have all scans and reports over-read and be restricted from making management decisions based on their scans until appropriately credentialed.

In the USA, graduating fellows are often granted critical care privileges solely based upon the statement of their fellowship program director that they are competent to perform typical ICU procedures such as CCUS. Credentialing committees accept the program directors' letter as prima facie evidence that the graduating fellow is competent, if the program director asserts that

S. Abraham · D. Brotherston · P. H. Mayo (✉)
Zucker School of Medicine at Hofstra/Northwell, Hempstead, NY, USA

M. J. Lanspa, A. T. Levinson (eds.), *Echocardiography and Ultrasonography in the ICU*, Respiratory Medicine, https://doi.org/10.1007/978-3-031-80038-2_70

this is the case. Full instruction in CCUS is not yet a mandatory component of critical care training. If a graduating fellow comes from a program with a strong faculty capability, they may be highly skilled at CCUS; while others with limited exposure to CCUS may have a marginal skill level.

Intensivists who are already at attending level may encounter difficulty in obtaining credentials to perform CCUS. In absence of a national standard, each credentialing committee defines criteria that must be met to grant privileges. One national society offers a comprehensive series of courses with a logbook requirement and board type examination that results in a so-called certification of completion. Some credentialing committees accept this qualification as strong evidence of competence.

While the granting of privileges for CCUS allows the intensivist to perform it, the granting of privileges does not assure that the clinician has competence in the field. Credentialing committees may be comprised of physicians who have no experience in CCUS and may grant privileges when the clinician is not competent. Alternatively, the committee may have strong representation with subspecialties who have prejudice against CCUS with the resulting denial of privileges when the applicant is competent. The granting of privileges to perform CCUS does not guarantee that the clinician is competent or vice versa. We advise that the ICU team develops an internal method to ascertain whether new team members are competent in CCUS, as credentialing committees may grant privileges based upon perceived competence which may be quite different from actual bedside capability.

Advanced critical care echocardiography is a subcomponent of CCUS; where there is a national standard that, if met, assures that the intensivist is competent. The National Board of Echocardiography (NBE) offers certification in ACCE. The process includes a challenging board examination [6] and a major logbook requirement. Intensivists who achieve the NBE certification should be regarded by credentialing committees and ICU team members as being competent in ACCE. Critical care clinicians must await the development of a similarly rigorous certification for all components of CCUS that would provide them with strong evidence of competence. Until that time, initial assurance of competence remains under the inexact purview of credentialing committees and internal assessment of skill by the ICU team. Ongoing determination of competence may be achieved through a QA process.

Quality Assurance

From a patient safety standpoint, QA serves to mitigate risks of missed or errant diagnoses leading to harm. It serves to assure that providers are operating within their scope of practice, that there is an enduring record of findings and interpretations, to identify when it is necessary to intervene with additional training, and to identify failures in image acquisition and interpretation. It can be used to verify competence for granting and maintenance of privileges to perform CCUS. It has value in training programs where there may be a wide variability in skill among trainees who are in the process of acquiring skill in CCUS, to track progress, and to identify failure points that require specific educational intervention.

The importance of CCUS QA is stressed by guidelines from the American College of Emergency Physicians (ACEP), Society of Critical Care Medicine (SCCM), and the European Society of Intensive Care Medicine. The SCCM Ultrasound Certification Task Force recommends that QA be overseen by an Ultrasound Director [7]. Both ACEP and SCCM recommend QA programs have the following basic processes: a digital archiving system that includes demographic data (e.g., name, medical record number, date-of-birth) and interpretation, image review by the Ultrasound Director or designee, for technical quality and accuracy of interpretation, and study documentation in the patient chart that is permanently archived [8].

It is instructive to describe a well-designed QA program. The University of Western Ontario's CCUS program is an example of an operational

QA process in a tertiary care hospital system [9]. There, critical care trainees undergo a minimum of 1 month of CCUS training. While on rotation, they are directly overseen; and all studies undergo quality assurance by the ultrasound program director or ultrasound fellows who are independently practicing physicians designated by the director. Ultrasound fellows are granted QA privileges once they have demonstrated expert level capability in ultrasound performance and interpretation by the ultrasound director.

All images are archived and reported in a database that is linked to the electronic medical record. Each exam type has a standardized report form which includes a summary of the patient's presentation, relevant history, pertinent US findings, quantitative measurements (using standardized checklists), and a global assessment with management recommendations section.

All QA feedback is documented using a standardized form. On occasion, feedback may be delivered in person through direct one-on-one review of images and the draft report written by the trainee. The reviewer indicates whether improvements to image acquisition and/or interpretation are required and records suggested improvements in a free text field. In the case of important deficiencies in interpretation, the reviewer will directly amend the report. A global assessment is then made assigning a value of standards either having been met, met with improvement suggestions, not met with concerns, or not met with serious concerns. A note is made of whether report editing was required, and the final report is placed in the medical record. The clinician performing the examination is notified by email that feedback about their study is available. Trainees and others attending who have demonstrated competence are granted the ability to publish reports independently but receive periodic feedback which can be self-initiated or is initiated by the ultrasound director or designee.

The described QA process has been in operation since 2012, indicating that it is sustainable and realistic in design. It should be regarded as a gold standard for CCUS QA, and yet it remains aspirational for the typical ICU team. In attempting to reach this high standard, the ICU team faces predictable challenges.

1. The QA process requires a well-designed archiving system for durable storage of CCUS video clips. There are several available video archiving systems that vary in cost and ease of use. Most picture archiving and communication systems (PACS) used by radiology services are not designed for a high volume of video image sets, so they have limited utility for CCUS QA which requires video clips. The QA process may require a separate system in parallel with the hospital wide PACS.
2. An effective QA program requires a significant time commitment by the ICU team. A busy ICU team can be overwhelmed by a high volume of CCUS studies, each of which requires analysis and feedback to the operator. This is particularly problematic in a training program, where a significant proportion of studies may be suboptimal. Due to competing clinical duties and economic pressures, it may be difficult for the ICU team to commit the time required for a sustained comprehensive QA process. Although suboptimal, a work around for this problem is to assess only a proportion of CCUS studies.
3. The ICU team needs to avoid performing CCUS without image storage and formal reporting of results. There is a natural inclination for a busy ICU team to perform CCUS studies without image storage or formal reporting of results, given the time required for documentation. This problem may be aggravated by the proliferation of low-cost handheld units. The ICU team commits to the principle that, unless under extreme clinical pressure, every study needs to be saved to the archiving system with formal interpretation and QA. Bar code scanning capability of patient information into the ultrasonography machine is a useful adjunct to improve adherence to this standard.

Summary Points

- There are several statements that define competence in CCUS which are useful in the initial and ongoing determination of competence. Lacking a national level certification process for CCUS, initial determination of competence is often handled by a hospital credentialing committee. As this is an imperfect process, a well-designed QA program may be used to assure that the ICU team maintains competence in CCUS.
- The main challenge with CCUS QA relates to the difficulty that the ICU team may encounter in allocating the time required to review studies and to provide constructive feedback to the clinician. Quality assurance activity and its associated teaching function are not income generating, reimbursement rates for CCUS are low, and ICU team members may be under pressure from administrative entities to be economically productive. The time required and the lack of support for QA activities may impact the sustainability of a QA program by a well-intentioned ICU group. Typically, the QA program fails due to inadequate resource allocation in terms of time allotment and economic support.

References

1. Mayo PH, Beaulieu Y, Doelken P, et al. American College of Chest Physicians/La Société de Reanimation de Langue Française statement on competence in critical care ultrasonography. Chest. 2009;135(4):1050–60.
2. Cholley B. International expert statement on training standards for critical care ultrasonography Expert Round Table on Ultrasound in ICU. Intensive Care Med. 2011;37:1077–83.
3. International consensus statement on training standards for advanced critical care echocardiography. Expert Round Table on Echocardiography in ICU. Intensive Care Med. 2014;40:654–66.
4. Robba C, Wong A, Poole D, Al Tayar A, et al. Basic ultrasound head-to-toe skills for intensivists in the general and neuro intensive care unit population: consensus and expert recommendations of the European Society of Intensive Care Medicine. Intensive Care Med. 2021;47(12):1347–67.
5. American Medical Association. Privileging for Ultrasound Imaging H-230.960; 2020. https://policysearch.ama-assn.org/policyfinder/detail/Ultrasoundimaging?uri=%2FAMADoc%2FHOD.xml-0-1591.xml
6. Panebianco NL, Mayo PH, Arntfield RT, et al. Assessing competence in critical care echocardiography: development and initial results of an examination and certification processes. Crit Care Med. 2021;49(8):1285–92.
7. Pustavoitau A, Blaivas M, Brown S, et al. Recommendations for achieving and maintaining competence and credentialing in critical care ultrasound with focused cardiac ultrasound and advanced critical care echocardiography. Official Statement of the Society of Critical Care Medicine. Available at: https://journals.lww.com/ccmjournal/Documents/CriticalCareUltrasound.pdf. Accessed August 1, 2025.
8. Ultrasound guidelines: emergency, point-of-care and clinical ultrasound guidelines in medicine. Ann Emerg Med. 2017;69(5):e27–54. https://doi.org/10.1016/j.annemergmed.2016.08.457.
9. Arntfield RT. The utility of remote supervision with feedback as a method to deliver high-volume critical care ultrasound training. J Crit Care. 2015;30(2):441–e1.

71 Accreditation, Credentialing, and Privileging

Gregory A. Schmidt and James Leatherman

Learning Objectives

1. Describe the pros and cons of various credentialing and privileging strategies.
2. 2.Discuss key issues related to accreditation, credentialing, and privileging of POCUS.

Healthcare organizations share with healthcare professionals the responsibility to assure that care is high-quality, safe, and effective. Among the mechanisms for ensuring quality care are accreditation, credentialing, and privileging. Accreditation has two broad meanings when applied to POCUS. Programs involved in training may seek official recognition from external entities (typically professional organizations or private companies). Accreditation signals that the training program meets minimum standards for administration, education, performance, interpretation, equipment management, transducer disinfection, image acquisition, archiving, and confidentiality. Accreditation also applies to individual practitioners and ranges from a certificate of course completion to board certification based on training, extensive logbook documentation, and written and practical exams. Credentialing is the process of obtaining, verifying, and assessing the qualifications of a practitioner to provide care or services. Privileging is the process of authorizing a specific scope of practice based on the practitioner's credentials and performance. The rapid adoption of point of care ultrasound and echocardiography has challenged healthcare organizations in each of these domains (Table 71.1).

At the heart of current debates regarding the need for accreditation, credentialing, and privileging of POCUS is whether diagnostic use constitutes a "special" skill, requiring specific oversight and regulation, separate from those skills expected of a reasonably trained and competent practitioner in the field [1, 2]. For example, diagnostic right heart catheterization, bronchoscopy, and percutaneous tracheostomy are judged "special" in this regard, so that practitioners are expected to have privileges to perform these procedures. In contrast, cardiac auscultation, funduscopic examination, interpretation of hemodynamic waveforms, and analysis of ventilator graphics are not judged "special": practitioners are not expected to provide evidence of accreditation and institutions make no effort to give credential or privilege to these skills. Competence is assumed based on a training pathway. What distinguishes those procedures requiring special privileges from those that do

G. A. Schmidt (✉)
Division of Pulmonary Diseases, Critical Care, and Occupational Medicine, University of Iowa, Iowa City, IA, USA
e-mail: Gregory-a-schmidt@uiowa.edu

J. Leatherman
Division of Pulmonary and Critical Care, Hennepin County Medical Center, University of Minnesota, Minneapolis, MN, USA
e-mail: James.Leatherman@hcmed.org

M. J. Lanspa, A. T. Levinson (eds.), *Echocardiography and Ultrasonography in the ICU*, Respiratory Medicine, https://doi.org/10.1007/978-3-031-80038-2_71

Table 71.2 Programs for training and credentialing in point-of-care ultrasound (POCUS)

	CHAMP ultrasound program[a]	Cleveland Clinic (ED)[b]	ACCP[c]	SCCM[d]	ACEP[e]	LUCC initiative[f]
Educational program	1) Online module 2) 3 day in-person course –9 h hands-on	6–8 h knowledge and hands-on with CME credit	In-person 2-day course with hands-on training and 1 online module	20 h, including hands-on training	Core knowledge can be acquired largely online, with hands-on training for image acquisition	In-person or online courses to acquire basic knowledge; hands-on for image acquisition
Portfolio/ logbook	BCUS 20 Thoracic 5, Abdominal 5 Deep leg veins 3	FAST 25 AAA 25 Central line 10	BCUS 20 Thoracic 5 Abdominal 5 Deep leg veins 5	BCUS 30 Thoracic 20 Abdominal 30 Deep leg veins 20	25–50 quality-reviewed exams for each diagnostic application; 5 exams for procedural applications	3–5 BCUS per week for 3–6 months (minimum 40 exams) with review by mentor every 2 weeks
Studies review by POCUS expert	Yes	Yes	Yes	Yes	Yes	Yes
Assessment	Written exam and skills assessment	Review of submitted scans for image acquisition and interpretation	Written and hands-on exam	Not specified- variable for credentialing, outside bodies for certification	By review of submitted exams by designated ED POCUS expert	Bedside assessment of 1–3 exams for adequacy of acquisition/interpretation by POCUS expert
Additional features	Optional monthly scanning sessions			To ensure maintenance of competence by at least 10 h of CME regarding US and performance of at least 50 US exams per year	After credentialing, periodic review of provider's exams to ensure competence maintained (~10% of exams)	Re-certification every 5 years by submission or logbook, 1 day refresher course with re-assessment of skills, regular institutional image review sessions

Abbreviations: *CHAMP* comprehensive hospitalist assessment and mentorship with porfolios; *ACCP* American College of Chest Physicians; *SCCM* Society of Critical Care Medicine; *ACEP* American College of Emergency Physicians; *LUCC* Learning Ultrasound in Critical Care; *BCUS* basic cardiac ultrasound; *FAST* focused assessment with sonography in trauma; *AAA* abdominal aortic aneurysm

[a]reference # 11; [b]reference # 9; [c]references # 6,12; [d]reference # 7; [e]reference # 4; [f]reference # 13

thrombosis (DVT). In contrast, applications that are essential for EM such as musculoskeletal imaging, evaluation of intrauterine pregnancy, and ocular exams could be omitted. Content might be delivered by local POCUS experts, national or regional 1–2 day courses, or by online programs that allow self-study at the practitioner's individual pace, with easy repetition to help cement key concepts. Hands-on imaging of easy-to-image volunteers, supplemented by simulation models if available, provides an introduction to image acquisition. Second, each of the published guidelines recommends creation of a portfolio of exams that can be reviewed by an established POCUS expert to assess adequacy of imaging acquisition and interpretation. Acknowledging that individuals learn at different rates, a target of between 20 and 50 archived exams is most often recommended for diagnostic applications and from 5 to 10 exams for procedural applications (vascular access, thoracentesis, and paracentesis) [4, 7–13]. Finally, some have also recommended a summative assessment by written exam or bedside observation, or both [5, 10–13].

It should be appreciated, however, that there may be several challenges to implementation of a successful POCUS credentialing program (Table 71.1). One barrier may be the lack of a local POCUS expert to critique exams. Even if one is present, it is essential that the local institution allocates sufficient resources for oversight and review of the program by the dedicated POCUS experts given the considerable time commitment to review studies and provide feedback, and especially if a large number of providers are undergoing credentialing [9–11]. A second challenge in assessing the quality of image acquisition is that the latter depends not only on skill of the individual performing the POCUS, but also on individual patient characteristics and the instrument used for imaging, with the more expensive cart-based ultrasound machines often providing superior images than inexpensive hand-held devices. Ideally, competence in image acquisition is best assessed by having a POCUS expert at the bedside who would duplicate the exam with the same device for comparison, but as a practical matter this may not always be possible. Imaging interpretation and clinical application is also optimally evaluated at the bedside, but could alternatively be assessed by having the provider interpret a library of POCUS studies that include both normal and abnormal exams, an endeavor that could be done remotely. For this purpose, archived POCUS exams would be preferable to formal echocardiograms or radiology studies since the former would closely simulate the real-world of bedside ultrasound [14].

It should be acknowledged that requiring credentialing in POCUS is not without harm. In addition to substantial costs in both time and infrastructure, a credentialing requirement may act as a barrier to performing and disseminating POCUS. The existing evidence and experience of those routinely using POCUS strongly supports the view that unrestricted use regularly identifies clinically relevant and unsuspected findings. According to the ACEP, *the greatest risk in regards to emergency US is lack of its use in appropriate cases* [4].

A creative solution seeking to balance the pros and cons of credentialing and privileging might be to distinguish a category of POCUS exams for which privileging is required (and all exams are documented, reported, billed, and archived) and another category in which exams are considered exploratory. For these studies, there would be no expectation that the provider be privileged, expected to document (negative) findings, or permanently archive the images. Such an approach could parallel that applied to the radiology department studies versus clinical examination findings. However, it may be challenging to find agreement as to how to categorize POCUS studies and wide variation across health systems could be expected.

In summary, credentialing and privileging for POCUS by individual hospitals or health care systems can be accomplished, but has significant barriers to successful implementation and often requires significant time and effort by those who supervise and direct such programs. Although ensuring competence in POCUS may be a laudable goal, pathways to acquire POCUS privileges that are excessively burdensome may cause some providers who might otherwise use POCUS forego its use, to the potential detriment of their patients.

Key Points

- There is no consensus on required training for those using POCUS and privileges are generally not required.
- Requiring privileges for POCUS carries risks as well as benefits.
- Few institutions have implemented image archiving, routine reporting, and quality control for POCUS examinations.
- Several professional organizations have recommended the level of experience expected to assure competence.

References

1. Walter JM, Satterwhite L, Lyn-Kew KE. Should the use of diagnostic point-of-care ultrasound in patient care require hospital privileging/credentialing? Yes Chest. 2020;157:496–8.
2. Kruser JM, Schmidt GA, Kory PD. Should the use of diagnostic point-of-care ultrasound in patient care require hospital privileging/credentialing? No Chest. 2020;157:498–500.
3. American Medical Association. Ultrasound Imaging: Hospitals. Privileging for Ultrasound Imaging H-230.960, 2020. https://policysearch.ama-assn.org/policyfinder/detail/Ultrasound%20imaging?uri=%2FAMADoc%2FHOD.xml-0-1591.xml. Accessed 23 Jan 2022.
4. American College of Emergency Physicians. Ultrasound Guidelines: emergency, point-of-care, and clinical ultrasound guidelines in medicine. Ann Emerg Med. 2017;69:e27–54.
5. Sonie NJ, Schnobrich D, Matthews B, et al. Point-of-care ultrasound for hospitalists: a position statement of the society of hospital medicine. J Hosp Med. 2019;14:E1–6.
6. Mayo P, Beaulieu Y, Doelken P, et al. American College of Chest Physicians/La Societe de Reanimation de Langue Francaise statement on competence in critical care ultrasonography. Chest. 2009;135:1050–60.
7. Pustavoitau A, Blaivas M, Brown SM, et al. Recommendations for achieving and maintaining competence and credentialing in critical care ultrasound with focused cardiac ultrasound and advanced critical care echocardiography. http://journals.lww.com/ccmjournal/Documents/Critical%20Care%20Ultrasound.pdf.
8. Galarza L, Wong A, Malbrain M. The state of critical care ultrasound training in Europe: a survey of traineers and a comparison of available accreditation programmes. Anaesthesiol Intensive Ther. 2017;49:382–6.
9. Smalley CM, Fertel BS, Broderick E. Standardizing point-of-care ultrasound credentialing across a large health care system. Jt Comm J Qual Patient Saf. 2020;46:471–6.
10. Mathews B, Zwanck MD. Hosptial medicine ultrasound credentialing: an example protocol. J Hosp Med. 2017;12(9):767–72.
11. Mathews BK, Reierson K, Vuong K, et al. The design and evaluation of the comprehensive hospitalist assessment and mentorship with portfoloios (CHAMP) ultrasound program. J Hosp Med. 2018;13:544–50.
12. American College of Chest Physisicans Critical Care Ultrasonagraphy Program. http://www.chestnet.org/Education/Advanced-Clinical-Training/Certificate-of-Completion-Program/Critical-Care-Ultrasonagraphy
13. Rajamani A, Galarza L, Sanfillipo F, et al. Criteria, processes, and determination of competence in basic critical care echocardiography training. A Delphi process consensus statement by the Learning Ultrasound in Critical Care (LUCC) Initiative. Chest. 2022;161(2):492–503. https://doi.org/10.1016/j.chest.2021.08.077. Epub 2021 Sep 8. PMID: 34508739.
14. Spencer KT, Kimura BJ, Korcarz CE, et al. Focused cardiac ultrasound: recommendations from the American Society of Echocardiography. J Am Soc Echocardiogr. 2013;26:567–81.

72 Image Storage and Reporting

Keith Boniface and Aaran Drake

Learning Objectives
After reading this chapter, learners will be able to:

1. Explain the importance of documenting point-of-care ultrasound interpretations and archiving images.
2. Recognize documentation and archiving as essential features of a sustainable Intensive Care Unit (ICU) Point of Care Ultrasound (POCUS) program.
3. Define the processes comprising the "front-end" and "back-end" of the POCUS workflow.
4. Identify stakeholders critical to the success of an ICU POCUS program.

Point-of-care ultrasound (POCUS) in the intensive care unit (ICU) can rule in or rule out life-threatening conditions and provide information to guide the best course of treatment. A quality POCUS program includes the acquisition of adequate images for decision-making, documentation of the exam interpretation, and archiving of the images. Critical care society guidelines addressing POCUS [SCCM [1, 2], ACCP [3], ESICM [4]] have described clinical indications for the use of ultrasound in decision-making at the bedside but have not addressed documentation and reporting of the exam interpretation, nor the need for preservation of images for evaluation by other practitioners, quality assurance, medico-legal or billing purposes. Other specialties have addressed these issues and recommend interpretation documentation and archiving as best practice [5, 6].

Why Document Exam Interpretation and Archive Images?

The use of bedside ultrasound informs decision-making in real-time and does not necessarily require formal documentation or archiving. In this paradigm, ultrasound theoretically serves as an "extension of the physical exam." However, ultrasound is a technology that requires additional provider time and specialized training to perform safely for diagnostic testing or procedural guidance purposes. As a result, the practice of bedside performance and interpretation of ultrasound while consistently documenting findings or archiving images is best practice for several reasons:

1. *Communication with other providers*—Much like a patient's current neurologic exam, vasopressor requirements, or ventilator settings, POCUS is inherently a snapshot of a patient's

K. Boniface (✉) · A. Drake
Department of Emergency Medicine, George Washington University, Washington, DC, USA
e-mail: kboniface@mfa.gwu.edu; adrake@mfa.gwu.edu

M. J. Lanspa, A. T. Levinson (eds.), *Echocardiography and Ultrasonography in the ICU*, Respiratory Medicine, https://doi.org/10.1007/978-3-031-80038-2_72

anatomy and physiology at one point in time. Part of its virtue is that it can be easily repeated when a patient's status changes or to monitor response to therapy. As with other forms of imaging, direct comparison of serial exams is the best way to assess interval change, but without POCUS image storage, only the bedside practitioner at the time of the exam will have access to the findings. The importance of image accessibility is highlighted by the shift-work coverage of ICUs, with patients receiving care from multiple providers throughout their course. Similarly, a baseline or previous study may prove useful in case a patient returns for care in the future. Stored images also improve the ability of the primary team to communicate with consulting services regarding the findings.

2. *Quality assurance* (QA)—Image storage plays a key role in ensuring quality use of ultrasound in the hands of appropriately skilled operators. By reviewing a subset of images, ultrasound leaders can ensure technical competence and interpretation accuracy of clinician sonographers and improve the quality of care provided.
3. *Billing*—POCUS alters management at the bedside and requires provider time and expertise. In many practice settings, this utility makes it eligible for billing and reimbursement. Image archiving and documentation of interpretation is necessary for reimbursement by private and government payors. Reimbursement enables support for training providers, updating machinery and software, and ensures continued availability of ultrasound technology to critically ill patients.

The Workflow

The process of image acquisition, interpretation, documentation, and archiving can be broken into front-end and back-end workflows. The bedside steps of image acquisition and interpretation represent the front-end, while the "behind the scenes" processes, or back-end workflow, is comprised of image storage (to specialized archival software, a Picture Archiving and Communication System (PACS), or a local computer) and creating a report in the electronic health record (EHR) [7].

Front-End: Entering Demographics, Acquiring Images

To begin the front-end processes, patient identifiers are entered into the demographics page of a new exam. Required information includes the patient's first and last name, medical record number, and the sonographer's name. Some systems will allow population of the patient's demographics via a worklist on the ultrasound machine generated by orders for POCUS exams in the EHR. In such systems, the operator would place an order in the EHR and select the patient from the worklist to begin the exam. Other systems do not require an order to be placed for patients to appear on the worklist; instead, the worklist is wirelessly updated periodically from the admission-discharge-transfer (ADT) system to reflect the unit census. On systems that do not offer selection of a patient from a worklist, patient demographics can be manually entered using the keyboard. A barcode reader can improve the speed and accuracy of patient and provider information entry in these systems.

To acquire images, the examination preset and probe type are selected to initiate the ultrasound scan. The images, clips, and measurements required by your institution for the given exam type are then obtained. Some machines' software will allow the user to enter interpretation directly into a worksheet on the machine after images are obtained. After image acquisition is complete, ending the exam initiates transfer of images from Wi-Fi-enabled ultrasound machines to the storage software. Beware—machines need to remain in the ON position for this transfer to take place, so they should be returned to their storage area and plugged into a power outlet.

Back-End: Archiving, Interpreting, and Documenting

Ideally, completed studies will transfer through a wireless network from the ultrasound machine to a specialized archival software (see Appendix A) [8]. Alternatively, ultrasound images and their interpretation may be transferred to the hospital's PACS system, siloed off from radiology and cardiology images to avoid confusion about the origin of the images. A cost-free solution is to archive images by periodically downloading them from the machine onto a hard drive, though there is a risk of data loss from the machine between manual downloads as well as more limited access to the images.

Users document their exam interpretations, either on the ultrasound machine, in the archival software, or in the EHR directly as a templated procedure note (see Appendix B). Templated documentation of POCUS provides a uniform language to communicate findings and interpretation among providers with specific details necessary for QA and billing. Solely documenting interpretations in the progress note does not demonstrate the additional skill and time required to obtain the valuable clinical information gleaned from POCUS and makes identifying previous ultrasound documentation more challenging.

It is important to separate exams performed by credentialed providers for diagnostic purposes and those performed by trainees upon which no decisions are based. These "educational images" should not be imported into the EHR and should remain in the archival software only for credentialing and QA purposes.

Billing, QA, and Credentialing

Billers/coders identify "billable" exams (those performed by credentialed providers for clinically indicated reasons) via archival software tags or templated notes in the EHR and subsequently submit requests to the appropriate payor. Archiving studies and interpretations is required for at least 5 years for potential audits.

QA should be performed on images in a regular, timely fashion to identify missed findings or inaccurate interpretations and provide feedback to providers. The QA and archiving of a provider's credentialing quality (adequate true positive or true negative) studies enable the development of a log to demonstrate competence, for both initial hospital credentialing and ongoing Focused Professional Practice Evaluation.

Partners

The maintenance of an ultrasound system involves multiple professionals in a typical hospital environment, from biomedical engineering, Information Services and Technology (IS&T) (including network engineers as well as those responsible for the EHR and archiver/PACS software), clinical operations staff, and billing and coding professionals. Most of these professionals have some understanding of ultrasound, but may need to gain understanding of the significant differences between clinician-performed ultrasound and consultative (radiology-performed) ultrasound. For instance, in radiology-performed ultrasound, no images are obtained without an antecedent order, and no (or few) images are obtained without submitting charges. In addition to radiology and cardiology, colleagues utilizing POCUS at your institution in obstetrics and gynecology, emergency medicine, internal medicine, or anesthesia may have solutions already in place that may fit your ICU's needs.

Summary Points

- Ultrasound images obtained in the critical care environment should be saved with patient and sonographer identifiers.
- These images should be stored in an accessible format for communication with other

8. Marin J, Abo A, Chilstrom M, Leo M, Liu R, Strony R. System Wide Clinical Ultrasound Program Development. White paper, American College of Emergency Physicians, Emergency Ultrasound Section. [Internet]; 2019 [cited 2022 Jan 13]. Available from: https://www.acep.org/globalassets/uploads/uploaded-files/acep/membership/sections-of-membership/ultra/subcommittees/swcus_section-3_082119.pdf.

Correction to: Mitral and Tricuspid Regurgitation

Maxwell Hockstein and Karuna Puttur Rajkumar

Correction to:
Chapter 20 in: M. J. Lanspa, A. T. Levinson (eds.), *Echocardiography and Ultrasonography in the ICU*, Respiratory Medicine, https://doi.org/10.1007/978-3-031-80038-2_20

The original version of the chapter, "Mitral and Tricuspid Regurgitation," was inadvertently published with incorrect authorship.

The correct authors are as follows:
Maxwell Hockstein and Karuna Puttur Rajkumar

The updated version of this chapter can be found at
https://doi.org/10.1007/978-3-031-80038-2_20

M. J. Lanspa, A. T. Levinson (eds.), *Echocardiography and Ultrasonography in the ICU*,
Respiratory Medicine, https://doi.org/10.1007/978-3-031-80038-2_73

Index

M. J. Lanspa, A. T. Levinson (eds.), *Echocardiography and Ultrasonography in the ICU*, Respiratory Medicine, https://doi.org/10.1007/978-3-031-80038-2

GPSR Compliance

The European Union's (EU) General Product Safety Regulation (GPSR) is a set of rules that requires consumer products to be safe and our obligations to ensure this.

If you have any concerns about our products, you can contact us on ProductSafety@springernature.com

In case Publisher is established outside the EU, the EU authorized representative is:

Springer Nature Customer Service Center GmbH
Europaplatz 3
69115 Heidelberg, Germany

Batch number: 10296502

Printed by Printforce, the Netherlands